Herbal Medicines

Herbal Medicines

THIRD EDITION

Joanne Barnes

BPharm, PhD, MRPharmS, RegPharmNZ, MPSNZ, FLS

Associate Professor in Herbal Medicines
School of Pharmacy
University of Auckland
New Zealand

Linda A Anderson

BPharm, PhD, FRPharmS

Principal Pharmaceutical Assessor
Medicines and Healthcare products Regulatory Agency
London, UK

J David Phillipson

BSc (Pharm), MSc, PhD, DSc, FRPharmS, FLS

Emeritus Professor
Centre for Pharmacognosy & Phytotherapy
The School of Pharmacy
University of London, UK

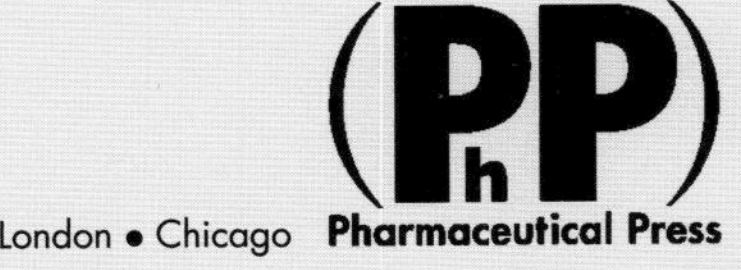

London • Chicago Pharmaceutical Press

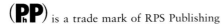

Published by the Pharmaceutical Press
An imprint of RPS Publishing

1 Lambeth High Street, London SE1 7JN, UK
100 South Atkinson Road, Suite 200, Grayslake, IL 60030-7820, USA

RPS Publishing is the publishing organisation of the Royal Pharmaceutical Society of Great Britain

First edition 1996
Second edition 2002
Reprinted 2003, 2006
Third edition 2007

Text design by Eric Drewery, East Molesey, Surrey
Typeset by Data Standards Ltd, Frome, Somerset
Printed in Great Britain by Butler and Tanner, Frome, Somerset

ISBN 978 0 85369 623 0

A catalogue record for this book is available from the British Library

Front cover images (from top l–r): Echinacea, Hops, Calendula, Echinacea root (dry), Milk Thistle, Calendula (dry), Passionflower, German Chamomile (dry), German chamomile

Disclaimer
Inclusion of a substance or preparation in *Herbal Medicines* is not to be considered a recommendation for use, nor does it confer any status on the substance or preparation. Although considerable efforts have been made to check the material in *Herbal Medicines*, the authors and publisher make no representation, express or implied, with regard to the accuracy of the information contained in this book and cannot accept any legal responsibility or liability for any errors or omissions that may be made. Also, the reader is assumed to possess the necessary knowledge to interpret the information provided.

The views expressed in this book are those of the authors and do not represent those of the UK Medicines and Healthcare products Regulatory Agency, European Medicines Agency, World Health Organization, or any other institution or organisation mentioned. Mention of specific product names is for clarity and identification purposes and does not represent endorsement.

Contents

This book is dedicated to the memory of
the late Dr W Gwynne Thomas,
former Director of Pharmaceutical Sciences at the
Royal Pharmaceutical Society of Great Britain.
The inspiration for the book came from him and
it is due to his efforts that the necessary funding
was obtained.

Preface to the Third Edition

This third edition of *Herbal Medicines: A guide for healthcare professionals* comes a little over ten years after publication of the first edition, and reflects continuing public, professional, research, commercial and other interests in medicinal plants. At the same time, there have been ongoing concerns surrounding the quality, safety and efficacy of herbal medicinal products, and heightened awareness of the need to protect the public against poor-quality and unsafe products. Pharmacists, doctors, nurses, herbal-medicine practitioners and other healthcare providers should be knowledgeable about these issues and should be able to advise patients and the public on the safe, effective and appropriate use of herbal preparations; this book aims to provide pharmacists and other healthcare professionals with summarised, yet sufficiently detailed, scientific information to enable them to do so.

Herbal medicines continue to be a popular healthcare choice with the general public not only for health maintenance and well-being, minor ailments (e.g. coughs and colds), chronic conditions (e.g. back pain) and serious chronic diseases (e.g. asthma, cancer, depression, diabetes), but also for 'enhancement' of functions or processes, such as the use of *Ginkgo biloba* products for memory enhancement. The general public receives information on herbal medicines through various sources, including popular magazines and newspaper articles, as well as television, internet and other sources of advertising literature provided by manufacturers. Much of this information is presented uncritically, and targeted to the consumer along with details of substantial price reductions on products, including continuous sales promotions, that often are the main recommendations for the products. There is an increasing number of products that respond to the public demand for so-called 'lifestyle' medicines, and manufacturers market, for example, herbal alternatives to Viagra (sildenafil), 'slimming/weight-loss' preparations, 'hangover' cures, and breast-enlargement products. Typically, these types of products are sold over the internet without any assurance of their quality, safety and efficacy.

The last decade has seen several important developments with respect to herbal medicines. The most significant of these has been the introduction of a new regulatory framework for traditional herbal medicines in the UK and the 27 other member states of the European Union (EU) following the implementation in 2005 of the EU Directive on Traditional Herbal Medicinal Products. Several other countries worldwide have introduced new legislation to regulate herbal medicinal products: Australia and Canada, for example, have been particularly active in this respect. That the regulatory landscape for herbal medicines has changed substantially has required a full revision of the 'Introduction to the Monographs', which in this edition can be found under 'How to Use *Herbal Medicines*'; this now includes details of new legislation in Europe and a summary of regulations for herbal medicines in several other countries.

Although there are new regulations, in Europe there is a transitional period until 2011 to allow manufacturers time to comply with the new requirements, so issues relating to the quality, safety and efficacy of herbal medicines are likely to continue, even beyond the next edition of this book! Therefore, with respect to quality, consumers and healthcare professionals should be aware that the labels of unlicensed (unregulated) herbal medicines may not reflect their actual contents, and that the precise constituents of herbal medicines containing the same herbal ingredient(s) but produced by different manufacturers are likely to differ. The quality of herbal medicines (i.e. uniformity of dose) is important for their efficacy: clinical trial results for a particular herbal medicinal product cannot necessarily be extrapolated to other products containing the same ingredient, since their precise contents may differ. Details of herbal medicinal products tested in clinical trials are provided in individual monographs in this book. There is an increasing amount of research comprising qualitative (i.e. the profile of chemical constituents) and quantitative (quantity of chemical constituents) analysis of herbal medicines and showing variations in the contents of different manufacturers' products. For those herbal ingredients for which there is substantial information, and for commonly encountered herbal ingredients, we have summarised the findings of these analyses in a new section in some monographs on *Quality of plant material and commercial products* (for examples, see the monographs on St John's wort and Echinacea).

The quality of herbal medicines is also important as regards their safety, and safety concerns with herbal medicines, including intrinsic toxicity as well as problems due to adulteration and contamination, continue to arise. This edition includes new monographs on kava (*Piper methysticum*) and greater celandine (*Chelidonium majus*) and a fully revised monograph on black cohosh (*Cimicifuga racemosa*), all of which have been associated with hepatotoxic reactions. The concurrent use of herbal and other medicines remains a major concern for healthcare professionals because of the potential for important drug interactions. Evidence of pharmacokinetic and pharmacodynamic interactions between St John's wort (*Hypericum perforatum*) and 'conventional' medicines emerged in the year 2000 and, since then, reports have been made of interactions between other herbal medicines and conventional medicines, typically those with a low therapeutic index. At present though, there has been little formal clinical research into interactions between herbal and other medicines, and information relies mainly on spontaneous reports and, to some extent, findings of *in-vitro* studies of the effects of certain herbal medicines on cytochrome P450 drug-metabolising enzymes. Information on known and potential interactions is summarised in the Appendices to this book, and further information and detail is provided in the individual monographs.

Continual vigilance and reporting of adverse effects, including interactions and problems related to poor quality, associated with herbal medicines is essential in order to detect safety issues as soon as possible. In the UK, pharmacists and other state-registered healthcare providers and, since 2005, patients and consumers, can report suspected adverse drug reactions (ADRs) associated with herbal medicines directly to the Medicines and Healthcare products Regulatory Agency (MHRA) using 'yellow card' report forms. These forms are included in the *British National Formulary* and available on-line (*see* www.mhra.gov.uk), and for the first time several are included in this book so that they may be more readily at hand to healthcare professionals using this book for information on adverse effects experienced and reported to them by consumers and patients. Many other countries have an ADR reporting scheme similar to that of the UK and encourage reporting of suspected herbal ADRs, at least by healthcare professionals. The World Health Organization's Uppsala Monitoring Centre in Sweden receives such reports from over 70 countries, including Australia, Canada, France, Germany, New Zealand, UK and the USA, and we have summarised this information for a number of herbal medicines for which there have been important safety concerns (see individual monographs).

The effects of herbal medicines are, of course, brought about by their chemical constituents. It may not be fully recognised by some individuals that while, for example, aspirin tablets contain a measured quantity (within narrow limits) of a single active chemical compound, tablets (and indeed other dosage forms) of a herbal medicine typically contain a complex mixture of many (hundreds or more) chemical compounds. In order to appreciate the quality control and quality assurance procedures that are essential for herbal medicinal products and to understand their pharmacological and toxicological effects, it is necessary to be aware of the different types of chemical constituents, e.g. alkaloids, glycosides, flavonoids, etc, that may be present, as well as the individual constituents in specific herbal medicines. This edition includes two new features which provide this information: chemical structural formulae are included with virtually every monograph to supplement the textual information on constituents, and a new chapter 'Chemical Constituents of Plants Used as Herbal Medicines' has been added, which summarises the different groups of natural product compounds (e.g. alkaloids, glycosides, flavonoids, terpenes) that are present in medicinal plants.

The first edition of this book provided information on herbal medicines available in pharmacies in the UK, whereas we have expanded the scope of this third edition to include new monographs on herbal medicines that may not necessarily be found in UK pharmacies but which are of public or professional interest. Hence, this edition includes new monographs on butterbur (*Petasites hybridus*), greater celandine (*Chelidonium majus*), kava (*Piper methysticum*) and rhodiola (*Rhodiola rosea*). Kava has been prohibited in the UK since 2002 because of its association with hepatotoxic reactions; we include a monograph here as it is possible that consumers and patients in the UK may obtain supplies from overseas. At least 10 existing monographs on popular herbal medicines have been completely revised, substantial updates and revisions have been made to over 20 other monographs, and minor amendments have been made to all remaining monographs. In addition, in response to comments from practising pharmacists, academics and other users of this book, this edition includes photographs of the crude herbal drugs which feature in the monographs as well as, for many monographs, the plants from which they originate. Also for the first time the individual monographs contain information from several countries on marketed products containing the respective herbal ingredients. We hope that these new features will be both useful and pleasing to the eye! As always, keeping a book up to date is a never-ending task, and the explosion in the scientific literature on herbal medicines makes this ever more difficult. In the last five years, there have been over 500 scientific papers published on St John's wort alone, and it is impossible and undesirable to describe each of them. The need for a book that reviews and summarises all this information has, perhaps, never been greater and we hope that this edition will provide healthcare professionals with the information they need to be able to advise their patients, competently and confidently, on the safe, effective and appropriate use of herbal medicines.

Constructive criticism of the contents of *Herbal Medicines* is welcome and may be used to assist in the preparation of any future editions. The reader is asked to send any comments to the publisher by post or email (pharmpress@rpsgb.org).

Joanne Barnes, Linda Anderson, David Phillipson
Auckland and London
May 2007

Acknowledgements

We are grateful to the following Pharmaceutical Press staff for their active help and encouragement with this book: Tamsin Cousins, Simon Dunton, Louise McIndoe, Karl Parsons, Linda Paulus, Paul Weller and John Wilson. We also thank Marion Edsall for her proofreading work, and Lida Teng, PhD student at the School of Pharmacy, University of London, for administrative assistance.

Photographs are included with kind permission of Thomas Brendler (www.plantaphile.com, Germany). Some of the photographs were supplied to Plantaphile by Larry Allain, Pierre Cabalion, Alvin Diamond, Ulrich Feiter, Trish Flaster, Nigel Gericke, Michael Guiry, MJ Hatfield, Gary Kauffman, Diane Robertson, Joachim Schmitz, Stan Shebs and Michael Wink.

In addition, the photograph of blue flag is reproduced with kind permission of Brian Mathew, Royal Botanic Gardens, Kew, UK, Honorary Research Associate, and the photograph of nettle with kind permission of Dr Tom Cope, Royal Botanic Gardens, Kew, UK.

Most of the herbal plant photographs were taken in major European botanical gardens. Photographs of the drug material were taken from materials supplied by reputable German herbal medicinal product suppliers.

We are also very grateful to Dr Christine Leon (Royal Botanic Gardens, Kew, UK), who provided helpful advice and suggestions on appropriate botanical names and synonyms to include. Dr Leon was able to call on the specialist advice of the following colleagues, whom we thank. Staff at the Royal Botanic Gardens, Kew, UK: Dr Tom Cope, Dr Aaron Davis, Dr Nicholas Hind, Dr Sven Landrein, Dr Gwilym Lewis, Eve Lucas, Dr Alan Paton, Dr Nigel Taylor. Kew Honorary Research Associates: Jill Cowley, Dr Phillip Cribb, Dr David Frodin, Brian Mathew. Dr Leon and colleagues also provided helpful comments on the photographs.

We thank all of the above individuals for their support with this publication. If there are any errors or omissions in the content of this book, then they are our responsibility.

About the Authors

Dr Joanne Barnes

BPharm, PhD, MRPharmS, RegPharmNZ, MPSNZ, FLS

Joanne Barnes obtained a degree in Pharmacy from the University of Nottingham in 1988, a postgraduate Certificate in Pharmacovigilance and Pharmacoepidemiology from the London School of Hygiene and Tropical Medicine in 1999, and a PhD in Pharmacy from the School of Pharmacy, University of London in 2001. She has been registered as a pharmacist with the Royal Pharmaceutical Society of Great Britain since 1989, was made a Fellow of the Linnean Society of London in 2003 and achieved registration as a pharmacist in New Zealand in 2007. She was Research Fellow in Complementary Medicines in the Department of Complementary Medicine, University of Exeter (1996–1999), Research Fellow (1999–2002) and Lecturer in Phytopharmacy (2002–2005) in the Centre for Pharmacognosy and Phytotherapy, School of Pharmacy, University of London, UK and, since 2005, has been Associate Professor in Herbal Medicines, School of Pharmacy, Faculty of Medical and Health Sciences, University of Auckland, New Zealand. Her research focuses on the utilisation, efficacy and safety of herbal medicines, particularly in exploring issues related to pharmacovigilance. Before embarking on an academic career, she practised as a hospital clinical pharmacist, as a medical information pharmacist in the pharmaceutical industry and worked in pharmaceutical publishing.

She was Editor (1996–1999) and a co-founder of the journal *Focus on Alternative and Complementary Therapies* (FACT), Co-editor (2003–2005) of *Complementary Therapies in Medicine* and is an Associate Editor of *Phytochemistry Letters* and a member of the editorial boards of *Phytotherapy Research*, *Drug Safety* and the *International Journal of Pharmacy Practice*. She is a member of the Health Canada Natural Health Product Directorate's Expert Resource Group, the RPSGB's complementary medicine working group, and was a member of the UK Medicines and Healthcare products Regulatory Agency's Independent Review Panel for the Classification of Borderline Products (2000–2005).

Dr Linda A Anderson

BPharm, PhD, FRPharmS

Linda Anderson obtained her first degree in Pharmacy and her PhD in Pharmacognosy at the Welsh School of Pharmacy in Cardiff. She was a postdoctoral research and teaching fellow at the School of Pharmacy, University of London from 1981 to 1987.

Dr Anderson joined the Medicines and Healthcare products Regulatory Agency (MHRA, Department of Health, UK; formerly Medicines Control Agency) in 1987.

Within the MHRA, she was initially involved in the assessment of new chemical entities and is now mainly involved with abridged applications and has specific responsibility for herbal products. She is Principal Assessor to the Committee on Safety of Medicine's (CSM) Expert Advisory Group on Chemistry, Pharmacy and Standards (CPS) and is UK delegate to the European Committee on Human Medicinal Products (CHMP) Quality Working Party. Dr Anderson is also UK Delegate to the European Medicines Agency (EMEA) Committee on Herbal Medicinal Products (HMPC), a member of the Herbal Medicines Advisory Committee (HMAC) of the MHRA, and is Vice-Chair of the British Pharmacopoeia Expert Advisory Group on Herbals and Complementary Medicines. She is a member of the Royal Pharmaceutical Society's Science Committee's working group on complementary/alternative medicine.

Linda Anderson has been awarded a Fellowship of the Royal Pharmaceutical Society of Great Britain (2001).

Professor J David Phillipson

BSc(Pharm), MSc, PhD, DSc, FRPharmS, FLS

David Phillipson graduated BSc in Pharmacy (1956), MSc (1959), and DSc (1979) from the University of Manchester, and PhD (1965) from the University of London. He was Lecturer in Pharmacognosy (1961–1972) at the Department of Pharmacy, Chelsea College, London, and Senior Lecturer (1973–1979), Reader in Phytochemistry (1979–1981), and Professor and Head of the Department of Pharmacognosy (1981–1994) at the School of Pharmacy, University of London. On retirement he became Emeritus Professor of Pharmacognosy. In 1995 he was appointed as Wilson T S Wang Distinguished International Visiting Professor at the Chinese University of Hong Kong from January to June. His research included investigations of the chemistry and biological activities of natural products from higher plants with special interests in indole and isoquinoline alkaloids, and plants used in traditional medicines for the treatment of malaria and other protozoal diseases. Collaboration with the pharmaceutical industry included the application of radioligand–receptor binding assays in the search for natural products with activity in the central nervous system.

David Phillipson has received awards from the Phytochemical Society of Europe including the Tate and Lyle Award (1982), Medal (1994), and the Pergamon Prize for Creativity in Plant Biochemistry (1996). He was awarded the Korber Foundation Prize for Achievement in European Science (1989) in collaboration with Professor MH Zenk of the University of Munich and four other European colleagues, was presented with the Harrison Memorial Medal of the Royal Pharmaceutical Society of Great Britain (1999), and with the Sir Hans Sloane Medal of the Faculty of the History and Philosophy of Medicine and Pharmacy, Society of Apothecaries (2001). In 1985 he was Science Chairman of the British Pharmaceutical Conference and has been Secretary (1977–1982), Vice-Chairman (1982–1984, 1986–1988) and Chairman (1984–1986) of the Phytochemical Society of Europe. He has been awarded Fellowships of the Royal Pharmaceutical Society of Great Britain (1980) and of the School of Pharmacy, University of London (1998).

He has supervised 33 PhD students and 11 postdoctoral researchers, publishing some 222 full research papers, 150 short communications, 42 review articles, and has edited six books on natural products. Collaborative research was established with scientists in many countries world-wide and in 1989 he was appointed Honorary Professor of the Chinese Academy of Medical Sciences at the Institute of Medicinal Plant Research and Development, Beijing, China. For 19 years he was a member of the Natural Products Group of the International Foundation for Science, Sweden, helping to award research grants to individual young scientists in developing countries. He has been a member of a number of national and international committees, including the Herbal Medicines Advisory Committee (HMAC) of the MHRA.

How to Use *Herbal Medicines*

Purpose and Scope

Herbal Medicines is intended to serve as a reference work for pharmacists, doctors, nurses and other healthcare professionals, assisting in their provision of advice on the use of herbal medicines to members of the public. *Herbal Medicines* is not intended to represent a guide to self-diagnosis and self-treatment with herbal medicines, and should not be used as such.

The term 'herbal medicine' or 'herbal medicinal product' (or, less frequently, 'herbal remedy') is used to describe a marketed product, whereas 'herbal ingredient' refers to an individual herb that is present in a herbal medicine. 'Herbal constituent' is used to describe a specific chemical constituent of a herbal ingredient. Thus, as examples, Valerian Tablets are a herbal product, valerian root is a herbal ingredient, and valtrate is a herbal constituent of valerian.

The main criterion for inclusion of a herbal ingredient in the text is its presence in herbal medicines that are used in the UK, particularly those which are sold through pharmacies. In addition, herbs that have recently been the subject of media or scientific interest have been included. The aim of *Herbal Medicines* is to draw the attention of the reader to the reputed actions and uses of herbal ingredients, and to whether or not these have been substantiated by evidence from preclinical and/or clinical studies. In addition, any known or potential toxicities of herbal ingredients, and how these may influence the suitability for inclusion in herbal medicines or for use with conventional medicines, are also discussed.

Introduction to the Monographs

The introductory section to the 152 monographs on the individual herbal ingredients contained in *Herbal Medicines* discusses the legal aspects of herbal medicines including licensed medicines and non-licensed products in the UK and within the European Union (EU). All medicines are assessed for their quality, safety and efficacy and, in the context of herbal medicines, there are often specific criteria which are not encountered in the assessment of other medicines. As a first line in ensuring the safety and efficacy of herbal medicines there is a series of guidelines for quality assessment and this is briefly discussed. In terms of safety, it is a popular conception that because herbs are 'natural' then they must also be safe. This is a misconception, and it is emphasised that some herbal ingredients have the capability to cause adverse effects, whilst some are decidedly toxic. Within the context of the 152 monographs on herbal ingredients, most have documented adverse effects, or the potential to interact with other medication, and few can be recommended for use during pregnancy.

Tables in the Introduction and appendices at the end of the monographs summarise the safety aspects of these herbal ingredients and give information on biologically active herbal ingredients and their active principles. Clinical efficacy has not been established for the majority of the herbal ingredients described in this handbook and, in some instances, there is a lack of documentation for chemical constituents and for pharmacological actions.

The Herbal Monographs

Some 152 monographs on individual herbal ingredients found in herbal products are included, the title used for the monograph being their preferred common name. A data sheet-type format was chosen for the monographs because it was felt important to arrange the relevant information in a format familiar to pharmacists, doctors, nurses and other healthcare professionals. Although conventional data sheets are written for products, it was decided to draw up the data sheets for herbal ingredients and not for specific products, although where possible details are provided of the specific products assessed in the studies discussed.

The headings used in the herbal monographs are listed below with a brief explanation of the information provided under them.

Monograph title	Common name for the herbal ingredient; if more than one common name exists, this is the chosen preferred name.
Summary and Pharmaceutical Comment	This section is designed to give the reader an overall summary of the monograph contents, indicating the extent of phytochemical, pharmacological and clinical data available for the herbal ingredient, whether or not proposed herbal uses are justified, concerns over safety and, based on this information, whether or not the herbal ingredient is considered suitable for use as a herbal medicine
Species (Family)	Preferred botanical name with authority, together with the plant family.
Synonym(s)	Other common or botanical names.
Part(s) Used	Plant part(s) traditionally used in herbal medicine.
Pharmacopoeial and Other Monographs	Key pharmacopoeial monographs and texts on herbal medicines.
UK Legal Category	Legal category of the herb with respect to licensed products. For the majority of herbal ingredients this will be the General Sales List (GSL).
Constituents	Main documented chemical constituents grouped into categories such as alkaloids (type specified), flavonoids, iridoid glycosides, saponins, tannins, triterpenes, volatile oil and other constituents for miscellaneous and minor chemical components.

table continues

Chemical structural formulae	Chemical structural formulae are included for key constituents of herbal ingredients for virtually every monograph. This information supplements the textual information on constituents.
Quality of plant material and commercial products	This section has been included for several herbal ingredients commonly encountered in commercial products. It describes studies examining the variation in phytochemical content of crude plant material and marketed products and other aspects relating to product quality, such as differences between actual and labelled content of commercial products.
Food Use	Provides an indication as to whether the herbal ingredient is used in foods. The Council of Europe (COE) category, which reflects the opinion of the COE on the suitability of the herbal ingredient for use as a food flavouring, is quoted where applicable.
Herbal Use	States the reputed actions and uses of the herbal ingredients, based on information from several sources. In some instances, current investigations of particular interest are included.
Photographs	Provided for most of the monographs for the crude drug substance and the plant from which it originates. As we do not provide botanical, macroscopical or microscopical descriptions, these photographs are for illustrative purposes only and are not intended to be used for identification purposes.
Dosage	States the traditional dose of the herbal ingredient, mainly from the British Herbal Pharmacopoeia (BHP), German Commission E and European Scientific Co-operative on Phytotherapy (ESCOP) monographs, giving doses for plant part used (e.g. herb, rhizome, leaf), liquid extract and infusion. Where possible, dosages typically used in clinical trials are included.
Pharmacological Actions	Describes any documented pharmacological actions for the herbal ingredient. This is further divided into a section on *In vitro and animal studies* and a *Clinical studies* section, which describes studies involving humans.
Side-effects, Toxicity	Details documented side-effects to the herbal ingredient and toxicological studies. If side-effects or toxicity are generally associated with any of the constituents in the herbal ingredient, or with its plant family, then these are mentioned here. *See also* Table 1 and Table 2 in the Introduction.
Contra-indications, Warnings	Describes potential contra-indications and potential side-effects, and individuals who may be more susceptible to a particular side-effect. This section should be used in conjunction with Appendices 1–3. Comments on Pregnancy and lactation are included; a summary is provided in Table 3 of the Introduction.
Preparations	Describes product information from over 35 countries. Arranged in two sections, the first section lists by country the proprietary names (product names) of preparations containing the single herbal ingredient described in the monograph. The second section lists by country products that contain multiple ingredients including the herbal ingredient described in the monograph. Specific suppliers of preparations are shown in Appendix 4 along with the supplier contact information in Appendix 5.
References	References are included at the end of the text on each monograph. There is considerable literature on herbal plants and general references have been selected for use with the handbook. These General References, referred to as G1 to G88, are listed after the Introduction. For some well-known herbal ingredients only general references are cited. The majority of the monographs also contain specific references which are cited at the end of each monograph.

Introduction

A general disillusionment with conventional medicines, coupled with the desire for a 'natural' lifestyle has resulted in an increasing utilisation of complementary and alternative medicine (CAM) across the developed world.

A study of long-term trends in the use of CAM therapies in the United States of America reported that the use of CAM therapies has increased steadily since the 1950s.[1] Use of CAM has increased independent of gender, ethnicity and level of education, but is more common in younger people. The use of herbal medicine increased particularly in the 1970s and then again in the 1990s. The report concluded that the continuing demand for CAM will affect delivery of healthcare for the foreseeable future. More recent studies have confirmed that the prevalence of CAM use has remained stable with about a third of US adults reported to use CAM therapies.[2,3] The ten top-selling herbal products in the US in 2004 have been reported as garlic, echinacea, saw palmetto, ginkgo, soy, cranberry, ginseng, black cohosh, St John's wort and milk thistle.[4] The continuing use of CAM has also been reported in South Australia where in 2004, CAMs were reportedly used by over 50% of the population.[5] Several other studies have documented the growing use of CAM in the United Kingdom, with the most common complementary therapies reported as acupuncture, homeopathy, herbal medicine and manipulative therapies, chiropractic and osteopathy.[6]

Estimates of the prevalence of CAM utilisation amongst the general population in the UK range from 10.6%, for use of a limited list of CAM therapies, to 46.6% for use of CAM therapies or over-the-counter (OTC) CAM products.[7,8] In its report on complementary and alternative medicine, the House of Lords Select Committee on Science and Technology's Subcommittee on Complementary and Alternative Medicine highlighted the lack of comprehensive information on the use of herbal medicines in the UK.[9] Estimates of herbal medicine use are available, but it is difficult to gauge usage accurately as many products are considered to be food supplements. Nevertheless, a national telephone survey of a nationally representative sample of 1204 British adults found that around 7% of those contacted had used herbal medicines in the previous year.[10] In another cross-sectional study, over 5000 randomly selected adults in England were sent a postal questionnaire on their use of CAM.[7] Around 20% of the respondents had bought an over-the-counter herbal remedy in the previous 12 months.

Estimates of expenditure on herbal medicines vary, but data generally show that the global market for herbal products has grown rapidly in the past decade. In the USA, annual retail sales of herbal medicines were estimated to be US$ 1.6 billion in 1994,[11] and almost US$ 4 billion in 1998.[12] However, since then there have been reports that the US market has levelled off and in some cases declined.[13] Retail sales of herbal products in the European Union (EU) were estimated to be US$ 7000 million in 1996.[14] A detailed analysis of the European herbal medicines market reported that Germany and France make up more than 70% of the market share.[15] In 1997, total sales of herbal products (using wholesale prices) were US$1.8 billion in Germany and US $1.1 billion in France. In the UK, retail sales of herbal products are reported to have increased by 43% in the period from 1994 to 1998, with retail sales of licensed herbal medicinal products reported to be £50 million in 1998.[9]

Market reports from 2003 indicated a growth in the UK sales of complementary medicines of almost 60% over the previous five years with an estimated value of £130 million. Herbal medicines were reported to represent 60% of the market.[16] Recent reports indicate that the UK market has continued to expand by 45% from 1999 to 2004, with sales of herbal medicines accounting for more than 50%, having risen by 16% since 2002.[17]

These figures demonstrate that herbal medicinal products are being used increasingly by the general public on a self-selection basis to either replace or complement conventional medicines. Against this background of increasing usage of herbal medicines by the public, a number of major public health issues have raised concerns about these products and have highlighted the need for healthcare professionals to have up-to-date scientific information on the quality, safety and efficacy of these products. The substitution of toxic *Aristolochia* species in traditional Chinese medicines (TCM) has resulted in cases of serious renal toxicity and renal cancer in Europe, China and America.[18] The emergence of interactions between *Hypericum perforatum* (*see* St John's wort) and certain prescription medicines has necessitated regulatory action world-wide.[19]

Serious cases of liver damage including a number of fatalities associated with the use of *Piper methysticum* (*see* Kava) have led to restrictions on its use in many countries.[20] Frequent reports of the presence of toxic heavy metals and pharmaceutical substances in Ayurvedic and traditional Chinese medicines reflect a global problem of poor quality of many herbal products.[21,22]

Pharmacists need to be able to advise the consumer on the rational and safe use of all medicines. Studies in the UK, Australia and the US show that pharmacists are frequently involved in the supply of herbal medicines.[23–26]

In order to fulfil this role, pharmacists need to be knowledgeable about herbal medicines and should have access to reliable information in order to advise patients and the public on the safe, effective and appropriate use of herbal preparations. The need to be reliably informed of the quality, safety and efficacy of herbal medicines has been highlighted.[27–29] Also, many other healthcare professionals are becoming increasingly aware of their patients' use of herbal medicines and need to be informed of the suitability of these products for use as medicines.

This handbook brings together in one text a series of monographs on 152 herbs commonly present in herbal medicinal products sold through pharmacies in the UK. Three appendices are also presented, grouping together herbs with specific actions, and highlighting potential interactions with conventional medicines.

As a preface to the monographs, an overview of UK and European legislation concerning herbal products is provided, together with issues pertaining to their quality, safety and efficacy. In addition to retail purchase, herbs can be obtained by picking the wild plant or from a herbal practitioner. This handbook does not discuss the self-collection of plant material for use as a herbal remedy or the prescribing of herbal medicines by herbal practitioners.

Herbal Medicines and Phytotherapy

Herbal medicines are also referred to as herbal remedies, herbal products, herbal medicinal products, phytomedicines, phytotherapeutic agents and phytopharmaceuticals. The use of herbal medicines in an evidence- or science-based approach for the treatment and prevention of disease is known as (rational) phytotherapy. This approach to the use of herbal medicines contrasts with traditional medical herbalism which uses herbal medicines in a holistic manner and mainly on the basis of their empirical and traditional uses. Although these two approaches – traditional/holistic and rational/evidence-based – are entirely different, in some instances they use the same terminology. For example, traditional herbalism is also described as 'phytotherapy' and refers to preparations of plant material as 'herbal medicines'. Today, a continuum between these approaches exists and many herbalists also use scientific evidence to support their traditional use of herbal medicines. Plants have been used medicinally for thousands of years by cultures all over the world. According to the World Health Organization, 80% of the world's population uses plant-based remedies as their primary form of healthcare;[30] in some countries, herbal medicines are still a central part of the medical system, such as Ayurvedic medicine in India and traditional Chinese medicine in China. Herbal medicine has a long history and tradition in Europe.

Herbal medicines and homeopathic remedies are often mistaken by the layperson to be similar. However, homeopathy is based on the principle of 'like should be treated by like', and involves the administration of minute doses of remedies that, in larger doses, produce symptoms in a healthy person mimicking those expressed by people who are ill. Many, but not all, homeopathic remedies originate from plants. By contrast, herbal medicine (phytotherapy) involves the use of dried plant material or extracts of plant parts in therapeutic doses to treat the symptoms exhibited. In this latter respect, it is similar to conventional medicine.

Regulatory Controls on Herbal Medicines

Herbal medicinal products in Europe

Herbal products are available in all Member States of the European Union (EU), although the relative size of their markets varies between countries. Since the late 1980s, the regulation of herbal products has been a major issue within the EU because of the differences between Member States in the way herbal products are classified and the difficulties this might present in the completion of the single market for pharmaceuticals.

According to Council Directive 2001/83/EEC, as amended, a medicinal product is defined as 'any substance or combination of substances presented as having properties for treating or preventing disease in human beings or any substance or combination of substances which may be administered to human beings with a view to restoring, correcting or modifying physiological functions by exerting a pharmacological, immunological or metabolic action, or to making a diagnosis.'[31]

Herbal products are considered as medicinal products if they fall within the definition of the Directive. However, the legal classification is complicated by the fact that in most Member States herbal products are available both as medicinal products with therapeutic claims and also as food/dietary supplements without medicinal claims. The situation is further complicated in that some Member States, including the UK (*see* Current regulatory position of herbal products in the UK), have national provisions which permit certain herbal medicinal products to be exempt from the licensing provisions under specific conditions. In general, in all Member States, herbal products are classified as medicinal products if they claim therapeutic or prophylactic indications.

The advent of the new pan-European marketing authorisation system in 1993 raised questions with regard to herbal products and, in particular, concerns that major differences in their classification/assessment would hinder free circulation within the EU. The new systems for marketing authorisations involve three procedures: centralised, decentralised (mutual recognition) and national.[32,33] The centralised procedure is mandatory for biotechnology products and since November 2005 was mandatory for orphan medicinal products and any medicinal product for human use containing new active substances (i.e. one not previously authorised in the Community) for the treatment of AIDS, cancer, neuro-degenerative disease and diabetes.[34] The decentralised procedure or mutual recognition system involves agreement of assessment between the Member States involved; this procedure became compulsory from January 1998, for products requesting authorisation in more than one Member State. Since then, simultaneous national applications have been possible, but the mutual recognition system automatically becomes involved once an authorisation has been granted in the first Member State. The original intention was to retain existing national procedures for medicinal products requesting authorisation in a single Member State only. However, the European Commission agreed that national procedures could continue for bibliographic applications, including those for herbal products until the harmonisation issues could be resolved.

In 1997, upon the initiative of the European Parliament, the European Commission and the (then) European Medicines Evaluation Agency (EMEA), now European Medicines Agency, an *ad hoc* Working Group on Herbal Medicinal Products (HMPWG) was established at the EMEA. The main thrust of the HMPWG was the protection of public health by preparing guidance to help facilitate mutual recognition of marketing authorisations in the field of herbal medicines, and to minimise CHMP (Committee on Human Medicinal Products) formerly the Committee on Proprietary Medicinal Products (CPMP) arbitrations.

A major study undertaken by the AESGP (Association of the European Self-medication Industry) in 1998 at the request of the European Commission confirmed the different approaches taken by Member States in the regulation of herbal medicinal products.[35] Different traditions in the therapeutic use of herbal preparations, coupled with different national approaches to their assessment, have resulted in differences in the availability of some herbal medicines. For example, ginkgo (*Ginkgo biloba*) is available as a prescription-only medicine in some EU countries, but as a food supplement in others. Similarly, St John's wort (*Hypericum perforatum*) is accepted as a treatment for depression in some Member States, but not in others.

The AESGP study revealed that, in general, herbal medicinal products were either fully licensed with efficacy proven by clinical trials or by bibliography (in accordance with Article 10.1 a (i) of Council Directive 2001/83/EC), or that herbal products had a more or less simplified proof of efficacy, according to their national use. Furthermore, the study found major discrepancies between Member States in the classification of individual herbal preparations and products into one of these categories, as well as in the requirements for obtaining a marketing authorisation (product licence). The report highlighted the need for clarification of the regulatory framework and harmonisation of the regulatory requirements to ensure that herbal medicinal products could have access to the single market for pharmaceuticals.

An important initiative in the harmonisation process has been the formation of the European Scientific Cooperative on Phytotherapy (ESCOP), an organisation representing national associations for phytotherapy. ESCOP was founded in 1989 by six EU national scientific associations with the objective of establishing a scientific umbrella organisation to provide harmonised criteria for the assessment of herbal medicinal products, to support scientific research and contribute to the acceptance of phytotherapy in Europe.[36, 37]

ESCOP now comprises 13 national associations across Europe, and the American Botanical Council. The ESCOP Scientific Committee has published 80 monographs for individual herbal drugs; the monographs follow the European Summary of Product Characteristics (SPC) format.[38] The EMEA Herbal Medicinal Products Working Party (HMPWP) formerly used the ESCOP monographs as a basis for its work in developing core SPCs from ESCOP monographs. The HMPWP has now been superseded by the Herbal Medicinal Products Committee (HMPC) as discussed below and the collaboration with ESCOP continues in accordance with the new EU regulations.

New regulations for traditional herbal medicinal products in the EU

From the late 1980s, the need for a new regulatory framework for herbal products has been under discussion supported by the European Parliament and the European Commission. It was generally accepted that a significant number of herbal medicinal products did not fulfil the requirements for marketing authorizations. In September 1999, the European Pharmaceutical Committee set up a working group of Member States to investigate the possibility of a directive for traditionally used medicines. Work commenced in April 2000 and a new EU Directive on Traditional Herbal Medicinal Products 2004/24/EC came into force in April 2004 requiring Member States to implement registration schemes by October 2005.[39] The aim is to remove the differences which create obstacles to the free movement of medicinal products in the EU, while ensuring protection for public health. For unlicensed herbal medicines legally on the market on 30 April 2004, the Directive provides a seven-year transitional period to allow companies time to meet the new requirements. The new Directive provides a framework for the regulation of traditionally used herbal medicinal products requiring them to meet specific and appropriate standards of safety and quality and for the product to be accompanied by suitable information to ensure its safe use. Registered products are required to be suitable for self-medication without the need for the intervention of a medical practitioner. The normal requirement for medicines to be proven to be efficacious, as required under Directive 2001/83/EC for a marketing authorisation, is replaced by a requirement to demonstrate 30 years' traditional use for the required medicinal indication; at least 15 years of this usage must have been within the EU.

Registration applications have to include a bibliographic review of the safety data associated with the use of the herbal product in a particular indication. In addition, this review will need to be accompanied by an expert report on the safety data submitted. The normal quality requirements applicable to licensed medicines will apply, including good manufacturing practice (GMP) and European Pharmacopoeia standards. Labelling and package leaflets for registered products will be required to include information and instructions about the safe use of the product and will include a statement to the effect that the product is based on long-standing use. In addition to the herbal ingredients, vitamins and minerals can be added provided that they are ancillary to the herbal active ingredients. Manufacturers will be required to have in place an adequate pharmacovigilance system to maintain records of all suspected adverse drug reactions (ADRs) occurring world-wide and will have to report all ADRs to the national regulatory licensing authority.

The Directive established a new European Committee at the EMEA, the Committee on Herbal Medicinal Products (HMPC) with responsibilities to prepare Community monographs and a Community list of herbal substances. A Community herbal monograph comprises the committee's scientific opinion on a given herbal medicinal product, based on its evaluation of available scientific data (well-established use) or on the historic use of that product in the European Community (traditional use). For some herbal medicinal products, the Community monograph will cover both well-established use and traditional use. The Community monographs are intended to assist harmonisation of requirements for 'bibliographic' marketing authorisation applications. When the HMPC has produced a draft Community monograph it is released for public consultation on the EMEA website, usually for a period of three months. The comments received are subsequently reviewed and the final version of the Community herbal monograph is published.

The Community list will contain, for each herbal substance or preparation, the indication, the specified strength and the posology, the route of administration and any other information necessary for the safe use of the herbal substance or preparation used as an ingredient of a traditional medicinal product. The Community list will provide a harmonised approach at EU level for providing information on substance(s) or preparation(s) that constitute traditional herbal medicinal products. The list will cover substances and preparations that have been in medicinal use for a sufficiently long time, and therefore considered not to be harmful under normal conditions of use. List entries are also released for public consultation on the EMEA website, usually for a period of three months. Applicants for traditional registrations can refer to the list rather than have to provide evidence of traditional use and safety thus further simplifying the registration procedure. Draft and adopted Community monographs are available on the EMEA website.[40]

A simplified registration scheme was introduced in the UK in October 2005 for traditional herbal medicinal products. A new advisory committee, the Herbal Medicines Advisory Committee (HMAC), has been established to advise Health Ministers on issues relating to registration of traditional herbal medicinal products and the safety and quality of unlicensed herbal remedies.

Current regulatory position of herbal products in the UK

Herbal products are available in the UK through various retail outlets, such as pharmacies, health-food shops, mail order companies, supermarkets, department stores and, increasingly, via the internet. Some herbal products consist solely of loose, dried plant material; others are presented as pre-packaged formulated products in a variety of pharmaceutical forms for both internal (tablets, capsules, liquids) and external use (creams, ointments) and may contain one or several herbal ingredients which may be dried herbs or their extracts. The current regulatory position is complicated by the fact that herbal products can fall into one of three categories: licensed herbal products, those exempt from licensing and those marketed as food supplements. In addition, from November 2005, the registration procedure for traditional herbal medicinal products has introduced a further category, that of 'registered products'.

The majority of herbal products are marketed without medicinal claims either exempt from licensing (*see* Herbal remedies exempt from licensing) or as food supplements. Those supplied as food supplements are controlled under food legislation whilst those exempt from licensing are controlled under medicines legislation. Difficulties in defining the status of products occupying the borderline between medicines and foods have resulted in similar products being marketed in both these categories. Provided the products were marketed without reference to medicinal claims, the Medicines and Healthcare products Regulatory Agency (MHRA; formerly Medicines Control Agency (MCA)), the government body responsible for regulating medicinal products has, in the past, generally been satisfied that the products were not subject to medicines legislation.[41] However, implementation of the definition of a medicinal product in accordance with EC Directives has meant that greater emphasis is now being placed on the nature of the herbal ingredients being supplied as food supplements.

Licensed herbal medicinal products

Almost all of the licensed herbal medicines on the UK market have been available for some time and most originally held Product Licences of Right (PLR). Following the implementation of the UK Medicines Act in 1971, Product Licences of Right were issued to all medicinal products already on the market in September 1971, however, scientific assessment was not undertaken at the time the PLR was granted. A subsequent review of all PLRs for safety, quality and efficacy took place culminating in 1990. During the UK review of herbal medicinal products holding a PLR, the Licensing Authority agreed to accept bibliographic evidence of efficacy for herbal medicinal products which were indicated for minor, self-limiting conditions.[42] No evidence was required from new clinical trials provided the manufacturers agreed to label their products as 'a traditional herbal remedy for the symptomatic relief of ...' and to include the statement 'if symptoms persist consult your doctor'. The Licensing Authority considered it inappropriate to relax the requirements for proof of efficacy for herbal medicinal products indicated for more serious conditions. Thus, evidence was required from controlled clinical trials for herbal medicinal products indicated for conditions considered inappropriate for self-diagnosis and treatment. Many features of the new traditional use registration scheme are similar to those applied during the review of PLRs.

The MHRA regulates medicinal products for human use in accordance with The Medicines (Marketing Authorisations etc.) Amendment Regulations 2005, (The Regulations)[43] and the Medicines Act 1968.[44] The Medicines Act and secondary legislation made under it remain the legal basis for other aspects of medicines control including manufacturer and wholesale dealers' authorisations, controls on sale and supply and controls on promotion. Further explanation may be obtained by reference to a chapter on herbal remedies in *Dale and Appelbe's Pharmacy Law and Ethics*.[45]

Applications for marketing authorisations (product licences) for new herbal products are assessed by the MHRA for quality, safety and efficacy in accordance with EC and UK legislation. Specific EC guidelines exist on the quality, specifications and manufacture of herbal medicinal products.[46–48] Few applications for new marketing authorisations are successful and the difficulties faced by herbal manufacturers in fulfilling the regulatory requirements have led to the development of the new simplified traditional use registration scheme outlined above. It will continue to be possible to obtain a marketing authorisation for a herbal medicinal product provided that the required data on safety, quality and efficacy can be demonstrated.

Herbal remedies exempt from licensing

Under the Medicines Act, herbal remedies manufactured and sold or supplied in accordance with specific exemptions set out in Sections 12(1) or (2) or Article 2 of the Medicines (Exemptions from Licences) (Special and Transitional Cases) Order 1971 (SI 1450)[49] are exempt from the requirement to hold product licences. The exempt products are those compounded and supplied by herbalists on their own recommendation, those comprised solely of dried, crushed or comminuted plants sold under their botanical name with no written recommendations as to their use, and those made by a holder of a Specials Manufacturing Licence on behalf of a herbalist.

The exemptions are intended, for example, to give herbal practitioners the flexibility they need to prepare their own remedies for individual patients without the burden of licensing, and to enable simple dried herbs to be readily available to the public. Supply of herbal remedies by herbal practitioners is not affected by the new regulations on traditional medicines. Proposals for the reform of the regulation of unlicensed herbal remedies made up to meet the needs of individual patients are currently under consideration.[50]

At the present time, most manufactured over-the-counter herbal medicines in the UK are sold under the exemptions provided for by Section 12(2) of the Medicines Act. It has been recognised for some time that the arrangements for unlicensed herbal medicinal products do not afford sufficient protection for public health and that there is a need to improve the regulatory position. The MHRA is now of the view that the present regulatory arrangements for unlicensed herbal medicines have significant weaknesses.[9] The regime for unlicensed herbal products is considered not to provide sufficient protection or information for the public and there are no specific safeguards in place to ensure adequate product quality and safety.[51]

The all party House of Lords Select Committee on Science and Technology concluded: *'We are concerned about the safety implications of an unregulated herbal sector and we urge that all legislative avenues be explored to ensure better control of this unregulated sector in the interests of public health.'*[9]

Evidence of the risks to public health have continued to emerge and in September 2004 the Committee on Safety of Medicines (CSM) repeated an earlier warning about their concerns in relation to the poor quality of some traditional Chinese medicines on the UK market.[52]

The MHRA has indicated that it is the Government's intention that, following the transitional period of the Traditional Use Directive, Section 12 (2) would cease to provide a regulatory route by which manufactured herbal medicinal products can reach the market place without a traditional registration or product licence.[53]

Control of herbal ingredients in the UK

Most of the herbal ingredients used in licensed herbal medicines have been used as traditional remedies for centuries without major safety problems, and the majority is included in the General Sales List (GSL).[54] Potentially hazardous plants such as digitalis, rauwolfia and nux vomica are specifically controlled under the Medicines Act as prescription only medicines (POM),[55] and thus are not available other than via a registered medical practitioner. In addition, certain herbal ingredients are controlled under The Medicines (Retail Sale and Supply of Herbal Remedies) Order 1977 SI 2130.[56] This Order (Part I) specifies 25 plants which cannot be supplied except via a pharmacy, and includes well-known toxic species, such as *Areca*, *Crotalaria*, *Dryopteris* and *Strophanthus*. In Part II, the Order specifies plant species, such as *Aconitum*, *Atropa*, *Ephedra* and *Hyoscyamus*, which can be supplied by 'herbal practitioners', and in Part III defines the dosages and routes of administration permitted.

Legislation has been introduced to prohibit the use of *Aristolochia* species or species likely to be confused with *Aristolochia* in unlicensed medicines.[57] These measures were introduced in the wake of cases of serious toxicity and evidence showing widespread substitution of certain ingredients in traditional Chinese medicines with *Aristolochia* (*see* Quality, Safety and Efficacy of Herbal Medicines).

Following cases of serious liver damage suspected to be associated with its consumption *Piper methysticum* (*see* Kava) was prohibited in unlicensed herbal medicines in January 2003.[58] The MHRA has also announced the need to update the list of herbal ingredients subject to restrictions or prohibitions in use in unlicensed medicines to take account of the herbal ingredients used in traditional Chinese and Ayurvedic medicines.[59]

Regulatory control of herbal medicines world-wide

The World Health Organization (WHO) has conducted a recent global survey on the regulatory control of herbal medicines and has reported findings from 141 countries.[60] This work provides a valuable update to the earlier WHO reviews and illustrates the wide differences in the approach to regulation between these countries[61, 62] The recent survey confirms that during the past four years many countries have established, or initiated, the process of establishing national policy and regulations regarding herbal medicines. The most important challenges faced by countries were those related to regulatory status, assessment of safety and efficacy, quality control and safety monitoring. In response to requests from Member States, WHO has resolved to provide technical support for the development of methodology to monitor or ensure product safety, efficacy and quality, preparation of guidelines, and promotion of information exchange. WHO guidelines have recently been developed in a number of important areas including consumer information, pharmacovigilance and good agricultural and collection practices (GACP).[63–65]

Herbal products are well established as phytomedicines in some countries, whereas in others they are regarded as foods, and therapeutic claims are not allowed. In the context of this book, it should be noted that many of the herbs included in the monographs are of economic importance in some non-European countries, particularly Australia, Canada and the USA.

In Australia, therapeutic goods for human use which are imported or manufactured are subject to the Therapeutic Goods Act, 1989 and all therapeutic goods imported into, supplied in or exported from Australia must be included in the Australian Register of Therapeutic Goods (ARTG).[66] Herbal medicines, including traditional medicines such as Ayurvedic medicines and traditional Chinese medicines (TCM) are regulated as complementary medicines. For the purpose of labelling requirements, herbs are included in the List of Australian Approved Names for Pharmaceutical Substances, which is published by the Therapeutic Goods Administration. The Australian system has a two-tiered approach based on risk. Low risk medicines, which include most complementary medicines, are included in the ARTG as listed medicines. These medicines are not evaluated before they are released on to the market, but are checked to ensure that they comply with certain legislative requirements. Listed medicines have limited therapeutic indications, for example health enhancement, reduction in risk of a disease, disorder or condition, reduction in frequency of a discrete event, aiding or assisting management of a symptom, disease, disorder or condition, relief of symptoms. Indications and claims referring to treatment, management, cure or prevention of a disease, disorder, or condition or reference to a serious form of a disease are generally not permitted for listed medicines. Those medicines deemed to be higher risk are assessed individually for safety, quality and efficacy prior to marketing.

In Canada, new regulations, the Natural Health Products Regulations, came into force in January 2004.[67] Products that fall within the new regulations include herbal remedies, homeopathic medicines, vitamins, minerals, traditional medicines, probiotics, amino acids and essential fatty acids. The new regulations introduce a system of product licensing, site licensing, GMP, adverse reaction reporting and requirements for labelling. Persons marketing products before January 2004 have a transition period of two years to comply with the site licence requirements of the regulations and those products with a valid Drug Identification Number, from the previous regulatory regime, have six years to obtain a product licence under the new regulations. Product licence applications are assessed for safety and efficacy and different types of claims can be proposed, e.g. therapeutic claims, risk reduction claims or structure–function claims supported by traditional use or non-traditional use.

In the USA, the majority of medicinal herbs and their products are regulated like foods as dietary supplements, under the 1994 Dietary Supplement Health and Education Act (DSHEA).[68, 69] Whilst medicinal claims cannot be made for the products, labelling may describe effects on general well-being. Unlike new medicines, dietary supplements do not generally have to go through review by the Food and Drug Administration for safety and effectiveness or be approved before they can be marketed. However, manufacturers must provide premarket notice and evidence of safety for any supplements they plan to sell that contain dietary ingredients that were not on the market before DSHEA was passed. Concerns have been raised about the effectiveness of the DSHEA legislation following the emergence of major safety issues arising with unsafe ingredients e.g. ephedra, lack of GMP, poor labelling and inadequate reporting of adverse reactions.[69, 70] In response, the FDA has announced the development of strategies to monitor and evaluate product and ingredient safety; to assure product quality (current good manufacturing practice regulations (cGMP); and to improve product labelling.[71, 72]

It is apparent that not only is the regulation of medicinal herbs different from one country to another, but also that the regulatory processes are not necessarily ideal and are under current review.

Quality, Safety and Efficacy of Herbal Medicines

In order to ensure public health, medicinal products must be safe, efficacious and of suitable quality for use. To obtain a marketing authorisation (product licence) within the EU, manufacturers of herbal medicinal products are required to demonstrate that their products meet acceptable standards of quality, safety and efficacy.

Quality

Over the past decade the quality of herbal products has continued to be a major concern. The importance of quality in ensuring the safety and efficacy of herbal products has been reviewed extensively.[22, 73–78]

Problems with unregulated herbal products

The vast majority of quality-related problems are associated with unregulated herbal products. There is substantial evidence that many ethnic medicines, in particular, those used in traditional Chinese medicine (TCM) and traditional Asian medicines (Ayurvedic and Unani), lack effective quality controls and may give rise to serious public health concerns. The problems include deliberate or accidental inclusion of prohibited or restricted ingredients, substitution of ingredients, contamination with toxic substances and differences between the labelled and actual contents. These problems are further compounded by demand outstripping supply of good quality ingredients, confusing nomenclature over plant species, cultural differences of view over toxicity and traditional practices such as substituting one ingredient for another having a reportedly similar action.

Although individual herbs present in traditional Chinese medicines and traditional Asian medicines are not the subject of monographs in this book, they do illustrate the problems that may be associated with the quality and safety of herbal medicines.

Substitution and adulteration

Aristolochia Exposure to *Aristolochia* species in unlicensed herbal medicines has resulted in cases of nephrotoxicity and carcinogenicity in Europe, China, Japan and the USA.[18] Concerns were first raised about the effects of products containing aristolochic acids in Belgium where, since 1993, over 100 cases of irreversible nephropathy have been reported in young women using a preparation claimed to aid weight loss. The nephrotoxicity was traced to the inadvertent use of the toxic *Aristolochia fangchi* root in the formulation as a substitute for *Stephania tetrandra*. Aristolochic acids, the toxic components of *Aristolochia* species, are known to be nephrotoxic, carcinogenic and mutagenic. The International Agency for Research on Cancer classifies products containing *Aristolochia* species as human carcinogens.[79] Several of the Belgian patients have subsequently developed urothelial cancer as a result of exposure to the toxic aristolochic acids.[80–84]

Seven cases of nephropathy involving substitution of *Aristolochia fangchi* and *Stephania tetrandra* have been reported in France.[18] Toxicity has also resulted from the substitution of *Aristolochia manshuriensis* stem for the stem of *Clematis* and *Akebia* species.[18] In the UK, two such cases of end-stage renal failure were reported in 1999.[85, 86] Other cases have been reported in China (17 cases with 12 fatalities) and Japan (ten cases of renal failure).[18] Also, the FDA has reported two cases of serious renal disease due to *Aristolochia* being substituted for *Clematis* species in a dietary supplement.[87]

Substitution of one plant species for another, often of a completely different genus, is an established practice in TCM. Furthermore, herbal ingredients are traded using their common Chinese Pin Yin names, and this can lead to confusion. For example, the name Fang ji can be used to describe the roots of *Aristolochia fangchi*, *Stephania tetrandra* or *Cocculus* species, and the name Mu Tong can be used to describe the stem of *Aristolochia manshuriensis*, *Clematis* or *Akebia* species. The widespread substitution with *Aristolochia* species in TCM products available in the UK was shown in a MHRA study which reported the presence of aristolochic acids in at least 40% of TCM products containing Fang ji and Mu Tong.[88]

The problems associated with *Aristolochia* have prompted regulatory action world-wide and new legislation has been introduced in the UK to prohibit the use of *Aristolochia* species in unlicensed medicines in the UK.[57]

Despite warnings and an import alert issued by the US FDA in 2001, products containing aristolochic acid were found to be available on US websites in 2003.[89] The MHRA has reported that it continues to find products containing *Aristolochia* on the UK market. In 2003, a product called Xie Gan Wan was found to contain aristolochic acids and in December 2004, tablets called Jingzhi Kesou Tanchuan were found to contain *Aristolochia* fructus.[90] Also in December 2004, the Hong Kong authorities alerted other health authorities to a product Shen Yi Qian Lie Hui Chin that contained aristolochic acids. In December 2005, MHRA issued a warning about the possible presence of *Aristolochia* species in African herbal remedies available in the UK.

Digitalis Cases of serious cardiac arrhythmias were reported in the USA in 1997 following the accidental substitution of plantain with *Digitalis lanata*.[91] Subsequent investigation revealed that large quantities of the contaminated plantain had been shipped to more than 150 manufacturers, distributors and retailers over a two-year period.

Podophyllum Fourteen cases of podophyllum poisoning have been reported from Hong Kong following the inadvertent use of the roots *Podophyllum hexandrum* instead of *Gentiana* and *Clematis* species.[92] It is reported that this accidental substitution arose because of the apparent similarity in morphology of the roots.

Aconitum Cases of cardiotoxicity resulting from the ingestion of *Aconitum* species used in TCM have been reported from Hong Kong.[93] In TCM, *Aconitum* rootstocks are processed by soaking or boiling them in water in order to hydrolyse the aconite alkaloids into their less toxic aconine derivatives. Toxicity can, however, result when such processes are uncontrolled and unvalidated. In the UK, the internal use of aconite is restricted to prescription only.

Star Anise The dangers of confusing Chinese (*Illicium verum* Hook.f.) and Japanese star anise (*Illicium anisatum* L.), have been known for many years as the dried fruits cannot be distinguished through visual examination. Japanese star anise is similar to the Chinese variety but has been reported to cause neurologic and gastrointestinal toxicities due to the presence of anisatin.[94, 95] In 2001 cases of poisoning were reported in the Netherlands, Spain and France where Japanese star anise had been accidentally used in place of Chinese star anise.[96–98] Several cases were epileptic-type seizures in babies who had been given star anise infusions. This led to over 50 cases of poisoning being reported, but there was no evidence that the affected products had been imported into the UK. In the US, seven cases of adverse neurologic reactions have been reported among infants aged two weeks to three months who were exposed to star anise tea.[99]

Adulteration with heavy metals/toxic elements and synthetic drugs

The adulteration of ethnic medicines with heavy metals/toxic elements and synthetic drugs continues to be a major international problem. A comprehensive review in 1992 summarised test results on products and case histories of patients who had experienced toxic effects.[72] Similar findings continue to be reported and the potential impact on public health is significant.[22] In most cases involving synthetic drugs, the drugs are undeclared in the product and only come to light when the user experiences adverse effects which are sufficiently serious to warrant medical intervention. Exposure to the undeclared drug is revealed in the subsequent investigation of the clinical case. Of particular concern is the deliberate addition of closely related derivatives of pharmaceutical drugs, for example the use of nitrosofenfluramine instead of fenfluramine in weight-loss products.[22]

The situation with the heavy metals/toxic elements differs in that whilst these ingredients may arise from the plant ingredients themselves or be introduced as trace contaminants during processing, they are also frequently added intentionally and declared as ingredients within some TCM and Asian medicine formulations. The Chinese Pharmacopoeia, for example, includes monographs for realgar (arsenic disulfide), calomel (mercurous chloride), cinnabaris (mercuric sulfide) and hydrargyri oxydum rubrum (red mercuric oxide), and includes formulations for nearly 50 products that include one or more of these substances.[100]

A US survey in 1998 reported widespread inconsistencies and adulterations in imported Asian medicines.[101] Of 260 imported products tested, at least 83 (32%) contained undeclared pharmaceuticals (most commonly ephedrine, chlorphenamine, methyltestosterone and phenacetin) or heavy metals (lead, arsenic or mercury). Another survey found evidence of a continuing problem, with 10% of 500 OTC products testing positive for undeclared drugs and/or toxic amounts of lead, mercury or arsenic.[102]

Elsewhere, health departments have reported similar conclusions based on their findings. A survey conducted in Singapore between 1990 and 1997 on TCM products reported that 42 different products were found to contain excessive amounts of heavy metals (mercury, lead, arsenic) and that 32 different TCM products were found to contain a total of 19 drugs.[103] In total, 93 cases of excessive content of toxic heavy metals and undeclared drugs were detected. The drugs detected included berberine, antihistamines (chlorphenamine, promethazine, cyproheptadine), non-steroidal anti-inflammatory drugs (diclofenac, indometacin, ibuprofen), analgesic antipyretics (paracetamol, dipyrone), corticosteroids (prednisolone, dexamethasone, fluocinonide), sympathomimetics agents (ephedrine), bronchodilators (theophylline), diuretics (hydrochlorthiazide) and the antidiabetic phenformin. A study in Taiwan found that more than 20% of 2609 products were found to be adulterated with synthetic drugs, most commonly caffeine, paracetamol, indometacin and hydrochlorthiazide.[104]

Other examples of adulterated products come from a report from the Singapore Ministry of Health which identified sildenafil in two Chinese proprietary medicines,[105] and a report from the USA FDA which described the recall of a herbal product after traces of chlordiazepoxide were found in the capsules.[106] In 2001, the UK MCA reported presence of mercury (due to the inclusion of cinnabaris) in samples of the product Shugan Wan on the UK market.[90]

Cases of toxicity associated with synthetic drugs present in ethnic medicines include a case of poisoning in Hong Kong resulting from the use of a TCM product containing anticonvulsant agents (phenytoin, carbamazepine and valproate).[107] In 2000, the USA FDA issued a public health warning on five herbal products following adverse effects in patients.[108] The products were found to contain the antihyperglycaemic prescription drugs glibenclamide and phenformin. In March 2001, the UK MCA reported a serious case of hypoglycaemic coma in a patient who had taken a TCM product, Xiaoke Wan, which contained glibenclamide.[109]

Cases of toxicity associated with heavy metals in ethnic medicines include a patient from Taiwan who developed a unique syndrome of multiple renal tubular dysfunction after taking a Chinese herbal medicine contaminated with cadmium.[110] In the USA, two cases of alopecia and sensory polyneuropathy resulting from thallium in a TCM product have been reported.[111] In the UK, cases have been reported of two patients with heavy metal intoxication following ingestion of an Indian remedy containing inorganic arsenic and mercury,[112] and of a patient with lead poisoning after exposure to an Indian medicine containing toxic amounts of lead, arsenic and mercury.[113] In a case reported from Macau, death of a 13-year-old girl from arsenic poisoning has been linked with a Chinese herbal product Niu Huang Chieh Tu Pien.[114]

Evidence of this international problem continues to grow and a substantial body of literature is now available. The adulteration of Chinese and Ayurvedic herbal medicines with synthetic drugs and toxic metals has been extensively reviewed.[21, 22, 115–119]

A survey of 70 Ayurvedic herbal medicinal products available in Boston-area stores (US) found that 20% contained potentially harmful concentrations of lead, mercury and/or arsenic.[120] In response to the many issues arising with herbal products the MHRA has introduced a specific web page Herbal Safety News to provide information on safety alerts.[90] Regular notifications concerning the presence of heavy metals/toxic elements and pharmaceutical drugs in TCM/Ayurvedic products and steroids in dermatological preparations are posted. Of particular concern in recent years has been the discovery of TCM slimming products containing potentially harmful ingredients such as fenfluramine, nitrosofenfluramine, sibutramine, methylphenidate. In March 2004, the Agency was made aware of a UK case of irreversible liver failure suspected to be caused by a product called 'Shubao-Slimming Capsules'. The patient required a liver transplant. The product was labelled as only containing botanical ingredients but was found to contain undeclared nitrosofenfluramine, a drug closely related to the prescription only medicine (POM), fenfluramine. Nitrosofenfluramine is known to be toxic to the liver. Other samples of Shubao tested were found to contain nitrosofenfluramine and/or fenfluramine.

The MHRA has issued guidance to the public alerting them to the specific concerns with TCM slimming products.[90] In September 2004, MHRA issued a press statement warning consumers that the poor quality of some TCM products could pose a health risk to those using them. The MHRA emphasised that it continued to find examples of products containing the prohibited ingredients *Aristolochia* and *Ephedra* as well as products containing heavy metals/ toxic elements, prescription drugs as well as human placenta and bat excreta.[52]

Quality of regulated herbal products

Compared with conventional preparations, herbal medicinal products present a number of unique problems when quality aspects are considered. These arise because of the nature of the herbal ingredients, which are complex mixtures of constituents, and it is well documented that concentrations of plant constituents can vary considerably depending on environmental and genetic factors. Furthermore, the constituents responsible for the claimed therapeutic effects are frequently unknown or only partly explained and this precludes the level of control which can routinely be achieved with synthetic drug substances in conventional pharmaceuticals. The position is further complicated by the traditional practice of using combinations of herbal ingredients, and it is not uncommon to have five herbal ingredients or more in one product.

In recognition of the special problems associated with herbal medicinal products, the CHMP (formerly CPMP) has issued specific guidelines dealing with quality, specifications and manufacture. These guidelines have recently been updated.[46–48] The EMEA HMPC has also issued guidance on Good Agricultural and Collection Practice (GACP) for starting materials of herbal origin.[121] The CHMP guidelines highlight the need for good control of both the starting materials and the finished product, and emphasise the importance of good manufacturing practice in the manufacture of herbal medicinal products.

The WHO has also published guidelines dealing with the quality control of medicinal plant materials and on good agricultural and collection practices (GACP).[65, 122]

European Pharmacopoeia

Since its creation in 1964, the European Pharmacopoeia (Ph Eur) has devoted part of its work to the establishment of monographs on herbal drugs which are used either in their natural state after drying or extraction, or for the isolation of natural active ingredients. The Ph Eur includes over 120 monographs on herbal drugs, and a similar number of monographs are under development. Many general methods of analysis are also described in the Ph Eur, including tests for pesticides and for microbial contamination.[123]

Herbal ingredients

Control of the starting materials is essential in order to ensure reproducible quality of herbal medicinal products.[22, 78, 124] The following points are to be considered in the control of starting materials.

Authentication and reproducibility of herbal ingredients The problems associated with unregulated herbal products, as illustrated above, highlight the major public health issues that can arise when their herbal ingredients have not been authenticated correctly. Herbal ingredients must be accurately identified by macroscopical and microscopical comparison with authentic material or accurate descriptions of authentic herbs.[125] It is essential that herbal ingredients are referred to by their binomial Latin names of genus and species; only permitted synonyms should be used. Even when correctly authenticated, it is important to realise that different batches of the same herbal ingredient may differ in quality due to a number of factors.

Inter- or intraspecies variation For many plants, there is considerable inter- and intraspecies variation in constituents, which is genetically controlled and may be related to the country of origin.

Environmental factors The quality of a herbal ingredient can be affected by environmental factors, such as climate, altitude and growing conditions.

Time of harvesting For some herbs the optimum time of harvesting should be specified as it is known that the concentrations of constituents in a plant can vary during the growing cycle or even during the course of a day.

Plant part used Active constituents usually vary between plant parts and it is not uncommon for a herbal ingredient to be adulterated with parts of the plant not normally utilised. In addition, plant material that has been previously subjected to extraction and is therefore 'exhausted' is sometimes used to increase the weight of a batch of herbal ingredient.

Post-harvesting factors Storage conditions and processing treatments can greatly affect the quality of a herbal ingredient. Inappropriate storage after harvesting can result in microbial contamination, and processes such as drying may result in a loss of thermolabile active constituents.

Adulteration/substitution Instances of herbal remedies adulterated with other plant material and conventional medicines, and the consequences of this, have been discussed above. In particular, the serious public health consequences that may arise from the substitution of herbal ingredients by toxic *Aristolochia* species have been highlighted. Reports of herbal products devoid of known active constituents have reinforced the need for adequate quality control of herbal remedies.

Identity tests In order to try to ensure the quality of licensed herbal medicines, it is essential not only to establish the botanical identity of a herbal ingredient but also to ensure batch-to-batch reproducibility. Thus, in addition to macroscopical and microscopical evaluation, identity tests are necessary. Such tests include simple chemical tests, e.g. colour or precipitation and chromatographic tests. Thin-layer chromatography is commonly used for identification purposes but for herbal ingredients containing volatile oils a gas–liquid chromatographic test may be used. Although the aim of such tests is to confirm the presence of active principle(s), it is frequently the case that the nature of the active principle has not been established. In such instances chemical and chromatographic tests help to provide batch-to-batch comparability and the chromatogram may be used as a 'fingerprint' for the herbal ingredient by demonstrating the profile of some common plant constituents such as flavonoids.

Assay For those herbal ingredients with known active principles, an assay should be established in order to set the criterion for the minimum accepted percentage of active substance(s). Such assays should, wherever possible, be specific for individual chemical substances and high-pressure liquid chromatography or gas–liquid chromatography are the methods of choice. Where such assays have not been established then non-specific methods such as titration or colorimetric assays may be used to determine the total content of a group of closely related compounds.

Contaminants of herbal ingredients Herbal ingredients should be of high quality and free from insects, other animal matter and excreta. It is not possible to remove completely all contaminants and hence specifications should be set in order to limit them:

Ash values Incineration of a herbal ingredient produces ash which constitutes inorganic matter. Treatment of the ash with hydrochloric acid results in acid-insoluble ash which consists mainly of silica and may be used to act as a measure of soil present. Limits may be set for ash and acid-insoluble ash of herbal ingredients.

Foreign organic matter It is not possible to collect a herbal ingredient without small amounts of related parts of plant or other plants. Standards should be set in order to limit the percentage of such unwanted plant contaminants.

Microbial contamination Aerobic bacteria and fungi are normally present in plant material and may increase due to faulty growing, harvesting, storage or processing. Herbal ingredients, particularly those with high starch content, may be prone to increased microbial growth. It is not uncommon for herbal ingredients to have aerobic bacteria present at 10^2–10^8 colony forming units per gram. Pathogenic organisms including *Enterobacter*, *Enterococcus*, *Clostridium*, *Pseudomonas*, *Shigella* and *Streptococcus* have been shown to contaminate herbal ingredients. It is essential that limits be set for microbial contamination and the Ph Eur now gives non-mandatory guidance on acceptable limits.[123]

Pesticides Herbal ingredients, particularly those grown as cultivated crops, may be contaminated by DDT (dichlorodiphenyltrichloroethane) or other chlorinated hydrocarbons, organophosphates, carbamates or polychlorinated biphenyls. Limit tests are necessary for acceptable levels of pesticide contamination of herbal ingredients. The Ph Eur includes details of test methods together with mandatory limits for 34 potential pesticide residues.[123]

Fumigants Ethylene oxide, methyl bromide and phosphine have been used to control pests which contaminate herbal ingredients. The use of ethylene oxide as a fumigant with herbal drugs is no longer permitted in Europe.

Toxic metals Lead, cadmium, mercury, thallium and arsenic have been shown to be contaminants of some herbal ingredients. Limit tests for such toxic metals are essential for herbal ingredients.

Other contaminants As standards increase for the quality of herbal ingredients it is possible that tests to limit other contaminants such as endotoxins, mycotoxins and radionuclides will be utilised to ensure high quality for medicinal purposes.

Herbal products

Quality assurance of herbal products may be ensured by control of the herbal ingredients and by adherence to good manufacturing practice standards. Some herbal products have many herbal ingredients with only small amounts of individual herbs being present. Chemical and chromatographic tests are useful for developing finished product specifications. Stability and shelf life of herbal products should be established by manufacturers. There should be no differences in standards set for the quality of dosage forms, such as tablets or capsules, of herbal medicines from those of other pharmaceutical preparations.

The quality of an unregulated herbal remedy will not have been assessed by a Regulatory Authority and may thus potentially affect the safety and efficacy of the product. In view of this, it may be concluded that a pharmacist should only sell or recommend herbal medicinal products that hold a product licence or a traditional herbal medicine registration. However, the majority of herbal medicinal products are only available as unlicensed products. When deciding upon the suitability of such products, a pharmacist should consider the intended use and the manufacturer. It is highly likely that unlicensed herbal remedies manufactured by an established pharmaceutical company will have been subjected to suitable in-house quality control procedures.

Safety

As with all forms of self-treatment, the use of herbal medicinal products presents a potential risk to human health.[22, 126] There are concerns that the patient may be exposed to potentially toxic substances either from the herbal ingredients themselves or as a result of exposure to contaminants present in the herbal product. Furthermore, self-administration of any therapy in preference to orthodox treatment may delay a patient seeking qualified advice, or cause a patient to abandon conventional treatment without first seeking appropriate advice. Emerging evidence suggests that herbal medicinal products may in some cases compromise the efficacy of conventional medicines, for example through herb–drug interactions.

The safety of all medicinal products is of the utmost importance. All applications for marketing authorisations for new medicines undergo extensive evaluation of their risks and benefits and, once granted, licensed products are closely monitored for the occurrence of suspected adverse effects. The safety of herbal medicinal products is of particular importance as the majority of these products is self-prescribed and is used to treat minor and often chronic conditions.

The extensive traditional use of plants as medicines has enabled those medicines with acute and obvious signs of toxicity to be well recognised and their use avoided. However, the premise that traditional use of a plant for perhaps many hundreds of years establishes its safety does not necessarily hold true.[22, 126, 127] The more subtle and chronic forms of toxicity, such as carcinogenicity, mutagenicity and hepatotoxicity, may well have been overlooked by previous generations and it is these types of toxicities that are of most concern when assessing the safety of herbal remedies.

A UK Medical Toxicology Unit conducted a study of potentially serious adverse reactions associated with exposure to traditional medicines and food supplements during 1991 to 1995.[128] Of 1297 enquiries from healthcare professionals, a total of 785 cases were identified as possible (n = 738), probable (n = 35) or confirmed (n = 12) cases of poisoning caused by traditional medicines or food supplements. The report concluded that the overall risk to public health from these types of products was low. However, clusters of cases were identified that gave cause for concern. Twenty-one cases of liver toxicity, including two deaths, were associated with the use of traditional Chinese medicines, although no causative agent was identified.

Potential hepatotoxicity associated with herbal medicines has been discussed for some time.[129, 130] Hepatotoxicity has been reported with a number of herbal medicines (*see* monographs on Black Cohosh, Chaparral, Comfrey, Ephedra, Kava). *Teucrium* species (*see* Scullcap) have also been implicated in hepatotoxicity. Following reports of serious cases of liver toxicity associated with the use of *Piper methysticum* (*see* Kava), *P. methysticum* has been prohibited in unlicensed medicinal products in the UK since January 2003.[58]

At the time of writing, MHRA was aware of 79 cases of liver damage associated with the consumption of kava that have been reported worldwide.[90] Cases of hepatotoxicity associated with the use of Black Cohosh have also been reported (*see* Black Cohosh).[90]

Intrinsically toxic constituents of herbal ingredients

Limited toxicological data are available on medicinal plants. However, there exists a considerable overlap between those herbs used for medicinal purposes and those used for cosmetic or culinary purposes, for which a significant body of information exists. For many culinary herbs used in herbal remedies, there is no reason to doubt their safety providing the intended dose and route of administration is in line with their food use. When intended for use in larger therapeutic doses the safety of culinary herbs requires re-evaluation.

Culinary herbs Some culinary herbs contain potentially toxic constituents. The safe use of these herbs is ensured by limiting the amount of constituent permitted in a food product to a concentration not considered to represent a health hazard.

Apiole The irritant principle present in the volatile oil of parsley is held to be responsible for the abortifacient action.[131] Apiole is also hepatotoxic and liver damage has been documented as a result of excessive ingestion of parsley, far exceeding normal dietary consumption, over a prolonged period (*see* Parsley).[131]

β-*Asarone* Calamus rhizome oil contains β-asarone as the major component, which has been shown to be carcinogenic in animal studies.[131] Many other culinary herbs contain low levels of β-asarone in their volatile oils and therefore the level of β-asarone permitted in foods as a flavouring is restricted. The EMEA HMPC has concluded that in view of the toxicity of α-and β-asarone, their concentration in herbal medicinal products should be reduced to minimum and diploid varieties should always be preferred. In analogy with the food regulation (limitation of the intake of β-asarone from food and alcoholic beverages), a limit of exposure from herbal medicinal products of approximately 115 μg/day, i.e. about 2 μg/kg body weight/day could be accepted temporarily until a full benefit–risk assessment has been carried out.[132]

Estragole (Methylchavicol) Estragole is a constituent of many culinary herbs but is a major component of the oils of tarragon, fennel, sweet basil and chervil. Estragole has been reported to be carcinogenic in animals.[131] The level of estragole permitted in food products as a flavouring is restricted. The EMEA HMPC has concluded that the present exposure to estragole resulting from consumption of herbal medicinal products (short time use in adults at recommended posology) does not pose a significant cancer risk. Nevertheless, further studies are needed to define both the nature and implications of the dose–response curve in rats at low levels of exposure to estragole. In the meantime exposure of estragole to sensitive groups such as young children, pregnant and breastfeeding women should be minimised. Toxicological assessment of preparations for topical and external use needs further investigation because data on absorption through the skin are missing.[133]

Safrole Animal studies involving safrole, the major component of sassafras oil, have shown it to be hepatotoxic and carcinogenic.[131] The permitted level of safrole as a flavouring in foods is 0.1 mg/kg.

Methyleugenol Methyleugenol is a constituent of many culinary herbs and is present in small amounts in cassia bark oil and clove oil (*see* Cassia, Clove). Chronic toxicity data on methyleugenol show the compound to be a genotoxic carcinogen. The EMEA HMPC has concluded that the present exposure to methyleugenol resulting from consumption of herbal medicinal products (short time use in adults at recommended posology) does not pose a significant cancer risk. Nevertheless, further studies are needed to define both the nature and implications of the dose–response curve in rats at low levels of exposure to methyleugenol. In the meantime, exposure of sensitive groups, such as young children, pregnant and breastfeeding women, to methyleugenol should be minimised. Toxicological assessment of preparations for topical and external use needs further investigation because data on absorption through the skin are missing.[134]

Other intrinsically toxic constituents *Aristolochic acids* are reported to occur only in the Aristolochiaceae family. They have been reported in *Aristolochia* species, and appear to occur throughout the plant in the roots, stem, herb and fruit. The aristolochic acids are a series of substituted nitrophenanthrene carboxylic acids. The main constituents are 3,4-methylene-dioxy-8-methoxy-10-nitrophenanthrene-1-carboxylic acid. Low concentrations of aristolochic acids have been reported in *Asarum* species, another member of the Aristolochiaceae family. Aristolochic acids have been shown to be nephrotoxic, carcinogenic and mutagenic.[135]

Pyrrolizidine alkaloids are present in a number of plant genera, notably *Crotalaria*, *Heliotropium* and *Senecio*. Many of these plants have been used in African, Caribbean and South American countries as food sources and as medicinal 'bush teas'. Hepatotoxicity associated with their consumption is well documented and has been attributed to the pyrrolizidine alkaloid constituents.[136, 137] Pyrrolizidine alkaloids can be divided into two categories based on their structure, namely those with an unsaturated nucleus (toxic) and those with a saturated nucleus (considered to be non-toxic).

Several herbs currently used in herbal remedies contain pyrrolizidines; they include liferoot, borage, comfrey, coltsfoot and echinacea (*see* individual monographs).

In addition to preclinical data, cases of human hepatotoxicity associated with the ingestion of comfrey have been documented (*see* Comfrey). The concentrations of pyrrolizidine alkaloids present in borage and coltsfoot are thought to be too low to be of clinical significance, although the dangers associated with long-term low-dose exposure are unclear. The use of borage oil as a source of gamma-linolenic acid and as an alternative to evening primrose oil is currently very popular. The pyrrolizidine alkaloids identified in echinacea to date have been of the non-toxic saturated type. In 2002, MHRA raised concerns about a TCM product known as Qianbai Biyan Pian available on the UK market containing *Senecio scandens* which is reported to contain the unsaturated pyrrolizidine alkaloids, senecionine and seneciphylline.[90]

Benzophenanthridine alkaloids are present in bloodroot and in prickly ash. Although some of these alkaloids have exhibited cytotoxic properties in animal studies, their toxicity to humans has been refuted (*see* Bloodroot).

Lectins are plant proteins that possess haemagglutinating and potent mitogenic properties. Both mistletoe and pokeroot contain lectins. Systemic exposure to pokeroot has resulted in haematological aberrations. Mistletoe lectins may also inhibit protein synthesis.[138] (*see* Mistletoe and Pokeroot).

Viscotoxins, constituents of mistletoe, are low molecular weight proteins which possess cytotoxic and cardiotoxic properties.[138] For many years, mistletoe preparations have been used in Europe as cancer treatments. Clinical trials carried out with Iscador, a product produced from the naturally fermented plant juice of mistletoe, have concluded that Iscador may exhibit some weak antitumour effects but should only be used alongside conventional therapy in the long-term treatment of cancer.

Lignans. Hepatotoxic reactions reported for chaparral have been associated with the lignan constituents (*see* Chaparral).

Table 1 Examples of adverse effects that may occur with herbal ingredients

Potential adverse effect	Constituent/Herbal ingredient
Allergic (*see* Appendix 2, Table 11)	
Hypersensitive	Sesquiterpene lactones: arnica, chamomile, feverfew, yarrow
Phototoxic	Furanocoumarins: angelica, celery, wild carrot
Immune	Canavanine: alfalfa
Cardiac (*see* Appendix 2, Table 2)	Cardiac glycosides: pleurisy root, squill
Endocrine	
Hypoglycaemic (*see* Appendix 2, Table 8)	Alfalfa, fenugreek
Hyperthyroid	Iodine: fucus
Hormonal (*see* Appendix 2, Table 9)	
Mineralocorticoid	Triterpenoids: liquorice
Oestrogenic; Anti-androgen	Isoflavonoids: alfalfa; red clover Saponins: ginseng, saw palmetto
Irritant (*see* Appendix 2, Table 12)	
Gastrointestinal	Numerous compounds including anthraquinones (purgative), capsaicinoids, diterpenes, saponins, terpene-rich volatile oils
Renal	Aescin: horse-chestnut; terpene-rich volatile oils
Toxic	
Hepatotoxic/carcinogenic	Pyrrolizidine alkaloids: comfrey, liferoot; β-asarone: calamus; lignans: chaparral; safrole: sassafras; hepatotoxic constituents unconfirmed: black cohosh, kava
Mitogenic	Proteins: mistletoe, pokeroot
Cyanide poisoning	Cyanogenetic glycosides: apricot
Convulsant	Camphor/thujone-rich volatile oils

Saponins. Pokeroot also contains irritant saponins which have produced severe gastrointestinal irritation involving intense abdominal cramping and haematemesis. Systemic exposure to these saponins has resulted in hypotension and tachycardia. In May 1979, the US Herb Trade Association requested that all its members should stop selling pokeroot as a herbal beverage or food because of its toxicity.[139]

Diterpenes. The irritant properties of many diterpenes are well documented and queen's delight contains diterpene esters which are extremely irritant to all mucosal surfaces (*see* Queen's Delight).

Cyanogenetic glycosides are present in the kernels of a number of fruits including apricot, bitter almond, cherry, pear and plum seeds. Gastric hydrolysis of these compounds following oral ingestion results in the release of hydrogen cyanide (HCN), which is rapidly absorbed from the upper gastrointestinal tract and which can lead to respiratory failure. It has been estimated that oral doses of 50 mg of HCN, equivalent to about 50–60 apricot kernels, can be fatal[140] (*see* Apricot). However, variation in cyanogenetic glycoside content of the kernels could reduce or increase the number required for a fatal reaction. In the early 1980s a substance called amygdalin was promoted as a 'natural' non-toxic cure for cancer. Amygdalin is a cyanogenetic glycoside that is also referred to as laetrile and 'vitamin B_{17}'. Two near-fatal episodes of HCN poisoning were recorded in which the patients had consumed apricot kernels as an alternative source of amygdalin, due to the poor availability of laetrile. Scientific research did not support the claims made for laetrile, although a small number of anecdotal reports suggested that laetrile may have some slight anticancer activity. As a result, legislation drawn up in 1984[141] restricted the availability of cyanogenetic substances so that amygdalin can only be administered under medical supervision.

Furanocoumarins are found predominantly in the families Umbelliferae (e.g. parsley, celery), Rutaceae (e.g. bergamot, *Citrus* species), Moraceae and Leguminosae. The furanocoumarins occur as linear and branched forms: the most commonly reported linear furanocoumarins are 8-methoxypsoralen, 5-methoxypsoralen (bergapten) and psoralen. The furanocoumarins are phototoxic. Severe phototoxic reactions have been reported in humans following the use of bergamot oil in topical preparations. Severe phototoxic burns have been reported in a Swedish patient following a visit to a suntan parlour after ingestion of a large quantity of celery soup.[142] In the UK, a patient developed severe phototoxicity during oral photochemotherapy with psoralen and ultraviolet A (PUVA) after eating a large quantity of soup made from celery, parsley and parsnip.[143] The authors highlighted the potential hazards of eating foods containing psoralens during PUVA therapy. In the UK, the MCA received two reports describing severe skin burns in patients who had been treated with TCM preparations derived from *Psoralea corylifolia* fruit.[144]

Volatile oils. See Precautions in specific patient groups, Pregnant/breastfeeding mothers, below.

Herbal ingredients that may cause adverse effects

Examples of adverse effects that have been documented in humans or animals for the herbal ingredients described in the monographs are summarised in Table 1. These adverse effects include allergic,

Table 2 Potential adverse effects of herbal ingredients listed in the monographs

Herb	Adverse effect	Reasons/Comments
Agnus Castus	Allergic reactions	–
Alfalfa	Systemic lupus erythematosus syndrome	Canavanine, toxic amino acid
Aloes	Purgative, irritant to GI tract	Anthraquinones
Angelica	Phototoxic dermatitis	Furanocoumarins
Aniseed	Contact dermatitis	Anethole in volatile oil
Apricot[(a)]	Cyanide poisoning, seed	Cyanogenetic glycosides
Arnica[(a)]	Dermatitis, irritant to GI tract	Sesquiterpene lactones
Artichoke	Allergenic, dermatitis	Sesquiterpene lactones
Asafoetida	Dermatitis, irritant	Gum, related species
Bayberry	Carcinogenic to rats	–
Blue Flag	Nausea, vomiting, irritant to GI tract and eyes	Fresh root, furfural (volatile oil)
Bogbean	Purgative, vomiting	In large doses
Boldo	Toxicity, irritant	Volatile oil
Borage[(a)]	Genotoxic, carcinogenic, hepatotoxic	Pyrrolizidine alkaloids
Broom	Cardiac depressant	Sparteine (alkaloid)
Buchu	Irritant to GI tract, kidney	Volatile oil
Butterbur	Genotoxic, carcinogenic, hepatotoxic	Pyrrolizidine alkaloids
Calamus[(a)]	Carcinogenic, nephrotoxic, convulsions	β-Asarone in oil
Capsicum	Irritant	Capsaicinoids
Cascara	Purgative, irritant to GI tract	Anthraquinones
Cassia	Allergenic, irritant	Cinnamaldehyde in volatile oil
Celery	Phototoxic, dermatitis	Furanocoumarins
Cereus	Irritant to GI tract	Fresh juice
Chamomile, German	Allergic reactions	Sesquiterpene lactones
Chamomile, Roman	Allergic reactions	Sesquiterpene lactones
Chaparral	Dermatitis, hepatotoxic	Lignans
Cinnamon	Allergenic, irritant	Cinnamaldehyde in volatile oil
Clove	Irritant	Eugenol in volatile oil
Cohosh, Blue	Irritant to GI tract	Seeds poisonous
Cola	Sleeplessness, anxiety, tremor	Caffeine
Coltsfoot[(a)]	Genotoxic, carcinogenic, hepatotoxic	Pyrrolizidine alkaloids
Comfrey[(a)]	Genotoxic, carcinogenic, hepatotoxic	Pyrrolizidine alkaloids
Corn Silk	Allergenic, dermatitis	–
Cowslip	Allergenic	Quinones
Damiana	Convulsions	High dose (one report only), quinones, cyanogenetic glycosides
Dandelion	Allergenic, dermatitis	Sesquiterpene lactones
Echinacea	Allergenic, irritant	Polysaccharide
Elecampane	Allergenic, irritant	Sesquiterpene lactones
Eucalyptus	Nausea, vomiting	Volatile oil
Evening Primrose Oil	Mild indigestion, increased risk of epilepsy	Schizophrenic patients taking phenothiazines
Eyebright	Mental confusion, raised intraocular pressure	Tincture
Feverfew	Allergenic, dermatitis	Sesquiterpene lactones
Frangula	Purgative, irritant to GI tract	Anthraquinones

table continues

Table 2 *continued*

Herb	Adverse effect	Reasons/Comments
Fucus	Hyperthyroidism	Iodine content
Garlic	Irritant to GI tract, dermatitis	Sulfides
Ginseng	Mastalgia, vaginal bleeding, insomnia	Various effects reported but species unconfirmed (*see* Ginseng, Eleutherococcus)
Golden Seal	Gastric upset	Berberine, potentially poisonous
Gravel Root[(a)]	Genotoxic, carcinogenic, hepatotoxic	Pyrrolizidine alkaloids
Greater Celandine	Hepatotoxic	Alkaloids
Ground Ivy	Irritant to GI tract, kidneys	Pulegone in volatile oil
Guaiacum	Allergenic, dermatitis	Lignans
Hops	Allergenic, dermatitis	Oleo-resin
Horehound, White	Dermatitis, irritant	Plant juice
Horse-chestnut	Nephrotoxic	Aescin
Horseradish	Allergenic, irritant	Glucosinolates
Hydrangea	Dermatitis, irritant to GI tract	–
Hydrocotyle	Phototoxic, dermatitis	–
Ispaghula	Oesophageal obstruction, flatulence	If swallowed with insufficient liquid
Jamaica Dogwood	Irritant, numbness, tremors	High doses
Juniper	Irritant, abortifacient	Volatile oil, confusion with savin
Lady's Slipper	Allergenic, dermatitis, hallucinations	–
Liferoot[(a)]	Genotoxic, carcinogenic, hepatotoxic	Pyrrolizidine alkaloids
Liquorice	Hyperaldosteronism	Excessive ingestion
Lobelia	Nausea, vomiting, diarrhoea	Lobeline (alkaloid)
Maté	Sleeplessness, anxiety, tremor	Caffeine
Mistletoe	Hepatitis, hypotension, poisonous	Mixed herbal preparation
Motherwort	Phototoxic dermatitis	Volatile oil
Nettle	Irritant	Amines
Parsley	Irritant, hepatitis, phototoxic, abortifacient	Apiole in volatile oil, excessive ingestion
Pennyroyal	Irritant, nephrotoxic, hepatotoxic	Pulegone in volatile oil
Pilewort[(a)]	Irritant	Protoanemonin
Plantain	Allergenic, dermatitis, irritant	Mustard-type oil
Pleurisy Root	Dermatitis, irritant, cardiac activity	Cardenolides
Pokeroot	Mitogenic, toxic, nausea, vomiting, cramp	Lectins
Prickly Ash, Southern	Toxic to animals	–
Pulsatilla[(a)]	Allergenic, irritant	Protanemonin
Queen's Delight[(a)]	Irritant to GI tract	Diterpenes
Red Clover	Oestrogenic	Isoflavonoids
Rhubarb	Purgative, irritant to GI tract	Anthraquinones
Rosemary	Convulsions	Camphor in volatile oil
Sage	Toxic, convulsant	Thujone, camphor in volatile oil
Sassafras[(a)]	Carcinogenic, genotoxic	Safrole in volatile oil
Scullcap	Hepatotoxicity	Due to adulteration with hepatotoxic *Teucrium* spp.
Senega	Irritant to GI tract	Saponins
Senna	Purgative, irritant to GI tract	Anthraquinones
Shepherd's Purse	Irritant	Isothiocyanates
Skunk Cabbage	Itch, inflammation	–

table continues

Table 2 *continued*

Herb	Adverse effect	Reasons/Comments
Squill	Irritant, cardioactive	Saponins
St. John's Wort	Phototoxic	Hypericin
Tansy[a]	Severe gastritis, convulsions	Thujone in volatile oil
Thyme	Irritant to GI tract	Thymol in volatile oil
Wild Carrot	Phototoxic, dermatitis	Furanocoumarins
Yarrow	Allergenic, dermatitis	Sesquiterpene lactones
Yellow Dock	Purgative, irritant to GI tract	Anthraquinones

[a]Not recommended for internal use.

cardiac, hepatic, hormonal, irritant and purgative effects, and a range of toxicities. Some of the potential adverse effects of the herbal ingredients which are the subject of the 152 monographs are listed in Table 2. For further detailed information, including literature references, the reader should consult individual monographs. The following few examples are illustrative of some of the adverse effects caused by herbal ingredients.

Comfrey, coltsfoot Hepatotoxic reactions have been documented for comfrey and coltsfoot. Both of these herbal ingredients contain pyrrolizidine alkaloids, compounds known to be hepatotoxic. However, it was later reported that the reaction documented for coltsfoot may have in fact involved a herbal tea containing a *Senecio* species rather than coltsfoot.[73] The *Senecio* genus is characterised by its pyrrolizidine alkaloid constituents.

Mistletoe, scullcap A case of hepatitis has been reported for a woman who was taking a multi-constituent herbal product (*see* Mistletoe). Based on the known toxic constituents of mistletoe and other herbal ingredients present in the product, it was concluded that mistletoe was the component responsible for the hepatitis. Lectins and viscotoxins, the toxic constituents in mistletoe, are not known to be hepatotoxic and no other reports of liver damage associated with mistletoe ingestion have been documented. The product also contained scullcap, which is recognised to be frequently adulterated with a *Teucrium* species. Hepatotoxic reactions have been associated with germander (*Teucrium chamaedrys*) (*see* Scullcap).

Pokeroot Severe gastrointestinal irritation and haematological abnormalities documented for pokeroot can be directly related to the saponin and lectin constituents of pokeroot.[73]

Sassafras Hepatotoxicity has been associated with the consumption of a herbal tea containing sassafras. The principal component of sassafras volatile oil is safrole, which is known to be hepatotoxic and carcinogenic.[127]

Excessive ingestion

Ginseng Excessive doses of ginseng have been reported to cause agitation, insomnia, and raised blood pressure and have been referred to as abuse of the remedy. Side-effects have also been reported for ginseng following the ingestion of recommended doses, and include mastalgia and vaginal bleeding. However, the reports are in the older literature, the products are poorly described and a causal association with ginseng has not been established (*see* Ginseng, Panax).

Liquorice Excessive ingestion of liquorice has resulted in typical corticosteroid-type side-effects of oedema and hypertension (*see* Liquorice).

Parsley Parsley volatile oil contains apiole which is structurally related to the recognised hepatocarcinogen, safrole. Ingestion of apiole has resulted in a number of cases of fatal poisoning.[131]

Hypersensitivity reactions

Chamomile Sesquiterpene lactones are known to possess allergenic properties. They occur predominantly in herbs of the Compositae (Asteraceae) family, of which chamomile is a member. Hypersensitivity reactions have been reported for chamomile and other plants from the same family (*see* Chamomile, German, Chamomile, Roman). Cross-sensitivity to other members of the Compositae family is well recognised. The EMEA HMPC has issued a public statement proposing the following SPC statement for chamomile products: 'Hypersensitivity reactions to (German) chamomile (e.g. contact dermatitis) are very rare. Cross reactions may occur in people with allergy to compositae (e.g. artemisia/mugwort). Very rarely severe allergic reactions (anaphylactic shock, asthma, facial oedema and urticaria) following internal use have been reported.'[145]

Feverfew The sesquiterpene lactones present in feverfew are considered to be the active principles in the herb. It is unknown whether documented side-effects for feverfew, such as mouth ulcers and swollen tongue, are also attributable to these constituents (*see* Feverfew).

Phototoxic reactions

Parsley Furanocoumarins, compounds known to cause phototoxic reactions, are constituents of parsley. Excessive ingestion of parsley has been associated with the development of photosensitive rash which resolved once parsley consumption ceased (*see* Parsley).[131]

Precautions in specific patient groups

Pregnant/breastfeeding mothers Few conventional medicines have been established as safe to take during pregnancy and it is generally recognised that no medicine should be taken unless the benefit to the mother outweighs any possible risk to the foetus. This rule should also be applied to herbal medicinal products. However, one of the major problems is that herbal products are often promoted to the public as being 'natural' and completely 'safe' alternatives to conventional medicines. A survey of 400 pregnant Norwegian women found that 36% had used herbal products during pregnancy.[146] This finding was higher than in other published studies from western countries. Of those women having used herbal products in pregnancy, nearly 40% used herbal products that the authors considered possibly harmful or where information on safety in pregnancy was missing. Interestingly, 43% of the women used herbal galactagogues and this is of concern as there is limited information on the safety of such products to the mother or infant (*see* Breastfeeding mothers below). The lack of information about the safety of herbal medicines during pregnancy is recognised.[147]

Table 3 Herbal ingredients best avoided or used with caution during pregnancy. Absence of a herbal ingredient from this list does not signify safety and, as with all medicines, herbal remedies should only be used where the perceived benefit outweighs any possible risk. For a number of herbs the chemistry and pharmacology are poorly documented and their use in pregnancy should be avoided. Some of the herbs listed are reputed to be abortifacient or to affect the menstrual cycle although no recent clinical or experimental data exist. In view of the potential serious effects caution in their use is advised.

Herb	Effect
Agnus Castus	Hormonal action
Aloes	Cathartic, reputed abortifacient
Apricot	Cyanide toxicity
Asafoetida	Reputed abortifacient and to affect menstrual cycle
Avens	Reputed to affect menstrual cycle
Blue Flag	Irritant oil
Bogbean	Irritant, possible purgative
Boldo	Irritant oil
Boneset	Cytotoxic constituents (related species)
Borage	Pyrrolizidine alkaloids
Broom	Sparteine is oxytoxic
Buchu	Irritant oil
Burdock	Uterine stimulant, *in vivo*
Butterbur	Pyrrolizidine alkaloids
Calendula	Reputed to affect menstrual cycle, uterine stimulant, *in vitro*
Cascara	Anthraquinones, non-standardised preparations to be avoided
Chamomile, German	Reputed to affect menstrual cycle, uterine stimulant with excessive use
Chamomile, Roman	Reputed abortifacient and to affect menstrual cycle with excessive use
Chaparral	Uterine activity, hepatotoxic
Cohosh, Black	Uterine oestrogen receptor binding *in vitro*, potential hepatotoxicity
Cohosh, Blue	Reputed abortifacient and to affect menstrual cycle
Cola	Caffeine, consumption should be restricted
Coltsfoot	Pyrrolizidine alkaloids
Comfrey	Pyrrolizidine alkaloids
Cornsilk	Uterine stimulant, *in vivo*
Damiana	Cyanogenetic glycosides, risk of cyanide toxicity in high doses
Eucalyptus	Oil should not be taken internally during pregnancy
Euphorbia	Smooth muscle activity, *in vitro*
Fenugreek	Oxytoxic, uterine stimulant, *in vitro*
Feverfew	Reputed abortifacient and to affect menstrual cycle
Frangula	Anthraquinones, non-standardised preparations to be avoided
Fucus	Thyroid gland activity, possible heavy metal contamination
Gentian	Reputed to affect menstrual cycle
Ginseng, Eleutherococcus	Hormonal activity
Ginseng, Panax	Hormonal activity
Golden Seal	Alkaloids with uterine stimulant activity, *in vitro*
Ground Ivy	Irritant oil
Hawthorn	Uterine activity, *in vivo*, *in vitro*
Hops	Uterine activity, *in vitro*
Horehound, Black	Reputed to affect menstrual cycle
Horehound, White	Reputed abortifacient and to affect menstrual cycle
Horseradish	Irritant oil; avoid excessive ingestion

table continues

Table 3 *continued*

Herb	Effect
Hydrocotyle	Reputed abortifacient and to affect menstrual cycle
Greater Celandine	Hepatotoxic
Jamaica Dogwood	Uterine activity, *in vitro*, *in vivo*; irritant
Juniper	Reputed abortifacient and to affect menstrual cycle. Confusion over whether oil is toxic
Kava	Hepatotoxic
Liferoot	Pyrrolizidine alkaloids
Liquorice	Oestrogenic activity, reputed abortifacient
Lobelia	Lobeline, toxicity
Maté	Caffeine, consumption should be restricted
Meadowsweet	Uterine activity, *in vitro*
Mistletoe	Toxic constituents, uterine stimulant, *in vivo*
Motherwort	Uterine activity, *in vitro*, reputed to affect menstrual cycle
Myrrh	Reputed to affect menstrual cycle
Nettle	Reputed abortifacient and to affect menstrual cycle
Passionflower	Harman, harmaline uterine stimulants, *in vivo*
Pennyroyal	Abortifacient, irritant oil (pulegone)
Plantain	Uterine activity, *in vitro*; laxative
Pleurisy Root	Uterine activity, *in vivo*; cardioactive constituents
Pokeroot	Toxic constituents, uterine stimulant, reputed to affect menstrual cycle
Poplar	Conflicting reports over use of aspirin in pregnancy; salicylates excreted in breast milk may cause rashes in babies
Prickly Ash, Northern	Pharmacologically active alkaloids and coumarins
Prickly Ash, Southern	Pharmacologically active alkaloids
Pulsatilla	Reputed to affect menstrual cycle, uterine activity, *in vitro*, *in vivo*; irritant (fresh plant)
Queen's Delight	Irritant diterpenes
Raspberry	Uterine activity, *in vitro*, traditional use to ease parturition
Red Clover	Oestrogenic activity
Rhubarb	Anthraquinones, non-standardised preparations to be avoided
Sage	Reputed abortifacient
Sassafras	Abortifacient (oil), hepatotoxic (safrole)
Scullcap	Traditional use to eliminate afterbirth and promote menstruation; potential hepatotoxicity
Senna	Anthraquinones, non-standardised preparations to be avoided
Shepherd's Purse	Reputed abortifacient and to affect menstrual cycle
Skunk Cabbage	Reputed to affect menstrual cycle
Squill	Reputed abortifacient and to affect menstrual cycle
St John's Wort	Slight uterine activity, *in vitro*
Tansy	Uterine activity, abortifacient (thujone in oil)
Uva-Ursi	Large doses, oxytocic
Vervain	Reputed abortifacient, oxytocic, utero-activity *in vivo*
Wild Carrot	Oestrogenic activity, irritant oil
Willow	Conflicting reports over use of aspirin in pregnancy; salicylates excreted in breast milk may cause rashes in babies
Yarrow	Reputed abortifacient and to affect menstrual cycle (thujone in oil)
Yellow Dock	Anthraquinones, non-standardised preparations to be avoided

Table 3 lists some herbal ingredients taken from the following 152 monographs that specifically should be avoided or used with caution during pregnancy. As with conventional medicines, no herbal products should be taken during pregnancy unless the benefit outweighs the potential risk.

Volatile oils Many herbs are traditionally reputed to be abortifacient and for some this reputation can be attributed to their volatile oil component.[131] Several volatile oils are irritant to the genito-urinary tract if ingested and may induce uterine contractions. Herbs that contain irritant volatile oils include ground ivy, juniper, parsley, pennyroyal, sage, tansy and yarrow. Some of these oils contain the terpenoid constituent, thujone, which is known to be abortifacient. Pennyroyal oil also contains the hepatotoxic terpenoid constituent, pulegone. A case of liver failure in a woman who ingested pennyroyal oil as an abortifacient has been documented (*see* Pennyroyal).

Utero-activity A stimulant or spasmolytic action on uterine muscle has been documented for some herbal ingredients including blue cohosh, burdock, fenugreek, golden seal, hawthorn, Jamaica dogwood, motherwort, nettle, raspberry and vervain. Raspberry is a popular remedy taken during pregnancy to help promote an easier labour by relaxing the uterine muscles. The pharmacological activity exhibited by raspberry may vary between different preparations and from one individual to another. Raspberry should not be used during pregnancy unless under medical supervision (*see* Raspberry).

Herbal teas Increased awareness of the harmful effects associated with excessive tea and coffee consumption has prompted many individuals to switch to herbal teas. Whilst some herbal teas may offer pleasant alternatives to tea and coffee, some contain pharmacologically active herbal ingredients, which may have unpredictable effects depending on the quantity of tea consumed and strength of the brew. Some herbal teas contain laxative herbal ingredients such as senna, frangula and cascara. In general stimulant laxative preparations are not recommended during pregnancy and the use of unstandardised laxative preparations is particularly unsuitable. A case of hepatotoxicity in a newborn baby has been documented in which the mother consumed a herbal tea during pregnancy as an expectorant.[148] Following analysis the herbal tea was reported to contain pyrrolizidine alkaloids which are known to be hepatotoxic.

Breastfeeding mothers A medicinal product taken by a breastfeeding mother presents a hazard if it is transferred to the breast milk in pharmacologically or toxicologically significant amounts. Limited information is available regarding the safety of conventional medicines taken during breastfeeding. Much less information exists for herbal ingredients, and generally the use of herbal remedies is not recommended during lactation.

Paediatric use Herbal medicines have traditionally been used to treat both adults and children. The belief that natural remedies may be safer than conventional medicines may influence parents in choosing herbal medicines for their children. Herbal medicines may offer a milder alternative to some conventional medicines, although the suitability of a herbal remedy needs to be carefully considered with respect to quality, safety and efficacy. Herbal medicines should be used with caution in children and medical advice should be sought if in doubt. The administration of herbal teas to children is generally unwise unless used according to professional advice.[149] Several surveys indicate that herbal use in children is increasing and it has been estimated that 28–40% of children may be exposed to herbal preparations for the management of asthma, anxiety, attention deficit hyperactivity disorders, insomnia and respiratory infections.[150, 151]

A survey of 503 children attending the Royal Children's Hospital, Melbourne, found that the use of CAM by children is common. Herbal products were used by 12% of the group surveyed and a further 8% were taking echinacea products Sixty-three percent of those reporting CAM use had not discussed this with their treating doctor. The authors concluded that given the potential risk of adverse events associated with the use of CAM or interactions with conventional management, doctors should ask about their use as a part of routine history taking.[152]

A review has been carried out of some of the most commonly used herbal products subjected to randomised controlled clinical trials in children including *Andrographis paniculata*, cranberry, echinacea, evening primrose oil, garlic, ivy leaf, and valerian. The authors concluded that whilst some of the studies showed promising results others suffered from methodological flaws such as small sample size, lack of product quality control, improper placebo and dose issues. Further well-designed randomised, controlled clinical trials are needed to evaluate these therapies for the paediatric population.[153]

Systematic reviews of the risks associated with the use of herbal medicines in children and adolescents have been carried out.[154, 155] The findings show that many of the reports of adverse effects are associated with products of poor quality where the adverse effect is caused by adulteration with heavy metals or conventional pharmaceutical drugs. In many cases it is not possible to demonstrate a causal relationship between the product taken and the adverse effect. The need for further investigations in the paediatric population is clear.

Older patients Surveys show that the use of herbal medicinal products by older patients is increasing and that typically more than one herbal product is used at a time, often concomitantly with prescription medicines. Older patients are reluctant to tell their doctor that they are taking herbal products and so are at risk of potential drug–herb interactions.[156–158]

A review has considered the available evidence on the use of several herbal medicinal products (St John's wort, valerian, ginkgo, horse-chestnut, saw palmetto and yohimbe) by older patients.[159] Whilst the treatments may offer considerable benefits for a range of conditions, there is a need for caution, particularly with regard to potential drug–herb interactions and possible adverse effects, when herbal medicinal products are used by older patients.

Patients with cardiovascular disease Concerns have been raised about the use of herbal medicinal products for the treatment of (and by patients with) cardiovascular disease, in particular, because of the lack of scientific assessment and the potential for toxic effects and major drug–herb interactions (*see* Herb–drug interactions).[160]

A systematic review of the literature covering 1990–2001 found evidence mostly from case reports and case series that herbal medicinal products could lead to serious cardiovascular adverse events. The adverse effects were attributed not only to the toxicity of the herbal products but in some cases to contamination of the products with substances such as prescription medicines, as well as to drug–herb interactions.[161]

A systematic review of the literature between January 1996 and February 2003 has been undertaken to determine the possible interactions between herbal medicines and cardiovascular drugs. Forty-three case reports and eight clinical trials were identified. Warfarin was the most common cardiovascular drug involved. It was found to interact with boldo, curbicin, fenugreek, garlic, danshen, devil's claw, dong quai, ginkgo, papaya, lycium, mango, PC-SPES (resulting in over-anticoagulation) and with ginseng, green tea, soy and St John's wort (causing decreased anticoagulant effect). Gum guar, St John's wort, Siberian ginseng and wheat bran were found to decrease plasma digoxin concentration; aspirin interactions include spontaneous hyphema when used concurrently with ginkgo and increased bioavailability if combined with tamarind. Decreased plasma concentration of simvastatin or lovastatin was observed after co-administration with St John's wort and wheat bran, respectively. Other adverse events reported were hypertension after co-administration of ginkgo and a diuretic thiazide, hypokalaemia after liquorice and antihypertensives and anticoagulation after phenprocoumon and St John's wort. The authors concluded that interaction between herbal medicines and cardiovascular drugs is a potentially important safety issue with patients taking anticoagulants at the highest risk.[162] The potential for herb–drug interactions is discussed further below (*see* Herb–drug interactions).

The British Heart Foundation has produced a Factfile entitled *Herbs and the Heart* in association with the British Cardiac Society which informs patients about the use of herbal products. The Factfile highlights possible cardiotoxicity that might occur with certain herbal ingredients, such as black hellebore, figwort, hawthorn, ephedra and yohimbe. The potential for drug–herb interactions is also discussed, in particular with warfarin, simvastatin, ciclosporin and digoxin.[163]

Patients with cancer Studies have shown that CAM use in patients with cancer is high in many countries.[164–168] Surveys indicate that this use is increasing and, interestingly, that patients with breast cancer appear to use more CAMs than individuals with other types of malignancy.[169] Studies in Europe have reported use of CAM in 23.6% of lung cancer patients, 32% of colorectal cancer patients and 44.7% of breast cancer patients after the diagnosis of cancer. In all of these surveys use of herbal medicine was the most common therapy used in over 40% of patients using CAM.[170–173] A survey carried out at the Royal Marsden Hospital in 2004 found that 164 (51.6%) of 318 patients were taking some complementary alternative medicine during their cancer treatment. Of these, 10.4% were taking herbal medicines, 42.1% were taking food supplements and 47.6% were taking a combination of the two. Of these patients, 30% were unsure why they were taking the remedies and 50% had not discussed the use with their doctor.[174]

In view of the prevalence of use of herbal products by cancer patients it is essential that healthcare professionals are aware and seek information from patients. It is well known that patients are often reluctant to discuss their use of CAM with their doctors.[175] In most cases the impact of herbal medicines on the patient's treatment is unknown and the potential for drug–herb interactions exists as shown by the effect of St John's wort on irinotecan used in the treatment of colon cancer.[176] There is also potential for other herbal ingredients such as garlic, ginkgo, echinacea, ginseng and kava to interact with anticancer agents (*see also* Herb–drug interactions).[177]

Peri-operative use Concerns about the need for patients to discontinue herbal medicinal products prior to surgery have been highlighted.[178, 179] Studies in the US have shown that the use of herbal medicines is common among surgical patients.[180] In one study of 2186 patients, 38% had taken herbal medicines in the two years before surgery and 16% continued the use of herbal medicines in the month of surgery. Herbal medicine use was found to be higher in patients undergoing gynaecologic (52%) and urologic (45%) procedures and lower amongst patients undergoing vascular (10%) surgical procedures.[180] A study of herbal medication use in paediatric surgical patients found that the prevalence of use was higher in children of parents who used herbal medications and children whose parents considered them to be chronically ill.[181] Whilst 21% of the parents were users of herbal medicines only 4% of their children used them. The most common herbal medicines used were echinacea, chamomile and aloe. Forty-two per cent of the children using herbal medicines were also taking prescription medicines concurrently. Interestingly, the study found that only 10% of parents reported that the surgeon enquired about patient herbal medication use.

From the available evidence, it has been suggested that the potential exists for direct pharmacological effects, pharmacodynamic interactions and pharmacokinetic interactions with eight commonly used herbal medicinal products (echinacea, ephedra, garlic, ginkgo, ginseng, kava, St John's wort, valerian). The need for physicians to have a clear understanding of the herbal medicinal products being used by patients and to take a detailed history was highlighted.[179] The American Society of Anesthesiologists (ASA) has reported that several anaesthesiologists have noted significant changes in heart rate or blood pressure in some patients who have been taking herbal medicinal products, including St John's Wort, ginkgo and ginseng. The ASA has produced information leaflets for both patients and physicians advising patients to tell their doctor if they are taking herbal products before surgery and emphasising the need for physicians to specifically ask patients if they are using herbal medicines.[182, 183]

The Royal College of Anaesthetists (RCA) and The Association of Anaesthetists of Great Britain and Ireland (AAGBI) has produced an information leaflet specifically targeted for patients which advises patients to bring any herbal remedies along with them to hospital. Patients are advised that they may need to discontinue the use of herbal remedies prior to their operation.[184] The MHRA has advised patients due to have a surgical operation to always tell their doctor about any herbal remedy they are taking.[90]

Menopausal women Many studies show that use of herbal medicines by women is greater than men and in some recent surveys this use appears to be increasing significantly.[3, 5] Women often try herbal medicines around the time of their menopause.[185–187] Use of conventional hormone replacement therapy (HRT) products has declined since 2002 following reports that HRT increases the risk of venous thromboembolism, stroke, endometrial cancer and breast cancer. In the wake of these reports, the use of herbal products for the relief of menopausal symptoms has increased substantially. Results of a national survey in the USA of 750 women aged 40 to 65 years revealed that 29% of the women had taken herbal remedies or soya products to ease menopause symptoms. The vast majority of the women had not discussed the use of the herbal products with their doctors but many were frustrated that their doctors did not provide enough information about herbal and dietary supplements to relieve menopause symptoms. Some 70% of the women expressed at least some concern or uncertainty about the safety of the products they were taking. The researchers highlighted the lack of patient–physician communication and called for more education for women about these treatments.[188]

The main herbal ingredients found in products for menopausal symptoms are those containing isoflavones (red clover, soya), black cohosh, dong quai, ginseng, evening primrose oil and wild yam.[189] Isoflavones are members of a group of polyphenolic non-steroidal plant compounds known as phytoestrogens. Other phytoestrogens include flavonoids, stilbenes and lignans. Epidemiological and experimental studies have shown that the consumption of phytoestrogen-rich diets may have protective effects on menopausal symptoms, diseases such as prostate and breast cancers, osteoporosis and cardiovascular diseases.[190]

Concerns have been raised about the use of isoflavone containing herbal medicines particularly in women with oestrogen-sensitive cancers. Limited data are available but some studies have shown that certain extracts of red clover and soya may induce cell proliferation in MCF-7 cells, an established *in vitro* oestrogen-dependent mammary tumour model.[191] In the same study, extracts of black cohosh tested did not cause cell proliferation. The authors concluded that preparations containing red clover and soya should be used with caution in the treatment of menopausal symptoms in women at risk of, or with a history of, oestrogen-sensitive breast cancer. Similar advice has been included in a fact sheet, *Herbal Medicines and Breast Cancer Risk* prepared by the US Program on Breast Cancer and Environmental Risk Factors (BCERF) at Cornell University.[192] A recent study of 452 women with family histories of breast cancer who were enrolled in a cancer risk assessment programme found that 32% reported soy food consumption.[193] The authors concluded that these women would benefit from clear messages regarding the health effects of soy.

Concerns have been raised about the potential for drug–herb interactions, known or theoretically associated with herbal medicines commonly used by women for the relief of menopausal symptoms.[194]

Herb–drug interactions

The evidence of significant problems associated with the ingestion of grapefruit juice concurrently with certain medicines has emphasised the fact that clinically relevant interactions between drugs and natural products, both herbs and foods, may occur.[195–197] The potential for interactions between herbal and conventional medicines has been recognised for some time but awareness has increased considerably since the emergence of clinically significant interactions between St John's Wort and a range of prescribed medicines.[198–201] The potential for drug–herb interactions has been reviewed extensively.[19, 202–206]

Concerns have been raised in the literature about herbal medicines interfering with breast cancer treatment, antirheumatic treatment and potential interactions between herbal products and cardiac drugs.[207–210]

Generally, information on herb–drug interactions, particularly in the clinical setting, is limited and in most cases there has been little formal clinical investigation. Instances of drug interactions have been tentatively linked, retrospectively, to the concurrent use of herbal medicines. The rationale for such interactions is often difficult to explain if knowledge regarding the phytochemical constituents of the herbal product, their pharmacological activity and metabolism are poorly understood. As with conventional drug interactions, herb–drug interactions may be pharmacodynamic or pharmacokinetic. Pharmacodynamic interactions could result when a herbal drug and a conventional drug have similar or antagonistic pharmacological effects or adverse effects. These interactions are usually predictable from a knowledge of the pharmacology of the interacting herb and drug. Pharmacokinetic interactions could occur when a herb alters the absorption, distribution, metabolism or elimination of a drug (and vice versa). These interactions are not easy to predict. In addition, there is also the potential issue of herb–herb interactions where combinations of herbal ingredients are used or where patients take a number of herbal products together. Little is known about the pharmacokinetics of herbal ingredients and whether or not they can, for example, induce their own metabolism.

As with all potential drug interactions there are particular concerns when patients are stabilised on conventional medicines, such as warfarin, digoxin, anticonvulsants (e.g. phenytoin) and ciclosporin that are known to have a narrow therapeutic window. Potential herb–drug interactions are considered for each herb under the individual monographs.

A recent review has illustrated the difficulties in assessing the significance of herb-drug interactions using four commonly used herbal substances, namely St John's wort, ginseng, ginkgo and liquorice.[211] The authors concluded that conclusive evidence of herb–drug interactions is often lacking and where clinical observations have been made or studies conducted, issues with respect to the type, quality and content of the herbal products are often not described. There is a need for rigorous studies to assess the mechanism and clinical significance of potential interactions in order to guide healthcare professionals and consumers.

In the absence of a comprehensive evidence base, patients receiving drugs with a narrow safety margin (e.g. immunosuppressants, anticoagulants, digoxin,) and those patients most at risk of serious drug interactions (i.e. patients who are elderly, have chronic illness, have organ dysfunction and those receiving multiple medicines) should be closely monitored to avoid the possible adverse consequences of herb–drug interactions. As highlighted in this review, the importance of the quality of the herbal product in terms of its phytochemical profiles should be emphasised. In view of the significant variability in herbal products, extrapolation of findings with a specific extract to other extracts may not be valid. For example, recent investigations reporting no alteration in bleeding time in elderly patients and no interactions with anticoagulant medicines with the specific ginkgo extract EGB 761 may not be valid for other ginkgo extracts.[212, 213]

St John's wort Since 1998 evidence has emerged from spontaneous reports and published case reports of the interactions between St John's wort and certain prescribed medicines leading to a loss of or reduction in therapeutic effect of these prescribed medicines (*see* St John's Wort).[19, 204] Drugs that may be affected include indinavir, warfarin, ciclosporin, digoxin, theophylline and oral contraceptives. There have also been reports of increased serotonergic effects in patients taking St John's wort concurrently with selective serotonin reuptake inhibitors (e.g. sertraline, paroxetine). Results of drug interaction studies have provided some evidence that St John's Wort may induce some cytochrome P450 (CYP) drug-metabolising enzymes in the liver as well as affecting P-glycoprotein (a transport protein). Regulatory Authorities throughout the EU and elsewhere have issued advice to patients and healthcare professionals.

Interactions with warfarin Several herbal ingredients have been reported to potentially interfere with warfarin, including devil's claw, dong quai, feverfew, garlic, ginkgo, ginseng and St John's wort.[202, 210, 214]

A survey of 1360 patients in the UK found that 8.8% were taking one or more herbal remedies thought to interact with warfarin. Complementary or homeopathic treatments not specified in the survey questionnaire were taken by 14.3% of responders.[215] Overall, 19.2% of the patients were taking one or more such medicines. Of these patients, 28.3% thought that herbal medicines might or definitely could interfere with other drugs prescribed by their doctor, however, patients taking any non-prescribed medication were less likely to believe this The use of herbal medicines had not been discussed with a conventional healthcare professional by 92.2% of patients.

Another UK study which conducted a retrospective analysis of the pharmaceutical care plans for 631 patients attending an outpatient anticoagulation clinic found that 26.9% of patients were using some form of CAM; of the CAM users, 58% were taking a CAM that could interfere with warfarin. The authors stressed the importance of taking a full drug history to avoid CAM–warfarin interactions.[216]

The CSM has issued advice to health professionals about the possibility of interaction between warfarin and cranberry juice.[217, 218] By October 2004, the MHRA had received 12 reports of suspected interactions involving warfarin and cranberry juice; eight cases involved increases in INR and/or bleeding episodes, in three cases the INR was reported to be unstable and in one case the INR decreased. The CSM has advised that it is not possible to define a safe quantity or brand of cranberry juice and therefore patients taking warfarin should avoid this drink unless the health benefits are considered to outweigh any risks (which is unlikely). It is not known whether other cranberry products, such as capsules or concentrates, might also interact with warfarin. Therefore similar caution should be observed with these products.

The evidence for and understanding of most drug–herb interactions is limited. An attempt can be made, however, to identify herbal ingredients that have the potential to interfere with specific categories of conventional drugs, based on known phytochemical information and pharmacological properties of the constituents of the herb, and on any documented adverse effects. For example, prolonged or excessive use of a herbal diuretic may potentiate existing diuretic therapy, interfere with existing hypo-/hypertensive therapy, or potentiate the effect of certain cardioactive drugs due to hypokalaemia. Herbs which have been documented to lower blood sugar concentrations may cause hypoglycaemia if taken in sufficient amounts and interfere with existing hypoglycaemic therapy. An individual receiving antihypertensive therapy may be more susceptible to the hypertensive adverse effects that have been documented with, for example, ginseng or which are associated with the excessive ingestion of plants such as liquorice. This approach has been used in drawing up Appendix 1, Table 1 and Appendix 2, Tables 1–12, which provide information on potential drug–herb interactions. Appendix 1, Table 1 groups together various therapeutic categories of medicines that may be affected by a particular herb or group of herbs. Appendix 2, Tables 1–12 list herbal ingredients that are claimed to have a specific activity alphabetically within each table, including laxative, cardioactive, diuretic, hypo-/hypertensive, anticoagulant/coagulant, hypo-/hyperlipidaemic, sedative, hypo-/hyperglycaemic, hormonal, immunostimulant, allergenic or irritant. Some commonly occurring groups of natural products found within these 152 herbal ingredients contribute towards their activities, toxicities or adverse effects. Appendix 2, Tables 13–21 list those herbal ingredients that contain amines, alkaloids or have sympathomimetic anti-inflammatory or antispasmodic activities, coumarins, flavonoids, iridoids, saponins, tannins or volatile oils.

Interactions of herbal products in therapeutic drug monitoring

There are also examples of herbal medicinal products which appear to cross-react with diagnostic markers in therapeutic drug monitoring, e.g. with a digoxin assay (*see* Ginseng, Eleutherococcus).[200]

Reporting of adverse reactions to herbal medicinal products

It is essential that information on the risks associated with the use of herbal products is systematically collected and analysed in order to protect public health. There is an increasing awareness of the need to develop pharmacovigilance practices for herbal medicines.[22, 219] The WHO has recently produced guidelines on safety monitoring of herbal medicines in pharmacovigilance systems.[64] The current arrangements for pharmcovigilance of herbal medicinal products in the UK have been reviewed.[219]

In 1996, the UK MHRA extended its 'Yellow Card Scheme' for adverse drug reaction reporting to include reporting of suspected adverse reactions to unlicensed herbal products. This followed a report from a UK Medical Toxicology Unit on potentially serious adverse reactions associated with herbal remedies. Twenty-one cases of liver toxicity, including two deaths, were associated with the use of TCMs.[128]

The need to further improve pharmacovigilance on herbal products was highlighted in a study of patients' perceived behaviour towards reporting adverse reactions.[6] The study found that patients would be less likely to consult their doctor for suspected adverse drug reactions (minor or severe) to herbal remedies than for similar adverse reactions to conventional over-the-counter medicines. This illustrates the need for greater public awareness that adverse reactions can occur and that such reactions should be reported. It also highlights the need for healthcare professionals to take a detailed medical history including use of herbal products and to be aware that patients may be reluctant to provide information. The UK Yellow Card scheme has recently been extended to include reporting from patients and carers for prescribed and OTC medicines as well as herbal and complementary medicines.[220] The Uppsala Monitoring Centre (UMC) of the World Health Organization plays an important role in the international monitoring of adverse health effects associated with herbal medicines.[221]

The UMC recognises the problems inherent in adverse drug reaction reporting for herbal medicines and has established a Traditional Medicines project to stimulate reporting in this area and to standardise information on herbal medicines, particularly with regard to nomenclature. For example, a special set of herbal anatomical–therapeutic–chemical (ATC) codes has been developed which is fully compatible with the regular ATC classification system for conventional medicines.[222] Another important project has focused on developing a herbal substance register for use in the international drug monitoring programme.[223] Comprehensive guidelines issued by UMC for setting up and running a pharmacovigilance centre are included in the recent WHO publication.[64]

Efficacy

Despite the growing popularity of herbal medicines world-wide there is a dearth of scientific evidence of efficacy for most herbal medicines. Indeed, many of the herbs used medicinally in Europe have a traditional reputation for their uses, but there is little scientific documentation of their active constituents, pharmacological actions or clinical efficacy.[224–231] Examples of this group include avens, boneset, burdock, clivers, damiana, Jamaica dogwood, parsley piert, pulsatilla and wild lettuce. For other herbs, documented phytochemical data or pharmacological data from animal studies may provide a plausible basis for their traditional uses, but evidence of efficacy from clinical studies is limited.

The current emphasis on evidence-based medicine requires evidence of efficacy from rigorous randomised controlled trials. Where possible, the evidence is best evaluated by systematic reviews and meta-analyses of available clinical trial data, as such approaches minimise both selection bias and random error.

Such approaches are now being applied to herbal medicines. Systematic reviews have been undertaken for a number of herbal ingredients, e.g. aloe vera, artichoke, echinacea, evening primrose, feverfew, garlic, ginger, ginkgo, ginseng, hawthorn, horse-chestnut, mistletoe, peppermint, saw palmetto, St John's wort and valerian[231–236] (*see* individual monographs). Several reviews have been prepared by the Cochrane Collaboration (the international association dedicated to preparing and maintaining systematic reviews of the effects of healthcare interventions).[237] Most reviews highlight that, in many cases, the evidence base is weak and studies are often flawed.[235, 236] In other cases, studies have been methodologically sound and evidence of efficacy is strong.

St John's wort, a widely used herbal product, has been investigated in many clinical studies (*see* St John's Wort).[19] A recent systematic review of the evidence from 37 randomised controlled trials has concluded that extracts seem more effective than placebo and as effective as standard antidepressants for treating mild-to-moderate depression. However, the authors highlighted that these findings apply only to the preparations tested in the trials as marketed preparations vary considerably.[238] There is, however, a need for further studies to evaluate efficacy compared with that of standard treatments, particularly newer antidepressant agents, in well-defined patient groups and conducted over longer time periods.

One of the fundamental problems characteristic of herbal medicinal products is that the individual herbal ingredients contain a vast array of chemical constituents. Further, herbal medicines traditionally involve mixtures of different herbal ingredients, although in developed countries, recent trends indicate that single-ingredient herbal products are becoming increasingly popular. Herbalists would argue that combinations of ingredients are designed to provide the best therapeutic outcome while reducing adverse effects and toxicity. Evidence is emerging that different constituents within a herbal preparation may contribute to the overall therapeutic effect of the product and that in some cases synergistic and additive effects play an important role.[239, 240]

In most cases there is a lack of knowledge of the phytochemical constituents responsible for the claimed therapeutic effects of many herbal ingredients. To further complicate matters, it is well known that herbal products derived from the same herbal drug can vary considerably in terms of their phytochemical constituents depending on the source of plant material, the manufacture of the extracts and formulation of the dosage forms. As a result, efforts to establish clinical efficacy are hampered by how far results for a specific product can be extrapolated to other products containing the same plant but different extracts. Where the active constituents of a herbal ingredient are known it is possible and, in most cases, desirable to standardise the extract/product. The aim of standardisation is to obtain an optimum and consistent quality of a herbal drug preparation by adjusting it to give a defined content of a constituent or a group of constituents with known therapeutic activity. Examples of herbal drugs with constituents with accepted, known therapeutic activity are few. Herbs with documented activities (and known active constituents) include: senna, frangula (hydroxyanthracenes); belladonna (alkaloids) and horse-chestnut (saponins).

In the case of St John's wort, early studies concentrated on the hypericin constituents but more recent work suggests that hyperforin and possibly flavonoids also contribute to the antidepressant properties.[19] Studies analysing St John's wort products have reported differing contents of hypericin and hyperforin.[241–243] Furthermore, some products showed consistent batch-to-batch concentrations of hypericin and hyperforin, whilst others exhibited significant interbatch variability.[241]

Despite the dearth of documented clinical evidence for the effects of the majority of herbal ingredients, there is no reason why herbal medicinal products should not be available for use in minor conditions, providing that these are consistent with traditional uses and that the herbal ingredients are of suitable quality and safety. It would seem to be more appropriate to use those herbal ingredients for which documented phytochemical and pharmacological data support the traditional use. Herbal medicines intended for use in more serious medical conditions require evidence of efficacy to support their use.

Conclusion

The use of herbal medicinal products continues to increase and there is growing evidence that herbal medicines are used widely by all groups of society including children, pregnant and breastfeeding mothers, women, especially during the menopause, and the elderly. Of particular importance is the use of herbal medicines by patients with a wide range of conditions many of whom are stabilised on prescription medicines and findings that patients are reluctant to tell their doctors about herbal products they are taking. Over the last five years the significance of herb–drug interactions has been recognised and with this the realisation that healthcare professionals need to be aware that patients may be taking herbal medicinal products, and need to understand their effects and be aware of the potential problems associated with their use. This handbook provides the reader with factual information on 152 herbal ingredients present in herbal medicinal products in European and other developed countries. Herbal medicinal products can offer an alternative to conventional medicines in non-life-threatening conditions, providing they are of adequate quality and safety, and are used in an appropriate manner.

References

1 Kessler RC *et al*. Long-term trends in the use of complementary and alternative medical therapies in the United States. *Ann Intern Med* 2001; 135: 262–268.

2 Barnes P *et al*. Complementary and alternative medicine among adults: United States, 2002. *Adv Data* 2004; 343: 1–19.
3 Tindle HA *et al*. Trends in use of complementary and alternative medicine by US adults: 1997–2002. *Alt Ther Health Med* 2005; 11(1): 42–49.
4 Blumenthal M. Herb sales down 7.4 percent in mainstream market. *Herbalgram* 2005; 66: 63.
5 MacLennan AH *et al*. The continuing use of complementary and alternative medicine in South Australia: costs and beliefs in 2004. *MJA* 2006; 184: 27–31.
6 Barnes J. Herbal medicine. *Pharm J* 1998; 260: 344–348.
7 Thomas KJ *et al*. Use and expenditure on complementary medicine in England: a population based survey. *Complement Ther Med* 2001; 9: 2–11.
8 Dixon A. *et al*. Complementary and Alternative Medicine in the UK and Germany – research and evidence on supply and demand. Anglo-German Foundation for the Study of Industrial Society 2003. http://www.agf.org.uk December 2005.
9 House of Lords Select Committee on Science and Technology Session 1999–2000, 6th Report. Complementary and Alternative Medicine. 21 November 2000.
10 Ernst E, White AR. The BBC survey of complementary medicine use in the UK. *Complement Ther Med* 2000; 8: 32–36.
11 Brevoort P. The US botanical market – an overview. *Herbalgram* 1996; 36: 49–57.
12 Brevoort P. The booming US botanical market. A new overview. *Herbalgram* 1998; 44: 33–46.
13 Rogers G. Herb consumers' attitudes, preferences profiled in new market study. *Herbalgram* 2005; 65: 60–61.
14 Blumenthal M. Herbs and phytomedicines in the European Community. In: Blumenthal M, ed. *The Complete German Commission E Monographs. Therapeutic Guide to Herbal Medicines*. Austin, Texas: American Botanical Council, 1998.
15 Institute of Medical Statistics (IMS) Self-Medication International. *Herbals in Europe*. London: IMS Self-Medication International, 1998.
16 *Complementary Medicines – UK*. Mintel International Group Ltd. April 2003.
17 *Complementary Medicines – UK*. Mintel International Group Ltd. March 2005.
18 EMEA Herbal Medicinal Products Committee. Public statement on the risks associated with the use of herbal products containing *Aristolochia* species. www.emea.europa.eu/pdfs/human/hmpc/13838105en.pdf November 2005.
19 Barnes J *et al*. St. John's Wort (*Hypericum perforatum* L.): a review of its chemistry, pharmacology and clinical properties. *J Pharm Pharmacol* 2001; 53: 583–600.
20 O'Sullivan HM, Lum K. The poisoning of 'awa: the non-traditional use of an ancient remedy. *Pac Health Dialog*. 2004; 11(2): 211–215.
21 Ernst E. Contamination of herbal medicines. *Pharm J* 2005; 275: 167–168.
22 De Smet PAGM. Health risks of herbal remedies: An update. *Clinical Pharmacology Therapeutics* 2004; 76(1): 1–17.
23 Barnes J, Abbot NC. Experiences with complementary remedies: a survey of community pharmacists. *Pharm J* 1999; 263 (Suppl. Suppl.) R37–R43.
24 Kayne S. A helping hand? *Chemist and Druggist* 2002; 12: 26–28.
25 Naidu S *et al*. Attitudes of Australian pharmacists toward complementary and alternative medicines. *Annals Pharmacotherapy* 2005; 39: 1456–1461.
26 Welna EM *et al*. Pharmacists' personal use, professional practice behaviours, and perceptions regarding herbal and other natural products. *Journal American Pharmacists Association* 2003; 43(5): 602–611.
27 Ernst E. Complementary medicine pharmacist. *Pharm J* 2004; 273: 197–198.
28 Ernst E. Recommended information sources. *Pharm J* 2005; 275: 348.
29 Nathan JP *et al*. Availability of and attitudes toward resources on alternative medicine products in the community pharmacy setting. *J Am Pharm Assoc* 2005; 45(6): 734–739.
30 Evans WC. *Trease and Evans' Pharmacognosy*, 15th edn. London: WB Saunders, 2001.
31 Council Directive 2001/83/EC. *Official Journal of the European Communities* 2001; 311: 67–128.
32 Britt R. The New EC Systems in the UK, *Regulatory Affairs J* 1995; 6: 380–384.
33 Gaedcke F, Steinhoff B. The European marketing authorisation system. In: *Herbal Medicinal Products*. Stuttgart: medpharm GmbH Scientific Publishers, 2003: 81–88.
34 Regulation (EC) No 726/2004 of the European Parliament and of the Council *Official Journal of the European Communities* 2004; 136: 1–33.
35 AESGP (Association of the European Self-medication Industry). Herbal Medicinal Products in the European Union, 15 March 1999. http://www.aesgp.be
36 Steinhoff B. The contribution of the European Scientific Cooperative on Phytotherapy and World Health Organisation monographs. *Drug Inform J* 1999; 33: 17–22.
37 Gaedcke F, Steinhoff B. Legal provisions relating to the efficacy and safety of herbal medicinal products: Attempts to harmonise the assessment criteria. In: *Herbal Medicinal Products*. Stuttgart: medpharm GmbH Scientific Publishers, 2003:117–130.
38 *ESCOP Monographs (European Scientific Cooperative on Phytotherapy)*. The Scientific Foundation for Herbal Medicinal Products, Exeter. 2nd edition (2003).
39 Council Directive 2004/24/EC. *Official Journal of the European Communities* 2004, 136: 85–90.
40 EMEA Committee for Herbal Medicinal Products (HMPC). Community Herbal Monographs. www.emea.europa.eu/htms/human/hmpc/hmpcmonographsadopt.htm March 2007.
41 *Medicines Act Leaflet (MAL) 8. A Guide to the Status under the Medicines Act of Borderline Products for Human Use*. London: Medicines Control Agency.
42 *Medicines Act Leaflet (MAL 2). Guidelines on Safety and Efficacy Requirements for Herbal Medicinal Products. Guidance Notes on Applications for Product Licences*; 1989, 53–54.
43 Statutory Instrument (SI) 2005:2759. The Medicines (Marketing Authorisations etc.) Amendment Regulations 2005.
44 *The Medicines Act, 1968*. London: HM Stationery Office.
45 Appelbe GE, Wingfield J. *Dale and Appelbe's Pharmacy Law and Ethics*, 8th edn. London: Pharmaceutical Press, 2005.
46 CPMP/QWP 2819/00 (EMEA/CVMP 814/00) Guideline on Quality of Herbal Medicinal Products. EMEA website: www.emea.europa.eu/pdfs/human/qwp/281900en.pdf October 2006.
47 CPMP/QWP 2820/00 (EMEA/CVMP 814/00) Guideline on Specifications: test procedures and acceptance criteria for herbal drugs, herbal drug preparations and herbal medicinal products. EMEA website: www.emea.europa.eu/pdfs/human/qwp/282000en.pdf October 2006.
48 *CPMP/CVMP Note for Guidance on Manufacture of Herbal Medicinal. Products. The Rules Governing Medicinal Products in the European Union 1992*, vol. IV: 127–129.
49 Statutory Instrument (SI) 1971: 1450. The Medicines (Exemptions from Licences) (Special and Transitional Cases) Order.
50 MHRA Consultation Letter MLX 299. Proposals for the reform of the regulation of unlicensed herbal remedies in the United Kingdom made up to meet the needs of individual patients. March 2004.
51 Holder S. Regulatory aspects of herbal medicines: a global view. *The Regulatory Review* 2001; 4: 13–17.
52 Reminder: Safety of Traditional Chinese Medicines and herbal remedies. *Current Problems* 2004; 30: 10.
53 Traditional Herbal Medicines Registration Scheme: Future changes to Section 12(2) of the Medicines Act? MHRA website: http://www.mhra.gov.uk February 2006.
54 Statutory Instrument (SI) 1984: 769, The Medicines (Products Other than Veterinary Drugs) (General Sales List) Order, 1984, as amended by SI 1985:1540, SI 1987: 910, SI 1989: 969 and SI 1990: 1129.
55 Statutory Instrument (SI) 1983: 1212, The Medicines (Products Other than Veterinary Drugs) (Prescription Only) Order 1983, as amended.
56 Statutory Instrument (SI) 1977: 2130, The Medicines Retail Sale or Supply of Herbal Remedies Order, 1977.
57 Statutory Instrument (SI) 2001:1841, The Medicines (Aristolochia and Mu Tong etc) (Prohibition) Order, 2001.
58 Statutory Instrument (SI) 2002:3170, The Medicines for Human Use (Kava-kava) (Prohibition) Order, 2002.

59 Medicines Control Agency. Review of herbal ingredients for use in unlicensed herbal medicinal products.. www.mhra.gov.uk September 2001
60 Anon. *National Policy on Traditional Medicine and Regulation of Herbal Medicines: Report of a WHO global survey.* Geneva: WHO, 2005.
61 Anon. *Regulatory Situation of Herbal Medicines – a Worldwide Review.* Geneva: WHO, 1998.
62 Anon. *Legal Status of Traditional Medicine and Complementary/ Alternative Medicine: A Worldwide Review.* Geneva: WHO, 2001.
63 World Health Organization. *WHO Guidelines for Developing Consumer Information on Proper Use of Traditional Medicines and Complementary/Alternative Medicines.* Geneva, Switzerland: World Health Organization, 2004.
64 World Health Organization.*WHO Guidelines on Safety Monitoring of Herbal Medicines in Pharmacovigilance Systems.* Geneva, Switzerland: World Health Organization, 2004.
65 World Health Organization. *WHO Guidelines on Good Agricultural and Collection Practices (GACP) for Medicinal Plants.* Geneva, Switzerland: World Health Organization, 2003.
66 Briggs D. The regulation of herbal medicines in Australia. *Toxicology* 2002; 181–182: 565–570.
67 Natural Health Products Directorate. A Regulatory Framework for Natural Health Products. www.hc-sc.gc.ca/dhp-mps/prodnatur/about-apropos/glance-apercu_e.html February 2006.
68 The Dietary Supplement Health and Education Act 1994 Pub L No. 103-417 Washington.
69 FDA Centre for Food Safety and Applied Nutrition. Dietary supplements. http://vm.cfsan.fda.gov/~dms/supplmnt.html
70 Marcus DM, Grollman AP. Botanical medicines – the need for new regulations. *N Engl J Med* 2002; 347(25): 2073–2076.
71 Wechsler J. Standards for supplements. *Pharmaceutical Technology Europe* 2003; March: 18–20.
72 Food and Drug Administration. FDA announces major initiatives for dietary supplements. 4 November 2004. www.fda.gov/bbs/topics/news/ 2004/NEW01130.html
73 De Smet PAGM. Toxicological outlook on quality assurance of herbal remedies. In: *Adverse Effects of Herbal Drugs*, vol 1. Berlin: Springer Verlag, 1992.
74 De Smet PAGM. Overview of herbal quality control. *Drug Inform J* 1999; 33: 717–724.
75 Bauer R. Quality criteria and standardization of phytopharmaceuticals: Can acceptable drug standards be achieved? *Drug Inform J* 1998, 32: 101–110.
76 Busse W. The significance of quality for efficacy and safety of herbal medicinal products. *Drug Inform J* 2000, 34: 15–23.
77 Corbin Winslow L. Herbs as medicines. *Arch Intern Med* 1998: 158: 2192–2199.
78 Gaedcke F, Steinhoff B. Quality assurance of herbal medicinal products. In: *Herbal Medicinal Products.* Stuttgart: medpharm GmbH Scientific Publishers, 2003: 37–66.
79 *IARC Monographs on the Evaluation of Carcinogenic Risk of Chemicals to Humans.* Lyons, France: IARC Press, 2002 Volume 82.
80 Vanherweghem JL, *et al.* Rapidly progressive interstitial renal fibrosis in young women: association with slimming regimen including Chinese herbs. *Lancet* 1993; 341: 135–139.
81 Cosyns JP *et al.* Chinese herbs nephropathy: A clue to Balkan endemic nephropathy. *Kidney Int* 1994; 45: 1680–1688.
82 Van Ypersele C, Vanherweghem JL. The tragic paradigm of Chinese herb nephropathy. *Nephrol Dial Transplant* 1995; 10: 157–160.
83 Cosyns J-P *et al.* Urothelial lesions in Chinese-herb nephropathy. *Am J Kidney Dis* 1999; 33: 1011–1017.
84 Nortier JL *et al.* Urothelial carcinoma associated with the use of a Chinese herb (*Aristolochia fangchi*). *N Engl J Med* 2000; 342: 1686–1692.
85 Lord G *et al.* Nephropathy caused by Chinese herbs in the UK. *Lancet* 1999; 354: 481–482.
86 Lord GM *et al.* Urothelial malignant disease and Chinese herbal nephropathy. *Lancet* 2001; 358: 1515–1516.
87 FDA Press Release. Vital Nutrients Recalls Joint Ease & Verified Quality Brand Joint Comfort Complex because of adverse health risk associated with aristolochic acid. www.fda.gov-USA June 2001.
88 Charvill A. *Investigation of formulated Traditional Chinese Medicines (TCM) and raw herbs for the presence of* Aristolochia *species.* British Pharmaceutical Conference Science Proceedings 2001. London: Pharmaceutical Press, 2001: 295.
89 Gold LS, Slone TH Aristolochic acid, an herbal carcinogen, sold on the Web after FDA alert. *N Engl J Med* 2003; 349: 1576–1577.
90 Medicines and Healthcare products Regulatory Agency (MHRA). Herbal Safety News. www.mhra.gov.uk
91 Slifman NR. Contamination of botanical dietary supplements by *Digitalis lanata. N Engl J Med* 1998; 339: 806–811.
92 But PPH *et al.* Adulterants of herbal products can cause poisoning. *BMJ* 1996; 313: 117.
93 Tai YT *et al.* Cardiotoxicity after accidental herb-induced aconite poisoning. *Lancet* 1992; 340: 1254–1256.
94 Read BE Bastard anise poisoning and its antidotal measures. *Chinese J Physiol* 1926; 1: 15–22.
95 Biessels GJ *et al.* Epileptic seizure after a cup of tea: intoxication with Japanese star anise. *Ned Tijdschr Geneeskd* 2002; 146: 808–811.
96 L'Agence française de sécurité sanitaire des produits de santé (Afssaps). Badiane et risque convulsive, 2001. Available at: http:// agmed.sante.gouv.fr/htm/10/filcoprs/011103c.htm February 2006.
97 Laboratoires de la DGCCRF. Mise en évidence de la contamination de la badiane de Chine (Illicium verum Hoocker f.) par d'autres espèces de badiane, Marseille, France; 2003. Available at: www.finances.gouv. fr/DGCCRF/activites/labos/2001/badiane.htm. Accessed April 22, 2003.
98 2002/75/EC: Commission Decision of 1 February 2002 laying down special conditions on the import from third countries of star anise (text with EEA relevance) (notified under document number C(2002) 379). *Off J Eur Commun* 2002; L: 33–34.
99 Diego Ize-Ludlow MD *et al.* Neurotoxicities in infants seen with consumption of star anise tea. *Pediatrics* 2004; 114 (5): e653–e656.
100 *Pharmacopoeia of the People's Republic of China* (English edition). Chemical Industry Press, 2005.
101 Ko R. Adulterants in Asian patent medicines. *N Engl J Med* 1998; 339: 847.
102 Au AM *et al.* Screening methods for drugs and heavy metals in Chinese patent medicines. *Bull Environ Contam Toxicol* 2000; 65: 112–119.
103 Koh H-L, Woo S-O. Chinese Proprietary Medicine in Singapore: Regulatory control of toxic heavy metals and undeclared drugs. *Drug Safety* 2000; 23: 351–362.
104 Huang WF *et al.* Adulteration by synthetic substances of traditional Chinese medicines in Taiwan. *J Clin Pharmacol* 1997; 37: 344–350.
105 Singapore Ministry of Health Press Statement. Chinese Proprietary Medicine Found Adulterated with Sildenafil. 3 March 2001.
106 FDA Press Release. Anso Comfort Capsules Recalled by Distributor. 13 February 2001. www.fda.gov-USA.
107 Lau KK *et al.* Phenytoin poisoning after using Chinese proprietary medicines. *Hum Exp Toxicol* 2000; 19: 385–386.
108 FDA Press Release. State Health Director Warns Consumers about Prescription Drugs in Herbal Products. 15 February 2000. www.fda. gov-USA.
109 Medicines Control Agency. Hypoglycaemia following the use of Chinese herbal medicine Xiaoke Wan. *Curr Probl Pharmacovigilance* 2001; 27: 8.
110 Wu M-S. Multiple tubular dysfunction induced by mixed Chinese herbal medicines containing cadmium. *Nephrol Dialysis Transplant* 1996; 11: 867–870.
111 Schaumburg HH *et al.* Alopecia and sensory polyneuropathy from thallium in a Chinese herbal medication. *JAMA.* 1992; 268: 3430–3431.
112 Kew J *et al.* Arsenic and mercury intoxication due to Indian ethnic remedies. *BMJ* 1993; 306: 506–507.
113 Sheerin NS *et al.* Simultaneous exposure to lead, arsenic and mercury from Indian ethnic medicines. *Br J Clin Pharmacol* 1994; 48: 332–333.
114 Cuncha J *et al.* Arsenic and acute lethal intoxication. *Hong Kong Pharm J* 1998; 7: 50–53.
115 Ernst E. Adulteration of Chinese herbal medicines with synthetic drugs: a systematic review. *Journal of Internal Medicine* 2002; 252: 107–113.
116 Ernst E. Heavy metals in traditional Indian remedies. *Eur J Clin Phar* 2002; 57: 891–896.

117 Ernst E. Toxic heavy metals and undeclared drugs in Asian herbal medicines. *Trends Pharmacol Sci* 2002; 23(3): 136–139.
118 Cole MR, Fetrow CW. Adulteration of dietary supplements. *Am J Health-Syst Pharm* 2003; 60: 1576–1580.
119 Ernst E. Risks of herbal medicinal products. *Pharmacoepidemiology Drug Safety* 2004; 13: 767–771
120 Saper RB *et al.* Heavy metal content of Ayurvedic herbal medicine products. *JAMA* 2004; 292: 2868–2873.
121 EMEA Committee for Herbal Medicinal Products (HMPC). Guideline on Good Agricultural and Collection Practice for starting materials of herbal origin. www.emea.europa.eu/pdfs/human/hmpc/24681605en.pdf August 2006.
122 World Health Organization. *Quality Control of Medicinal Plant Materials.* Geneva: World Health Organization, 1998.
123 *European Pharmacopoeia*, 5th edn. 2005. Strasbourg: Council of Europe, 2005.
124 Phillipson JD. Quality assurance of medicinal plants. In: Franz C *et al.* First World Congress on medicinal and aromatic plants for human welfare, WOCMAP, quality, phytochemistry, industrial aspects, economic aspects. *Acta Horticult* 1993; 333: 117–122.
125 Houghton P. Establishing identification criteria for botanicals. *Drug Inform J* 1998; 32: 461–469.
126 De Smet PAGM. Health risks of herbal remedies. *Drug Safety* 1995; 13: 81–93.
127 De Smet PAGM. Adverse effects of herbal remedies. *Adverse Drug React Bull* 1997; 183: 695–698.
128 Shaw D *et al.* Traditional remedies and food supplements. A 5-year toxicological study (1991–1995). *Drug Safety* 1997; 17: 342–356.
129 Chitturi S, Farrell GC. Herbal hepatotoxicity: an expanding but poorly defined problem. *Journal Gastroenterology and Hepatology* 2000; 15: 1093–1099.
130 Pittler MH, Ernst E. Systematic review: hepatotoxic events associated with herbal medicinal products. *Aliment Pharmacol Ther* 2003; 18: 451–471.
131 Tisserand R, Balacs T. *Essential Oil Safety.* Edinburgh: Churchill Livingstone, 1995.
132 EMEA HMPC. *Public Statement on the use of herbal medicinal products containing asarone.* www.emea.europa.eu/pdfs/human/hmpc/13921505en.pdf November 2005.
133 EMEA HMPC. *Public Statement on the use of herbal medicinal products containing estragole.* www.emea.europa.eu/pdfs/human/hmpc/13721205en.pdf November 2005.
134 EMEA HMPC. *Public Statement on the use of herbal medicinal products containing methyleugenol.* www.emea.europa.eu/pdfs/human/hmpc/13836305en.pdf November 2005.
135 De Smet PAGM. Aristolochia species. In: *Adverse Effects of Herbal Drugs*, vol 1. Berlin: Springer Verlag, 1992.
136 D'Arcy PF. Adverse reactions and interactions with herbal medicines. Part 1. Adverse reactions. *Adverse Drug React Toxicol Rev* 1991; 10: 189–208.
137 Mattocks AR. *Chemistry and Toxicology of Pyrrolizidine Alkaloids.* New York: Academic Press, 1986.
138 Anderson LA, Phillipson JD. Mistletoe – the magic herb. *Pharm J* 1982; 229: 437–439.
139 Tyler VE. *The Honest Herbal*, 3rd edn. New York: Howarth Press, 1993.
140 Chandler RF *et al.* Controversial laetrile. *Pharm J* 1984; 232: 330–332.
141 Statutory Instrument (SI) 1984:87. The Medicines (Cyanogenetic Substances) Order 1984.
142 Ljunggren B. Severe phototoxic burn following celery ingestion. *Arch Dermatol* 1990; 126: 1334–1336.
143 Boffa MJ *et al.* Celery soup causing severe phototoxicity during PUVA therapy. *Br J Dermatol* 1996; 135: 330–345.
144 Medicines Control Agency. *Psoralea corylifolia* fruit in Traditional Chinese Medicines causing severe skin reaction. *Curr Probl Pharmacovigilance* 2001; 27: 12.
145 EMEA HMPC. *Public statement on chamomilla containing herbal medicinal products.* www.emea.europa.eu/pdfs/human/hmpc/13830905en.pdf March 2006.
146 Nordeng H, Havnen G. Use of herbal drugs in pregnancy: a survey among 400 Norwegian women. *Pharmacoepidemiology and Drug safety* 2004; 13: 371–380.
147 Gallo M *et al.* The use of herbal medicine in pregnancy and lactation. In: Koren G, ed. *Maternal-fetal toxicology. A clinician's guide.* 3rd ed. New York: Marcel Dekker; 2001; 569–601.
148 Roulet M *et al.* Hepatic veno-occlusive disease in newborn infant of a woman drinking herbal tea. *J Pediatr* 1988; 112: 433–436.
149 Allen JR *et al.* Are herbal teas safe for infants and children? *Aust Family Physician* 1989; 18: 1017–1019.
150 Sawini-Sikand A *et al.* Use of complementary/alternative therapies among children in primary care pediatrics. *Ambul Pediatr* 2002; 2: 99–103.
151 OttoliniMC *et al.* Complementary and alternative medicine use among children in Washington, DC area. *Ambul Pediatr* 2000; 1: 122–125.
152 Lim A *et al.* Survey of complementary and alternative medicine use at a tertiary children's hospital. *Journal of Paediatrics and Child Health* 2005; 41(8): 424–427.
153 Hrastinger A *et al.* Is there clinical evidence supporting the use of botanical dietary supplements in children? *Journal of Pediatrics* 2005; 146: 311–317.
154 Ernst E. Herbal medicines for children. *Clin Pediatr* 2003; 42: 193–196.
155 Ernst E. Serious adverse effects of unconventional therapies for children and adolescents: a systematic review of recent evidence. *Eur J Pediatr* 2003; 162: 72–80.
156 Foster D *et al.* Alternative medicine use in older Americans. *J Am Geriatr Soc* 2000; 48: 1560–1565.
157 Canter PH, Ernst E. Herbal supplement use by persons aged over 50 years in Britain. *Drugs Aging* 2004; 21(9): 597–605.
158 Raji MA *et al.* Ethnic differences in herb and vitamin/mineral use in the elderly. *Annals of Pharmacotherapy* 2005; 39: 1019–1023.
159 Ernst E. Herbal Medications for common ailments in the elderly. *Drugs Ageing* 1999; 15: 423–428.
160 Mashour NH. Herbal medicine for the treatment of cardiovascular disease. *Arch Intern Med* 1998; 158: 2225–2234.
161 Ernst E. Cardiovascular adverse effects of herbal medicines: a systematic review of recent literature. *Canadian Journal of Cardiology* 2003; 19(7): 818–827.
162 Izzo AA *et al.* Cardiovascular pharmacotherapy and herbal medicines: the risk of drug interaction. *Int J Cardiol* 2005; 98(1):1–14.
163 British Heart Foundation. Herbs and the heart. 28 July 2003 (www.bhf.org.uk January 2006).
164 Ernst E. A primer of CAM commonly used by cancer patients. *MJA* 2001; 174: 88–92.
165 Richardson MA, Straus SE. Complementary and alternative medicine: Opportunities and challenges for cancer management and research. *Semin Oncol* 2002; 29: 531–545.
166 Lowenthal RM. Public illness: how the community recommended CAM for a prominent politician with cancer. *MJA* 2005; 183 (11/12): 576–579.
167 DiGianni LM *et al.* Complementary and alternative medicine use among women with breast cancer. *J Clin Oncol* 2002 (Suppl. Suppl.18); 20: 34S–38S.
168 Girgis A *et al.* The use of complementary and alternative therapies by patients with cancer. *Oncol Res* 2005; 15(5): 281–289.
169 Morris KT *et al.* A comparison of complementary therapy use between breast cancer patients and patients with other primary tumor sites. *Am J Surg* 2000; 179: 407–411.
170 Scott JA *et al.* Use of complementary and alternative medicine in patients with cancer: a UK survey. *Eur J Oncol Nurs* 2005; 9(2): 131–137.
171 Molassiotis A *et al.* Complementary and alternative medicine use in lung cancer patients in eight European countries. *Complement Ther Clin Pract* 2006; 12(1): 34–39.
172 Molassiotis A *et al.* Complementary and alternative medicine use in colorectal cancer patients in seven European countries. *Complement Ther Med* 2005; 13(4): 251–257.
173 Molassiotis A *et al.* Complementary and alternative medicine use in breast cancer patients in Europe. *Support Care Cancer* 2006; 14(3): 260–267.
174 Werneke U *et al.* Potential health risks of complementary alternative medicines in cancer patients. *British Journal of Cancer* 2004; 90: 408–413.
175 Richardson MA *et al.* Discrepant views of oncologists and cancer patients on CAM. *Support Care Cancer* 2004; 12: 797–804.

176 Mathijssen RH *et al*. Effects of St John's Wort on irinotecan metabolism. *J Natl Cancer Inst* 2002; 94: 1247–1249.
177 Sparreboom A *et al*. Herbal remedies in the United States: Potential adverse interactions with anticancer agents. *J Clin Oncol* 2004; 22: 2489–2503.
178 McLesky CH *et al*. The incidence of herbal and selected nutraceutical use in surgical patients. *Anaesthesiology* 1999; 91 (3A): A1168.
179 Ang-lee MK *et al*. Herbal medicines and peri operative care. *JAMA* 2001; 286: 208–216.
180 Adusumilli P *et al*. The prevalence and predictors of herbal medicine use in surgical patients. *J Am Coll Surg* 2004: 198(4): 583–590.
181 Noonan K *et al*. Herbal medication use in the pediatric surgical patient. *Journal Pediatric Surgery* 2004; 39(3): 500–503.
182 American Society of Anesthesiologists (ASA). What you should know about herbal and dietary supplement use and anesthesia. www.asahq.org/patientEducation/herbPatient.pdf February 2006.
183 American Society of Anesthesiologists (ASA). What you should know about your patients' use of herbal medicines and other dietary supplements. www.asahq.org/patientEducation/herbPhysician.pdf February 2006.
184 Royal College of Anaesthetists. You and Your Anaesthetic. 2nd edition. www.rcoa.ac.uk/docs/yaya.doc January 2003.
185 Armato P, Marcus DM. Review of alternative therapies for the treatment of menopausal symptoms. *Climacteric* 2003; 6: 278–284.
186 Mahady GB *et al*. Botanical dietary supplements usage in peri- and postmenopausal women. *Menopause* 2003; 10: 65–72.
187 Barnes J. Women's health. *Pharm J* 2003; 270: 16–18.
188 Stafford RS *et al*. Women's decision-making concerning alternative menopause treatments post WHI: Results from national on-line survey [abstract]. Washington, DC: North American Menopause Society 2004 Annual Meeting; October 6-9, 2004. Abstract P-125.
189 Mason P. How effective are complementary therapies for menopausal symptoms? *Pharm J* 2004; 273: 59–61.
190 Cos P *et al*. Phytoestrogens: recent developments. *Planta Medica* 2003; 69: 589–599.
191 Bodinet C, Freudenstein J. Influence of marketed herbal menopause preparations on MCF-7 cell proliferation. *Menopause* 2004; 11(3): 281–289.
192 Program on breast cancer and environmental risk factors. Herbal medicines and breast cancer risk. http://envirocancer.cornell.edu/factsheet/diet/fs53.herbal.cfm (accessed January 2006).
193 Fang CY *et al*. Correlates of soy food consumption in women at increased risk for breast cancer. *J Am Diet Assoc* 2005; 105(10):1552–1558.
194 Huntley A. Drug-herb interactions with herbal medicines for menopause. *Journal British Menopause Society* 2004; 10(4): 162–165.
195 Anon. Grapefruit and drug effects. *Drugs Q* 1999; 3: 25–28.
196 Huang SM *et al*. Drug interactions with herbal products and grapefruit juice: A conference report. *Clinical Pharmacology Therapeutics* 2004; 75(1): 112.
197 Fujita KI. Food-drug interactions via human cytochrome P450 3A (CYP3A). *Drug Metabol Drug Interact* 2004; 20(4): 195–217.
198 Ernst E. Possible interactions between synthetic and herbal medicinal products. *Perfusion* 2000; 13: 4–15.
199 Fugh-Berman A. Herb–drug interactions. *Lancet* 2000; 355: 134–138.
200 Miller L. Selected clinical considerations focusing on known and potential drug–herb interactions. *Arch Intern Med* 1998; 158: 2200–2211.
201 Brown R. Potential interactions of herbal medicines with antipsychotics, antidepressants and hypnotics. *Eur J Herb Med* 1997; 3: 25–28.
202 Barnes J *et al*. Herbal interactions. *Pharm J* 2003; 270: 118–121.
203 Williamson EM. Drug interactions between herbal and prescription medicines. *Drug Safety* 2003; 26(15): 1075–1092.
204 Mannel M. Drug interactions with St John's Wort. *Drug Safety* 2004; 27(11): 773–797.
205 Hu Z *et al*. Herb-drug interactions. *Drugs*. 2005; 65(9); 1239–1282.
206 Williamson EM. Interactions between herbal and conventional medicines. *Expert Opinion Drug Safety*. 2005; 4(2): 355–378.
207 Boyle F. Herbal medicines can interfere with breast cancer treatment. *Med J Aust* 1997; 167: 286.
208 Holden W. Use of herbal remedies and potential drug interactions in rheumatology outpatients. *Ann Rheum Dis* 2005; 64: 790.
209 Cheng TO. Herbal interactions with cardiac drugs. *Arch Intern Med* 2000; 160: 870–871.
210 Izzo AA, Ernst E. Interactions between herbal medicines and prescribed drugs. A systematic review. *Drugs* 2001; 61(15): 2163–2175.
211 Coxeter PD *et al*. Herb-drug interactions: an evidence based approach. *Current Medicinal Chemistry* 2004; 11: 1513–1525.
212 Halil M *et al*. No alteration in the PFA-100 in vitro bleeding time induced by the Ginkgo biloba special extract, Egb 761, in elderly patents with mild cognitive impairment. *Blood Coagul Fibrinolysis* 2005; 16: 349–353.
213 Gaus W *et al*. Identification of adverse drug reactions by evaluation of a prescription database, demonstrated for 'risk of bleeding'. *Methods Inf Med* 2005; 44: 697–703.
214 Stenton SB *et al*. Interactions between warfarin and herbal products, minerals and vitamins: a pharmacist's guide. *Can J Hosp Pharm* 2001; 54: 184–190.
215 Smith L *et al*. Co-ingestion of herbal medicines and warfarin. *Br J Gen Pract* 2004; 54(503): 439–441.
216 Ramsay NA. Complementary and alternative medicine use among patients starting warfarin. *British Journal Haematology* 2005; 130(5): 777–780.
217 Medicines and Healthcare products Regulatory Agency. Possible interaction between warfarin and cranberry juice. *Curr Probl Pharmacovigilance* 2003; 29: 8.
218 Medicines and Healthcare products Regulatory Agency. Interaction between warfarin and cranberry juice: new advice *Curr Probl Pharmacovigilance* 2004; 30: 10.
219 Barnes J. Pharmacovigilance of herbal medicines: a UK perspective. *Drug Safety* 2003; 26(12): 829–851.
220 Medicines and Healthcare products Regulatory Agency. Patient reporting of suspected adverse drug reactions. www.mhra.gov.uk February 2006.
221 Farah MH *et al*. International reporting of adverse health effects associated with herbal medicines. *Pharmacoepidemiol Drug Safety* 2000; 9: 105–112.
222 World Health Organization Collaborating Centre for International Drug Monitoring. Draft guidelines for herbal ATC classification. Uppsala: The Uppsala Monitoring Centre, 2002.
223 Fucik H *et al*. Building a computerised herbal substance register for implementation and use in the WHO international drug monitoring programme. *Drug Information Journal* 2002; 36: 839–854.
224 Barnes J. Herbal therapeutics (1). An introduction to herbal medicinal products. *Pharm J* 2002; 268: 804–806.
225 Barnes J. Herbal therapeutics (2). Depression. *Pharm J* 2002; 268: 908–910.
226 Barnes J. Herbal therapeutics (3). Cognitive deficiency and dementia. *Pharm J*, 2002; 269: 160–162.
227 Barnes J. Herbal therapeutics (4). Hyperlipidaemia. *Pharm J* 2002; 269: 193–195.
228 Barnes J. Herbal therapeutics (5). Insomnia. *Pharm J* 2002; 269: 219–221.
229 Barnes J. Herbal therapeutics (6). Benign prostatic hyperplasia. *Pharm J* 2002; 269: 250–252.
230 Barnes J. Herbal therapeutics (7). Colds. *Pharm J* 2002; 269: 716–718.
231 Barnes J. Herbal therapeutics (8). Gastrointestinal system and liver disorders *Pharm J* 2002; 269: 848–850.
232 Ernst E, Pittler MH. The efficacy of herbal drugs. In: *Herbal Medicine: a Concise Overview for Professionals*. London: Butterworth-Heinemann, 2000: 69–81.
233 Ernst E. The clinical efficacy of herbal treatments: an overview of recent systematic reviews. *Pharm J* 1999; 262: 85–87.
234 Ernst E. Herbal medicines: where is the evidence? *BMJ* 2000; 321: 395–396.
235 Linde K *et al*. Systematic reviews of herbal medicines – an annotated bibliography.: *Forsch Komplementarmed Klass Naturheilkd* 2003; 10 (Suppl. Suppl.1): 17–27.
236 Ernst E. The efficacy of herbal medicine – an overview. *Fundam Clin Pharmacol* 2005; 19(4): 405–409.
237 The Cochrane Library. www.update-software.com/cochrane/
238 Linde K *et al*. *St John's Wort for depression*. The Cochrane Database of Systematic Reviews 2006 Issue 1.

239 Williamson EM. Synergy – myth or reality? In: *Herbal Medicine: a Concise Overview for Professionals*. London: Butterworth-Heinemann, 2000: 43–58.
240 Williamson EM. Synergy and other interactions in phytomedicines. *Phytomedicine* 2001; 8(5): 401–409.
241 Wurglics M *et al*. Comparison of German St John's wort products according to hyperforin and total hypericin content. *J Am Pharm Assoc* 2001; 41: 560–566.
242 Bergonzi MC *et al*. Variability in the content of the constituents *of Hypericum perforatum* L. and some commercial extracts. *Drug Dev Indust Pharm* 2001; 26: 491–497.
243 Chandrasekera DH *et al*. Quantitative analysis of the major constituents of St John's wort with HPLC-ESI-MS. *J Pharm Pharmacol* 2005; 57(12):1645–1652.

Chemical Constituents of Plants Used as Herbal Medicines

All living organisms produce numerous chemical substances that are termed natural products. Those natural products that are common to all life forms are known collectively as primary metabolites and are exemplified by carbohydrates, proteins and fats. Thus, many of the chemical building blocks of primary metabolism are found in all medicinal plants (e.g. amino acids, common sugars, such as glucose, and fatty acids). In addition to primary metabolites, plants also produce other compounds with a more restricted distribution and these are referred to collectively as secondary metabolites. Plants are a rich source of secondary metabolites and some of these are of such limited distribution that they are found only in a particular genus (e.g. *Papaver*), or even in only a single species (e.g. *Papaver somniferum*). On the other hand, some secondary metabolites are widely distributed throughout many of the plant families. It is not always understood why particular plants produce specific secondary metabolites, but some of them are known to have definite functions; for example, some are toxic and form a defence against predators, while some are attractive to insects and aid pollination. W hatever their roles are within plants, many of them have pharmacological actions and this has been exploited to provide medicinal drugs such as codeine, morphine, digoxin and quinine. Some secondary metabolites have proved to be too toxic for human use (e.g. aconitine from aconite), but investigations of their mode of action have stimulated research into synthetic analogues as potential therapeutic agents.

For more details of plant secondary metabolites, the reader is recommended to consult specialist texts, for example on the biosynthesis of medicinal natural products (e.g. Dewick, 2002[(1)]), on scientific background to herbal medicines (e.g. Evans, 2002;[(2)] Heinrich *et al.*, 2003[(3)]) and on specific chemical structures (e.g. Harborne and Baxter, 1993;[(4)] *Dictionary of Natural Products* CD-ROM[(5)]).

Numerous secondary metabolites are derived from a common biosynthetic precursor; for example, shikimic acid is involved in the formation of coumarins, lignans, phenylpropanes and tannins. Although each of these groups of secondary metabolites is different chemically they all contain a common structural feature, namely a C6–C3 moiety. Among the most prevalent of secondary metabolites are alkaloids, glycosides and phenols. Examples of these types of secondary metabolite can be found in many of the medicinal plants.

Alkaloids

A typical alkaloid is chemically basic (alkaline) and contains a secondary or tertiary amine function within a heterocyclic ring (e.g. codeine). Alkaloids may be classified by their chemical skeleta (Figure 1) into the following major types: pyrrolidine (e.g. betonicine from white horehound); pyridine (e.g. gentianine from gentian); piperidine (e.g. lobeline from lobelia); pyrrolizidine (e.g. symphytine from comfrey); quinolizidine (e.g. sparteine from broom); quinoline (e.g. quinine from cinchona); isoquinoline (e.g. boldine from boldo); indole (e.g. harman from passionflower); tropane (e.g. hyoscine from belladonna); imidazole (e.g. pilocarpine from jaborandi); and xanthine (e.g. caffeine from maté). Biosynthetically related compounds that do not follow the above definition of an alkaloid may also be referred to as alkaloids, for example phenylalkylamines that do not contain an *N*-heterocyclic ring (e.g. ephedrine from ephedra), or that are not basic (e.g. colchicine from colchicum). Examples of medicinal plants that contain alkaloids are given in Appendix 2, Table 15. For further information on alkaloids the reader is referred to other texts (e.g. references 1, 3 and 6).

Glycosides

A glycoside consists of two components, an aglycone (non-sugar) part and a sugar part. The aglycone portion may be of several different types of secondary metabolite (Figure 2), including coumarin (e.g. scopolin from horse-chestnut, *see also* Appendix 2, Table 16), flavonoid (e.g. rutin from buchu, *see also* Appendix 2, Table 17), or hydroxyanthracene (e.g. cascaroside A from cascara, *see also* Appendix 2, Table 1). The sugar moiety is linked to the aglycone by a direct carbon-to-carbon bond (C-glycoside), or through an oxygen-to-carbon bond (O-glycoside). Cyanide glycosides, (e.g. amygdalin from apricot) release toxic hydrogen cyanide when cells are damaged and act as a defence mechanism. Glucosinolates (e.g. sinigrin from horseradish) contain nitrogen and sulfur and are pungent. Hydroxyanthracene glycosides are the active principles of the laxative herbs cascara and senna (*see also* Appendix 2, Table 1).

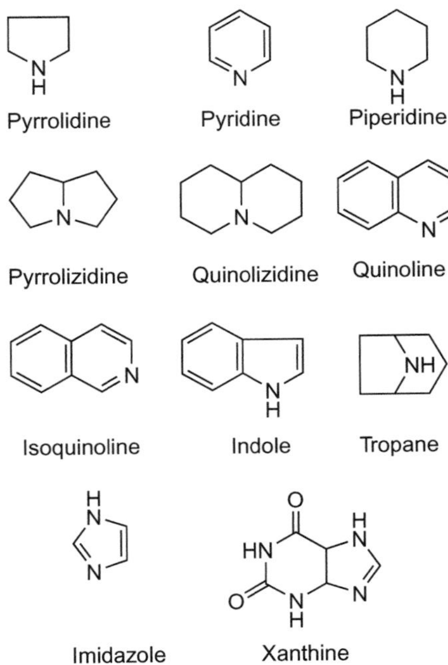

Figure 1 Examples of alkaloid skeleta.

Scopolin

Rutin

Cascaroside A

Figure 2 Examples of glycosides.

Phenolics

Many of the aromatic constituents of plants contain hydroxy substituents and are phenolic. There is a wide variety of phenolics in medicinal plants and they range in chemical structure from simple phenolic acids (Figure 3), e.g. caffeic acid from artichoke, to complex tannins (*see* Appendix 2, Table 20).

Where chemical structures are included in a monograph they may be the active principles or they may be compounds that can be used as chemical markers for that plant, i.e. they are present in significant quantities or are otherwise characteristic for a particular plant. As some compounds are of common occurrence in medicinal plants, their chemical structures are not necessarily included within a monograph. Some of the commonly encountered natural products, including mono-, sesqui-, di- and triterpenes, flavonoids and tannins, are briefly summarised below.

	R^1	R^2	R^3
p-Hydroxybenzoic acid	H	OH	H
Protocatechuic acid	OH	OH	H
Vanillic acid	OCH_3	OH	H
Gallic acid	OH	OH	OH

	R^1	R^2
p-Coumaric acid	H	OH
Caffeic acid	OH	OH
Ferulic acid	OCH_3	OH

Figure 3 Examples of simple phenolic acids.

Terpenes

Terpenes are derived from two C5 units (isopentane), dimethylallylpyrophosphate and isopentenylpyrophosphate. The monoterpenes contain two isopentane units (C10) and are constituents of many volatile oils (*see* Appendix 2, Table 21). Some of the more common monoterpenes are shown in Figure 4. Sesquiterpenes contain three isopentane units (C15) and occur as different skeletal types, e.g. eudesmane, germacrene, guaiane (Figure 5). A large number of sesquiterpenes contain a γ-lactone ring and these are known as sesquiterpene lactones. Some sesquiterpene lactones are allergenic (*see* Appendix 2, Table 11). Examples of different skeletal types of molecule, including eudesmolide, germacranolide and guaianolide (e.g. constituents of comfrey) and pseudoguaianolide (e.g. matricine, chamomile), are illustrated in Figure 5. Diterpenes are derived from four isopentane units (C20) and examples of abietane (e.g. carnosic acid from sage), daphnane, kaurene, labdane (e.g. rotundifarine from agnus castus), taxane and tigliane are given in Figure 6. The ginkgolides from ginkgo are examples of complex diterpenes. Triterpenes are derived from six isopentane units (C30), and some commonly occurring compounds are illustrated in Figure 7, e.g. campesterol, β-sitosterol, stigmasterol, α- and β-amyrin, oleanoic and ursolic acids. Cardiac glycosides (cardenolides, *see* Appendix 2, Table 2) and saponins (*see* Appendix 2, Table 19) are examples of triterpenes that are less widely distributed in plants than the triterpenes illustrated in Figure 7.

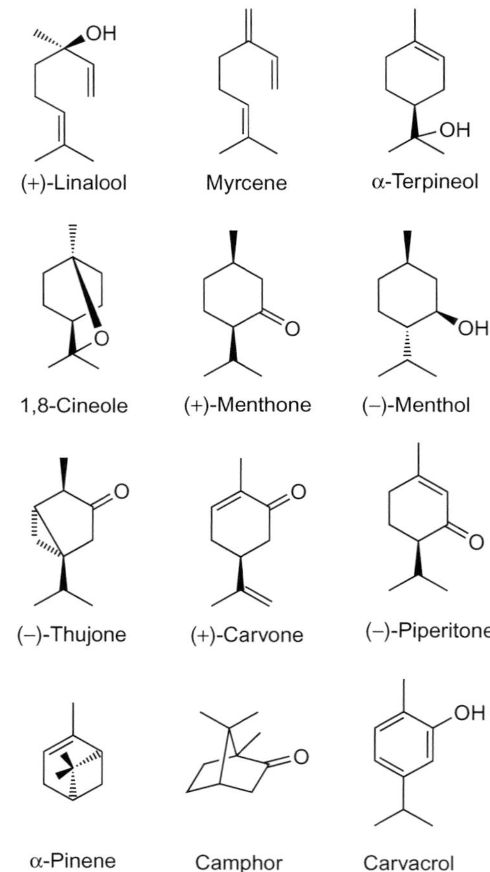

Figure 4 Some common monoterpenes from volatile oils.

Flavonoids

Flavonoids are biosynthesised from a phenylpropane unit (C6–C3), derived via shikimic acid and phenylalanine, and a C6 unit from three molecules of malonyl–CoA. They are widely distributed in the plant kingdom and occur in many medicinal plants (*see* Appendix 2, Table 17). There are five major types: chalcones, flavanones, flavones, flavonols and anthocyanins (Figure 8). The flavones and their 3-hydroxy analogues (flavonols) are the most widespread. The five aglycones kaempferol, quercetin, myricetin, apigenin and luteolin, as well as the quercetin glycosides quercitrin and rutin are among the most commonly present in medicinal plants (Figure 9).

Tannins

Tannins are also common constituents of many medicinal plants (*see* Appendix 2, Table 20) and they occur as two major types – the hydrolysable tannins and the non-hydrolysable (condensed) tannins. The hydrolysable tannins are esters of sugars with phenolic acids and they are either gallotannins (galloyl esters of glucose), e.g. pentagalloyl glucose, or ellagitannins (hexahydrodiphenic acid, derived from two units of gallic acid, esters with glucose), e.g. agrimoniin from agrimony. Non-hydrolysable tannins, also known as condensed tannins or proanthocyanidins, are polymers of catechin or gallocatechin linked by C–C bonds (e.g. cola tannins). Examples of some chemical structures of hydrolysable and non-hydrolysable tannins are given in Figure 10.

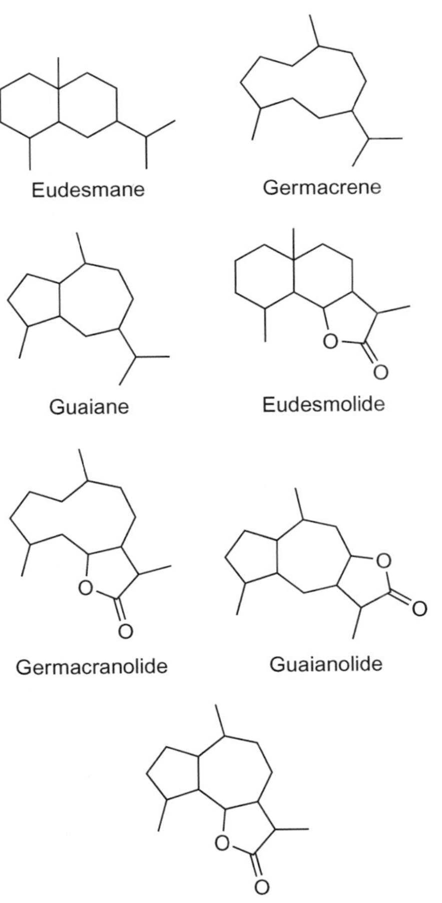

Figure 5 Some skeletal types of sesquiterpenes and sesquiterpene lactones.

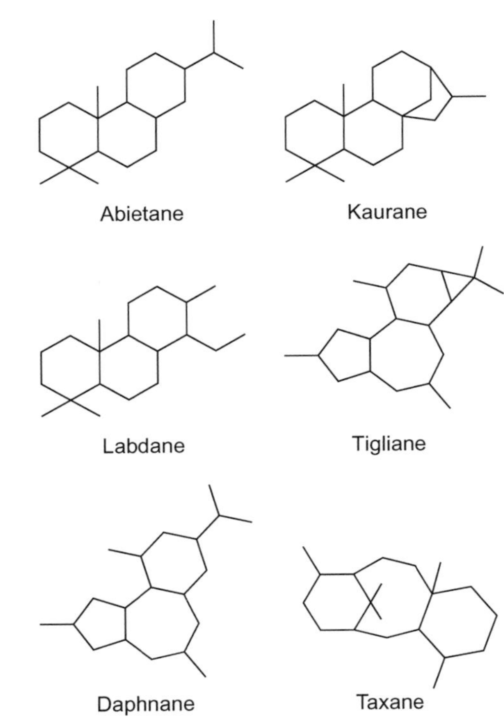

Figure 6 Examples of some different skeletal types of diterpenes.

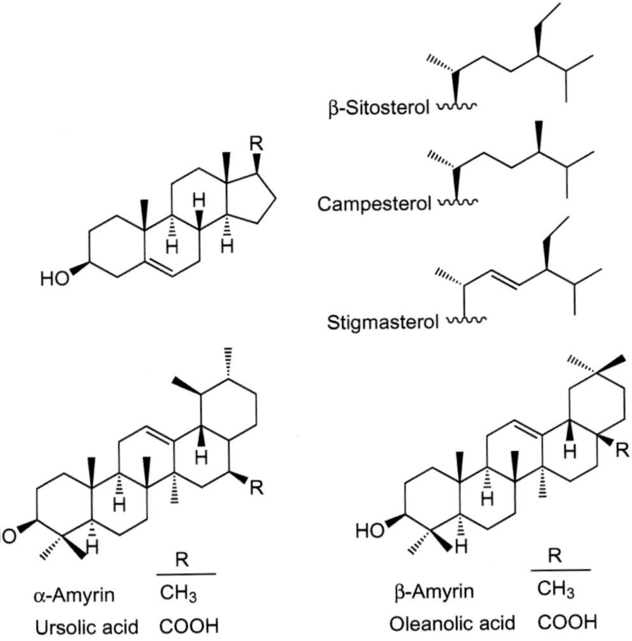

Figure 7 Examples of some common triterpenes.

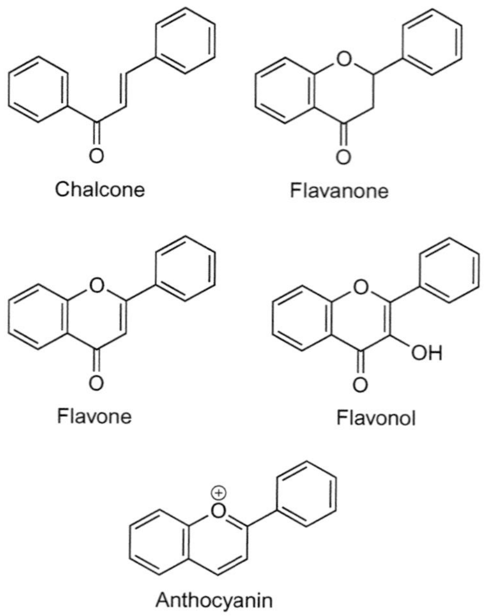

O O
Chalcone Flavanone

O O OH
Flavone Flavonol

Anthocyanin

Figure 8 Examples of some flavonoid skeleta.

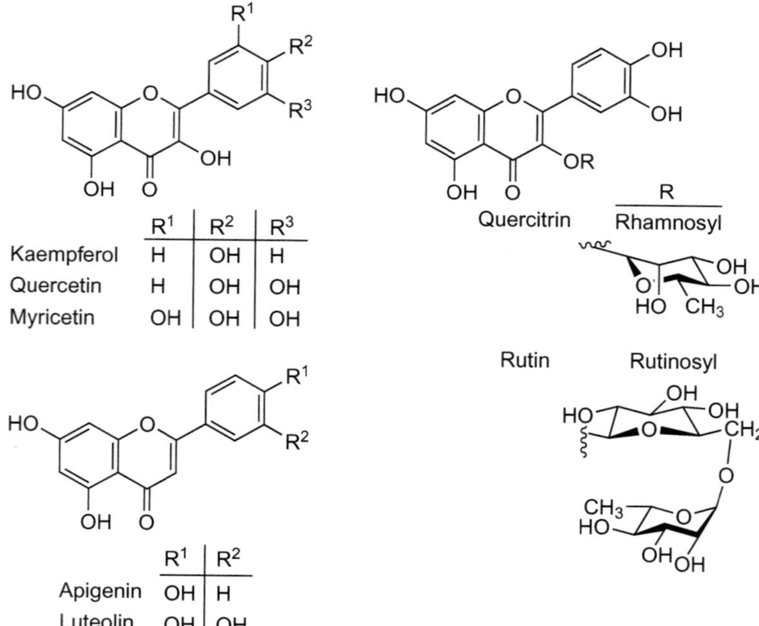

Figure 9 Examples of some common flavonoids.

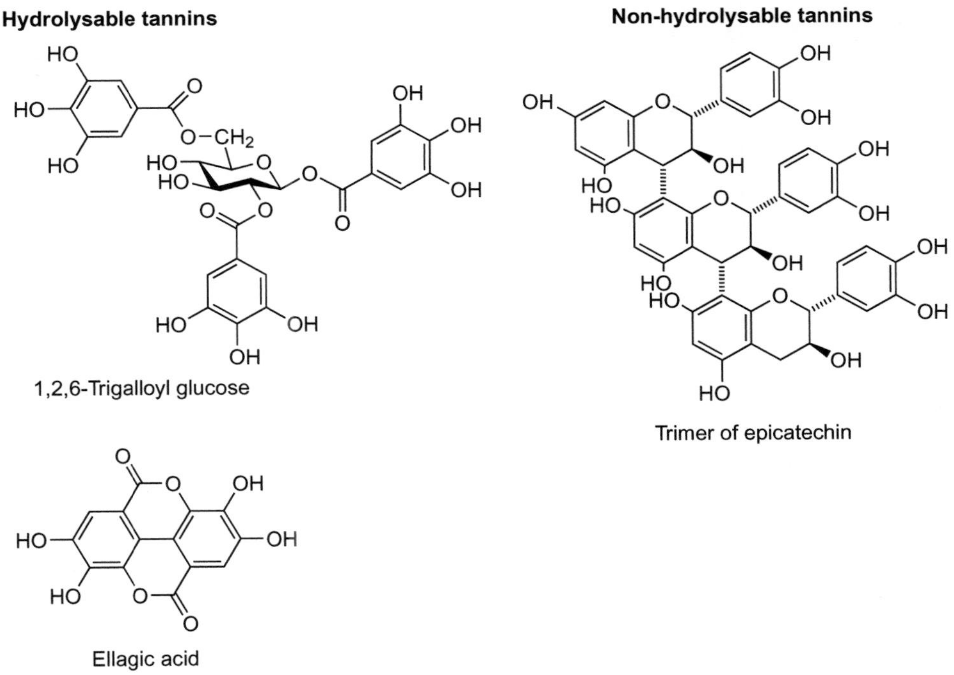

Hydrolysable tannins

1,2,6-Trigalloyl glucose

Non-hydrolysable tannins

Trimer of epicatechin

Ellagic acid

Figure 10 Examples of components of tannins.

References

1 Dewick PM. *Medicinal Natural Products. A Biosynthetic Approach*, 2nd edn. Chichester: John Wiley and Sons, 2002.

2 Evans WC. *Trease and Evans Pharmacognosy*, 15th edn. Edinburgh, London: WB Saunders, 2002.

3 Heinrich M *et al*. *Fundamentals of Pharmacognosy and Phytotherapy*. Edinburgh, London: Churchill Livingstone, 2004.

4 Harborne JB, Baxter H. *Phytochemical Dictionary*. London: Taylor and Francis, 1993.

5 *Dictionary of Natural Products* (CD-ROM). London: Chapman & Hall/CRC, 2003.

6 Cordell GA. *Introduction to Alkaloids: a Biogenetic Approach*. New York: Wiley Interscience, 1981

General References

General references are cited with the prefix 'G' in the monographs (e.g. 'G1').

1 *American Herbal Pharmacopoeia and Therapeutic Compendium.* Analytical, quality control and therapeutic monographs. Santa Cruz, California: American Herbal Pharmacopoeia, 1997–2005.
2 Bisset NG, ed. *Herbal Drugs and Phytopharmaceuticals* (Wichtl M, ed., German edition). Stuttgart: medpharm, 1994.
3 Blumenthal M *et al.*, eds. *The Complete German Commission E Monographs.* Austin, Texas: American Botanical Council, 1998.
4 Blumenthal M *et al.*, eds. *Herbal Medicine.* Expanded Commission E Monographs. Austin, Texas: American Botanical Council, 2000.
5 Boon H, Smith M. *The Botanical Pharmacy.* The Pharmacology of 47 Common Herbs. Kingston: Quarry Press, 1999.
6 Bradley PR, ed. *British Herbal Compendium*, vol 1. Bournemouth: British Herbal Medicine Association, 1992.
7 *British Herbal Pharmacopoeia.* Keighley: British Herbal Medicine Association, 1983.
8 *British Herbal Pharmacopoeia, 1990*, vol 1. Bournemouth: British Herbal Medicine Association, 1990.
9 *British Herbal Pharmacopoeia, 1996.* Exeter: British Herbal Medicine Association, 1996
10 *British Pharmaceutical Codex 1934.* London: Pharmaceutical Press, 1934.
11 *British Pharmaceutical Codex 1949.* London: Pharmaceutical Press, 1949.
12 *British Pharmaceutical Codex 1973.* London: Pharmaceutical Press, 1973.
13 *British Pharmacopoeia 1993.* London: HMSO, 1993.
14 *British Pharmacopoeia 1999.* London: The Stationery Office, 1999
15 *British Pharmacopoeia 2001.* London: The Stationery Office, 2001.
16 Council of Europe. *Flavouring Substances and Natural Sources of Flavourings*, 3rd edn. Strasbourg: Maisonneuve, 1981.
17 Council of Europe. *Natural Sources of Flavourings.* Report No. 1. Strasbourg: Council of Europe, 2000.
18 Cupp MJ, ed. *Toxicology and Clinical Pharmacology of Herbal Products.* Totawa, New Jersey: Humana Press, 2000.
19 De Smet PAGM *et al.*, eds. *Adverse Effects of Herbal Drugs*, vol 1. Berlin: Springer-Verlag, 1992.
20 De Smet PAGM *et al.*, eds. *Adverse Effects of Herbal Drugs*, vol 2. Berlin: Springer-Verlag, 1993.
21 De Smet PAGM *et al.*, eds. *Adverse Effects of Herbal Drugs*, vol 3. Berlin: Springer-Verlag, 1997.
22 Duke JA. *Handbook of Medicinal Herbs.* Boca Raton: CRC, 1985.
23 European Medicines Evaluation Agency. Herbal Medicinal Products Working Party Draft Core Summary of Product Characteristics for Valerian and Ispaghula (accessed 20 February 2002).
24 *European Pharmacopoeia*, 2nd edn. Strasbourg: Maisonneuve, 1980.
25 *European Pharmacopoeia*, 3rd edn. Strasbourg: Council of Europe, 1997.
26 *European Pharmacopoeia*, 3rd edn, 1998 Supplement. Strasbourg: Council of Europe, 1998.
27 *European Pharmacopoeia*, 3rd edn, 1999 Supplement. Strasbourg: Council of Europe, 1999.
28 *European Pharmacopoeia*, 4th edn, 2002. Strasbourg: Council of Europe, 2002.
29 Evans WC. *Trease and Evans' Pharmacognosy*, 14th edn. London: WB Saunders Company, 1998.
30 Farnsworth NR. Potential value of plants as sources of new antifertility agents I. *J Pharm Sci* 1975; 64: 535–598.
31 Fetrow CW, Avila JR. *Professional's Handbook of Complementary and Alternative Medicines.* Springhouse: Springhouse Corporation, 1999.
32 Foster S, Tyler VE. *Tyler's Honest Herbal*, 4th edn. New York: The Haworth Herbal Press, 1999.
33 Frohne D, Pfänder HJ. *A Colour Atlas of Poisonous Plants.* London: Wolfe, 1984.
34 Grieve M. *A Modern Herbal.* Thetford, Norfolk: Lowe and Brydon, 1979.
35 Gruenwald J *et al.*, eds. *PDR for Herbal Medicines*, 1st edn. Montvale: Medical Economics Company, 1998.
36 Gruenwald J *et al.*, eds. *PDR for Herbal Medicines*, 2nd edn. Montvale: Medical Economics Company Inc, 2000.
37 The Medicines (Products other than Veterinary Drugs) (General Sales List), SI No.769: 1984, as amended SI No.1540: 1985; SI No.1129: 1990; and SI No.2410: 1994.
38 Guenther E. *The Essential Oils*, six volumes. New York: Van Nostrand, 1948–1952.
39 Hamon NW, Blackburn JL. *Herbal Products – A Factual Appraisal for the Health Care Professional.* Winnipeg: Cantext, 1985.
40 Hoppe HA. *Taschenbuch der Drogenkunde.* Berlin: de Gruyter, 1981.
41 Leung AY. *Encyclopedia of Common Natural Ingredients Used in Food, Drugs and Cosmetics.* New York-Chichester: Wiley, 1980.
42 Mabey R., ed. *The Complete New Herbal.* London: Elm Tree Books, 1988.
43 *Martindale. The Complete Drug Reference*, 32nd edn. (Parfitt K, ed.). London: The Pharmaceutical Press, 1999.
44 *Martindale: The Extra Pharmacopoeia*, 28th edn. (Reynolds JEF, ed.). London: The Pharmaceutical Press, 1982.
45 *Martindale: The Extra Pharmacopoeia*, 29th edn. (Reynolds JEF, ed.). London: The Pharmaceutical Press, 1989.
46 *Martindale, The Extra Pharmacopoeia*: 30th edn. (Reynolds JEF, ed.). London: The Pharmaceutical Press, 1993.
47 *Martindale. The Extra Pharmacopoeia*, 31st edn. (Reynolds JEF, ed.). London: The Pharmaceutical Press, 1996.
48 *The Merck Index. An Encyclopedia of Chemicals, Drugs and Biologicals*, 11th edn. Rahway, NJ: Merck, 1989.
49 Mills SY. *The Dictionary of Modern Herbalism.* Wellingborough: Thorsons, 1985.
50 Mills S, Bone K. *Principles and Practice of Phytotherapy.* Edinburgh: Churchill Livingstone, 2000.
51 Mitchell J, Rook A. *Botanical Dermatology – Plants and Plant Products Injurious to the Skin.* Vancouver: Greengrass, 1979.
52 *Monographs on the Medicinal Uses of Plant Drugs*, Fascicules 1 and 2 (1996), Fascicules 3, 4 and 5 (1997), Fascicule 6 (1999). Exeter: European Scientific Cooperative on Phytotherapy.
53 Morelli I *et al. Selected Medicinal Plants.* Rome: FAO, 1983.
54 Robbers JE, Tyler VE. *Tyler's Herbs of Choice.* New York: The Haworth Herbal Press, 1999.
55 Schulz V, Hänsel R, Tyler V. *Rational Phytotherapy. A Physicians' Guide to Herbal Medicine.* Berlin: Springer-Verlag, 1998.
56 Schulz V, Hänsel R, Tyler V. *Rational Phytotherapy. A Physicians' Guide to Herbal Medicine*, 4th edn. Berlin: Springer-Verlag, 2000.
57 Simon JE *et al. Herbs – An Indexed Bibliography, 1971–80.* Oxford: Elsevier, 1984.
58 Tisserand R, Balacs T. *Essential Oil Safety.* Edinburgh: Churchill Livingstone, 1995.
59 Trease GE, Evans WC. *Pharmacognosy*, 13th edn. London: Baillière Tindall, 1989.
60 Tyler VE. *The Honest Herbal*, 3rd edn. Philadelphia: Strickley, 1993.
61 *United States Pharmacopeia 24 and National Formulary 19 and Supplements.* Rockville, Maryland, US: United States Pharmacopeial Convention, 2000.
62 Wagner H *et al. Plant Drug Analysis.* Berlin: Springer-Verlag, 1983.
63 World Health Organization. *WHO Monographs on Selected Medicinal Plants*, vol 1. Geneva: World Health Organization, 1999.
64 Wren RC. *Potter's New Cyclopedia of Botanical Drugs and Preparations* (revised, Williamson EW, Evans FJ). Saffron Walden: Daniel, 1988.

65 www.cfsan.fda.gov/~dms/eafus.html (US Food and Drug Administration).
66 British Herbal Medicine Association. *A Guide to Traditional Herbal Medicines* Bournemouth: British Herbal Medicine Association Publishing, 2003.
67 *Martindale. The Complete Drug Reference*, 33nd edn. (Sweetman S, ed.). London: The Pharmaceutical Press, 2002.
68 Evans WC. *Trease and Evans Pharmacognosy*, 15nd edn. Edinburgh: WB Saunders, 2002.
69 Williamson EM. *Potter's Herbal Cyclopaedia*. Saffron Walden: CW Daniel Co., 2003.
70 World Health Organization. *WHO Monographs on Selected Medicinal Plants*, vol 2. Geneva: World Health Organization, 2002.
71 *British Pharmacopoeia 2002*. London: The Stationery Office, 2002.
72 *European Pharmacopoeia*, 4th edn, 2004 Supplement. Strasbourg: Council of Europe, 2004.
73 *United States Pharmacopoeia 26 and National Formulary 21 and Supplements*. Rockville, Maryland, US: United States Pharmacopeial Convention, 2003.
74 *British Pharmacopoeia 2004*. London: The Stationery Office, 2004.
75 Wichtl M (ed.). *Herbal Drugs and Phytopharmaceuticals. A handbook for practice on a scientific basis*. 3rd edition. Stuttgart: medpharm Scientific publishers, 2004.
76 European Scientific Co-operative on Phytotherapy. *ESCOP monographs*. 2nd edition. Exeter, Stuttgart, New York: ESCOP, Georg Thieme Verlag, Thieme New York, 2003.
77 *Martindale. The complete drug reference*. 34th edn. (Sweetman S, ed.) London: Pharmaceutical Press, 2005.
78 *British National Formulary 49*. London: British Medical Association and Royal Pharmaceutical Society of Great Britain, 2005.
79 Stockley IH (editor in chief). *Stockley's Drug Interactions*. 6th edn. London: Pharmaceutical Press, 2002.
80 European Medicines Agency. Committee on Herbal Medicinal Products. *Community Herbal Monograph on* Valeriana officinalis *L., radix*. London, 26 October 2006. Doc. Ref. EMEA/HMPC/340719/2005.
81 *European Pharmacopoeia*, 5th edn, and Supplements 5.1–5.7. Strasbourg: Council of Europe, 2004–2007.
82 European Medicines Agency. Committee on Herbal Medicinal Products. *Community Herbal Monograph on* Plantago ovata *Forssk., seminis tegumentum*. London, 26 October 2006. Doc. Ref. EMEA/HMPC/340857/2005.
83 European Medicines Agency. Committee on Herbal Medicinal Products. *Community Herbal Monograph on* Plantago ovata *Forssk., semen*. London, 26 October 2006. Doc. Ref. EMEA/HMPC/340861/2005.
84 *British Pharmacopoeia 2007*. London: The Stationery Office, 2007.
85 *Martindale. The Complete Drug Reference*, 35th edn. (Sweetman S, ed.) London: Pharmaceutical Press, 2007.
86 *United States Pharmacopeia 29 and National Formulary 24 and Supplements*. Rockville, Maryland, US, United States Pharmacopeial Convention, 2006.
87 Majerus PW, Tollefsen DM. Anticoagulant, thrombolytic and antiplatelet drugs. In: Hardman JG, Limbird LE (eds). *Goodman & Gilman's The Pharmacological Basis of Therapeutics*, 10th edn. New York: McGraw-Hill, 2001: 1519–1538.
88 European Medicines Agency. Committee on Herbal Medicinal Products. *Community Herbal Monograph on* Aloe barbadensis *Miller and on Aloe (various species, mainly* Aloe ferox *Miller and its hybrids)*. London, 26 October 2006. Doc. Ref. EMEA/HMPC/76310/2006.

A

Agnus Castus

Summary and Pharmaceutical Comment

The chemistry of agnus castus is well-documented; the active constituents have not been established definitely, although the diterpene constituents are considered to be important, at least for dopaminergic activity. Dopaminergic activity has been documented in preclinical studies, and this provides some supporting evidence for the traditional uses of agnus castus. At present, there is conflicting evidence from *in vitro* studies regarding oestrogenic effects of agnus castus fruit extract and its constituents, and this requires further investigation.

Clinical trials of agnus castus preparations have focused on assessing effects in premenstrual syndrome and mastalgia, although rigorous clinical investigations are limited. In addition, studies have tested different agnus castus preparations, including combination herbal preparations containing agnus castus extract. Therefore, at present there is insufficient evidence to support definitively the efficacy of specific agnus castus products. Preliminary uncontrolled clinical studies involving women with hyperprolactinaemia and/or menstrual disorders have reported reductions in serum prolactin concentrations following treatment with certain agnus castus preparations, although further research is needed to confirm these findings.

Similarly, only limited data relating to the safety of agnus castus preparations are available, and further investigation of safety aspects is required. The available evidence indicates that certain agnus castus preparations are well-tolerated when used according to recommended dosage regimens. In view of the lack of data, the use of agnus castus preparations should be avoided in pregnancy and breastfeeding. As there is pharmacological evidence that agnus castus has dopaminergic activity, agnus castus should not be used with dopamine receptor agonists or antagonists.

Species (Family)

Vitex agnus-castus L. (Verbenaceae)

Synonym(s)

Agni Casti, Chasteberry, Chaste Tree, Monk's Pepper

Part(s) Used

Fruit

Pharmacopoeial and Other Monographs

American Herbal Pharmacopoeia[G1]
BHP 1996[G9]
BP 2007[G84]
BHMA 2003[G66]
Complete German Commission E[G3]
ESCOP 2003[G76]
Martindale 35th edition[G85]
PhEur 2007[G81]

Legal Category (Licensed Products)

GSL[G37]

Constituents

The following is compiled from several sources, including General Reference G75.

Diterpenes Labdane-type, including rotundifuran 0.04–0.3%, vitexilactone 0.02–0.17%, 6β,7β-diacetoxy-13-hydroxy-labda-8,14-diene 0.02–0.15%,[1, 2] vitexlactam A (6β-acetoxy-9α-hydroxy-13(14)-labden-16,15-amide.[3]

Flavonoids Casticin (3',5-dihydroxy-3,6,7,4'-tetramethoxy-flavone) 0.02–2.0%, penduletin, chrysoplenol. C-glycosides orientin, isoorientin and isovitexin.[4–6, G75, G76] The total flavonoid content of three Croatian samples varied from 0.05 to 0.08%.[7]

Iridoids Agnuside (*p*-hydroxybenzoylaucubin) 0.6% and aucubin 0.3%.[8, 9] The agnuside content of eight samples of dried fruits varied from 0.01–0.21%[10] and a standard of 0.02–0.40% has been proposed.[G76]

Polyphenols Seven Croatian samples analysed contained tannin 0.24–1.6% and total polyphenols 6.92–13.24%.[11]

Essential oil 0.8–1.8%; 85 compounds identified.[12] There are two distinct chemotypes, one containing α-pinene and the other α-terpinylacetate.[13] Comminution, maturity of fruit, length of distillation and extraction method markedly affect yields and composition of the oil: sabinene 16.4–44.1%, 1,8-cineole 8.4–15.2%, β-caryophyllene 2.1–5.0% and *trans*-β-farnesene 5.0–11.7%.[14] A yield of 0.5% volatile oil containing 35% monoterpenes (mainly α-pinene, sabinene, β-phellandrene and 4-terpineol) and 52% sesquiterpenes (mainly β-caryophyllene, allo-aromadendrene, germacrene B, spathulenol and τ-cadinol) has been reported.[15–17]

Other constituents Fatty acids, including oleic, stearic, palmitic, α-linolenic and linoleic acids.[G76]

Other parts of the plant The flowering stems contain the iridoids 6′-O-foliomenthoyl-mussaenosidic acid (agnucastoside A), 6′-O-(6,7-dihydro-foliomenthoyl-mussaenosidic acid (agnucastoside B), 7-*O-trans-p*-coumaroyl-6′-*O-trans*-caffeoyl-8-epiloganic acid (agnucastoside C), aucubin, agnuside, mussaenosidic acid and 6′-*O-p*-hydroxybenzoylmussaenosidic acid together with a phenylbutanone glucoside (myzodendrone).[18]

Material from agnus castus contains the flavonoids luteolin, artemetin, isorhamnetin, luteolin-6-C-(4″-methyl-6″-*O-trans*-caffeoylglucoside), luteolin-6-C-(6″-*O-trans*-caffeoylglucoside), luteolin-6-C-(2″-*O-trans*-caffeoylglucoside) and luteolin-7-*O*-(6″-*p*-hydroxy-benzoylglucoside).[19] The source of the material concerned is unclear: the experimental section of the paper refers to the fruit, whereas other sections of the paper mention the root bark.

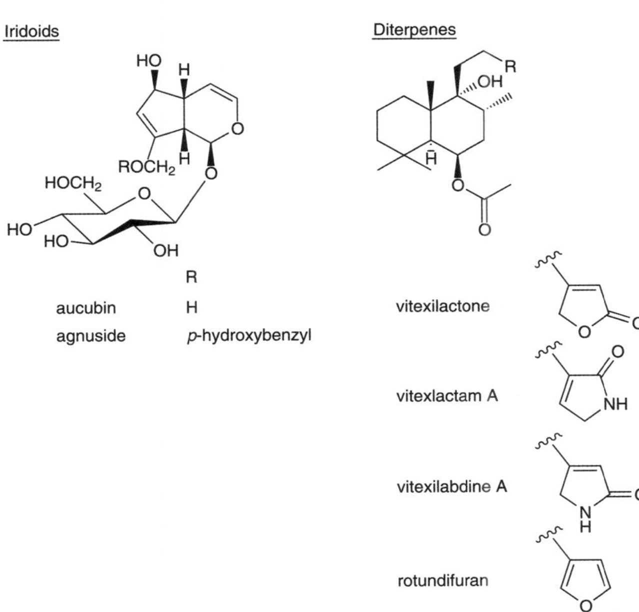

Figure 1 Selected constituents of agnus castus.

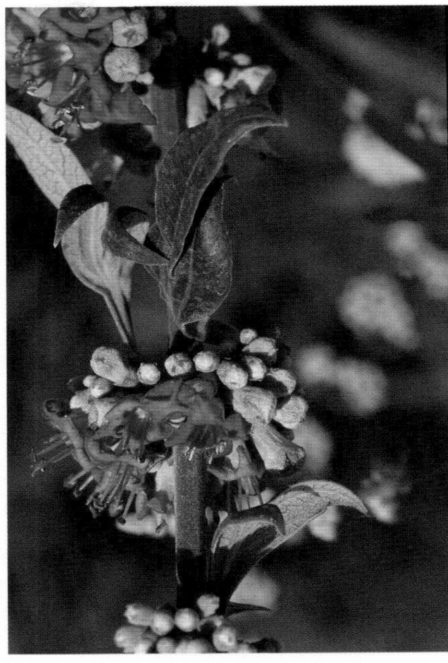

Figure 2 Agnus castus (*Vitex agnus-castus*).

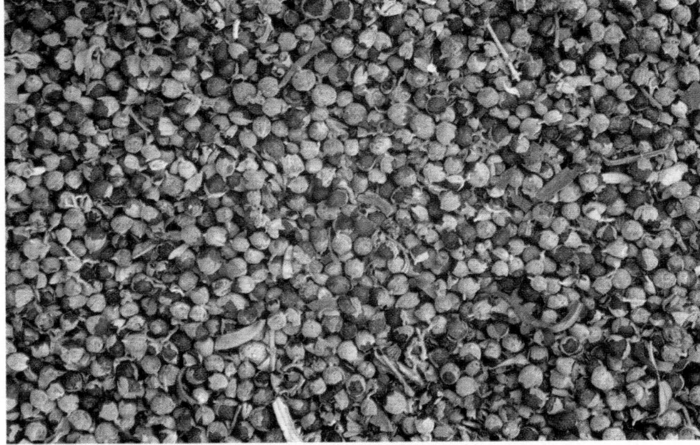

Figure 3 Agnus castus – dried drug substance (fruit).

Food Use

Agnus castus is not used in foods.

Herbal Use

Traditionally, agnus castus has been used for menstrual problems resulting from corpus luteum deficiency, including premenstrual symptoms and spasmodic dysmenorrhoea, for certain menopausal conditions, and for insufficient lactation.[G4, G49] The German Commission E approved it for internal use for irregularities of the menstrual cycle, premenstrual complaints and mastodynia.[G3]

Dosage

Dosages for oral administration (adults) recommended in older standard herbal reference texts are given below.

Fruit 0.5–1.0 g three times daily;[G49] aqueous–alcoholic extracts corresponding to 30–40 mg daily of dried crushed fruit.[G3]

Tincture 1 : 5 (g/mL), 50–70% ethanol (v/v) 0.15–0.2 mL.[G4]

Pharmacological Actions

In vitro and animal studies

Previously it was thought that agnus castus does not contain any oestrogenic constituents, although new findings are conflicting on this point. In an *in vitro* assay, a methanol extract of *V. agnus-castus* fruits showed competitive binding to both oestrogen receptors of the α- (ER-α) and β-subtypes (ER-β), with mean (standard deviation) IC_{50} values of 46 (3) and 64 (4) μg/mL, respectively.[20] *In vitro* ligand binding assays showed that a 68% ethanol extract of *V. agnus-castus* dried fresh fruits bound to ER-β in a concentration-dependent manner with an EC_{50} of around 10 μg/mL, but binding to ER-α was not observed.[21] Bioassay-guided fractionation revealed that apigenin was the constituent with the greatest affinity for ER-β (EC_{50} = 0.08 μg/mL), whereas penduletin and vitexin had EC_{50} values of 0.25 and 10 μg/mL, respectively. The compounds were all found to be selective for ER-β. In contrast, in *in vitro* experiments using a recombinant cell bioassay, a methanol extract of agnus castus (not further specified) had no measurable oestrogenic activity.[22]

Extracts of agnus castus act at dopamine receptors and affect prolactin release. Dopamine D_2-receptor binding of extracts has been demonstrated for three different dopamine receptors (rat striatum, calf striatum and human recombinant receptors) and for two separate ligands (sulpiridine and spiroperidol).[1,23,24] The active compounds acted as dopamine agonists and were characterised as labdane diterpenes. The two most active diterpenes, rotundifuran and 6β,7β-diacetoxy-13-hydroxy-labda-8,14-diene, had IC_{50} values (calf striatum preparation, ^{3}H-spiroperidol ligand) of 45 μg/mL (124 nmol/mL) and 79 μg/mL (194 nmol/mL), respectively.[24] A lyophilised extract of agnus castus (5 mg/mL) was similar in activity to 10^{-4} mol/L dopamine in receptor–ligand binding assays, displacing ^{3}H-spiroperidol from calf brain striatal preparations.[23]

An extract of agnus castus inhibited release of acetylcholine from ^{3}H-choline loaded rat brain striatal cells on electrical stimulation, and had an IC_{50} value of 30 μg/mL.[24]

Hexane fractions of agnus castus bind to human opiate receptors with IC_{50} values of 20 μg/mL (μ-receptors) and 10 μg/mL (κ-receptors).[25]

Similar properties have been described for several different 60% ethanol extracts of *Vitex agnus-castus* dried fruits that contained at least 0.08% casticin. In radioligand binding studies, mean IC_{50} values for binding to dopamine-D_2 receptors ranged from 40 to 70 μg/mL for the five ethanolic extracts tested, and the IC_{50} value was 32 μg/mL for a hexane subfraction (containing diterpenes and fatty acids) of an 80% methanol extract.[26] The chemical profile of the ethanolic extracts varied quantitatively and extracts were characterised with respect to the constituents casticin (0.54–1.22%), rotundifuran (1.04–2.23%), vitexilactone (0.34–1.01) and 6β,7β-diacetoxy-13-hydroxy-labda-8,14-diene (0.18–0.80%).

In *in vitro* experiments using rat pituitary cells, an ethanolic extract of agnus castus (not further specified) inhibited basal and thyroxine releasing hormone-stimulated prolactin secretion in a concentration-dependent manner at concentrations of 115–460 μg/mL.[27] The effect was blocked by addition of a dopamine receptor agonist to the system, indicating that the inhibition of prolactin secretion by agnus castus was brought about through a dopaminergic effect of constituents of the agnus castus extract. Other experiments using rat pituitary cells have demonstrated inhibition of basal and thyroxine releasing hormone-stimulated prolactin secretion by a 60% ethanol extract of agnus castus seeds.[28] Further experiments showed that the inhibition of prolactin release was not due to a cytotoxic effect on rat pituitary cells, and that the agnus castus extract had no effect on gonadotrophin release.

An ethanol extract of *V. agnus-castus* fruit significantly inhibited phorbol-ester-promoted Epstein–Barr virus early antigen (EBV-EA) activation *in vitro*.[29] This assay is used to identify potential cancer chemopreventive substances. Cytotoxic effects have been described for an ethanol extract of *V. agnus-castus* fruit against various non-cancer (human uterine cervical canal fibroblast, HCF) and cancer cell lines (gastric signet ring carcinoma (KATO-III), colon cancer (COLO-201), small-cell lung carcinoma (Lu-134-A-H), ovarian cancer (MCF-7), cervical carcinoma (SKG-3a) and breast carcinoma (SKOV-3)). The cytotoxic effect correlated significantly with the growth rate of the respective cells and, therefore, was greatest in those cells with a higher growth rate (HCF, MCF-7, SKG-3a and SKOV-3); cytotoxic activity did not appear to be selective for cancer cells.[30] Further work using KATO-III cells suggested that *V. agnus-castus* extract may bring about apoptosis through a mechanism involving oxidative stress.[31] These findings, however, cannot be extrapolated to the clinical setting, and further investigation of the potential cytotoxic effects of *V. agnus-castus* fruit extract, including with respect to normal cells, is required. Several flavonoid compounds with cytotoxic activity against P388 lymphocytic leukaemia cells have been isolated from the root bark of *V. agnus castus*.[19]

Antimicrobial activity has been described for extracts of *V. agnus-castus* fruits in *in vitro* assays using a disc-diffusion method. Ethanol, methanol, *n*-hexane and aqueous extracts inhibited the growth of *Escherichia coli* ATCC29998, *E. coli* ATCC11230, *Staphylococcus aureus* ATCC29213, *S. epidermidis* ATCC12228 and *Salmonella typhimurium* CCM5445 (zone of inhibition including disc >6 mm).[32] The ethanol, *n*-hexane and aqueous extracts also inhibited the growth of *S. aureus* ATCC6538P and *Pseudomonas aeruginosa* ATCC27853. None of the extracts, however, was active against the yeast *Candida albicans*. Ether and ethanol extracts of the leaves of *V. agnus-castus* have also shown antibacterial activity *in vitro*.[33]

A carbon dioxide extract of the seeds of *V. agnus-castus* at a concentration of 1–3% in a formulation containing human skin care substances provides protection against ticks, fleas, mosquitoes and biting flies in various animal models for up to eight hours,[34] according to a preliminary report.

Clinical studies

Clinical trials of agnus castus preparations have focused on assessing effects in premenstrual syndrome (PMS) and mastalgia, although rigorous clinical investigations are limited. In addition, studies have tested different agnus castus preparations, including combination herbal preparations containing agnus castus extract. At present there is insufficient evidence to support definitively the efficacy of specific agnus castus products.

One of the most robust studies was a randomised, double-blind, placebo-controlled trial in which 170 women with PMS received a casticin-standardised agnus castus extract (ZE-440) 20 mg daily, or placebo, for three menstrual cycles. At the end of the third menstrual cycle, self-assessed improvements in PMS symptoms (irritability, mood alteration, anger, headache, breast fullness, bloating) were significantly greater in the agnus castus group, compared with the placebo group ($p < 0.001$). Clinical global impression (CGI) scores for severity of condition, global improvement and the overall benefit–harm profile were also significantly better for agnus castus, compared with placebo ($p < 0.001$).[35]

In a double-blind, placebo-controlled trial, 37 women with deficiencies in corpus luteal phase and latent hyperprolactinaemia received an agnus castus preparation ($n = 17$) or placebo ($n = 20$) for three menstrual cycles. In the treated group, the luteal phase was extended to 10.5 days from an initial 3.4–5.5 days.[36]

A small number of other trials has compared the effects of agnus castus preparations with those of other agents. In a randomised, double-blind trial, 41 women aged 24–45 years with regular menstrual cycles and who were diagnosed with premenstrual dysphoric disorder received a *V. agnus-castus* extract 20–40 mg daily (not further specified), or fluoxetine 20–40 mg daily, for eight weeks. At the end of the study, daily symptom record scores, Hamilton depression scale scores and psychiatrist-assessed clinical global impression scores were significantly improved for both groups, compared with baseline values, and there were no statistically significant differences between the two groups ($p > 0.05$ for all at the 8-week endpoint).[37] However, these findings can only be considered preliminary as the study has several methodological limitations: at present, there is insufficient evidence that fluoxetine is efficacious in premenstrual dysphoric disorder and, as a placebo arm was not included in the study, a placebo response in both the fluoxetine and the agnus castus groups cannot be excluded; a sample size calculation does not appear to have been carried out; the statistical analysis appears to have been carried out with the 'per protocol' population, and an intention-to-treat analysis using last available measurements for participants who withdrew was not reported; and the study involved treatment over two menstrual cycles only. Further randomised, controlled trials that include a placebo arm and have sufficient statistical power are required.

Another randomised, double-blind, controlled trial involving women with PMS (n = 175) compared the effects of an agnus castus fruit extract (Agnolyt capsules; drug to extract ratio 9.6–11.5:1, equivalent to 3.5–4.2 mg extract per capsule) two capsules daily with those of pyridoxine (vitamin B_6) over three menstrual cycles. Similar reductions in self-assessed and physician-assessed PMS scores were reported for both groups.[38] However, the results of this study should be interpreted with caution as evidence for pyridoxine in reducing PMS symptoms is at present inconclusive, therefore, a placebo response in both groups cannot be excluded.

Results of randomised, double-blind, placebo-controlled trials involving women with mastalgia alone who received a combination preparation (Mastodynon) containing agnus castus extract and five other herbal ingredients (at various dilutions) have provided some evidence of efficacy for this product although definitive studies are still required. One such study which involved 104 women who received the preparation formulated as a solution, or as tablets, or placebo, for three menstrual cycles found that breast pain was reduced to a significantly greater extent with agnus castus than with placebo (p = 0.0067 and p = 0.0076 for solution and tablets, respectively, versus placebo).[39] Basal prolactin concentrations were reduced significantly in the agnus castus groups, compared with the placebo group (reductions of 4.35, 3.7 and 0.57 ng/mL for the solution, tablets and placebo group; p = 0.04 and 0.02 for solution versus placebo and tablets versus placebo, respectively).

A similar trial involving 97 women with cyclic mastalgia who received Mastodynon solution 30 drops twice daily (equivalent to 32.4 mg *V. agnus-castus* fruit extract daily), or placebo, found statistically significant differences in reduction of breast pain intensity as measured by visual analogue scale scores between treatment and placebo after one and two menstrual cycles (p = 0.018 and p = 0.006, respectively), but no statistically significant difference (p = 0.064) after three menstrual cycles.[40]

In a randomised, double-blind, placebo-controlled pilot study, 30 women aged 24–46 years who had tried unsuccessfully to conceive for 6–36 months received a combination preparation containing extracts of agnus castus and green tea (not further specified), L-arginine and several vitamins and minerals, three capsules daily, or placebo, for three menstrual cycles.[41] After three months, four women in the treatment group had become pregnant whereas none had done so in the placebo group (p = 0.02). During an open-label extension in which all participants received the combination preparation, another woman became pregnant. The pregnancies resulted in four healthy live births; one pregnancy resulted in a miscarriage.

Several open, uncontrolled studies involving small numbers of women with fertility disorders, hyperprolactinaemia and menstrual disorders have explored the effects of treatment with preparations containing extracts of agnus castus (e.g. Mastodynon and Agnucaston; Bionorica), administered orally, generally at doses equivalent to 30–40 mg drug daily for several months. These studies report decreased prolactin concentrations at the end of treatment, compared with baseline values.[42, 43] By contrast, in an open-label study involving 50 women who received a casticin-standardised preparation of agnus castus (Ze-440, containing 20 mg of a 60% ethanol extract of *V. agnus-castus* fruit; drug to extract ratio 6–12:1) during three menstrual cycles, there was no statistically significant difference in plasma concentrations of prolactin at the end of treatment, compared with baseline values ($p > 0.05$).[44] However, the design of these studies does not allow the observed effects to be attributed definitively to the intervention.

The effects of agnus castus have also been investigated in men. In an open, placebo-controlled, crossover study, 20 healthy men were given a commercial preparation of agnus castus fruit extract (BP-1095E1) at doses of 120, 240 and 480 mg extract (3–12 times higher than doses used in women) for 14 days, with a wash-out period of at least one week between each study phase.[45] A statistically significant increase in serum prolactin concentrations was observed with the lowest dose tested, compared with placebo (p = 0.033) whereas the higher dose decreased prolactin concentrations (p = 0.016).

In an open, placebo-controlled, crossover study designed to assess effects on melatonin secretion, 20 healthy male volunteers received a 70% ethanol–water extract of *V. agnus-castus* fruit 120, 240 and 480 mg daily in three divided doses for 14 days, with a wash-out period of at least one week between each treatment phase.[46] During treatment with agnus castus extract, the area under the serum concentration curve of melatonin was significantly higher than during placebo administration ($p < 0.005$). The effects of agnus castus on melatonin secretion require further investigation in randomised, double-blind, controlled experiments.

Preliminary reports describe the use of agnus castus preparations in the treatment of acne,[47] although randomised controlled trials assessing the effects of agnus castus in this indication are required.

Side-effects, Toxicity

Clinical data

Clinical data relating to safety aspects of *V. agnus-castus* preparations are available from several sources, including controlled clinical trials, post-marketing surveillance studies and spontaneous reports of suspected adverse reactions associated with agnus castus preparations.

Only limited data relating to the safety of agnus castus preparations are available from randomised controlled trials. In a randomised, double-blind, controlled trial in which 170 women with PMS received a casticin-standardised agnus castus extract (ZE-440) 20 mg daily, or placebo, for three menstrual cycles, the frequency of adverse events was similar in the agnus castus and the placebo groups (4.7 and 4.8%, respectively).[35] Adverse events reported for agnus castus were acne, multiple abscesses, intermenstrual bleeding and urticaria, and for placebo, acne, early menstrual period and gastric upset; all adverse events were considered to be mild and resolved without discontinuation of treatment. Adverse events were either not observed or not reported in other placebo-controlled trials of agnus castus preparations.

In a randomised, double-blind trial, 41 women aged 24–45 years with regular menstrual cycles and who were diagnosed with premenstrual dysphoric disorder received a *V. agnus-castus* extract 20–40 mg daily (not further specified), or fluoxetine 20–40 mg daily, for eight weeks.[37] During the study, 17 participants (nine in the fluoxetine group and eight in the agnus castus group) reported a total of 36 adverse events (20 and 16 with fluoxetine and agnus castus, respectively), most commonly nausea and headache in both groups. Another randomised, double-blind, controlled trial involving women with PMS (n = 175) compared the effects of an agnus castus fruit extract (Agnolyt capsules; drug to extract ratio 9.6–11.5:1, equivalent to 3.5–4.2 mg extract) with those of pyridoxine (vitamin B_6) over three menstrual cycles.[38] Adverse events were reported for five agnus castus recipients (persistent gastroenteritis, nausea, acneiform facial inflammation, allergic rashes (2)), and four placebo recipients (sensation of a lump in the throat, abdominal discomfort, recurrence of ulcerative colitis, persistent bleeding of unknown origin). Although current desire to conceive was an exclusion criterion for the study, five women, all from the agnus castus group, became pregnant during the trial.[38]

A systematic review of publications containing data relating to adverse events associated with agnus castus preparations included five post-marketing surveillance studies of an agnus castus fruit extract (Agnolyt) formulated as a tincture.[48] The studies involved a total of over 7500 patients who received the agnus castus preparation at a dose of around 40 drops daily, typically for around four to six months, although in one study the duration of administration ranged from one week to 19 months. Four studies, involving a total of 7152 participants, reported the number of participants withdrawing from the respective studies because of adverse events (total n = 71; 1.0%). Adverse events reported most frequently included nausea and other gastrointestinal disturbances, such as diarrhoea.

In another post-marketing surveillance study in Germany in which 1634 women with premenstrual syndrome received a dried extract of *V. agnus-castus* fruit (Femicur capsules containing 1.6–3.0 mg extract, corresponding to 20 mg drug; drug to extract ratio, 6.7–12.5:1) for around three months, 37 participants reported a total of 45 adverse events, most commonly skin complaints and hair loss (n = 13) and gastrointestinal symptoms (n = 6), none of which were considered serious. Of these, 23 adverse events occurring in 20 participants were considered to be related to treatment with agnus castus.[49] During treatment with the agnus castus preparation, 23 participants became pregnant and for 12 of these women treatment with agnus castus was stopped because of the pregnancy. A report of the study does not state whether pregnancy was intended or unintended (although it was stated that 19 of the 23 women had previously tried unsuccessfully to become pregnant), whether or not they were concurrently taking oral contraceptives, for how long during pregnancy agnus castus was taken, or what were the outcomes of the pregnancies in women who consumed agnus castus while pregnant.

In an open-label study, 50 women received a casticin-standardised preparation of agnus castus (Ze-440, containing 20 mg of a 60% ethanol extract of *V. agnus-castus* fruit; drug to extract ratio 6–12:1) during three menstrual cycles.[44] During the study, 20 participants reported 37 adverse events, most commonly acne (n = 7), headache (6), 'spotting' (5) and gastrointestinal symptoms (5).

Preclinical data

Cytotoxic effects have been described for an ethanol extract of *V. agnus-castus* fruit against various non-cancer (human uterine cervical canal fibroblast, HCF) and cancer cell lines (*see* Pharmacological Actions, *In vitro* and animal studies).[30]

Contra-indications, Warnings

Drug interactions None have been described for agnus castus preparations. However, as there is pharmacological evidence that agnus castus has dopaminergic activity, agnus castus should not be used with dopamine receptor agonists or antagonists. As with other herbal medicines, the potential for preparations of *V. agnus castus* to interact with other medicines administered concurrently should be considered.

Pregnancy and lactation In view of the documented pharmacological actions and lack of toxicity data, the use of agnus castus during pregnancy should be avoided. Agnus castus has been reported to stimulate milk secretion without altering the composition of the breast milk.[50] Nevertheless, agnus castus should be avoided during breastfeeding until further information is available.

In a randomised, double-blind, placebo-controlled pilot study, 30 women aged 24–46 years who had tried unsuccessfully to conceive for 6–36 months received a combination preparation containing extracts of agnus castus and green tea (not further specified), L-arginine and several vitamins and minerals, three capsules daily, or placebo, for three menstrual cycles.[41] After three months, four women in the treatment group had become pregnant whereas none had done so in the placebo group (p = 0.02). During an open-label extension in which all participants received the combination preparation, a further woman became pregnant. The pregnancies resulted in four healthy live births; one pregnancy resulted in a miscarriage. In another placebo-controlled study, current desire to conceive was an exclusion criterion for the study, yet five women, all from the agnus castus group, became pregnant during the trial.[38] The effects of agnus castus containing preparations on fertility and on resulting pregnancies require further investigation.

An isolated case report describes a 32-year-old woman with tubal infertility who was undergoing unstimulated *in vitro* fertilisation (IVF) treatment and who took a *V. agnus-castus* preparation at the beginning of a fourth IVF treatment cycle.[51] The woman developed multiple follicles (n = 4), whereas previous IVF treatment cycles, and two subsequent cycles, resulted in the development of a single follicle. In addition, the woman's serum gonadotrophin and ovarian hormone concentrations were disordered during ingestion of agnus castus. None of the six cycles of IVF treatment (i.e. three before the woman took agnus castus, one during and two afterwards) resulted in a pregnancy.

Preparations

Proprietary single-ingredient preparations

Austria: Agnofem; Agnucaston; Agnumens. *Brazil:* Lutene; Regulatum; Tenag; Vitenon; Vitex. *Czech Republic:* Agnucaston; Evana. *Germany:* Agno-Sabona; Agnolyt; Agnucaston; Agnufemil; Biofem; Castufemin; Cefanorm; Femicur N; Feminon A; Femisana mens; Gynocastus; Hevertogyn; Sarai; Strotan; Valverde Monchspfeffer bei Menstruationsbeschwerden. *Hungary:* Agnucaston; Cefanorm; PreMens. *Mexico:* Cicloplant. *Russia:* Agnucaston (Агнукастон). *Spain:* Dismegyn; Femiplante. *Switzerland:* Agnolyt; Emoton; Oprane; Prefemine; PreMens. *Thailand:* Agnucaston. *UK:* Herbal Premens.

Proprietary multi-ingredient preparations

Australia: Dong Quai Complex; Feminine Herbal Complex; Lifesystem Herbal Formula 4 Women's Formula; PMT Complex; Women's Formula Herbal Formula 3. *Canada:* Natural HRT. *Singapore:* Phytoestrin. *USA:* Women's Menopause Formula.

References

1 Hoberg E *et al.* Diterpene aus agni-casti fructus und ihre analytik. *Z Phytother* 1999; 20: 140–158.
2 Hoberg E *et al.* Quantitative high performance liquid chromatographic analysis of diterpenoids in Agni-Casti Fructus. *Planta Med* 2000; 66: 352–355.
3 Li S-H *et al.* Vitexlactam A, a novel labdane diterpene lactam from the fruits of *Vitex agnus-castus. Tetrahedron Lett* 2002; 43: 5131–5134.
4 Belic I *et al.* Constituents of *Vitex agnus castus* seeds. Part 1. Casticin. *J Chem Soc* 1961; 2523–2525.
5 Gomaa CS *et al.* Flavonoids and iridoids from *Vitex agnus castus. Planta Med* 1978; 33: 277.
6 Wollenweber E, Mann K. Flavonols from fruits of *Vitex agnus castus. Planta Med* 1983; 48: 126–127.
7 Maleš Ž. Determination of the content of the polyphenols of *Vitex agnus-castus* L. f. rosea. *Acta Pharm* 1998; 48: 215–218.
8 Rimpler H. Verbenaceae. Iridoids and ecdysones from *Vitex* species. *Phytochemistry* 1972; 11: 2653–2654.
9 Görler K, *et al.* Iridoidführung von Vitex agnus-castus. *Planta Med* 1985; 530–531.
10 Hoberg E *et al.* An analytical high performance liquid chromatographic method for the determination of agnuside and p-hydroxybenzoic acid contents in Agni-casti fructus. *Phytochem Anal* 2000; 11: 327–329.
11 Antolić A, Maleš Ž. Quantitative analysis of the polyphenols and tannins of *Vitex agnus-castus* L. *Acta Pharm* 1997; 47: 207–211.
12 Senatore F *et al.* Constituents of *Vitex agnus-castus* L. essential oil. *Flav Frag Journal* 1996; 11: 179–182.
13 Novak J *et al.* Essential oil composition of *Vitex agnus-castus* – comparison of accessions and different plant organs. *Flav Frag Journal* 2005; 20: 186–192.
14 Sørensen JM, Katsiotis STh. Parameters influencing the yield and composition of the essential oil from Cretan *Vitex agnus-castus* fruits. *Planta Med* 2000; 66: 245–250.
15 Kustrak D *et al.* The composition of the volatile oil of *Vitex agnus castus. Planta Med* 1992; 58 (Suppl. Suppl.1): A681.
16 Zwaving JH, Bos R. Composition of the essential fruit oil of *Vitex agnus castus. Pharm World Sci* 1993; 15 (Suppl. Suppl.H): H15.
17 Zwaving JH, Bos R. Composition of the essential fruit oil of *Vitex agnus-castus. Planta Med* 1996; 62: 83–84.
18 Kuruüzüm-Uz A *et al.* Glucosides from *Vitex agnus-castus. Phytochemistry* 2003; 63: 959–964.
19 Hirobe C *et al.* Cytotoxic flavonoids from *Vitex agnus-castus. Phytochemistry* 1997; 46: 521–524.
20 Liu J *et al.* Evaluation of estrogenic activity of plant extracts for the potential treatment of menopausal symptoms. *J Agric Food Chem* 2001; 49: 2472–2479.
21 Jarry H *et al.* Evidence for estrogen receptor β-selective activity of *Vitex agnus-castus* and isolated flavones. *Planta Med* 2003; 69: 945–947.
22 Oerter Klein K *et al.* Estrogen bioactivity in Fo-Ti and other herbs used for their estrogen-like effects as determined by a recombinant cell bioassay. *J Clin Endocrinol Metab* 2003; 88: 4077–4079.
23 Jarry H *et al.* Auf der suche nach dopaminergen substanzen in agni-casti-fructus-präparaten: warum eigentlich? *Z Phytother* 1999; 20: 140–158.
24 Berger D *et al.* Rezeptorbindungsstudien mit extrakten und daraus isolierten substanzen. *Z Phytother* 1999; 20: 140–158.
25 Brugisser R *et al.* Untersuchungen an opioid-rezeptoren mit *Vitex agnus-castus* L. *Z Phytother* 1999; 20: 140–158.
26 Meier B *et al.* Pharmacological activities of *Vitex agnus-castus* extracts *in vitro. Phytomedicine* 2000; 7: 373–381.
27 Sliutz G *et al.* Agnus castus extracts inhibit prolactin secretion of rat pituitary cells. *Horm Metab Res* 1993; 25: 253–255.
28 Jarry H *et al.* In vitro prolactin but not LH and FSH release is inhibited by compounds in extracts of agnus castus: direct evidence for a dopaminergic principle by the dopamine receptor assay. *Exp Clin Endocrinol* 1994; 102: 448–454.
29 Kapadia GJ *et al.* Inhibitory effect of herbal remedies on 12-O-tetradecanoylphorbol-13-acetate-promoted Epstein-Barr virus early antigen activation. *Pharmacol Res* 2002; 45(3): 213–220.11884218
30 Ohyama K *et al.* Cytotoxicity and apoptotic inducibility of *Vitex agnus-castus* fruit extract in cultured human normal and cancer cells and effect on growth. *Biol Pharm Bull* 2003; 26: 10–18.
31 Ohyama K *et al.* Human gastric signet ring carcinoma (KATO-III) cell apoptosis induced by *Vitex agnus-castus* fruit extract through intracellular oxidative stress. *Int J Biochem Cell Biol* 2005; 37: 1496–1510.
32 Kivçak B *et al.* Antimicrobial and cytotoxic activities of *Vitex agnus-castus* L. *J Fac Pharm Gazi* 2002; 19: 55–59.
33 Pepeljnjak S *et al.* Antibacterial and antifungal activities of the *Vitex agnus-castus* L. extracts. *Acta Pharm* 1996; 46: 201–206.
34 Mehlhorn H *et al.* Extract of the seeds of the plant *Vitex agnus castus* proven to be highly efficacious as a repellent against ticks, fleas, mosquitoes and biting flies. *Parasitol Res* 2005; 95: 363–365.
35 Schellenberg R. Treatment for the premenstrual syndrome with agnus castus fruit extract: prospective, randomised, placebo controlled study. *BMJ* 2001; 322: 134–137.
36 Milewicz A *et al.* *Vitex agnus castus* extract in the treatment of luteal phase defects due to latent hyperprolactinaemia. Results of a randomized placebo-controlled double blind study. *ArnzneimittelForsch* 1993; 43: 752–756.
37 Atmaca M *et al.* Fluoxetine versus *Vitex agnus castus* extract in the treatment of premenstrual dysphoric disorder. *Human Psychopharmacol Clin Exp* 2003; 18: 191–195.
38 Lauritzen CH *et al.* Treatment of premenstrual tension syndrome with *Vitex agnus castus* – Controlled, double-blind study versus pyridoxine. *Phytomedicine* 1997; 4: 183–189.
39 Wuttke W *et al.* Behandlung zyklusabhängiger Brustschmerzen mit einem Agnus-castus-haltigen Arzneimittel. *Geburtshilfe Frauenheilkd* 1997; 57: 1–14.
40 Halaška M *et al.* Treatment of cyclical mastalgia with a solution containing a *Vitex agnus castus* extract: results of a placebo-controlled double-blind study. *The Breast* 1999; 8: 175.
41 Westphal LM *et al.* A nutritional supplement for improving fertility in women. A pilot study. *J Reproductive Med* 2004; 49: 289–293.
42 Gorkow C. Klinischer Kenntnisstand von Agni-casti fructus: Klinisch-pharmakologische Untersuchungen und Wirksamkeitsbelege. *Z Phytother* 1999; 20: 159–168.
43 Gorkow C *et al.* Evidence of efficacy of *Vitex agnus castus* preparations. In: Loew D, Blume H, Dingermann TH, eds. *Phytopharmaka V, Forschung und Klinische Anwendung.* Darmstadt: Steinkopf Verlag, 1999: 189–208.
44 Berger D *et al.* Efficacy of *Vitex agnus-castus* L. extract Ze 440 in patients with pre-menstrual syndrome (PMS). *Arch Gynecol Obstet* 2000; 264: 150–153.
45 Merz PG *et al.* The effects of a special *Agnus castus* (BP1095E1) on prolactin secretion in healthy male subjects. *Exp Clin Endrocrinol Diabetes* 1996; 104: 447–453.
46 Dericks-Tan JSE *et al.* Dose-dependent stimulation of melatonin secretion after administration of agnus castus. *Exp Clin Endocrinol Diabetes* 2003; 111: 44–46.
47 Amann W. Akne vulgaris und *Agnus castus* (Agnolyt^{R}). *Z Allg Med* 1975; 51: 1645–1648.
48 Daniele C *et al.* *Vitex agnus castus*: a systematic review of adverse events. *Drug Safety* 2005; 28: 319–332.
49 Loch E-G *et al.* Treatment of premenstrual syndrome with a phytopharmaceutical formulation containing *Vitex agnus castus. J Women's Health Gender-Based Med* 2000; 9: 315–320.
50 Bruckner C. In mitteleuropa genutzte heilpflanzen mit milchsekretionsfördernder wirkung (galactagoga). *Gleditschia* 1989; 17: 189–201.
51 Cahill DJ *et al.* Multiple follicular development associated with herbal medicine. *Hum Reprod* 1994; 9: 1469–1470.

A

Agrimony

Summary and Pharmaceutical Comment

Limited information is available on the chemistry and pharmacological properties of agrimony. Clinical investigation of agrimony is extremely limited and rigorous studies are needed to establish the efficacy of agrimony. The tannin constituents may justify the astringent activity attributed to the herb. In view of the lack of toxicity data, excessive use of agrimony and use during pregnancy and breastfeeding should be avoided. The potential for preparations of agrimony to interfere with other medicines administered concurrently, particularly those with similar or opposing effects, should be considered.

Species (Family)

Agrimonia eupatoria L. (Rosaceae)

Synonym(s)

Agrimonia

Part(s) Used

Herb

Pharmacopoeial and Other Monographs

BHP 1996 [G9]
BP 2007[G84]
Complete German Commission E[G3]
Martindale 35th edition[G85]
Ph Eur 2007[G81]

Legal Category (Licensed Products)

GSL[G37]

Constituents

The following is compiled from several sources, including References 1 and 2, and General Reference G2.

Acids Palmitic acid, salicylic acid, silicic acid and stearic acid.

Flavonoids Apigenin, luteolin, luteolin-7-glucoside, quercetin, quercitrin, kaempferol and glycosides.[3]

Tannins 3–21%. Condensed tannins in herb; hydrolysable tannins (e.g. ellagitannin).

Vitamins Ascorbic acid (vitamin C), nicotinamide complex (about 100–300 μg/g leaf), thiamine (about 2 μg/g leaf) and vitamin K.

Other constituents Bitter principle, triterpenes (e.g. α-amyrin, ursolic acid, euscapic acid), phytosterols and volatile oil 0.2%.

Food Use

Agrimony is listed by the Council of Europe as a natural source of food flavouring (category N2). This category indicates that agrimony can be added to foodstuffs in small quantities, with a possible limitation of an active principle (as yet unspecified) in the final product.[G16]

Herbal Use

Agrimony is stated to possess mild astringent and diuretic properties.[1] It has been used for diarrhoea in children, mucous colitis, grumbling appendicitis, urinary incontinence, cystitis, and as a gargle for acute sore throat and chronic nasopharyngeal catarrh.[G2, G7]

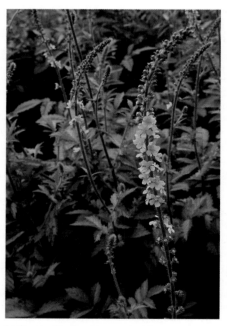

Figure 1 Agrimony (*Agrimonia eupatoria*).

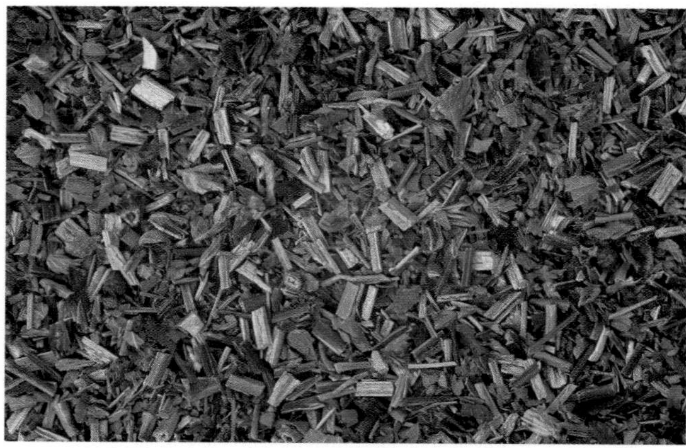

Figure 2 Agrimony – dried drug substance (herb).

Dosage

Dosages for oral administration (adults) for traditional uses recommended in older standard herbal reference texts are given below.

Dried herb 2–4 g by infusion three times daily.[G7]

Liquid extract 1–3 mL (1 : 1 in 25% alcohol) three times daily.[G7]

Tincture 1–4 mL (1 : 5 in 45% alcohol) three times daily.[G7]

Pharmacological Actions

In vitro and animal studies

Significant uricolytic activity has been documented for agrimony infusions and decoctions (15% w/v), following their oral administration to male rats at a dose of 20 mL/kg body weight (equivalent to 3 g dry drug).[4] Diuretic activity was stated to be minimal and elimination of urea unchanged. A hypotensive effect in anaesthetised cats has been documented for an agrimony extract given by intravenous injection; blood pressure was lowered by more than 40%.[5]

Marked antibacterial activity against *Staphylococcus aureus* and α-haemolytic streptococci has been reported for agrimony.[6]

An aqueous ethanol extract of the herb was tested for immunomodulative activity in the peritoneal cavities of mice.[7] Immunostimulant activity resulted in an increase in phagocytic activity and increases in the activities of lysozyme and peroxidase. *Agrimonia eupatoria* given in the diet of mice for 12 days prior to intraperitoneal administration of streptozotocin resulted in a reduction in hyperglycaemia.[8] Further investigation revealed stimulation of 2-deoxyglucose transport, glucose oxidation and incorporation of glucose into glycogen in mouse abdominal muscle. An aqueous extract (0.25–1 mg/mL) stimulated insulin secretion from a BRIN-BD11 pancreatic B cell line.[9] These findings demonstrate that *A. eupatoria* aqueous extract given orally to mice has antihyperglycaemic, insulin-releasing and insulin-like activity.[9]

A related species, *A. pilosa*, has also been investigated. *In vivo* antitumour activity in mice has been attributed to the tannin agrimoniin[10] which has not been reported as a constituent of *A. eupatoria*. Agrimoniin was administered intraperitoneally into ascites-type and solid tumours in rodents.[11] At doses of greater than 10 mg/kg, given before or after intraperitoneal inoculation with MM2 cells, it completely rejected tumour growth in mice.[11] Solid tumours of MH134 and Meth-A were inhibited by agrimoniin, and the number of peripheral blood cells was increased, indicating that agrimoniin has antitumour activity and that it exerts its effect by enhancing the immune response. *In vitro* studies have reported that agrimoniin induces the cytotoxicity of murine peritoneal exudate cells,[12] and that it induces interleukin 1 in human peripheral blood mononuclear cells and in mouse adherent peritoneal exudate cells *in vivo*.[13] Several phloroglucinols isolated from *A. pilosa* have demonstrated activity against *Staphylococcus aureus*,[14] and a methanol extract of the herb inhibited HIV-1 protease activity.[15] An aqueous suspension of *A. pilosa* herb (1 mg/kg and 5 mg/kg) given orally or intraperitoneally significantly reduced blood glucose concentrations in streptozotocin-induced diabetic rats.[16]

An aqueous extract of the aerial parts of *A. eupatoria* inhibited the secretion of hepatitis surface antigen in an *in vitro* system using HepG2.2.15 cells, which produce complete virion particles and viral proteins.[17]

Clinical studies

Clinical investigation of the effects of agrimony is extremely limited and rigorous randomised controlled clinical trials are needed. The use of agrimony infusions to treat cutaneous porphyria in a group of 20 patients has been described. Improvements in skin eruptions, and a decrease in serum iron concentrations and urinary porphyrins were observed,[18] although the methodological limitations of this small, uncontrolled study do not allow any conclusions to be made on the effects of agrimony.

A combination herbal preparation containing agrimony has been used in 35 patients suffering from chronic gastroduodenitis.[19] After 25 days of therapy, 75% of patients claimed to be free from pain, 95% from dyspeptic symptoms and 76% from palpitation pains. Gastroscopy was said to indicate that previous erosion and haemorrhagic mucous changes had healed. However, the methodological limitations of this small, uncontrolled study do not allow any conclusions to be made on the effects of agrimony.

Side-effects, Toxicity

None documented for *A. eupatoria*. A polar fraction containing flavonoids and triterpenes, but not tannins, produced a negative result in the Ames test.[1]

In mice, agrimoniin has been documented to cause stretching and writhing reactions when administered by intraperitoneal injection, and cyanosis and necrosis at the site of intravenous injection.[11] These reactions were considered to be inflammatory reactions. The LD_{50} of agrimoniin in mice has been estimated as 33 mg/kg (by intravenous injection), 101 mg/kg (by intraperitoneal injection), and greater than 1 g/kg (by mouth).[11] Cytotoxic activity has been reported for *A. pilosa*[10] (*see* Pharmacological Actions, *In vitro* and animal studies).

Contra-indications, Warnings

In view of the tannin constituents, excessive use of agrimony should be avoided.

Drug interactions In view of the documented pharmacological actions of agrimony, the potential for preparations of agrimony to interfere with other medicines administered concurrently (particularly those with similar or opposing effects) should be considered.

Pregnancy and lactation Agrimony is reputed to affect the menstrual cycle.[G22] In view of the lack of toxicity data, use of agrimony should be avoided during pregnancy and lactation.

Preparations

Proprietary single-ingredient preparations

Czech Republic: Nat Repiku Lekarskeho; Repik Lekarsky; Repikovy Caj, Repikova Nat.

Proprietary multi-ingredient preparations

Austria: Amersan; Gallen- und Lebertee St Severin; Novocholin. *Czech Republic:* Amersan; Cynarosan; Eugastrin; Hemoral; Naturland Grosser Swedenbitter; Nontusyl; Species Cholagogae Planta; Stomaran; The Salvat; Ungolen; Zlucnikova Cajova Smes. *France:* Tisane Hepatique de Hoerdt. *Russia:* Herbion Drops for the Gallbladder (Гербион Капли Желчегонные). *Spain:* Natusor Astringel; Natusor Farinol. *UK:* Piletabs.

A

References

1 Bilia AR *et al*. Constituents and biological assay of *Agrimonia eupatoria*. *Fitoterapia* 1993; 64: 549–550.
2 Carnat A *et al*. L'aigremoine: étude comparée d'*Agrimonia eupatoria* L. et *Agrimonia procera* Wallr. *Plantes médicinales et phytothérapie* 1991; 25: 202–211.
3 Sendra J, Zieba J. Flavonoids from *Agrimonia eupatoria* L. *Diss Pharm Pharmacol* 1971; 24: 79–83.
4 Giachetti D *et al*. Ricerche sull'attivita diuretica ed uricosurica di *Agrimonia eupatoria*. *Boll Soc Ital Biol Sper* 1986; 62: 705–711.
5 Petkov V. Plants with hypotensive, antiatheromatous and coronarodilatating action. *Am J Chin Med* 1979; 7: 197–236.
6 Petkov V. Bulgarian traditional medicine: A source of ideas for phytopharmacological investigations. *J Ethnopharmacol* 1986; 15: 121–132.
7 Bukovsky M, Blanárik P. Immunomodulative effects of ethanolic-aqueous extracts of herba Agrimoniae, flos Chamomillae and flos Calendulae cum calyce. *Farmaceutiky Obzor* 1994; 63: 149–156.
8 Swanston-Flatt SK *et al*. Traditional plant treatments for diabetes in normal and streptozotocin diabetic rats. *Diabetologia* 1990; 33: 462–464.
9 Gray AM, Flatt PR. Actions of the traditional anti-diabetic plant, *Agrimonia eupatoria* (agrimony): effects on hyperglycaemia, cellular glucose metabolism and insulin secretion. *Br J Nutr* 1998; 80: 109–114.
10 Miyamoto K *et al*. Isolation of agrimoniin, an antitumour constituent, from the roots of *Agrimonia pilosa* Ledeb. *Chem Pharm Bull (Tokyo)* 1985; 33: 3977–3981.
11 Miyamoto K *et al*. Antitumour effect of agrimoniin, a tannin of *Agrimonia pilosa* Ledeb., on transplantable rodent tumors. *Jpn J Pharmacol* 1987; 43: 187–195.
12 Miyamoto K *et al*. Induction of cytotoxicity of peritoneal exudate cells by agrimoniin, a novel immunomodulatory tannin of *Agrimonia pilosa* Ledeb. *Cancer Immunol Immunother* 1988; 27: 59–62.
13 Murayama T *et al*. Agrimoniin, an antitumour tannin of *Agrimonia pilosa* Ledeb., induces interleukin-1. *Anticancer Res* 1992; 12: 1471–1474.
14 Yamaki M *et al*. Antimicrobial activity of naturally occurring and synthetic phloroglucinols against *Staphylococcus aureus*. *Phytother Res* 1994; 8: 112–114.
15 Min BS *et al*. Screening of Korean plants against human immunodeficiency virus type 1 protease. *Phytother Res* 1999; 13: 680–682.
16 Hsu F-L, Cheng J-T. Investigation in rats of the antihyperglycaemic effect of plant extracts used in Taiwan for the treatment of diabetes mellitus. *Phytother Res* 1992; 6: 108–111.
17 KwonDH *et al*. Inhibition of hepatitis B virus by an aqueous extract of *Agrimonia eupatoria* L. *Phytother Res* 2005; 19: 355–358.
18 Patrascu V *et al*. Rezultate terapeutice favorabile in porfiria cutanata cu *Agrimonia eupatoria*. *Dermato-venerologia* 1984; 29: 153–157.
19 Chakarski I *et al*. Clinical study of a herb combination consisting of *Agrimonia eupatoria*, *Hipericum perforatum*, *Plantago major*, *Mentha piperita*, *Matricaria chamomila* for the treatment of patients with chronic gastroduodenitis. *Probl Vatr Med* 1982; 10: 78–84.

Alfalfa

Summary and Pharmaceutical Comment

The chemistry of alfalfa is well documented and it does appear to be a good source of vitamins and minerals, thereby supporting the herbal uses. However, normal human dietary intake of alfalfa is low and excessive ingestion should be avoided in view of the many pharmacologically active constituents (e.g. canavanine, isoflavones and saponins), which may give rise to unwanted effects if taken to excess. Oestrogenic effects are generally associated with the ingestion of large amounts of the herb, such as in fodder for poultry and cattle. Reports of a possible systemic lupus erythematosus (SLE) inducing capacity for alfalfa, particularly the seeds, also suggests that excessive ingestion is not advisable. In view of the reports of arthralgia, alfalfa should not be recommended for the treatment of arthritis. Coumarin compounds detected so far in alfalfa do not possess the minimum structural requirements (a C-4 hydroxyl substituent and a C-3 non-polar carbon substituent)[G87] for anticoagulant activity.

Species (Family)

Medicago sativa L. (Fabaceae/Leguminosae)

Synonym(s)

Lucerne, Medicago, *M. afganica* (Bord.) Vass, *M. grandiflora* (Grossh.) Vass, *M. ladak* Vass, *M. mesopotanica* Vass, *M. orientalis* Vass, *M. polia* (Brand) Vassi, *M. praesativa* Sinsk, *M. sogdiana* (Brand) Vass, Purple Medick, *Trigonella upendrae* Chowdh. and Rao

Part(s) Used

Herb

Pharmacopoeial and Other Monographs

BHP 1996[G9]
Martindale 35th edition[G85]

Legal Category (Licensed Products)

GSL[G37]

Constituents

The following is compiled from several sources, including General References G19, G22 and G41.

Acids Lauric acid, maleic acid, malic acid, malonic acid, myristic acid, oxalic acid, palmitic acid and quinic acid.

Alkaloids Pyrrolidine-type (e.g. stachydrine, homostachydrine); pyridine-type (e.g. trigonelline) in the seeds only.

Amino acids Arginine, asparagine (high concentration in seeds), cystine, histidine, isoleucine, leucine, lysine, methionine, phenylalanine, threonine, tryptophan and valine. The non-protein toxic amino acid canavanine is present in leaves (0.9–1.2 mg/g), stems (0.6–0.9 mg/g) and seeds (5–14 mg/g).[G19]

Coumarins Medicagol.

Isoflavonoids Coumestrol, biochanin A, daidzein, formononetin and genistein.

Saponins 2–3%. Hydrolysis yields aglycones, medicagenic acid, soyasapogenols A–F and hederagenin.[1] Sugar chain components include arabinose, galactose, glucuronic acid, glucose, rhamnose and xylose.

Steroids Campesterol, cycloartenol, β-sitosterol (major component), α-spinasterol and stigmasterol.

Other constituents Carbohydrates (e.g. arabinose, fructose, sucrose, xylose), vitamins (A, B_1, B_6, B_{12}, C, E, K), pectin methylesterase, pigments (e.g. chlorophyll, xanthophyll, β-carotene, anthocyanins), proteins, minerals and trace elements.

Food Use

Alfalfa is widely used in foods and is listed by the Council of Europe as a source of natural food flavouring (categories N2 and N3). These categories indicate that alfalfa can be added to

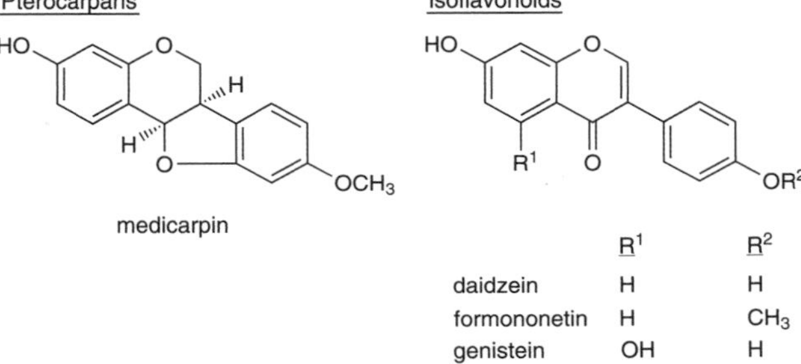

Figure 1 Selected constituents of alfalfa.

foodstuffs in small quantities, with a possible limitation of an active principle (as yet unspecified) in the final product.[G16] Previously, alfalfa has been listed as GRAS (Generally Recognised As Safe).[G41]

Herbal Use

The herb was not valued by ancient civilisations and is not detailed in classical herbals. Herbal use probably developed in the USA where claims have been made for it in the treatment of arthritis, high cholesterol, diabetes and peptic ulcers.[2, G19, G32] Reputedly, the herb has bactericidal, cardiotonic, diuretic, emetic, emmenagogue and oestrogenic properties.[2] Commercial preparations including teas, tablets and capsules are available.[G19] Alfalfa is stated to be a source of vitamins A, C, E and K, and of the minerals calcium, potassium, phosphorus and iron. It has been used for avitaminosis A, C, E or K, hypoprothrombinaemic purpura, and debility of convalescence.[G7, G64]

Dosage

Dosages for oral administration (adults) for traditional uses recommended in older standard herbal reference texts are given below.

Dried herb 5–10 g as an infusion three times daily.[G7]

Liquid extract 5–10 mL (1 : 1 in 25% alcohol) three times daily.[G7]

Pharmacological Actions

In vitro and animal studies

Alfalfa top (stem and leaves) saponins have been reported to decrease plasma cholesterol concentrations without changing high-density lipoprotein (HDL) cholesterol concentrations, decrease intestinal absorption of cholesterol, increase excretion of neutral steroids and bile acids, prevent atherosclerosis and induce the regression of atherosclerosis.[3]

Hypocholesterolaemic activity has been reported for root saponins, when given to monkeys receiving a high-cholesterol diet.[4] Alfalfa herb fed to monkeys reduced hypercholesterolaemia and atherosclerosis; the effect may be partially due to the saponin constituents.[G19] In mice fed with alfalfa (6.25% of diet) for 12 days before administration of streptozotocin, hyperglycaemia was reduced compared with values for control animals.[5]

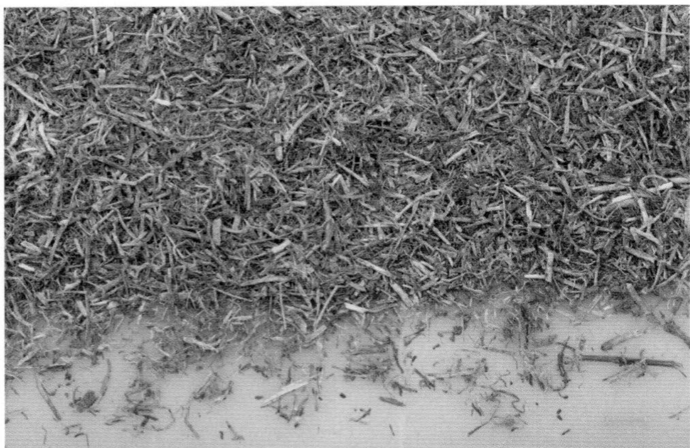

Figure 2 Alfalfa – dried drug substance (herb).

Oestrogenic activity in ruminants has been documented for coumestrol and the isoflavone constituents.[G22, G41]

An investigation into the effect of various herbs on hepatic drug metabolising enzymes in the rat, showed that alfalfa potentiated the activity of aminopyrine *N*-demethylase but had no effect on glutathione *S*-transferase or epoxide hydrolase activities.[6]

The seeds are reported to contain trypsin inhibitors.[G41] Saponins isolated from the aerial parts have been reported to stimulate the lipolytic activity of neopancreatinum (a mixture of porcine pancreatic enzymes including lipase, amylase and proteases).[7]

Alfalfa root saponins have been documented to exhibit selective toxicity towards fungi.[1, 8, 9] A medicagenic acid glycoside with low haemolytic activity, isolated from alfalfa root, was found to exhibit both strong inhibitory and fungitoxic activities towards several medically important yeasts including *Candida* species, *Torulopsis* species, *Geotrichum canadidum* and *Rhodotorula glutinis*.[8] It has been proposed that the antimycotic activity of alfalfa saponins is related to their ability to complex steroids and that fungi sensitive to the saponins may contain relatively more steroids in their membranes.[8] Antifungal properties have also been documented for alfalfa.[G41]

The saponin constituents are documented to be haemolytic and to interfere with vitamin E utilisation, and are believed to be one of the causes of ruminant bloat.[G41] Haemolytic activity is associated with the medicagenic acid glycosides and not the hederagenin and soyasapogenol glycosides.

The effects of polysaccharides from alfalfa on mice lymphocytes *in vitro* indicated immunopotentiating activity.[10]

Clinical studies

Clinical investigation of the effects of alfalfa is extremely limited and rigorous randomised controlled clinical trials are required. In a short-term study involving three normolipidaemic individuals given alfalfa seeds (60–80 g daily), serum cholesterol concentrations were reported to be reduced.[G19] In another small study in which heat-treated alfalfa seeds (40 g three times daily for eight weeks) were taken by eight type-IIA hyperlipoproteinaemic patients and three type IIB patients, a significant decrease was noted in total serum cholesterol concentrations, low-density lipoprotein (LDL) cholesterol and apolipoprotein B. The LDL cholesterol concentration fell by less than 5% in two of the 11 patients.[11] The methodological limitations of this small, uncontrolled study do not allow any conclusions to be made on the effects of alfalfa.

The manganese content of alfalfa (45.5 mg/kg) is reported to be the active principle responsible for a hypoglycaemic effect documented for the herb.[12] A case report descibes a diabetic patient, treated with soluble insulin but poorly controlled, in whom control of diabetes was achieved following use of an alfalfa extract. When administered separately, only small doses of manganese chloride (5–10 mg) were required to have a hypoglycaemic effect. However, no effect was seen on the blood sugar concentrations of non-diabetic controls or of other diabetic patients, who were also administered manganese.[12]

Side-effects, Toxicity

Both alfalfa seed and herb have been reported to induce a systemic lupus erythematosus (SLE)-like syndrome in female monkeys.[3, 13, G19, G32] This activity has been attributed to canavanine, a non-protein amino acid constituent which has been found to have effects on human immunoregulatory cells *in vitro*.[14] Reactivation of quiescent SLE in humans has been associated with the ingestion of alfalfa tablets which, following analysis, were found to contain canavanine.[15] It was not stated whether the tablets contained seed or herb material. Canavanine is known to be toxic to all animal species because it is a structural analogue of arginine and may interfere with the binding of this amino acid to enzymes and its incorporation into proteins.[16, G19] Alfalfa seeds are reported to contain substantial quantities of canavanine (8.33–13.6 mg/kg), whereas the herb contains considerably less.[16, 17]

Pancytopenia has been associated with human ingestion of ground alfalfa seeds (80–160 g/day), which were taken to lower plasma cholesterol concentrations.[18]

Dietary studies using alfalfa top saponins (ATS) in the diet of rats and monkeys showed no evidence of toxicity and serum lipid concentrations were lowered.[3, 19, 20] In addition, when ATS were given to cholesterol-fed animals, a reduction in serum lipid concentrations was observed.[3, 19, 20] ATS are reported to be free of the SLE-inducing substance that is present in the seeds.[3]

Coumarin compounds detected so far in alfalfa do not possess the minimum structural requirements (a C-4 hydroxyl substituent and a C-3 non-polar carbon substituent)[G87] for anticoagulant activity.

Negative results were documented for alfalfa when tested for mutagenicity using *Salmonella* strains TA98 and TA100.[21]

Contra-indications, Warnings

Individuals with a history of SLE should avoid ingesting alfalfa. Ingestion of large amounts of alfalfa (exceeding amounts normally consumed in the diet) should be avoided in view of the documented pharmacological activities. Alfalfa may affect blood sugar concentrations in diabetic patients because of the manganese content.

Drug interactions In view of the documented pharmacological actions of alfalfa the potential for preparations of alfalfa to interfere with those of other medicines administered concurrently, particularly those with similar or opposing effects, such as medicines with hormonal activity, should be considered.

Pregnancy and lactation Alfalfa seeds are reputed to affect the menstrual cycle and to be lactogenic.[G30] Although the safety of alfalfa herb has not been established, it is probably acceptable for use during pregnancy and lactation provided that doses do not exceed the amounts normally ingested as a food. Alfalfa seeds should not be ingested during pregnancy or lactation.

Preparations

Proprietary multi-ingredient preparations

Australia: Neo-Cleanse; Panax Complex; Plantiodine Plus; Zinc Zenith. *Chile:* Calcio 520. *France:* Gonaxine; Gynosoja. *USA:* B-100 Complex; My Favorite Multiple Energizer; My Favorite Multiple Take One; My Favorite Multiple Take One Iron-Free; Natural Herbal Water Tablets; Zero Flush Niacin 400mg.

References

1 Oleszek W, Jurzysta M. Isolation, chemical characterization and biological activity of alfalfa (*Medicago media* Pers.) root saponins. *Acta Soc Bot Pol* 1986; 55: 23–33.

2 Berry M. Alfalfa. *Pharm J* 1995; 255: 353–354.

3 Malinow MR *et al.* Lack of toxicity of alfalfa saponins in cynomolgus macaques. *J Med Primatol* 1982; 11: 106–118.

4 Malinow MR *et al.* Prevention of elevated cholesterolemia in monkeys by alfalfa saponins. *Steroids* 1977; 29: 105–110.

5 Swanston-Flatt SK *et al.* Traditional plant treatments for diabetes in normal and streptozotocin-diabetic mice. *Diabetologia* 1990; 33: 462–464.

6 Garrett BJ *et al.* Consumption of poisonous plants (*Senecio jacobaea*, *Symphytum officinale*, *Pteridium aquilinum*, *Hypericum perforatum*) by rats: chronic toxicity, mineral metabolism, and hepatic drug-metabolizing enzymes. *Toxicol Lett* 1982; 10: 183–188.

7 Sroka Z *et al.* Stimulation of pancreatic lipase activity by saponins isolated from *Medicago sativa* L. *Z Naturforschung, Section C, J Biosci* 1997; 52: 235–239.

8 Polacheck I *et al.* Activity of compound G2 isolated from alfalfa roots against medically important yeasts. *Antimicrob Agents Chemother* 1986; 30: 290–294.

9 Jurzysta M, Waller GR. Antifungal and haemolytic activity of aerial parts of alfalfa (*Medicago*) species in relation to saponin composition. *Adv Expl Med Biol* 1996; 404: 565–574.

10 Zhao WS *et al.* Immunopotentiating effects of polysaccharides isolated from *Medicago sativa* L. *Acta Pharmacol Sinica* 1993; 14: 273–276.

11 Mölgaard J *et al.* Alfalfa seeds lower low density lipoprotein cholesterol and apolipoprotein B concentrations in patients with type II hyperlipo proteinemia. *Atherosclerosis* 1987; 65: 173–179.

12 Rubenstein AH *et al.* Manganese-induced hypoglycaemia. *Lancet* 1962; ii: 1348–1351.

13 Malinow MR *et al.* Systemic lupus erythematosus-like syndrome in monkeys fed alfalfa sprouts: role of a nonprotein amino acid. *Science* 1982; 216: 415–417.

14 Alcocer-Varela J *et al.* Effects of L-canavanine on T cells may explain the induction of systemic lupus erythematosus by alfalfa. *Arthritis Rheum* 1985; 28: 52–57.

15 Roberts JL, Hayashi JA. Exacerbation of SLE associated with alfalfa ingestion. *N Engl J Med* 1983; 308: 1361.

16 Natelson S. Canavanine to arginine ratio in alfalfa (*Medicago sativa*), clover (*Trifolium*), and the jack bean (*Canavalia ensiformis*). *J Agric Food Chem* 1985; 33: 413–419.

17 Natelson S. Canavanine in alfalfa (*Medicago sativa*). *Experientia* 1985; 41: 257–259.

18 Malinow MR *et al.* Pancytopenia during ingestion of alfalfa seeds. *Lancet* 1981; i: 615.

19 Malinow MR *et al.* The toxicity of alfalfa saponins in rats. *Food Cosmet Toxicol* 1981; 19: 443–445.

20 René M *et al.* Lack of toxicity of alfalfa saponins in rats. *Cholesterol Metab* 1981; 40: 349.

21 White RD *et al.* An evaluation of acetone extracts from six plants in the Ames mutagenicity test. *Toxicol Lett* 1983; 15: 25–31.

Aloe Vera

Summary and Pharmaceutical Comment

Aloe vera is obtained from the mucilaginous tissue in the centre of the *Aloe vera* leaf and consists mainly of polysaccharides and lipids. It should not be confused with aloes, which is obtained by evaporation of water from the bitter yellow juice that is drained from the leaf. Unlike aloes, aloe vera does not contain any anthraquinone compounds and does not, therefore, exert any laxative action. Studies have reported an anti-inflammatory and anti-arthritic action for total leaf extracts but the activity seems to be associated with anthraquinone compounds. Hypoglycaemic activity has been reported for aloe vera extract. Aloe vera is a source of gamolenic acid. The literature on burn management with aloe vera gel preparations is confused and further studies are required.

Species (Family)

**Aloe vera* (L.) Burm.f., (Xanthorrhoeaceae)
A. africana Mill.

Synonym(s)

**Aloe barbadensis* Mill.,
Aloe Gel

Part(s) Used

Leaf gel

Pharmacopoeial and Other Monographs

Martindale 35th edition[G85]
WHO volume 1 1999[G63]

Legal Category (Licensed Products)

Aloe vera is not included in the GSL.

Constituents

The following is compiled from several sources, including General References G2 and G6.

Aloe vera is reported to contain mono- and polysaccharides, tannins, sterols, organic acids, enzymes (including cyclooxygenase),[1] saponins, vitamins and minerals.[2]

Carbohydrates Glucomannan and other polysaccharides containing arabinose, galactose and xylose.

Lipids Includes cholesterol, gamolenic acid and arachidonic acid.[1]

Food Use

Aloe vera is not used in foods.

Herbal Use

Traditionally, aloe vera has been used in ointments and creams to assist the healing of wounds, burns, eczema and psoriasis.[G2, G6, G41, G64]

Dosage

None documented.

Pharmacological Actions

Aloe vera refers to the mucilaginous tissue located in the leaf parenchyma of *Aloe vera* or related *Aloe* species. However, many documented studies for *Aloe vera* have utilised homogenised leaf extracts which therefore combine aloe vera with aloes, the laxative preparation obtained from the bitter, yellow juice also found in the leaf (*see* Aloes). Unless otherwise specified, the following refers to a total leaf extract.

In vitro and animal studies

Gel preparations have been reported to be effective against radiation burns, skin ulcers and peptic ulcers.[2] However, the gel was also found to be ineffective against drug- and stress-induced gastric and peptic ulcers in rats.[2]

Anti-inflammatory activity has been observed in various rat and mouse models that received subcutaneous injections of *Aloe vera*

Figure 1 Aloe vera (*Aloe vera*).

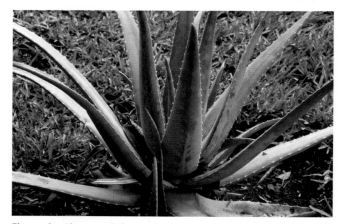

Figure 2 Aloe vera – dried drug substance (leaf gel).

leaf extract.[3] A positive response was noted in wound-healing (10 mg/kg, rat; 100 mg/kg, mouse), mustard oedema (10 mg/kg, rat) and polymorphonuclear leukocyte infiltration (2 mg/kg, mouse) tests, although no activity was demonstrated in the antifibrosis test (cotton pellet granuloma) (400 mg/kg, rat).

Anti-arthritic and anti-inflammatory activity have been documented for a cream containing homogenised *Aloe africana* leaves, ribonucleic acid, and ascorbic acid, following topical application to rats which had been injected (day 0) with *Mycobacterium butyricum* to cause adjuvant arthritis.[4] This model is considered a good experimental tool for studying rheumatoid arthritis.[4] The cream was found to be active when applied both as a prevention (days 1–13) and as a regression (days 21–35) treatment.[4] Subsequent work suggested that anthraquinone compounds (anthraquinone, anthracene and anthranilic acid) may be the active components in the aloe leaf mixture.[5] These compounds are, however, constituents of aloes rather than aloe vera (*see* Aloes). Aloe vera juice (presumably containing the anthraquinones contained in aloe preparation) has been applied directly to open pressure sores to assist in their healing.[6] The aloe vera extract exhibited an anaesthetic reaction, antibacterial action and increased local microcirculation.[6]

Endogenous cyclooxygenase in *Aloe vera* has been found to convert endogenous arachidonate to various prostanoids, namely PGE_2 (major), TXB_2, PGD_2, $PGF_{2\alpha}$, and 6-keto-$PGF_{1b\alpha}$.[1] The production of these compounds, especially PGE_2, has been associated with the beneficial effect of an aloe vera extract on human bronchial asthma[8] (*see* Clinical studies).

Hypoglycaemic actions have been documented for aloes extracts (*see* Aloes).

Clinical studies

Enhancement of phagocytosis in adult bronchial asthma has been attributed to a non-dialysable fraction of the extract, consisting of active components that are a mixture of polysaccharide and protein or glycoprotein.[7] Despite the nature of these proposed active components, it has been proposed that activity of the fraction may be related to the previous observation that aloe vera synthesises prostaglandins from endogenous arachidonic acid using endogenous cyclooxygenase.[1] In this study,[7] activity of the aloe vera extract required dark storage at 4–30°C for a period of 3–10 days.[3] These conditions are reported to be favourable for the hydrolysis of phospholipids, thus releasing arachidonic acid for synthesis of prostanoids.[1] In addition, activity was dependent on patients not having received prior treatment with a corticosteroid.[8]

The gel has been reported to be effective in the treatment of mouth ulcers.[8]

The literature on burn management with aloe vera gel preparations is confused and further studies are required.[9]

Side-effects, Toxicity

None documented.

Contra-indications, Warnings

Hypoglycaemic activity has been documented for an aloe vera extract, although it is unclear whether this is associated with the true aloe vera gel or aloes extract.[10]

Pregnancy and lactation The external application of aloe vera gel during pregnancy is not thought to be any cause for concern. However, products stated to contain aloes extracts or aloe vera may well contain gastrointestinal stimulant anthraquinone components that are well recognised as the active constituents in aloes (laxative). As such, ingestion of such preparations during pregnancy and lactation should be avoided.

Preparations

Proprietary single-ingredient preparations

Argentina: Bio-Dermis; Biorevit Gel; Capson. *Brazil:* Probeks. *France:* Veraskin. *Italy:* Epitaloe. *New Zealand:* Solarcaine Aloe Vera.

Proprietary multi-ingredient preparations

Argentina: Abanta; Acuaderm; Aloebel; Aristaloe; Brunavera; Controlacne; Dermaloe; Dermvien; Eurocolor Post Solar; Europrotec Post Solar; KW; Negacne; Odontobiotic; Pedicrem; Puraloe; Refrane P; Refrane Plus; Sadeltan F; Snella Vag; Solenil Post Solar; Talowin; Yuyo. *Australia:* Aloe Vera Plus; Percutane; Psor-Asist. *Brazil:* Derm'attive Solaire. *Chile:* Ac-Sal; Fray Romano; Nenegloss; Solarcaine Aloe Vera Gel. *Czech Republic:* After Burn. *France:* Postopyl; Rhinodoron. *Germany:* Rhinodoron. *India:* Elovera-SPF; Elovera; Sofderm. *Israel:* Aphtagone; Aptha-X. *Italy:* Capso; Ektrofil; Ginoxil Ecoschiuma; Ninfagin; Vicks Baby Balsam; Vulnopur. *Malaysia:* Lorasil Feminine Hygeine; Neo-Healar. *Mexico:* Gelconordin; Hipoglos Cremoso. *New Zealand:* Chap Stick; Odor Eze. *Portugal:* Alkagin; Antiacneicos Ac-Sal; Multi-Mam Compressas. *Singapore:* Desitin Creamy. *UK:* Herbal Laxative Tablets. *USA:* Aloe Grande; Biotene with Calcium; Bodi Kleen; Dermtex HC with Aloe; Entertainer's Secret; Geri-Lav Free; Gold Bond Medicated Triple Action Relief; Hawaiian Tropic Cool Aloe with I.C.E.; Hemorid For Women; MSM with Glucosamine Creme; Maximum Strength Flexall 454; Nasal-Ease; OraMagicRx; Solarcaine Aloe Extra Burn Relief.

References

1 Afzal M *et al.* Identification of some prostanoids in *Aloe vera* extracts. *Planta Med* 1991; 57: 38–40.
2 Parmar NS *et al.* Evaluation of *Aloe vera* leaf exudate and gel for gastric and duodenal anti-ulcer activity. *Fitoterapia* 1986; 57: 380–381.
3 Davis RH *et al.* Biological activity of *Aloe vera*. *Med Sci Res* 1987; 15: 235.
4 Davis RH *et al.* Topical effect of aloe with ribonucleic and vitamin C on adjuvant arthritis. *J Am Pod Med Assoc* 1985; 75: 229–237.
5 Davis RH *et al.* Antiarthritic activity of anthraquinones found in aloe for podiatric medicine. *J Am Pod Med Assoc* 1986; 76: 61–66.
6 Cuzzell JZ. Readers' remedies for pressure sores. *Am J Nurs* 1986; 86: 923–924.
7 Shida T *et al.* Effect of Aloe extract on peripheral phagocytosis in adult bronchial asthma. *Planta Med* 1985; 51: 273–275.
8 Plemons JM *et al.* Evaluation of acemannan in the treatment of aphthous stomatitis. *Wounds* 1994; 6: 40–45.
9 Marshall JM. Aloe vera gel: What is the evidence? *Pharm J* 1990; 244: 360–362.
10 Ghanam N *et al.* The antidiabetic activity of aloes: preliminary clinical and experimental observations. *Hormone Res* 1986; 24: 288–294.

Aloes

Summary and Pharmaceutical Comment

Aloes and aloe gel are often confused with each other. Aloes is obtained by evaporation of water from the bitter yellow juice drained from the leaves of *A. vera*. Commercial 'aloin' is a concentrated form of aloes.[G41] Aloe gel is prepared by many methods, but is obtained from the mucilaginous tissue in the centre of the leaf and does not contain anthraquinones (*see* Aloe Vera). Aloes is a potent purgative which has been superseded by less toxic drugs such as senna and cascara. Generally, the use of unstandardised preparations containing anthraquinone glycosides should be avoided, since their pharmacological effect is unpredictable and they may cause abdominal cramp and diarrhoea. In particular, the use of products containing combinations of anthraquinone laxatives should be avoided.

Species (Family)

**Aloe vera* (L.) Burm. f.
Aloe ferox Mill. (Xanthorrhoeaceae)

Synonym(s)

**Aloe barbadensis* Mill.

Part(s) Used

Dried leaf juice

Pharmacopoeial and Other Monographs

BHC 1992[G6]
BHP 1996[G9]
BP 2007[G84]
Complete German Commission E[G3]
ESCOP 1997 (Cape Aloes)[G52]
Martindale 35th edition[G85]
Ph Eur 2007[G81]
USP29/NF24[G86]
WHO volume 1 1999[G63]

Legal Category (Licensed Products)

GSL[G37]

Constituents

The following is compiled from several sources, including References 1–7, and General References G2, G20 and G52.

Anthranoids Cape aloes anthranoids are qualitatively identical to leaf exudate of *A. ferox*.[4] Anthrones (up to 30%), mainly the C-glycosides aloins A and B (= barbaloin, isobarbaloin, stereo isomers of 10-glucosyl-aloe-emodin anthrone); other glycosides include 8-O-methyl-7-hydroxy aloins A and B, aloinosides A and B (aloin-11-O-α-L-rhamnosides). Small quantities of 1,8-dihydroxyanthraquinoid aglycones, including aloe-emodin and chrysophanol are also present.

Chromones Major constituents are aloesin (2-acetonyl-5-methyl-8-glucosyl chromone) and aloeresin E. Lesser quantities of isoaloeresin D, 8-C-glucosyl-7-O-methyl-aloesol and related glycosides, which may be esterified at the glucose moiety by either cinnamic, *p*-coumaric or ferulic acids, are also present. Non-glycosylated chromones include 7-hydroxy-2,5-dimethylchromone, furoaloesone, 2-acetonyl-7-hydroxy-8-(3-hydroxyacetonyl)-5-methyl chromone and 2-acetonyl-8-(2-furoylmethyl)-7-hydroxy-5-methylchromone.[8,9]

Phenyl pyrones Glycosides include aloenin and aloenin B.[1,2]

Other constituents Cinnamic acid and 1-methyltetralin.[G52]

Food Use

Aloes is listed by the Council of Europe as a natural source of food flavouring (category N3).[G16] This category indicates that aloes can be added to foodstuffs in the traditionally accepted manner, although there is insufficient information available for an adequate assessment of potential toxicity. The concentration of aloin present in the final product is limited to 0.1 mg/kg; 50 mg/kg in alcoholic beverages.[G16] Previously, aloes has been listed as GRAS (Generally Recognised As Safe).[G41]

Herbal Use

Aloes is recommended for the treatment of atonic constipation and suppressed menstruation.[G2, G49, G64]

Dosage

Dosages for oral administration (adults) for traditional uses recommended in older and contemporary standard herbal reference texts are given below.

Dried juice 50–200 mg or equivalent three times daily.[G6, G49]

In view of potential adverse effects, the dose recommended for adults and children aged over 10 years is 10–30 mg of hydroxyanthracene derivatives (calculated as barbaloin) once daily at night.[G52] Use of aloes as a laxative in self-treatment of constipation for more than two weeks is not recommended.[G52]

Pharmacological Actions

The activity of aloes can be attributed to the anthranoid glycoside content. The glycosides are metabolised by glycosidases in the intestinal flora to form active anthrones. The laxative action is due to an increase in motility of the large intestine by inhibition of the Na^+/K^+ pump and chloride ion channels; enhanced fluid secretion occurs due to stimulation of mucus and chloride ion secretion.[G52]

In vitro and animal studies

Nine hours after oral administration, aloes produced diarrhoea at doses of 5 g/kg (in 20% of rats) and 20 g/kg (in 100% of rats).[10] Pretreatment of rats with the nitric oxide (NO) synthase inhibitor *N*-nitro-L-arginine methyl ester given intraperitoneally reduced diarrhoea induced by aloes (20 g/kg) nine hours after oral administration. The results suggest that endogenous NO modulates the diarrhoeal effects of Cape aloes.[10]

Inhibitory effects of aqueous extracts of five species of *Aloe*, including *A. ferox* and *A. barbadensis*, and aloe powder (Japanese Pharmacopoeia) on histamine release from rat peritoneal mast cells induced by antigen were investigated *in vitro*.[11] All extracts tested inhibited histamine release in a concentration-dependent manner under the test conditions. *Aloe ferox* extract, Japanese Pharmacopoeia aloes and barbaloin strongly inhibited histamine release (IC_{50} 0.16, 0.07 and 0.02 μg/mL, respectively).[11]

Aqueous extracts of aloes are said to elevate the rate of ethanol oxidation *in vivo*.[12] Oral administration of aloin (300 mg/kg) to rats 12 hours prior to administration of alcohol (3 g/kg) resulted in a significant decrease (40%) in blood alcohol concentration.[12] Treatment with intraperitoneal aloe-emodin two hours prior to alcohol administration significantly reduced blood alcohol concentrations; it was hypothesised that aloin is metabolised to aloe-emodin which exerts its effect on alcohol metabolism.[12] Activity-guided fractionation of the leaves of *A. aborescens* resulted in the isolation and characterisation of elgonica-dimers A and B (dimeric *C*-glycosides of anthrone emodin-10′-C-β-D-glucopyranoside and aloe-emodin) as potent inhibitors of cytosolic alcohol dehydrogenase and aldehyde dehydrogenase activities *in vitro*.[13]

Aloe-emodin and an alcoholic extract of aloes have been reported to possess antitumour activity.[G41]

Hypoglycaemic activity has been shown in alloxan-diabetic mice for aloes[14] and in diabetic rats for an aloe gum extract.[15, 16]

Barbaloin is active *in vitro* against *Mycobacterium tuberculosis* and *Bacillus subtilis* (minimum inhibitory concentration 0.125 mg/mL and 0.25 mg/mL, respectively).[G18]

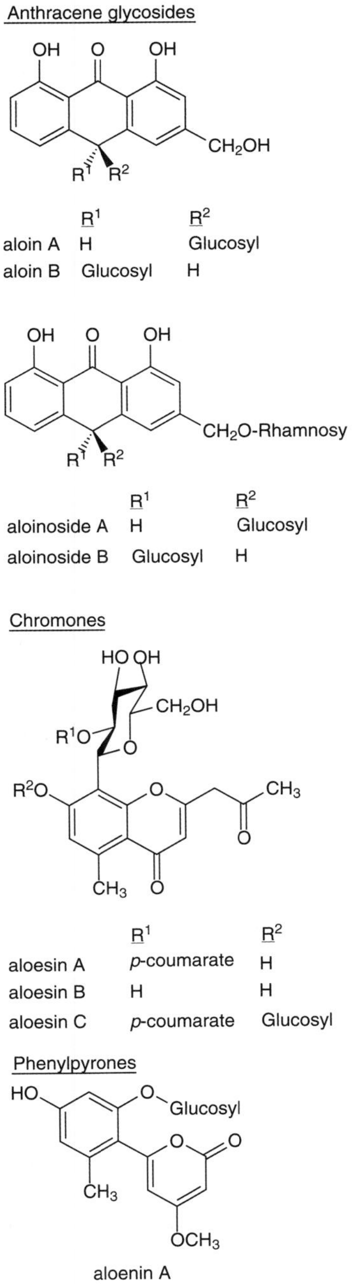

Clinical studies

The purgative action of the anthraquinone glycosides is well recognised (*see* Senna), although aloes is reported to be more potent than both senna and cascara.[G41, G45] Orally ingested anthranoid glycosides are not metabolised until they reach the colon. In humans, the intestinal flora break down *O*-glycosides readily and *C*-glycosides to some extent. The main active metabolite is aloe-emodin-9-anthrone.[G52]

An aloes extract in doses too small to cause abdominal cramps or diarrhoea had a significant hypoglycaemic effect in five patients with non-insulin-dependent diabetes.[14] However, the methodological limitations of this small, uncontrolled study do not allow any conclusions to be drawn on the effects of aloes.

Side-effects, Toxicity

Aloes is a potent purgative that may cause abdominal pains, gastrointestinal irritation leading to pelvic congestion and, in large doses, may result in nephritis, bloody diarrhoea and haemorrhagic gastritis.[G41, G44] Like all stimulant purgatives, prolonged use of aloes may produce watery diarrhoea with excessive loss of water and electrolytes (particularly potassium), muscular weakness and weight loss.[G44]

Tests of the possible carcinogenicity of hydroxyanthraquinones and their glycosides showed that exposure to certain aglycones and glycosides may represent a human cancer risk.[17] Most of the aglycones tested were found to be mutagenic and some, such as emodin and aloe-emodin, were genotoxic in mammalian cells.

Administration of dried aloes extract 50 mg/kg per day for 12 weeks to mice did not result in the development of severe pathological symptoms, although a raised sorbitol dehydrogenase concentration was suggested to be indicative of liver damage.[G20] No mutagenic effects in *Salmonella typhimurium* and Va7 cells, or DNA repair induction in rat hepatocytes, were observed. These negative results are due to the inability of the test systems to release mutagenic anthranoids from the *C*-glycosides.[G20] Retrospective and prospective studies have shown no causal relationship between anthranoid laxative use and colorectal cancer.[G20]

Contra-indications, Warnings

Aloes has been superseded by less toxic laxatives.[G45] The drastic purgative action of aloes contra-indicates its use in individuals with haemorrhoids and existing kidney disease. In common with

Anthracene glycosides

	R^1	R^2
aloin A	H	Glucosyl
aloin B	Glucosyl	H

	R^1	R^2
aloinoside A	H	Glucosyl
aloinoside B	Glucosyl	H

Chromones

	R^1	R^2
aloesin A	*p*-coumarate	H
aloesin B	H	H
aloesin C	*p*-coumarate	Glucosyl

Phenylpyrones

aloenin A

Figure 1 Selected constituents of aloes.

all purgatives, aloes should not be given to patients with inflammatory disease of the colon (e.g. Crohn's disease, ulcerative colitis), appendicitis, intestinal obstruction, abdominal pain, nausea or vomiting. Aloes colours alkaline urine red. Long-term use should be avoided and a doctor should be consulted within two weeks of treatment initiation if symptoms persist.

Drug interactions Hypokalaemia resulting from laxative abuse potentiates the action of cardiac glycosides, interacts with anti-arrhythmic drugs, and with drugs which induce reversion to sinus rhythm, e.g. quinidine. Concomitant use with thiazide diuretics, adrenocorticosteroids and liquorice may aggregate electrolyte imbalance.

Pregnancy and lactation In view of the irritant and cathartic properties documented for aloes, its use is contra-indicated during pregnancy.(G44) Anthraquinones may be secreted into breast milk and, therefore, aloes should be avoided during lactation (*see* Senna).

Aloes is reputed to be an abortifacient and to affect the menstrual cycle.(G22)

Preparations

Proprietary single-ingredient preparations

France: Contre-Coups de l'Abbe Perdrigeon. *Germany:* Krauterlax; Rheogen. *Italy:* Vulcase. *Monaco:* Akipic.

Proprietary multi-ingredient preparations

Argentina: Genolaxante. *Australia:* Herbal Cleanse; Lexat; Peritone. *Austria:* Artin; Waldheim Abfuhrdragees forte; Waldheim Abfuhrdragees mild. *Belgium:* Grains de Vals. *Brazil:* Paratonico. *Canada:* Laxative. *Chile:* Aloelax; Bulgarolax. *Czech Republic:* Dr Theiss Rheuma Creme; Dr Theiss Schweden Krauter; Dr Theiss Schwedenbitter. *France:* Ideolaxyl; Opobyl; Petites Pilules Carters. *Germany:* Chol-Kugeletten Neu; Cholhepan N. *Israel:* Laxative Comp. *Italy:* Grani di Vals; Lassativi Vetegali; Puntualax. *Russia:* Doktor Mom (Доктор Мом); Original Grosser Bittner Balsam (Оригинальный Большой Бальзам Биттнера). *South Africa:* Helmontskruie; Lewensessens; Moultons Herbal Extract; Turulington Tincture; Wonderkroonessens. *Spain:* Alofedina; Crislaxo; Cynaro Bilina; Laxante Sanatorium; Nico Hepatocyn; Opobyl; Pildoras Zeninas. *Switzerland:* Padma-Lax; Padmed Laxan; Phytolaxin; Schweden-Mixtur H nouvelle formulation. *UK:* Constipation Tablets; Dual-Lax Normal Strength; Laxative Tablets; Natural Herb Tablets; Out-of-Sorts; Sure-Lax (Herbal). *USA:* Diaparene Corn Starch; Vagisil.

References

1 Park MK *et al.* Analysis of 13 phenolic compounds in *Aloe* species by high performance liquid chromatography. *Phytochem Anal* 1998; 9: 186–191.
2 Okamura N *et al.* High-performance liquid chromatographic determination of phenolic compounds in *Aloe* species. *J Chromatogr A* 1996; 746: 225–231.
3 Van Wyk E-E *et al.* Geographical variation in the major compounds of *Aloe ferox* leaf exudate. *Planta Med* 1995; 61: 250–253.
4 Reynolds T. Chromatographic examination of some old samples of drug aloes. *Pharmazie* 1994; 49: 524–529.
5 Rauwald HW, Sigler A. Simultaneous determination of 18 polyketides typical of *Aloe* by high performance liquid chromatography and photodiode array detection. *Phytochem Anal* 1994; 5: 266–270.
6 Rauwald HW, Beil A. High-performance liquid chromatographic separation and determination of diastereomeric anthrone-C-glucosyls in Cape aloes. *J Chromatogr* 1993; 639: 359–362.
7 Rauwald HW *et al.* Three 8-C-glucosyl-5-methyl-chromones from *Aloe barbadensis* (Ph. Eur. 1997). *Pharmazie* 1997; 52: 962–964.
8 Speranza G *et al.* Studies on aloe, 12. Furoaloesone, a new 5-methylchromone from Cape aloe. *J Nat Prod* 1993; 56: 1089–1094.
9 Speranza G *et al.* Studies on aloe, 15. Two new 5-methylchromones from Cape aloe. *J Nat Prod* 1997; 60: 692–694.
10 Izzo AA *et al.* The role of nitric oxide in aloe-induced diarrhoea in the rat. *Eur J Pharmacol* 1999; 368: 43–48.
11 Yamamoto M *et al.* Inhibitory effects of aloe extracts on antigen- and compound 48/80-induced histamine release from rat peritoneal mast cells. *Jpn J Toxicol Environ Health* 1993; 39: 395–400.
12 Chung J-H *et al.* Acceleration of the alcohol oxidation rate in rats with aloin, a quinone derivative of aloe. *Biochem Pharmacol* 1996; 52: 1461–1468.
13 Shin KH *et al.* Elongica-dimers A and B, two potent alcohol metabolism inhibitory constituents of *Aloe arborescens. J Nat Prod* 1997; 60: 1180–1182.
14 Ghannam N *et al.* The antidiabetic activity of aloes: preliminary and experimental observations. *Horm Res* 1986; 24: 288–294.
15 Al-Awadi FM, Gumaa KA. Studies on the activity of individual plants of an antidiabetic plant mixture. *Acta Diabetol Lat* 1987; 24: 37–41.
16 Al-Awadi FM *et al.* On the mechanism of the hypoglycaemic effect of a plant extract. *Diabetologia* 1985; 28: 432–434.
17 Westendorf J *et al.* Possible carcinogenicity of anthraquinone-containing medical plants. *Planta Med* 1988; 54: 562.

Angelica

Summary and Pharmaceutical Comment

The chemistry of angelica is well documented. Although the traditional use of Chinese angelica species, such as *A. sinensis* (often referred to as dong quai or dang gui) and *A. acutiloba*, is well established in oriental medicine, there is limited documented pharmacological information available for *A. archangelica*, the species most commonly used in Europe, to justify its herbal uses. In view of the presence of known pharmacologically active constituents, especially bergapten, consumption of amounts exceeding normal human dietary intake should be avoided. Angelica contains furanocoumarins which are known to possess photosensitising properties. Coumarin compounds detected so far in *A. archangelica* do not possess the minimum structural requirements (a C-4 hydroxyl substituent and a C-3 non-polar carbon substituent)[G87] for anticoagulant activity.

Species (Family)

Angelica archangelica L. (Apiaceae/Umbelliferae)

Synonym(s)

Angelicae Radix, *Archangelica officinalis* Hoffm., Garden Angelica

Part(s) Used

Fruit, leaf, rhizome, root

Pharmacopoeial and Other Monographs

BHP 1996[G9]
BP 2007[G84]
Complete German Commission E[G3]
Martindale 35th edition[G85]
Ph Eur 2007[G81]

Legal Category (Licensed Products)

GSL[G37]

Constituents

The following is compiled from several sources, including General Reference G2.

The literature mainly refers to constituents of the root.

Coumarins Over 20 furanocoumarins, including angelicin, archangelicin, bergapten, isoimperatorin and xanthotoxin.[1,G2] Also the coumarins osthol (major constituent in rhizome/root, 0.2%) and umbelliferone.[G2] The root also contains the furanocoumarins 2′-angeloyl-3′-isovaleryl vaginate,[2] heraclenol-2′-O-senecioate and heraclenol-2′-O-isovalerate.[3]

Volatile oils 0.35–1.3% in root and fruit. 80–90% monoterpenes, including α- and β-phellandrene, α- and β-pinene, sabinene, α-thujene, limonene, linalool, borneol[1,4] and four macrocyclic lactones.

Other constituents Archangelenone (a flavonoid), palmitic acid, caffeic and chlorogenic acids, sugars (fructose, glucose, sucrose, umbelliferose).

The chemistry of *A. sinensis* is similar to that of *A. archangelica*, with coumarins and volatile oil being major components.[5] In addition, a series of phthalides (e.g. ligustilide, butylphthalide, butylidenephthalide) have been isolated.

Food Use

Angelica is widely used in foods.[1,G32] Angelica is listed by the Council of Europe as a natural source of food flavouring (stem: category 1; other parts and preparations: category 4, with limits on coumarin and furanocoumarin) (*see* Appendix 3).[G17] Previously, angelica has been listed as GRAS (Generally Recognised As Safe).[G41]

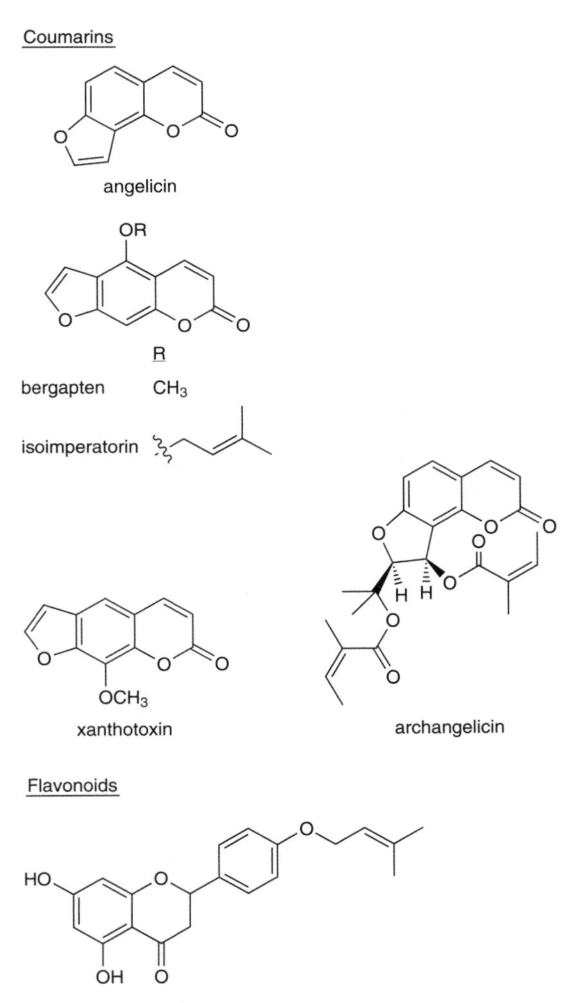

Figure 1 Selected constituents of angelica.

A

Herbal Use

Angelica is stated to possess antispasmodic, diaphoretic, expectorant, bitter aromatic, carminative, diuretic and local anti-inflammatory properties. It has been used for respiratory catarrh, psychogenic asthma, flatulent dyspepsia, anorexia nervosa, rheumatic diseases, peripheral vascular disease, and specifically for pleurisy and bronchitis, applied as a compress, and for bronchitis associated with vascular deficiency.[G7, G49, G64, G75] The German Commission E monograph states that angelica can be used for lack of appetite and dyspeptic complaints such as mild stomach cramps and flatulence.[G4]

Many related species, including *A. sinensis* (dong quai), are traditionally used in Chinese medicine.[G57] *A. sinensis* occurs in about 70% of all traditional Chinese medicine prescriptions to treat dysmenorrhoea, postnatal disturbances, anaemia, constipation and chronic pelvic infections.[5] Western naturopaths recommend the use of dong quai in hypertension, for modification of high blood sugar concentrations, regulation of the immune system, liver detoxification, anaemia and to relieve allergic conditions. Several unlicensed over-the-counter (OTC) products containing dong quai are readily available.

Dosage

Dosages for oral administration (adults) for traditional uses recommended in older standard herbal reference texts are given below.

Dried leaf 2–5 g by infusion three times daily.[G7]

Leaf liquid extract 2–5 mL (1 : 1 in 25% alcohol) three times daily.[G7]

Leaf tincture 2–5 mL (1 : 5 in 45% alcohol) three times daily.[G7]

Dried rhizome/root Daily dose 4.5 g[G2] or 1–2 g by infusion three times daily.[G4, G7]

Rhizome/root liquid extract 0.5–2.0 mL (1 : 1 in 25% alcohol) three times daily.[G7]

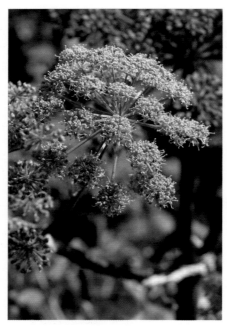

Figure 2 Angelica (*Angelica archangelica*).

Rhizome/root tincture 0.5–2 mL (1 : 5 in 50% alcohol) three times daily.[G7]

Fruit 1–2 g.[G49]

Pharmacological Actions

In vitro and animal studies

Minimal anti-inflammatory activity (1% inhibition of carrageenan-induced rat paw oedema) has been documented for fruit extracts (100 mg/kg body weight by mouth) given 45 minutes before eliciting oedema.[6] This was compared with 45% inhibition by indometacin (5 mg/kg by mouth).

Angelica is reported to possess antibacterial and antifungal properties.[G41, G46] Antibacterial activity against *Mycobacterium avium* has been documented, with no activity exhibited against *Escherichia coli*, *Bacillus subtilis*, *Streptococcus faecalis* or *Salmonella typhi*.[7] Antifungal activity was reported in 14 of 15 fungi tested.[7]

A methanolic extract of *A. archangelica* root showed antispasmodic activity against spontaneous contractions of circular smooth muscle (IC_{50} 265 μg/mL) and inhibited acetylcholine- and barium chloride-induced contractions of longitudinal smooth muscle (IC_{50} values 242 and 146 μg/mL, respectively).[8]

Extracts of *A. archangelica* root exhibit calcium channel-blocking activity.[9] A series of isolated coumarins showed activity, the most active being archangelicin with an IC_{50} 1.2 μg/mL (verapamil 2.0 μg/mL) as a calcium channel antagonist as assessed by inhibition of depolarisation in GH_4C_1 rat pituitary cells.[10]

Sixteen coumarin compounds isolated from *A. archangelica* were tested for activity in cyclooxygenase-1 (COX-1) and 5-lipoxygenase (5-LO) inhibition assays *in vitro*.[11] None of the compounds demonstrated activity against COX-1, but osthol and oxypeucedanin isovalerate were active in the 5-LO assay.

In rabbits, a uterotonic action has been documented for Japanese angelica root following intraduodenal administration of a methanolic extract (3 g/kg).[12] *A. sinensis* is reported to have induced uterine contraction and relaxation.[G57] Pharmacological investigations have shown that phthalides and coumarins found in *A. sinensis* have antispasmodic activity. The volatile constituents generally exert a hypotensive effect. A polysaccharide component is active against Ehrlich ascites tumours in mice and has immunostimulating activity,[13] and protects the gastric mucosa against ethanol- and indometacin-induced damage.[14]

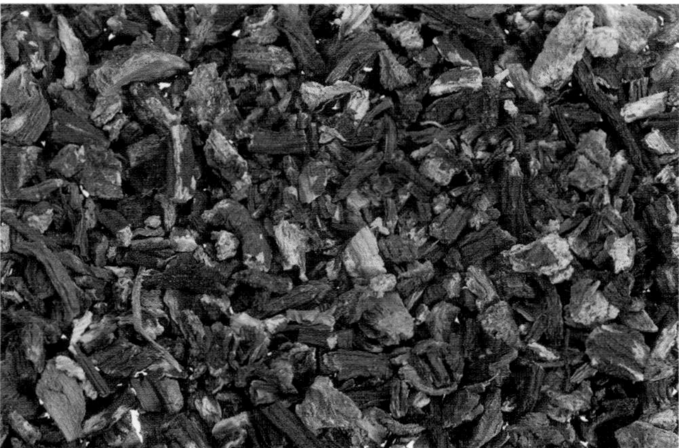

Figure 3 Angelica – dried drug substance (root).

Clinical studies

None documented for angelica (*A. archangelica*). The furanocoumarin constituent bergapten (5-methoxypsoralen) has been used in the PUVA (psoralen (P) and high-intensity long-wavelength ultraviolet irradiation) treatment of psoriasis.[G45]

Clinical investigation has failed to support the claims for *A. sinensis* with respect to relieving menopausal symptoms.[15] *A. sinensis* has been reported to be effective in improving abnormal protein metabolism in patients with chronic hepatitis or hepatic cirrhosis.[16]

Side-effects, Toxicity

Both angelica and the root oil have been reported to cause photodermatitis and phototoxicity, respectively, following external contact.[7, G22, G33, G58] Angelica contains furanocoumarin constituents which are known to cause photosensitisation. Concern has been expressed at the possible carcinogenic risk of the furanocoumarin bergapten. Seven species of plants known to cause dermatitis were analysed for psoralen, 8-methoxypsoralen (xanthotoxin) and 5-methoxypsoralen (bergapten). The highest total yield was obtained from *A. archangelica*.[17]

The root oil has been reported to be non-irritant and non-sensitising on animal and human skin.[7]

Root and fruit oils obtained by steam distillation are claimed to be devoid of furanocoumarins, although extracts may contain them.[G41]

Coumarin compounds detected so far in *A. archangelica* do not possess the minimum structural requirements (a C-4 hydroxyl substituent and a C-3 non-polar carbon substituent)[G87] for anticoagulant activity.

Toxicity studies have been documented for the root oil.[7] Acute LD_{50} values have been reported as 2.2 g/kg body weight (mouse, by mouth) and 11.16 g/kg (rat, by mouth). Death was attributed to liver and kidney damage, although animals surviving for three days completely recovered with a reversal of organ damage. An acute LD_{50} (rabbit, dermal) value was reported to be greater than 5 g/kg. Subacute toxicity studies, lasting eight weeks, suggested that the tolerated dose in the rat was 1.5 g/kg, although at lower doses the animals weighed less than the controls.[7]

Furanocoumarins isolated from another related Chinese species, *Angelica koreana*, have been reported to affect the hepatic metabolism of hexobarbitone. The compounds were found to cause a marked inhibition of drug metabolism in the first phase and an acceleration in the second phase, and were thought to be drug-metabolising enzyme inhibitors rather than enzyme inducers. Furanocoumarins investigated included imperatorin and oxypeucedanin, which are also documented as constituents of *A. archangelica*.

An extract of dong quai administered subcutaneously to rabbits did not affect prothrombin time given alone, but did after concurrent administration of a single dose of warfarin.[18] Elevation of prothrombin time was noted in a patient stabilised on warfarin who began taking dong quai.[19] Coagulation values returned to normal one month after discontinuing use of dong quai.

Contra-indications, Warnings

Angelica may provoke a photosensitive allergic reaction because of the furanocoumarin constituents.

The use of bergapten in cosmetic and suntan preparations is stated to be ill-advised by some regulatory authorities,[G45] in view of the concerns regarding the risk of skin cancer. The International Fragrance Association recommended that angelica root oil be limited to a maximum of 0.78% in products applied to skin which is then exposed to sunshine.[G58]

Drug interactions None documented. However, the potential for preparations of angelica to interact with other medicines administered concurrently, particularly those with similar or opposing effects, should be considered.

Pregnancy and lactation Angelica root is reputed to be an abortifacient and to affect the menstrual cycle. In view of this and the photosensitising constituents, the use of angelica during pregnancy and lactation in amounts exceeding those used in foods should be avoided.

Preparations

Proprietary multi-ingredient preparations

Argentina: Sigmafem. *Australia:* Infant Tonic; Irontona; Lifesystem Herbal Formula 4 Women's Formula; Medinat Esten; Vitatona; Women's Formula Herbal Formula 3. *Austria:* Abdomilon N; Original Schwedenbitter. *Czech Republic:* Dr Theiss Rheuma Creme; Dr Theiss Schweden Krauter; Dr Theiss Schwedenbitter; Stomaran; Valofyt Neo. *France:* Dystolise; Mediflor Tisane Digestive No 3. *Germany:* Abdomilon; Abdomilon N; Gastritol; Iberogast; Klosterfrau Melisana; Melissengeist; Schwedentrunk Elixier. *Italy:* Florelax. *Russia:* Doppelherz Melissa (Доппельгерц Мелисса); Original Grosser Bittner Balsam (Оригинальный Большой Бальзам Биттнера). *South Africa:* Melissengeist; Spiritus Contra Tussim Drops. *Spain:* Agua del Carmen; Himelan. *Switzerland:* Gastrosan; Iberogast. *UK:* Melissa Comp..

References

1 Czygan F-C. (Root of the holy ghost or Angelica root – *Angelica archangelica*). *Z Phytother* 1998; 19: 342–348.

2 Harmala P *et al.* A furanocoumarin from *Angelica archangelica*. *Planta Med* 1992; 58: 287–289.

3 Sun H, Jakupovic J. Further heraclenol derivatives from *Angelica archangelica*. *Pharmazie* 1986; 41: 888–889.

4 Holm Y *et al.* Enantiomeric composition of monoterpene hydrocarbons in n-hexane extracts of *Angelica archangelica* L. roots and seeds. *Flavour Fragrance J* 1997; 12: 397–400.

5 Awang DVC. Dong quai. *Can Pharm J* 1999; 132: 38–41.

6 Zielinska-Jenczylik J *et al.* Effect of plant extracts on the *in vitro* interferon synthesis. *Arch Immunol Ther Exp* 1984; 32: 577.

7 Opdyke DLJ. Angelica root oil. *Food Cosmet Toxicol* 1975; 13 (Suppl. Suppl.): 713.

8 Izzo AA *et al.* Spasmolytic activity of medicinal plants used for the treatment of disorders involving smooth muscles. *Phytother Res* 1996; 10: S107–S108.

9 Harmala P *et al.* Choice of solvent in the extraction of *Angelica archangelica* roots with reference to calcium blocking activity. *Planta Med* 1992; 58: 176–183.

10 Harmala P *et al.* Isolation and testing of calcium blocking activity of furanocoumarins from *Angelica archangelica*. *Planta Med* 1991; 57: A58–A59.

11 Roos G *et al.* Isolation, identification and screening for COX-1 and 5-LO inhibition of coumarins from *Angelica archangelica*. *Pharmaceut Pharmacol Lett* 1997; 7: 157–160.

12 Harada M *et al.* Effect of Japanese angelica root and peony root on uterine contraction in the rabbit *in situ*. *J Pharm Dyn* 1984; 7: 304–311.

13 Choy YM *et al*. Immunological studies of low molecular weight polysaccharide from *Angelica sinensis*. *Am J Chin Med* 1994; 22: 137–145.

14 Cho CH *et al*. Study of the gastrointestinal protective effects of polysaccharides from *Angelica sinensis* in rats. *Planta Med* 2000; 66: 348–351.

15 Hirata JD *et al*. Does dong quai have oestrogenic effects in postmenopausal women? A double-blind, placebo-controlled trial. *Fertil Steril* 1997; 68: 981–986.

16 Chang H-M, But PP-H. *Pharmacology and Applications of Chinese Materia Medica*, vol 1. Singapore: World Scientific, 1986: 499.

17 Zobel AM, Brown SA. Dermatitis-inducing psoralens on the surface of seven medicinal plant species. *J Toxicol Cutan Ocul Toxicol* 1991; 10: 223–231.

18 Lo ACT *et al*. Dong quai (*Angelica sinensis*) effects the pharmacodynamics but not the pharmacokinetics of warfarin in rabbits. *Eur J Drug Metab Pharmacokinet* 1995; 20: 55–60.

19 Page RL, Lawrence JD. Potentiation of warfarin by dong quai. *Pharmacotherapy* 1999; 19: 870–876.

Aniseed

Summary and Pharmaceutical Comment

The chemistry of aniseed is well studied and documented pharmacological activities support some of the herbal uses. Aniseed is used extensively as a spice and is widely used in conventional pharmaceuticals for its carminative, expectorant and flavouring properties. Aniseed contains anethole and estragole which are structurally related to safrole, a known hepatotoxin and carcinogen. Although both anethole and estragole have been shown to cause hepatotoxicity in rodents, aniseed is not thought to represent a risk to human health when it is consumed in amounts normally encountered in foods. Anethole was reaffirmed as GRAS (Generally Regarded As Safe) in 1997 on the basis of the recognised metabolic detoxication of *trans*-anethole in humans at low levels of exposure (1 mg/kg body weight).[(1)] For medicinal use, it is recommended that treatment should not be continued for extended periods.

Species (Family)

Pimpinella anisum L. (Apiaceae/Umbelliferae)

Synonym(s)

Anise, Anisi Fructus, Anisum, *Anisum officinarum* Moench., *Anisum vulgare* Gaertn.

Part(s) Used

Fruit

Pharmacopoeial and Other Monographs

BHP 1996[(G9)]
BP 2007[(G84)]
Complete German Commission E[(G3)]
ESCOP 1997[(G52)]
Martindale 35th edition[(G85)]
Ph Eur 2007[(G81)]

Legal Category (Licensed Products)

GSL[(G37)]

Constituents

The following is compiled from several sources, including General References G2 and G52.

Coumarins Scopoletin, umbelliferone, umbelliprenine; bergapten (furanocoumarin).

Flavonoids Flavonol (quercetin) and flavone (apigenin, luteolin) glycosides, e.g. quercetin-3-glucuronide, rutin, luteolin-7-glucoside, apigenin-7-glucoside; isoorientin and isovitexin (C-glucosides).

Volatile oils 2–6%. Major components are *trans*-anethole (80–95%), with smaller amounts of estragole (methyl chavicol),[(G52)] anise ketone (*p*-methoxyphenylacetone) and β-caryophyllene. Minor components include anisaldehyde and anisic acid (oxidation products of anethole), linalool, limonene, α-pinene, pseudoisoeugenol-2-methyl butyrate, acetaldehyde, *p*-cresol, cresol, hydroquinone, β-farnesene, α-, β- and γ-himachalene, bisabolene, *d*-elemene, *ar*-curcumene and myristicin.[(2)]

Other constituents Carbohydrate (50%), lipids 16% (saturated and unsaturated), β-amyrin (triterpene), stigmasterol (phytosterol) and its palmitate and stearate salts.

Food Use

Aniseed is used extensively as a spice and is listed by the Council of Europe as a natural source of food flavouring (category N2). This category allows small quantities of aniseed to be added to foodstuffs, with a possible limitation of an active principle (as yet unspecified) in the final product.[(G16)] Previously, aniseed has been listed as GRAS.[(1, G41)]

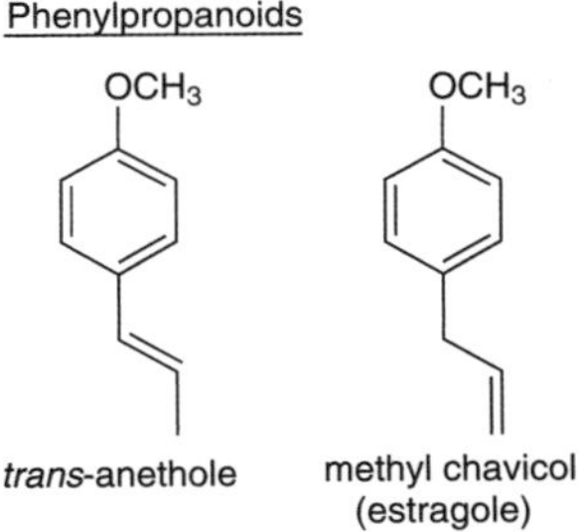

Aromatic aldehyde

OCH_3

CHO

anisaldehyde

Coumarins

	R^1	R^2
umbelliferone	H	OH
scopoletin	OCH_3	OH

OCH_3

bergapten

Figure 1 Selected constituents of aniseed.

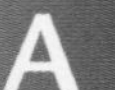

Herbal Use

Aniseed is stated to possess expectorant, antispasmodic, carminative and parasiticide properties. Traditionally, it has been used for bronchial catarrh, pertussis, spasmodic cough, flatulent colic; topically for pediculosis and scabies; its most specific use is for bronchitis, tracheitis with persistent cough, and as an aromatic adjuvant to prevent colic following the use of cathartics.[G2, G7, G64] Modern use of aniseed is mainly for the treatment of dyspeptic complaints and catarrh of the upper respiratory tract.[G41, G52, G75]

Aniseed has been used as an oestrogenic agent.[3] It has been reputed to increase milk secretion, promote menstruation, facilitate birth, alleviate symptoms of the male climacteric and increase libido.[3]

Dosage

Dosages for oral administration (adults, unless otherwise stated) for traditional uses recommended in older and contemporary standard herbal reference texts are given below.

Dried fruit Adults: 1.0–5.0 g crushed fruits in 150 mL water as an infusion several times daily.[G52] Children: 0–1 year old, 1.0 g of crushed fruits as an infusion; 1–4 years of age, 2.0 g; over four years, use adult dose.[G52]

Oil 0.05–0.2 mL three times daily.[G7]

Spirit of anise (BPC 1949) 0.3–1.0 mL three times daily.

Distilled anise water (BPC 1934) 15–30 mL three times daily.

Pharmacological Actions

The pharmacological effects of aniseed are largely due to the presence of anethole, which is structurally related to the catecholamines adrenaline, noradrenaline and dopamine. Anethole dimers closely resemble the oestrogenic agents stilbene and diethylstilbestrol.[3]

In vitro and animal studies

Antimicrobial, antifungal and insecticidal activities The volatile oil has antibacterial, antifungal and insecticidal activities.[G41, G52] Anethole, anisaldehyde and myristicin have exhibited mild insecticidal properties.[G41]

Antispasmodic activity Anise oil (200 mg/L) was shown to antagonise carbachol-induced spasms in a guinea-pig tracheal muscle preparation.[G52]

Secretolytic and expectorant effect Application of aniseed (6.4 g/140 mL) to isolated ciliated epithelium of frog trachea induces small increases in transport velocity.[G52] Dilutions of anise oil increased respiratory tract fluid in anaesthetised guinea-pigs, rats and cats. A similar action was observed in anaesthetised rabbits inhaling anise oil.[G52] The reputed lactogogic action of anise has been attributed to anethole, which exerts a competitive antagonism at dopamine receptor sites (dopamine inhibits prolactin secretion), and to the action of polymerised anethole, which is structurally related to the oestrogenic compounds stilbene and diethylstilbestrol.[3]

CNS activities Whole plant aqueous infusions have been reported to delay (but not prevent) the onset of picrotoxin-induced seizures and to reduce the mortality rate in mice following intraperitoneal injection.[4] Aniseed has also been found to slightly elevate γ-aminobutyric acid (GABA) concentrations in brain tissue.[4] The anticonvulsant effect is much weaker with aniseed than with conventional drug treatment and therefore its use as an anticonvulsant in Arabic folklore is not supported.[4] Anise oil diluted in sesame oil (0.25–1.0 mL/kg) given intraperitoneally to mice increased in a dose-dependent manner the dose of pentylenetetrazole needed to induce clonic and tonic seizures.[5] Activity was also observed against tonic seizures induced by maximal electric shock. Motor impairment was observed at higher doses of anise oil. Pentobarbital-induced sleeping time was prolonged by intraperitoneal administration of anise oil (50 mg/kg) to mice.[G52]

Other activities Oral administration of anethole (250–1000 mg/kg) to Swiss albino mice with Ehrlich ascites tumour in the paws indicated antitumour activity.[6] The conclusions were based on biochemical changes (nucleic acids, proteins, malondialdehyde, glutathione), survival rate and tumour weight. Anise oil given to rats (100 mg/kg given subcutaneously) stimulated liver regeneration after partial hepatectomy.[G52]

Clinical studies

There is a lack of documented clinical research involving aniseed and rigorous randomised controlled clinical trials are required.

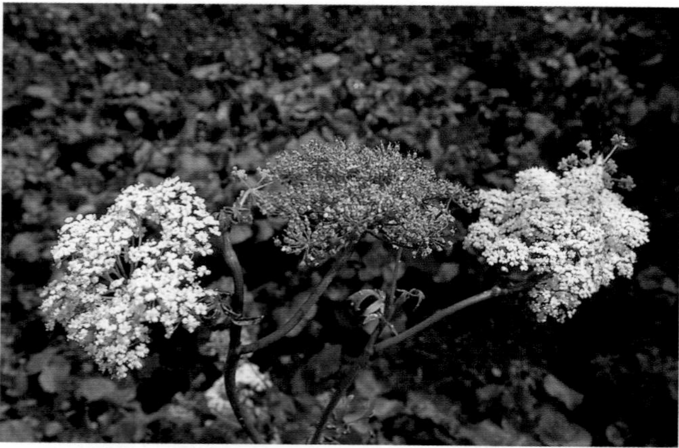

Figure 2 Aniseed (*Pimpinella anisum*).

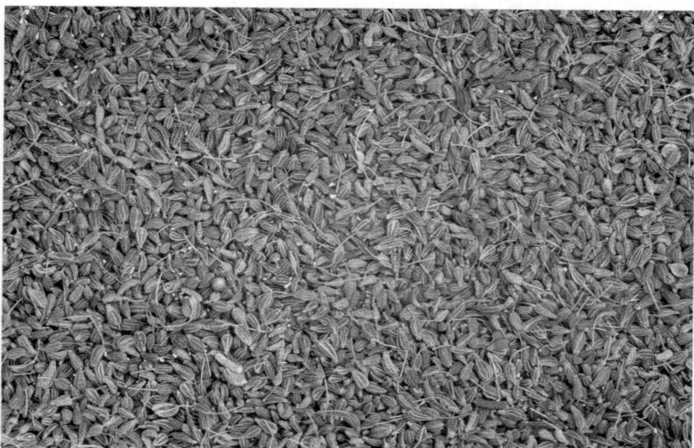

Figure 3 Aniseed – dried drug substance (fruit).

A

Side-effects, Toxicity

Contact dermatitis reactions to aniseed and aniseed oil have been attributed to anethole.[7, G31, G51] Reactions have been reported with products, such as creams and toothpastes, flavoured with aniseed oil.[G51] The volatile oil and anethole have been stated to be both irritant and sensitising.[G31, G51] Two female workers in a cake factory developed severe dermatitis, and patch tests indicated sensitivity to anise oil and to anethole.[8] Soreness, dryness and cracking of lips and perioral skin occurred in an individual using a herbal (fennel) toothpaste; anethole was reported to be the sensitising agent.[9] Bergapten is known to cause photosensitivity reactions and concern has been expressed over the possible carcinogenic risk of bergapten.[G45]

Ingestion of as little as 1–5 mL of anise oil can result in nausea, vomiting, seizures, and pulmonary oedema.[7]

The LD_{50} values per kg body weight for anise oil and *trans*-anethole are 2.7 g and 2–3 g, respectively.[G52] Mild liver lesions were observed in rats fed repeated anethole doses (695 mg/kg) for an unspecified duration.[3] Hepatic changes have been described in rats fed anethole in their daily diet (1%) for 15 weeks,[G22] although at a level of 0.25% there were no changes after one year. Rats fed with 0.1% *trans*-anethole in their diet for 90 days showed no toxic effects, but higher concentrations (0.3%, 1.0% and 3.0%) resulted in liver oedema.[G52] In therapeutic doses, anethole is reported to cause minimal hepatotoxicity.[G22] *Trans*-anethole given orally to rats (50–80 mg/kg) resulted in dose-dependent anti-implantation activity.[10] Significant oestrogenic activity was observed, but no anti-oestrogenic, progestational, anti-progestational, androgenic or antiandrogenic activity.[10]

Oral administration (1% of diet) of *trans*-anethole to rats resulted in induction of parathion-degrading drug enzymes.[G52] Male Wistar rats were treated with *trans*-anethole (125 or 250 mg/kg) by gavage for 10 days and the activities of liver microsome and cytosol phase I and II biotransformation enzymes were determined.[11] There was no effect on cytochrome P450, but UDP-glucuronyltransferase activity in the cytosol towards the substrates 4-chlorophenol and 4-hydroxyphenol was significantly increased for both doses. It was concluded that *trans*-anethole preferentially induces phase II biotransformation in rat liver *in vivo*.[11]

The safety of *trans*-anethole (4-methoxy propenylbenzene) has been reviewed by the Expert Panel of the Flavour and Extract Manufacturer Association (FEMA).[2] The evaluation was based on whether the hepatotoxic metabolite anethole epoxide is produced. At low levels of exposure, *trans*-anethole is efficiently detoxicated in rodents and humans, primarily by *O*-demethylation and ω-oxidation, respectively, while epoxidation is only a minor pathway. At higher doses in rats, a metabolic shift occurs resulting in epoxidation and formation of anethole epoxide. The continuous intake of high doses of *trans*-anethole induces a continuum of cytotoxicity, cell necrosis and cell proliferation. In chronic dietary studies in rats, hepatotoxicity resulted when the daily production of anethole epoxide exceeded 30 mg anethole epoxide per kg body weight. Neither *trans*-anethole nor anethole epoxide showed any evidence of genotoxicity. The Expert Panel concluded that the hepatocarcinogenic effects in female rats occur via a non-genotoxic mechanism and are secondary to hepatotoxicity caused by continuous exposures to high hepatocellular concentrations of anethole epoxide. *Trans*-anethole was reaffirmed as GRAS, based on a thorough study of the scientific literature.[1] Because *trans*-anethole undergoes efficient metabolic detoxication in humans at low levels of exposure, the neoplastic effects in rats associated with dose-dependent hepatotoxicity are not indicators of any significant risk to human health from the use of *trans*-anethole as a flavouring substance.[1]

Coumarin compounds detected so far in aniseed do not possess the minimum structural requirements (a C-4 hydroxyl substituent and a C-3 non-polar carbon substituent)[G87] for anticoagulant activity.

Contra-indications, Warnings

Aniseed may cause an allergic reaction. It is recommended that the use of aniseed oil should be avoided in dermatitis, and inflammatory or allergic skin conditions.[G31, G58] Aniseed should be avoided by persons with known sensitivity to anethole.[G52] Bergapten may cause photosensitivity in sensitive individuals. In view of the structural similarity reported between anethole and myristicin, consumption of large amounts of aniseed may cause neurological effects similar to those documented for nutmeg.

Drug interactions None documented. However, the potential for preparations of aniseed to interact with other medicines administered concurrently, particularly those with similar (e.g. hormonal therapies) or opposing effects, should be considered.

Pregnancy and lactation Traditionally, aniseed is reputed to be an abortifacient[G22] and also to promote lactation. The safety of aniseed taken during pregnancy and lactation has not been established; however, there are no known problems provided that doses taken do not greatly exceed the amounts used in foods. It has been proposed that aniseed and preparations used at recommended dosages may be used during pregnancy and lactation.[G52]

Preparations

Proprietary multi-ingredient preparations

Australia: Neo-Cleanse. *Austria:* Asthmatee EF-EM-ES; Brady's-Magentropfen; Euka; Nesthakchen. *Brazil:* Balsamo Branco. *Chile:* Paltomiel. *Czech Republic:* Blahungstee N. *France:* Elixir Bonjean; Herbesan; Mediflor Tisane Digestive No 3; Mucinum a l'Extrait de Cascara. *Germany:* Em-medical; Floradix Multipretten N; Majocarmin-Tee; Ramend Krauter. *Hong Kong:* Mucinum Cascara. *Israel:* Jungborn. *Italy:* Cadifen; Cadimint; Dicalmir; Lassatina; Tisana Kelemata. *Russia:* Original Grosser Bittner Balsam (Оригинальный Большой Бальзам Биттнера). *South Africa:* Clairo; Cough Elixir. *Spain:* Crislaxo; Digestovital; Laxante Sanatorium; Laxomax. *Switzerland:* Kernosan Elixir; Kernosan Heidelberger Poudre; Tisane favorisant l'allaitement. *UK:* Herb and Honey Cough Elixir; Revitonil. *Venezuela:* Neo-Atropan.

References

1 Newberne P *et al*. The FEMA GRAS assessment of trans-anethole used as a flavouring substance. *Food Chem Toxicol* 1999; 37: 789–811.

2 Burkhardt G *et al*. Terpene hydrocarbons in *Pimpinella anisum* L. *Pharm Weekbl (Sci)* 1986; 8: 190–193.

3 Albert-Puleo M. Fennel and anise as estrogenic agents. *J Ethnopharmacol* 1980; 2: 337–344.

4 Abdul-Ghani A-S *et al*. Anticonvulsant effects of some Arab medicinal plants. *Int J Crude Drug Res* 1987; 25: 39–43.

5 Pourgholami MH *et al*. The fruit essential oil of *Pimpinella anisum* exerts anticonvulsant effects in mice. *J Ethnopharmacol* 1999; 66: 211–215.

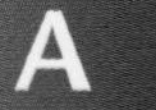

6 Al-Harbi MM *et al*. Influence of anethole treatment on the tumour induced by Ehrlich ascites carcinoma cells in paw of Swiss albino mice. *Eur J Cancer Prevent* 1995; 4: 307–318.
7 Chandler RF, Hawkes D. Aniseed – a spice, a flavor, a drug. *Can Pharm J* 1984; 117: 28–29.
8 Garcia-Bravo B *et al*. Occupational contact dermatitis from anethole in food handlers. *Contact Dermatitis* 1997; 37: 38.
9 Franks A. Contact allergy to anethole in toothpaste associated with loss of taste. *Contact Dermatitis* 1998; 38: 354–355.
10 Dhar SK. Anti-fertility activity and hormonal profile of trans-anethole in rats. *Indian J Physiol Pharmacol* 1995; 39: 63–67.
11 Rompelberg CJM *et al*. Effects of the naturally occurring alkenylbenzenes eugenol and trans-anethole on drug-metabolising enzymes in the rat liver. *Food Chem Toxicol* 1993; 31: 637–645.

Apricot

Summary and Pharmaceutical Comment

Interest in apricot kernels was generated as a result of claims in the late 1970s that laetrile, a semi-synthetic derivative of the naturally occurring constituent amygdalin, was a natural, non-toxic cure for cancer. Apricot kernels were seen as an alternative source for this miracle cure. These claims have since been disproved and it has been established that laetrile (amygdalin) is toxic, particularly if administered orally. Fatal cases of cyanide poisoning have been reported following the ingestion of apricot kernels. Amygdalin was made a prescription-only medicine in the UK in 1984.[1]

Species (Family)

Armeniaca vulgaris Lam. var. *vulgaris*

Synonym(s)

Ku Xing Ren (seed/kernel), *Prunus armeniaca* L., *Prunus tiliifolia* Salisb.

Part(s) Used

Kernel (seed), expressed oil

Pharmacopoeial and Other Monographs

Martindale 35th edition[G85]

Legal Category (Licensed Products)

Apricot is not included in the GSL. Amygdalin (a cyanogenetic glycoside) is classified as a POM.[1]

Constituents

Acids Phenolic. Various quinic acid esters of caffeic, *p*-coumaric and ferulic acids.[2] Neochlorogenic acid major in kernel, chlorogenic in fruit.[3]

Glycosides Cyanogenetic. Amygdalin (mandelonitrile diglucoside). Cyanide content of kernel varies from 2 to 200 mg/100 g.[3]

Tannins Catechins, proanthocyanidins (condensed).[4]

Other constituents Cholesterol, an oestrogenic fraction (0.09%) containing estrone (both free and conjugated) and α-estradiol.[5]

Other plant parts

Leaves and fruit contain various flavonol (kaempferol, quercetin) glycosides including rutin (major).[5]

Food Use

Apricot fruit is commonly eaten. Apricot is listed by the Council of Europe as a natural source of food flavouring (categories N1 and N2). These categories limit the total amount of hydrocyanic acid permitted in the final product to 1 mg/kg. Exceptions to this are 25 mg/kg for confectionery, 50 mg/kg for marzipan and 5 mg/kg for fruit juices.[G16] Previously, apricot kernel extract has been listed as GRAS (Generally Recognised As Safe).[G65]

Herbal Use

Traditionally, the oil has been incorporated into cosmetic and perfumery products such as soaps and creams.[G34]

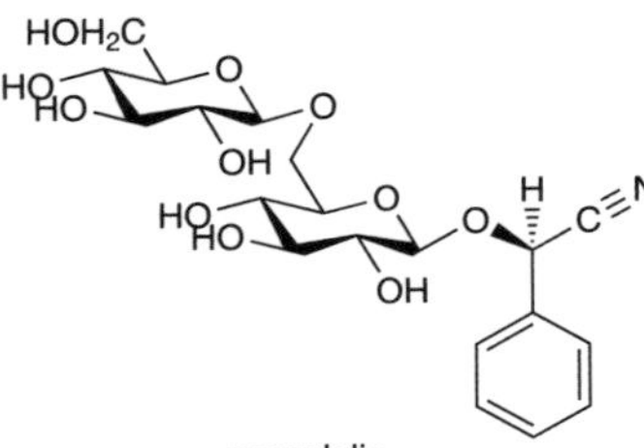

Figure 1 Selected constituents of apricot.

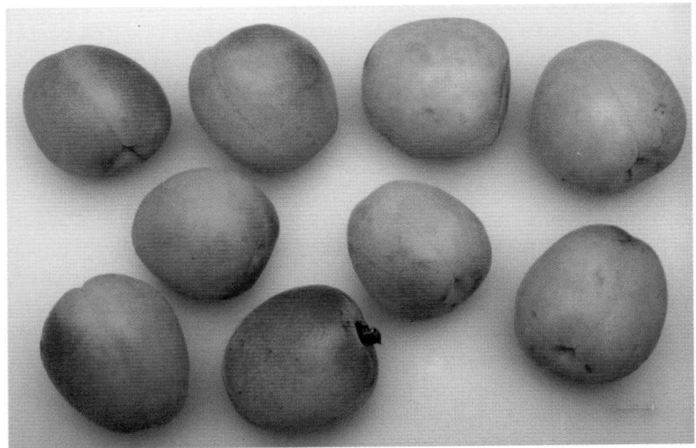

Figure 2 Apricot (fruit).

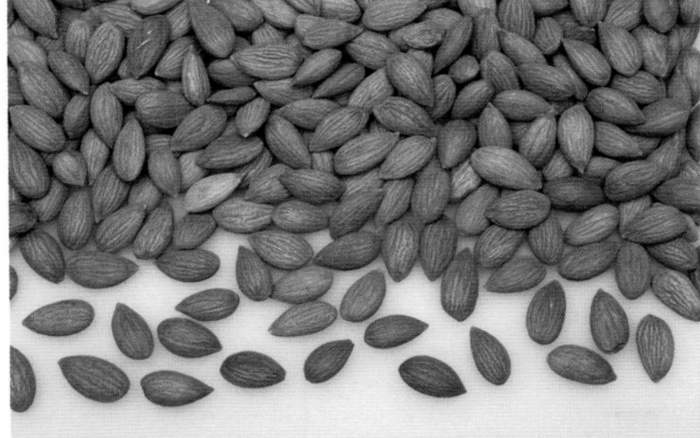

Figure 3 Apricot – dried drug substance (kernel).

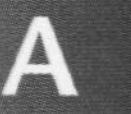

Dosage

None documented. Traditionally, apricot kernels have not been utilised as a herbal remedy.

Pharmacological Actions

During the late 1970s and early 1980s considerable interest was generated in apricot from claims that laetrile (a semi-synthetic derivative of amygdalin) was an effective treatment for cancer. Two review papers[6,7] discuss these claims for laetrile together with its chemistry, metabolism and potential toxicity.

The claims for laetrile were based on three different theories. The first claimed that cancerous cells contained abundant quantities of β-glucosidases, enzymes which release hydrogen cyanide from the laetrile molecule as a result of hydrolysis. Normal cells were said to be protected because they contained low concentrations of β-glucosidases and high concentrations of rhodanese, an enzyme which converts cyanide to the less toxic thiocyanate. However, this theory was disproved when it was shown that both cancerous and normal cells contain only trace amounts of β-glucosidases, and similar amounts of rhodanese. In addition, it was thought that amygdalin was not absorbed intact from the gastrointestinal tract.[6,7]

The second theory proposed that following ingestion, amygdalin was hydrolysed to mandelonitrile, transported intact to the liver and converted to a β-glucuronide complex. This complex was then carried to the cancerous cells, hydrolysed by β-glucuronidases to release mandelonitrile and subsequently hydrogen cyanide. This theory was considered to be untenable.[7]

A third theory proposed that laetrile is vitamin B_{17}, that cancer is a result of a deficiency of this vitamin, and that chronic administration of laetrile would prevent cancer. Again this was not substantiated by any scientific evidence.[7]

Clinical studies

A Cochrane systematic review that aimed to assess the efficacy of laetrile in cancer reported that there were no controlled clinical trials available in this indication.[8] The review concluded, therefore, that there is no evidence from controlled clinical trials to support the alleged beneficial effects of laetrile as an anticancer agent, or as an adjunctive agent in cancer chemotherapy.

A retrospective analysis of the use of laetrile by cancer patients reported that it may have slight activity.[6,7] However, a subsequent clinical trial concluded that laetrile was ineffective in cancer treatment. Furthermore, it was claimed that patients taking laetrile reduced their life expectancy as a result of lack of proper medical care and chronic cyanide poisoning.[6,7]

Side-effects, Toxicity

Laetrile and apricot kernel ingestion are the most common sources of cyanide poisoning, with more than 20 deaths reported.[6,7] Apricot kernels are toxic because of their amygdalin content. Hydrolysis of the amygdalin molecule by β-glucosidases, heat, mineral acids or high doses of ascorbic acid (vitamin C) yields hydrogen cyanide (HCN), benzaldehyde, and glucose. β-Glucosidases are not generally abundant in the gastrointestinal tract, but they are present in the kernels themselves as well as certain foods including beansprouts, carrots, celery, green peppers, lettuce, mushrooms and sweet almonds. Hydrolysis of the amygdalin molecule is slow in an acid environment but much more rapid in an alkaline pH. There may therefore be a delay in the onset of symptoms of HCN poisoning as a result of the transit time from the acid pH of the stomach to the alkaline environment of the small intestine.

Acute poisoning

Cyanide is rapidly absorbed from the upper gastrointestinal tract, diffuses readily throughout the body and promptly causes respiratory failure if untreated. Symptoms of cyanide toxicity progress rapidly from dizziness, headache, nausea, vomiting and drowsiness to dyspnoea, palpitations, marked hypotension, convulsions, paralysis, coma and death, which may occur from 1–15 minutes after ingestion. Antidotes for cyanide poisoning include nitrite, thiosulfate, hydroxocobalamin, cobalt edetate and aminophenol.[6,7]

Chronic poisoning

Principal symptoms include increased blood thiocyanate, goitre, thyroid cancer, lesions of the optic nerve, blindness, ataxia, hypertonia, cretinism and mental retardation.[6] These symptoms may develop as a result of ingesting significant amounts of cyanide, cyanogenetic precursors in the diet, or cyanogenetic drugs such as laetrile. Demyelinating lesions and other neuromyopathies reportedly occur secondary to chronic cyanide exposure, including long-term therapy with laetrile. Agranulocytosis has also been attributed to long-term laetrile therapy.[6,7]

Individual reports of adverse reactions and cyanide poisoning in patients using laetrile have been documented.[G45]

Normally, low concentrations of ingested cyanide are controlled naturally by exhalation or by rapid conversion to the less toxic thiocyanate by the enzyme rhodanese. Oral doses of 50 mg of hydrogen cyanide (HCN) can be fatal. This is equivalent to approximately 30 g kernels which represents about 50–60 kernels, and approximately 2 mg HCN/g kernel. Apricot seed has also been reported to contain 2.92 mg HCN/g.[9] A 500-mg laetrile tablet was found to contain between 5 and 51 mg HCN/g.

There may be considerable variation in the number of kernels required to be toxic, depending on the concentration of amygdalin and β-glucosidases present in the kernels, the timespan of ingestion, the degree of maceration of the kernels, individual variation in hydrolysing, and detoxifying abilities.

Systemic concentrations of β-glucosidases are low and therefore toxicity following parenteral absorption of amygdalin is low. However, cyanide poisoning has been reported in rats following intraperitoneal administration of laetrile, suggesting another mechanism of hydrolysis had occurred.[6,7]

It is thought that cyanogenetic glycosides may possess carcinogenic properties. Mandelonitrile (amygdalin = mandelonitrile diglucoside) is mutagenic and stimulates guanylate cyclase.[6,7]

Contra-indications, Warnings

Apricot kernels are toxic due to their amygdalin content. Following ingestion hydrogen cyanide is released and may result in cyanide poisoning. Fatalities have been reported following the ingestion of apricot kernels. Contact dermatitis has been reported following contact with apricot kernels.[10]

Drug interactions None documented.

Pregnancy and lactation Apricot kernels are toxic and should not be ingested. The ingestion of cyanogenetic substances may result in teratogenic effects.[6] However, one case has been reported where no acute toxicity was noted in the infant when laetrile was used during the third term of pregnancy. It was unknown whether chronic effects would be manifested at a later date.[6] Breeding rats fed ground apricot kernels had pups with normal birth weights, but with lower survival rates and lower weaning weights.[3]

References

1 The Medicines (Cyanogenetic Substances) Order, SI 1984 No. 187, London: HMSO, 1984.
2 Möller B, Herrmann K. Quinic acid esters of hydroxycinnamic acids in stone and pome fruit. *Phytochemistry* 1983; 22: 477–481.
3 Miller KW *et al*. Amygdalin metabolism and effect on reproduction of rats fed apricot kernels. *J Toxicol Environ Health* 1981; 7: 457–467.
4 Awad O. Steroidal estrogens of *Prunus armeniaca* seeds. *Phytochemistry* 1973; 13: 678–690.
5 Henning W, Herrmann K. Flavonol glycosides of apricots (*Prunus armeniaca* L.) and peaches (*Prunus persica* Batch). 13. Phenolics of fruits. *Z Lebensm Unters Forsch* 1980; 171: 183–188.
6 Chandler RF *et al*. Laetrile in perspective. *Can Pharm J* 1984; 117: 517–520.
7 Chandler RF *et al*. Controversial laetrile. *Pharm J* 1984; 232: 330–332.
8 Milazzo S *et al*. Laetrile treatment for cancer. Cochrane Database of Systematic Reviews, issue 2, 2006. London: Macmillan.
9 Holzbecher MD *et al*. The cyanide content of laetrile preparations, apricot, peach and apple seeds. *Clin Toxicol* 1984; 22: 341–347.
10 Göransson K. Contact urticaria to apricot stone. *Contact Dermatitis* 1981; 7: 282.

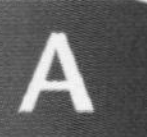

Arnica

Summary and Pharmaceutical Comment

The chemistry and pharmacology of arnica are well documented, but there is a paucity of clinical data. Anti-inflammatory properties associated with sesquiterpene lactones justify the herbal uses, although allergenic and cytotoxic properties are also associated with this class of constituents. Arnica is not suitable for internal use, although it is present in some homeopathic products. External use of arnica tincture, which is included as an ingredient in some cosmetics, hair shampoos and bath preparations, may cause an allergic reaction. The pyrrolizidine alkaloids tussilagine and isotussilagine, reportedly present in arnica, are non-toxic. Moreover, they are artefacts produced during the extraction process with methanol.

Species (Family)

Arnica montana L. (Asteraceae/Compositae)

Arnica chamissonis Less. subsp. *foliosa* (Nutt.) Maguire also allowed in German Pharmacopoeia.[G52]

Synonym(s)

Arnicae Flos, Leopard's Bane, Mountain Tobacco, Wolf's Bane

Part(s) Used

Flower

Pharmacopoeial and Other Monographs

BHP 1996[G9]
BP 2007[G84]
ESCOP 1997[G52]
Martindale 35th edition[G85]
Ph Eur 2007[G81]

Legal Category (Licensed Products)

GSL, for external use only.[G37]

Constituents

The following is compiled from several sources, including References 1–3, and General References G2 and G52.

Alkaloids Traces of non-toxic alkaloids tussilagine and isotussilagine[4] but these are reportedly artefacts produced during extraction.[5]

Amines Betaine, choline and trimethylamine.

Carbohydrates Mucilage, polysaccharides including inulin.

Coumarins Scopoletin and umbelliferone.

Flavonoids Betuletol, eupafolin, flavonol glucuronides,[1–3] hispidulin, isorhamnetin, kaempferol, laciniatin, luteolin, patuletin, quercetin, spinacetin, tricin and 3,5,7-trihydroxy-6,3′,4′-trimethoxyflavone.

Terpenoids Sesquiterpene lactones of the pseudoguaianolide-type, 0.2–0.8%.[G52] Pharmacopoeial standard not less than 0.4%.[G81, G85] Helenalin,[6] 11α,13-dihydrohelenalin and their esters with acetic, isobutyric, methacrylic, tiglic and other carboxylic acids.[G52] Diterpenes including *z*-labda-13-ene-8α,15-diol.[7]

Volatile oils Up to 1%, normally about 0.3%. Thymol and thymol derivatives.

Other constituents Amino acid (2-pyrrolidine acetic), bitter principle (arnicin), caffeic acid, carotenoids, fatty acids, phytosterols, polyacetylenes, resin, tannin (unspecified).

Food Use

Arnica is listed by the Council of Europe as a natural source of food flavouring (category N2). This category indicates that arnica can be added to foodstuffs in small quantities, with a possible limitation of an active principle (as yet unspecified) in the final product.[G16] Previously, arnica has been listed by the Food and Drugs Administration (FDA) as an 'unsafe herb',[G22] and is only approved for food use in alcoholic beverages.[G41]

Herbal Use

Arnica is stated to possess topical counter-irritant properties. It has been used for unbroken chilblains, alopecia neurotica, insect bites, gingivitis, aphthous ulcers, rheumatoid complaints and specifically for sprains and bruises.[G2, G7, G52, G64]

German Commission E approved external use for injuries and consequences of accidents, e.g. haematoma, dislocation, contusions, oedema due to fracture, rheumatoid muscle and joint pains, inflammation of oral and throat region, furuncolosis, inflammation caused by insect bites and superficial phlebitis.[G3, G4]

Arnica is mainly used in homeopathic preparations; it is used to a lesser extent in herbal products.

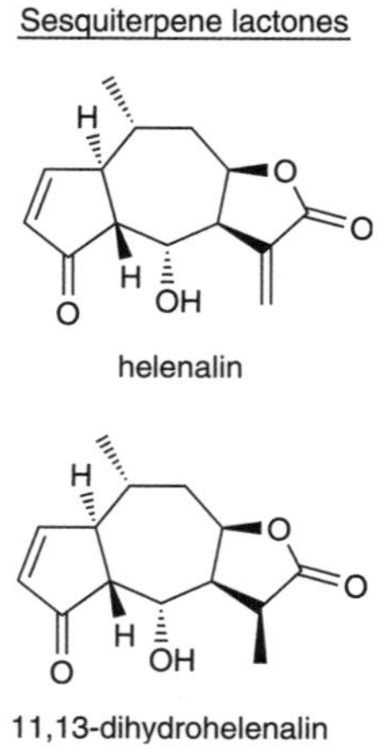

Figure 1 Selected constituents of arnica.

Dosage

Recommendations for external use (adults) for traditional uses recommended in older standard herbal reference texts are given below.

Tincture of arnica flower (BPC 1949) 2–4 mL for external application only.

Preparations Ointments, creams, gels, compresses made with 5–25% v/v tinctures, 5–25% v/v fluid extracts, diluted tinctures or fluid extract (1 : 3–1 : 10), decoctions 2.0 g drug/100 mL water.[G3, G4]

Pharmacological Actions

In vitro and animal studies

Antimicrobial activity Arnica has been reported to exhibit bactericidal properties against *Listeria monocytogenes* and *Salmonella typhimurium*.[G41] Helenalin and related sesquiterpenes from arnica have antimicrobial activity against *Bacillus subtilis* and *Staphylococcus aureus*,[8] *Corynebacterium insidosum*, *Micrococcus roseus*, *Mycobacterium phlei*, *Sarcinia lutea* and *Proteus vulgaris*.[G52] Antifungal activity against *Trichophyton mentagrophytes*, *Epidermaphyton* spp. and *Botrytis cinerea* is reported for helenalin.[8, G52]

Antitumour activity The cytotoxicity of 21 flavonoids and five sesquiterpene lactones from *Arnica* spp. has been investigated *in vitro* in studies using GLC_4 (a human small cell lung carcinoma) and COLO 320 (a human colorectal cancer) cell lines.[9] The most potent compound, helenalin, had an IC_{50} value of 0.44 μmol/L against GLC_4 and 1.0 μmol/L against COLO 320 after two hours' exposure.[9] Some of the individual flavonols and flavones of arnica at non-toxic concentrations significantly reduced helenalin-induced cytotoxicity *in vitro*.[10]

Anti-inflammatory activity Moderate (29%) anti-inflammatory effect in the carageenan rat paw model has been reported for arnica.[11] Helenalin is a potent inhibitor in this test and in chronic adjuvant arthritis tests in rats.[12] The α-methylene-γ-lactone moiety of sesquiterpenes is required for activity, and the potency of helenalin is enhanced by the presence of the 6-hydroxy group.[13] The mode of action of sesquiterpene lactones as anti-inflammatory agents is at multiple sites. At a concentration of 5×10^{-4} mol/L, the compounds uncoupled oxidative phosphorylation of human polymorphoneutrophils, elevated cyclic adenosine monophosphate (cAMP) levels of rat neutrophils, and rat and mouse liver cells, and inhibited free and total lysosymal enzyme activity.[12] Human polymorphonuclear neutrophil chemotaxis was inhibited at 5×10^{-4} mol/L, whereas prostaglandin synthetase activity was inhibited at concentrations of 10^{-3} mol/L. Helenalin and 11α-13-dihydrohelenalin inhibited collagen-induced platelet aggregation, thromboxane formation and 5-hydroxytryptamine secretion in a concentration-dependent manner.[14]

Other activities Helenalin has potent activity in the hotplate tail flick analgesic test in mice.[13]

Helenalin has also been reported to possess immunostimulant activity *in vitro*,[15] while high molecular weight polysaccharides have been found to exhibit immunostimulant activity *in vivo* in the carbon clearance test in mice.[15, 16]

Arnica contains an adrenaline-like pressor substance and a cardiotonic substance.[G24]

Clinical studies

Clinical investigation of the effects of arnica is limited, and rigorous randomised controlled clinical trials are required. A gel preparation of arnica flowers applied externally to the limbs of 12 male volunteers was more effective than placebo in the treatment of muscle ache.[G50, G52] In a randomised, double-blind, placebo-controlled study, 89 patients with venous insufficiency received arnica gel (20% tincture) or placebo.[G50] It was reported that arnica treatment produced improvements in venous tone, oedema and in feeling of heaviness in the legs.

Side-effects, Toxicity

Arnica is poisonous if taken internally. It is irritant to mucous membranes and ingestion may result in fatal gastroenteritis, muscle paralysis (voluntary and cardiac), increase or decrease in pulse rate, palpitation of the heart, shortness of breath, and may even lead to death.[G33, G41] Helenalin is stated to be the toxic principle responsible for these effects.[G33] Thirty millilitres of a 20% arnica tincture, taken by mouth, was reported to produce serious, but not fatal, symptoms.[G41] The topical application of arnica has been documented to cause dermatitis.[17, G51] Arnica is a strong sensitiser, with the sesquiterpene lactone constituents implicated as the contact allergens: they possess an α-methylene group exocyclic to a γ-lactone ring, which is recognised as an immunological prerequisite for contact allergy.[17, 18] Helenalin is also reported to possess cytotoxic activity and this has been

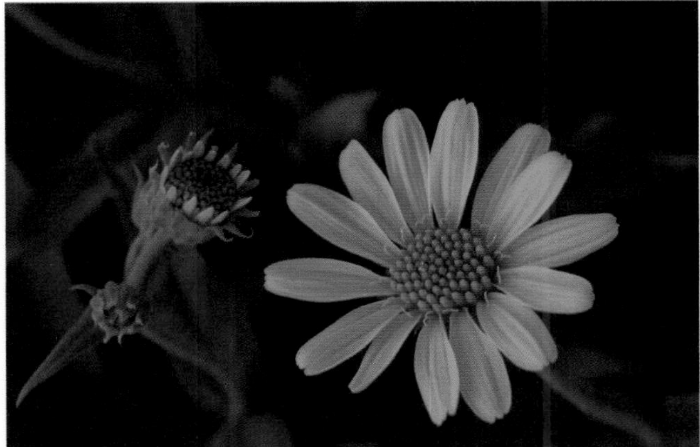

Figure 2 Arnica (*Arnica montana*).

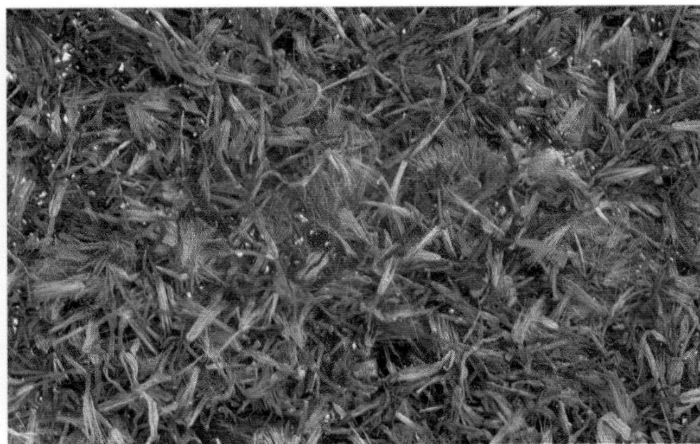

Figure 3 Arnica – dried drug substance (flower).

A

attributed to its ability to alkylate with sulfhydryl groups.(G33) Helenalin was not mutagenic in the *Salmonella typhimurium* assay.(G52)

Contra-indications, Warnings

Arnica should not be taken internally except in suitable homeopathic dilutions.(G42)

Externally, arnica is poorly tolerated by some people, precipitating allergic reactions in sensitive individuals.(G42) It should only be applied to unbroken skin and withdrawn at the first sign of reaction.(G7) Toxic allergic skin reactions have occurred following application of the tincture.(G33)

Pregnancy and lactation There are insufficient data on the use of arnica preparations during pregnancy and breastfeeding, and their use should be avoided during these periods.

Preparations

Proprietary single-ingredient preparations

Chile: Arnikaderm. *France:* Arnican; Pharmadose teinture d'arnica. *Germany:* Arnikatinktur; Arthrosenex AR; Doc; Enelbin-Salbe; Hyzum N. *Mexico:* Balsamo Nordin; Estimul. *Portugal:* Arnigel.

Proprietary multi-ingredient preparations

Argentina: Fluido. *Australia:* Joint & Muscle Relief Cream; Percutane. *Austria:* Arnicet; Asthmatee EF-EM-ES; Berggeist; Cional; Dynexan; Heparin Comp; Rheuma. *Brazil:* Dermol; Traumed. *Chile:* Lefkaflam; Matikomp. *Czech Republic:* Arnidol; Heparin-Gel. *France:* Arnicadol; Creme Rap; Dermocica; Evarose. *Germany:* Cefawell; Combudoron; Dolo-cyl; Gothaplast Rheumamed AC; Heparin Comp; Lindofluid N; Retterspitz Ausserlich; Retterspitz Quick; Sportino Akut; Stullmaton; Trauma-cyl; Varicylum-S; Venengel. *Hong Kong:* New Patecs A. *Italy:* Flebolider. *Mexico:* Reudol. *South Africa:* Combudoron; Dynexan; Lotio Pruni Comp cum Cupro; Muscle Rub; Wecesin. *Spain:* Arnicon. *Switzerland:* Combudoron; Euceta avec camomille et arnica; Fortacet; Onguent aux herbes Keller; Perskindol Cool Arnica; Topaceta. *UK:* Hansaplast Herbal Heat Plaster; Profelan. *USA:* MSM with Glucosamine Creme. *Venezuela:* Biomicovo.

References

1 Merfort I, Wendisch D. Flavonoidglycoside aus *Arnica montana* und *Arnica chamissonis*. *Planta Med* 1987; 53: 434–437.

2 Merfort I. Flavonol glycosides of Arnicae flos DAB 9. *Planta Med* 1986; 52: 427.

3 Merfort I, Wendisch D. Flavonolglucuronide aus den blüten von *Arnica montana*. *Planta Med* 1988; 54: 247–250.

4 Passreiter CM *et al*. Tussilagine and isotussilagine: two pyrrolizidine alkaloids in the genus *Arnica*. *Planta Med* 1992; 58: 556–557.

5 Passreiter CM. Co-occurrence of 2-pyrrolidine acetic acid with the pyrrolizidines tussilaginic acid and isotussilaginic acid and their 1-epimers in *Arnica* species and *Tussilago farfara*. *Phytochem* 1992; 31: 4135–4137.

6 Leven W, Willuhn G. Spectrophotometric determination of sesquiterpenlactone (S1) in 'Arnicae flos DAB 9' with m-dinitrobenzene. *Planta Med* 1986; 52: 537–538.

7 Schmidt Th *et al*. First diterpenes from *Arnica*. *Planta Med* 1992; 58: A713.

8 Lee K-H *et al*. Structure–antimicrobial activity relationships among the sesquiterpene lactones and related compounds. *Phytochemistry* 1977; 16: 117–118.

9 Woerdenbag HJ *et al*. Cytotoxicity of flavonoids and sesquiterpene lactones from *Arnica* species against the GLC_4 and the COLO 320 cell lines. *Planta Med* 1994; 60: 434–437.

10 Woerdenbag HJ *et al*. Decreased helenalin-induced cytotoxicity by flavonoids from *Arnica* as studied in a human lung carcinoma cell line. *Phytomedicine* 1995; 2: 127–132.

11 Mascolo N *et al*. Biological screening of Italian medicinal plants for anti-inflammatory activity. *Phytother Res* 1987; 1: 28–31.

12 Hall IH *et al*. Mode of action of sesquiterpene lactones as anti-inflammatory agents. *J Pharm Sci* 1980; 69: 537–543.

13 Hall IH *et al*. Anti-inflammatory activity of sesquiterpene lactones and related compounds. *J Pharm Sci* 1979; 68: 537–542.

14 Schröder H *et al*. Helenalin and 11α,13-dihydrohelenalin, two constituents from *Arnica montana* L., inhibit human platelet function via thiol-dependent pathways. *Thrombosis Res* 1990; 57: 839–845.

15 Chang HM *et al*. *Advances in Chinese Medicinal Materials Research*. Philadelphia: World Scientific, 1985.

16 Puhlmann J, Wagner H. Immunologically active polysaccharides from *Arnica montana* herbs and tissue cultures. *Planta Med* 1989; 55: 99.

17 Rudzki E, Grzywa Z. Dermatitis from *Arnica montana*. *Contact Dermatitis* 1977; 3: 281–282.

18 Hausen BM. Identification of the allergens of *Arnica montana* L. *Contact Dermatitis* 1978; 4: 308.

Artichoke

Summary and Pharmaceutical Comment

Globe artichoke is characterised by the phenolic acid constituents, in particular cynarin. Experimental studies (*in vitro* and *in vivo*) support some of the reputed uses of artichoke. Traditionally, the choleretic and cholesterol-lowering activities of globe artichoke have been attributed to cynarin. However, studies in animals and humans have suggested that these effects may in fact be due to the monocaffeoylquinic acids present in globe artichoke (e.g. chlorogenic and neochlorogenic acids). Clinical trials investigating the use of globe artichoke and cynarin in the treatment of hyperlipidaemia generally report positive results. However, further rigorous clinical trials are required to establish the benefit of globe artichoke leaf extract as a lipid- and cholesterol-lowering agent. Hepatoprotective and hepatoregenerating activities have been documented for cynarin *in vitro* and in animals (rats). However, these effects have not yet been documented in clinical studies.

Species (Family)

Cynara scolymus L. (Asteraceae/Compositae)

Synonym(s)

Globe Artichoke.

Globe artichoke should not be confused with Jerusalem artichoke, which is the tuber of *Helianthus tuberosus* L.

Part(s) Used

Leaf

Pharmacopoeial and Other Monographs

BHP 1996[G9]
BP 2007[G84]
Complete German Commission E[G3]
Martindale 35th edition[G85]
Ph Eur 2007[G81]

Legal Category (Licensed Products)

GSL[G37]

Constituents

The following is compiled from several sources, including References 1 and 2, and General Reference G41.

Acids Phenolic, up to 2%. Caffeic acid, mono- and dicaffeoylquinic acid derivatives, e.g. cynarin (1,5-di-O-caffeoylquinic acids) and chlorogenic acid (mono derivative).

Flavonoids 0.1–1%. Flavone glycosides, e.g. luteolin-7β-rutinoside (scolymoside), luteolin-7β-D-glucoside and luteolin-4β-D-glucoside.

Volatile oils Sesquiterpenes β-selinene and caryophyllene (major); also eugenol, phenylacetaldehyde, decanal, oct-1-en-3-one, hex-1-en-3-one, and non-*trans*-2-enal.

Other constituents Phytosterols (taraxasterol and β-taraxasterol), tannins, glycolic and glyceric acids, sugars, inulin, enzymes including peroxidases,[3] cynaropicrin and other sesquiterpene lactones, e.g. grosheimin, cynarotriol.[4,5] The root and fully developed fruits and flowers are devoid of cynaropicrin; highest content reported in young leaves.[6]

Food Use

Artichoke is listed by the Council of Europe as a natural source of food flavouring (category N2). This category indicates that artichoke can be added to foodstuffs in small quantities, with a possible limitation of an active principle (as yet unspecified) in the

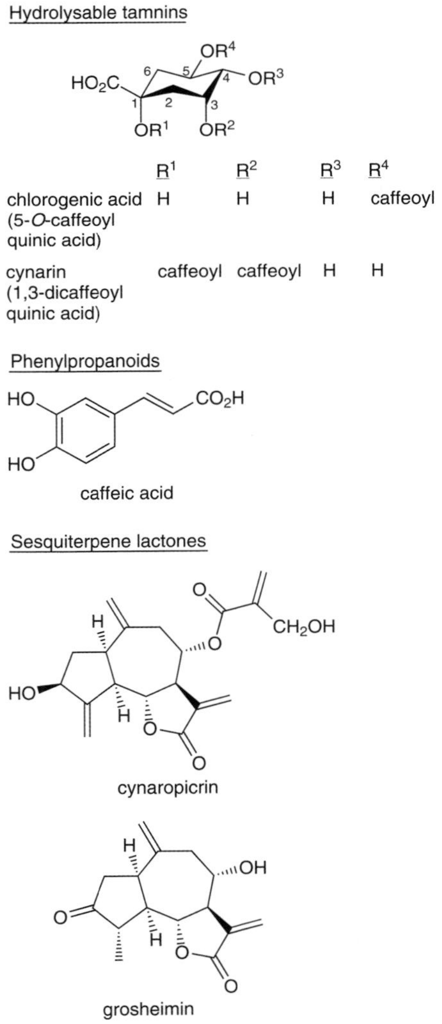

Hydrolysable tamnins

	R^1	R^2	R^3	R^4
chlorogenic acid (5-*O*-caffeoyl quinic acid)	H	H	H	caffeoyl
cynarin (1,3-dicaffeoyl quinic acid)	caffeoyl	caffeoyl	H	H

Phenylpropanoids

caffeic acid

Sesquiterpene lactones

cynaropicrin

grosheimin

Figure 1 Selected constituents of artichoke.

final product.[G16] Previously, in the USA, artichoke leaves were approved for use in alcoholic beverages only, with an average maximum concentration of 0.0016% (16 ppm).[G41]

Herbal Use

Artichoke is stated to possess diuretic, choleretic, hypocholesterolaemic, hypolipidaemic, and hepatostimulating properties.[7–9] Modern use of artichoke is focused on its use in the treatment of hyperlipidaemia, hyperlipoproteinaemia, non-ulcer dyspepsia and conditions requiring an increase in choleresis. There is also interest in the potential hepatoprotective properties of globe artichoke, although this has not yet been tested in controlled clinical trials.[10,11]

Dosage

The German Commission E recommended an average daily dose of 6 g drug, or an equivalent dose of extract (based on the herb-to-extract ratio) or other preparations, for dyspeptic problems.[G3,G56] A recommended dosage regimen for liquid extract (1 : 2) is 3–8 mL daily.[G50]

Dosages used in clinical trials of globe artichoke leaf extract have assessed the effects of dosages of up to 1.92 g daily in divided doses for up to six months.[12]

Pharmacological Actions

Several pharmacological properties have been documented for artichoke leaf, including inhibition of cholesterol biosynthesis, hypolipidaemic, antioxidant and hepatoprotective activity. It remains unclear which of the constituents of artichoke are responsible for its pharmacological activities. The dicaffeoylquinic acids, which include cynarin, are likely to be an important group of constituents in this respect.[11,G50] The sesquiterpene lactones, such as cynaropicrin, and flavonoids, such as luteolin glycoside, may also exert biological effects.[11]

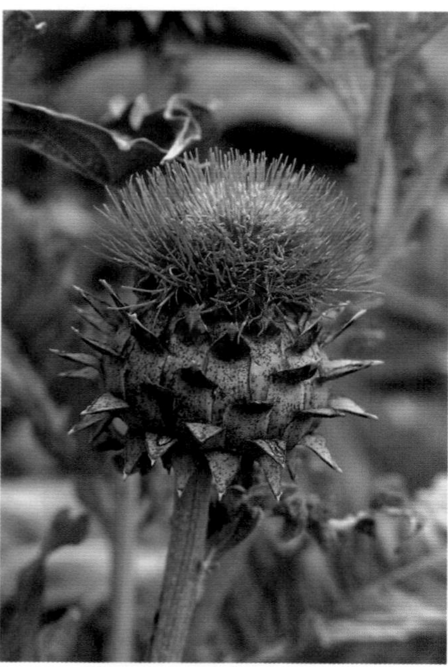

Figure 2 Artichoke (*Cynara scolymus*).

In vitro and animal studies

Hypolipidaemic, hypocholesterolaemic and choleretic activity

Hypolipidaemic, hypocholesterolaemic and choleretic activities are well documented for globe artichoke leaf extract and particularly for the constituent cynarin.[10,11] Globe artichoke leaf extract not only increases choleresis and, therefore, cholesterol elimination, but also has been shown to inhibit cholesterol biosynthesis.[10] Preparations of globe artichoke leaf extract inhibit cholesterol biosynthesis in a concentration-dependent manner in studies in cultured rat hepatocytes.[13,14] Low concentrations (<0.1 mg/mL) of globe artichoke extract achieved around 20% inhibition, whereas 65% inhibition was noted with concentrations of 1 mg/mL. Luteolin was considered to be one of the most important constituents for this effect, and it was suggested that a possible mechanism of action might be indirect inhibition of hydroxymethylglutaryl-CoA reductase (HMG-CoA).[14] Other *in vitro* studies have documented a concentration-dependent inhibition of *de novo* cholesterol biosynthesis in cultured rat and human hepatocytes for globe artichoke leaf extract 0.03–0.1 mg/mL.[15]

Several other experimental studies have documented lipid-lowering effects for globe artichoke leaf extract and cynarin *in vivo*.[10,11] A study in rats explored the hypocholesterolaemic, hypolipidaemic and choleretic effects of purified (containing 46% caffeoylquinic acids, calculated as chlorogenic acid) and total extracts of globe artichoke leaf (containing 19% caffeoylquinic

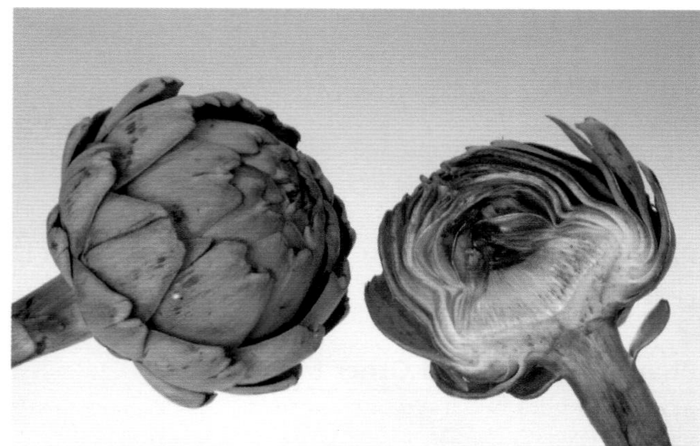

Figure 3 Artichoke.

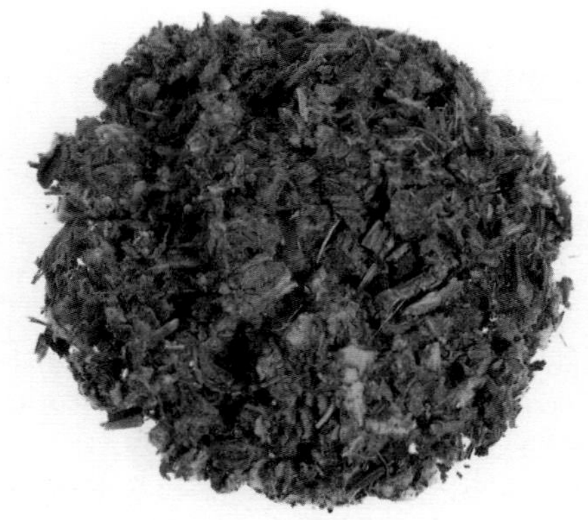

Figure 4 Artichoke – dried drug substance (leaf).

acids, calculated as chlorogenic acid).[7] The purified extract was found to be more potent than the total artichoke extract: purified extract 25 mg/kg intraperitoneally reduced plasma triglyceride and cholesterol concentrations by 33% and 45%, respectively, whereas reductions of only 18% and 14%, respectively, were observed with the total extract (100 mg/kg intraperitoneally).[7] Both purified (25 mg/kg intraperitoneally) and total extract (200 mg/kg intraperitoneally) significantly enhanced bile secretion following treatment, compared with baseline values; the increase in bile secretion seen with the purified extract was still statistically significant three hours after treatment. The more potent pharmacological activities observed with the purified extract were attributed to the higher concentration of monocaffeoylquinic acids (e.g. chlorogenic, neochlorogenic) compared with dicaffeoylquinic acids (e.g. cynarin) present.

Another study investigated the effects of cynarin on total cholesterol concentrations in serum and liver of rats given ethanol (6 g/kg/day by gavage over three days).[16] In rats given ethanol alone, serum cholesterol concentrations rose significantly by 44%, compared with controls ($p < 0.01$). Rats given ethanol plus cynarin (30 mg/kg intraperitoneally 30 minutes before gavage) showed a significant reduction in serum cholesterol concentrations, compared with controls ($p < 0.05$).

Antioxidant and hepatoprotective activity *In vitro*, a luteolin-rich globe artichoke leaf aqueous extract (flavonoid content around 0.4% w/w) retarded low-density lipoprotein (LDL) oxidation in a concentration-dependent manner (determined by a prolongation of the lag phase to conjugated diene formation).[17] The same tests carried out with the pure aglycone luteolin at concentrations of 0.1–1 μmol/L showed that this constituent had a similar concentration-dependent effect on LDL oxidation in this model. Luteolin-7-O-glucoside also demonstrated a concentration-dependent reduction in LDL oxidation, but was less potent than luteolin.

Several *in vitro* and *in vivo* studies have investigated the antioxidative and hepatoprotective properties of globe artichoke leaf extracts, and their constituents, against liver cell damage induced by different hepatotoxins.

The hepatoprotective effect of polyphenolic compounds isolated from artichoke has been investigated *in vitro* using rat hepatocytes.[8] Cynarin was the only compound reported to exhibit significant cytoprotective activity, with a lesser action demonstrated by caffeic acid. A standardised extract of globe artichoke (Hepar-SL forte) significantly inhibited the formation of malondialdehyde induced by *tert*-butylhydroperoxide (*t*-BHP) in a concentration-dependent manner within 40 minutes of incubation, compared with control.[18] The protective antioxidant effect of globe artichoke was reported to be significant, compared with control, even at a concentration of 1 μg/mL. A reduction in *t*-BHP-induced cell death with globe artichoke extract was also observed. Further studies assessed the antioxidative and protective potential of the same extract (Hepar-SL forte) in cultures of primary rat hepatocytes exposed to *t*-BHP.[19] Incubation of cultured hepatocytes with globe artichoke extract and *t*-BHP inhibited *t*-BHP-induced malondialdehyde formation in a concentration-dependent manner. Globe artichoke extract was significantly effective, compared with control, at concentrations down to 0.001 mg/mL. Furthermore, concentrations of globe artichoke extract down to 0.005 mg/mL significantly enhanced hepatocyte survival. The antioxidative effect of the extract was not affected by various pretreatments (including tryptic digestion, boiling and acidification), although it was sensitive to alkalinisation. Incubation with the globe artichoke constituents chlorogenic acid and cynarin resulted in significant inhibition, and incubation with both compounds was reported to have a synergistic effect, although an additive effect may be a more accurate description of the findings. Chlorogenic acid and cynarin were not solely responsible for the antioxidant effect, as reduction of malondialdehyde formation by the extract was at least twofold that seen with the chlorogenic acid and cynarin.[19] The antioxidative and hepatoprotective potential of globe artichoke extract was confirmed in other studies which also indicated that several constituents of the extract may contribute to the effects.[20]

The effects of globe artichoke leaf extract and its constituents have also been investigated for activity against oxidative stress in studies using human leukocytes.[21] Globe artichoke leaf extract demonstrated a concentration-dependent inhibition of oxidative stress induced by several agents, such as hydrogen peroxide and phorbol-12-myristate-13-acetate, that generate reactive oxygen species. The constituents cynarin, caffeic acid, chlorogenic acid and luteolin also showed concentration-dependent inhibitory activity in these models.

In vivo hepatoprotectivity against tetrachloromethane-induced hepatitis has been documented for globe artichoke leaf extract (500 mg/kg) administered orally to rats 48 hours, 24 hours and one hour before intoxication.[9] Concentrations of liver transaminases were significantly lower in rats given globe artichoke leaf extract, compared with those in controls. A hepatoregenerating effect has also been described for an aqueous extract of globe artichoke leaf administered orally to rats for three weeks following partial hepatectomy.[22] Regeneration was determined by stimulation of mitosis and increased weight in the residual liver when animals were sacrificed in globe artichoke-treated rats, compared with controls. In a similar study, aqueous extract of globe artichoke leaf (0.5 mL daily for five days preceding hepatectomy) was found to be more potent than a root extract.[23]

Clinical studies

Several clinical trials have explored the choleretic and hypolipidaemic properties of globe artichoke leaf extract, and its effects in patients with symptoms of dyspepsia. A randomised, double-blind, placebo-controlled, crossover trial involving 20 male volunteers assessed the choleretic effects of a single intraduodenal dose (1.92 g in 300 mL water) of the globe artichoke leaf extract Hepar-SL forte.[24] Intraduodenal bile secretion, the primary outcome variable, was measured using multichannel probes starting 30 minutes after drug administration and continuing for up to four hours afterwards. An increase in bile secretion was observed in both groups; maximal increases for globe artichoke leaf extract and placebo were 152% at 60 minutes after drug administration, and 40% at 30 minutes, respectively. Differences between globe artichoke leaf extract and placebo were statistically significant at 30, 60 and 90 minutes after drug administration ($p < 0.01$) and at 120 and 150 minutes after drug administration ($p < 0.05$). In another randomised controlled trial, 60 patients with dyspepsia received a combination preparation containing extracts of globe artichoke 50 mg, boldo (*Peumus boldus*) 30 mg and chelidonium (*Chelidonium majus*) 20 mg per tablet, or placebo, three times daily for 14 days.[25] The volume of bile secreted, measured using a duodenal probe, increased significantly in the treatment group, compared with the placebo group ($p < 0.01$). Also, an improvement in symptoms was reported for 50% of the treatment group, compared with 38% of the placebo group. There are also clinical studies in the older literature (some of which were placebo-controlled trials, whereas others were open, uncontrolled studies) which report choleretic effects with globe artichoke leaf extract. These trials have been summarised in several reviews.[10, 24, G50]

The effects of globe artichoke leaf extract have also been monitored in several postmarketing surveillance (phase IV) studies in patients with non-specific gastrointestinal complaints, including dyspepsia,[12] functional biliary tract complaints, constipation and gastric irritation.[11] The studies monitored the effects of globe artichoke leaf extract (Hepar-SL forte; one capsule contains 320 mg standardised aqueous extract; drug–extract ratio: 3.5 to 5.5 : 1) up to six capsules daily for six weeks[11] or six months.[12] Both studies reported improvements in clinical symptoms and reductions in serum total cholesterol and triglyceride concentrations, compared with baseline values. A subgroup analysis of 279 patients with at least three of five symptoms of irritable bowel syndrome reported significant reductions in the severity of symptoms and favourable evaluations of overall effectiveness by both physicians and participants.[26] The findings from postmarketing surveillance studies provide supporting data for the effects of globe artichoke leaf extract, but these are open studies and do not include a control group and, therefore, are not designed to assess efficacy.

The efficacy of globe artichoke leaf extract in patients with hyperlipoproteinaemia has been assessed in a randomised, double-blind, placebo-controlled, multicentre trial involving 143 patients with initial total cholesterol concentrations of >7.3 mmol/L (>280 mg/dL).[27] Participants received globe artichoke leaf extract (CY450; drug–extract ratio: 25 to 35 : 1) 1800 mg daily in two divided doses, or placebo, for six weeks. At the end of the study, mean total cholesterol concentrations had decreased by 18.5% to 6.31 mmol/L and by 8.6% to 7.03 mmol/L in the CY450 and placebo groups, respectively ($p < 0.0001$). CY450 treatment also led to a significant reduction in LDL cholesterol, compared with placebo ($p = 0.0001$). There was no difference between CY450 recipients and placebo recipients in blood concentrations of the liver enzyme gamma-glutamyltransferase (GGT).

A published abstract reports the findings of a previous randomised, double-blind, placebo-controlled trial of a globe artichoke leaf extract (Hepar-SL forte; 640 mg three times daily for 12 weeks) involving 44 healthy volunteers.[15] Mean baseline total cholesterol concentrations for participants in this study were low (placebo group: 203.0 mg/dL; globe artichoke extract group: 204.2 mg/dL). Subgroup analysis suggested lipid-lowering effects with globe artichoke extract for participants with baseline total cholesterol concentrations of >200 mg/dL. However, numbers of participants included in this analysis were small. The study indicates only that trials in patients with hyperlipoproteinaemia are required.

A series of three open, uncontrolled studies involved the administration of pressed globe artichoke juice (obtained from fresh leaves and flower buds) 10 mL three times daily for up to 12 weeks to a total of 84 patients with secondary hyperlipidaemia (total cholesterol ⩾260 mg/dL).[28] After six weeks' treatment, total cholesterol, LDL cholesterol and triglyceride concentrations decreased, whereas high-density lipoprotein cholesterol tended to increase. Another uncontrolled study involved the administration of cynarin to 17 patients with familial type IIa or type IIb hyperlipoproteinaemia for whom blood lipid concentrations were maintained with dietary treatment alone.[29] Cynarin was taken 15 minutes before meals at either 250 mg or 750 mg daily dose. Over a period of three months, cynarin was reported to have no effect on mean serum cholesterol and triglyceride concentrations.[29] The results were in agreement with the findings of some previous workers, but also in contrast to other studies that have reported cynarin to be effective in lowering serum concentrations of cholesterol and triglycerides when taken in daily doses ranging from 60 mg to 1500 mg.[29]

A Cochrane systematic review[30] of randomised, double-blind, placebo-controlled studies of artichoke preparations for hypercholesterolaemia included two studies (see above).[15, 27] The review concluded that there is limited evidence from randomised controlled trials to support the use of artichoke leaf preparations in hypercholesterolaemia and that such preparations cannot be recommended as a treatment option.

Side-effects, Toxicity

A randomised, double-blind, placebo-controlled trial involving 143 patients with hyperlipoproteinaemia reported a similar frequency of adverse events for globe artichoke leaf extract (CY450) and placebo groups.[27] A total of 28 adverse events were reported during the study, 26 of which related to mild changes in laboratory values. The relationship to the globe artichoke was considered to be 'unlikely' in all cases.

Postmarketing surveillance (phase IV) studies have monitored patients with non-specific gastrointestinal complaints receiving treatment with globe artichoke leaf extract (Hepar-SL forte; up to 1.92 g daily for six weeks[11] or six months[12]). In one study involving 533 patients with non-specific gastrointestinal complaints, including dyspepsia, functional biliary tract complaints, constipation and gastric irritation, seven adverse events (weakness, hunger, flatulence) were reported (1.3% of participants).[11] No serious adverse events were reported. A second postmarketing surveillance study involved 203 patients with symptoms of dyspepsia who received globe artichoke leaf extract up to 1.92 g daily for up to six months.[12] It was reported that no adverse events were recorded during the study, and that the physician's overall judgement of tolerability was given as 'good' or 'excellent' in 98.5% of cases.

Allergic contact dermatitis, with cross-sensitivity to other Compositae plants, has been documented for globe artichoke.[31, G51] A case of occupational contact urticaria syndrome in a 20-year-old woman has been reported in association with globe artichoke. The woman developed acute generalised urticaria, angioedema of the hands, forearms and face, and respiratory symptoms after handling globe artichokes. The clinical history and results of skin-prick tests indicated that the woman had developed type I allergy to globe artichoke antigen(s).[32] An isolated case of allergy to ingested globe artichoke has also been described.[33]

Cynaropicrin and other sesquiterpene lactones with allergenic potential have been isolated from globe artichoke.[31, G53] Purified globe artichoke extract is more toxic than a total extract. LD_{50} values (rat, by intraperitoneal injection) have been documented as greater than 1000 mg/kg (total extract) and 265 mg/kg (purified extract).[7]

Contra-indications, Warnings

Globe artichoke yields cynaropicrin, a potentially allergenic sesquiterpene lactone.[G51] Individuals with an existing hypersensitivity to any member of the Compositae family may develop an allergic reaction to globe artichoke.

Drug interactions None documented. However, the potential for preparations of artichoke to interact with other medicines administered concurrently, particularly those with similar or opposing effects, should be considered.

Pregnancy and lactation In view of the lack of toxicity data, excessive use of globe artichoke should be avoided during pregnancy and lactation.

Preparations

Proprietary single-ingredient preparations

Argentina: Alcachofa Plus; Chofitol; Cynarex. *Austria:* Cynarix; Hepar-POS. *Belgium:* Hebucol. *Brazil:* Chophytol. *France:* Chophytol; Hepanephrol. *Germany:* aar gamma N; Ardeycholan; Cefacynar; Cholagogum; Cynacur; Cynalip duo; Cynarix N; Hepagallin N; Hepar SL; Hepar-POS; Heparstad; Hewechol Artischockendragees; Lipei; Losapan; Natu-Hepa; Naturreiner; Valverde Artischocke. *Russia:* Chophytol (Хофитол). *Switzerland:* Chophytol; Hepa-S; Natu-Hepa.

Proprietary multi-ingredient preparations

Argentina: Arceligasol; Bagohepat; Bilidren; Biliosan Compuesto; Boldina; Dioxicolagol; HDG; Hepacur; Hepatalgina; Hepatalgina; Hepatodirectol; Metiogen; Palatrobil; Palatrobil. *Australia:* Extralife Liva-Care; Lifesystem Herbal Formula 7 Liver Tonic; Liver Tonic Herbal Formula 6; Livstim; Livton Complex. *Austria:* Cynarix comp. *Brazil:* Alcafelol; Alcaflor; Chofranina; Colachofra; Composto Emagrecedor; Digestron; Emagrevit; Figatil; Hecrosine B12; Hepatoregius; Jurubileno; Lisotox; Olocynan; Prinachol; Solvobil. *Canada:* Milk Thistle. *Czech Republic:* Cynarosan. *France:* Actibil; Canol; Elixir Spark; Hepaclem; Hepax. *Germany:* Carmol Magen-Galle-Darm; Cynarzym N; Gallexier; Gallexier. *Hong Kong:* Hepatofalk. *Italy:* Colax; Digelax; Epagest. *Malaysia:* Dandelion Complex. *Mexico:* Chofabol; Hepedren; Ifuchol. *Russia:* Herbion Drops for the Gallbladder (Гербион Капли Желчегонные). *Spain:* Cynaro Bilina; Lipograsil; Menabil Complex; Nico Hepatocyn. *Switzerland:* Bilifuge; Boldocynara; Demonatur Gouttes pour le foie et la bile; Heparfelien; Strath Gouttes pour le foie et la bile; Tisane hepatique et biliaire. *UK:* Bio-Strath Artichoke Formula; Boots Alternatives Easy Digest. *USA:* Ultimate Antioxidant Formula.

References

1 Brand N. Cynara scolymus L. – Die Artischocke. *Z Phytother* 1990; 11: 169–175.
2 Hammouda FM *et al.* Quantitative determination of the active constituents in Egyptian cultivated *Cynara scolymus*. *Int J Pharmacog* 1993; 31: 299–304.
3 Kamel MY, Ghazy AM. Peroxidases of *Cyanara scolymus* (global artichoke) leaves: purification and properties. *Acta Biol Med Germ* 1973; 31: 39–49.
4 Jouany JM *et al.* Dosage indirect de la cynaropicrine dans la *Cynara scolymus* (Compositae) par libération de sa chaîne latérale hydroxyméthylacrylique. *Plant Méd Phytothér* 1975; 9: 72–78.
5 Barbetti P *et al.* Grosulfeimin and new related guaianolides from *Cynara scolymus* L. *Ars Pharmac* 1992; 33: 433–439.
6 Schneider G, Thiele Kl. Die Verteilung des Bitterstoffes Cynaropicrin in der Artischocke. *Planta Med* 1974; 26: 174–183.
7 Lietti A. Choleretic and cholesterol lowering properties of two artichoke extracts. *Fitoterapia* 1977; 48: 153–158.
8 Adzet T *et al.* Hepatoprotective activity of polyphenolic compounds from *Cynara scolymus* against CCl_4 toxicity in isolated rat hepatocytes. *J Nat Prod* 1987; 50: 612–617.
9 Adzet T *et al.* Action of an artichoke extract against CCl_4-induced heptotoxicity in rats. *Acta Pharm Jugosl* 1987; 37: 183–187.
10 Kraft K. Artichoke leaf extract – recent findings reflecting effects on lipid metabolism, liver and gastrointestinal tracts. *Phytomedicine* 1997; 4: 369–378.
11 Fintelmann V, Menssen HG. Artichoke leaf extract. Current knowledge concerning its efficacy as a lipid-reducer and antidyspeptic agent. *Dtsch Apoth Ztg* 1996; 136: 1405–1414.
12 Fintelmann V, Petrowicz O. Long-term administration of an artichoke extract for dyspepsia symptoms. Results of an observational study. *Natura Med* 1998; 13: 17–26.
13 Gebhardt R. Artischockenextrakt. In vitro Nachweis einer Hemmwirkung auf die Cholesterin-Biosynthese. *Med Welt* 1995; 46: 348–350.
14 Gebhardt R. Inhibition of cholesterol biosynthesis in primary cultured rat hepatocytes by artichoke (*Cynara scolymus* L.) extracts. *J Pharmacol Exp Ther* 1998; 286: 1122–1128.
15 Petrowicz O *et al.* Effects of artichoke leaf extract (ALE) on lipoprotein metabolism *in vitro* and *in vivo*. *Atherosclerosis* 1997; 129: 147.
16 Wójcicki J. Effect of 1,5-dicaffeylquinic acid (Cynarine) on cholesterol levels in serum and liver of acute ethanol-treated rats. *Drug Alcohol Depend* 1978; 3: 143–145.
17 Brown JE, Rice-Evans CA. Luteolin-rich artichoke extract protects low density lipoprotein from oxidation *in vitro*. *Free Radic Res* 1998; 29: 247–255.
18 Gebhardt R. Protektive antioxidative Wirkungen von Artischocken-extrakt an der Leberzelle. *Med Welt* 1995; 46: 393–395.
19 Gebhardt R. Antioxidative and protective properties of extracts from leaves of the artichoke (*Cynara scolymus* L.) against hydroperoxide-induced oxidative stress in cultured rat hepatocytes. *Toxicol Appl Pharmacol* 1997; 144: 279–286.
20 Gebhardt R, Fausel M. Antioxidant and hepatoprotective effects of artichoke extracts and constituents in cultured rat hepatocytes. *Toxicology in Vitro* 1997; 11: 669–672.
21 Perez-Garcia F *et al.* Activity of artichoke leaf extract on reactive oxygen species in human leukocytes. *Free Radic Res* 2000; 33: 661–665.
22 Maros T *et al.* Wirkungen der *Cynara scolymus*-Extrakte auf die Regeneration der Rattenleber. *Arzneimittelforschung* 1966; 16: 127–129.
23 Maros T *et al.* Wirkungen der *Cynara scolymus*-extrakte auf die Regeneration der Rattenleber. *Arzneimittelforschung* 1968; 18: 884–886.
24 Kirchhoff R *et al.* Increase in choleresis by means of artichoke extract. *Phytomedicine* 1994; 1: 107–115.
25 Kupke D *et al.* Prüfung der choleretischen Aktivität eines pflanzlichen Cholagogums. *Z Allg Med* 1991; 67: 1046–1058.
26 Walker A *et al.* Artichoke leaf extract reduces symptoms of irritable bowel syndrome in a post-marketing surveillance study. *Phytother Res* 2001; 15: 58–61.
27 Englisch W *et al.* Efficacy of artichoke dry extract in patients with hyperlipoproteinemia. *Arzneim-Forsch/Drug Res* 2000; 50: 260–265.
28 Dorn M. Improvement in raised lipid levels with artichoke juice (*Cynara scolymus* L.). *Br J Phytother* 1995/96; 4: 21–26.
29 Heckers H *et al.* Inefficiency of cynarin as therapeutic regimen in familial type II hyperlipoproteinaemia. *Atherosclerosis* 1977; 26: 249–253.
30 Pittler MH *et al.* Artichoke leaf extract for treating hypercholesterolaemia (Review). Cochrane Database of Systematic Reviews issue 3, 2002. London: Macmillan.
31 Meding B. Allergic contact dermatitis from artichoke, *Cynara scolymus*. *Contact Dermatitis* 1983; 9: 314.
32 Quirce S *et al.* Occupational contact urticaria syndrome caused by globe artichoke (*Cynara scolymus*). *J Allergy Clin Immunol* 1996; 97: 710–711.
33 Romano C *et al.* A case of allergy to globe artichoke and other clinical cases of rare food allergy. *J Invest Allergol Clin Immunol* 2000; 10: 102–104.

Asafoetida

Summary and Pharmaceutical Comment

Asafoetida is a complex oleo gum resin consisting of many constituents that vary according to the different species used. Asafoetida is commonly used in foods but little scientific evidence is available to justify the herbal uses. In view of the known pharmacologically active constituents, asafoetida should not be taken in amounts exceeding those used in foods.

Species (Family)

There are reportedly 172 species of *Ferula*. The main source is believed to be from *Ferula assafoetida* L. and *Ferula foetida* (Bunge) Regel.

Synonym(s)

Asafetida, Asant, Devil's Dung, *Ferula foetida* (Bunge) Regel, Gum Asafetida

Part(s) Used

Oleo gum resin obtained by incising the living rhizomes and roots.

Pharmacopoeial and Other Monographs

BHC 1992[G6]
BHP 1996[G9]
Martindale 35th edition[G85]

Legal Category (Licensed Products)

GSL[G37]

Constituents

The following is compiled from several sources, including General References G6, G59 and G62.

Gum fraction 25%. Glucose, galactose, L-arabinose, rhamnose and glucuronic acid.

Resins 40–64%. Ferulic acid esters (60%), free ferulic acid (1.3%), asaresinotannols and farnesiferols A, B and C, coumarin derivatives (e.g. umbelliferone), coumarin–sesquiterpene complexes (e.g. asacoumarin A and asacoumarin B).[1] Free ferulic acid is converted to coumarin during dry distillation.

Volatile oils 3–17%. Sulfur-containing compounds with disulfides as major components, various monoterpenes.[1]

The oleo gum resins of different *Ferula* species are not identical and many papers have documented their phytochemistry,[2–11] reporting polysulfanes,[2–11] complex acetylenes,[3] phenylpropanoids[7] and many sesquiterpene derivatives.[2, 4–6, 8, 9]

C-3 prenylated 4-hydroxycoumarin derivatives (e.g. ferulenol) are thought to represent the toxic principles in the species *Ferula communis*.[12]

Food Use

Asafoetida is used widely in foods. Asafoetida (essential oil, fluid extract and gommo-oleoresin) is listed by the Council of Europe as a source of natural food flavouring (category 5) (*see* Appendix 3).[G17] Previously, asafoetida was approved for food use in the USA.[G41]

Herbal Use

Asafoetida is stated to possess carminative, antispasmodic and expectorant properties. It has been used for chronic bronchitis, pertussis, laryngismus stridulus, hysteria and specifically for intestinal flatulent colic.[G6, G7]

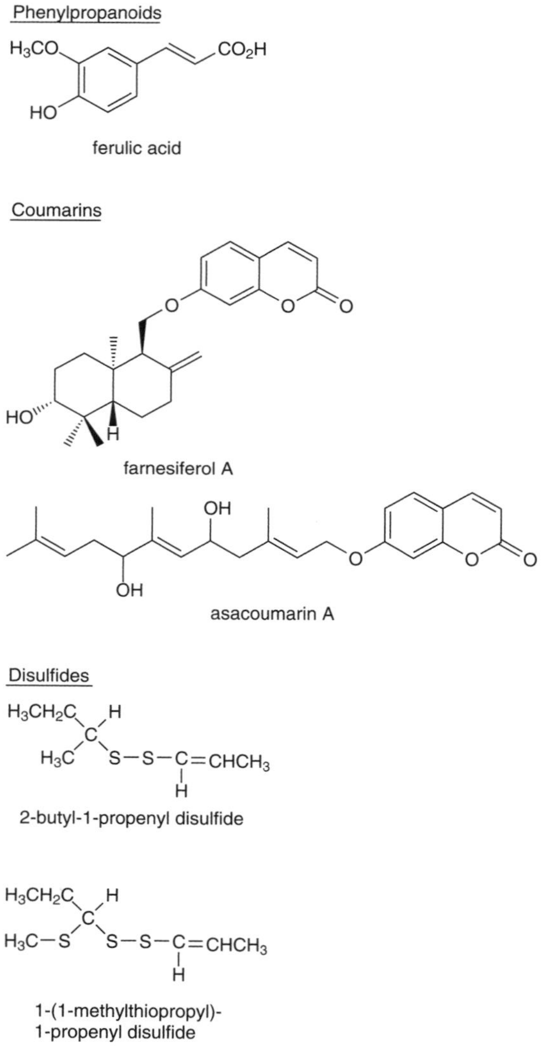

Phenylpropanoids
ferulic acid

Coumarins
farnesiferol A
asacoumarin A

Disulfides
2-butyl-1-propenyl disulfide
1-(1-methylthiopropyl)-1-propenyl disulfide

Figure 1 Selected constituents of asafoetida.

Dosage

Dosages for oral administration (adults) for traditional uses recommended in older standard herbal and pharmaceutical reference texts are given below.

Powdered resin 0.3–1 g three times daily[G6, G7]

Tincture of asafoetida (BPC 1949) 2–4 mL

Pharmacological Actions

In vitro and animal studies

Asafoetida has been reported to possess anticoagulant and hypotensive properties,[G41] although the scientific basis for these statements is not clear; coumarin constituents detected so far in asafoetida do not possess minimum structural requirements for anticoagulant activity. Asafoetida is an ingredient of a plant mixture reported to have antidiabetic properties in rats.[13] However, when the individual components of the mixture were studied asafoetida was devoid of antidiabetic effect with myrrh and aloe gum extracts representing the active hypoglycaemic principles.[14]

Oestrogenic activity in rats has been documented for carotane sesquiterpenes and ferujol (a coumarin) isolated from *Ferula jaeschkeana*.[15, 16]

Clinical studies

Clinical investigation of asafoetida is limited and rigorous randomised controlled clinical trials are required. A protective action against fat-induced hyperlipidaemia has been documented for asafoetida and attributed to the sulfur compounds in the volatile oil fraction of the resin.[17] Two double-blind studies have reported significant effects for asafoetida in the treatment of irritable bowel syndrome[18, 19]

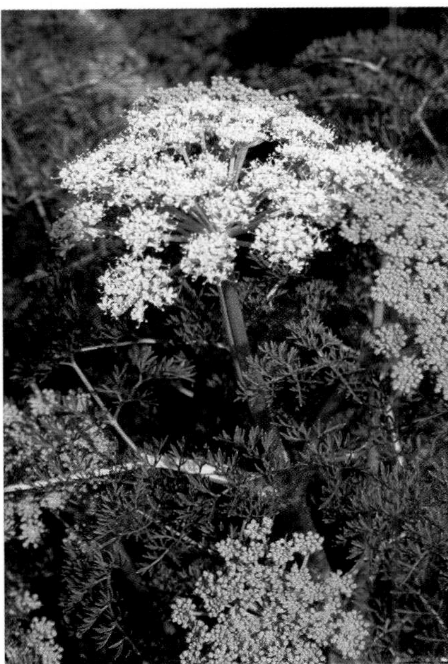

Figure 2 Asafoetida (*Ferula assafoetida*).

Side-effects, Toxicity

Asafoetida is documented to be relatively non-toxic; ingestion of 15 g produced no untoward effects.[G45] A report of methaemoglobinaemia has been associated with the administration of asafoetida (in milk) to a five-week-old infant for the treatment of colic.[20] Asafoetida was found to exert an oxidising effect on fetal haemoglobin but not on adult haemoglobin.

Coumarin constituents detected so far in asafoetida do not possess minimum structural requirements (a C-4 hydroxyl substituent and a C-3 non-polar carbon substituent)[G87] for anticoagulant activity.

A weak sister chromatid exchange-inducing effect in mouse spermatogonia[21] and clastogenicity in mouse spermatocytes[22] has been documented for asafoetida. Chromosomal damage by asafoetida has been associated with the coumarin constituents.

Toxic coumarin constituents of a related species, *Ferula communis*, have been documented to reduce prothrombin concentrations and to cause haemorrhaging in livestock.[23, G51]

Two other species, *Ferula galbaniflua* and *Ferula rubicaulis*, are stated to contain a gum that is rubefacient and irritant, causing contact dermatitis in sensitive individuals.[G51, G58]

Contra-indications, Warnings

Asafoetida should not be given to infants because of the oxidising effect on fetal haemoglobin resulting in methaemoglobinaemia.[20] The gum of some *Ferula* species is reported to be irritant and therefore may cause gastrointestinal irritation or induce contact dermatitis in some individuals.

Drug interactions None documented. However, the potential for preparations of asafoetida to interact with other medicines administered concurrently, particularly those with similar or opposing effects, should be considered.

Pregnancy and lactation Asafoetida has a folkloric reputation as an abortifacient and an emmenagogue.[G30] However the use of asafoetida during pregnancy is probably acceptable, provided doses do not exceed amounts normally ingested in foods. In view of the toxic effect to infants (e.g. methaemoglobinaemia), asafoetida should be avoided during breastfeeding.

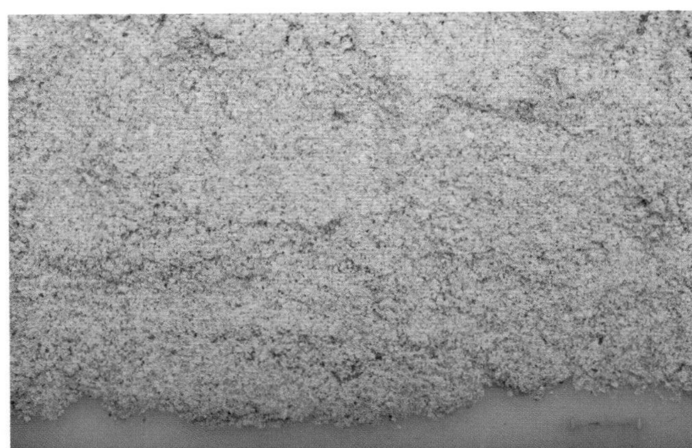

Figure 3 Asafoetida – dried drug substance (resin).

A

Preparations

Proprietary single-ingredient preparations

South Africa: Duiwelsdrekdruppels.

Proprietary multi-ingredient preparations

India: Tummy Ease. *South Africa:* Entressdruppels HM; Stuidruppels. *Thailand:* Flatulence Gastulence. *UK:* Daily Tension & Strain Relief; Nerfood Tablets.

References

1 Kajimoto T *et al.* Sesquiterpenoid and disulphide derivatives from *Ferula assa-foetida. Phytochemistry* 1989; 28: 1761–1763.

2 Dawidar A-A *et al.* Marmaricin, a new sesquiterpenoid coumarin from *Ferula marmarica* L. *Chem Pharm Bull* 1979; 27: 3153–3155.

3 de Pascual Teresa J *et al.* Complex acetylenes from the roots of *Ferula communis. Planta Med* 1986; 52: 458–462.

4 Miski M. Fercoperol, an unusual cyclic-endoperoxynerolidol derivative from *Ferula communis* subsp. *communis. J Nat Prod* 1986; 49: 916–918.

5 Garg SN *et al.* Feruginidin and ferugin, two new sesquiterpenoids based on the carotane skeleton from *Ferula jaeschkeana. J Nat Prod* 1987; 50: 253–255.

6 Garg SN *et al.* New sesquiterpenes from *Ferula jaeschkeana. Planta Med* 1987; 53: 341–342.

7 Gonzalez AG *et al.* Phenylpropanoid and stilbene compounds from *Ferula latipinna. Planta Med* 1988; 54: 184–185.

8 Miski M. New daucane and germacrane esters from *Ferula orientalis* var. *orientalis. J Nat Prod* 1987; 50: 829–834.

9 Miski M. New daucane esters from *Ferula tingitana. J Nat Prod* 1986; 49: 657–660.

10 Samimi MN and Unger W. Die gummiharze afghanischer asa foetida-liefernder ferula-arten. Beobachtungen zur herkunft und qualität afghanischer asa foetida. *Planta Med* 1979; 36: 128–133.

11 Zhi-da M *et al.* Polysulfanes in the volatile oils of *Ferula* species. *Planta Med* 1987; 53: 300–302.

12 Valle MG *et al.* Prenylated coumarins and sesquiterpenoids from *Ferula communis. Phytochemistry* 1987; 26: 253–256.

13 Al-Awadi FM *et al.* On the mechanism of the hypoglycaemic effect of a plant extract. *Diabetologia* 1985; 28: 432–434.

14 Al-Awadi FM, Gumaa KA. Studies on the activity of individual plants of an antidiabetic plant mixture. *Acta Diabetol Lat* 1987; 24: 37–41.

15 Singh MM *et al.* Contraceptive efficacy and hormonal profile of ferujol: a new coumarin from *Ferula jaeschkeana. Planta Med* 1985; 51: 268–270.

16 Singh MM *et al.* Antifertility and hormonal properties of certain carotane sesquiterpenes of *Ferula jaeschkeana. Planta Med* 1988; 54: 492–494.

17 Bordia A, Arora SK. The effect of essential oil (active principle) of asafoetida on alimentary lipemia. *Indian J Med Res* 1975; 63: 707–711.

18 Rahlfs VW, Mössinger P. Zur Behandlung des Colon irritabile. *Arzneimittelforschung* 1976; 26: 2230–2234.

19 Rahlfs VW, Mössinger P. Asafoetida bei colon irritabile. *Dtsch med Wochenschr* 1978; 104: 140–143.

20 Kelly KJ *et al.* Methemoglobinemia in an infant treated with the folk remedy glycerited asafoetida. *Pediatrics* 1984; 73: 717–719.

21 Abraham SK, Kesavan PC. Genotoxicity of garlic, turmeric and asafoetida in mice. *Mutat Res* 1984; 136: 85–88.

22 Walia K. Effect of asafoetida (7-hydroxycoumarin) on mouse spermatocytes. *Cytologia* 1973; 38: 719–724.

23 Aragno M *et al.* Experimental studies on the toxicity of *Ferula communis* in the rat. *Res Commun Chem Pathol Pharmacol* 1973; 59: 399–402.

Avens

Summary and Pharmaceutical Comment

Limited phytochemical or pharmacological data are available for avens, although reported tannin constituents would indicate an astringent action thus supporting the traditional use in diarrhoea and haemorrhage. In view of the lack of toxicity data, excessive use should be avoided.

Species (Family)

Geum urbanum L. (Rosaceae)

Synonym(s)

Benedict's Herb, Colewort, Geum, Herb Bennet, Wood Avens

Part(s) Used

Herb

Pharmacopoeial and Other Monographs

BHP 1983[G7]

Legal Category (Licensed Products)

Avens is not included in the GSL.[G37]

Constituents

The following is compiled from several sources, including General References G40, G49, G64.

Limited information is available on the herb. Constituents reported include bitter principles, resin, tannins and volatile oil.

Other plant parts

The root has been more extensively studied and is reported to contain a phenolic glycoside (gein), yielding eugenol as the aglycone and vicianose (disaccharide) as the sugar component;[1] 30% tannin, including gallic, caffeic and chlorogenic acids (pseudotannins generally associated with condensed tannins);[1] a bitter substance, a flavonoid, and volatile oil.

Food Use

Avens is listed by the Council of Europe as a natural source of food flavouring (category N2). This category indicates that avens can be added to foodstuffs in small quantities, with a possible limitation of an active principle (as yet unspecified) in the final product.[G16]

Phenylpropanoids

H_3CO, HO

eugenol

Figure 1 Selected constituents of avens.

Herbal Use

Avens is stated to possess antidiarrhoeal, antihaemorrhagic, and febrifugal properties. It has been used for diarrhoea, catarrhal colitis, passive uterine haemorrhage, intermittent fevers, and specifically for ulcerative colitis.[G7, G64]

Dosage

Dosages for oral administration (adults) for traditional uses recommended in older standard herbal reference texts are given below.

Dried herb 1–4 g as an infusion three times daily.[G7]

Liquid extract 1–4 mL (1 : 1 in 25% alcohol) three times daily.[G7]

Pharmacological Actions

In vitro and animal studies

A 20% aqueous decoction of avens, administered by intravenous injection, has been reported to produce a reduction in blood

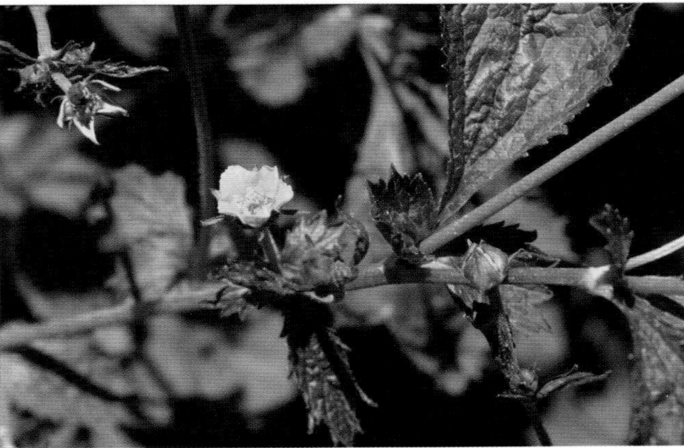

Figure 2 Avens (*Geum urbanum*).

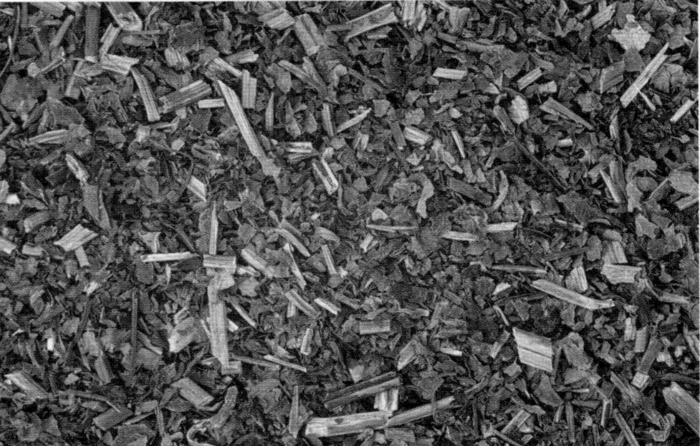

Figure 3 Avens – dried drug substance (herb).

pressure in cats.[2] Tannins are generally known to possess astringent properties.

Clinical studies

None documented.

Side-effects, Toxicity

None documented.

Contra-indications, Warnings

In view of the reported tannin constituents and the lack of toxicity data, it is advisable to avoid excessive use of avens.

Drug interactions None documented.

Pregnancy and lactation Avens is reputed to affect the menstrual cycle.[G30] In view of the lack of phytochemical, pharmacological and toxicological data, the use of avens during pregnancy should be avoided.

References

1 Psenák M *et al*. Biochemical Study on *Geum urbanum*. *Planta Med* 1970; 19: 154–159.

2 Petkov V. Plants and hypotensive, antiatheromatous and coronarodilating action. *Am J Chin Med* 1979; 7: 197–236.

Bayberry

Summary and Pharmaceutical Comment

Limited chemical information is available for bayberry. Documented tannin constituents justify some of the herbal uses. In addition, mineralocorticoid activity has been reported for one of the triterpene constituents. In view of this and the tannin constituents, excessive use of bayberry should be avoided.

Species (Family)

Myrica cerifera L. (Myricaceae)

Synonym(s)

Candleberry Bark, Myrica, Southern Bayberry, Southern Wax Myrtle, Wax Myrtle Bark

Part(s) Used

Root bark

Pharmacopoeial and Other Monographs

BHP 1996[(G9)]
Martindale 35th edition[(G85)]

Legal Category (Licensed Products)

GSL[(G37)]

Constituents

The following is compiled from several sources, including General References G22, G41, G48 and G64.

Flavonoids Myricitrin.

Tannins 3.9% (bark), 34.82% (total aqueous extract).

Terpenoids Myricadiol, taraxerol and taraxerone.[(1)]

Other constituents Albumen, red dye, gum, resin, starch, wax containing palmitic, myristic and lauric acid esters.

Food Use

Bayberry is not used in foods.

Herbal Use

Bayberry is stated to possess antipyretic, circulatory stimulant, emetic and mild diaphoretic properties. It has been used for diarrhoea, colds and specifically for mucous colitis. An infusion has been used as a gargle for a sore throat, and as a douche for leucorrhoea. Powdered root bark has been applied topically for the management of indolent ulcers.[(G7, G41, G64)]

Dosage

Dosages for oral administration (adults) for traditional uses recommended in older standard herbal reference texts are given below.

Powdered bark 0.6–2.0 g by infusion or decoction three times daily.[(G7)]

Liquid extract 0.6–2.0 mL (1 : 1 in 45% alcohol) three times daily.[(G7)]

Pharmacological Actions

In vitro and animal studies

Myricitrin has been reported to exhibit choleretic, bactericidal, paramecicidal, and spermatocidal activity; myricadiol has mineralocorticoid activity.[(G41)] Tannins are known to possess astringent properties.

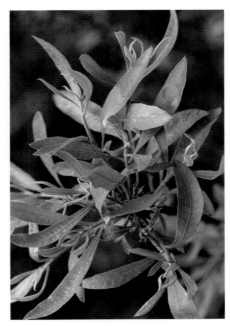

Figure 1 Bayberry (*Myrica cerifera*).

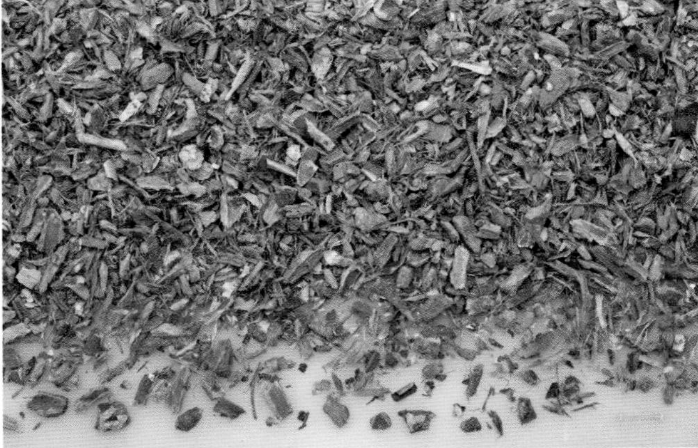

Figure 2 Bayberry – dried drug substance (root bark).

B

Clinical studies

There is a lack of clinical investigation with bayberry and rigorous randomised controlled clinical trials are required.

Side-effects, Toxicity

A total aqueous extract, tannin fraction, and tannin-free fraction from bayberry were all reported to produce tumours in NIH black rats, following weekly subcutaneous injections for up to 75 weeks.[2,3] The number of tumours that developed were stated to be statistically significant for the tannin fraction and tannin-free fraction. Analysis of the tannin-free fraction revealed the presence of four phenolic compounds, one of which was identified as myricitrin. No tumours were reported in a later study, in which rats were given subcutaneous injections of total aqueous extract for 78 weeks.

Large doses may cause typical mineralocorticoid side-effects (e.g. sodium and water retention, hypertension).

Contra-indications, Warnings

Excessive use of tannin-containing herbs is not recommended.

Drug interactions None documented. However, the potential for preparations of bayberry to interact with other medicines administered concurrently, particularly those with similar or opposing effects (e.g. steroids or those with hypo-/hypertensive activity), should be considered.

Pregnancy and lactation The safety of bayberry has not been established. In view of the possible mineralocorticoid activity and the reported carcinogenic activity, the use of bayberry during pregnancy and lactation should be avoided.

Preparations

Proprietary multi-ingredient preparations

UK: EP&C Essence; Peerless Composition Essence.

References

1 Paul BD *et al*. Isolation of myricadiol, myricitrin, taraxerol, and taraxerone from *Myrica cerifera* L. root bark. *J Pharm Sci* 1974; 63: 958–959.
2 Kapadia GJ *et al*. Carcinogenicity of *Camellia sinensis* (tea) and some tannin-containing folk medicinal herbs administered subcutaneously in rats. *J Natl Cancer Inst* 1976; 57: 207–209.
3 Kapadia GJ *et al*. Carcinogenicity of some folk medicinal herbs in rats. *J Natl Cancer Inst* 1978; 60: 683–686.

Bilberry

Summary and Pharmaceutical Comment

The chemistry of bilberry is well documented and there is good evidence that the anthocyanin constituents are responsible for the pharmacological effects of bilberry.

Data from *in vitro* and animal studies provide supportive evidence for some of the uses of bilberry. There have been several clinical studies investigating the effects of bilberry in a range of conditions. However, many studies have been uncontrolled, involved only small numbers of patients and had other methodological flaws. Further, well-designed clinical trials are required to establish the efficacy of bilberry.

There are some limited toxicity and safety data for bilberry which together with data on adverse effects reported in clinical trials provide some support for the safety of bilberry when used at recommended doses in the short term. However, further data on the long-term safety of bilberry use are required and, therefore, excessive use of bilberry should be avoided.

Several of the intended uses of bilberry are not suitable for unsupervised self-treatment.

Species (Family)

Vaccinium myrtillus L. (Ericaceae)

Synonym(s)

Blueberry, bogberry, huckleberry, *Myrtilus niger* Gilib., whortleberry

Part(s) Used

Fruit (berries), leaves

Pharmacopoeial and Other Monographs

American Herbal Pharmacopoeia[G1]
BP 2007[G84]
Complete German Commission E[G3]
Martindale 35th edition (Myrtillus)[G85]
Ph Eur 2007[G81]

Legal Category (Licensed Products)

Bilberry is not included in the GSL.

Constituents

The following is compiled from several sources, including General References G2 and G55.

Berries

Flavonoid glycosides Anthocyanins (particularly glycosides of delphinidin, cyanidin, petunidin, peonidin, malvidin),[1,2] quercetin-3-glucuronide and hyperoside.[3]

Polyphenols Catechin, epicatechin and tannins.

Other constituents Pectins[1] and vitamin C.

Leaves

Flavonoids Quercetin and its glycosides (hyperoside, quercitrin).[1]

Phenolic acids Caffeic, *p*-coumaric, *p*-hydroxybenzoic, protocatechuic and melilotic.[4]

Other constituents Tannins and iridoids.[1]

Food Use

Bilberries are used in foods.[1] Bilberry is listed by the Council of Europe as a natural source of food flavouring (category N1). This category indicates that there are no restrictions on the use of bilberry in foods.[G16]

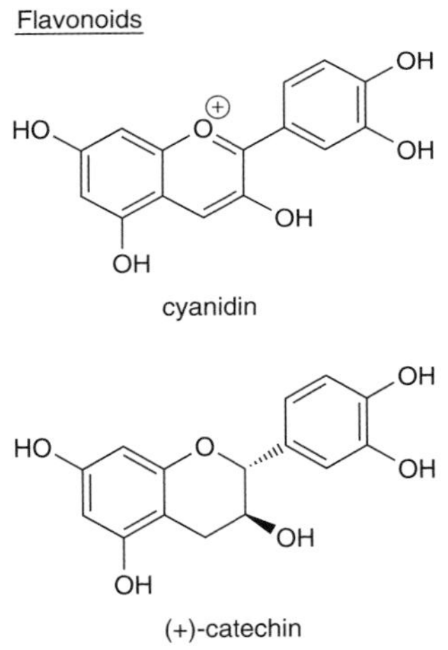

Flavonoids

cyanidin

(+)-catechin

Figure 1 Selected constituents of bilberry.

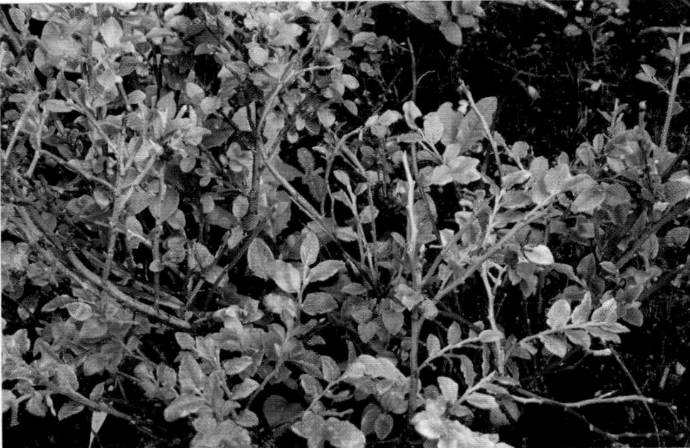

Figure 2 Bilberry (*Vaccinium myrtillus*).

Herbal Use

Bilberry is stated to possess astringent, tonic and antiseptic properties and has traditionally been used in the treatment of diarrhoea, dysentry, haemorrhoids, gastrointestinal inflammations, mouth infections, scurvy and urinary complaints.[1] It has also been used in diabetes, gout and rheumatism and applied locally in eye inflammation, burns and skin infections.[1]

Dosage

Dosages for oral administration (adults) for traditional uses recommended in standard herbal reference texts are given below.

Dried fruit 20–60 g daily as a decoction for the treatment of diarrhoea.[G2]

Pharmacological Actions

Several pharmacological activities have been documented for bilberry, including ophthalmic activity and anti-inflammatory, wound-healing, anti-ulcer, anti-atherosclerotic and vasoprotective properties.[1]

In vitro and animal studies

An anthocyanidin extract of *V. myrtillus* has been reported to act as a superoxide anion scavenger[1, 5] and as an inhibitor of lipid peroxidation in rat liver microsomes[1, 5, 6] and in mouse liver tissue *in vivo*,[5] and to inhibit potassium ion loss induced by free radicals in human erythrocytes.[1] *V. myrtillus* extract is stated to have a potent protective antioxidant action on human low-density lipoproteins (LDLs) *in vitro* during copper-mediated oxidation.[7] Oxidative activity is recognised as a major process in tissue damage in a variety of pathological conditions, such as atherosclerosis and carcinogenesis. In addition, oxidative stress is thought to be involved in brain ageing and age-related neurodegenerative disease. A study in rats reported that, compared with rats fed a control diet, dietary supplementation of blueberry (bilberry) extract for eight weeks reversed age-related deficits in several neuronal and behavioural parameters, such as enhancement of dopamine release from striatal slices and a water maze performance test.[8]

V. myrtillus anthocyanins inhibit aggregation of human platelets *in vitro* in a concentration-dependent manner[9] and, in rats, *V. myrtillus* anthocyanins administered orally at doses ranging from 5–400 mg/kg prolong bleeding time markedly.[10] Inhibition of platelet aggregation has also been reported in humans treated with *V. myrtillus* anthocyanins (*see* Clinical studies).[11]

In vitro inhibition of elastase, a proteolytic enzyme involved with elastic fibre and connective tissue degeneration and with some pathological vascular conditions, has been demonstrated in studies using anthocyanins extracted from *V. myrtillus*.[12]

The hypolipidaemic activity of oral administration of extracts of *V. myrtillus* leaves has been demonstrated in rats.[13, 14] In genetically hyperlipidaemic rats, plasma triglyceride and cholesterol concentrations, but not free fatty acids, decreased significantly.[13] In streptozotocin-induced diabetic rats, plasma glucose concentrations as well as plasma triglyceride concentrations decreased significantly compared with values in control rats.[14] In further experiments using bilberry and clofibrate, both preparations reduced plasma triglyceride concentrations in a dose-dependent manner in rats fed a hyperlipidaemic diet and in ethanol-treated normolipidaemic rats.[14] Bilberry, however, did not prevent fructose-elicited increases in plasma triglyceride concentrations. Other studies in glucose-loaded mice failed to demonstrate hypoglycaemic activity following oral administration of bilberry leaf extract.[15]

Several *in vitro* studies have demonstrated the relaxing effects of *V. myrtillus* anthocyanins on isolated vascular smooth muscle preparations, including the thoracic vein and splenic and coronary arteries.[16–18] There is evidence that the mechanism for this smooth muscle relaxant effect is via stimulation of prostaglandin release within vessel walls.[19]

Effects of *V. myrtillus* anthocyanins on enhancing arterial vasomotion (rhythmic variation of arteriole diameter in the microvasular network which influences microvascular blood flow and the formation of interstitial fluid) have been shown in experimental models, including the cheek pouch microcirculation of hamsters.[20] This model has also been used to investigate the effects of *V. myrtillus* anthocyanins on ischaemia–reperfusion injury.[21] Oral administration for two and four weeks of Myrtocyan, a commercially available product comprising bilberry anthocyanin complex, reduced the increase in capillary permeability, decreased leukocyte adhesion and improved capillary perfusion compared with controls. In rats, oral administration of *V. myrtillus* anthocyanins for 12 days before the induction of hypertension (by ligature of the abdominal aorta) limited the increase in vascular permeability and maintained a normal blood–brain barrier permeability.[22]

Components of bilberry exhibit potential anticarcinogenic activity *in vitro* as demonstrated by inhibition of the induction

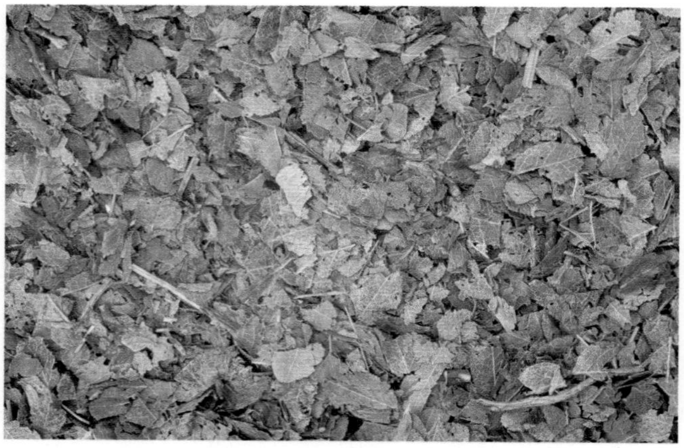

Figure 3 Bilberry – dried drug substance (leaves).

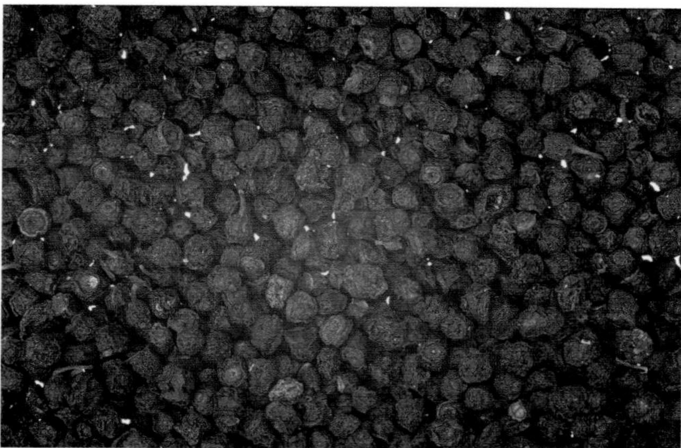

Figure 4 Bilberry – dried drug substance (fruit).

of ornithine decarboxylase (ODC) by the tumour promoter phorbol 12-myristate 13-acetate (TPA).[23]

Myrtocyan and one of its anthocyanin constituents have displayed anti-ulcer activity in various experimental models of acute gastric ulcer and in chronic ulcer induced by acetic acid.[24] The mechanism for this may be by potentiation of the defensive barriers of the gastrointestinal mucosa, such as the secretion of gastric mucus or stimulation of cellular regeneration.[24]

Extracts of *V. myrtillus* leaves have antibacterial activity against several species, including *Staphylococcus aureus* and *Escherichia coli*, as determined by the hole-plate diffusion method and the microdilution broth method.[25] *V. myrtillus* fruit extracts were less active.

The pharmacokinetics of *V. myrtillus* anthocyanins have been studied in rats.[26] Following a single oral administration, plasma anthocyanin concentrations peaked after 15 minutes and declined rapidly within two hours. No hepatic first-pass effect was observed; elimination occurred mostly through the urine and bile.

Clinical studies

Clinical studies with extracts of *V. myrtillus* fruits (berries) have focused mainly on its therapeutic applications in certain ophthalmological conditions and in altered microcirculation and peripheral venous insufficiency.[1]

A study involving 30 healthy subjects with normal platelet aggregation investigated the effects of administration of *V. myrtillus* anthocyanins (Myrtocyan) (480 mg) daily, ascorbic acid 3 g daily and *V. myrtillus* anthocyanins plus ascorbic acid on collagen- and ADP-induced platelet aggregation.[11] Platelet aggregation in blood samples taken from participants after 30 and 60 days' treatment was reduced in all subjects compared with baseline values. The reduction in platelet aggregation was greater in subjects who received *V. myrtillus* anthocyanins alone than in those who received ascorbic acid alone and was most marked in subjects who received both preparations. Platelet aggregation returned to baseline values when tested 120 days after discontinuation of treatment.[11]

Early studies involving healthy subjects and patients with visual disorders who received *V. myrtillus* extracts alone or in combination with β-carotene and vitamin E reported improvements in night vision and faster adjustment to darkness and restoration of visual acuity following exposure to a bright flash of light.[1] Other studies reported improvements in retinal sensitivity and the visual field in patients with myopia or glaucoma following short- or long-term (six months) treatment with *V. myrtillus* anthocyanins.[1] However, none of these studies included a control group, and so the observed effects cannot be attributed to bilberry treatment. Other uncontrolled studies in small numbers of patients with retinal pathologies have reported improvements in retinal function, compared with pretreatment values (e.g. ref. 27).

In a randomised, double-blind, placebo-controlled trial, 40 patients with diabetic and/or hypertensive retinopathy received Myrtocyan (160 mg) twice daily or placebo for one month.[28] At the end of the study, the placebo group received Myrtocyan for one month. It was reported that 77–90% of treated patients experienced improvement compared with the pretreatment period, as determined by ophthalmoscopy and fluorescein fundus angiography.[28] However, there does not appear to have been a statistical comparison between the treatment and placebo groups. A similar placebo-controlled trial involving 40 patients with early-phase diabetic retinopathy who received Myrtocyan for 12 months also reported improvements in Myrtocyan-treated patients.[29]

In a randomised, double-blind trial involving 51 patients with mild senile cortical cataract who received *V. myrtillus* anthocyanins plus vitamin E twice daily for four months, treated patients showed significant improvements in lens opacity compared with placebo recipients.[30]

Studies involving patients with peripheral vascular disorders of various origins are stated to have demonstrated clinical benefits with *V. myrtillus* extracts.[1] Other studies in patients with ulcerative dermatitis secondary to post-thrombotic or venous varicose stasis, capillary fragility secondary to liver disorders and other conditions, or chronic venous insufficiency have been reported to have shown improvements in clinical signs and symptoms.[1] However, several of these studies appear to have been uncontrolled (e.g. refs 31–33) and/or included only small numbers of patients (e.g. refs 31 and 32). A double-blind, placebo-controlled study involving 47 patients with peripheral vascular disorders reported reductions in subjective symptoms, such as paraesthesia, pain and heaviness and improved oedema in patients treated with Myrtocyan (480 mg/day) for 30 days.[1] A single-blind study involving 60 patients with venous insufficiency who received Myrtocyan (480 mg/day) or placebo for 30 days reported significant improvements in oedema, paraesthesia, cramp-like pain and pressure sensation in Myrtocyan-treated patients compared with pretreatment values in these patients.[1]

V. myrtillus anthocyanins have been investigated in a variety of other disorders.

A randomised, double-blind, placebo-controlled trial of *V. myrtillus* anthocyanins (320 mg/day) taken for three days before menstruation was conducted involving 30 patients with chronic primary dysmenorrhoea.[34] Significant differences between the active treatment and placebo groups were reported for several symptoms investigated, including nausea and vomiting and breast tenderness; there was no effect on headache.

In a trial involving 60 patients who had undergone haemorrhoidectomy, participants were randomised to receive *V. myrtillus* anthocyanins (320–480 mg/day) postoperatively in addition to usual medical care or to no additional treatment. Reductions in itch and oedema occurred in bilberry recipients, but there were no effects on other symptoms.[35]

Other studies, all of which were uncontrolled, have reported beneficial effects following administration of *V. myrtillus* extracts in patients with fibrocystic mastopathy[36] and type II diabetes mellitus,[37] in infantile dyspepsia[38] and in pregnant women with lower limb venous insufficiency and acute-phase haemorrhoids.[39]

Side-effects, Toxicity

A review of clinical trials of *V. myrtillus* extracts stated that no adverse effects had been observed, even following prolonged treatment.[1] However, most trials involved relatively small numbers of patients and, therefore, would only be able to detect very common acute adverse effects.

The same review summarised the results of an unpublished postmarketing surveillance study which had involved 2295 subjects who had taken Myrtocyan, usually 160 mg twice daily for 1–2 months, for lower limb venous insufficiency, capillary fragility, functional changes in retinal microcirculation or haemorrhoids. Ninety-four subjects reported side-effects, mainly relating to the skin and gastrointestinal and nervous systems.[1]

Long-term consumption of bilberry leaves may lead to toxicity. Chronic administration of doses of 1.5 g/kg per day or more to animals has been reported to be fatal.[G2]

B

Animal toxicity data indicate that in mice and rats, the LD_{50} for Myrtocyan is over 2 g/kg and, in dogs, single doses of 3 g/kg produced no adverse effects other than marked darkening of urine and faeces (demonstrating absorption).[1] Oral daily doses to rats and dogs of 125–500 mg/kg and 80–320 mg/kg, respectively, for six months did not induce mortality or toxic effects.[1] Pharmacokinetic studies of *V. myrtillus* anthocyanins in rats demonstrated that anthocyanins are removed rapidly from the systemic circulation within two hours of oral administration.[26]

Contra-indications, Warnings

Drug interactions None documented. However, the potential for preparations of bilberry to interact with other medicines administered concurrently, particularly those with similar or opposing effects, should be considered. For example, there is evidence from preclinical studies that *V. myrtillus* anthocyanins inhibit platelet aggregation and prolong bleeding time, although clinical evidence is limited. It is not known whether or not the use of bilberry preparations concurrently with antiplatelet or anticoagulant agents carries an increased risk of bleeding; concurrent use of bilberry with such agents, and initiation or cessation of bilberry treatments, should be monitored

Pregnancy and lactation In an uncontrolled study, *V. myrtillus* anthocyanin extract (Tegens) (80 or 160 mg) twice or three times daily for three months was administered to pregnant women with lower limb venous insufficiency and acute-phase haemorrhoids with no apparent adverse effects.[39] However, the safety of bilberry has not been established and, in view of the lack of toxicity data, the use of bilberry during pregnancy and lactation should be avoided.

Preparations

Proprietary single-ingredient preparations

Australia: Herbal Eye Care Formula. *Brazil:* Miralis. *Germany:* Difrarel. *Italy:* Alcodin; Mirtilene Forte; Tegens. *Portugal:* Difrarel; Varison. *Russia:* Mirtilene Forte (Миртилене Форте). *Switzerland:* Myrtaven.

Proprietary multi-ingredient preparations

Australia: Bilberry Plus Eye Health; Bioglan Pygno-Vite; Bioglan Vision-Eze; Extralife Eye-Care; Extralife Leg-Care; Herbal PMS Formula; Prophthal; Pykno; St Mary's Thistle Plus. *Austria:* Amersan. *Czech Republic:* Amersan; Diabetan; Diabeticka Cajova Smes-Megadiabetin; Tormentan; Urcyston Planta. *France:* Diacure; Difrarel E; Difrarel; Flebior; Klorane Shampooing Antipelliculaire; Stomargil. *Hungary:* Difrarel E. *Italy:* Alvear con Ginseng; Angioton; Api Baby; Bebimix; Biolactine; Capill; Dermilia Flebozin; Evamilk; Memovisus; Mirtilene; Mirtilux; Mirtilux; Neomyrt Plus; Nerex; Pik Gel; Retinovit; Tussol; Ultravisin; Varicofit. *Netherlands:* Difrarel. *Spain:* Antomiopic; Mirtilus. *UK:* I-Sight; Nature's Garden; Se-Power. *USA:* Bilbery 40mg; Eye Support Formula Herbal Blend; Healthy Eyes; Mental Clarity; My Favorite Multiple Iron-Free; My Favorite Multiple Original; My Favorite Multiple Prime Multi Vitamin; My Favorite Multiple Take One; My Favorite Multiple Take One Iron-Free; Ultimate Antioxidant Formula; Ocusense.

References

1 Morazzoni P, Bombardelli E. *Vaccinium myrtillus* L. *Fitoterapia* 1996; 66: 3–29.

2 Di Pierro F, Morazzoni P. Reaping the benefits: the role of two edible plants (*Vaccinium myrtillus* and *Glycine max*). Proceedings of the Herbal Medicine in the New Millennium Conference, Lismore, NSW, Australia, 1999: 146–150.

3 Fraisse D *et al*. Composition polyphénolique de la feuille de myrtille. *Ann Pharm Fr* 1996; 54: 280–283.

4 Dombrowicz E *et al*. Phenolic acids in leaves of *Arctostaphylos uva ursi* L., *Vaccinium vitis idaea* L. and *Vaccinium myrtillus* L. *Pharmazie* 1991; 46: 680–681.

5 Martín-Aragon S *et al*. *In vitro* and *in vivo* antioxidant properties of *Vaccinium myrtillus*. *Pharm Biol* 1999; 37: 109–113.

6 Martín-Aragon S *et al*. Antioxidant action of *Vaccinium myrtillus* L. *Phytother Res* 1998; 12 (Suppl. Suppl.): S104–S106.

7 Laplaud PM *et al*. Antioxidant action of *Vaccinium myrtillus* extract on human low-density lipoproteins *in vitro*: initial observations. *Fund Clin Pharmacol* 1997; 11: 35–40.

8 Joseph JA *et al*. Reversals of age-related declines in neuronal signal transduction, cognitive, and motor behavioral deficits with blueberry, spinach, or strawberry dietary supplementation. *J Neurosci* 1999; 19: 8114–8121.

9 Bottecchia D *et al*. Preliminary report on the inhibitory effect of *Vaccinium myrtillus* anthocyanosides on platelet aggregation and clot retraction. *Fitoterapia* 1987; 58: 3–8.

10 Morazzoni P, Magistretti MJ. Activity of Myrtocyan, an anthocyanin complex from *Vaccinium myrtillus* (VMA), on platelet aggregation and adhesiveness. *Fitoterapia* 1990; 61: 13–21.

11 Pulliero G *et al*. *Ex vivo* study of the inhibitory effects of *Vaccinium myrtillus* anthocyanosides on human platelet aggregation. *Fitoterapia* 1989; 60: 69–75.

12 Jonadet M *et al*. Anthocyanosides extraits de *Vitis vinifera*, de *Vaccinium myrtillus* et de *Pinus maritimus*. *J Pharm Belg* 1983; 38: 41–46.

13 Cignarella A *et al*. Hypolipidaemic activity of *Vaccinium myrtillus* leaves on a new model of genetically hyperlipidaemic rat. *Planta Med* 1992; 58 (Suppl. Suppl.1): A581–A582.

14 Cignarella A *et al*. Novel lipid-lowering properties of *Vaccinium myrtillus* L. leaves, a traditional antidiabetic treatment, in several models of rat dyslipidaemia: a comparison with clofibrate. *Thromb Res* 1996; 84: 311–322.

15 Neef H *et al*. Hypogylcaemic activity of selected European plants. *Phytother Res* 1995; 9: 45–48.

16 Bettini V *et al*. Effects of *Vaccinium myrtillus* anthocyanosides on vascular smooth muscle. *Fitoterapia* 1984; 55: 265–272.

17 Bettini V *et al*. Interactions between *Vaccinium myrtillus* anthocyanosides and serotonin on splenic artery smooth muscle. *Fitoterapia* 1984; 55: 201–208.

18 Bettini V *et al*. Mechanical responses of isolated coronary arteries to barium in the presence of *Vaccinium myrtillus* anthocyanosides. *Fitoterapia* 1985; 56: 3–10.

19 Morazzoni P, Magistretti MJ. Effects of *Vaccinium myrtillus* anthocyanosides on prostacyclin-like activity in rat arterial tissue. *Fitoterapia* 1986; 57: 11–14.

20 Colantuoni A *et al*. Effects of *Vaccinium myrtillus* anthocyanosides on arterial vasomotion. *Arzneimittelforschung* 1991; 41: 905–909.

21 Bertuglia S *et al*. Effect of *Vaccinium myrtillus* anthocyanosides on ischaemia reperfusion injury in hamster cheek pouch microcirculation. *Pharmacol Res* 1995; 31: 183–187.

22 Detre Z *et al*. Studies on vascular permeability in hypertension: action of anthocyanosides. *Clin Physiol Biochem* 1986; 4: 143–149.

23 Bomser J *et al*. *In vitro* anticancer activity of fruit extracts from *Vaccinium* species. *Planta Med* 1996; 62: 212–216.

24 Magistretti MJ *et al*. Antiulcer activity of an anthocyanidin from *Vaccinium myrtillus*. *Arzneimittelforschung* 1988; 38: 686–690.

25 Brantner A, Grein E. Antibacterial activity of plant extracts used externally in traditional medicine. *J Ethnopharmacol* 1994; 44: 35–40.

26 Morazzoni P *et al*. *Vaccinium myrtillus* anthocyanosides pharmacokinetics in rats. *Arzneimmittelforschung* 1991; 41: 128–131.

27 Forte R *et al*. Fitotherapy and ophthalmology: considerations on dynamized myrtillus retinal effects with low luminance visual acuity. *Ann Ottal Clin Ocul* 1996; 122: 325–333.

28 Perossini M *et al*. Diabetic and hypertensive retinopathy therapy with *Vaccinium myrtillus* anthocianosides (Tegens) double-blind placebo-controlled clinical trial. *Ann Ottal Clin Ocul* 1988; 113: 1173–1190.

29 Repossi P *et al*. The role of anthocyanosides on vascular permeability in diabetic retinopathy. *Ann Ottal Clin Ocul* 1987; 113: 357–361.

30 Bravetti GO *et al*. Preventive medical treatment of senile cataract with vitamin E and *Vaccinium myrtillus* anthocianosides: clinical evaluation. *Ann Ottal Clin Ocul* 1989; 115: 109–116.

31 Coget J, Merlen JF. Étude clinique d'un nouvel agent de protection vasculaire le difrarel 20, composé d'anthocyanosides extraits du *Vaccinum myrtillus*. *Phlebologie* 1968; 21: 221–228.

32 Piovella F *et al*. Impiego di antocianosidi da *Vaccinium myrtillus* al 25% come antocianidine nel trattamento della diatesi emorragica da deficit dell'emostasi primaria. *Gaz Med It* 1981; 140: 445–449.

33 Tori A, D'Errico F. Gli antocianosidi da *Vaccinium myrtillus* nella cura delle flebopatie da stasi degli arti inferiori. *Gaz Med It* 1980; 139: 217–224.

34 Colombo D, Vescovini R. Studio clinico controllato sull'efficacia degli antocianosidi del mirtillo cel trattamento della dismenorrea essenziale. *Giorn It Ost Gin* 1985; 7: 1033–1038.

35 Pezzangora V *et al*. La terapia medica con antocianosidi del mirtillo nei pazienti operati di emorroidectomia. *Gaz Med It* 1984; 143: 405–409.

36 Leonardi M. Il trattamento della mastopatia fibrosa con antocianosidi di mirtillo. *Minerva Ginecol* 1993; 45: 617–621.

37 Ionescu-Tirgoviste C *et al*. Efectul unui amestec pe plante asupra echilibrului metabolic la bolnavii cu diabet zaharat de tip 2. *Med Intern* 1989; 41: 185–192.

38 Tolan L *et al*. Utilizarea prafului de afine in dispepsiile sugarului. *Pediatria* 1969; 18: 375–379.

39 Teglio L *et al*. *Vaccinium myrtillus* anthocyanosides in the treatment of venous insufficiency of inferior limbs and acute piles in pregnancy. *Quaderni Clin Osterica Ginecol* 1987; 42: 221–231.

Bloodroot

Summary and Pharmaceutical Comment

Bloodroot is characterised by isoquinoline alkaloid constituents (benzophenanthridine-type), predominantly sanguinarine. A wide range of pharmacological activities has been documented for this class of compounds including antimicrobial, anti-inflammatory, antihistaminic, cardiotonic and antiplaque. Other benzophenanthridine alkaloids have been associated with cytotoxic activities. However, recent interest over the potential use of bloodroot in oral hygiene has stimulated considerable research into both sanguinarine and bloodroot extracts. Results have indicated that products such as oral rinses and toothpastes containing either sanguinaria extracts or sanguinarine may be of value in dental hygiene.

Species (Family)

Sanguinaria canadensis L. (Papaveraceae)

Synonym(s)

Red Indian Paint, Red Root, Sanguinaria, *S. australis* Greene, *S. canadensis* var. *rotundifolia* (Greene) Fedde, *S. dilleniana* Greene, Tetterwort

Part(s) Used

Rhizome

Pharmacopoeial and Other Monographs

BHP 1983[G7]
Martindale 35th edition[G85]

Alkaloids

	R^1	R^2
sanguinarine	—CH_2—	
chelerythrine	CH_3	CH_3

protopine

Figure 1 Selected constituents of bloodroot.

Legal Category (Licensed Products)

Bloodroot is not included in the GSL.[G37]

Constituents

The following is compiled from several sources, including General References G22 and G41.

Alkaloids Isoquinoline type. 3.0–7.0%.[1] Sanguinarine (approx. 1%), sanguidimerine, chelerythrine, protopine; others include oxysanguinarine, α- and β-allocryptopine, sanguilutine, dihydrosanguilutine, berberine, coptisine and homochelidonine.

Other constituents Resin, starch, organic acids (citric, malic).

Alkaloid content of other plant parts recorded as 0.08% (leaf), 1.8% (root).

Food Use

Bloodroot is listed by the Council of Europe as a natural source of food flavouring (category N3). This category indicates that bloodroot can be added to foodstuffs in the traditionally accepted manner, although there is insufficient information available for an adequate assessment of potential toxicity.[G16]

Herbal Use

Bloodroot is stated to act as an expectorant, spasmolytic, emetic, cathartic, antiseptic, cardioactive, topical irritant and escharotic (scab-producing). Traditionally it is indicated for bronchitis (subacute or chronic), asthma, croup, laryngitis, pharyngitis, deficient capillary circulation, nasal polyps (as a snuff), and specifically for asthma and bronchitis with feeble peripheral circulation.[G7]

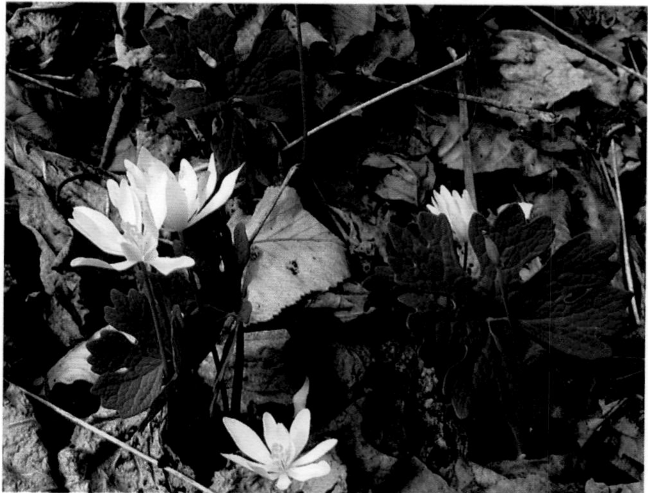

Figure 2 Bloodroot (*Sanguinaria canadensis*).

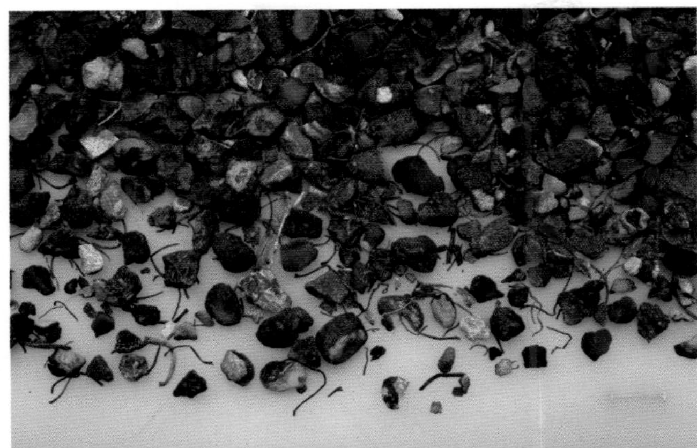

Figure 3 Bloodroot – dried drug substance (rhizome).

Dosage

Dosages for oral administration (adults) for traditional uses recommended in older standard herbal reference texts are given below.

Rhizome 0.06–0.5 g (1–2 g for emetic dose) three times daily.[G7]

Liquid extract 0.06–0.3 mL (1 : 1 in 60% alcohol) (1–2 mL for emetic dose) three times daily.[G7]

Tincture 0.3–2 mL (1 : 5 in 60% alcohol) (2–8 mL for emetic dose) three times daily.[G7]

Pharmacological Actions

Activities documented for bloodroot are principally attributable to the isoquinoline alkaloid constituents, in particular sanguinarine. Interest has focused on the use of sanguinarine in dental hygiene products. Unless otherwise stated, the following actions refer to sanguinarine.

In vitro and animal studies

Considerable antimicrobial activity has been documented against both Gram-positive and Gram-negative bacteria, *Candida* and dermatophytes (fungi), and *Trichomonas* (protozoa).[2] In addition, anti-inflammatory activity has been described against carrageenan-induced rat paw oedema.[3]

Prolongation of the ventricular refractory period has been attributed to an inhibition of $Na^{+}K^{+}$ ATPase.[4,5] However, a single intravenous injection of sanguinarine to anaesthetised dogs reportedly exerted no effect on cardiovascular parameters monitored.[4]

In vitro inhibition of bone resorption and collagenase has been documented.[2]

Clinical studies

Many studies have investigated the efficacy of bloodroot extracts in oral hygiene.[2] Preparations containing bloodroot extracts, such as oral rinses and toothpastes, have been reported to significantly lower plaque, gingival and bleeding indices.[2] Alteration of the oral microbial flora, or development of resistant microbial strains has not been observed with the use of bloodroot extracts.[2]

Side-Effects, Toxicity

None documented for bloodroot. Much has been documented concerning the potential toxicity of the alkaloid constituents in bloodroot, in particular of sanguinarine.

Conclusions reached in the 1960s over the carcinogenic potential of sanguinarine have more recently been disproved.[6] In addition, negative mutagenic activity has been observed in the Ames test (microbial, with and without activation).[6]

Sanguinarine is poorly absorbed from the gastrointestinal tract. This is reflected in stated acute oral LD_{50} values (rat) of 1.7 g/kg (sanguinarine) and 1.4 g/kg (sanguinaria extract), compared with an acute intravenous LD_{50} (rat) value of 28.7 mg/kg (sanguinarine).[1] Symptoms of diarrhoea, ataxia and reduced activity were observed in animals receiving high oral doses of sanguinarine.[5] The acute dermal toxicity (LD_{50}) of sanguinarine is stated to be greater than 200 mg/kg in rabbits.[1] The first experimental study of sanguinarine toxicity (1876) reported prostration and severe respiratory distress as the most marked signs of oral toxicity.[1] However, in more recent short-term toxicity studies no toxic signs were observed in the fetuses of rats following maternal administration of 5–30 mg/kg/day of sanguinarine. [1]

The reproductive and developmental toxicity potential of an *S. canadensis* extract has been evaluated in rats and rabbits.[6] Developmental toxicity (increase in postimplantation loss, slight decrease in fetal and pup body weights) was only evident at maternally toxic doses. No effect was reported on reproductive capabilities, on parturition or on lactation. It was concluded that oral ingestion of sanguinaria extract has no selective effect on fertility, reproduction, or on fetal or neonatal development.[6]

Hepatotoxicity has been documented in rats following a single intraperitoneal administration (10 mg/kg) of sanguinarine.[5] Toxicity was indicated by an increase in serum alanine aminotransferase and serum asparate aminotransferase activity, and by a significant reduction in microsomal cytochrome P450 and benzfetamine *N*-demethylase activities.[5] Macroscopic lesions were also observed but the authors stated that the two events could not be conclusively directly related.[5] No hepatotoxicity has been observed in short-term toxicity studies involving oral administration of sanguinarine.[1]

Animal studies have indicated sanguinarine to be non-irritant and to exhibit no allergenic or anaphylactic potential.[4] Human patch tests have shown sanguinarine to be non-irritant and non-sensitising.[4]

Contra-indications, Warnings

Drug interactions None documented. However, the potential for preparations of bloodroot to interact with other medicines administered concurrently, particularly those with similar or opposing effects, should be considered.

Pregnancy and lactation There is limited evidence from animal studies that bloodroot is non-toxic during pregnancy (see above). However, in view of its pharmacologically active constituents and lack of clinical data on safety, use of bloodroot during pregnancy and lactation should be avoided.

Preparations

Proprietary multi-ingredient preparations

Australia: Lexat. *Canada:* Mielocol; Viadent; Wampole Bronchial Cough Syrup. *Italy:* Dentosan Carie & Alito.

B

References

1 Becci PJ *et al*. Short-term toxicity studies of sanguinarine and of two alkaloid extracts of *Sanguinaria canadensis*. *J Toxicol Environ Health* 1987; 20: 199–208.
2 Godowski KC. Antimicrobial action of sanguinarine. *J Clin Dent* 1989; 1: 96–101.
3 Lenfield J *et al*. Antiinflammatory activity of quaternary benzophenanthridine alkaloids from *Chelidonium majus*. *Planta Med* 1981; 43: 161–165.
4 Schwartz HG. Safety profile of sanguinarine and sanguinaria extract. *Compend Cont Educ Dent Suppl* 1986; 7: S212–S217.
5 Dalvi RR. Sanguinarine: its potential as a liver toxic alkaloid present in the seeds of *Argemone mexicana*. *Experientia* 1985; 41: 77–78.
6 Keller KA. Reproductive and developmental toxicological evaluation of Sanguinaria extract. *J Clin Dent* 1989; 1: 59–66.

Blue Flag

Summary and Pharmaceutical Comment

Little is known about the phytochemical, pharmacological or toxicological properties of blue flag and its constituents, although related species are known to be toxic. In view of these factors, the use of blue flag is not recommended.

Species (Family)

Iris versicolor L.

Synonym(s)

Iris caroliniana Watson, *Iris virginica* L.

Part(s) Used

Rhizome

Pharmacopoeial and Other Monographs

BHC 1992[G6]
BHP 1996[G9]
Martindale 35th edition[G85]

Legal Category (Licensed Products)

GSL[G37]

Constituents

The following is compiled from several sources, including General References G22, G40, G48 and G64.

Acids Isophthalic acid 0.002%, salicylic acid, lauric acid, stearic acid, palmitic acid and 1-triacontanol.

Volatile oils 0.025%. Furfural.

Other constituents Iridin, β-sitosterol, iriversical[1] and tannin.

Food Use

Blue flag is not used in foods.

Herbal Use

Blue flag is stated to possess cholagogue, laxative, diuretic, dermatological, anti-inflammatory and antiemetic properties. It has been used for skin diseases, biliousness with constipation and liver dysfunction, and specifically for cutaneous eruptions.[G7, G64]

Triterpenes

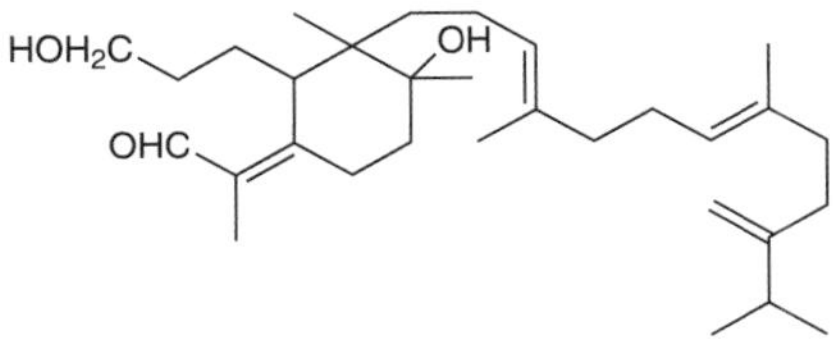

HOH$_2$C, OHC, OH

iriversical

Figure 1 Selected constituents of blue flag.

Dosage

Dosages for oral administration (adults) for traditional uses recommended in older standard herbal and pharmaceutical reference texts are given below.

Dried rhizome 0.6–2.0 g as a decoction three times daily.[G6, G7, G10]

Liquid extract 1–2 mL (1 : 1 in 45% alcohol) three times daily.[G6, G7, G10]

Pharmacological Actions

None documented.

Side-effects, Toxicity

It has been stated that the fresh root of blue flag can cause nausea and vomiting.[G42] Therefore, dosage recommendations relate to small doses of dried root.

Furfural, a volatile oil constituent, is known to be irritant to mucous membranes causing lachrymation, inflammation of the

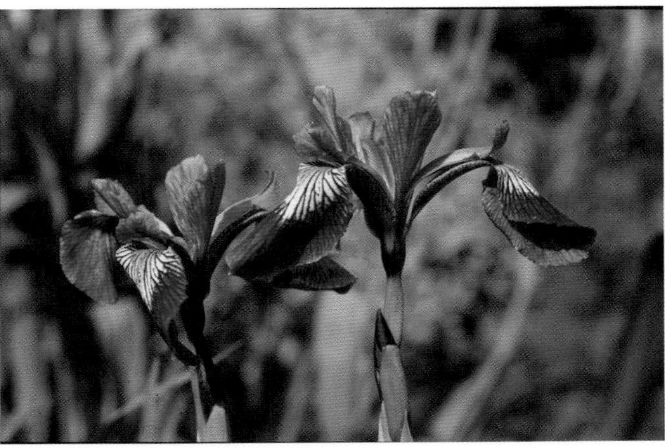

Figure 2 Blue flag (*Iris versicolor*).

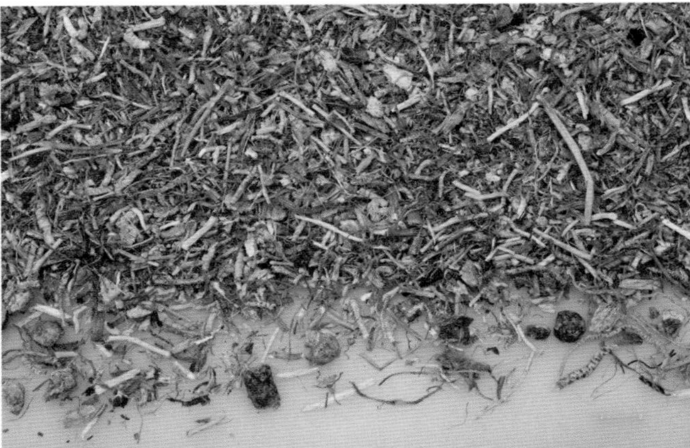

Figure 3 Blue flag – dried drug substance (rhizome).

eyes, irritation of the throat, and headache.[G48] Whether these irritant properties are attributable to the volatile oil of blue flag has not been established. Acute oral toxicity (rat, LD_{50}) for furfural has been documented as 127 mg/kg body weight.[G48] Iridin has been reported to be poisonous in both humans and livestock.[G22] However, it is unclear whether this substance is the same iridin documented as a constituent of blue flag.

Contra-indications, Warnings

In view of the possible irritant nature of the volatile oil, blue flag may not be suitable for internal use.

Drug interactions None documented.

Pregnancy and lactation The safety of blue flag has not been established. In view of this, together with the documented irritant properties of some of the constituents, blue flag should not be taken during pregnancy.

Preparations

Proprietary multi-ingredient preparations

UK: Catarrh Mixture; HRI Clear Complexion; Napiers Skin Tablets; Skin Eruptions Mixture.

References

1 Krick W *et al*. Isolation and structural determination of a new methylated triterpenoid from rhizomes of *Iris versicolor* L. *Z Naturforsch* 1983; 38: 689–692.

Bogbean

Summary and Pharmaceutical Comment

The chemistry of bogbean is well studied, but no pharmacological information is available to justify the herbal uses. In view of the lack of toxicity data, excessive doses should be avoided.

Species (Family)

Menyanthes trifoliata L. (Menyanthaceae)

Synonym(s)

Buckbean, Marsh Trefoil, Menyanthes

Part(s) Used

Leaf

Pharmacopoeial and Other Monographs

BHP 1996[G9]
BP 2007[G84]
Complete German Commission E[G3]
Martindale 35th edition[G85]
Ph Eur 2007[G81]

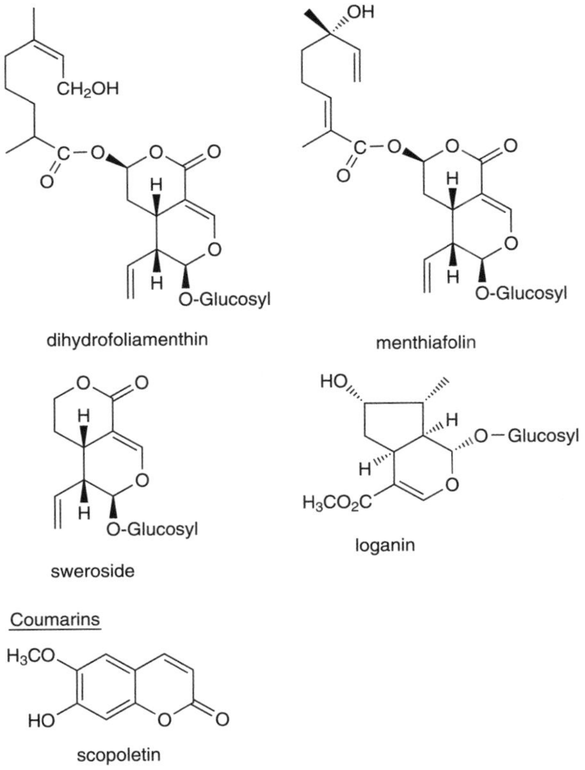

Iridoids

dihydrofoliamenthin

menthiafolin

sweroside

loganin

Coumarins

scopoletin

Figure 1 Selected constituents of bogbean.

Legal Category (Licensed Products)

GSL[G37]

Constituents

The following is compiled from several sources, including General References G2, G62 and G64.

Acid Caffeic acid, chlorogenic acid, ferulic acid, *p*-hydroxybenzoic acid, protocatechuic acid, salicylic acid, vanillic acid;[1,2] folic acid and palmitic acid.[2]

Alkaloids Gentianin and gentianidine (pyridine-type); choline.[2]

Coumarins Scopoletin.[2]

Flavonoids Hyperin, kaempferol, quercetin, rutin and trifolioside.[1,2]

Iridoids 7′,8′-Dihydrofoliamenthin, foliamenthin, loganin, menthiafolin and sweroside.[2–4]

Other constituents Carotene, ceryl alcohol, enzymes (e.g. emulsin, invertin), α-spinasterol, an unidentified substance with haemolytic properties.[2] α-Spinasterol has been reported to be a mixture of five sterols with α-spinasterol and stigmast-7-enol as major components.[5]

Food Use

Bogbean is listed by the Council of Europe as a natural source of food flavouring (category N2). This category indicates that bogbean can be added to foodstuffs in small quantities, with a possible limitation of an active principle (as yet unspecified) in the final product.[G16]

Herbal Use

Bogbean is stated to possess bitter and diuretic properties. It has been used for rheumatism, rheumatoid arthritis, and specifically for muscular rheumatism associated with general asthenia.[G2, G7, G8, G64]

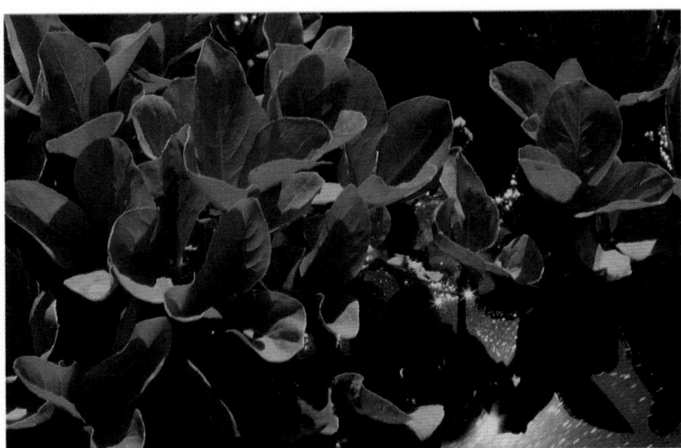

Figure 2 Bogbean (*Menyanthes trifoliata*).

B

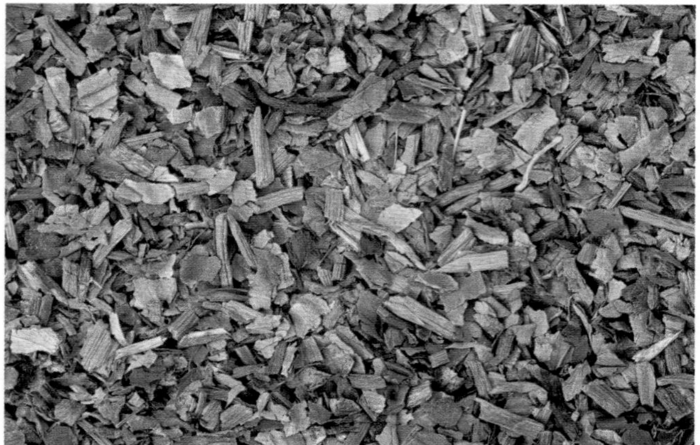

Figure 3 Bogbean – dried drug substance (leaf).

Dosage

Dosages for oral administration (adults) for traditional uses recommended in older and contemporary standard herbal reference texts are given below.

Dried leaf 1–2 g or by infusion three times daily.(G7)

Liquid extract 1–2 mL (1 : 1 in 25% alcohol) three times daily.(G7)

Tincture 1–3 mL (1 : 5 in 45% alcohol) three times daily.(G7)

Pharmacological Actions

In vitro and animal studies

A choleretic action has been described for caffeic acid and ferulic acid; a stomachic secretive action has been reported for protocatechuic acid and *p*-hydroxybenzoic acid. The iridoids possess bitter properties.(1) The bitter index (BI) of bogbean is stated to be 4000–10 000 (compared to gentian BI 10 000–30 000).(G62) Bogbean extracts have antibacterial activities.(6, 7)

Side-effects, Toxicity

Large doses of bogbean are stated to be purgative and may cause vomiting.(8) An unidentified substance with haemolytic activity has been isolated from bogbean.(2)

Contra-indications, Warnings

Excessive doses may be irritant to the gastrointestinal tract, causing diarrhoea, griping pains, nausea and vomiting.(8)

Drug interactions None documented. However, the potential for bogbean to interact with other medicines administered concurrently, particularly those with similar or opposing effects, should be considered.

Pregnancy and lactation The safety of bogbean has not been established. In view of the lack of toxicity data and possible purgative action, the use of bogbean during pregnancy and lactation should be avoided.

Preparations

Proprietary single-ingredient preparations

Czech Republic: List Vachty Trojliste.

Proprietary multi-ingredient preparations

Austria: Mariazeller. *Czech Republic:* Naturland Grosser Swedenbitter. *France:* Tisane Hepatique de Hoerdt. *Germany:* Gallexier. *Russia:* Original Grosser Bittner Balsam (Оригинальный Большой Бальзам Биттнера). *UK:* Modern Herbals Rheumatic Pain; Rheumatic Pain; Rheumatic Pain Relief; Rheumatic Pain Remedy; Rheumatic Pain Tablets; Sciatica Tablets; Vegetex.

References

1 Swiatek L *et al.* Content of phenolic acids in leaves of *Menyanthes trifoliata. Planta Med* 1986; 52: 530.
2 Giaceri G. Chromatographic identification of coumarin derivatives in *Menyanthes trifoliata* L. *Fitoterapia* 1972; 43: 134–138.
3 Battersby AR *et al.* Seco-cyclopentane glucosides from *Menyanthes trifoliata*: foliamenthin, dihydrofoliamenthin, and menthiafolin. *Chem Commun* 1968; 1277–1280.
4 Loew P *et al.* The structure and biosynthesis of foliamenthin. *Chem Commun* 1968; 1276–1277.
5 Popov S. Sterols of the Gentianaceae family. *Dokl Bolg Akad Nauk* 1969; 22: 293–296.
6 Moskalenko SA. Preliminary screening of Far-Eastern ethnomedicinal plants for antibacterial activity. *J Ethnopharmacol* 1986; 15: 231–259.
7 Bishop CJ, MacDonald RE. A survey of higher plants for antibacterial substances. *Can J Bot* 1951; 29: 260–269.
8 Todd RG, ed. *Martindale: The Extra Pharmacopoeia*, 25th edn. London: Pharmaceutical Press, 1967.

Boldo

Summary and Pharmaceutical Comment

The chemistry of boldo is well documented, and some pharmacological data are available. Clinical studies have described choleretic activity, although further well-designed studies are required to establish this. The reputed diuretic and mild urinary antiseptic properties of boldo are probably attributable to the irritant volatile oil. In view of the toxicity data and the irritant nature of the volatile oil, excessive and/or long-term use of boldo should be avoided.[G56]

Species (Family)

Peumus boldus Molina (Monimiaceae)

Synonym(s)

Boldi Folium, Boldus

Part(s) Used

Leaf

Pharmacopoeial and Other Monographs

BHP 1996[G9]
BP 2007[G84]
Complete German Commission E[G3]
ESCOP 1996[G52]
Martindale 35th edition[G85]
Ph Eur 2007[G81]
WHO volume 1 1999[G63]

Legal Category (Licensed Products)

GSL[G37]

Constituents

The following is compiled from several sources, including General References G2, G52 and G62.

Alkaloids Isoquinoline-type. 0.25–0.7%. Pharmacopoeial standard not less than 0.1% alkaloid calculated as boldine.[G81, G84] Boldine 0.06% (major, disputed), isoboldine, 6a,7-dehydroboldine, isocorydine, isocorydine-*N*-oxide, norisocorydine, laurolitsine, laurotetanine, *N*-methyllaurotetanine (aporphines), reticuline; (−)-pronuciferine (proaporphine) and sinoacutine (morphinandienone).[1–4]

Flavonoids Flavonols (e.g. isorhamnetin) and their glycosides.[5, 6]

Volatile oils 2.5%. Some 38 components have been identified, including *p*-cymene 28.6%, ascaridole 16.1%, 1,8-cineole 16.0%, linalool 9.1%, terpinen-4-o1 2.6%, α-terpineol 0.9%, fenchone 0.8% and terpinolene 0.4%.

Other constituents Coumarin 0.5%, resin and tannin.

Food Use

Boldo is listed by the Council of Europe as a natural source of food flavouring (category N3). This category indicates that boldo can be added to foodstuffs in the traditionally accepted manner, although insufficient information is available for an adequate assessment of potential toxicity.[G16] Previously, in the USA, boldo was approved for food use in alcoholic beverages only.[G64]

Herbal Use

Boldo is stated to possess cholagogue, liver stimulant, sedative, diuretic, mild urinary demulcent, and antiseptic properties. It has been used for mild digestive disturbances, constipation, gallstones, pain in the liver or gall bladder, cystitis, rheumatism, and specifically for cholelithiasis with pain.[G2, G7, G64] The German Commission E approved use for treatment of dyspepsia and mild spastic gastrointestinal complaints.[G3]

Dosage

Dosages for oral administration (adults) for traditional uses recommended in older and contemporary standard herbal reference texts are given below.

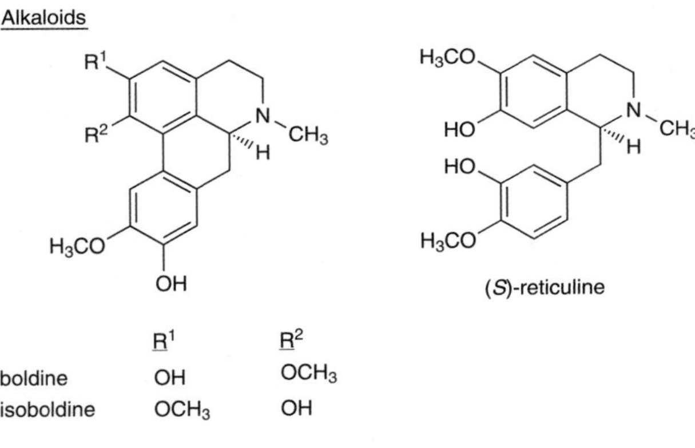

Monoterpenes

p-cymene

1,8-cineole

linalool

ascaridole

Figure 1 Selected constituents of boldo.

Dried leaf 60–200 mg as an infusion three times daily;[(G7)] 2–5 g as a tea.[(G52)]

Liquid extract 0.1–0.3 mL (1 : 1 in 45% alcohol) three times daily.[(G7)]

Tincture 0.5–2.0 mL (1 : 10 in 60% alcohol) three times daily.[(G7)]

Pharmacological Actions

In vitro and animal studies

Boldo has exhibited choleretic (highest activity in rats), diuretic, stomachic and cholagogic properties.[(G41, G52)] The choleretic activity may be due to synergy between flavonoids and alkaloids.[(G52)] Experiments in rats have failed to demonstrate choleretic activity after oral administration of 400 or 800 mg/kg aqueous ethanolic extract, intraduodenal administration of 200 mg or 800 mg/kg, and intravenous administration of 32.5–130 mg/kg of a dry ethanolic extract.[(7)]

An aqueous ethanolic extract (equivalent to 0.5–1.0 mg/mL dried ethanolic extract) and also boldine (33 μg/mL) gave significant hepatoprotection against *t*-butyl hydroperoxide-induced hepatotoxicity in rat hepatocytes *in vitro*.[(7)] Boldine at a concentration of 0.015 mol/L inhibited microsomal lipid peroxidation in a rat liver preparation by 50%.[(8)] A dried aqueous ethanolic extract (0.06–0.115%) of boldine at a dose of 500 mg/kg gave 70% protection against carbon tetrachloride-induced hepatotoxicity in mice, and boldine alone (10 mg/kg) gave 49% protection.[(7)] An aqueous ethanolic extract of boldo at doses of 50 and 100 mg/kg administered intraperitoneally showed anti-inflammatory activity in the rat paw carrageenan-induced oedema test, whereas boldine alone appeared to be inactive.[(7)]

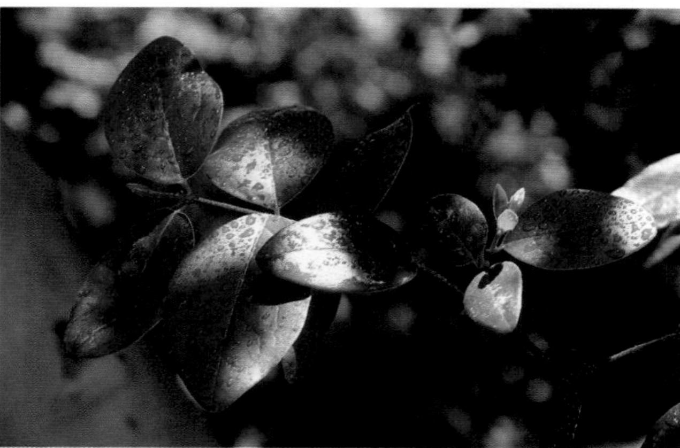

Figure 2 Boldo (*Peumus boldus*).

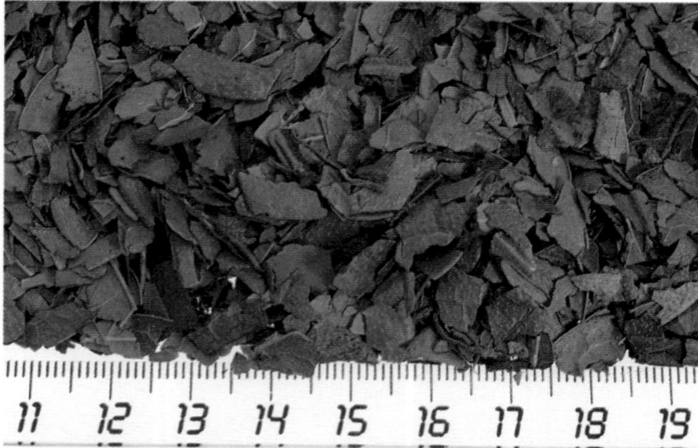

Figure 3 Boldo – dried drug substance (leaf).

Boldine showed concentration-dependent relaxant activity on isolated rat ileum (EC_{50} 1.7 × 10^{-4} mol/L), and acted as a competitive antagonist of acetylcholine and as a non-competitive antagonist of barium.[(9)] Boldine at low micromolar concentrations prevented oxidation in rat brain homogenate and lipid peroxidation of red cell plasma membranes, led to inactivation of lysozymes, indicating high reactivity of free radicals.[(10)]

Boldo essential oil contains terpinen-4-ol, the irritant and diuretic principle in juniper oil.

Clinical studies

Clinical investigation of the effects of boldo is extremely limited and rigorous randomized controlled clinical trials are required. In a controlled trial, boldo, in combination with cascara, rhubarb and gentian, had a beneficial effect on a variety of symptoms such as loss of appetite, digestion difficulties, constipation, flatulence and itching.[(11, 12)] Rhubarb and gentian were found to be more effective with respect to appetite-loss related symptoms, and boldo and cascara more effective in relieving constipation-related symptoms.

Two preparations containing extracts of boldo and cascara have been documented to increase biliary flow without altering the lithogenic index or bile composition.[(13)] Treatment of 12 human volunteers with boldo dry extract resulted in prolongation of intestinal transit time.[(G4)] However, the methodological limitations of this small, uncontrolled study do not allow any conclusions to be drawn on the effects of boldo.

Ascaridole, a component of the volatile oil, previously found a clinical use as an anthelmintic agent.[(14)] However, this use has declined with the development of synthetic compounds with lower toxicity and a wider range of activity.

Side-effects, Toxicity

Boldo volatile oil is stated to be one of the most toxic oils.[(G58)] Application of the undiluted oil to the hairless backs of mice has an irritant effect.[(15)] The oil contains irritant terpenes, including terpinen-4-ol, the irritant principle in juniper oil.

An acute oral LD_{50} value for boldo oil has been given as 0.13 g/kg body weight in rats, with doses of 0.07 g/kg causing convulsions.[(15)] The acute dermal LD_{50} in rabbits has been reported as 0.625–1.25 g/kg.[(15)] No acute toxicity was observed in rats given oral doses of 3 g/kg of dry aqueous ethanolic extract, and in mice, an aqueous ethanolic extract (1 : 1) had an LD_{50} of 6 g/kg (intraperitoneal administration).[(G52)] The LD_{50} values of total alkaloids and of boldine in mice were 420 and 250 mg/kg (intraperitoneal administration), respectively.[(G52)] Total alkaloids (intraperitoneal administration) given to dogs produced vomiting, diarrhoea and epileptic symptoms with a recovery after 50 minutes.[(G52)]

Boldine was not genotoxic as indicated by the SOS chromotest with *Escherichia coli*, or in the Ames test, and did not induce mutations in *Saccharomyces cerevisiae*.[(16)] Boldine did not induce an increase in the frequency of chromosome aberrations in human lymphocytes *in vitro*, or in mouse bone marrow cells *in vivo*. There were no signs of genotoxicity in mouse bone marrow, as assessed by the micro nucleus test.[(16)]

Contra-indications, Warnings

Excessive doses of boldo may cause renal irritation, because of the volatile oil, and should be avoided by individuals with an existing kidney disorder. Boldo is contra-indicated in individuals with obstruction of bile duct or severe liver disease. Boldo should only be used in patients with gallstones after consultation with a physician.(G3) Ascaridole is toxic and use of the oil is not recommended.(G58)

Drug interactions None documented. However, the potential for preparations of boldo to interact with other medicines administered concurrently, particularly those with similar or opposing effects, should be considered.

Pregnancy and lactation The safety of boldo taken during pregnancy has not been established. In view of the potential irritant nature of the volatile oil, the use of boldo during pregnancy should be avoided.

Preparations

Proprietary multi-ingredient preparations

Argentina: Biliosan Compuesto; Boldina; Dioxicolagol; Drenocol; Hepacur; Hepatalgina; Hepatodirectol; Metiogen; Opobyl; Radicura. *Australia:* Berberis Complex; Lexat. *Austria:* St Bonifatius-Tee. *Brazil:* Alcafelol; Alcaflor; Bilifel; Boldopeptan; Boljuprima; Colachofra; Ductoveran; Emagrevit; Eparema; Figatil; Gotas Digestivas; Hepatoregius; Jurubileno; Prinachol; Solvobil. *Chile:* Hepabil; Nature Complex Reduct-Te; Reduc-Te. *Czech Republic:* The Salvat. *France:* Bolcitol; Drainactil; Elixir Spark; Grains de Vals; Hepaclem; Hepax; Jecopeptol; Mediflor no 11 Draineur Renal et Digestif; Mediflor Tisane Hepatique No 5; Mucinum a l'Extrait de Cascara; Opobyl; Solution Stago Diluee; Tisane Hepatique de Hoerdt. *Germany:* Cynarzym N; Heumann Verdauungstee Solu-Lipar. *Hong Kong:* Mucinum Cascara. *Italy:* Amaro Medicinale; Caramelle alle Erbe Digestive; Coladren; Colax; Confetti Lassativi CM; Critichol; Digelax; Dis-Cinil Complex; Eparema-Levul; Eparema; Eupatol; Hepatos B12; Hepatos; Magisbile; Mepalax; Solvobil. *Mexico:* Chofabol; Hepedren Ifuchol; Peptochol. *Spain:* Natusor Hepavesical; Nico Hepatocyn; Odisor; Opobyl; Resolutivo Regium; Solucion Schoum. *Switzerland:* Boldocynara; Heparfelien; Tisane hepatique et biliaire. *UK:* Adios; Boldex; Fenneherb Slim Aid; HealthAid Boldo-Plus; Napiers Slimming Tablets; Reducing (Slimming) Tablets; Weight Loss Aid.

References

1 Urzúa A, Acuña P. Alkaloids from the bark of *Peumus boldus*. *Fitoterapia* 1983; 4: 175–177.
2 Urzúa A, Torres R. 6a,7-Dehydroboldine from the bark of *Peumus boldus*. *J Nat Prod* 1984; 47: 525–526.
3 Hughes DW *et al*. Alkaloids of *Peumus boldus*. Isolation of laurotetatine and laurolitsine. *J Pharm Sci* 1968; 57: 1619–1620.
4 Hughes DW *et al*. Alkaloids of *Peumus boldus*. Isolation of (+)-reticuline and isoboldine. *J Pharm Sci* 1968; 57: 1023–1025.
5 Bombardelli E *et al*. A new flavonol glycoside from *Peumus boldus*. *Fitoterapia* 1976; 46: 3–5.
6 Krug H, Borkowski B. Neue Flavonol-Glykoside aus den Blättern von Peumus boldus Molina. *Pharmazie* 1965; 20: 692–698.
7 Lanhers MC *et al*. Hepatoprotective and anti-inflammatory effects of a traditional medicinal plant of Chile, *Pneumus boldo*. *Planta Med* 1991; 57:110–115.
8 Cederbaum AI *et al*. Inhibition of rat liver microsomal lipid peroxidation by boldine. *Biochem Pharmacol* 1992; 44: 1765–1772.
9 Speisky H *et al*. Activity of boldine on rat ileum. *Planta Med* 1991; 57: 519–522.
10 Speisky H *et al*. Antioxidant properties of the alkaloid boldine in systems undergoing lipid peroxidation and enzyme inactivation. *Biochem Pharmacol* 1991; 41: 1575–1581.
11 Borgia M *et al*. Pharmacological activity of a herbs extract: A controlled clinical study. *Curr Ther Res* 1981; 29: 525–536.
12 Borgia M *et al*. Studio policentrico doppio-cieco doppio-controllato sull'attività terapeutica di una nota associazione di erbe medicamentose. *Clin Ter* 1985; 114: 401–409.
13 Salati R *et al*. Valutazione delle proprietà coleretiche di due preparati contenenti estratti di boldo e cascara. *Minerva Dietol Gastroenterol* 1984; 30: 269–272.
14 Wagner H, Wolff P, eds. *New Natural Products and Plant Drugs with Pharmacological, Biological or Therapeutical Activity.* Berlin: Springer-Verlag, 1977.
15 Boldo leaf oil. *Food Chem Toxicol* 1982; 20 (Suppl. Suppl.B): 643.
16 Moreno PRH *et al*. Genotoxicity of the boldine aporphine alkaloid in prokaryotic and eukaryotic organisms. *Mutat Res* 1991; 260: 145–152.

Boneset

Summary and Pharmaceutical Comment

The constituents of boneset are fairly well documented and include many pharmacologically active classes such as flavonoids, sesquiterpene lactones (typical for the Asteraceae family) and triterpenes. Immunostimulant activity (*in vitro*) has been reported for sesquiterpene lactone and polysaccharide components, but there is a lack of rigorous clinical research assessing the efficacy of boneset. Many pharmacological studies have focused on the cytotoxic/antitumour actions of sesquiterpene lactone components of various *Eupatorium* species, although these actions have not been reported for sesquiterpene lactones isolated from boneset. Little is known regarding the toxicity of boneset. Hepatotoxic pyrrolizidine alkaloids, which have been documented for other *Eupatorium* species, have not been reported for boneset.

Species (Family)

Eupatorium perfoliatum L. (Asteraceae/Compositae)

Synonym(s)

Common Boneset, *Eupatorium chapmanii* Small, Feverwort, Thoroughwort. Snakeroot has been used to describe poisonous *Eupatorium* species.

Part(s) Used

Herb

Pharmacopoeial and Other Monographs

BHP 1983[G7]
Martindale 35th edition[G85]

Legal Category (Licensed Products)

GSL – as Boneset and Eupatorium.[G37]

Constituents

The following is compiled from several sources, including General References G22, G41 and G48.

Flavonoids Flavonol (kaempferol, quercetin) glycosides including astragalin, hyperoside and rutin; eupatorin (flavone) and dihydroflavonols.[1]

Terpenoids Sesquiterpene lactones including euperfolin and euperfolitin (germacranolides), eufoliatin (guianolide), eufoliatorin (dilactone guaiane) and euperfolide.[2] Sesquiterpenes, diterpenes (dendroidinic acid, hebeclinolide), triterpenes (α-amyrin, dotriacontane) and sterols (sitosterol, stigmasterol).

Other constituents Volatile oil, resin, wax, tannic and gallic acids, bitter glucoside, inulin, polysaccharides and sugars.

Food Use

Boneset is not used in foods.

Herbal Use

Boneset is stated to possess diaphoretic and aperient properties. Traditionally, it has been used for influenza, acute bronchitis, nasopharyngeal catarrh, and specifically for influenza with deep aching, and congestion of the respiratory mucosa.[G7, G64]

Dosage

Dosages for oral administration (adults) for traditional uses recommended in older standard herbal reference texts are given below.

Herb 1–2 g as an infusion three times daily.[G7]

Liquid extract 1–2 mL (1 : 1 in 25% alcohol) three times daily.[G7]

Tincture 1–4 mL (1 : 5 in 45% alcohol) three times daily.[G7]

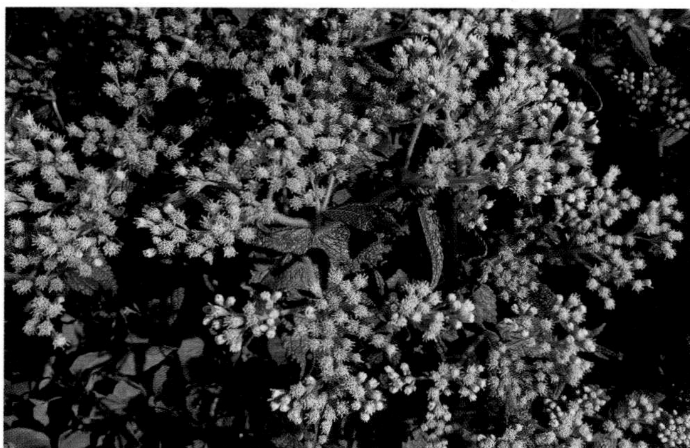

Figure 1 Boneset (*Eupatorium perfoliatum*).

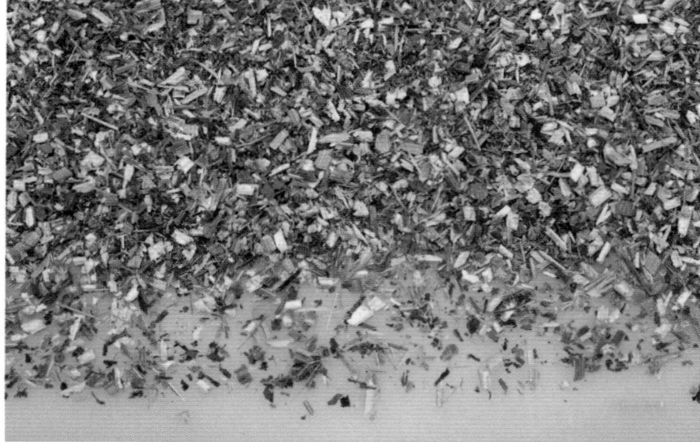

Figure 2 Boneset – dried drug substance (herb).

Pharmacological Actions

In vitro and animal studies

Immunostimulant activity (*in vitro* stimulation of granulocyte phagocytic activity) has been demonstrated by high dilutions (10^{-5}–10^{-7} g/100 mL) of various sesquiterpene lactones isolated from *E. perfoliatum*.[3] In addition, immunostimulating actions (granulocyte, macrophage and carbon clearance tests) have been documented for polysaccharide fractions from *E. perfoliatum*.[3,4]

An ethanol extract of the whole plant has exhibited weak anti-inflammatory activity in rats.[G41] Many activities, including anti-inflammatory activity, have been documented for flavonoid compounds.

Clinical studies

None documented. Rigorous randomised controlled clinical trials assessing the effects of boneset are required.

Side-effects, Toxicity

Contact dermatitis has been reported for *Eupatorium* species, but not specifically for boneset (*E. perfoliatum*).[G51] Cytotoxic properties have been documented for a related species, *E. cannabinum*, and are attributed to the sesquiterpene lactone eupatoriopicrin. This compound has not been documented as a constituent of boneset. Hepatotoxic pyrrolizidine alkaloids (PAs) have been isolated from various *Eupatorium* species, although none have been documented as constituents of boneset (*E. perfoliatum*).[5]

Instances of allergic and anaphylactic reactions have been associated with the sesquiterpene lactone constituents in German chamomile, although no reactions specifically involving boneset have been documented.

The US Food and Drugs Administration (FDA) has classified boneset as a herb of undefined safety.[G22]

Contra-indications, Warnings

The allergenic potential of sesquiterpene lactones is well recognised. Individuals with a known hypersensitivity to other members of the Asteraceae family (e.g. chamomile, feverfew, ragwort, tansy) should avoid using boneset. Individuals with existing hypersensitivities/allergies should use boneset with caution.

Drug interactions None documented. However, the potential for preparations of boneset to interact with other medicines administered concurrently, particularly those with similar or opposing effects, should be considered.

Pregnancy and lactation The safety of boneset taken during pregnancy has not been established. In view of the lack of toxicity data and the possibility of constituents with allergenic activity, the use of boneset during pregnancy and lactation should be avoided.

Preparations

Proprietary multi-ingredient preparations

Australia: Flavons. *UK:* Catarrh Mixture.

References

1 Herz W *et al*. Dihydroflavonols and other flavonoids of *Eupatorium* species. *Phytochemistry* 1972; 11: 2859–2863.
2 Herz W *et al*. Sesquiterpene lactones of *Eupatorium perfoliatum*. *J Org Chem* 1977; 42: 2264–2271.
3 Wagner H. Immunostimulants from medicinal plants. In: Chang HM *et al*, eds. *Advances in Chinese Medicinal Materials Research*. Singapore: World Scientific, 1985: 159–170.
4 Wagner H *et al*. Immunostimulating polysaccharides (heteroglycans) of higher plants. *Arzneimittelforschung* 1985; 35: 1069.
5 *Pyrrolizidine Alkaloids*. Environmental Health Criteria 80. Geneva: World Health Organization, 1988.

Borage

Summary and Pharmaceutical Comment

Limited information is available on the constituents of borage. No documented pharmacological data were located to support the traditional uses, although the mucilage content supports the use of borage as a demulcent. Interest has focused on the volatile oil as a source of gamolenic acid. Borage contains known toxic pyrrolizidine alkaloids, although at concentrations considerably lower than those found in comfrey for which human toxicity has been documented. However, it would seem wise to avoid excessive or prolonged ingestion of borage. It is unclear whether borage oil, currently available in food supplements, contains any pyrrolizidine alkaloids.

Species (Family)

Borago officinalis L. (Boraginaceae)

Synonym(s)

Beebread, Bee Plant, Burrage, Starflower (oil)

Part(s) Used

Herb

Pharmacopoeial and Other Monographs

BP 2007[G84]
Martindale 35th edition[G85]
Ph Eur 2007[G81]

Legal Category (Licensed Product)

Borage is not included in the GSL.[G37]

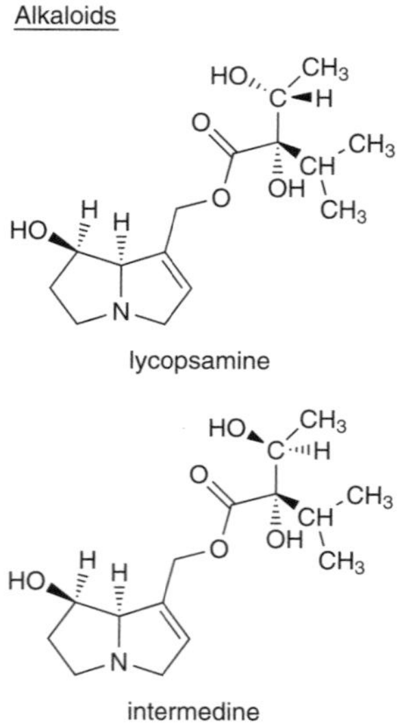

Alkaloids

lycopsamine

intermedine

Figure 1 Selected constituents of borage.

Constituents

The following is compiled from several sources, including General References G22 and G64.

Alkaloids Pyrrolizidine-type. Lycopsamine, intermedine, acetyllycopsamine, acetylintermedine, amabiline, supinine and thesinine (unsaturated).[1,2] Concentrations reported as 0.01% and 2–10 ppm for commercial dried samples. Alkaloid concentrations reportedly the same for fresh and dried samples; fresh samples revealed alkaloids as the free base in the roots and mainly as *N*-oxides in the leaves.

Mucilages 11.1%. Yielding glucose, galactose and arabinose.

Oil Rich in fatty acids, in particular gamolenic acid.

Other constituents Acids (acetic, lactic, malic, silicic), cyanogenetic compounds and tannins (up to 3%).

Food Use

Borage is occasionally used in salads and soups.

Herbal Use

Borage is stated to possess diaphoretic, expectorant, tonic, anti-inflammatory and galactogogue properties.[3] Traditionally, borage has been used to treat many ailments including fevers, coughs and depression.[3, G42, G64] Borage is also reputed to act as a restorative agent on the adrenal cortex.[3] Borage oil (starflower oil) is used as an alternative source to evening primrose oil for gamolenic acid.

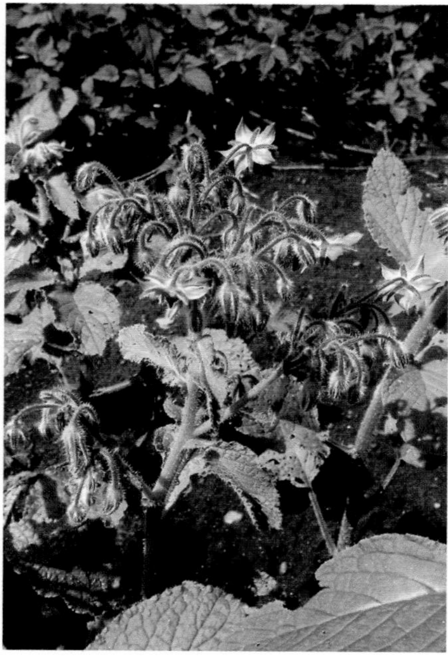

Figure 2 Borage (*Borago officinalis*).

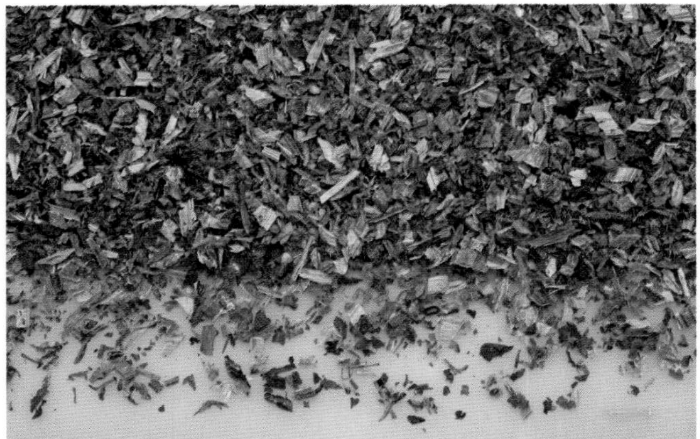

Figure 3 Borage – dried drug substance (herb).

Dosage

Dosages for oral administration (adults) for traditional uses recommended in older and contemporary standard herbal reference texts are given below.

Infusion Two 5-mL spoonfuls of dried herb to one cup boiling water three times daily.[3]

Tincture 1–4 mL three times daily.[3]

Pharmacological Actions

In vitro and animal studies

Borage oil has been reported to attenuate cardiovascular reactivity to stress in rats.[4]

Clinical studies

The effect of borage seed oil on the cardiovascular reactivity of humans to acute stress has been studied in 10 individuals, who each received a total daily dose of 1.3 g for 28 days.[4] The individuals were required to undertake an acute psychological task requiring sensory intake and vigilance (Stroop colour test). Borage oil was found to attenuate cardiovascular reactivity to stress, indicated by a reduction in systolic blood pressure and heart rate and by increased task performance. The specific mechanisms by which borage exerts this effect were unknown, but a central mechanism of action of the fatty acids was suggested in view of the simultaneous reduction in heart rate and blood pressure.[4]

Side-effects, Toxicity

None documented. However, borage contains low concentrations of unsaturated pyrrolizidine alkaloids, which are known to be hepatotoxic in both animals and humans (*see* Comfrey).[5]

B

Contra-indications, Warnings

Evening primrose oil is recommended to be used with caution in epileptic patients, especially in those with schizophrenia and/or those taking phenothiazines (*see* Evening Primrose); on the basis that borage oil, like evening primrose oil, also contains high concentrations of gamolenic acid, borage oil should also be used with caution in these patient groups. In view of the known toxic pyrrolizidine alkaloid constituents, excessive or prolonged ingestion of borage should be avoided. In particular, infusions (e.g. herbal teas) containing borage should be avoided.

Drug interactions None documented. However, the potential for preparations of borage to interact with other medicines administered concurrently, particularly those with similar or opposing effects, should be considered.

Pregnancy and lactation In view of the documented pyrrolizidine constituents and lack of toxicity data, borage should not be used during pregnancy or lactation.

Preparations

Proprietary single-ingredient preparations

Chile: Dexol.

Proprietary multi-ingredient preparations

Chile: Celltech Gold. *Italy:* Sclerovis H. *New Zealand:* Mr Nits. *USA:* Borage Oil; Omega-3 Complex; Omega-3 Glucosamine.

References

1 Luthry J *et al*. Pyrrolizidin-Alkaloide in Arzneipflanzen der Boraginaceen: *Borago officinalis* and *Pulmonaria officinalis*. *Pharm Acta Helv* 1984; 59: 242–246.
2 Larsen KM *et al*. Unsaturated pyrrolizidines from Borage (*Borage officinalis*) a common garden herb. *J Nat Prod* 1984; 47: 747–748.
3 Hoffman D. *The Herb Users Guide, the Basic Skills of Medical Herbalism*. Wellingborough: Thorsons, 1987.
4 Mills DE. Dietary fatty acid supplementation alters stress reactivity and performance in man. *J Hum Hypertens* 1989; 3: 111–116.
5 Mattock AR. *Chemistry and Toxicology of Pyrrolizidine Alkaloids*. London: Academic Press, 1986.

Broom

Summary and Pharmaceutical Comment

The chemistry of broom is reasonably well documented. The pharmacological actions are primarily due to the alkaloid constituents. Sparteine, the major alkaloid component, is a cardiac depressant with actions similar to those of quinidine. Although these actions support some of the documented traditional herbal uses, there is a lack of rigorous clinical research assessing the effects of broom. The intended uses of broom are not suitable for self-medication.

Species (Family)

Cytisus scoparius (L.) Link

Synonym(s)

Hogweed, *Sarothamnus scoparius* (L.) Koch, Scoparius, *Spartium scoparium* L.

Part(s) Used

Flowerhead

Pharmacopoeial and Other Monographs

BHC 1992[G6]
BHP 1996[G9]
Martindale 35th edition[G85]

Legal Category (Licensed Products)

Broom is not included in the GSL.[G37]

Constituents

The following is compiled from several sources, including General References G2, G40, G41, G48, G62 and G64.

Alkaloids Quinolizidine-type. 0.8–1.5%. Sparteine 0.3–0.8% (major component); minor alkaloids include cytisine (presence disputed), genisteine (*d*-α-isosparteine), lupanine, oxysparteine and sarothamine.

Figure 1 Selected constituents of broom.

Amines Epinine, hydroxytyramine and tyramine.

Flavonoids Scoparin and vitexin.

Other constituents Amino acids, bitter principles, carotenoids, fat, resin, sugars, tannin, wax and volatile oil.

Food Use

Broom is listed by the Council of Europe as a natural source of food flavouring (category N3). This category indicates that broom can be added to foodstuffs in the traditionally accepted manner, although there is insufficient information available for an adequate assessment of potential toxicity.[G16]

Herbal Use

Broom is stated to possess cardioactive, diuretic, peripheral vasoconstrictor and antihaemorrhagic properties. It has been used for cardiac dropsy, myocardial weakness, tachycardia, profuse menstruation and specifically for functional palpitation with lowered blood pressure.[G2, G7, G64] Broom is also reported to possess emetic and cathartic properties.[G41]

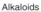

Figure 2 Broom (*Cytisus scoparius*).

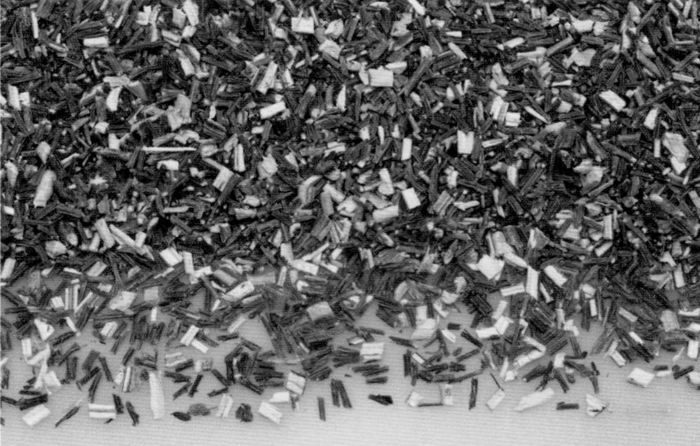

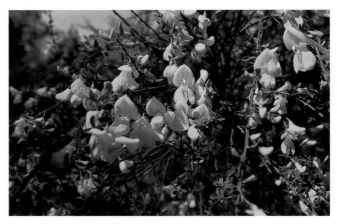

Figure 3 Broom – dried drug substance (herb).

Dosage

Dosages for oral administration (adults) for traditional uses recommended in older and contemporary standard herbal reference texts are given below.

Dried tops 1–2 g as a decoction.(G7)

Liquid extract 1–2 mL (1 : 1 in 25% alcohol).(G7)

Tincture 0.5–2.0 mL (1 : 5 in 45% alcohol).(G7)

Pharmacological Actions

The pharmacological actions of broom are primarily due to the alkaloid constituents.

In vitro and animal studies

Sparteine is reported to exhibit pharmacological actions similar to those of quinidine. Low doses administered to animals result in tachycardia, whereas high doses cause bradycardia and may lead to ventricular arrest. Sparteine has little effect on the central nervous system (CNS), but peripherally, paralyses motor nerve terminals and sympathetic ganglia as a result of a curare-like action.(G44)

Clinical studies

None documented for broom. The major alkaloid constituent sparteine is known to decrease the irritability and conductivity of cardiac muscle and has been used to treat cardiac arrhythmias,(G44) restoring normal rhythm in previously arrhythmic patients.(G2) Sparteine is reported to have a quinidine-like action rather than a digitalis-like action.(G2) Sparteine is also stated to be a powerful oxytocic drug, which was once used to stimulate uterine contractions.

Side-effects, Toxicity

The alkaloid constituents in broom are toxic. Sparteine sulfate has been reported to be a cardiac depressant and can also produce respiratory arrest.(G86) Symptoms of poisoning are characterised by tachycardia with circulatory collapse, nausea, diarrhoea, vertigo and stupor.

Contra-indications, Warnings

Broom is stated to be inappropriate for non-professional use.(G49) Its use is contra-indicated in individuals with high blood pressure(G49) or a cardiac disorder, because of the alkaloid constituents.

Drug interactions None documented. However, the potential for preparations of broom to interact with other medicines administered concurrently, particularly those with similar or opposing effects, should be considered.

Pregnancy and lactation Sparteine is contra-indicated during pregnancy; therefore, broom should not be used during pregnancy in view of its sparteine content.(G42) Sparteine is stated to be a powerful oxytocic drug and is cardiotoxic. Broom should not be taken during lactation.

Preparations

Proprietary single-ingredient preparations

Germany: Spartiol.

Proprietary multi-ingredient preparations

France: Creme Rap.

Buchu

Summary and Pharmaceutical Comment

Limited chemical data are available for buchu. No scientific evidence was found to justify the herbal uses, although reputed diuretic and anti-inflammatory activities may be attributable to the irritant nature of the volatile oil and the flavonoid components, respectively. In view of the lack of documented toxicity data, together with the presence of pulegone in the volatile oil, excessive use of buchu should be avoided.

Species (Family)

Agathosma betulina (Berg.) Pillans (Rutaceae)

Synonym(s)

Barosma betulina, Folia Bucco, *Hartogia betulina* Berg., Round Buchu, Short Buchu

Part(s) Used

Leaf

Pharmacopoeial and Other Monographs

BHC 1992[G6]
BHP 1996[G9]
Martindale 35th edition[G85]

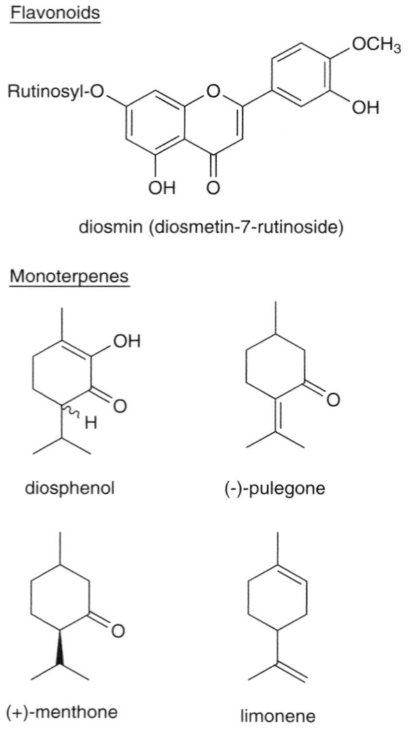

Flavonoids

Rutinosyl-O, OCH3, OH, O, OH, O

diosmin (diosmetin-7-rutinoside)

Monoterpenes

diosphenol

(-)-pulegone

(+)-menthone

limonene

Figure 1 Selected constituents of buchu.

Legal Category (Licensed Products)

GSL[G37]

Constituents

The following is compiled from several sources, including General References G2, G22, G41 and G48.

Flavonoids Diosmetin, quercetin, diosmin, quercetin-3,7-diglucoside, rutin.

Volatile oils 1.0–3.5%. Over 100 identified compounds, including diosphenol, limonene, menthone and pulegone as the major components.

Other constituents Mucilage, resin. Coumarins have been reported for many other *Agathosma* species.[1]

Food Use

Buchu is listed by the Council of Europe as a natural source of food flavouring (category N3). This category allows buchu to be added to foodstuffs in the traditionally accepted manner, although there is insufficient information available for an adequate assessment of potential toxicity.[G16] In the USA, buchu volatile oil is approved for food use with concentrations usually up to about 0.002% (15.4 ppm).[G16, G41]

Herbal Use

Buchu is stated to possess urinary antiseptic and diuretic properties. It has been used for cystitis, urethritis, prostatitis, and specifically for acute catarrhal cystitis.[G2, G7, G8, G64]

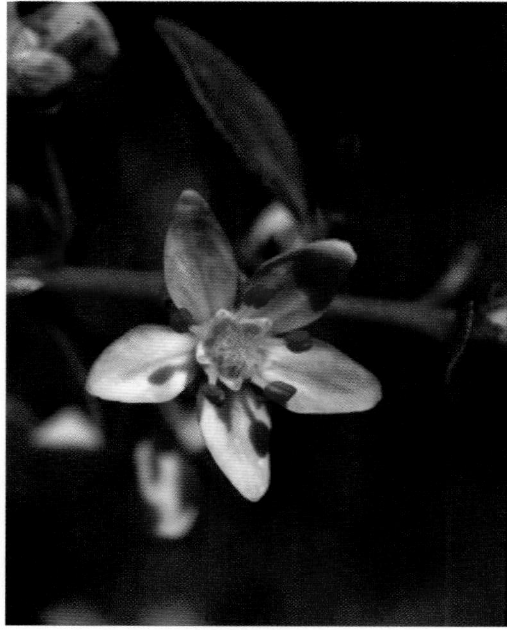

Figure 2 Buchu (*Agathosma betulina*).

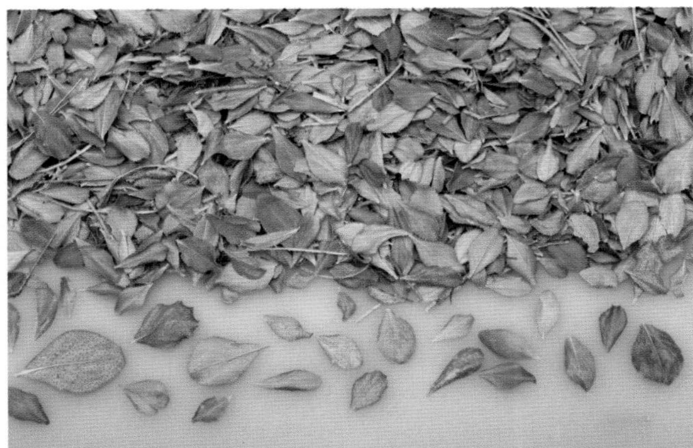

Figure 3 Buchu – dried drug substance (leaf).

Dosage

Dosages for oral administration (adults) for traditional uses recommended in older standard reference texts are given below.

Dried leaf 1–2 g by infusion three times daily.[G6, G7]

Liquid extract 0.3–1.2 mL (1 : 1 in 90% alcohol).[G6, G7]

Tincture 2–4 mL (1 : 5 in 60% alcohol).[G6, G7]

Pharmacological Actions

In vitro and animal studies

None documented for buchu. Diosmin has documented anti-inflammatory activity against carrageenan-induced rat paw oedema, at a dose of 600 mg/kg body weight.[2]

Clinical studies

None documented. Rigorous randomised controlled clinical trials assessing the effects of buchu are required.

Side-effects, Toxicity

None documented for buchu. The volatile oil contains pulegone, a known hepatotoxin (*see* Pennyroyal).[G20] The oil may cause gastrointestinal and renal irritation.

Contra-indications, Warnings

Excessive doses of buchu should not be taken in view of the potential toxicity of the volatile oil. It has been stated that buchu should be avoided in kidney infections, although the scientific basis for this is not clear.[G42]

Drug interactions None documented. However, the potential for preparations of buchu to interact with other medicines administered concurrently, particularly those with similar or opposing effects, should be considered.

Pregnancy and lactation The safety of buchu has not been established. In view of this, together with the potential toxicity and irritant action of the volatile oil, the use of buchu during pregnancy and lactation should be avoided.

Preparations

Proprietary multi-ingredient preparations

Australia: Althaea Complex; Bioglan Cranbiotic Super; Cranberry Complex; Cranberry Complex; De Witts New Pills; Extralife Uri-Care; Fluid Loss; Medinat PMT-Eze; PMS Support; Serenoa Complex; Urinase; Uva-Ursi Complex. *Canada:* Herbal Diuretic. *Czech Republic:* Epilobin. *France:* Urophytum. *New Zealand:* De Witts Pills. *South Africa:* Borstol Cough Remedy; Doans Backache Pills; Docrub. *Switzerland:* Heparfelien; Urinex. *UK:* Antitis; Backache; Backache Relief; Buchu Backache Compound Tablets; De Witt's K & B Pills; Diuretabs; Fenneherb Cystaid; HRI Water Balance; Kas-Bah; Roberts Black Willow Compound Tablets; Skin Eruptions Mixture; Watershed. *USA:* Water Pill.

References

1 Campbell WE *et al*. Coumarins of the Rutoideae: tribe Diosmeae. *Phytochemistry* 1986; 25: 655–657.

2 Farnsworth NR, Cordell GA. A review of some biologically active compounds isolated from plants as reported in the 1974–1975 literature. *Lloydia* 1976, 39: 420–455.

Burdock

Summary and Pharmaceutical Comment

The chemistry of burdock and related *Arctium* species is well documented. Various pharmacological activities have been reported in animals, although none support the reputed herbal uses and there is a lack of rigorous clinical research assessing the effects of burdock. Documented bitter constituents, however, may explain the traditional use of burdock as an orexigenic. In view of the lack of toxicity data, excessive use of burdock should be avoided.

Species (Family)

Arctium lappa L.

Synonym(s)

Arctium majus Bernh., Bardanae Radix, Greater Burdock

Part(s) Used

Root

Pharmacopoeial and Other Monographs

BHC 1992[G6]
BHP 1996[G9]
Martindale 35th edition[G85]

Legal Category (Licensed Products)

GSL[G37]

Constituents

The following is compiled from several sources, including General References G6 and G75.

Acids Acetic acid, butyric acid, caffeic acid, chlorogenic acid, gamma-guanidino-*n*-butyric acid, α-guanidino-*n*-isovaleric acid, *trans*-2-hexenoic acid, isovaleric acid, lauric acid, linoleic acid, linolenic acid, myristic acid, oleic acid, palmitic acid, propionic acid, stearic acid and tiglic acid.[1–3]

Aldehydes Acetaldehyde, benzaldehyde, butyraldehyde, caproicaldehyde, isovaleraldehyde, propionaldehyde and valeraldehyde.[1]

Carbohydrates Inulin (up to 45–50%), mucilage, pectin and sugars.

Polyacetylenes 0.001–0.002% dry weight. Fourteen identified compounds include 1,11-tridecadiene-3,5,7,9-tetrayne (50%), 1,3,11-tridecatriene-5,7,9-triyne (30%) and 1-tridecen-3,5,7,9,11-pentayne as the major components.[4]

Terpenoids Sesquiterpenes arctiol, β-eudesmol, fukinone, costus acid, dehydrocostus lactone, arctiopicrin.[5]

Thiophenes Arctinone-a, arctinone-b, arctinol-a, arctinol-b, arctinal, arctic acid-b, arctic acid-c, methyl arctate-b and arctinone-a acetate (sulfur-containing acetylenic compounds).[6,7]

Sesquiterpenes

arctiol β-eudesmol

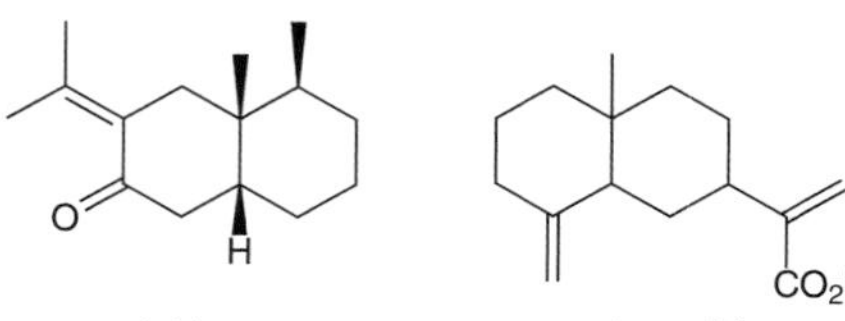

dehydrocostus lactone

Thiophenes

	R
arctinone-a	$-CH_2OH$
arctinol	$-CHOHCH_2OH$
arctinal	$-CHO$
arctic acid	$-COOH$

Polyenes

$H_3C-CH=CH-(C\equiv C)_4-CH=CH_2$

trideca-1,11-diene-3,5,7,9-tetrayne

Lignan

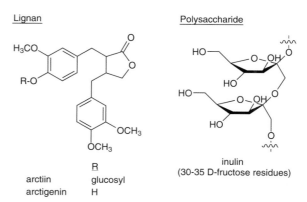

	R
arctiin	glucosyl
arctigenin	H

Polysaccharide

inulin (30-35 D-fructose residues)

Figure 1 Selected constituents of burdock.

Other constituents Fats (0.4–0.8%), fixed and volatile oils (0.07–0.18%), bitters (lappatin), resin, phytosterols (sitosterol and stigmasterol), tannin[8] and arctiin, arctigenin and other lignans.[9–12]

Other species Flavonol (kaempferol, quercetin) glycosides are present in *Arctium minus* (Hill) Bernh.[3]

Food Use

Burdock is listed by the Council of Europe as a natural source of food flavouring (category N2). This category indicates that burdock can be added to foodstuffs in small quantities, with a possible limitation of an active principle (as yet unspecified) in the final product.[G16]

Herbal Use

Burdock is stated to possess diuretic and orexigenic properties. It has been used for cutaneous eruptions, rheumatism, cystitis, gout, anorexia nervosa, and specifically for eczema and psoriasis.[G2, G6, G7, G8, G60]

Dosage

Dosages for oral administration (adults) for traditional uses recommended in older and contemporary standard herbal reference texts are given below.

Dried root 2–6 g by infusion three times daily.[G7]

Liquid extract 2–8 mL (1 : 1 in 25% alcohol) three times daily.[G7]

Tincture 8–12 mL (1 : 10 in 45% alcohol) three times daily.[G7]

Decoction 500 mL (1 : 20) per day.[G7]

Pharmacological Actions

In vitro and animal studies

The roots and leaves of burdock plants not yet flowering are stated to possess diuretic, hypoglycaemic and antifurunculous properties.[7] A burdock extract (plant part not stated) was reported to cause a sharp, long-lasting reduction in the blood sugar concentration in rats, together with an increase in carbohydrate tolerance and a reduction in toxicity.[13]

The antimicrobial activity documented for burdock has been attributed to the polyacetylene constituents,[4] although only traces of these compounds are found in the dried commercial herb.[G62] Furthermore, arctiopicrin is stated to be a bitter with antibiotic activity against Gram-positive bacteria.[7, 14] Antibacterial activity against Gram-positive (e.g. *Staphylococcus aureus*, *Bacillus subtilis*, *Mycobacterium smegmatis*) and Gram-negative (*Escherichia coli*, *Shigella flexneri*, *Shigella sonnei*) bacteria has been documented for burdock leaf and flower, whereas the root was only found to be active towards Gram-negative strains.[15]

In vivo uterine stimulant activity has been reported.[G30]

Protection against mutagenic activity has also been documented for burdock.[9, 16, 17] Burdock reduced the mutagenicity to *Salmonella typhimurium* (TA98, TA100) of mutagens both requiring and not requiring S9 metabolic activation.[10] A lignan-like structure was proposed for the desmutagenic factor.[9] *In vivo* studies have shown that fresh or boiled plant juice from burdock may cause a significant reduction in DMBA-induced chromosome aberrations.[17]

Burdock has been reported to exhibit antitumour activity.[18]

The addition of dietary fibre (5%) from burdock roots to the diet of rats has been documented to provide protection against the toxicity of various artificial food colours.[19]

Clinical studies

There is a lack of clinical research assessing the effects of burdock and rigorous randomised controlled clinical trials are required.

Side-effects, Toxicity

A single report of human poisoning initially associated with burdock has been documented.[20] The patient exhibited symptoms of atropine-like poisoning following the ingestion of a commercially packaged burdock root tea. However, atropine is not a constituent of burdock, and subsequent analysis indicated that the tea was contaminated with a herbal source of solanaceous alkaloids, possibly belladonna leaf. This report served to highlight the problems which may arise with inadequate quality control of herbal preparations.

The carcinogenicity of burdock was investigated in 12 rats fed dried roots (33% of diet) for 120 days, followed by a normal diet until 480 days.[21] Ten of the 12 rats survived 480 days and no tumours were detected. A urinary bladder papilloma and an oligodendroglioma were observed in one rat, but these were considered to have been induced spontaneously.

Burdock has been reported to exhibit antitumour properties (*see In vitro* and animal studies).

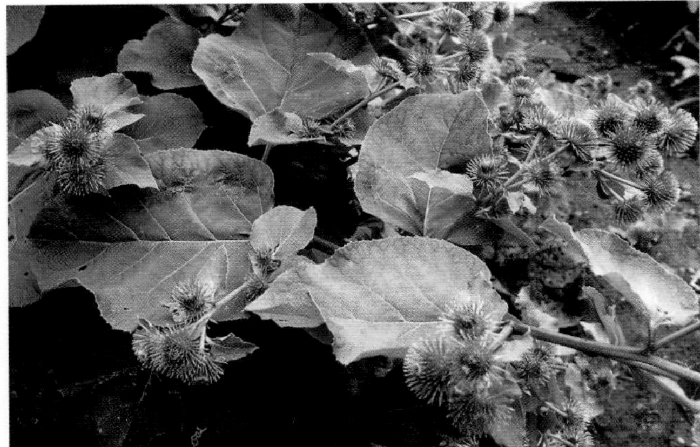

Figure 2 Burdock (*Arctium lappa*).

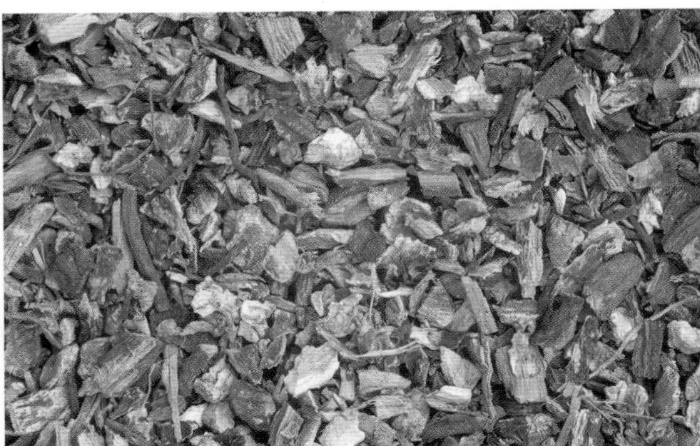

Figure 3 Burdock – dried drug substance (root).

B

Contra-indications, Warnings

Drug interactions None documented. However, the potential for burdock to interact with other medicines administered concurrently, particularly those with similar or opposing effects, should be considered. For example, there is limited evidence from preclinical studies that burdock (not further specified) has hypoglycaemic activity.

Pregnancy and lactation *In vivo* uterine stimulant action has been reported.[G30] In view of this, and the lack of toxicity data, the use of burdock during pregnancy and lactation should be avoided.

Preparations

Proprietary single-ingredient preparations

Mexico: Saforelle. *Portugal:* Saforelle.

Proprietary multi-ingredient preparations

Australia: Acne Oral Spray; Dermaco; Herbal Cleanse; Percutane; Trifolium Complex. *Canada:* Natural HRT. *Czech Republic:* Diabetan. *France:* Arbum; Depuratif Parnel; Fitacnol; Zeniac LP; Zeniac. *Malaysia:* Celery Plus; Cleansa Plus; Dandelion Complex. *South Africa:* Lotio Pruni Comp cum Cupro. *Spain:* Diabesor. *UK:* Aqua Ban Herbal; Backache; Cascade; Catarrh Mixture; GB Tablets; Gerard House Skin; Gerard House Water Relief Tablets; HRI Clear Complexion; Modern Herbals Water Retention; Napiers Skin Tablets; Rheumatic Pain Remedy; Skin Cleansing; Skin Eruptions Mixture; Tabritis; Tabritis Tablets; Water Naturtabs. *USA:* Liver Formula Herbal Blend; Skin Hair Nails.

References

1 Obata S *et al.* Studies on the components of the roots of *Arctium lappa* L. *Agric Biol Chem* 1970; 34: A31.
2 Yamada Y *et al.* γ-Guanidino-*n*-butyric acid from *Arctium lappa*. *Phytochemistry* 1975; 14: 582.
3 Saleh NAM, Bohm BA. Flavonoids of *Arctium minus* (Compositae). *Experientia* 1971; 27: 1494.
4 Schulte KE *et al.* Polyacetylenes in burdock root. *Arzneimittelforschung* 1967; 17: 829–833.
5 Bever BO, Zahnd GR. Plants with oral hypoglycaemic action. *Q J Crude Drug Res* 1979; 17: 139–196.
6 Washino T *et al.* New sulfur-containing acetylenic compounds from *Arctium lappa*. *Agric Biol Chem* 1986; 50: 263–269.
7 Washino T *et al.* Structures of lappaphen-a and lappaphen-b, new guaianolides linked with a sulfur-containing acetylenic compound, from *Arctium lappa* L. *Agric Biol Chem* 1987; 51: 1475–1480.
8 Nakabayashi T. Tannin of fruits and vegetables. III. Polyphenolic compounds and phenol-oxidising enzymes of edible burdock. *Nippon Shokuhin Kogyo Gakkaishi* 1968; 15: 199–206.
9 Morita K *et al.* Chemical nature of a desmutagenic factor from burdock (*A. lappa* L.). *Agric Biol Chem* 1985; 49: 925–932.
10 Ichihara A *et al.* Lappaol A and B, novel lignans from *Arctium lappa* L. *Tetrahedron Lett* 1976; 44: 3961–3964.
11 Ichihara A *et al.* New sesquilignans from *Arctium lappa* L. The structure of lappaol C, D and E. *Agric Biol Chem* 1977; 41: 1813–1814.
12 Liu S *et al.* Isolation and identification of arctiin and arctigenin in leaves of burdock (*Arctium lappa* L.) by polyamide column chromotography in combination with HPLC-ESI/MS. *Phytochemical Anal* 2005; 16: 86–89.
13 Lapinina LO, Sisoeva TF. Investigation of some plants to determine their sugar lowering action. *Farmatsevt Zh* 1964; 19: 52–58.
14 Cappelletti EM *et al.* External antirheumatic and antineuralgic herbal remedies in the traditional medicine of North-eastern Italy. *J Ethnopharmacol* 1982; 6: 161–190.
15 Moskalenko SA. Preliminary screening of far-eastern ethnomedicinal plants for antibacterial activity. *J Ethnopharmacol* 1986; 15: 231–259.
16 Morita K *et al.* Desmutagenic factor isolated from burdock (*Arctium lappa* L.). *Mutat Res* 1984; 129: 25–31.
17 Ito Y *et al.* Suppression of 7,12-dimethylbenz(a) anthracene-induced chromosome aberrations in rat bone marrow cells by vegetable juices. *Mutat Res* 1986; 172: 55–60.
18 Dombradi CA, Foldeak S. Anti-tumor activity of *A. lappa* ext. *Tumori* 1966; 52: 173–175.
19 Tsujita J *et al.* Comparison of protective activity of dietary fiber against the toxicities of various food colors in rats. *Nutr Rep Int* 1979; 20: 635–642.
20 Bryson PD *et al.* Burdock root tea poisoning. Case report involving a commercial preparation. *JAMA* 1978; 239: 2157–2158.
21 Hirono I *et al.* Safety examination of some edible plants, Part 2. *J Environ Pathol Toxicol* 1977; 1: 72–74.

Burnet

Summary and Pharmaceutical Comment

The chemistry of burnet herb does not appear to have been studied, although data are available for the underground plant parts. If present in the herb as well as the root, the tannin constituents would support the reputed astringent and antihaemorrhagic actions of burnet. In view of the lack of toxicity data and the possible high tannin content of the herb, excessive use of burnet should be avoided.

Species (Family)

Sanguisorba officinalis L. (Rosaceae)

Synonym(s)

Garden Burnet, Greater Burnet, *Poterium officinale* A. Gray, Sanguisorba, *Sanguisorba polygama* F. Nyl

Part(s) Used

Herb

Pharmacopoeial and Other Monographs

BHP 1983[G7]
Martindale 35th edition[G85]

Legal Category (Licensed Products)

GSL (Sanguisorba)[G37]

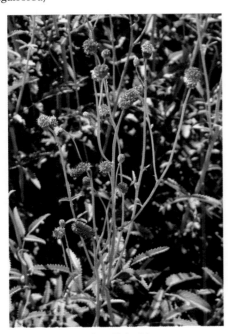

Figure 1 Burnet (*Sanguisorba officinalis*).

Constituents

The following is compiled from several sources, including General Reference G40.

All phytochemical data located refer to the underground plant parts and not to the herb.

Flavonoids Flavones, unstable flavonol derivatives.

Saponins Ziyu glycosides I and II (major glycosides),[1] pomolic acid as aglycone (not tomentosolic acid as documented in earlier work), sanguisorbin 2.5–4.0%.

Tannins Numerous compounds (condensed and hydrolysable) have been isolated, including 3,3,4-tri-*O*-methylellagic acid.[2–6]

Other constituents Volatile oil, ascorbic acid (vitamin C) in the fresh plant.

Food Use

Burnet is not used in foods.

Herbal Use

Burnet is stated to possess astringent, antihaemorrhagic, styptic and antihaemorrhoidal properties. It has been used for ulcerative colitis, metrorrhagia, and specifically for acute diarrhoea.[G7, G64]

Dosage

Dosages for oral administration (adults) for traditional uses recommended in older standard herbal reference texts are given below.

Dried herb 2–6 g as an infusion three times daily.[G7]

Liquid extract 2–6 mL (1 : 1 in 25% alcohol) three times daily.[G7]

Tincture 2–8 mL (1 : 5 in 45% alcohol) three times daily.[G7]

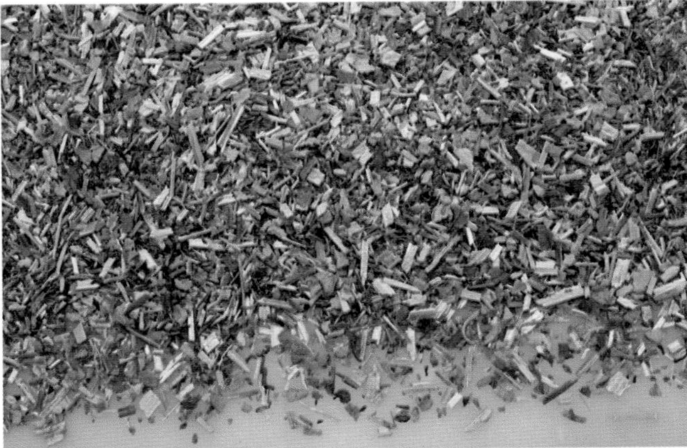

Figure 2 Burnet – dried drug substance (herb).

B

Pharmacological Actions

In vitro and animal studies

None documented for burnet. The roots have been reported to contain an antihaemorrhagic principle, 3,3,4-tri-O-methylellagic acid.[2]

Clinical studies

There is a lack of clinical research assessing the effects of burnet and rigorous randomised controlled clinical trials are required.

Side-effects, Toxicity

None documented. However, there is a lack of research assessing the safety and toxicity profile of burnet.

Contra-indications, Warnings

None documented. However, there is a lack of research assessing the safety and toxicity profile of burnet.

Drug interactions None documented. However, the potential for preparations of burnet to interact with other medicines administered concurrently, particularly those with similar or opposing effects, should be considered.

Pregnancy and lactation In view of the lack of phytochemical, pharmacological and toxicity data, the use of burnet during pregnancy and lactation should be avoided.

Preparations

Proprietary multi-ingredient preparations

Canada: Swiss Herb Cough Drops. *Czech Republic:* Tormentan.

References

1 Yosioka I *et al*. Soil bacterial hydrolysis leading to genuine aglycone. III. The structures of glycosides and genuine aglycone of *Sanguisorbae radix*. *Chem Pharm Bull* 1971; 19: 1700–1707.

2 Kosuge T *et al*. Studies on antihemorrhagic substances in herbs classified as hemostatics in Chinese medicine. III. On the antihemorrhagic principle in *Sanguisorba officinalis* L. *Chem Pharm Bull* 1984; 32: 4478–4481.

3 Nonaka G-I *et al*. Tannins and related compounds. XVII. Galloylhamameloses from *Castanea crenata* L. and *Sanguisorba officinalis* L. *Chem Pharm Bull* 1984; 32: 483–489.

4 Nonaka G-I *et al*. A dimeric hydrolyzable tannin, sanguiin H-6 from *Sanguisorba officinalis* L. *Chem Pharm Bull* 1982; 30: 2255–2257.

5 Tanaka T *et al*. Tannins and related compounds. XVI. Isolation and characterization of six methyl glucoside gallates and a gallic acid glucoside gallate from *Sanguisorba officinalis* L. *Chem Pharm Bull* 1984; 32: 117–121.

6 Tanaka T *et al*. 7-O-galloyl-(+)-catechin and 3-O-galloylprocyanidin B-3 from *Sanguisorba officinalis*. *Phytochemistry* 1983; 22: 2575–2578.

Butterbur

B

Summary and Pharmaceutical Comment

The chemistry of butterbur is well documented. There is evidence from preclinical studies to indicate that the eremophilane sesquiterpene constituents (e.g. petasin and isopetasin), found in the petasin chemovar, are important for activity. However, there are some conflicting reports and it is not clear precisely which constituents are most active. Furthermore, certain activities have been documented for the furanoeremophilane sesquiterpenes found in the furanopetasin chemovar of *Petasites hybridus*.

There is evidence from preclinical studies of the anti-inflammatory, anti-allergic and antispasmodic properties of butterbur extracts and/or their constituents, hence supporting some of the traditional uses. Precise mechanisms of action have not yet been elucidated, although inhibition of leukotriene synthesis, phospholipase A_2 activity and 5-lipoxygenase translocation, and effects on intracellular calcium ion concentrations have been documented in *in vitro* studies. The implications of binding of certain butterbur constituents at dopamine D_2, histamine H_1 and muscarinic receptors, described following *in vitro* studies, require further investigation.

There is a paucity of well-designed, randomised clinical trials of butterbur extracts. Existing trials generally have involved individuals with seasonal allergic rhinitis and migraine and have tested the effects of only a small number of herbal medicinal products containing butterbur extracts. While most of these studies have reported beneficial effects for butterbur extracts, methodologically rigorous investigation of efficacy in allergic rhinitis and migraine prophylaxis is limited and large, well-designed clinical trials are required. Similarly, at present, there is insufficient evidence from randomised clinical trials to support the use of butterbur extracts in patients with asthma and bronchitis.

There is also only limited information on the safety of butterbur extracts and further investigation in this area is required. On the basis of small, randomised clinical trials, certain butterbur extracts appear to be well-tolerated when taken at recommended doses for relatively short periods (clinical studies have involved ingestion for up to four months); adverse events reported most frequently are gastrointestinal symptoms. Chronic toxicity studies are lacking, and there is a lack of clinical information on the safety of long-term use. Against this background, butterbur should not be used for long periods, nor at higher than recommended doses (see below). Spontaneous reports of liver damage associated with the use of a butterbur root extract have been received in Germany. On the basis of this information, the Swiss regulatory authority for medicines revoked the licences for certain butterbur products marketed in Switzerland.

No drug interactions have been reported for butterbur extracts. Based on data from preclinical studies, there is a theoretical possibility that butterbur extracts potentially could interact with hypertensive and antihypertensive medicines, leukotriene receptor antagonists and agonists/antagonists at dopamine D_2, histamine H_1 and muscarinic M_3 receptors.

Both chemotypes (petasin and furanopetasin) of *P. hybridus* contain unsaturated pyrrolizidine alkaloids, and these compounds occur in low concentrations throughout all parts of the plant.(G19) These constituents are known to be hepatotoxic in humans, and have been shown to be carcinogenic and mutagenic in preclinical studies (*see* Comfrey). Several manufacturers of products containing butterbur include in their manufacturing processes steps to remove the unsaturated pyrrolizidine alkaloids to concentrations below the detectable limit (e.g. <35 parts per billion). However, there remains the possibility that toxic quantities of unsaturated pyrrolizidine alkaloids may be present in poorly processed products, and any products which contain *Petasites* species as a result of botanical misidentification or adulteration.

There is a view that butterbur is unsuitable for use as a tea or infusion.(G69) This is because the *N*-oxides of unsaturated pyrrolizidine alkaloids, which can be formed from unsaturated pyrrolizidine alkaloids during storage of plant material but which can also be present in raw plant material, are more water soluble than the parent compounds and are, therefore, extracted more easily during preparations of herbal teas and infusions.(G19)

The dose of butterbur should be such that the daily intake of unsaturated pyrrolizidine alkaloids, including their *N*-oxides, is not greater than 1 µg.(G3) The duration of use of butterbur should not exceed a total of 4–6 weeks in a year.(G3)

Species (Family)

Petasites hybridus (L.) P. Gaertn., B. Meyer et Scherb. (Asteraceae/Compositae).

Synonym(s)

Blatterdock, Bogshorns, Bog rhubarb, Butterdock, Butterfly Dock, Capdockin, Flapperdock, *P. officinalis* Moench, *P. ovatus* Hill, *P. sabaudus* Beauv., *P. vulgaris* Desf., Umbrella Plant(G34)

Part(s) Used

Aerial parts, leaf, rhizome, root

Pharmacopoeial and Other Monographs

German Commission E (root and leaf).(G3)
Martindale 35th edition(G85)

Legal Category (Licensed Products)

Butterbur is not on the GSL. There are no licensed products containing butterbur available in the UK.

Constituents

Two chemovars of *P. hybridus* have been described, which differ markedly in the profile of sesquiterpenes present in the root/

B

rhizome and leaf. The furanopetasin chemovar contains furanoeremophilane sesquiterpenes, whereas the petasin chemovar contains esters of the eremophilane sesquiterpenes petasol, isopetasol and neopetasol.[1–3] The furanopetasin chemovar contains exclusively furanoeremophilane sesquiterpenes: petasin sesquiterpenes are not found in this chemovar.[2,4] Eremophilanlactones have been reported as constituents of the furanopetasin chemovar,[1] but it has been shown that they are produced by rearrangement of 9-hydroxy-furanoeremophilanes during storage of raw plant material.[5]

Both chemotypes contain unsaturated pyrrolizidine alkaloids,[6] and these compounds occur throughout all parts of the plant.[G19]

Leaf

Alkaloids Pyrrolizidine type, mainly senecionine and integerrimine.[7] Content may vary from 0.02–1.50 parts per million (ppm),[8] or <0.1–3.9 or 27.7 ppm (for leaves and leafstalks, respectively).[7]

Flavonoids Astragalin, isoquercitrin, quercetin.[G2]

Sesquiterpenes Furanopetasin chemovar: furanoeremophilane type, including 9-hydroxy-furanoeremophilanes and 9-oxo-furanoeremophilanes.[2] Petasin chemovar: eremophilane type, mainly petasin and neopetasin (2.8 and 1.9 mg/g of dried plant material, respectively), also isopetasin, and the sulfur-containing compounds neo-*S*-petasin, *S*-petasin and iso-*S*-petasin (= *S*-isopetasin; trace).[3]

Other constituents Tannins, mucilage, volatile oil (about 0.1%), triterpenoid saponins (traces).[G2]

Rhizome, root

Alkaloids Pyrrolizidine type, mainly senecionine, its isomer integerrimine and senkirkine.[9] Concentration can vary from 2–500 ppm.[10] Values reported following specific investigations include 5–90 ppm[8] and 6–105 (mean 49.2) ppm (calculated as senecionine);[7] concentrations of senecionine and senkirkine have been reported as 11.3 and 25.8 ppm, respectively.[11]

Sesquiterpenes Furanopetasin chemovar: furanoeremophilane type,[1] mainly furanopetasin and 9-hydroxy-furanoeremophilane (approximately 16–21% and 30–37%, respectively),[2] as well as furanoeremophilane, 2-senecioyl-furanopetasol, 2-tigloyl-furanopetasol and 2-methylthioacryloyl-furanopetasol (6–10%).[2] Petasin chemovar: eremophilane type, mainly petasin (9.4, 7.0 and 7.0 mg/g of dried plant material for rhizomes, roots and runners, respectively), also isopetasin, neopetasin, iso-*S*-petasin, neo-*S*-petasin and *S*-petasin.[3] Minor compounds include 3-methylcrotonyl- and methacryloyl-esters of petasol, neopetasol, isopetasol, 3-desoxyneopetasol and 3-desoxyisopetasol.[12]

Volatile oil A mixture of at least 26 compounds of which 1-nonene, 1-undecene, albene, furanoeremophilane and fukinanolide are major components; minor compounds include the novel sesquiterpene hydrocarbons petasitene and pethybrene.[13]

Quality of crude material and marketed products

As with other medicinal plants, the profile of constituents in different parts of *P. hybridus* can vary both qualitatively and quantitatively depending on various factors, and this has implications for safety and efficacy. The petasin content of the underground parts of plants (petasin chemovar) grown in four different locations in Switzerland ranged from 6.6–13.8 mg/g across regions.[14] Furthermore, although plants showed an approximately similar relative distribution of the six main petasin sesquiterpenes (petasin, isopetasin, neopetasin, iso-*S*-petasin, neo-*S*-petasin and *S*-petasin), there were exceptions: for example, in plants grown in the Krauchthal region, the content of *S*-petasin was approximately half that of neo-*S*-petasin, whereas in plants grown in the Chessiloch region, *S*-petasin content was greater than that of neo-*S*-petasin. Raised temperatures and storage conditions also affect the profile of constituents in *P. hybridus* (petasin chemovar) roots. Under moderate drying conditions (40°C in the dark), isomerisation occurs: sesquiterpene esters with petasol and neopetasol skeletons form the corresponding esters with isopetasin skeletons.[15] The isomerisation of neopetasin to petasin occurs more readily than that of petasin to isopetasin (half-life for neopetasin and petasin: 49 and 205 days, respectively). In the furanopetasin chemovar, 9-hydroxy-furanoeremophilanes rearrange to the corresponding eremophilanlactones during drying and storage of raw plant material.[5]

Some manufacturers of herbal medicinal products containing butterbur state that the unsaturated pyrrolizidine alkaloids are removed from the product before it is released for sale.[16] One method used to achieve acceptably low concentrations (the German Commission E advised that the maximum daily intake is 1 μg)[G3] of these alkaloids is by multiple applications of a method involving a cation-exchange resin;[17] other methods of separating pyrrolizidine alkaloids from several plants, including *P. hybridus*, containing these compounds have been described.[11] A different approach to achieving extremely low concentrations of pyrrolizidine alkaloids is to cultivate clones of wild-type plants previously selected for almost absence of these constituents. Achievement of an initial step – *in vitro* propagation of wild-type plants – in this approach has been documented.[18]

Food Use

Butterbur is not used in foods.

Herbal Use

Butterbur root has been used traditionally for the treatment of fevers, wheezing and colds and as a diuretic and vermifuge.[19, G34] It is also reputed to be a heart stimulant, cardiac tonic and antispasmodic, and to promote menstruation. It has been used externally for treating persistent sores and other skin problems.

Butterbur root was approved by the German Commission E for use as supportive therapy for acute spastic pain in the urinary tract, particularly if urinary stones were present.[G3] Modern-day use of butterbur and clinical trials of products containing butterbur have focused on its use in seasonal allergic rhinitis and migraine prophylaxis.

Dosage

The German Commission E advised that the dose of butterbur should be such that the daily intake of unsaturated pyrrolizidine alkaloids, including their *N*-oxides, is not greater than 1 μg.[G3] The duration of use of butterbur should not exceed a total of 4–6 weeks in a year.[G3]

As an antispasmodic and for other traditional uses

Dosages described in the herbal literature are typically preparations equivalent to 4.5–7 g dried butterbur root daily in the form of an ethanolic or lipophilic extract.[G3, G69]

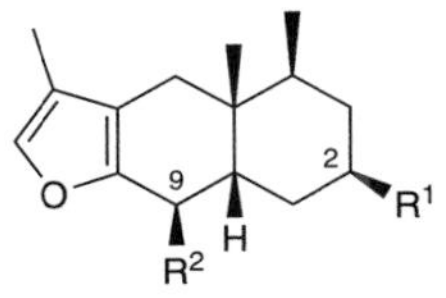

	R1	R2
furanoeremophilane	H	H
9-hydroxyeremophilane	H	OH
furanopetasin	ang	OH
2-senecioylfuranopetasol	sen	OH
2-tigloylfuranopetasol	tig	OH
2-methylthioacryloylpetasol	mta	OH
9-oxofuranoeremophilane	H	O
9-oxofuranopetasin	ang	O

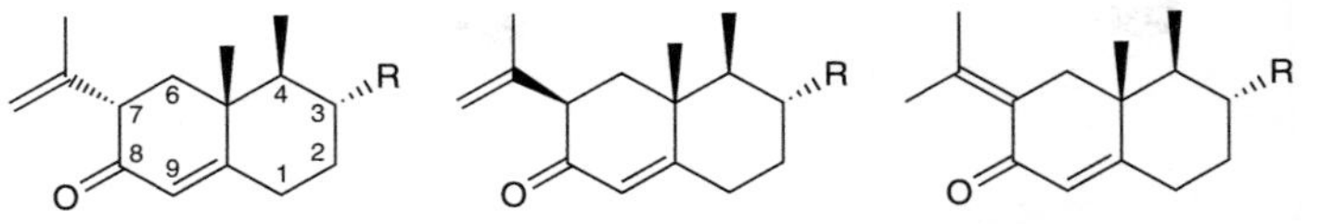

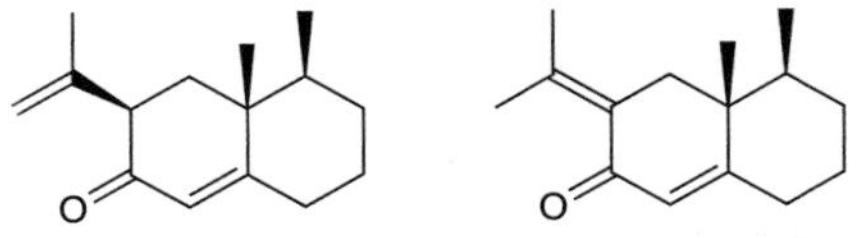

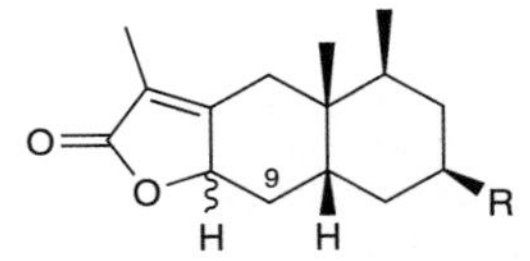

Figure 1 Selected constituents of butterbur.

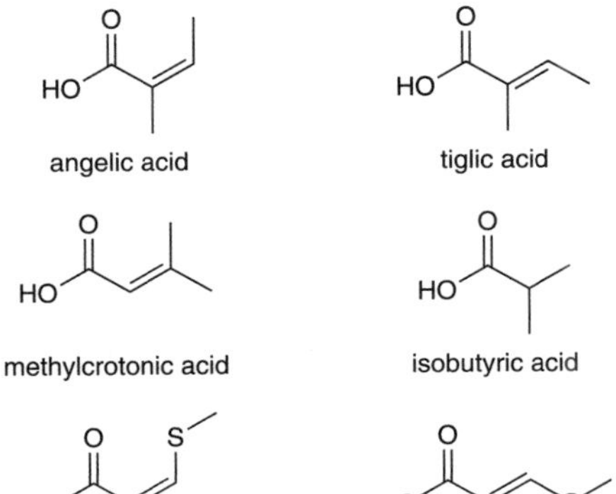

Figure 2 Selected constituents of butterbur.

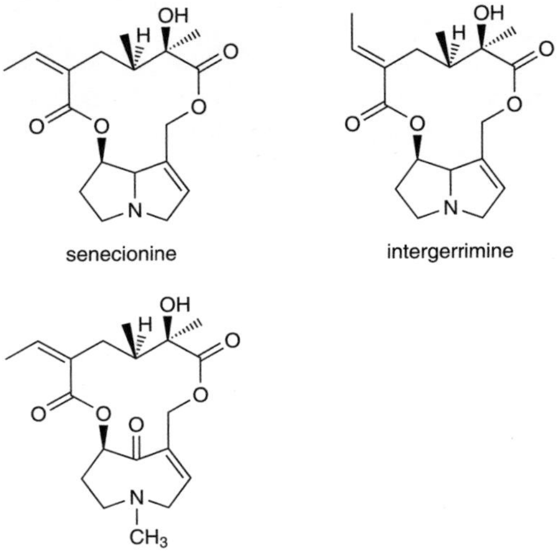

Figure 3 Selected constituents of butterbur.

B

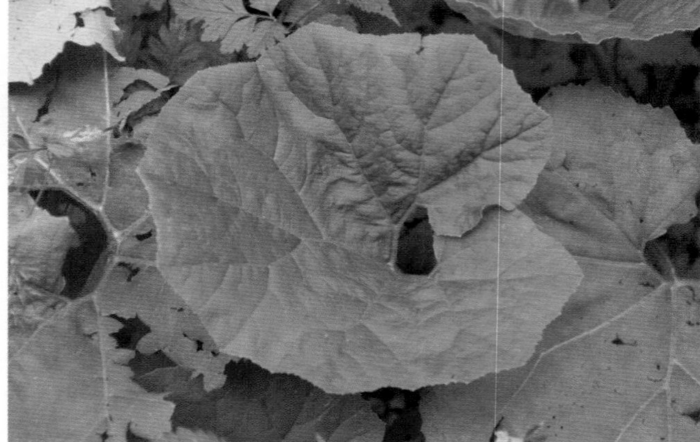

Figure 4 Butterbur (*Petasites hybridus*).

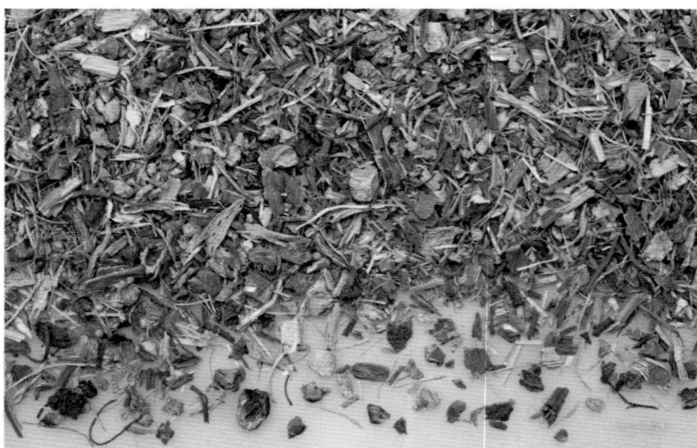

Figure 5 Butterbur – dried drug substance (root)

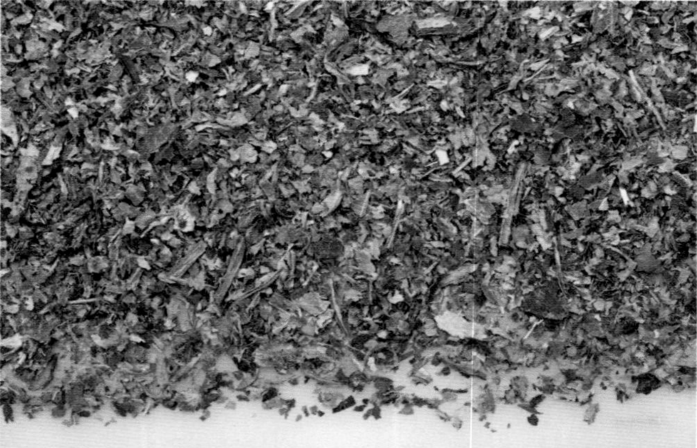

Figure 6 Butterbur – dried drug substance (leaf)

Dosages of butterbur extract used in clinical trials have varied. In trials involving adults with seasonal allergic rhinitis, one study used a butterbur root extract (containing not less than 15% petasins calculated as isopetasin; Petaforce) (D Martin, Bioforce (UK) Ltd, personal communication, 10 June 2004) 50 mg twice daily for two weeks,[20] whereas another study tested a butterbur leaf extract (ZE-339) one tablet four times daily (equivalent to 32 mg petasins daily) for two weeks.[21] Trials of butterbur in migraine prophylaxis have tested a carbon dioxide extract of butterbur rhizome (Petadolex) at doses of 50 or 75 mg twice daily (equivalent to at least 15 or 22.5 mg petasins daily, respectively) for 12 or 16 weeks.[22,23]

Pharmacological Actions

Several pharmacological activities, including anti-inflammatory, anti-allergic and antispasmodic effects, have been described for butterbur root/rhizome and leaf following preclinical studies. Extracts of butterbur have been tested clinically in patients with seasonal and perennial allergic rhinitis (hayfever), bronchial asthma and chronic obstructive bronchitis, and in prophylaxis of migraine headaches. The precise chemical constituents responsible for the documented effects of butterbur are not clearly understood, although several preclinical studies have shown that the petasin constituents, such as petasin and isopetasin, are important for certain pharmacological activities. These compounds may have several intracellular targets, and there is some evidence that the stereoisomers may have different affinities at these, even bringing about different effects.[24] However, other *in vitro* studies have reported that petasin is inactive,[25] and activities for the furanoeremophilane and eremophilanlactone constituents have been documented.[26]

Published papers and texts often use the words root and rhizome interchangeably, although this is not strictly correct. This monograph uses terms exactly as published in the reference material, since it is not possible to say otherwise with certainty precisely which plant part was meant. Published reports also often fail to state which chemovar of *P. hybridus* was used.

In vitro and animal studies

Pharmacokinetics Petasins have been shown to be bioavailable following studies in rabbits fed butterbur leaf extract (containing 50 mg petasin) twice daily for seven days; petasins were detected by gas chromatography-mass spectrometry (GC-MS) within the low nanogram range.[27]

Anti-allergic and anti-inflammatory properties Inhibition of peptido-leukotriene (LT) biosynthesis in murine peritoneal macrophages has been documented following *in vitro* experiments using several different extracts of butterbur root and leaf.[25,28] A petroleum ether extract of *P. hybridus* ground root showed the greatest inhibitory activity of LT synthesis from mouse peritoneal macrophages stimulated with calcium ionophore A23187 (10^{-6} mol/L): 12.6, 95.1 and 100% inhibition at concentrations of *P. hybridus* extract of 6.3, 31.0 and 94.0 µg/mL, respectively ($p < 0.01$ versus control).[25] By contrast, a pyrrolizidine alkaloid-free extract showed no activity in this assay, and the addition of the pyrrolizidine alkaloids senkirkine and senecionine to this extract and to the macrophage-containing tissue culture system also failed to result in inhibition of LT synthesis.[25] A report of this work does not describe the constituents of the pyrrolizidine alkaloid-free extract, so the latter results for lack of activity are difficult to interpret.

Further work involving fractions of the active *P. hybridus* root extract indicated that isopetasin and the oxopetasan esters (= eremophilanlactones, the presence of these is due to rearrangement of 9-hydroxy-furanoeremophilanes during drying and storage as stated above) were important for activity: the content of isopetasin and oxopetasan esters in the fractions correlated with inhibition of LT synthesis in a concentration-dependent manner.[25] By contrast, petasin was not important for activity, but appeared to reduce the activity of isopetasin in this assay.

B

Other *in vitro* studies, however, have reported that petasin is one of the major active compounds of *P. hybridus* extract. Isolated petasin and a standardised high-pressure carbon dioxide extract of *P. hybridus* (containing 14.1% petasin; ZE-339, Zeller) inhibited the synthesis of cysteinyl-LTs in eosinophils and LTB_4 in neutrophils which had been primed with granulocyte-macrophage colony-stimulating factor and subsequently stimulated with platelet-activating factor (PAF) or the anaphylatoxin C5a.[29] Petasin, ZE-339 and the positive control zileuton (a 5-lipoxygenase inhibitor) achieved similar inhibition of cysteinyl-LTs and LTB_4 in eosinophils and neutrophils, respectively, in these models (IC_{50} (concentration for 50% inhibition) $\leqslant$ 24 µg/mL in each case).

In other *in vitro* studies using a similar model of eosinophil stimulation, ZE-339 showed greater inhibition of cysteinyl-LT synthesis than did a fraction containing petasin, isopetasin and neopetasin.[30] When each of these latter compounds was tested separately in this model, all inhibited C5a- and PAF-induced cysteinyl-LT synthesis in a concentration-dependent manner and to the same extent as zileuton (positive control). However, the release of eosinophil cationic protein (ECP) from eosinophils (a measure of eosinophil degranulation) was inhibited by petasin, but not by isopetasin, neopetasin or zileuton. Similarly, petasin, but not isopetasin, neopetasin or zileuton, suppressed cytosolic phospholipase A_2 activity, 5-lipoxygenase translocation and PAF- and C5a-induced increases in intracellular calcium ion concentrations. These findings suggest that the different petasin constituents of butterbur may act upon different intracellular signalling molecules.[30] Extracts of *P. hybridus* rhizomes with different petasin and isopetasin contents (2.1 and 0.4, 0.2 and 0.1, 12.1 and 6.1, and 21.9 and 9.4% petasin and isopetasin respectively) are weak inhibitors of cyclo-oxygenase 1 (COX-1) *in vitro* (IC_{50} > 400 µg/mL) and strong inhibitors of the inducible isoform COX-2 (IC_{50} 20 to 30.4 µg/mL), apart from the extract with the lowest petasin and isopetasin content (IC_{50} 60.6 µg/mL).[31] The former three extracts also inhibited lipopolysaccharide-induced and, therefore, COX-2-mediated prostaglandin E_2 release in primary rat microglial cells in a concentration-dependent manner (IC_{50} < 6 µg/mL); this effect was also independent of the petasin and isopetasin contents. The extract containing petasin 12.1% and isopetasin 6.1% completely inhibited COX-2 synthesis in microglia at a concentration of 5 µg/mL whereas COX-1 synthesis was unaffected. Overall, these findings suggest selective inhibition of COX-2 and its expression.[31]

Gastroprotective effects A petroleum ether extract of *P. hybridus* ground root protects against gastrointestinal damage induced by ethanol and indometacin (indomethacin) *in vivo*.[28] *P. hybridus* root extract 0.83, 2.5 and 7.5 mg/kg administered intragastrally to fasted rats 30 minutes before intragastral administration of 1.5 mL ethanol significantly reduced gastric mucosal damage in a dose-dependent manner, compared with control ($p < 0.05$). In an experiment involving normally fed rats, indometacin (8 mg/kg orally) was administered with *P. hybridus* root extract (6.3, 12.5 or 25 mg/kg orally), cimetidine (50 mg/kg orally) or control, followed by a second dose six hours later, and sacrifice after a further 16 hours. Compared with control, all doses of *P. hybridus* root extract significantly inhibited indometacin-induced intestinal damage ($p < 0.05$), and *P. hybridus* root extract 2 × 25 mg/kg inhibited intestinal damage to a greater extent than did cimetidine ($p < 0.05$).[28]

Other activities Extracts of butterbur rhizome from both petasin and furanopetasin chemovars of *P. hybridus* have been reported to inhibit the binding of radioactive ligands at dopamine D_2 and histamine H_1 receptors to a similar extent. The greatest inhibition was observed for extracts with the highest content (>60%) of eremophilane constituents. For example, for a rhizome extract from the petasin chemovar, mean (standard error of mean; SEM) IC_{50} values for inhibition of dopamine D_2 and histamine H_1 radioligand binding were 38 (3) and 155 (52), respectively.[26] Fractions of the petasin chemovar extract inhibited radioligand binding in a concentration-dependent manner, with the highest affinities displayed by the petasin and desoxyneopetasol fractions. This was confirmed in assays with individual constituents in which the lowest IC_{50} values were determined for petasin and isopetasin. The furanopetasin chemovar constituents hydroxyfuranoeremophilane and furanopetasin also inhibited radioligand binding, as did the eremophilanlactones eremophilanolide and hydroxy-eremophilanolide, albeit with markedly lower affinities than the eremophilanes.[26]

Petasin, isopetasin, *S*-petasin and iso-*S*-petasin, isolated from *Petasites formosanus*, a species related to *P. hybridus*, relaxed histamine-, carbachol-, potassium chloride- and LTD_4-induced precontractions of isolated guinea-pig trachea in a concentration-dependent manner.[32] *S*-Petasin was more potent than petasin and isopetasin for precontractions induced by all four reagents. *S*-Petasin relaxed the precontractions induced by all four reagents in a non-selective manner, with IC_{50} values of <10 µmol/L, whereas iso-*S*-petasin selectively relaxed precontractions induced by carbachol and potassium chloride, with IC_{50} values of around 10 µmol/L for each. The reason for these differences in the respective profiles of activity, and the influence of isomerisation (*S*-petasin to iso-*S*-petasin) is not clear. The documented relaxant effects of *S*-petasin and iso-*S*-petasin from *P. formosanus* on precontracted guinea-pig trachea may be due to antispasmodic and antimuscarinic properties, respectively.[33] Following a study using isolated guinea-pig atria, it has been reported that iso-*S*-petasin may act preferentially on tracheal muscarinic M_3 receptors, rather than cardiac M_2 receptors.[34]

Hypotensive activity has been documented for *S*-petasin and iso-*S*-petasin isolated from *P. formosanus*. In rats, a dose-dependent hypotensive effect occurred following intravenous administration of *S*-petasin or iso-*S*-petasin (0.1–1.5 mg/kg body weight for each); *in vitro* experiments indicated that these compounds have a relaxant effect on precontracted rat aortic ring segments and that this may be due in part to blockade of calcium ion (Ca^{2+}) channels in vascular smooth muscle cells by *S*-petasin and iso-*S*-petasin.[35,36]

S-Petasin from *P. formosanus* has been shown to have negative chronotropic activity *in vivo*. In anaesthetised rats, *S*-petasin (1.0–1.5 mg/kg body weight, intravenously) induced bradycardia in a dose-dependent manner within a few seconds of administration and the effect persisted for up to 11 minutes after administration.[37] The highest administered dose of *S*-petasin (1.5 mg/kg body weight intravenously) evoked a maximal reduction in heart rate of approximately 25%. *S*-Petasin had a negative inotropic effect in isolated rat atria and depressed the amplitude of contraction of rat cardiac myocytes. Iso-*S*-petasin also depresses cardiac contraction as demonstrated by *in vitro* studies involving ventricular myocytes.[38] The mechanism for the observed negative cardiac chronotropic and inotropic effects of *S*-petasin and iso-*S*-petasin may be through inhibition of cardiac L-type voltage-dependent Ca^{2+} channels.[37,38] Further work has shown that *S*-petasin decreases the amplitude of L-type Ca^{2+} currents in NG108-15 cells (a mouse neuroblastoma and rat glioma hybrid cell line) in a concentration-dependent manner (IC_{50} = 11 µmol/L).[39]

B

Clinical studies

Several clinical trials of butterbur extracts have been conducted and have involved individuals with, for example, seasonal and perennial allergic rhinitis and migraine. While many of these studies have reported beneficial effects with butterbur, rigorous investigation of the efficacy of butterbur extracts is limited and further large, well-designed clinical trials are required.

Pharmacokinetics There are limited pharmacokinetic data for the constituents of butterbur extracts. The bioavailability of petasin has been reported following a study involving healthy volunteers who received a single dose of two (n = 24) or four tablets (n = 24) of butterbur leaf extract (ZE-339) orally; each tablet contained 8 mg petasins.[27] The time to maximal petasin concentrations (t_{max}) was around 1.6 hours in each group (mean (standard deviation, SD): 1.62 (0.50) and 1.61 (0.93) hours for the lower and higher dose groups, respectively), whereas the mean (SD) half-life was 7.16 (4.61) and 7.62 (3.34) hours for the lower and higher dose group, respectively. Maximal mean (SD) petasin concentrations were 25.5 (14.8) and 58.1 (26.7) ng/mL for the lower and higher dose groups, respectively.[27] In a proof-of-principle study in which six patients with seasonal (n = 4) and perennial (n = 2) allergic rhinitis each received butterbur extract (ZE-339) three tablets twice daily, serum petasin concentrations reached steady state after five days' treatment (mean (SD) 15.1 (2.3) ng/mL (A Brattström, Zeller AG, personal communication, 19 July 2004).

Another study described monitoring compliance by measuring serum petasin concentrations using an enzyme-linked immunosorbent assay,[40] but these results were not reported.

Therapeutic effects

Seasonal and perennial allergic rhinitis In a randomised, double-blind, double-dummy, parallel-group study involving 125 individuals with seasonal allergic rhinitis, the effects of a carbon dioxide extract of butterbur leaf (ZE-339) one tablet four times daily (equivalent to 32 mg petasins daily) were compared with those of the non-sedating antihistamine cetirizine 10 mg each evening. At the end of the two-week study, butterbur recipients (n = 61) achieved similar scores to cetirizine recipients on the SF-36 (Short Form 36; a self-assessment scale for medical and health outcomes), the primary outcome measure.[21] There were also no differences between groups with respect to secondary outcome measures, including the clinical global impression score. The overall frequency of adverse events was similar in both groups (*see* Side-effects, Toxicity).

The statistical power of the study only allowed the conclusion to be drawn that butterbur was not inferior to cetirizine (i.e. the study does not demonstrate equivalence of the two preparations),[41] and the study has been criticised for its choice of subjective outcome measures and interpretation.[42,43]

A subsequent study used an objective outcome measure – the adenosine monophosphate (AMP) nasal provocation test (AMP is important in the pathway leading to the release of allergic inflammatory mediators, such as histamine, cysteinyl leukotrienes and prostaglandins) – to assess the effects of butterbur. In a randomised, double-blind, crossover trial, 20 individuals with seasonal allergic rhinitis ceased any existing treatment for the condition (antihistamines and/or intranasal corticosteroids) one week before starting treatment with butterbur 50 mg (Petaforce; Bioforce), or placebo, twice daily for two weeks.[20] No further details of the preparation were provided in the report of the study, although Petaforce marketed in the UK contains butterbur root extract 25 mg per capsule (containing not less than 15% petasins calculated as isopetasin).

At the end of each treatment period, participants underwent AMP challenge (described as two applications to each nostril of a 400 mg/mL solution delivered via a pump actuator spray device) and spontaneous recovery was monitored by measuring peak nasal inspiratory flow (PNIF) at regular intervals over one hour. Time to recovery was significantly attenuated and the maximum fall in PNIF was significantly less in butterbur recipients compared with placebo recipients (p = 0.028 and 0.036, respectively).[20] The study design did not incorporate a wash-out period between the two phases of the study, and it is not clear whether there could have been any carry-over effect in patients who received butterbur during the first phase of the study and what influence, if any, this may have had on the results.

In a randomised, double-blind, parallel group, controlled trial, 330 individuals with seasonal allergic rhinitis and a history of seasonal allergic rhinitis for at least two seasons in consecutive years, received a carbon dioxide extract of butterbur leaves (ZE-339, tablets standardised for 8.0 mg total petasins per tablet) one tablet three times daily (n = 110), fexofenadine (Telfast) 180 mg each morning (n = 113), or placebo (n = 107), for two weeks; double dummy preparations were used to achieve blinding.[44] At the end of the study, both butterbur extract and fexofenadine were superior to placebo with respect to the primary outcome variable (the change in evening total symptom scores, determined for the previous 12-hour period, from baseline values to the 2-week endpoint) ($p <$ 0.001), and there was no statistically significant difference between the two active treatment groups (p = 0.37). With respect to secondary outcome variables, responder rates were significantly higher in the butterbur extract and fexofenadine groups ($p < 0.001$ for both versus placebo), and there was no statistically significant difference between the two active treatment groups (p = 0.88).[44] Outcomes of statistical analyses for the other secondary outcome variables were not reported. In a similar randomised, double-blind, parallel group trial, 186 individuals with seasonal allergic rhinitis and a history of seasonal allergic rhinitis for at least two seasons in consecutive years, received a carbon dioxide extract of butterbur leaves (ZE-339, tablets standardised for 8.0 mg total petasins per tablet) one tablet three times daily (n = 60), one tablet twice daily (n = 65), or placebo (n = 61), for two weeks to assess the relationship between dose and response.[45] At the end of the study, changes in symptom scores from baseline were significantly greater for both butterbur groups when compared with placebo ($p < 0.001$) and the change in symptom scores for the higher-dose butterbur group was significantly greater than that for the lower-dose butterbur group (p = 0.02). The effects of butterbur extract (Petaforce) 50 mg twice daily in perennial allergic rhinitis were compared with those of fexofenadine 180 mg daily in a randomised, double-blind, placebo-controlled, crossover study involving 16 individuals. Participants stopped their existing treatment for allergic rhinitis one week before starting their randomised treatment; treatments were taken for one week, with a one-week wash-out period between each randomised treatment. At the end of the study, the maximum percentage fall from baseline values in PNIF after nasal AMP challenge was significantly attenuated in the butterbur and fexofenadine groups, compared with the placebo group (mean (SEM) for butterbur, fexofenadine and placebo: 34 (3), 39 (3) and 46 (3), respectively; $p < 0.05$).[46] The total nasal symptom score, a secondary outcome measure, was also significantly improved for the butterbur and fexofenadine groups, compared with the placebo group ($p < 0.05$). This study is limited in that the duration of treatment was short, and the sample size calculation was not based on detecting differences in nasal symptom scores, so a larger study is needed to confirm the latter result.

Asthma and bronchitis At present, there is insufficient evidence from well-designed randomised controlled trials to support the efficacy of butterbur extracts in asthma and bronchitis.

In a randomised, double-blind, crossover study, 16 patients with atopic asthma who had been stabilised on inhaled corticosteroid therapy for at least three months before the study received butterbur (Petaforce) 25 mg twice daily (no further details stated in the report although Petaforce marketed in the UK contains not less than 15% petasins calculated as isopetasin), or placebo, for one week.[47] Participants stopped any treatment with long-acting β_2-agonists one week before and for the duration of the study. At the end of the study, bronchial hyper-responsiveness in response to AMP bronchial challenge was significantly improved in butterbur recipients compared with placebo recipients ($p < 0.05$), and concentrations of inflammatory markers (exhaled nitric oxide, serum eosinophil cationic protein and peripheral blood eosinophil count) were significantly suppressed in the butterbur group, compared with the placebo group ($p < 0.05$ for each).[47]

In a preliminary trial, 80 individuals (aged 6–85 years) with mild or moderate asthma received a lipophilic carbon dioxide extract of butterbur rhizome (Petadolex; standardised to contain at least 15% petasins) 50 mg three times daily (equivalent to 22.5 mg petasins daily; dose reduced for children depending on age) for a minimum of two months following a two-week run-in phase. A report of this study attributes several improvements to administration of butterbur, including reductions in the number, duration and severity of asthma attacks, increases in peak flow and forced expiratory volume in one second (FEV_1), and reduced use of existing asthma medications.[48] However, such conclusions may be flawed because of the design and methodological limitations of the study and because no statistical analysis was undertaken.

Allergic skin reactions A randomised, double-blind, double-dummy, controlled, crossover trial assessed the effects of butterbur on the histamine and allergen cutaneous response in 20 atopic patients with asthma or allergic rhinitis and sensitisation to at least one common household allergen, such as house dust mite, on skin prick testing.[49] Participants received butterbur (Petaforce) 50 mg twice daily (no further details given), fexofenadine 180 mg daily, montelukast 10 mg daily, or placebo, for one week; existing treatment with antihistamines and leukotriene receptor antagonists was stopped one week before and for the duration of the study, although existing treatment for asthma or allergic rhinitis was continued. Each day, approximately two hours after taking the first daily dose of study medication, each participant underwent skin prick testing with the allergen that had previously been shown to provoke the greatest response in that individual, as well as with histamine (1.7 mg/mL; no further details reported) and 0.9% sodium chloride as control. Mean histamine and allergen wheal and flare responses were significantly attenuated by fexofenadine, compared with placebo, but not by butterbur or montelukast.[49]

Migraine prophylaxis The rationale for the use of butterbur in migraine prophylaxis is centred around the understanding that vasoconstrictive and neurogenic inflammatory processes are involved in the generation of migraine headaches, and that butterbur and certain of its isolated constituents have been shown in preclinical studies to have anti-inflammatory properties.[22] However, at present, rigorous clinical investigation of the effects of butterbur extracts in preventing migraine is limited.

In a randomised, double-blind, parallel-group trial, 60 hospital outpatients with migraine (minimum of three attacks per month for the three months prior to the study and a minimum of two attacks in the four-week run-in phase) received a carbon dioxide extract of *P. hybridus* rhizome (Petadolex) two capsules twice daily (equivalent to 100 mg extract or 15 mg petasins daily), or placebo, for 12 weeks. None of the participants were previous users of the butterbur extract.[22] Inclusion and exclusion criteria for the study were in accordance with the International Headache Society guidelines.[50] The frequency of migraine attacks in the last four weeks of the study was significantly lower in the butterbur group, compared with the placebo group: the mean (SD) numbers of attacks during the month were 1.7 (0.9) and 2.6 (1.1), for the butterbur and placebo groups, respectively; $p < 0.05$). The number of days with migraine during the last four weeks of the study also decreased significantly in the butterbur group, compared with the placebo group (mean (SD) number of days at baseline and weeks 8–12: 3.4 (1.6) and 1.7 (0.9) versus 3.0 (1.3) and 2.6 (1.2), for butterbur and placebo, respectively; $p < 0.05$). There were no statistically significant differences between the two groups in the duration and intensity of migraine headaches at the end of the study.[22]

The study has several limitations which should be considered when interpreting the results. A sample size calculation was not carried out, baseline characteristics (apart from age and variables relating to migraine attacks) of participants were not provided in a report of the study, so it is not clear if the randomisation was successful (i.e. whether or not the two groups were similar at baseline) and differences at baseline in the frequency of migraine attacks are not considered in the analysis. There are further flaws in the statistical analysis, for example, the analysis was carried out only with those participants who adhered to the protocol (i.e. an intention-to-treat analysis was not carried out), efficacy parameters were not defined *a priori*,[51] the results are reported without 95% confidence intervals and precise *p*-values are not provided.

Against this background, an independent re-analysis of the data from this study was undertaken. Data entry from original case report forms was completely repeated under the principles of good clinical practice (which includes double data entry and consistency checks), and all four primary efficacy criteria and data from all three time points (four, eight and 12 weeks) were evaluated equally weighted in an attempt to avoid bias by post-hoc selections of efficacy criteria.[51] All analyses were undertaken with data from the intention-to-treat population (i.e. all patients who were randomised and took the study medication at least once).

The new analysis confirmed the findings of the original analysis and stated that all 12 primary efficacy criteria (number of attacks, number of days with attacks, mean duration and mean intensity of attacks at all three time points) were significantly reduced in the butterbur group, compared with the placebo group, and the most conservative analysis showed that seven of these 12 variables were still statistically significant.[51] However, the possibility of bias in this retrospective re-analysis cannot be excluded entirely, and other methodological issues remain, such as the lack of a sample size calculation.

A larger randomised, double-blind, placebo-controlled trial of a butterbur extract for migraine prophylaxis has since been conducted. In the trial, 245 patients with migraine (two of six attacks per month for the three months prior to the study and a minimum of two attacks in the four-week run-in phase; with or without aura and meeting International Headache Society criteria) received an extract of butterbur rhizome (Petadolex) 50 mg twice daily, 75 mg twice daily, or placebo, for 16 weeks.[23] Overall, 202 participants completed the study (per-protocol analysis) and 229 were included in the intention-to-treat analysis. At the end of the study, the mean number of migraine attacks was reduced by 45%, 32% and 28%, compared with baseline values, for the butterbur extract 150 mg daily, 100 mg daily and placebo groups, respectively. This finding was statistically significant for butterbur extract 150 mg daily versus placebo ($p = 0.005$; intention-to-treat analysis).[23] The proportion of 'responders' (proportion of participants with > 50% reduction in mean attack frequency per month relative to baseline) was significantly higher for the butterbur 150 mg group when compared with the placebo group ($p < 0.05$), but there was no statistically significant difference in this outcome for butterbur 100 mg, compared with placebo.

The effectiveness of a carbon-dioxide extract of *P. hybridus* rhizome (Petadolex) at doses ranging from 50–150 mg, depending on participant's age, were explored in 108 young people (aged 6–17 years) with a history of migraine for at least one year diagnosed according to International Headache Society criteria, in a prospective, open-label, multi-centre, four-month trial.[52] At the end of the study, the frequency of migraine attacks was reduced by 63%, compared with baseline values, and 77% of participants experienced a reduction in the frequency of migraine attacks of at least 50%. As this study did not involve a control group, the effects cannot be attributed to treatment with butterbur, and the hypothesis that butterbur rhizome extract reduces the frequency of migraine attacks in this patient population requires testing in rigorous randomised controlled trials involving sufficient numbers of participants.

Side-effects, Toxicity

As with many herbal medicines, the safety of butterbur preparations has not yet been adequately assessed: only limited preclinical and clinical safety and toxicity data are available (see below). One of the main issues regarding the clinical use of butterbur extracts concerns the unsaturated pyrrolizidine alkaloid constituents which are known to be hepatotoxic in humans, and have been shown to be carcinogenic and mutagenic in preclinical studies (*see* Comfrey). These alkaloids may be present in low concentrations in all parts of the plant (*see* Constituents).

Several manufacturers of products containing butterbur include in their manufacturing processes steps to remove the unsaturated pyrrolizidine alkaloids to concentrations below the detectable limit (e.g. <35 parts per billion).[53] However, there remains the possibility that toxic quantities of unsaturated pyrrolizidine alkaloids may be present in poorly processed products, and any products which contain *Petasites* species as a result of botanical misidentification or adulteration.

Butterbur is a member of the Asteraceae family, and members of this family may cause allergic reactions in sensitive individuals, especially those with an existing hypersensitivity to other members of the Asteraceae/Compositae. No reports of allergic reactions to butterbur were identified.

Clinical data

Swissmedic, the competent authority for licensing medicines in Switzerland, has revoked the licences for certain products containing butterbur root extract following spontaneous reports received in Germany of liver damage associated with their use.[54] At the time of writing, the German authority had not taken any regulatory action, but was monitoring the situation.

There is only limited information available for butterbur from long-term postmarketing surveillance studies. Clinical trials reported to date generally have involved only small numbers of participants, mostly with allergic rhinitis or migraine who are generally otherwise healthy, and have involved ingestion of butterbur preparations for relatively short periods of time (up to four months). Some clinical trials have not adequately reported data on safety, and two randomised, double-blind, placebo-controlled trials involving individuals with seasonal allergic rhinitis or asthma who received butterbur extracts and in which participants continued to take their existing medication (inhaled or intranasal corticosteroids, long-or short-acting β_2-agonists)[47,49] have either not assessed or not reported data on safety parameters at all.

In a randomised, double-blind, trial involving 125 individuals with seasonal allergic rhinitis who received butterbur extract (ZE-339) equivalent to 32 mg petasins daily, or cetirizine 10 mg daily, for two weeks, the frequency of adverse events was similar in both groups (proportions of butterbur and cetirizine recipients who reported adverse events were 10% and 11%, respectively).[21] Eight of the 12 adverse events reported by cetirizine recipients and two of the 10 adverse events reported by butterbur recipients were classified as fatigue or drowsiness. Raised liver enzyme activity (no further details provided) and pruritus were reported for one butterbur recipient each, but not for cetirizine recipients.

In a randomised, double-blind, placebo-controlled, crossover study, 20 patients with seasonal allergic rhinitis stopped taking any existing treatment one week before receiving butterbur (Petaforce) 50 mg twice daily for two weeks (no further details of the preparation were provided in a report of the study, although Petaforce marketed in the UK contains not less than 15% petasins calculated as isopetasin). At the end of the study, liver function test values (blood concentrations of alanine aminotransferase (ALT), bilirubin, alkaline phosphatase (ALP) and albumin) were reported to be similar for butterbur and placebo groups,[20] although no statistical analysis was carried out. Furthermore, this study involved only small numbers of participants and was conducted over a short time period and, therefore, cannot provide adequate data on safety.

In a randomised, double-blind, parallel group, controlled trial in which 330 individuals with seasonal allergic rhinitis received a carbon dioxide extract of butterbur leaves (ZE-339, tablets standardised for 8.0 mg total petasins per tablet) one tablet three times daily ($n = 110$), fexofenadine (Telfast) 180 mg each morning ($n = 113$), or placebo ($n = 107$), for two weeks, the frequency of adverse events was similar in all three groups (9.1, 7.1 and 6.5%

for the butterbur, fexofenadine and placebo groups, respectively).[44] There were no differences between the three groups with respect to changes in mean liver function test values at the end of treatment from baseline values,[44] although no statistical analyses were reported. This finding is of limited value because of the short treatment period. Furthermore, it would be more useful to know whether or not liver function test values were raised in any individual butterbur recipients, rather than reporting mean values for the group.

Open, uncontrolled studies of butterbur extracts (ZE-339 and Petadolex) in patients with seasonal and/or perennial allergic rhinitis or asthma have reported that butterbur was well tolerated,[40, 48] although the design of these studies renders them unsuitable for an adequate assessment of safety. In one of these studies, in which participants (aged 6–85 years) with mild or moderate asthma received a lipophilic carbon dioxide extract of butterbur rhizome (Petadolex; standardised to contain at least 15% petasins) 50 mg three times daily (reduced for children depending on age) for a minimum of two months, seven participants reported 11 adverse events.[48] These included abdominal pain, flatulence, sneezing, allergic conjunctivitis, allergic rhinitis and halitosis (reported by children) and hair loss, coughing, dyspnoea, difficulty exhaling and depression (reported by adults). None of these was judged by the study physician to be causally related to butterbur ingestion and none led to withdrawal of participants from the study.

In a randomised, double-blind, placebo-controlled trial involving 60 individuals with migraine who received a carbon dioxide extract of *P. hybridus* rhizome (Petadolex) two capsules twice daily (equivalent to 100 mg extract daily), or placebo, for 12 weeks, no adverse events were reported for the butterbur group and no statistically significant changes from baseline values were reported for vital signs and physical examination results.[22] However, two butterbur recipients withdrew from the study, one because of a suspected pregnancy; the other participant did not provide a reason. An independent re-analysis of the data from this trial added that, at the end of the study, three butterbur recipients had liver function test (ALT, aspartate transaminase (AST)) values which were higher than normal ranges and significantly higher than baseline values, and that bilirubin concentration and erythrocyte count were significantly higher than baseline values for the butterbur group, compared with the placebo group.[51] These changes were not regarded as being clinically relevant,[51] although no numerical data were provided to support this judgement.

In a larger randomised, double-blind, placebo-controlled trial, 245 patients with migraine received an extract of butterbur rhizome (Petadolex) 50 mg twice daily, 75 mg twice daily, or placebo, for 16 weeks.[23] Data from 230 participants were included in a safety analysis. The most frequently reported adverse events that were considered possibly related to treatment were gastrointestinal symptoms (not specified), which occurred in 22, 26 and 7% of participants in the butterbur extract 75 mg, butterbur extract 50 mg and placebo groups, respectively. There were no statistically significant differences in the frequencies of adverse events for the butterbur groups, compared with placebo, except for belching. No differences in liver function test values were observed between the three groups.[23]

A review of safety data for a specific preparation of butterbur rhizome – an extract (Petadolex) standardised to contain a minimum of 15% petasins and processed to achieve a concentration of unsaturated pyrrolizidine alkaloids of less than 0.08 ppm – includes data from four postmarketing surveillance studies involving a total of 188 patients (145 with migraine, including 50 children and adolescents aged 6–17 years). Adverse events deemed to be possibly or probably causally related to ingestion of the butterbur product included eructations (belching; $n = 7$), bad taste/smell of the product (2) and skin rash (1).[55] However, it is unclear why these four studies included such a small number of participants: a single postmarketing surveillance study would normally be expected to include many more participants.

The review also refers to 93 spontaneous suspected adverse drug reaction (ADR) reports (75 of which originated from Germany, where the manufacturer is located) received by the product manufacturer from 1976 to the end of June 2002. In total, 27 of these reports were determined to be possibly ($n = 19$) or probably (8) causally related to butterbur administration; the latter included one case of reversible cholestatic hepatitis.[55] The review states an overall frequency of suspected ADRs, calculated on the basis of sales figures and the total number of spontaneous ADR reports received by the manufacturer. However, for several reasons, these types of data should not be used to calculate frequencies of suspected ADRs.

The World Health Organization's Uppsala Monitoring Centre (WHO-UMC; Collaborating Centre for International Drug Monitoring) receives summary reports of spontaneous reports of suspected adverse drug reactions from national pharmacovigilance centres of over 70 countries worldwide. At the end of 2005, the WHO-UMC's Vigisearch database contained a total of 10 reports, describing a total of 22 adverse reactions, for products reported to contain *P. hybridus* only as the active ingredient.[56] Reactions reported included hepatic enzymes increased ($n = 2$), hepatic necrosis (2), hepatitis (1), cholestatic hepatitis (1) and hepatocellular damage (1) from three case reports. Nine of the reports originated from Germany and one from Switzerland. In six of the 10 reports, *P. hybridus* was the sole suspected drug. (These data were obtained from the Vigisearch database held by the WHO Collaborating Centre for International Drug Monitoring, Uppsala, Sweden. The information is not homogeneous at least with respect to origin or likelihood that the pharmaceutical product caused the adverse reaction. Any information included in this report does not represent the opinion of the World Health Organization.)

Preclinical data

There are limited data from animal toxicity studies for butterbur preparations, although a review[55] summarises data from unpublished toxicity studies. Acute toxicity studies in rats yielded LD_{50} values for a single-dose oral administration and single-dose intraperitoneal administration of $\geqslant 2.5$ and approximately 1 g/kg body weight, respectively. A chronic toxicity study in rats ($n = 200$) carried out over 26 weeks established a no adverse effect level for the lower dose range tested (oral administration; no further details provided).[55]

Information on mutagenicity and genotoxicity of butterbur extracts is limited to summaries of unpublished data. An extract of butterbur rhizome (Petadolex) produced a negative result in the Ames test for mutagenicity using several strains of *Salmonella typhimurium*.[57] In an *in vitro* test for clastogenic activity in which the butterbur extract was incubated with cultured human peripheral lymphocytes, the mean number of chromosomal aberrations was within the reference range of the negative control.[58] This result was obtained irrespective of whether or not the test included metabolic activation using a rat liver postmitochondrial fraction. In contrast, mitomycin C and

B

cyclophosphamide, as positive controls, induced chromosomal damage.

There is some evidence from preclinical studies that *S*-petasin, a constituent of butterbur root, rhizome and leaf, has effects on certain endocrine systems. In rats, *S*-petasin (10 μg/kg body weight, intravenously) reduced basal plasma corticosterone concentrations to a significantly greater extent than did control at 30 minutes after administration ($p < 0.05$), although there were no statistically significant differences between groups when corticosterone concentrations were measured at one, two and three hours after administration.[59] The same dose of *S*-petasin also significantly reduced adrenocorticotrophin (ACTH)-induced increases in plasma corticosterone concentrations at 30 minutes, but not longer intervals, after administration, compared with control. Similar effects were observed following *in vitro* experiments: *S*-petasin significantly reduced basal, ACTH- and forskolin (an adenylyl cyclase activator)-stimulated corticosterone release from rat adrenal gland cells (zona fasciculata reticularis) in a concentration-dependent manner. Results of further *in vitro* experiments suggested that the mechanism for the observed effects is in part through inhibition by *S*-petasin of the enzymes adenylyl cyclase (which catalyses the formation of cyclic AMP), and cytochrome P450 side-chain cleavage and 11β-hydroxylase, which are important in the biosynthesis of corticosterone.[59, 60]

S-Petasin (1 μg/kg body weight, intravenously) administered as a single dose to small numbers of adult male rats reduced basal plasma testosterone concentrations, compared with control (mean (SEM): 0.81 (0.06) and 1.31 (0.21) ng/mL for *S*-petasin and control, respectively; $p < 0.05$).[61] Incubation of *S*-petasin at concentrations of 0.14–14.4 μg/mL with rat testicular interstitial cells led to a concentration-dependent inhibition of testosterone release. *S*-Petasin also inhibited forskolin-, human chorionic gonadotrophin- and androstenidione-induced stimulation of testosterone secretion from rat testicular interstitial cells *in vitro*.

Contra-indications, Warnings

In view of the known toxicity, the German Commission E recommended that the maximum daily intake of unsaturated pyrrolizidine alkaloids is 1 μg, and that the duration of use should not exceed 4–6 weeks in a year.[G3] In Switzerland, there are concerns regarding reports in Germany of hepatotoxicity associated with the use of certain products containing butterbur root extract (*see* Side-effects, Toxicity).

Drug interactions No reports of drug interactions with butterbur extracts were identified. Certain constituents of butterbur have been documented in preclinical studies to have hypotensive activity and negative chronotropic and negative inotropic effects. Against this background, and on a theoretical basis, the possibility of interactions with hypertensive and antihypertensive medicines should be considered. Likewise, several constituents of butterbur have been documented to displace the binding of ligands at dopamine D_2 and histamine H_1 receptors, so there is a theoretical possibility of interactions with medicinal agents acting at these receptors.

Pregnancy and lactation In view of the lack of safety data and the possible hepatotoxic effects of poorly processed butterbur extracts, the use of products containing butterbur is contra-indicated in pregnancy and by breastfeeding women.

Preparations

Proprietary single-ingredient preparations

Germany: Petadolex; Petaforce V. *Switzerland:* Pollivita; Tesalin.

Proprietary multi-ingredient preparations

Switzerland: Dragees aux figues avec du sene; Dragees pour la detente nerveuse; Relaxane; Valverde Constipation dragees; Valverde Detente dragees; Wala Pulmonium suc contre la toux.

References

1 Novotny L *et al*. Substances from *Petasites officinalis* Moench. *Tetrahedron Lett* 1961; 20: 697–701.
2 Siegenthaler P, Neuenschwander M. Sesquiterpenes from *Petasites hybridus* (furanopetasin chemovar): separation, isolation and quantitation of compounds from fresh plant extracts. *Pharm Acta Helv* 1997; 72: 57–67.
3 Debrunner B *et al*. Sesquiterpenes of *Petasites hybridus* (L.) G.M. et Sch.: distribution of sesquiterpenes over plant organs. *Pharm Acta Helv* 1995; 70: 167–173.
4 Novotny L *et al*. Contribution to the chemotaxonomy of some European *Petasites* species. *Phytochemistry* 1966; 5: 1281–1287.
5 Siegenthaler P, Neuenschwander M. Analytic investigations of sesquiterpenes of *Petasites albus* (L.) and *Petasites hybridus* (furanopetasin chemovar). *Pharm Acta Helv* 1998; 72: 362–364.
6 Chizzola R. Distribution of the pyrrolizidine alkaloids senecionine and integerrimine within the *Petasites hybridus* plant. *Planta Med* 1992; 58 (Suppl. Suppl.1): A693–A694.
7 Langer T *et al*. A competitive enzyme immunoassay for the pyrrolizidine alkaloids of the senecionine type. *Planta Med* 1996; 62: 267–271.
8 Wildi E *et al*. Quantitative analysis of petasin and pyrrolizidine alkaloids in leaves and rhizomes of *in situ* grown *Petasites hybridus* plants. *Planta Med* 1998; 64: 264–267.
9 Lüthy J *et al*. Pyrrolizidin-Alkaloide in *Petasites hybridus* L. und *P. albus* L. *Pharm Acta Helv* 1983; 58: 98–100.
10 Chizzola R. Distribution of pyrrolizidine alkaloids in crossing progenies of *Petasites hybridus*. *J Herbs Spices Med Plants* 2002; 9: 39–44.
11 Mroczek T *et al*. Simultaneous determination of *N*-oxides and free bases of pyrrolizidine alkaloids by cation-exchange solid-phase extraction and ion-pair high-performance liquid chromatography. *J Chromatogr A* 2002; 949: 249–262.
12 Siegenthaler P, Neuenschwander M. Furanoeremophilane und Eremophilanlaktone. *Z Phytother* 1994; 15: 270–271.
13 Saritas Y *et al*. Sesquiterpene constituents in *Petasites hybridus*. *Phytochemistry* 2002; 59: 795–803.
14 Debrunner B *et al*. Sesquiterpenes of *Petasites hybridus* (L.) G.M. et Sch.: influence of locations and seasons on sesquiterpene distribution. *Pharm Acta Helv* 1995; 70: 315–323.
15 Debrunner B. Influence of temperature and storage on the stability of some eremophilane esters in *Petasites hybridus* (L.) G.M. et Sch. (petasin chemovar). *Pharm Acta Helv* 1998; 72: 364–365.
16 Anon. Safety concerns over butterbur. *Pharm J* 2002; 268: 126.
17 Mauz Ch *et al*. Methode zur Entfernung von Pyrrolizidin-Alkaloiden aus Arzneipflanzenextrakten. *Pharm Acta Helv* 1985; 60: 256–259.
18 Wildi E *et al*. In vitro propagation of *Petastites hybridus* with high petasin and low pyrrolizidine alkaloid content. *Pharm Acta Helv* 1998; 72: 371–373.
19 Tobyn G. *Culpeper's Medicine. A Practice of Western Holistic Medicine*. Shaftesbury: Element, 1997.
20 Lee DKC *et al*. Butterbur, a herbal remedy, attenuates adenosine monophosphate induced nasal responsiveness in seasonal allergic rhinitis. *Clin Exp Allergy* 2003; 33: 882–886.
21 Schapowal A for the Petasites Study Group. Randomised controlled trial of butterbur and cetirizine for treating seasonal allergic rhinitis. *BMJ* 2002; 324: 1–4.

22 Grossmann M, Schmidramsl H. An extract of *Petasites hybridus* is effective in the prophylaxis of migraine. *Int J Clin Pharmacol Ther* 2000; 38: 430–435.
23 Lipton RB *et al. Petasites hybridus* root is an effective preventive treatment for migraine. *Neurology* 2004; 63: 2240–2244.
24 Thomet OAR, Simon H-U. Petasins in the treatment of allergic diseases: results of preclinical and clinical studies. *Int Arch Allergy Immunol* 2002; 129: 108–112.
25 Bickel D *et al*. Identification and characterization of inhibitors of peptido-leukotriene synthesis from *Petasites hybridus. Planta Med* 1994; 60: 318–322.
26 Berger D *et al*. Influence of *Petasites hybridus* on dopamine-D_2 and histamine-H_1 receptors. *Pharm Acta Helv* 1998; 72: 373–375.
27 Brattström A. Mode of action and pharmacological data of Petasites extract Ze 339. In: Chrubasik S, Roufogalis B, eds. *Herbal Medicinal Products for the Treatment of Pain*. Lismore: Southern Cross University Press, 2000.
28 Brune K *et al*. Gastro-protective effects by extracts of *Petasites hybridus*: the role of inhibition of peptido-leukotriene synthesis. *Planta Med* 1993; 59: 494–496.
29 Thomet OA *et al*. Role of petasin in the potential anti-inflammatory activity of a plant extract of *Petasites hybridus. Biochem Pharmacol* 2001; 61: 1041–1047.
30 Thomet OA *et al*. Differential inhibition of inflammatory effector functions by petasin, isopetasin and neopetasin in human eosinophils. *Clin Exp Allergy* 2001; 31: 1310–1320.
31 Fiebich BL *et al. Petasites hybridus* extracts in vitro inhibit COX-2 and PGE2 release by direct interaction with the enzyme and by preventing p42/44 MAP kinase activation in rat primary microglial cells. *Planta Med* 2005; 71: 12–19.
32 Ko W-C *et al*. Relaxant effects of petasins in isolated guinea pig trachea and their structure-activity relationships. *Planta Med* 2000; 66: 650–652.
33 Ko W-C *et al*. Mechanisms of relaxant action of S-petasin and S-isopetasin, sesquiterpenes of *Petasites formosanus*, in isolated guinea pig trachea. *Planta Med* 2001; 67: 224–229.
34 Ko W-C *et al*. S-isopetasin, a sesquiterpene of *Petasites formosanus*, allosterically antagonized carbachol in isolated guinea pig atria. *Planta Med* 2002; 68: 652–655.
35 Wang G-J *et al*. Calcium channel blockade in vascular smooth muscle cells: major hypotensive mechanism of S-petasin, a hypotensive sesquiterpene from *Petasites formosanus. J Pharmacol Exp Ther* 2001; 297: 240–246.
36 Wang G-J *et al*. Ca^{2+} blocking effect of iso-S-petasin in rat aortic smooth muscle cells. *Eur J Pharmacol* 2002; 445: 239–245.
37 Wang G-J *et al*. Calcium-antagonizing activity of S-petasin, a hypotensive sesquiterpene from *Petasites formosanus*, on inotropic and chronotropic responses in isolated rat atria and cardiac myocytes. *Naunyn-Schmeideberg's Arch Pharmacol* 2004; 369: 322–329.
38 Esberg LB *et al*. Iso-S-petasin, a hypotensive sesquiterpene from *Petasites formosanus*, depresses cardiac contraction and intracellular Ca^{2+} transients in adult rat ventricular myocytes. *J Pharm Pharmacol* 2003; 55: 103–107.
39 Wu S-N *et al*. The mechanism of inhibitory actions of S-petasin, a sesquiterpene of *Petasites formosanus*, on L-type calcium current in NG108-15 neuronal cells. *Planta Med* 2003; 69: 118–124.
40 Thomet OAR *et al*. Anti-inflammatory activity of an extract of *Petasites hybridus* in allergic rhinitis. *Int Immunopharmacol* 2002; 2: 997–1006.
41 Schapowal A. Author's reply [letter]. *BMJ* 2002; 324: 1277.
42 Shuster S. Well designed experiments should have been used [letter]. *BMJ* 2002; 324: 1277.
43 McArthur CA, Arnott N. Trial does not show that there is no difference between butterbur and cetirizine [letter]. *BMJ* 2002; 324: 1277.
44 Schapowal A, on behalf of study group. Treating intermittent allergic rhinitis: a prospective, randomized, placebo and antihistamine-controlled study of butterbur extract Ze 339. *Phytotherapy Res* 2005; 19: 530–537.
45 Schapowal A, for the Petasites Study Group. Butterbur Ze339 for the treatment of intermittent allergic rhinitis. Dose-dependent efficacy in a prospective, randomized, double-blind, placebo-controlled study. *Arch Otolaryngol Head Neck Surg* 2004; 130: 1381–1386.
46 Lee DKC *et al*. A placebo-controlled evaluation of butterbur and fexofenadine on objective and subjective outcomes in perennial allergic rhinitis. *Clin Exp Allergy* 2004; 34: 646–649.
47 Lee DKC *et al*. Butterbur, a herbal remedy, confers complementary anti-inflammatory activity in asthmatic patients receiving inhaled corticosteroids. *Clin Exp Allergy* 2004; 34: 110–114.
48 Danesch U. *Petasites hybridus* (butterbur root) extract in the treatment of asthma – an open trial. *Altern Med Rev* 2004; 9: 54–62.
49 Jackson CM *et al*. The effects of butterbur on the histamine and allergen cutaneous response. *Ann Allergy Asthma Immunol* 2004; 92: 250–254.
50 Tfelt-Hansen P *et al*. for the International Headache Society Clinical Trials Subcommittee. Guidelines for controlled trials of drugs in migraine, second edition. *Cephalalgia* 2000; 20: 765–786.
51 Diener HC *et al*. The first placebo-controlled trial of a special butterbur root extract for the prevention of migraine: reanalysis of efficacy criteria. *Eur Neurol* 2004; 51: 89–97.
52 Pothmann R, Danesch U. Migraine prevention in children and adolescents: results of an open study with a special butterbur root extract. *Headache* 2005; 45: 196–203.
53 Brattström A. A newly developed extract (Ze 339) from butterbur (*Petasites hybridus* L.) is clinically efficient in allergic rhinitis (hay fever). *Phytomedicine* 2003; 10 (Suppl. Suppl.IV): 50–52.
54 NN. Präparate aus Petasitesrhizom in der Schweiz vom Markt. *Deutsche Apotheker Zeitung* 2004; 144: 64–66.
55 Danesch U, Rittinghausen R. Safety of a patented special butterbur root extract for migraine prevention. *Headache* 2003; 43: 76–78.
56 Vigibase. WHO Adverse Reactions database, Uppsala Monitoring Centre. (accessed January 13, 2006).
57 Koch V, Danesch U. Response to Fox and DeSousa [letter]. *Headache* 2001; 41: 325–326.
58 Danesch U, Rittinghausen R. Response from Danesch and Rittinghausen [letter]. *Headache* 2003; 43: 822–823.
59 Chang L-L *et al*. Effects of S-petasin on corticosterone release in rats. *Chin J Physiol* 2002; 45: 137–142.
60 Chang L-L *et al*. Effects of S-petasin on cyclic AMP production and enzyme activity of P450scc in rat zona fasciculata-reticularis cells. *Eur J Pharmacol* 2004; 489: 29–37.
61 Lin H *et al*. Inhibition of testosterone secretion by S-petasin in rat testicular interstitial cells. *Chin J Physiol* 2000; 43: 99–103.

Calamus

C

Summary and Pharmaceutical Comment

The phytochemistry of calamus, especially the oil, is well documentated. Three genotypes (diploid, triploid and tetraploid) have been identified which are chemically distinct with respect to the β-asarone content. Spasmolytic and anti-ulcer effects documented for the oil support the traditional herbal uses of calamus. In addition, bitter principles documented as constituents may account for the use of the root in anorexia. However, in view of the toxic properties documented for the oil and associated with β-asarone, it has been recommended that only β-asarone-free calamus root should be used in phytotherapy. Use of the oil is not recommended due to its carcinogenic activity and its ability to cause kidney damage, tremors and convulsions.[G58] Studies carried out to investigate the mutagenic potential of calamus have produced conflicting results.

Species (Family)

Acorus calamus L. (Acoraceae)

Various genetic species (n = 12): diploid North American, triploid European, tetraploid Asian, Eastern, Indian.

Synonym(s)

Sweet Flag

Part(s) Used

Rhizome

Pharmacopoeial and Other Monographs

BHP 1996[G9]
Martindale 35th edition[G85]

Legal Category (Licensed Products)

GSL[G37]

Constituents

The following is compiled from several sources, including General References G19, G22, G41 and G58.

Amines Dimethylamine, methylamine, trimethylamine and choline.

Volatile oil 1.5–3.5%. β-Asarone content varies between genetic species: 96% in tetraploid (Indian), 5% in triploid (European) and 0% in the diploid (North American) species.[1–4] Other identified components include calamenol (5%), calamene (4%), calamone (1%), methyl eugenol (1%), eugenol (0.3%) and the sesquiterpenes acolamone, acoragermacrone and isoacolamone. Considerable qualitative and quantitative differences have been reported between the volatile oil from different genetic species, and between the volatile fraction of an alcoholic extract and the essential oil from the same variety (European).[3,4]

Tannin 1.5%.

Other constituents Bitter principles (e.g. acorin), acoric and palmitic acids, resin (2.5%), mucilage, starch (25–40%), sugars.

Food Use

The level of β-asarone permitted in foods is restricted to 0.1 mg/kg in foods and beverages, 1 mg/kg in alcoholic beverages and in foods containing *Acorus calamus* or *Asarum europaeum*.[G16] Calamus is listed by the Council of Europe as a source of natural food flavouring (category N3). This category indicates that calamus can be added to foodstuffs in the traditionally accepted manner, although there is insufficient information available for an adequate assessment of potential toxicity.[G16] Previously, calamus was classified as an 'unsafe herb' by the US Food and Drugs Administration (FDA),[G22] and the use of the rhizome and its derivatives (oil, extracts) was prohibited from use in human food.[G41]

Herbal Use

Calamus is stated to act as a carminative, spasmolytic and diaphoretic. Traditionally it has been indicated for acute and

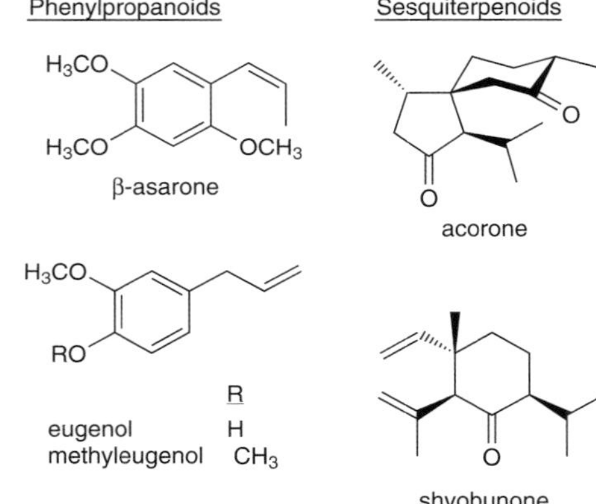

Figure 1 Selected constituents of calamus.

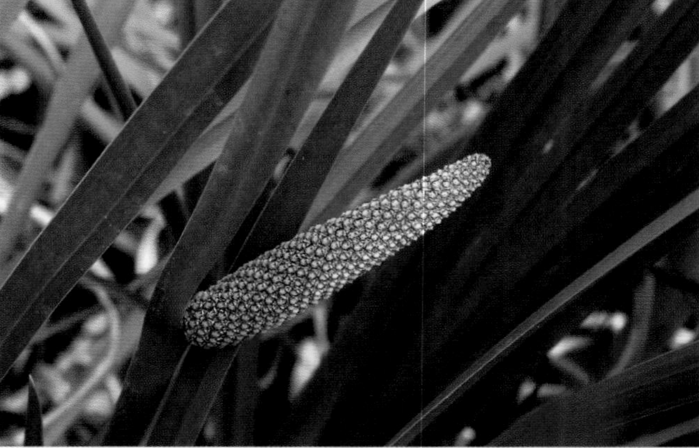

Figure 2 Calamus (*Acorus calumus*).

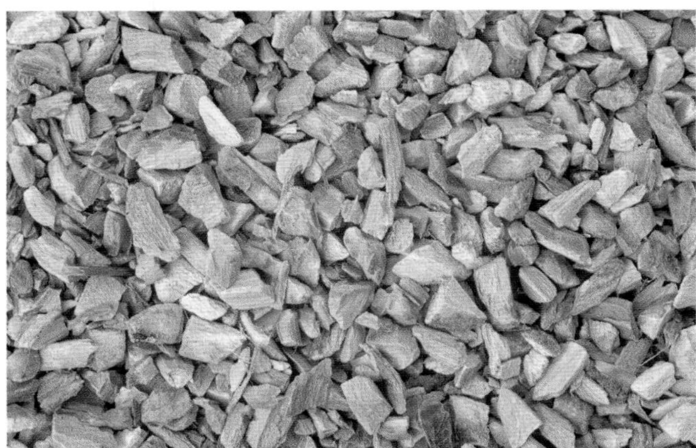

Figure 3 Calamus – dried drug substance (rhizome).

chronic dyspepsia, gastritis and gastric ulcer, intestinal colic and anorexia.[G7]

Dosage

Dosages for oral administration (adults) for traditional uses recommended in older standard herbal reference texts are given below.

Rhizome 1–3 g as an infusion three times daily.[G7]

Liquid extract 1–3 mL (1 : 1 in 60% alcohol) three times daily.[G7]

Tincture 2–4 mL (1 : 5 in 60% alcohol) three times daily.[G7]

Pharmacological Actions

In vitro and animal studies

Numerous documented studies have concentrated on activities associated with the oil.[5] Unless specified, all of the following actions refer to those exhibited by the oil.

Spasmolytic action *in vitro* versus various spasmogens in different smooth muscle preparations including tracheal, intestinal, uterine, bronchial and vascular has been reported for European and Indian varieties.[5–8] In one study, activity was associated with a lack of β-asarone,[6] whereas oils with either low or high concentrations of β-asarone have also exhibited activity.[5,7] The pattern of spasmolytic activity has been compared to that of papaverine, and a direct musculotropic action has been proposed.[8] Unlike papaverine, an acetylcholine-like action has also been observed with low dilutions of the oil and asarone.[8]

Inhibition of monoamine oxidase activity and a stimulation of D- and L-amino oxidase has been reported.[5] The mechanism for this activity, involving serotonin and adrenaline, has been disputed, and an alternative mechanism involving depression of hypothalamic function has been proposed.[9]

Oil rich in β-asarone has been reported to reduce phenylbutazone-induced ulcers in the rat by 5–60%, although no effect was observed on stress- or ethanol-induced ulcers.[7] No spasmolytic activity was reported for oil free from or containing only low concentrations of β-asarone.

A sedative action and a potentiation of barbiturate effect (increased sleeping time, reduction in body temperature) have been described in a number of small animals (mice, rats, rabbits and cats) following intravenous or intraperitoneal administration of European (alcoholic and aqueous extracts) and Indian varieties.[5] Dexamfetamine has been found to block the potentiating action of the Indian variety on barbiturate sleeping time.[5] Potentiation of morphine activity has been reported for the European variety.

The Indian oil has been reported to deplete serotonin and noradrenaline in the rat brain following intraperitoneal administration.[5] The mechanism of action was suggested as similar to that of reserpine, and a potentiation of the amfetamine-detoxifying effect of reserpine has also been described.[5] In contrast, the central action of the European variety has been stated not to resemble that of reserpine.[5] Anti-adrenergic activity demonstrated by antagonism of dexamfetamine-induced agitational symptoms has been reported for the Indian variety in various small animals.[5]

Anticonvulsant, anti-arrhythmic (like quinidine) and hypotensive (apparently not due to a nervous mechanism) activities in small animals have also been reported for the Indian variety.[5]

α-Asarone, isolated from *Asarum europaeum* (Aristolochiaceae), has a local anaesthetic activity similar to that of benzocaine.[10]

Weak antifungal activity has been documented for β-asarone[11] and for the oil.[5] Insecticidal and leech repellant properties have been reported for the oil and may be synergised by synthetic pine oil.[5] Antibacterial activity primarily versus organisms responsible for gut and throat infections has been documented,[12] although a lack of antibacterial activity has also been reported.[5]

Clinical studies

There is a lack of clinical research assessing the effects of calamus, and rigorous randomised controlled clinical trials are required.

Side-Effects, Toxicity[G19, G58]

Concerns over the toxicity of calamus centre around the volatile oil and in particular on the β-asarone content. The level of β-asarone in the oil varies considerably between the different genetic species of calamus (*see* Constituents).

Feeding studies (rat) using the Indian oil (high β-asarone concentration) have shown death, growth depression, hepatic and heart abnormalities, and serous effusion in abdominal and/or peritoneal cavities.[13, 14] A two-year study involving diet supplemented with calamus oil at 0, 500, 1000, 2500 and 5000 ppm, reported growth depression, and malignant duodenal tumours after 59 weeks at all levels of dietary supplementation.[13, 14] Tumours of the same type were not noted in the controls.

Genotoxic activity (strong induction of chromo somal aberrations, slight increase in the rate of sister chromatid exchanges) has been exhibited by β-asarone in human lymphocyte cultures in the presence of microsomal activation.[15] Mutagenic activity (Ames) has been documented for root extracts, a tincture and β-asarone in one (TA100) of the various *Salmonella typhimurium* strains (TA98, 100, 1535, 1537, 1538) tested, but only in the presence of a microsomal activation mix.[16] Lack of mutagenicity has also been reported for an organic extract, when tested in the above *Salmonella typhimurium* strains (except TA1538) with and without activation.[17]

Acute toxicities (LD_{50}) quoted for the volatile oil from the Indian variety (high β-asarone content) include 777 mg/kg (rat, oral), >5 g/kg (guinea-pig, dermal), 221 mg/kg (rat, intraperitoneal).[5] The oleoresin is stated to be toxic at 400 and 800 mg/kg (mouse, intraperitoneal).[5] The LD_{50} of asarone in mice is stated to be 417 mg/kg (oral) and 310 mg/kg (intraperitoneal).[9]

C

There is a lack of clinical safety and toxicity data for calamus and investigation of these aspects is required. Generally the oil is considered to be non-irritant, non-sensitising and non-phototoxic.[5, G58] However, bath preparations containing the oil have reportedly caused erythema, and dermatitis has been reported in hypersensitive individuals.[5]

Contra-indications, Warnings

The toxicity of calamus oil has been associated with the β-asarone content.[16] It has therefore been advised that only roots free from, or with a low content of β-asarone should be used in human phytotherapy.[16] In foods and beverages, the concentration of β-asarone permitted in the final product is restricted (*see* Food use).

Use of the isolated oil is not recommended.[G49, G58] In general, topical application of any undiluted volatile oil is not recommended; external contact with calamus oil may cause an irritant reaction in sensitive individuals.

Drug interactions None documentated. However, the potential for preparations of calamus to interact with other medicines administered concurrently, particularly those with similar or opposing effects, should be considered. For example, calamus has amine constituents, and there is limited evidence from *in vitro* studies that calamus has monamine oxidase inhibitory activity; however, the clinical significance of this, if any, is not clear.

Pregnancy and lactation In view of the toxic properties associated with calamus, it should not be used during pregnancy or lactation. It is not known whether β-asarone is excreted into the breast milk.

Preparations

Proprietary single-ingredient preparations

Czech Republic: Koren Puskvorce.

Proprietary multi-ingredient preparations

Austria: Abdomilon N; Original Schwedenbitter. *Czech Republic:* Dr Theiss Schwedenbitter; Eugastrin; Stomaran. *France:* Jouvence de l'Abbe Soury. *Germany:* Abdomilon; Abdomilon N; ventri-loges N. *Israel:* Rekiv. *Portugal:* Cholagutt. *Russia:* Original Grosser Bittner Balsam (Оригинальный Большой Бальзам Биттнера). *Switzerland:* Kernosan Elixir; Tisane pour l'estomac; Urinex. *UK:* Pegina.

References

1 Stahl E, Keller K. Zur Klassifizierung handelsüblicher Kalmusdrogen. *Planta Med* 1981; 43: 128–140.

2 Keller K, Stahl E. Zusammensetzung des ätherischen Öles von β-asaronfreiem Kalmus. *Planta Med* 1983; 47: 71–74.

3 Mazza G. Gas chromatographic and mass spectrometric studies of the constituents of the rhizome of calamus. I. The volatile constituents of the essential oil. *J Chromatogr* 1985; 328: 179–194.

4 Mazza G. Gas chromatographic and mass spectrometric studies of the constituents of the rhizome of calamus. II. The volatile constituents of alcoholic extracts. *J Chromatogr* 1985; 328: 195– 206.

5 Opdyke DJL. Calamus oil. *Food Cosmet Toxicol* 1977; 15: 623–626.

6 Keller K *et al.* Spasmolytische wirkung des isoasaronfreien kalmus. *Planta Med* 1985; 6–9.

7 Keller K *et al.* Pharmacological activity of calamus oil with different amount of cis-isoasaron. *Naunyn Schmiedeberg's Arch Pharmacol* 1983; 324 (Suppl. Suppl.): R55.

8 Das PK *et al.* Spasmolytic activity of asarone and essential oil of *Acorus calamus*, Linn. *Arch Int Pharmacodyn* 1962; 135: 167–177.

9 Calamus. *Lawrence Review of Natural Products.* St Louis, MO: JB Lippincott, 1989.

10 Gracza L. The active substances of *Asarum europaeum.* 16. The local anaesthetic activity of the phenylpropanoids. *Planta Med* 1983; 48: 153–157.

11 Ohmoto T, Sung Y-I. Antimycotic substances in the crude drugs II. *Shoyakugaku Zasshi* 1982; 36: 307–314.

12 Jain SR *et al.* Antibacterial evaluation of some indigenous volatile oils. *Planta Med* 1974; 26: 196–199.

13 Taylor JM *et al.* Toxicity of oil of calamus (Jammu Variety). *Toxicol Appl Pharmacol* 1967; 10: 405.

14 Gross MA *et al.* Carcinogenicity of oil of calamus. *Proc Am Assoc Cancer Res* 1967; 8: 24.

15 Abel G. Chromosome damaging effect on human lymphocytes by β-asarone. *Planta Med* 1987; 251–253.

16 Göggelmann W, Schimmer O. Mutagenicity testing of β-asarone and commercial calamus drugs with *Salmonella typhimurium. Mutat Res* 1983; 121: 191–194.

17 Riazuddin S *et al.* Mutagenicity testing of some medicinal herbs. *Environ Mol Mutagen* 1987; 10: 141–148.

Calendula

Summary and Pharmaceutical Comment

Phytochemical studies have reported four main groups of constituents, for calendula, namely flavonoids, polysaccharides, volatile oil and triterpenes. The latter seems to represent the principal group, with many compounds isolated, including pentacyclic alcohols, glycosides (saponins) and sterols. Animal studies have reported wound-healing and anti-inflammatory effects, supporting the traditional uses of calendula in various dermatological conditions. The anti-inflammatory effect is due to the triterpenoid constituents, although flavonoids may contribute to the activity. The reputed antispasmodic effect may be attributable to the volatile oil fraction. In addition, immunostimulant activity has been reported for high molecular weight polysaccharide components. Clinical research assessing the effects of calendula preparations is limited, and rigorous randomised controlled clinical trials are required.

Species (Family)

Calendula officinalis L. (Asteraceae)

Synonym(s)

Gold-bloom, Marigold, Marybud, Pot Marigold

Part(s) Used

Flower

Pharmacopoeial and Other Monographs

BHP 1996[(G9)]
BP 2007[(G84)]
Complete German Commission E[(G3)]
ESCOP 2003[(G76)]
Martindale 35th edition[(G85)]
Ph Eur 2007[(G81)]
WHO volume 1 1999[(G63)]

Legal Category (Licensed Products)

GSL (external use only)[(G37)]

Constituents

The following is compiled from several sources, including General References G2, G48, G62 and G76.

Flavonoids Pharmacopoeial standard not less than 0.4% flavonoids.[(G81, G84)] Flavonol (isorhamnetin, quercetin) glycosides including isoquercitrin, narcissin, neohesperidoside, and rutin.[(1)]

Polysaccharides Three polysaccharides PS-I, -II and –III have a (1→3)-β-D-galactan backbone with short side chains at C-6, comprising α-araban-(1→3)-araban, α-L-rhamnan-(1→3)-araban or simple α-L-rhamnan moieties.[(2)]

Terpenoids Many components, including α- and β-amyrin, lupeol, longispinogenin, oleanolic acid, arnidiol, brein, calenduladiol, erythrodiol, faradiol, faradiol-3-myristic acid ester, faradiol-3-palmitic acid ester,[(3)] helantriols A1, B0, B1 and B2, lupeol, maniladiol, urs-12-en-3,16,21-triol, ursadiol; oleanolic acid saponins including calendulosides C–H;[(4)] campesterol, cholesterol, sitosterol, stigmasterol and taraxasterol (sterols).[(5)]

Volatile oils Terpenoid components include menthone, isomenthone, caryophyllene and an epoxide and ketone derivative, pedunculatine, α- and β-ionone, a β-ionone epoxide derivative, dihydroactinidiolide.[(6)]

Other constituents Bitter (loliolide),[(7)] arvoside A (sesquiterpene glycoside),[(8)] carotenoid pigments[(9)] and calendulin (gum).[(9)]

Food Use

Calendula is not used in foods. Previously, calendula has been listed as GRAS (Generally Recognised As Safe).[(G65)]

Herbal Use

Calendula is stated to possess antispasmodic, mild diaphoretic, anti-inflammatory, anti-haemorrhagic, emmenagogue, vulnerary,

Saponins

RO OH

	R
faradiol-3-*O*-laurate	laurate
faradiol-3-*O*-myristate	myristate
faradiol-3-*O*-palmitate	palmitate

RO OH

	R
maniladiol-3-*O*-laurate	laurate
maniladiol-3-*O*-myristate	myristate

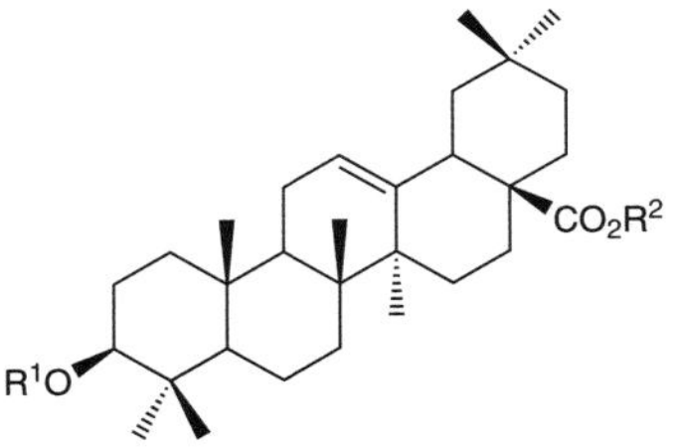

Calendulosides

R^1	R^2
glucose (1→4)— galactose (1→3)— glucuronic acid	glucose
glucose (1→4)— galactose (1→3)— glucuronic acid	H
galactose (1→3)—glucuronic acid	glucose
galactose (1→4)—glucuronic acid	H
glucose (1→4)—glucuronic acid	H
glucuronic acid	H

Figure 1 Selected constituents of calendula.

styptic and antiseptic properties. Traditionally, it has been used to treat gastric and duodenal ulcers, amenorrhoea, dysmenorrhoea and epistaxis; crural ulcers, varicose veins, haemorrhoids, anal eczema, proctitis, lymphadenoma, inflamed cutaneous lesions (topically) and conjunctivitis (as an eye lotion). The German Commission E approved internal and external use for inflammation of oral and pharyngeal mucosa and external use in treatment of poorly healing sores.[G3]

Dosage

Dosages for oral administration (adults) and directions for external use (where stated) for traditional uses recommended in older and contemporary standard herbal reference texts are given below.

Dried florets 1–4 g by infusion three times daily.[G7]

Liquid extract 0.5–1.0 mL (1 : 1 in 40% alcohol) three times daily.[G7]

Calendula Tincture (BPC 1934) 0.3–1.2 mL (1 : 5 in 90% alcohol) three times daily.[G7]

External use Tincture–liquid extract (1 : 1) in 40% alcohol or tincture 1 : 5 in 90% alcohol. Apply to wounds as such and dilute 1 : 3 with water for compresses. Ointment 2.5%.[G52]

Pharmacological Actions

In vitro and animal studies

Anti-inflammatory, antibacterial and antiviral activities have been reported for calendula.[10] Weak anti-inflammatory activity in rats (carrageenan-induced oedema) has been reported.[11,12] An aqueous ethanolic extract had mild dose-dependent action in the mouse croton oil test with 20% inhibition being reached at a dose of 1200 μg/ear, whereas a carbon dioxide extract exhibited 70% inhibition at the same concentration.[5,13] The activity was shown to be due to the triterpenoids, the most active being a monoester of faradiol. Further separation of the triterpenoids has shown that the three most active compounds in the croton oil mouse test are faradiol-3-myristic acid ester, faradiol-3-palmitic acid ester and 4-taraxosterol.[3]

A polysaccharide enriched extract showed strong concentration-dependent adhesive properties on porcine buccal membranes *ex vivo*.[14] Fluorescent labelled rhamnogalacturan indicated the presence of polysaccharide layers on buccal membranes, leading to the suggestion that irritated buccal membranes may be smoothed by mucilage.

The formation of new blood vessels is an essential part of the wound-healing process. Angiogenic activity has been shown for a freeze-dried aqueous extract of calendula utilising the chick chorioallantoic membrane (CAM) assay.[15] The number of microvessels in calendula-treated CAMs was significantly higher than in the control ($p < 0.0001$). Furthermore, calendula-treated CAMs were positive for the glycosaminoglycan hyaluronan (HA) associated with neovascularisation. The presence of HA was not demonstrated in control CAMs.

A combination of allantoin and calendula extract applied to surgically induced skin wounds in rats has been reported to stimulate physiological regeneration and epithelisation.[16] This effect was attributed to a more intensive metabolism of glycoproteins, nucleoproteins and collagen proteins during the regenerative period in the tissues.[16] Allantoin applied on its own was found to exert a much weaker action.[16]

A proprietary cream containing a combination of plant extracts, including calendula, has been reported to be effective in dextran and burn oedemas and in acute lymphoedema in rats. Activity against lymphoedema was primarily attributed to an enhancement of macrophage proteolytic activity.[17] Slight increases in foot oedema were attributed to a vasodilatory action.

The trichomonacidal activity of calendula has been associated with the essential oil terpenoid fraction.[6]

An *in vitro* uterotonic effect has been described for calendula extract on rabbit and guinea-pig preparations.[18]

Immunostimulant activity, assayed using granulocyte and carbon clearance tests, of calendula extracts has been attributed to polysaccharide fractions of high molecular weight.[19] Polysaccharides PS-I, -II and -III have immunostimulant activity at concentrations of 10^{-5} to 10^{-6} mg/mL, stimulating phagocytosis of human granulocytes *in vitro*.[2] A dry 70% ethanolic extract was not directly mitogenic, and was inhibitory in the mitogen-induced lymphocyte assay, causing stimulation at concentrations of 0.1–10 μg/mL, and inhibition at higher concentrations.[20]

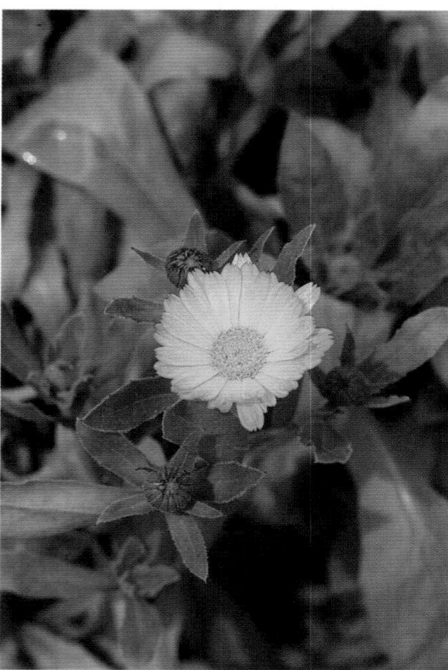

Figure 2 Calendula (*Calendula officinalis*).

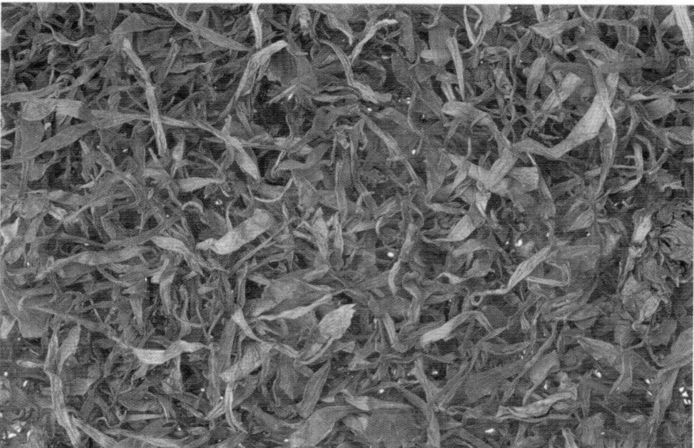

Figure 3 Calendula – dried drug substance (flower).

A 70% methanolic extract of calendula was successively extracted with ether, chloroform, ethyl acetate and *n*-butanol, leaving a residual aqueous extract. Each of the five extracts were concentrated and dissolved in 50% ethanol to produce 6% (w/v) solutions which were assessed for activity on liposomal lipid peroxidation induced by Fe^{2+} and ascorbic acid. The ether, butanol and water extracts showed antioxidant activity.[21]

The triterpenoid constituents of calendula are reported to be effective as spermicides and as antiblastocyst and abortion agents.[G53]

In vitro cytotoxic activity and *in vivo* antitumour activity (against mouse Ehrlich carcinoma) have been documented for calendula extracts.[7] The most active fraction *in vivo* (saponin-rich) was not the most active *in vitro*.[10]

A 70% aqueous ethanolic extract had marked antiviral activity against influenza virus and herpes simplex virus.[G52] A dichloromethane–methanol (1 : 1) extract exhibited potent anti-HIV activity in an *in vitro* MTT/tetrazolium-based assay.[22] Uninfected Molt-4 cells were completely protected for up to 24 hours from fusion and subsequent death caused by co-cultivation with persistently infected U-937/HIV-1 cells. The organic extract caused a significant concentration- and time-dependent reduction of HIV-1 reverse transcriptase.[22]

In a study in mice fed for three weeks with a diet containing either 0.1% or 0.4% of a calendula extract (containing 37% of esters of the carotenoid lutein), mammary tumour cells were infused into the mammary glands. Tumour latency increased, and tumour growth was inhibited in a dose-dependent manner by dietary lutein. In addition, dietary lutein was reported to enhance lymphocyte proliferation.[23]

Clinical studies

Clinical research assessing the effects of calendula preparations is limited, and rigorous randomised controlled clinical trials are required.

A proprietary cream preparation containing several plant extracts, including calendula, has been reported to reduce pain associated with postmastectomy lymphoedema, although there was no significant clinical difference in the reduction of oedema between controls and experimental groups.[17] Calendula tincture 20% has been used in the treatment of chronic suppurative otitis,[24] and calendula extracts are used to accelerate healing and to reduce inflammation.[9] However, the efficacy of calendula preparations in these indications has not been assessed in randomised controlled clinical trials. In an open, uncontrolled pilot study, 30 patients with burns or scalds were treated three times daily with a hydrogel containing 10% aqueous ethanolic extract of calendula for 14 days.[25] Improvement was noted for reddening, swelling, blistering, pain, soreness and heat sensitivity. However, the methodological limitations of this study do not allow any conclusions to be made on the effects of calendula.

Side-effects, Toxicity

An aqueous extract of calendula had an LD_{50} of 375 mg/kg (intravenous administration) and an LD_{100} of 580 mg/kg (intraperitoneal administration) in mice.[G52] Aqueous ethanolic extracts (drug/extract ratio 1 : 1 and 0.5 : 1, 30% ethanol) had LD_{50} values of 45 mg/mouse (subcutaneous administration) and 526 mg/100 g in rat (intravenous administration). An aqueous extract was not toxic following chronic administration to mice. Six saponins at doses of 400 µg were non-mutagenic in the Ames test using *Salmonella typhimurium* TA98 with and without S9 activation mixture.[G52] *In vitro* cytotoxicity has been reported for calendula extracts.[10] Extracts have been reported to be non-carcinogenic in rats and hamsters.[G52]

There is a lack of clinical safety and toxicity data for calendula and investigation of these aspects is required.

Contra-indications, Warnings

Calendula may cause an allergic reaction in sensitive individuals, especially those with an existing hypersensitivity to other members of the Asteraceae/Compositae.

Drug interactions None documentated. However, the potential for preparations of calendula to interact with other medicines administered concurrently, particularly those with similar or opposing effects, should be considered.

Pregnancy and lactation Calendula is traditionally reputed to affect the menstrual cycle. An uterotonic effect (*in vitro*) has been reported, and the triterpenoid constituents are reported to be effective as spermatocides and as antiblastocyst and abortion agents. In view of the lack of toxicity data, the use of calendula is best avoided during pregnancy and lactation.

Preparations

Proprietary single-ingredient preparations

Austria: Calendumed. *Czech Republic:* Dr Theiss Ringelblumen Salbe; Gallentee; Mesickovy. *France:* Calendulene. *Monaco:* Akipic. *UK:* Calendolon.

Proprietary multi-ingredient preparations

Argentina: Acnetrol; Brunavera; Bushi; Controlacne; Eurocolor Post Solar; Europrotec Post Solar; Lavandula Oligoplex; Odontobiotic. *Australia:* Eczema Relief; Galium Complex; Nappy Rash Relief Cream; Skin Healing Cream. *Austria:* The Chambard-Tee. *Brazil:* Calendula Concreta; Malvatricin Natural. *Chile:* Matikomp. *Czech Republic:* Abfuhr-Heilkrautertee; Blahungstee N; Blasen- und Nierentee; Cicaderma; Epilobin; Hertz- und Kreislauftee. *France:* Dioptec; Eryange; Hemorrogel. *Germany:* bioplant-Kamillenfluid; Cefawell; Nephronorm med; Unguentum lymphaticum. *Italy:* Alkagin; Babygella; Decon Ovuli; Lenirose; Nevril; Proctopure. *Mexico:* Sanicut; Supranettes Naturalag. *Portugal:* Alkagin; Alkagin; Alkagin; Cicaderma. *South Africa:* Heilsalbe; Oleum Rhinale Nasal Oil; Wecesin. *Spain:* Banoftal; Menstrunat. *Switzerland:* Gel a la consoude; Onguent aux herbes Keller; Urinex; Wala Echinacea. *UK:* Calendula Nappy Change Cream; Massage Balm with Calendula; Napiers Echinacea Tea. *USA:* Nasal-Ease; Ultimate Antioxidant Formula. *Venezuela:* Biomicovo; Supranettes.

References

1 Vidal-Ollivier E *et al.* Flavonol glycosides from *Calendula officinalis* flowers. *Planta Med* 1989; 55: 73.

2 Varljen J *et al.* Structural analysis of a rhamnoarabinogalactan and arabinogalactans with immuno-stimulating activity from *Calendula officinalis*. *Phytochemistry* 1989; 28: 2379–2383.

3 Zitterl-Eglseer K *et al.* Anti-oedematous activities of the main triterpendiol esters of marigold (*Calendula officinalis* L.). *J Ethnopharmacol* 1997; 57: 139–144.

4 Pizza C *et al.* Plant metabolites. Triterpenoid saponins from *Calendula arvensis*. *J Nat Prod* 1987; 50: 927–931.

C

5 Della Loggia R *et al.* The role of triterpenoids in the topical anti-inflammatory activity of *Calendula officinalis* flowers. *Planta Med* 1994; 60: 516–520.
6 Gracza L. Oxygen-containing terpene derivatives from *Calendula officinalis*. *Planta Med* 1987; 53: 227.
7 Willuhn G, Westhaus R-G. Loliolide (Calendin) from *Calendula officinalis*. *Planta Med* 1987; 53: 304.
8 Pizza C, de Tommasi N. Plants metabolites. A new sesquiterpene glycoside from *Calendula arvensis*. *J Nat Prod* 1987; 50: 784–789.
9 Fleischner AM. Plant extracts: To accelerate healing and reduce inflammation. *Cosmet Toilet* 1985; 100: 45.
10 Boucard-Maitre Y *et al.* Cytotoxic and antitumoral activity of *Calendula officinalis* extracts. *Pharmazie* 1988; 43: 220.
11 Peyroux J *et al.* Propriétés anti-oedémateuses et anti-hyperhémiantes du *Calendula officinalis* L. *Plant Méd Phytothér* 1981; 15: 210–216.
12 Mascolo N *et al.* Biological screening of Italian medicinal plants for anti-inflammatory activity. *Phytother Res* 1987; 1: 28–31.
13 Della Loggia R *et al.* Topical anti-inflammatory activity of *Calendula officinalis* extracts. *Planta Med* 1990; 56: 658.
14 Schmidgall J *et al.* Evidence for bioadhesive effects of polysaccharides and polysaccharide-containing herbs in a *ex vivo* bioadhesion assay on buccal membranes. *Planta Med* 2000; 66: 48–53.
15 Patrick KFM *et al.* Induction of vascularisation by an aqueous extract of the flowers of *Calendula officinalis* L. the European marigold. *Phytomedicine* 1996; 3: 11–18.
16 Kioucek-Popova E *et al.* Influence of the physiological regeneration and epithelization using fractions isolated from *Calendula officinalis*. *Acta Physiol Pharmacol Bulg* 1982; 8: 63–67.
17 Casley-Smith JR, Casley-Smith JR. The effect of 'Unguentum lymphaticum' on acute experimental lymphedema and other high-protein edemas. *Lymphology* 1983; 16: 150–156.
18 Shipochliev T. Extracts from a group of medicinal plants enhancing the uterine tonus. *Vet Med Nauki* 1981; 4: 94–98.
19 Wagner H *et al.* Immunostimulating polysaccharides (heteroglycans) of higher plants. *Arzneimittelforschung* 1985; 35: 1069.
20 Amirghofran Z *et al.* Evaluation of the immunomodulatory effects of five herbal plants. *J Ethnopharmacol* 2000; 72: 167–712.
21 Popović M *et al.* Combined effects of plant extracts and xenobiotics on liposomal lipid peroxidation. Part 1. Marigold extract-ciprofloxacin/pyralene. *Oxidation Commun* 1999; 22: 487–494.
22 Kalvatchev Z *et al.* Anti-HIV activity of extracts from *Calendula officinalis* flowers. *Biomed Pharmacother* 1997; 51: 176–180.
23 Chew BP *et al.* Effects of lutein from marigold extract on immunity and growth of mammary tumors in mice. *Anticancer Res* 1996; 16: 3689–3694.
24 Shaparenko BA. On use of medicinal plants for treatment of patients with chronic suppurative otitis. *Zh Ushn Gorl Bolezn* 1979; 39: 48–51.
25 Baranov von AP. Calendula – wie ist die wirksamkeit bei verbrennungen und verbrühungen? *Dtsch Apotheker Zeitung* 1999; 139: 2135–2138.

Capsicum

Summary and Pharmaceutical Comment

Capsicum is commonly used in both foods and medicinal products. The capsaicinoids are principally responsible for the biological activity of capsicum. These pungent principles are thought to stimulate and aid digestion and to act as a counter-irritant when applied externally. Capsaicin has also been used as a neurochemical tool for studying sensory neurotransmission. Topical creams containing capsaicin 0.025% and 0.075% are licensed in the UK for symptomatic relief of osteoarthritis, and post-herpetic neuralgia, respectively. Capsicum oleoresin and capsaicin are ingredients of a number of over-the-counter (OTC) topical preparations for relief of pain in muscle, tendon and joints.

Conflicting reports have been documented concerning the effect of capsicum on acid secretion and on ulcer healing. Capsaicin-sensitive areas of the gastric and duodenal mucosa are thought to provide protection against mucosal damage. It has been suggested that this protection is lost if the sensory fibres are desensitised. Whether oral consumption of capsicum by humans can cause desensitisation is unclear. The toxicity of capsicum extracts observed in animals is considered to be due to the capsaicinoid components. However, ingestion of capsicum in the diet is not thought to represent a health risk. Capsicum should not be ingested in doses greatly exceeding amounts normally used in foods.

Species (Family)

Capsicum species (Solanaceae) including *C. annum* L., *C. baccatum* L., *C. chinense* Jacq., *C. frutescens* L., *C. pubescens* Ruiz & Pavon, *C. minimum* Roxb.

Synonym(s)

Cayenne, Chilli Pepper, Hot Pepper, Paprika, Red Pepper, Tabasco Pepper

Part(s) Used

Fruit

Pharmacopoeial and Other Monographs

BHP 1996[(G9)]
BP 2007[(G84)]
Complete German Commission E (Paprika)[(G3)]
Martindale 35th edition[(G85)]
Ph Eur 2007[(G81)]
USP29/NF24[(G86)]

H_3CO HO O N H

capsaicin

Figure 1 Selected constituents of capsicum.

Legal Category (Licensed Products)

GSL[(G37)]

Constituents

The following is compiled from several sources, including General References G22 and G41.

Capsaicinoids Up to 1.5%, usually 0.11%. Major components capsaicin (48.6%), 6,7-dihydrocapsaicin (36%), nordihydrocapsaicin (7.4%), homodihydrocapsaicin (2%) and homocapsaicin (2%).

Volatile oils Trace. Over 125 components have been isolated with at least 24 characterised.

Other constituents Carotenoid pigments (capsanthin, capsorubin, carotene, lutein), proteins (12–15%), fats (9–17%), vitamins including A and C.

Other plant parts The plant material contains solanidine, solanine and solasodine (steroidal alkaloidal glycosides) and scopoletin (coumarin).

Food Use

Capsicum (chilli) peppers are widely used as a spice. Capsicum is listed by the Council of Europe as a natural source of food flavouring (category N2). This category indicates that capsicum can be added to foodstuffs in small quantities, with a possible limitation of an active principle (as yet unspecified) in the final product.[(G16)] Previously, capsicum has been stated to be GRAS (Generally Recognised As Safe).[(G41)]

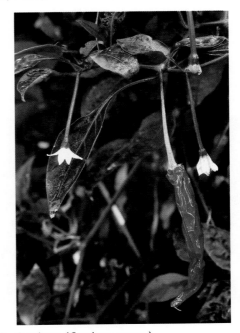

Figure 2 Capsicum (*Capsicum annum*).

C

Herbal Use

Capsicum is stated to possess stimulant, antispasmodic, carminative, diaphoretic, counterirritant, antiseptic and rubefacient properties.[G4, G7, G64] Traditionally, it has been used for colic, flatulent dyspepsia without inflammation, chronic laryngitis (as a gargle), insufficiency of peripheral circulation and externally for neuralgia including rheumatic pains and unbroken chilblains (as a lotion/ointment). The German Commission E approved external use for treatment of painful muscle spasms in shoulder, arm and spine; arthritis, rheumatism, lumbago and chilblains.[G3]

Dosage

Dosages for oral administration (adults) for traditional uses recommended in older and contemporary standard herbal reference texts are given below.

Fruit 30–120 mg three times daily.[G7]

Capsicum Tincture (BPC 1968) 0.3–1.0 mL; capsaicin content 0.005–0.01%.[G4]

Stronger Tincture of Capsicum (BPC 1934) 0.06–2.0 mL.

Oleoresin 0.6–2.0 mg.[G44]

Oleoresin, internal 1.2 mg (maximum dose), 1.8 mg (maximum daily dose).[G37]

Oleoresin, external 2.5% maximum strength.[G37]

Creams, ointments 0.02–0.05%.[G4]

Pharmacological Actions

Capsaicin has effects on nervous, cardiovascular, respiratory, thermoregulatory and gastrointestinal systems.[1] Capsaicin has been used as a neurochemical tool for studying sensory neurotransmission.[1]

In vitro and animal studies

Infusion of capsaicin (200 µg/kg, by intravenous injection) has been reported to evoke dose-dependent catecholamine secretion (adrenaline, noradrenaline) from the adrenal medulla of pentobarbitone-anaesthetised rats.[2]

The addition of capsaicin (0.014%) to a high-fat (30%) diet fed to rats was found to reduce serum-triglyceride concentrations but to have no effect on serum cholesterol or pre-β-lipoprotein concentrations.[3] Capsaicin was thought to stimulate lipid mobilisation from adipose tissue. Lipid absorption was unaffected by capsaicin supplementation.[3]

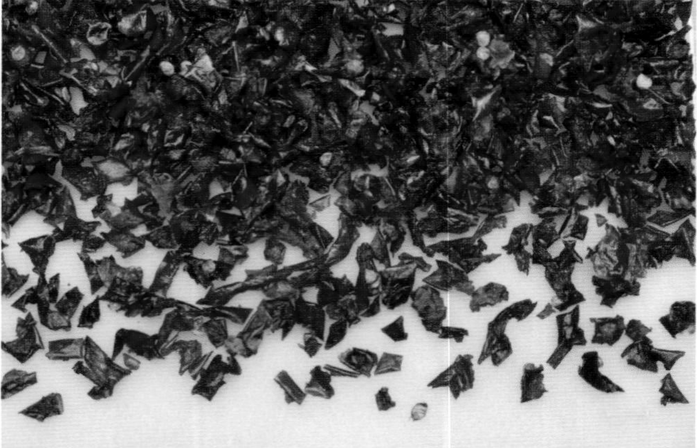

Figure 3 Capsicum – dried drug substance (fruit).

Activities of two hepatic enzymes, glucose-6-phosphate dehydrogenase and adipose lipoprotein lipase, were elevated in rats when capsaicin was added to the diet.[3] Capsicum extracts fed orally to hamsters have been reported to significantly decrease hepatic vitamin A concentrations.[4] Serum vitamin A concentrations were not affected.[4]

Both the gastric and duodenal mucosae are thought to contain 'capsaicin-sensitive' areas which afford protection against acid- and drug-induced ulcers when stimulated by hydrochloric acid or by capsaicin itself. Stimulation causes an increase in mucosal blood flow and/or vascular permeability, inhibits gastric motility, and activates duodenal motility.[5] Desensitisation of these areas, using a regimen involving subcutaneous or oral administration of capsaicin, is thought to remove the protection.[5] However, capsaicin desensitisation was found to have little effect on peripheral responses to stress (i.e. ulcer formation) but did enhance central responses (increase in plasma corticosterone concentration) in rats.[6] The increase in plasma corticosterone concentration observed in capsaicin-desensitised rats was similar in stressed and non-stressed animals.[6]

Capsaicin was found to influence adrenal cortical activity independently of the presence of a stress factor and may represent a stressor in itself.[6] Capsaicin desensitisation was not found to influence basal gastric acid secretion in non-stressed rats, but did lower pentagastrin-stimulated gastric output.[6] However, other results have reported that capsaicin desensitisation does increase acid secretion.[6]

Capsicum (leaf and stem) has been reported to exhibit uterine stimulant activity in animal studies.[G30]

Pharmacokinetic studies in rats have reported that capsaicin is readily transported via the gastrointestinal tract and absorbed through non-active transport into the portal vein.[2] Capsaicin is partly hydrolysed during absorption and the majority is excreted in the urine within 48 hours.[2, 7] Dihydrocapsaicin-hydrolysing enzyme is present in various organs of the rat but principally in the gastrointestinal tract and the liver. The biotransformation pathway of dihydrocapsaicin in the rat has been studied.[7] Metabolites are mainly excreted as glucuronide conjugates in the urine.[7]

Clinical studies

Ingestion of red chillies (10 g in wheatmeal) by patients with duodenal ulcers and by control patients does not have a significant effect on acid or pepsin secretion, or on sodium, potassium and chloride concentrations in the gastric aspirate.[8] No apparent change (qualitative or quantitative) in mucous and gastric mucosal erosion was evident.[8] However, in contrast, capsicum has been shown to increase acid concentration and DNA content (indicating exfoliation of epithelial cells) of gastric aspirates in both control subjects and patients with duodenal ulcers.[1] A study involving 18 healthy volunteers suggested that chilli (20 g in 200 mL water) protected against aspirin-induced gastroduodenal mucosal injury, compared with control (water).[9]

Capsicum is applied externally as a counter-irritant in many preparations used for rheumatism, arthritis, neuralgia and lumbago. Clinical studies of topical preparations containing capsaicin have investigated its effectiveness in the treatment of chronic post-herpetic neuralgia, shingles, diabetic neuropathy, rhinopathy and neuropathic pain in cancer patients.[G4] A systematic review of randomised, double-blind, placebo-controlled trials of topical capsaicin included 13 trials involving patients with diabetic neuropathy, osteoarthritis, post-herpetic neuralgia, postmastectomy pain and psoriasis.[10] All the included trials reported that capsaicin was superior to placebo. However, the review drew cautious conclusions because blinding may have been compromised by the irritant effects of capsaicin.

Side-effects, Toxicity

Capsicum contains pungent principles (capsaicinoids) that are strongly irritant to mucosal membranes. Inhalation of paprika can produce a form of allergic alveolitis.[G51]

Chronic administration of capsicum extract (0.5 μg capsaicin/kg body weight) to hamsters has been reported to be toxic.[4] Treated animals did not survive beyond 17 months whereas all untreated controls survived beyond this period. In addition, eye abnormalities were observed in the treated animals. This effect was attributed to the depletion of substance P in primary afferent neurons by capsaicin, causing a loss of corneal pain sensation and subsequently the loss of protective corneal reflexes.[4]

It is thought that metabolism of capsaicin and related analogues may reduce their acute toxicity.[7] LD_{50} values stated for capsaicin in mice include 0.56 mg/kg (intravenous), 7.56 mg/kg (intraperitoneal), 9.00 mg/kg (subcutaneous) and 190 mg/kg (oral). In rats, an intraperitoneal LD_{50} of 10 mg/kg has been reported for capsaicin.[7] The toxicity of capsaicinoids has reportedly not been ascribed to any one specific action but may be due to their causing respiratory failure, bradycardia and hypotension.[7]

Contra-indications, Warnings

Capsicum may cause gastrointestinal irritation, although it has been stated that capsicum does not influence the healing of duodenal ulcers and does not need to be avoided by patients with this condition.[1]

Drug interactions None documented. However, the potential for preparations of capsicum to interact with other medicines administered concurrently, particularly those with similar or opposing effects, should be considered.

There is limited evidence from preclinical studies that capsicum can stimulate catecholamine release and that it can induce activity of glucose-6-phosphate dehydrogenase and adipose lipoprotein lipase in the liver. However, the clinical significance of this, if any (particularly for topical preparations), is not known.

Pregnancy and lactation There are no known problems with the use of capsicum during pregnancy, although it may cause gastrointestinal irritation and should therefore be used with caution. Doses should not greatly exceed amounts normally ingested in foods. It is not known whether the pungent components in capsicum are secreted into breast milk.

Preparations

Proprietary single-ingredient preparations

Austria: ABC. *Chile:* Dolorub Capsico; Parche Leon Fortificante. *Germany:* Capsamol; Jucurba; Thermo Burger.

Proprietary multi-ingredient preparations

Argentina: Sebulex. *Australia:* Bioglan Joint Mobility; Bioglan The Blue One; Euphrasia Complex; Euphrasia Compound; For Peripheral Circulation Herbal Plus Formula 5; Lifesystem Herbal Formula 6 For Peripheral Circulation; Valerian. *Austria:* Mentopin; Salhumin; Trauma-Salbe warmend. *Belgium:* Thermocream. *Brazil:* Pilulas Ross. *Canada:* Absorbine Arthritis. *Germany:* Cremor Capsici compositus; Gothaplast Rheumamed AC. *India:* Flexi-muv. *Israel:* Mento-O-Cap. *Italy:* Gelovis. *Malaysia:* Dandelion Complex; Total Man. *Mexico:* Parche Negro Belladona. *Netherlands:* Cremor capsici comp; Kruidvat Spierbalsem. *Portugal:* Balsamo Analgesico Sanitas; Medalginan. *Russia:* Efcamon (Эфкамон); Espol (Эспол). *South Africa:* Muscle Rub; Tandpyndruppels. *Spain:* Dolokey; Embrocacion Gras; Linimento Naion. *Switzerland:* Midalgan. *Thailand:* Flatulence Gastulence; Meloids. *UK:* Allens Dry Tickly Cough; Buttercup Syrup; Catarrh Mixture; Hactos; Hansaplast Herbal Heat Plaster; Honey & Molasses; Indian Brandee; Indian Brandee; Indigestion Relief; Jamaican Sarsaparilla; Kilkof; Life Drops; Rheumatic Pain Relief; Sanderson's Throat Specific; Sanderson's Throat Specific; Vegetable Cough Remover. *USA:* MSM with Glucosamine Creme; Throat Discs. *Venezuela:* Ehrlich Balsamo.

References

1 Locock RA. Capsicum. *Can Pharm J* 1985; 118: 517–519.
2 Watanabe T *et al.* Capsaicin, a pungent principle of hot red pepper, evokes catecholamine secretion from the adrenal medulla of anesthetized rats. *Biochem Biophys Res Commun* 1987; 142: 259–264.
3 Kawada T *et al.* Effects of capsaicin on lipid metabolism in rats fed a high fat diet. *J Nutr* 1986; 116: 1272–1278.
4 Agrawal RC *et al.* Chilli extract treatment and induction of eye lesions in hamsters. *Toxicol Lett* 1985; 28: 1–7.
5 Maggi CA *et al.* Capsaicin-sensitive mechanisms and experimentally induced duodenal ulcers in rats. *J Pharm Pharmacol* 1987; 39: 559–561.
6 Dugani A, Glavin GB. Capsaicin effects on stress pathology and gastric acid secretion in rats. *Life Sci* 1986; 39: 1531–1538.
7 Kawada T, Iwai K. *In vivo* and *in vitro* metabolism of dihydrocapsaicin, a pungent principle of hot pepper in rats. *Agric Biol Chem* 1985; 49: 441–448.
8 Pimparkar BND *et al.* Effects of commonly used spices on human gastric secretion. *J Assoc Physicians India* 1972: 20: 901–910.
9 Yeoh KG *et al.* Chili protects against aspirin-induced gastroduodenal mucosal injury in humans. *Dig Dis Sci* 1995; 40: 580–583.
10 Zhang WY *et al.* The effectiveness of topically applied capsaicin. *Eur J Clin Pharmacol* 1994; 46: 517–522.

Cascara

Summary and Pharmaceutical Comment

The chemistry of cascara is characterised by the anthraquinone derivatives, especially the cascarosides. The laxative action of these compounds is well recognised. Cascara has been used extensively in conventional pharmaceutical preparations. Stimulant laxatives have largely been superseded by bulk-forming laxatives. However, the use of non-standardised anthraquinone-containing preparations should be avoided since their pharmacological effects will be variable and unpredictable. In particular, the use of products containing combinations of anthraquinone laxatives is not advisable.

Species (Family)

Rhamnus purshiana DC. (*Frangula purshiana* (DC). A. Gray ex J. C. Cooper) (Rhamnaceae)

Synonym(s)

Cascara Sagrada, Rhamni Purshianae Cortex, Rhamnus

Part(s) Used

Bark

Pharmacopoeial and Other Monographs

BHP 1996(G9)
BP 2007(G84)
Complete German Commission E(G3)
ESCOP 2003(G76)
Martindale 35th edition(G85)
Ph Eur 2007(G81)
USP29/NF24(G86)

Legal Category (Licensed Products)

GSL(G37)

Constituents

The following is compiled from several sources, including General References G2, G6, G52, G59 and G62.

Anthracene glycosides Pharmacopoeial standard, not less than 8% hydroxyanthracene glycosides.(G15, G28) Cascarosides A and B are anthrone C- and O-glycosides being 8-*O*-β-D-glucosides of 10-*S*-deoxyglucosyl aloe-emodin anthrone (aloin A) and of 10-*R*-deoxyglucosyl aloe-emodin anthrone (aloin B), respectively. Cascarosides C and D are the 8-*O*-β-D-glucosides of 10-(*R*)-(*S*)-deoxyglucosyl chrysophanol anthrone (chrysaloin A and B, respectively). Cascarosides E and F are the 8-*O*-β-D-glucosides of 10-deoxyglucosyl emodin-9-anthrone. The cascarosides comprise 60–70% of the total hydroxyanthracene complex. Aloins A and B, chrysaloins A and B account for 10–30% of the total hydroxyanthracene complex. The remaining 10–20% is a mixture of hydroxyanthracene *O*-glycosides including monoglucosides of aloe-emodin, chrysophanol, emodin and physcion.

Other constituents Linoleic acid, myristic acid, syringic acid, lipids, resin and tannin.

Food Use

Cascara is listed by the Council of Europe as a natural source of food flavouring (category N4). This category indicates that while the use of cascara for flavouring purposes is recognised, it cannot be classified into the categories N1, N2 or N3 because of insufficient information.(G16) Previously, in the USA, cascara has been approved for food use.(G41)

Herbal Use

Cascara is stated to possess mild purgative properties and has been used for constipation. The German Commission E approved use for treatment of constipation.(G3)

Anthracene glycosides

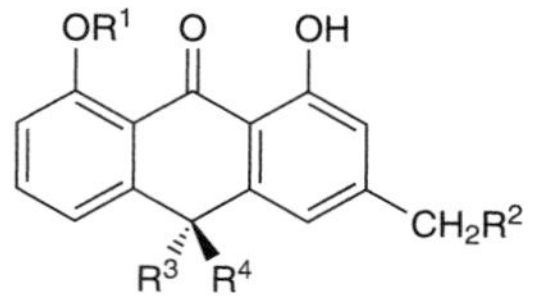

	R^1	R^2	R^3	R^4
cascaroside A	β-D-glucose	OH	H	β-D-glucose
cascaroside B	β-D-glucose	OH	β-D-glucose	H
cascaroside C	β-D-glucose	H	H	β-D-glucose
cascaroside D	β-D-glucose	H	β-D-glucose	H

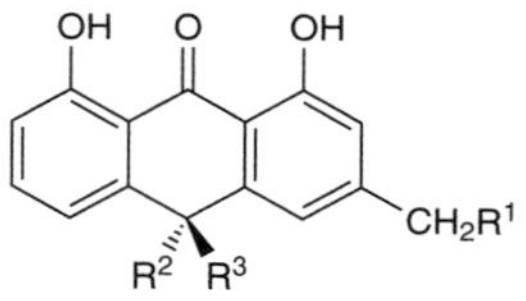

	R^1	R^2	R^3
aloin A	OH	H	β-D-glucose
aloin B	OH	β-D-glucose	H
(+)-11-desoxyaloin	H	H	β-D-glucose
(-)-11-desoxyaloin	H	β-D-glucose	H

Anthraquinones

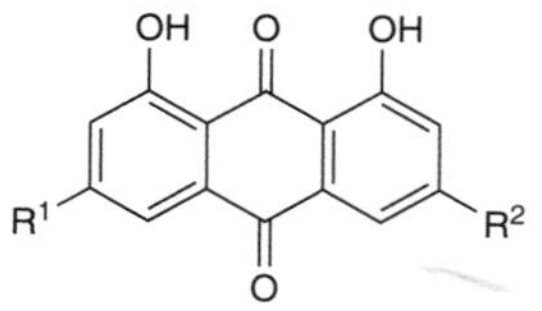

	R^1	R^2
emodin	OH	CH_3
aloe emodin	H	CH_2OH
chrysophanol	H	CH_3
physcion	OCH_3	CH_3

Figure 1 Selected constituents of cascara.

Dosage

Dosages for oral administration (adults) for traditional uses recommended in older and contemporary standard herbal reference texts are given below.

Dried bark 0.3–1 g as a single daily dose.[G3, G76]

Infusion 1.5–2 g of dried bark in 150 mL hot water.[G3, G76]

Cascara Liquid Extract (BP 1980) 2–5 mL.

Preparations Equivalent to 20–30 mg hydroxyanthracene derivatives calculated as cascaroside A, daily.[G3, G76]

Cascara is not recommended for use in children under 10 years of age.[G76]

Pharmacological Actions

The laxative action of anthraquinone glycosides is well recognised (*see* Senna). Cascara has a laxative action.[G45, G76]

Clinical studies

Studies involving elderly patients suggest that cascara treatment, compared with placebo, leads to relief of constipation and increased bowel movements.[1]

Side-effects, Toxicity

The side-effects and toxicity documented for anthraquinone glycosides are applicable (*see* Senna).

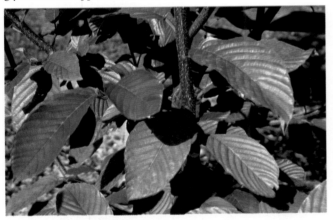

Figure 2 Cascara (*Rhamnus purshiana*).

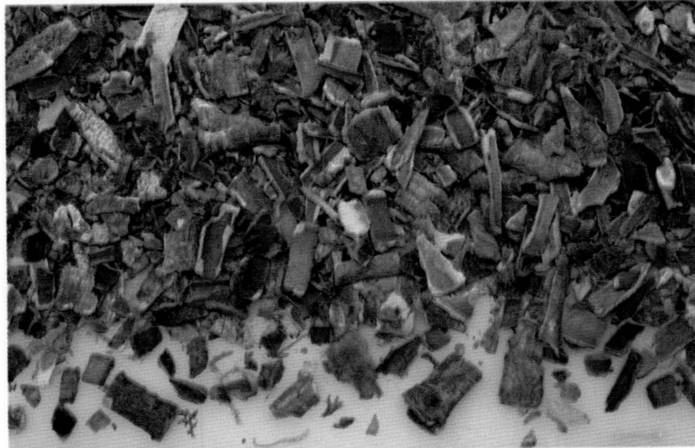

Figure 3 Cascara – dried drug substance (bark).

Contra-indications, Warnings

Contra-indications and warnings described for antraquinone glycosides are applicable (*see* Senna).

Cascara is contra-indicated for patients with intestinal obstruction and stenosis, atony, inflamatory diseases of the colon (e.g. Crohn's disease, colitis), appendicitis, abdominal pain of unknown origin, severe dehydration states with water and electrolyte depletion and in children under 10 years.[G76] Cascara should not be used over an extended period of time – use for more than two weeks requires medical supervision.

Drug interactions Hypokalaemia (resulting from long-term laxative abuse) potentiates the action of cardiac glycosides and interacts with antiarrhythmic drugs or with drugs that induce reversion to sinus rhythm (e.g. quinidine). Concomittant use of cascara with other drugs inducing hypokalaemia (e.g. thiazide-diuretics, andrenocorticosteroids, liquorice root) may aggravate electrolyte imbalance.[G76]

Pregnancy and lactation Cascara should not be used during pregnancy and lactation.

Preparations

Proprietary single-ingredient preparations

Argentina: Natulax. *France:* Peristaltine. *Germany:* Legapas. *Portugal:* Laxolen; Mucinum.

Proprietary multi-ingredient preparations

Argentina: Bilidren; Cascara Sagrada Bouzen; Veracolate; Yuyo. *Australia:* Colax; Colax; Peritone. *Austria:* Cascara-Salax; Silberne. *Belgium:* Grains de Vals; Vethoine. *Brazil:* Bilifel; Boldopeptan; Chofranina; Composto Emagrecedor; Emagrevit; Eparema; Jurubileno; Pilulas De Witt's; Prisoventril; Solvobil; Ventre Livre. *Canada:* Bicholate; Cholasyn II; Control; Doulax; Herbal Laxative; Herbalax; Herborex; Laxaco; Laxative; Mucinum. *Chile:* Bulgarolax. *France:* Dragees Fuca; Dragees Vegetales Rex; Grains de Vals; Imegul; Mucinum a l'Extrait de Cascara. *Hong Kong:* Mucinum Cascara. *Italy:* Amaro Medicinale; Coladren; Confetti Lassativi CM; Critichol; Digelax; Dis-Cinil Complex; Draverex; Eparema-Levul; Eparema; Eupatol; Fave di Fuca; Grani di Vals; Hepatos B12; Hepatos; Lassatina; Magisbile; Mepalax; Solvobil; Stimolfit. *Norway:* Cosylan. *South Africa:* Moultons Herbal Extract. *Spain:* Crislaxo; Lipograsil; Menabil Complex; Nico Hepatocyn; Pildoras Zeninas. *Sweden:* Emulax. *Switzerland:* Padma-Lax; Padmed Laxan. *Thailand:* Flatulence Gastulence; Hemolax; Veracolate. *UK:* Dual-Lax Extra Strong; Dual-Lax Normal Strength; Jacksons Herbal Laxative; Laxative Tablets; Modern Herbals Laxative; Modern Herbals Pile; Natural Herb Tablets; Out-of-Sorts; Pileabs; Piletabs; Rhuaka; Skin Eruptions Mixture. *USA:* Citrimax Plus with ChromeMate; Concentrated Milk of Magnesia-Cascara. *Venezuela:* Gameral.

Reference

1 Petticrew M *et al*. Epidemiology of constipation in the general adult population. *Health Technol Assess* 1997; 1: 1–52.

Cassia

Summary and Pharmaceutical Comment

Cassia is similar in composition to cinnamon and both are widely used as flavouring agents in foods, and in pharmaceutical and cosmetic preparations. Cassia oil is stated to be inferior in flavour to cinnamon oil. The reputed herbal uses of cassia have been attributed to the oil. Cassia contains an irritant and sensitising principle in the oil, cinnamaldehyde, and should not be used in amounts generally exceeding those used in foods. It has been recommended that the oil should never be applied topically.

Species (Family)

Cinnamomum cassia Pressl. (Lauraceae)

Synonym(s)

Cassia Bark, Cassia Lignea, Chinese Cinnamon, *Cinnamomum aromaticum* Nees, *Cinnamomum pseudomelastoma* auct. non Liao, False Cinnamon

Part(s) Used

Bark

Pharmacopoeial and Other Monographs

BHP 1996[G9]
BP 2007[G84]
Martindale 35th edition[G85]
PhEur 2007[G81]

Legal Category (Licensed Products)

GSL (oil)[G37]

Constituents

The following is compiled from several sources, including General References G41, G58, G59 and G62.

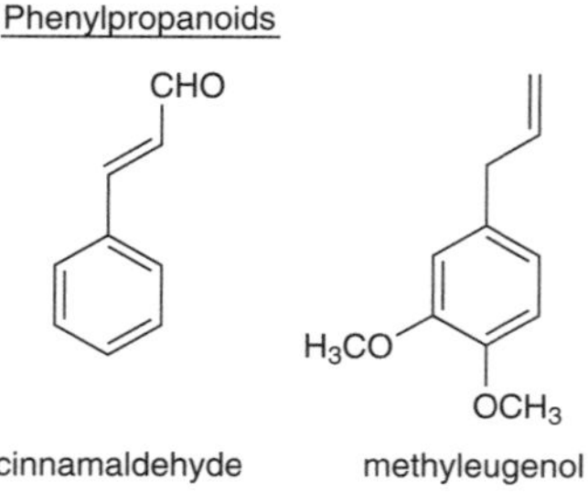

Figure 1 Selected constituents of cassia.

Volatile oils 1–2%. Mainly composed of cinnamaldehyde (75–90%). Other major components include salicylaldehyde, methylsalicylaldehyde, and methyleugenol. Eugenol is reported to be absent. Cassia oil contains no monoterpenoids or sesquiterpenoids.[1]

Other constituents Calcium oxalate, coumarin, mucilage (higher content compared to cinnamon), resins, sugars and tannins (condensed). Complex diterpenoids have been isolated from cinnamomi cortex, for which *C. cassia* is used as a source.[1]

Food Use

Cassia bark and oil are extensively used as food flavourings. A temporary estimated acceptable daily intake of cinnamaldehyde is 700 μg/kg body weight. Previously, cassia has been listed as GRAS (Generally Recognised As Safe).[G41]

Herbal Use

Cassia is stated to possess carminative, antispasmodic, anti-emetic, antidiarrhoeal and antimicrobial properties. It has been used for flatulent dyspepsia, flatulent colic, diarrhoea, the common cold, and specifically for colic or dyspepsia with flatulent distension and nausea.[G7] Cassia bark is also documented to possess astringent properties.[G41, G64] Carminative and antiseptic properties are documented for the oil.[G41]

Dosage

Dosages for oral administration (adults) for traditional uses recommended in older standard herbal reference texts are given below.

Dried bark 0.5–1 g as an infusion three times daily.[G7]

Oil of cassia (BPC 1949) 0.05–0.2 mL three times daily.[G7]

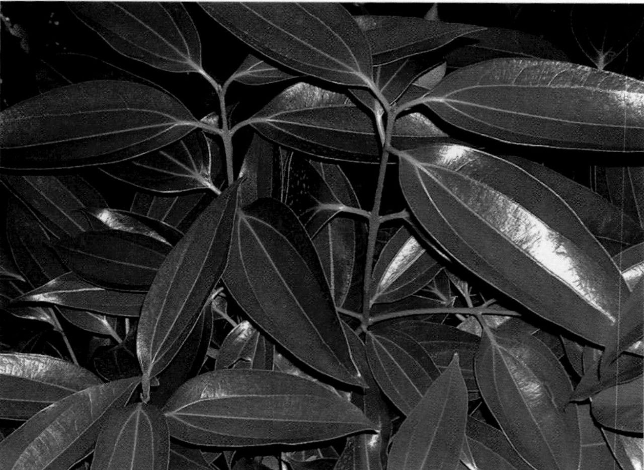

Figure 2 Cassia (*Cinnamomum cassia*).

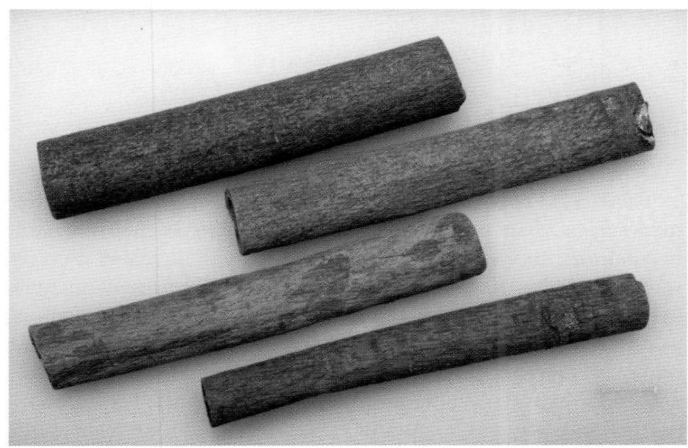

Figure 3 Cassia – dried drug substance (bark).

Pharmacological Actions

In vitro and animal studies

Anti-ulcerogenic properties have been described for two propionic derivatives isolated from cassia.[2] An *in vivo* study using rats reported activity against a variety of ulcerogens including serotonin, phenylbutazone, ethanol, water immersion and stress. The compounds were thought to act by improving gastric blood flow rather than by inhibiting gastric secretion.

Many pharmacological investigations have been carried out on cinnamomi cortex (bark), for which sources include *C. cassia* (cassia) and *Cinnamomum zeylanicum* (cinnamon). These studies have either examined the volatile oil, in particular the major constituent cinnamaldehyde, or parts excluding the oil.[1]

Activities documented for cinnamaldehyde include CNS stimulation (low dose), sedation (high dose), hypothermic and antipyretic actions;[1, G41] antibacterial and antifungal activity, acceleration of catecholamine (mainly adrenaline) release from the adrenal glands, weak papaverine-like action, increase in peripheral blood flow, hypotension, bradycardia and hyperglycaemia have also been reported.[1] However, these actions are of low potency and, in addition, much of the cinnamaldehyde content of cassia is thought to be lost by evaporation and auto-oxidation during decoction of the crude drug. The contribution of cinnamaldehyde to the overall therapeutic efficacy of cassia has, therefore, been questioned.[1]

Actions observed for essential oil-free aqueous extracts have been reported to be weak, and the only appreciable effects are prolongation of barbiturate-induced sedation and a slight reduction of acetic acid-induced writhing.[1]

In vivo inhibitory activity against complement formation has been documented and attributed to the diterpenoid and condensed tannin constituents.[1] Anti-inflammatory activity exhibited by the Japanese plant *Cinnamomum sieboldii* Meisn (also used as a source for cassia bark), has been attributed to a series of condensed tannin constituents.[1] Antiplatelet aggregation and antithrombotic actions have also been reported. These actions, together with the documented anti-inflammatory activity, are thought to contribute to the suppression of thrombus formation in certain diseases.[1]

Antitumour activity has been described and the activity depends on the plant source used.[1]

Clinical studies

There is a lack of clinical research assessing the effects of cassia and rigorous randomised controlled clinical trials are required.

Side-effects, Toxicity

Allergic reactions, mainly contact sensitivity, to cassia oil and bark have been reported.[G51, G58] Cinnamaldehyde in toothpastes and perfumes has also been reported to cause contact sensitivity.[G51] Cassia oil is stated to cause dermal and mucous membrane irritation.[G58] The irritant and sensitising properties of cassia oil have been attributed to cinnamaldehyde.[G58] The dermal LD_{50} value for cassia oil is stated as 320 mg/kg body weight.[G58]

There is a lack of clinical safety data and toxicity data for cassia and further investigation of these aspects is required.

Contra-indications, Warnings

Contact with cassia bark or oil may cause an allergic reaction. Cassia oil is stated to be one of the most hazardous oils and should not be used on the skin in concentrations of more than 0.2%.[G58]

Drug interactions None documented. However, the potential for preparations of cassia to interact with other medicines administered concurrently, particularly those with similar or opposing effects, should be considered.

Pregnancy and lactation There are no known problems with the use of cassia during pregnancy, provided that amounts taken do not exceed those generally used in foods. It is not known whether the constituents of cassia are secreted into breast milk.

References

1 Hikino H. Oriental medicinal plants. In: Wagner H *et al*., eds. *Economic and Medicinal Plants*, vol 1. London: Academic Press, 1985: 69–70.

2 Tanaka S *et al*. Antiulcerogenic compounds isolated from Chinese Cinnamon. *Planta Med* 1989; 55: 245–248.

C

Cat's Claw

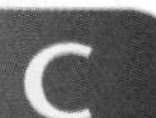

Summary and Pharmaceutical Comment

The chemistry of cat's claw is well documented. Reported pharmacological activities are mainly associated with the oxindole alkaloids and the quinovic acid glycosides.

The two species *Uncaria tomentosa* and *U. guianensis* may be confused. In addition, there are two chemotypes of *U. tomentosa*, one predominantly producing pentacyclic oxindole alkaloids, and the other tetracyclic oxindole alkaloids. Since the tetracyclic oxindole alkaloids have been reported to antagonise the immunostimulant effect of the pentacyclic oxindole alkaloids on human cells *in vitro*, it has been stated that mixtures of the two chemotypes of cat's claw are unsuitable for therapeutic use unless certified to contain less than 0.02% tetracyclic oxindole alkaloids.

Documented scientific evidence from *in vitro* and, to a lesser extent, animal studies provides some supportive evidence for some of the uses of cat's claw. However, there is a lack of clinical data, and well-designed clinical trials involving adequate numbers of patients and using standardised preparations manufactured from the appropriate chemotype are necessary.

In view of the lack of toxicity and safety data, excessive use of cat's claw should be avoided. Individuals wishing to use cat's claw concurrently with conventional medicines should first seek advice from an appropriate healthcare professional.

Species (Family)

Uncaria tomentosa (Willd. ex Schult.) DC., *Uncaria guianensis* (Aubl.) Gmel. (Rubiaceae)

Synonym(s)

Life-giving Vine of Peru, Savéntaro, Uña de gato

Part(s) Used

Roots, root bark, stem bark and leaves

Pharmacopoeial and Other Monographs

None

Legal Category (Licensed Products)

Cat's claw is not included in the GSL.[G37]

Constituents

Alkaloids Both *U. tomentosa* and *U. guianensis* yield oxindole alkaloids, including isorhynchophylline and rhynchophylline and their *N*-oxides, mitraphylline and the indole alkaloids dihydrocorynantheine, hirsutine and hirsuteine.[1] Glucoalkaloids including 3,4-dehydro-5-carboxystrictosidine, carboxystrictosidine and lyaloside are also present. *U. tomentosa* also contains isomitraphylline, its *N*-oxide, dihydrocorynantheine *N*-oxide and hirsutine *N*-oxide.[1]

There are two chemotypes of *U. tomentosa* which differ markedly in their patterns of alkaloids present in the root bark; in addition, the alkaloidal pattern of individual plants changes with time.[2,3] One chemotype primarily contains the pentacyclic oxindole alkaloids pteropodine, isopteropodine, mitraphylline, isomitraphylline, uncarine F and speciophylline,[4] whereas the other chemotype primarily contains the tetracyclic oxindole alkaloids rhynchophylline and isorhynchophylline.[1] Although a particular plant may contain either tetracyclic or pentacyclic oxindole alkaloids predominantly, both types of alkaloids can co-occur in the same plant.[3,5]

Other constituents Quinovic acid glycosides have been isolated from both species.[6–9] Polyhydroxylated triterpenes[10] and steroids (β-sitosterol, stigmasterol, campesterol)[11] occur in *U. tomentosa*. An unidentified South American species of *Uncaria* (presumably either *U. guianensis* or *U. tomentosa*) contains polyphenols ((−)-epicatechin and procyanidins).[4]

Food Use

Cat's claw is not used in foods.

Herbal Use

Cat's claw is stated to possess anti-inflammatory, antiviral, antioxidant, immunostimulating, antirheumatic and anticancer properties.[G32] It is native to the Amazon and has been used traditionally to treat gonorrhoea, dysentry, arthritis, rheumatism, gastric ulcers and various tumours.[12] It is also reputed to be a contraceptive.

Dosage

None documented in standard herbal and pharmaceutical reference texts.

Commercial products (tablets, capsules) contain varying amounts of material, ranging from 25–300 mg standardised extract and from 400 mg to 5 g of plant material.[G31]

Pharmacological Actions

Several pharmacological activities have been documented for cat's claw, including anti-inflammatory, antimutagenic, antitumour, antioxidant and immunostimulating properties.[12,13]

In vitro and animal studies

Certain oxindole alkaloids isolated from *U. tomentosa* (isopteropodine, pteropodine, isomitraphylline, isorhynchophylline) have been shown to enhance phagocytosis markedly *in vitro*.[14] Pentacyclic oxindole alkaloids from *U. tomentosa* have been reported to induce the release of a lymphocyte proliferation-regulating factor from human endothelial cells; tetracyclic oxindole alkaloids were found to reduce the activity of pentacyclic oxindole alkaloids on these cells in a concentration-dependent manner.[12,15] Stem bark extracts of *U. tomentosa* have also been shown to stimulate interleukin 1 (IL-1) and interleukin 6 (IL-6) production *in vitro* in rat alveolar macrophages in a concentra-

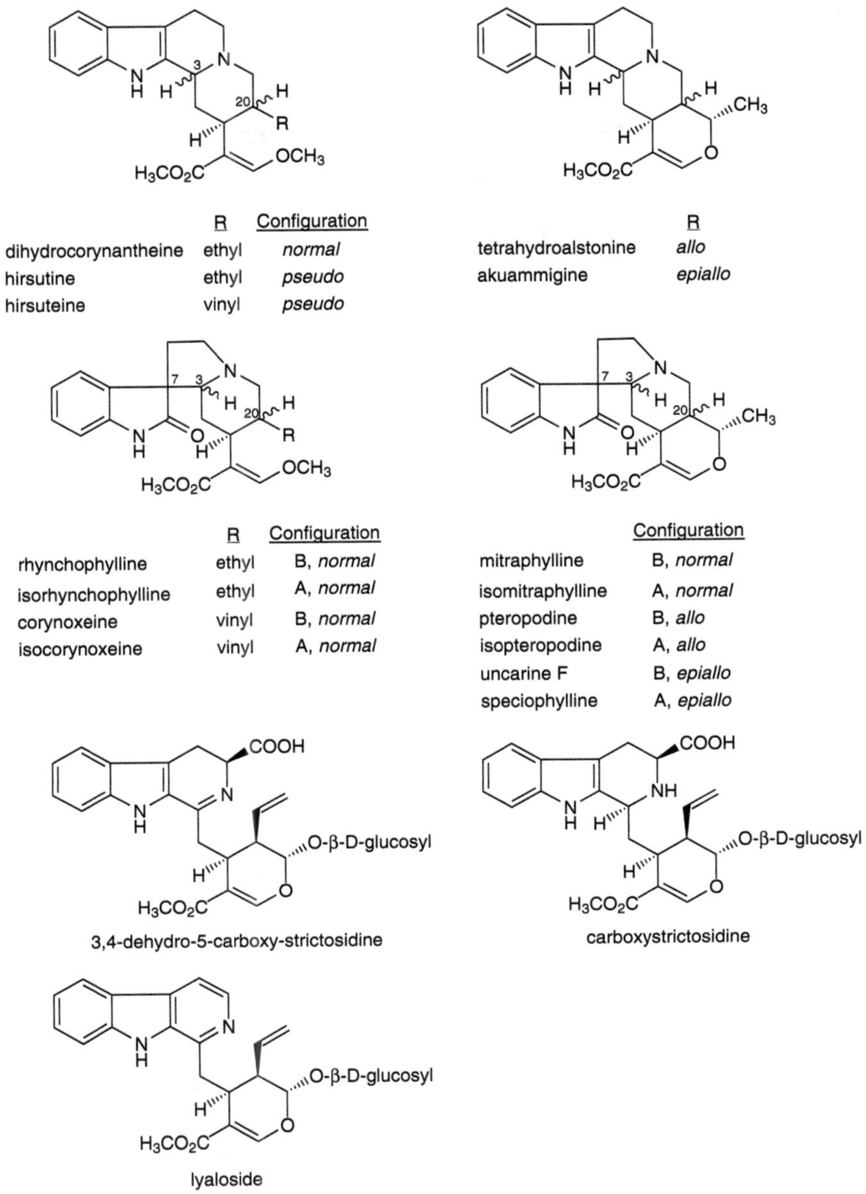

	R	Configuration
dihydrocorynantheine	ethyl	*normal*
hirsutine	ethyl	*pseudo*
hirsuteine	vinyl	*pseudo*

	R
tetrahydroalstonine	*allo*
akuammigine	*epiallo*

	R	Configuration
rhynchophylline	ethyl	B, *normal*
isorhynchophylline	ethyl	A, *normal*
corynoxeine	vinyl	B, *normal*
isocorynoxeine	vinyl	A, *normal*

	Configuration
mitraphylline	B, *normal*
isomitraphylline	A, *normal*
pteropodine	B, *allo*
isopteropodine	A, *allo*
uncarine F	B, *epiallo*
speciophylline	A, *epiallo*

3,4-dehydro-5-carboxy-strictosidine

carboxystrictosidine

lyaloside

Figure 1 Selected constituents of cat's claw.

tion-dependent manner (range 0.025–0.1 mg/mL) and to potentiate the production of IL-1 and IL-6 in lipopolysaccharide-stimulated macrophages.[16]

Extracts and fractions of *U. tomentosa* bark have shown no mutagenic effect but demonstrated a protective antimutagenic effect *in vitro* against 8-methoxypsoralen- and UVA-induced photomutagenesis in *Salmonella typhimurium* TA102.[17] This antimutagenic activity may be due to an antioxidant effect of *U. tomentosa*.[17]

In vitro antioxidant activity of stem bark and root extracts of *U. tomentosa* has been demonstrated in an assay using *tert*-butylhydroperoxide-initiated chemoluminescence in rat liver homogenates.[18] Extracts also prevented free radical-mediated DNA sugar damage.[18]

In vitro antitumour activity of water extracts of *U. tomentosa* (C-Med-100) has been shown in a human leukaemic cell line (HL-60) and a human Epstein–Barr virus (EBV)-transformed B lymphoma cell line (Raji).[19] The suppressive effect of *U. tomentosa* extracts on tumour cell growth appear to be mediated through induction of apoptosis.[19] The pentacyclic oxindole alkaloids uncarine C and uncarine E from *U. guianensis* have been identified as cytotoxic and DNA-damaging agents in a yeast-based assay.[20] These alkaloids also showed moderate cytotoxicity to several mammalian cell lines, including human lung carcinoma.[20] *In vitro*, aqueous extracts of *U. tomentosa* bark appear to interact with oestrogen receptor-binding sites.[21]

Rhynchophylline has been reported to inhibit rat[22] and rabbit platelet aggregation *ex vivo*.[23] Studies in cats and dogs have reported that rhynchophylline has a negative inotropic effect which can contribute to a hypotensive effect.[24] Rhynchophylline and isorhynchophylline have been reported to have negative chronotropic and inotropic effects in isolated guinea-pig atria.[25]

Isorhynchophylline has been reported to have hypotensive effects in rats and dogs.[26]

Trichloromethane/methanol and aqueous extracts of cat's claw (*U. tomentosa*) bark have demonstrated anti-inflammatory activity in the rat paw carrageenan-induced oedema test; a quinovic acid glycoside was identified as one of the active principles.[8] An aqueous extract of cat's claw (*U. tomentosa*) bark was reported to protect against oxidant-induced stress *in vitro* and to attenuate indometacin-induced chronic intestinal inflammation in rats.[27] Cat's claw extract was found to prevent the activation of the transcription factor NF-κB, which suggests a mechanism for the anti-inflammatory activity of cat's claw.[27]

Quinovic acid glycosides have demonstrated antiviral activity in *in vitro* tests against the RNA virus vesicular stomatitis virus.[7] Two quinovic acid glycosides also demonstrated *in vitro* activity against rhinovirus type 1B.[7]

Receptor-binding assays using dihydrocorynantheine isolated from the branchlet and hook of *Uncaria sinensis* (and also found in *U. tomentosa*) have shown that this alkaloid is a partial agonist for serotonin receptors.[28]

Triterpenes

$COOR^3$, $COOR^2$, R^1

	R^1	R^2	R^3
quinovic acid glycosides	Glc (3→1)-Fuc	Glc	H
	Glc (3→1)-Fuc	H	H
	Glc (3→1)-Fuc	H	Glc

(Glc = glucosyl; Fuc = fucosyl)

Procyanidins

epicatechin

cinchonain 1a	β-H
cinchonain 1b	α-H

Figure 2 Selected constituents of cat's claw.

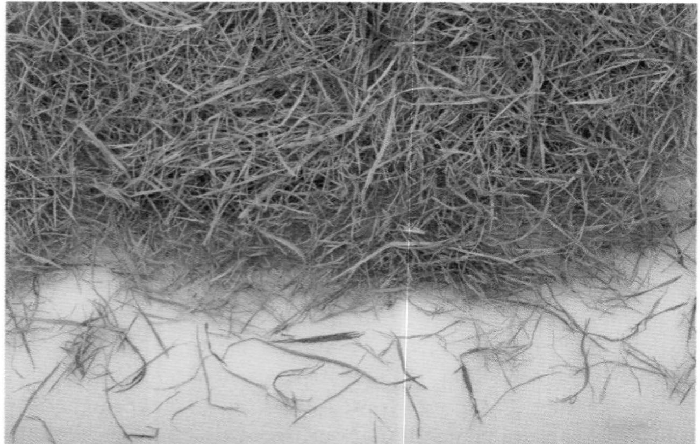

Figure 3 Cat's claw – dried drug substance (stem bark).

Clinical studies

There is a lack of clinical research assessing the effects of cat's claw and rigorous randomised controlled clinical trials are required.

A decoction of *U. tomentosa* bark ingested daily for 15 days by a smoker decreased the mutagenicity induced in *S. typhimurium* TA98 and TA100 by the subject's urine; urine from a non-smoker who ingested the same regimen of *U. tomentosa* did not show any mutagenic activity before, during or after treatment.[17]

In an uncontrolled study, 13 HIV-positive individuals who refused to receive other therapies ingested 20 mg daily of an extract of *U. tomentosa* root (containing 12 mg total pentacyclic oxindole alkaloids per gram) for 2.2–5 months.[12] The total leukocyte number in the group was unchanged, compared with pretreatment values, whereas the relative and absolute lymphocyte count increased significantly. No significant changes in T4/T8 cell ratios were observed.[12]

Side-effects, Toxicity

There is a lack of clinical safety and toxicity data for cat's claw and further investigation of these aspects is required.

There has been an isolated report of acute renal failure in a Peruvian woman with systemic lupus erythematosus who had added a product containing cat's claw (one capsule four times daily, obtained from a local herbal shop) to her regimen of prednisone, atenolol, metolazone, furosemide and nifedipine.[29] The patient had a serum creatinine concentration of 3.6 mg/dL and was diagnosed with acute allergic interstitial nephritis. She was advised to discontinue cat's claw and, one month later, her renal function had improved (serum creatinine 2.7 mg/dL).

Data on the acute oral toxicity of *U. tomentosa* aqueous root extract (containing 35 mg total pentacyclic oxindole alkaloids per gram) in mice and four-week oral toxicity of an aqueous extract of *U. tomentosa* root (containing 7.5 mg total oxindole alkaloids per gram) in rats administered 1000 mg/kg/day have been summarised.[12] The acute median LD_{50} to mice was found to be greater than 16 g/kg body weight. In the study in rats, a slight but statistically significant increase in the percentage of lymphocytes and a decrease in the percentage of neutrophil granulocytes were seen. In addition, an increase in the relative weight of the kidneys in rats of both sexes was noted, although kidney histology was normal.

In vitro, extracts of *U. tomentosa* have been shown to possess antitumour activity and to stimulate production of the cytokines IL-1 and IL-6, both of which are known to initiate a cascade of defence activities of the immune system. Oxindole alkaloids from *U. tomentosa* have been reported to enhance phago cytosis *in vitro* (*see* Pharmacological Actions, *In vitro* and animal studies).

The *in vitro* toxicity of aqueous extracts of *U. tomentosa* has been evaluated in bioassays using Chinese hamster ovary (CHO) cells and bacterial cells (*Photobacterium phosphoreum*).[30] At the concentrations used (10–100 mg/mL), the extracts did not show a significant cytotoxic effect in CHO cells and demonstrated a non-toxic effect in the bacterial cells used.

Contra-indications, Warnings

Drug interactions None documented. However, the potential for preparations of cat's claw to interact with other medicines administered concurrently, particularly those with similar or opposing effects, should be considered. There is limited evidence from preclinical studies that cat's claw has immunostimulant properties, and it is advised that extracts of the pentacyclic chemotype of *U. tomentosa* should be avoided where there is a risk of organ rejection in patients undergoing transplants; this includes bone marrow transplants.[13]

There is also limited evidence from preclinical studies that rhynchophylline inhibits platelet aggregation[22, 23] and that rhynchophylline[24] and isorhynchopylline[26] have hypertensive effects. However, the clinical significance of these, if any, is not known.

It has been stated that mixtures of the two chemotypes of cat's claw are unsuitable for therapeutic use unless certified to contain less than 0.02% tetracyclic oxindole alkaloids.[31]

Pregnancy and lactation The safety of cat's claw has not been established. In view of the lack of toxicity data, use of cat's claw during pregnancy and lactation should be avoided. In addition, use in children (<3 years) is not advised.

Preparations

Proprietary multi-ingredient preparations

USA: Cran Support.

References

1 Hemingway SR, Phillipson JD. Alkaloids from South American species of *Uncaria* (Rubiaceae). *J Pharm Pharmacol* 1974; 26 (Suppl. Suppl.): P113.
2 Laus G, Keplinger D. Separation of stereoisomeric oxindole alkaloids from *Uncaria tomentosa* by high performance liquid chromatography. *J Chromatogr* 1994; 662: 243–249.
3 Laus G *et al.* Alkaloids of Peruvian *Uncaria tomentosa*. *Phytochemistry* 1997; 45: 855–860.
4 Montenegro de Matta S *et al.* Alkaloids and procyanidins of an *Uncaria* sp. from Peru. *Il Farmaco-Ed Sci* 1976; 31: 5227–5235.
5 Phillipson JD *et al.* Alkaloids of *Uncaria*. Part V. Their occurrence and chemotaxonomy. *Lloydia* 1978; 41: 503–570.
6 Cerri R *et al.* New quinovic acid glycosides from *Uncaria tomentosa*. *J Nat Prod* 1988; 51: 257–261.
7 Aquino R *et al.* Plant metabolites. Structure and *in vitro* antiviral activity of quinovic acid glycosides from *Uncaria tomentosa* and *Guettarda platypoda*. *J Nat Prod* 1989; 52: 679–685.
8 Aquino R *et al.* Plant metabolites. New compounds and anti-inflammatory activity of *Uncaria tomentosa*. *J Nat Prod* 1991; 54: 453–459.
9 Yepez AM *et al.* Quinovic acid glycosides from *Uncaria guainensis*. *Phytochemistry* 1991; 30: 1635–1637.
10 Aquino R *et al.* New polyhydroxylated triterpenes from *Uncaria tomentosa*. *J Nat Prod* 1990; 53: 559–564.
11 Senatore A *et al.* Richerche fitochimiche e biologiche sull'*Uncaria tomentosa*. *Boll Soc It Biol Sper* 1989; 65: 517–520.
12 Keplinger K *et al.* *Uncaria tomentosa* (Willd.) DC. – ethnomedicinal use and new pharmacological, toxicological and botanical results. *J Ethnopharmacol* 1999; 64: 23–34.
13 Reinhard K-H. *Uncaria tomentosa* (Willd.) D.C.: cat's claw, Uña de gato, Savéntaro. *J Alt Complement Med* 1999; 5: 143–151.
14 Wagner H *et al.* Die alkaloide von *Uncaria tomentosa* und ihre Phagozytose-steigernde Wirkung. *Planta Med* 1985; 51: 419–423.
15 Wurm M *et al.* Pentacyclic oxindole alkaloids from *Uncaria tomentosa* induce human endothelial cells to release a lymphocyte-proliferation-regulating factor. *Planta Med* 1998; 64: 701–704.
16 Lemaire I *et al.* Stimulation of interleukin-1 and -6 production in alveolar macrophages by the Neotropical liana, *Uncaria tomentosa* (Uña de gato). *J Ethnopharmacol* 1999; 64: 109–115.
17 Rizzi R *et al.* Mutagenic and antimutagenic activities of *Uncaria tomentosa* and its extracts. *J Ethnopharmacol* 1993; 38: 63–77.
18 Desmarchelier C *et al.* Evaluation of the *in vitro* antioxidant activity in extracts of *Uncaria tomentosa* (Willd.) DC. *Phytother Res* 1997; 11: 254–256.
19 Sheng Y *et al.* Induction of apoptosis and inhibition of proliferation in human tumor cells treated with extracts of *Uncaria tomentosa*. *Anticancer Res* 1998; 18: 3363–3368.
20 Lee KK *et al.* Bioactive indole alkaloids from the bark of *Uncaria guianensis*. *Planta Med* 1999; 65: 759–760.
21 Salazar E, Jayme V. Depletion of specific binding sites for estrogen receptor by *Uncaria tomentosa*. *Proc Western Pharmacol Soc* 1998; 41: 123–124.
22 Jin RM *et al.* Effect of rhynchophylline on platelet aggregation and experimental thrombosis. *Acta Pharm Sin* 1991; 26: 246–249.
23 Chen C-X *et al.* Inhibitory effect of rhynchophylline on platelet aggregation and thrombosis. *Acta Pharmacol Sin* 1992; 13: 126–130.
24 Zhang W, Liu G-X. Effects of rhynchophylline on myocardial contractility in anesthetized dogs and cats. *Acta Pharmacol Sin* 1986; 7: 426–428.
25 Zhu Y *et al.* Negatively chronotropic and inotropic effects of rhynchophylline and isorhynchophylline on isolated guinea pig atria. *Chin J Pharmacol Toxicol* 1993; 7: 117–121.
26 Shi JS *et al.* Hypotensive and hemodynamic effects of isorhynchophylline in conscious rats and anesthetised dogs. *Chin J Pharmacol Toxicol* 1989; 3: 205–210.
27 Sandoval-Chacón M *et al.* Antiinflammatory actions of cat's claw: the role of NF-κB. *Aliment Pharmacol Ther* 1998; 12: 1279–1289.
28 Kanatani H *et al.* The active principles of the branchlet and hook of *Uncaria sinensis* Oliv. examined with a 5-hydroxytryptamine receptor binding assay. *J Pharm Pharmacol* 1985; 37: 401–404.
29 Hilepo JN *et al.* Acute renal failure caused by 'cat's claw' herbal remedy in a patient with systemic lupus erythematosus. *Nephron* 1997; 77: 361.
30 Santa Maria A *et al.* Evaluation of the toxicity of *Uncaria tomentosa* by bioassays *in vitro*. *J Ethnopharmacol* 1997; 57: 183–187.
31 Laus G, Keplinger K. Radix *Uncariae tomentosae* (Willd.) DC. *Z Phytother* 1997; 18: 122–126.

C

Celandine, Greater

C

Summary and Pharmaceutical Comment

The chemistry of *C. majus* aerial parts and root is well documented. The yellow-orange alkaloid-containing latex occurs throughout the entire plant, and it is the alkaloids which are considered to be the active principles. Precisely which of the alkaloid constituents are responsible for the documented pharmacological activities has not been determined. There is also evidence that, at least for certain activities, all components of the total extract (i.e. alkaloids plus other constituents, such as caffeic acid esters) are necessary, rather than a single constituent, or group of constituents.

Several pharmacological properties, including antispasmodic, choleretic, anti-inflammatory, cytotoxic and antimicrobial activities, have been described for preparations of *C. majus* following preclinical studies, providing some supporting evidence for the traditional uses. However, well-designed clinical trials of *C. majus* preparations are lacking and further studies are required to determine clinical efficacy and safety. To date, clinical investigations are limited to a small number of trials which has assessed the effects of proprietary products containing *C. majus*, often in combination with other herbal ingredients, in patients with functional epigastric disorders. These trials have involved relatively small numbers of participants (less than 80 per trial) and been of short duration (up to six weeks).

Information on the safety and toxicity of *C. majus* preparations is limited and, in view of this, excessive use (higher than recommended dosages and/or for long periods of time) of *C. majus* should be avoided. Numerous reports have described hepatotoxic effects, including severe hepatitis, severe cholestasis and fibrosis, associated with the use of preparations of *C. majus*. The majority of these reports has involved different German manufacturers' preparations of *C. majus*, several of which formulations include only *C. majus* extract as the active component; such preparations are usually standardised for content of chelidonine. A mechanism for *C. majus* induced hepatotoxicity has not been established, although because of the apparent lack of a dose-dependent effect and variable latent period in the reported cases, an idiosyncratic reaction may be the most plausible explanation.

On the basis of the available evidence, and in view of the intended uses for greater celandine, *C. majus* preparations appear to have a negative benefit–harm profile. In May 2003, the Complementary Medicines Evaluation Committee, which advises the Australian Government's Therapeutic Goods Administration, recommended that preparations of *C. majus* for oral administration should include on their label statements advising consumers to use such products only under the supervision of a healthcare professional, to seek advice from a healthcare professional before using the product if the potential user has a history of liver disease, and to stop using *C. majus* preparations if symptoms associated with liver disease occur.

Pharmacists and other healthcare professionals should be aware that herbal products containing *C. majus* are readily available over the internet and from retail outlets; such products are promoted as being beneficial in indigestion, dyspepsia, nervousness, restlessness, sleeplessness and for nervous headaches and menstrual complaints. There are no licensed *C. majus* products available in the UK, so the quality of commercially available products is not assured.

Species (Family)

Chelidonium majus L. (Papaveraceae)

Synonym(s)

Common celandine, garden celandine, swallow wort. Greater celandine should not be confused with Lesser celandine (*Ranunculus ficaria* L., Ranunculaceae) which is unrelated.

Part(s) Used

Aerial parts (herb), collected at the time of flowering, root, latex (juice/sap) from leaves, stems, roots.

Pharmacopoeial and Other Monographs

BHMA 2003[G66]
BP 2007 (herb) [G84]
Complete German Commission E [G3]
ESCOP 2003 [G76]
Martindale 35th edition [G85]
Ph Eur 2007 (aerial parts) [G81]

Legal Category (Licensed Products)

Greater celandine is not on the GSL. *Chelidonium majus* is listed in Parts 2 and 3 to the Medicines (Retail Sale or Supply of Herbal Remedies) Order 1977 (Statutory Instrument 1977/2130) which restricts its sale or supply to that by a registered pharmacist from a registered pharmacy, or that by a herbal practitioner in response to a one-to-one consultation, provided maximum daily dosage is not exceeded.[1]

Constituents

The plant is particularly well known for the presence of alkaloids which are located in laticiferous vessels. The latex is yellow-orange due to the presence of benzophenanthridine and protoberberine alkaloids.

Aerial parts

Acids Chelidonic, malic, citric;[G75] caffeic (0.4%), ferulic (0.02%), *p*-coumaric (0.06%), gentisic and *p*-hydroxybenzoic (traces, $< 0.01\%$).[2]

Hydroxycinnamic acid derivatives (-)-2-(*E*)-caffeoyl-D-glyceric acid, (-)-4-(*E*)-caffeoyl-L-threonic acid, (-)-2-(*E*)-caffeoyl threonic acid lactone, (+)-(*E*)-caffeoyl-L-malic acid).[2]

Alkaloids Benzylisoquinoline type, 0.1–1%.[G75] More than 20 have been identified including benzophenanthridines (e.g. chelerythrine, chelidonine, sanguinarine, isochelidonine), protoberberines (e.g. berberine, coptisine, sylopine), protopines (e.g. protopine).[3, G75]

Others A saponin, carotenoids,[G75] a phytocytostatin (chelidocystatin),[4] flavonoids.[2, G75]

Root

Alkaloids Benzylisoquinoline type, up to 3%,[G75] including benzophenanthridines (e.g. chelerythrine, sanguinarine, chelidonine (0.2–0.4%)), protoberberines (e.g. coptisine),[5] protopines (e.g. protopine, cryptopine,[6] α-allocryptopine =β-homochelidonine (0.01–0.06%)).

Others Choline, histamine, tyramine, saponins, flavonol, chelidoniol, vitamin C, carotene.[6]

Sap (from leaves/roots)

Glycoproteins, including a lectin.[7–9]

In addition to the above, the alkaloids (-)-turkiyenine[10] and (+)-norchelidonine[11] have been isolated from material comprising the whole plant.

Quality of plant material and commercial products

The European Pharmacopoeia defines greater celandine as consisting of the dried aerial parts collected during flowering and containing not less than 0.6% of total alkaloids, expressed as chelidonine and calculated with reference to the dried drug.[G81] The alkaloids are found in both the aerial parts and the roots, although there are differences in the total alkaloid content and the relative proportions of the individual alkaloid constituents.[12] The concentrations of the alkaloids chelerythrine, chelidonine, coptisine and sanguinarine in the latex undergo daily variations, reaching a maximum in the summer in the evening and in the middle of the day in the winter.[13] The increases in concentration during the day are probably due to light and temperature, and decreases in concentration during the night are probably due to catabolism rather than translocation.[13] In contrast, the concentration of berberine appears to be relatively stable.

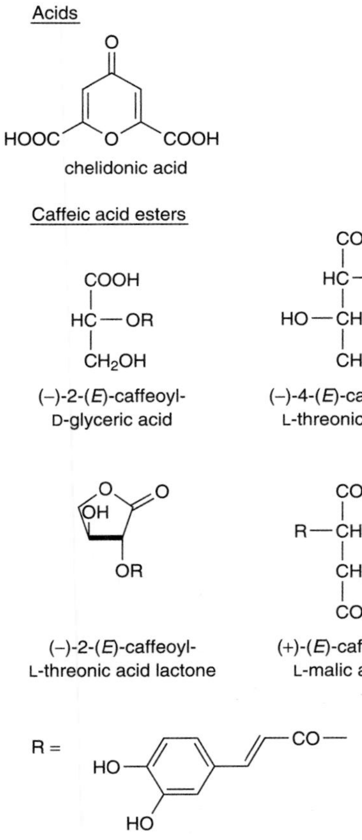

Figure 1 Selected constituents of greater celandine.

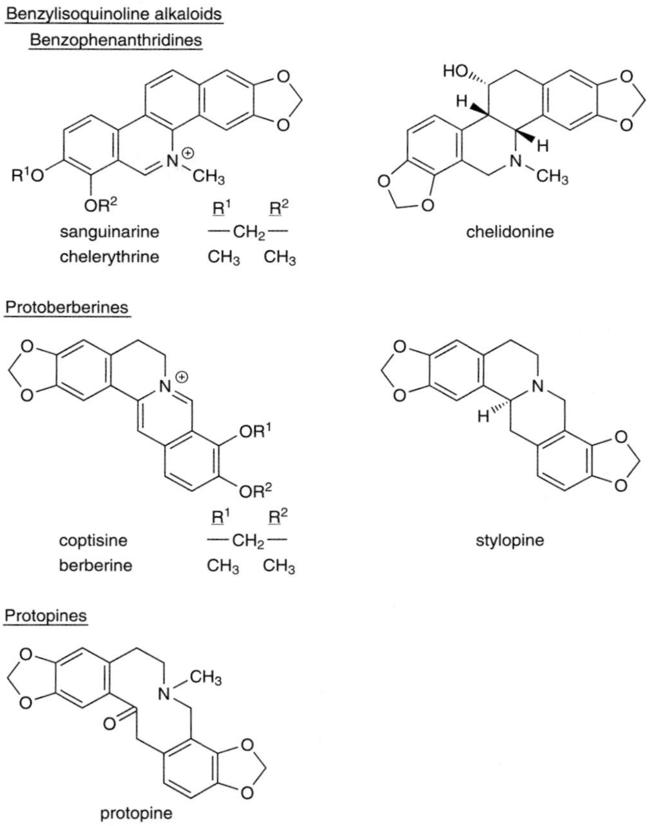

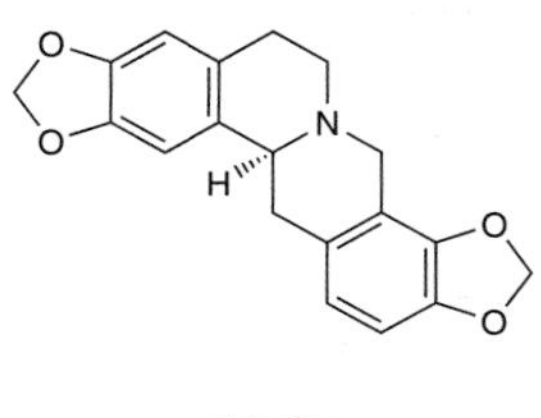

Figure 2 Selected constituents of greater celandine.

Food Use

Greater celandine is not used in foods.

Herbal Use

Greater celandine is stated to have antispasmodic, laxative, diuretic and alterative properties.[G34, G49] It has been used traditionally in Western countries in eczema and scurvy, as a cholagogue, in jaundice, gall bladder and biliary diseases, and in preparations intended to remove obstructions of the liver and gall bladder.[G34] The German Commission E approved greater celandine herb for use in spastic discomfort of the bile ducts and gastrointestinal tract.[G3] Topical preparations of the roots and aerial parts have been used in the treatment of piles.[G34] The fresh latex has been used externally for the treatment of warts and other skin conditions, such as corns, *Tinea* infections, eczema, and tumours of the skin.[G66]

Dosage

Dosages for oral administration (adults) recommended in older standard herbal reference texts for the traditional uses are given below.

Spastic discomfort of the bile ducts and gastrointestinal tract

Aerial parts Daily dosage 2–5 g, equivalent to 12–30 mg total alkaloids, calculated as chelidonine.[G3]

Gall stones, gall bladder and biliary diseases

Aerial parts 1–2 g dried herb three times daily.[G49] Modern standard herbal reference texts recommend the following dosages for oral administration (adults).

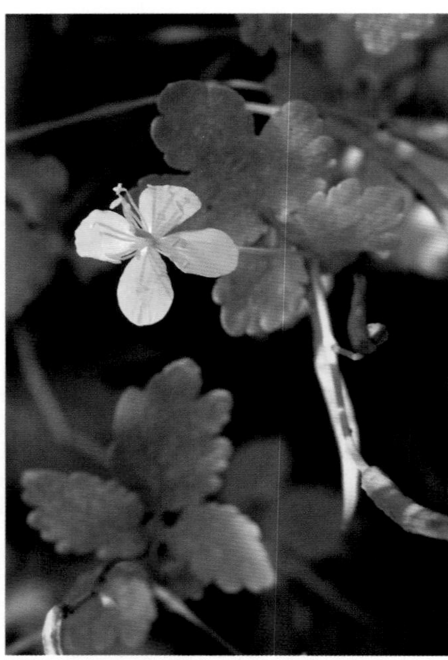

Figure 3 Greater celandine (*Chelidonium majus*).

Liver and gall bladder disorders, cramp-like pain of the gall ducts and gastrointestinal tract

Liquid extract 1–2 mL of a 1 : 2 preparation daily[G50] or 1–2 mL of a 1 : 1 preparation three times daily.[G76]

Tincture 2–4 mL of a 1 : 5 preparation daily[G50] or 2–4 mL of a 1 : 10 preparation three times daily.[G76]

A clinical trial of a monopreparation containing greater celandine (tablets containing 66–167.2 mg dry extract (5.3–7.5 : 1), equivalent to 4 mg total alkaloids calculated as chelidonine) tested the effects of two tablets taken three times daily (equivalent to 24 mg total alkaloids, calculated as chelidonine) in patients with functional epigastric complaints.[14]

Pharmacological Actions

Several pharmacological properties, including antispasmodic, choleretic, anti-inflammatory, cytotoxic and antimicrobial activities, have been described for preparations of *C. majus* following preclinical studies, providing some supporting evidence for the traditional uses. However, there has been little rigorous clinical investigation of *C. majus* and further studies are required to determine its clinical efficacy and safety.

In-vitro and animal studies

Pharmacokinetics No information on the pharmacokinetics of constituents following ingestion of *C. majus* preparations was found. However, there is a limited amount of data on the pharmacokinetics of individual constituents found in *C. majus*. In a randomised controlled experiment involving swine fed sanguinarine and chelerythrine (isolated from *Macleya cordata* (Wild.), Papaveraceae) in their feed (mean daily intake 0.1 or 5 mg/kg body weight), or a standard diet, for 90 days, plasma concentrations of the alkaloids remained constant during the study when assessed at days 30, 60 and 90,[15] although data to support this were not provided in a report of the study. At the 90-day time point for both groups of animals fed the alkaloids (i.e. 0.1 or 5 mg/kg body weight daily), sanguinarine was detected in plasma, faeces and all tissues tested (liver, gingival, tongue, stomach, intestine) with the exception of muscle tissue. Mean (standard deviation, SD) concentrations (ng/g) in plasma were 4 (1) and 108 (4) and in faeces 1180 (72) and 16 110 (2604) for the low and high intakes of alkaloids, respectively. Chelerythrine was detected in plasma (high alkaloid intake only), faeces, liver, gingival and intestinal tissues. Mean (standard deviation, SD) concentrations (ng/g) in plasma

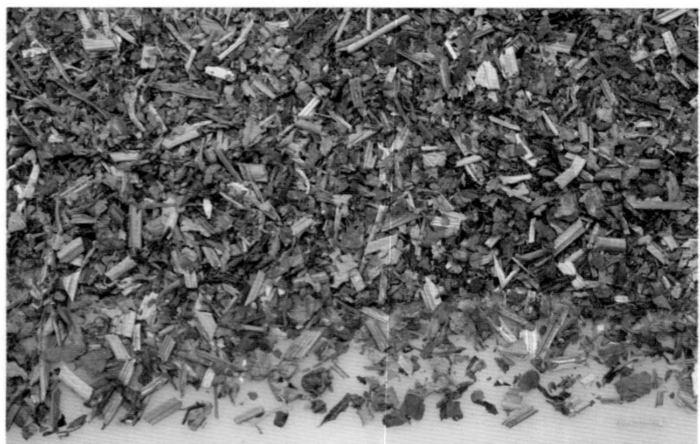

Figure 4 Greater celandine – dried drug substance (herb).

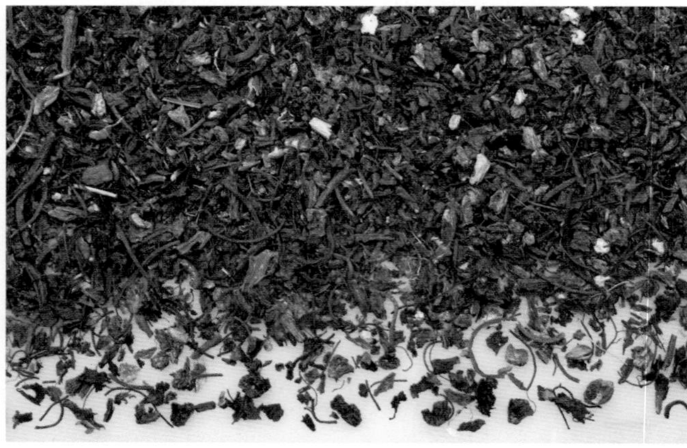

Figure 5 Greater celandine – dried drug substance (root).

were 24 (4) (not detected in low alkaloid intake group) and in faeces 834 (120) and 8412 (1705) for the low and high intakes of alkaloids, respectively. These results indicate that, in swine, sanguinarine and chelerythrine are mostly excreted in the faeces and that a small proportion is absorbed and retained to different extents by different tissues.[15]

Antispasmodic activity Antispasmodic activity has been documented for an aqueous-methanolic extract of the flowering aerial parts of *C. majus* and for the isolated constituents coptisine and (+)-caffeoylmalic acid following *in vitro* experiments involving isolated rat ileum.[16] The extract (containing 0.81% alkaloids, 2.00% flavonoids, 1.20% hydroxycinnamic acid derivatives and 0.06% (+)-caffeoylmalic acid) displayed a mean (standard error of mean; SEM) antispasmodic activity of 12.7% (4.0) relative to that of control (acetylcholine), whereas values for coptisine at a concentration of 1.0×10^{-5} g/mL organ bath and (+)-caffeoylmalic acid 2.5×10^{-5} g/mL organ bath were 16.5 (3.0) and 6.9 (standard error = 2.6), respectively, indicating that these two constituents contribute to the total antispasmodic activity of the extract. A lower concentration of coptisine (0.5×10^{-5} g/mL organ bath) did not exhibit any statistically significant antispasmodic activity,[16] although no p values for this, or any of the other results, were given.

In isolated guinea-pig ileum, two hydroalcoholic (ethanol 70% w/w) extracts of *C. majus* herb (at a concentration of 5×10^{-4} g/mL organ bath for both) relaxed barium-chloride (10^{-6} g/mL)-induced contractions: mean (SEM) per cent relaxation values were 53.5 (4.1) and 49.0 (3.7), for extracts one and two, respectively.[17] The alkaloid content, determined by high-pressure liquid chromatography, for extract one was chelidonine 0.38%, protopine 0.41% and coptisine 0.32% and for extract two, 0.59%, 0.48% and 0.26%, respectively. Mean (SEM) per cent relaxation values for the individual constituents chelidonine (both at a concentration of 1×10^{-5} g/mL organ bath) and protopine were 68.8 (11.2) and 54.8 (5.8), respectively, whereas coptisine (up to 3×10^{-5} g/mL) was ineffective. Values for papaverine hydrochloride (1×10^{-5} g/mL) under the same conditions were 87.2 (7.4). Further experiments using the two extracts and the individual alkaloids produced concentration-dependent reductions in carbachol- and electric-field-induced contractions. Together, these results indicate that the antispasmodic effects of *C. majus* herb preparations comprise both musculotropic and neurotropic mechanisms.[17]

In vitro studies have demonstrated effects of an extract of *C. majus* herb and certain constituent alkaloids at $GABA_A$ receptors. In radioreceptor assays, high concentrations (more than 160 µg/assay) of a dry ethanolic extract of *C. majus* herb inhibited 50% of specific [^3H]-muscimol binding, whereas at lower concentrations (around 90 µg/assay), specific binding of 115% was observed, indicating induction of positive co-operation.[18] The alkaloid content (mg/100 mg dry extract) of the extract was determined as: allocryptopine 0.076, chelerythrine 0.009, protopine 0.465, sanguinarine 0.003 and stylopine 0.154. Further binding studies indicated that the alkaloids allocryptopine, stylopine and protopine are responsible for the positive cooperative effect and that, of these, the effect is mainly due to protopine; the content of chelerythrine and sanguinarine was considered to be too low to account for the effect.[18]

The individual protopine-type alkaloids protopine, cryptopine and allocryptopine (plant or synthetic source not stated) enhance [^3H]-GABA binding to rat brain synaptic membrane receptors.[19]

Analgesic activity Several *in vitro* experiments have proposed mechanisms for analgesic activity for *C. majus*, although analgesic effects for *C. majus* preparations have yet to be demonstrated in preclinical (animal) studies. Furthermore, to date, studies have not explored which constituents of *C. majus* are involved in these mechanisms.

The effects of *C. majus* on GABA receptors have also been investigated with respect to determining analgesic activity. In patch-clamp experiments using fresh periaqueductal grey (PAG) neurons isolated from rats, an aqueous extract of *Chelidonii herba* (*C. majus*, and other details of authentication and preparation, not specified) applied every two minutes at concentrations of over 0.3–10 mg/mL elicited chloride ion current in a concentration-dependent manner.[20] This effect was inhibited in a reversible manner by the $GABA_A$ receptor antagonist bicuculline. Low concentrations of *Chelidonii herba* (0.03 and 0.1 mg/mL) inhibited GABA-activated chloride current; this effect was abolished by the application of the opioid antagonist naltrexone in a proportion of PAGs and potentiated by naltrexone in other PAGs. As inhibition of the inhibitory influence of GABA on neurons involved with descending antinociceptive pathways is a mechanism of action of opioid analgesics, the inhibitory action of *Chelidonii herba* on GABA may provide a mechanism for analgesic activity.[20]

Further experiments using similar methods have demonstrated that low concentrations (0.03 and 0.1 mg/mL) of an aqueous extract of *Chelidonii herba* (*C. majus*, and other details of authentication and preparation, not specified) suppress glycine-activated and increase glutamate-activated ion current in PAG neurons.[21] (Glycine is an inhibitory neurotransmitter and glutamate an excitatory neurotransmitter, so these effects are suggestive of increased PAG neuronal excitability and activation of antinociceptive pathways.) In these studies, the inhibitory effect of *Chelidonii herba* on glycine-activated ion current was partially abolished by naltrexone, and the effect on glutamate-activated ion current was not affected by naltrexone.

Choleretic activity A dry total extract (extraction solvent 70% ethanol) of the aerial parts of *C. majus* harvested during flowering (total alkaloid content 1.6%; caffeic acid esters 1.9%; after hydrolysis: caffeic acid 1.1%, *p*-coumaric acid 0.11%, ferulic acid 0.02%) administered at a concentration of 10 mg/mL/minute for 30 minutes led to a statistically significant increase in bile flow in isolated perfused rat liver, compared with control ($p < 0.025$).[22] There were no statistically significant increases in bile flow following administration of a phenolic fraction (1 mg/mL/minute) and an alkaloid fraction (0.4 mg/mL/minute), separately and in combination. This suggests that all components of the total extract are necessary for activity, rather than a single constituent, or group of constituents.

Anticancer activity There are some preliminary data suggesting that *C. majus* herb extract may have preventive effects against certain cancers, although this requires further research; there are conflicting results regarding cytotoxic properties and antitumour activity of *C. majus* preparations.

In an *in vivo* study, rats were given the carcinogenic agent *N*-methyl-*N*′-nitro-*N*-nitrosoguanidine (MNNG; 200 mg/kg body weight by gavage) and saturated sodium chloride solution (to mimic a high-salt diet), or 0.9% saline, over three weeks, followed by treatment with a water–methanol extract of *C. majus* herb (0.1 or 0.2% in the diet for 16 weeks), or no further treatment; animals were killed at 20 weeks.[23] At the end of the study, preneoplastic pepsinogen-1-altered glands (PPAGs) in the pyloric mucosa of the stomach occurred in all groups of rats, but the mean number of PPAGs was significantly lower in animals treated with 0.1% *C. majus* herb extract, compared with animals treated with MNNG and saturated sodium chloride alone ($p < 0.02$). However, there was no statistically significant difference in the mean number of PPAGs in animals treated with 0.2% *C. majus* herb extract, compared with this control group. There were also no statistically significant differences between any groups in the numbers of animals with papilloma and squamous cell carcinoma lesions of the forestomach.[23]

An ethanol–water (1 : 1) dry extract of *C. majus* roots and rhizomes was inactive in animal models of leukaemia (L-1210, mice) and carcinosarcoma (Walker 256, rats).[24] However, the extract did exhibit cytotoxic activity in an assay utilising Eagle's 9KB carcinoma of the nasopharynx ($ED_{50} < 15\,\mu g/mL$). Coptisine chloride and a second, unnamed, alkaloid were also shown to have cytotoxic activity.[24] A polysaccharide fraction (CM-Ala) from a water extract of *C. majus* 'herbs' inhibited the proliferation of several tumour cell lines *in vitro*. At a concentration of 100 μg/mL, CM-Ala showed over 50% cytotoxicity for the P815 and B16F10 cell lines.[25]

Sanguinarine intercalates with DNA,[26] and structure–activity relationship studies with alkaloids of the protoberberine and benzophenanthridine types have shown that intercalation is influenced by substitutions on rings C and D of the alkaloid molecules.[27] The antiproliferative effects of *C. majus* have been explored *in vitro* in studies using a rapidly multiplying human keratinocyte cell line (HaCaT cells). *C. majus* herb dry extract (containing 0.68% alkaloids, calculated as chelidonine) inhibited HaCaT cell growth, determined by direct counting of cells, with an IC_{50} value of 1.9 μmol/L. The alkaloids sanguinarine, chelerythrine and chelidonine gave IC_{50} values in the micromolar range (0.2, 3.2 and 3.3 μmol/L, respectively). The potency of sanguinarine was similar to that of the antipsoriatic agent anthralin ($IC_{50} = 0.7\,\mu mol/L$), whereas berberine showed a low potency ($IC_{50} = 30\,\mu mol/L$).[28] Further work (measurement of lactate dehydrogenase release into the culture medium as an indicator of plasma membrane damage) indicated that the mechanism of action of *C. majus* extract was due to cytostatic, rather than cytotoxic, activity.

A substantial amount of preclinical research has explored the effects of a preparation (Ukrain) comprising a semi-synthetic thiophosphoric (triaziridide) derivative of the purified alkaloid chelidonine isolated from *C. majus*. The molecule is reported to be a trimer of chelidonine, with the alkaloid linked to thiophosphoric acid; the chemical name of this preparation has been stated to be Tris{2{(5bS-(5bα,6β,12bα))-5b,6,7,12b,13,14-hexahydro-13-methyl(1,3)-benzo-dioxolo(5,6-c)-1,3-dioxolo(4,5-i)phenanthridinium-6-ol}ethane-aminyl}phosphine-sulphide.6hydrochloride.[29] However, chemical analyses of Ukrain using a range of techniques were unable to confirm the existence of the proposed trimeric molecule and indicated that the preparations tested simply contained a mixture of *C. majus* alkaloids, including chelidonine.[30]

It has been reported that Ukrain has antitumour activity *in vitro* against various cancer cell lines and *in vivo* in several experimental models of cancer, as well as immunomodulatory properties.[31] It has also been reported to induce cell cycle arrest and apoptosis in human epidermoid cancer cell lines, but not in normal human keratinocytes,[32] and to protect normal human fibroblasts, but not various types of human tumour cells, against ionising radiation in *in vitro* experiments;[33] radioprotective effects have also been reported following *in vivo* (preclinical) studies.[34] Other properties reported include effects on bone tissue *in vivo* (rats).[35]

Subsequent research in some of these areas has, however, failed to replicate the findings. *In vitro* studies using normal, transformed and malignant cell lines have shown that there was no difference in the effects of Ukrain on cell growth, cell cycle progression and morphology for the different cell lines, indicating that there is no selective toxicity towards malignant cells.[36] Other *in vitro* research by the same authors has also raised doubts about claims of a lack of adverse effects with Ukrain.[37]

Immunomodulatory activity Incubation of spleen cells with protein-bound polysaccharide fractions from a water extract of *C. majus* 'herbs' for 5 days increased the lytic activity of spleen lymphocytes to Yac-1 tumour cells from 0.9% to 30.0% and 34.2% for the fractions CM-Al and CM-Ala, respectively (*p* values not given).[25] The optimal concentration for generation of activated killer cells was 5 μg/mL for both fractions. Similarly, mouse peritoneal macrophages cultured with CM-Ala (10–100 μg/mL) show increased cytotoxicity, compared with control, as determined by the degree of inhibition of radiolabelled thymidine uptake by tumour cells. CM-Ala contains around 30% protein and 70% carbohydrate.[25]

Further work suggested that CM-A1a may have a radioprotective effect *in vivo*. In experiments involving mice given CM-A1a 50 mg/kg intraperitoneally 24 hours before sublethal doses of irradiation, platelet numbers were significantly increased in CM-A1a treated mice, compared with control, five days post-irradiation, and white blood cell count was significantly increased in CM-A1a treated mice, compared with control, nine days post-irradiation ($p < 0.001$ and < 0.01, respectively), indicating haematopoietic recovery.[38] In other experiments involving mice given lethal doses of irradiation (9 Gy), the survival rate for mice treated with CM-Ala 50 or 100 mg/kg intraperitoneally before irradiation was 80% at 30 days post-irradiation, whereas all mice in the control group were dead by day 15 post-irradiation.

Anti-inflammatory activity Various effects related to anti-inflammatory activity have been documented for *C. majus* extract and for certain alkaloids isolated from the plant.

In *in vitro* experiments using mouse peritoneal macrophages, nitric oxide production was significantly increased when cells were treated with a water extract of *C. majus* dried 'herbs' (plant part not stated precisely) at concentrations of 0.01, 0.1 and 1 mg/mL together with murine recombinant interferon-gamma (rIFN-γ), compared with treatment with rIFN-γ alone ($p < 0.05$), indicating a cooperative induction of NO production.[39] NO production in mouse peritoneal macrophages induced by *C. majus* extract plus rIFN-γ was progressively inhibited by incubation with increasing amounts ($p < 0.05$ for 0.01 and 0.1 mM, compared with control) of N^G-monomethyl-L-arginine (N^GMMA) and by addition of the antioxidant compound pyrrolidine dithiocarbamate (PDTC) at a concentration of 100 μM. Furthermore, incubation of mouse peritoneal macrophages with *C. majus* extract (1 mg/mL) plus rIFN-γ increased tumour-necrosis-factor-alpha (TNF-α) production in a concentration-dependent manner; adding the nuclear factor kappa B (NF-κB) inhibitor PDTC significantly decreased the production of TNF-α, indicating that *C. majus* extract increases TNF-α production via NF-κB activation.[39]

Anti-inflammatory activity has also been described for the alkaloids sanguinarine and chelerythrine isolated from *C. majus* root following studies involving the carrageenan-induced rat paw oedema test. Greatest inhibition of oedema was observed with subcutaneous (rather than oral) administration of sanguinarine (rather than chelerythrine) 5 and 10 mg/kg body weight, compared with control (no p values stated).[40]

An extract of *C. majus* herb and the alkaloids sanguinarine and chelerythrine (isolated from *C. majus* root in this study) inhibited 5-lipoxygenase (5-LO) in isolated bovine polymorphonuclear leukocytes (PMNL) with IC_{50} values of 1.9, 0.4 and 0.8 μmol/L, respectively.[41] Sanguinarine and chelerythrine also inhibited 12-lipoxygenase (12-LO) obtained from mouse epidermis (IC_{50} = 13 and 33 μmol/L, respectively), whereas *C. majus* herb extract (170 μg extract/mL test solution) was inactive. Chelidonine was inactive against both lipoxygenase enzymes (IC_{50} = >100 μmol/L for each). The enzymes 5-LO and 12-LO are involved with leukotriene B_4 and 12-hydroxyeicosatetraenoic acid synthesis.

Antimicrobial activity A glycoprotein isolated from the juice of *C. majus* leaves and roots is active against drug-resistant staphylococci and enterococci *in vitro*.[7] Minimum bactericidal concentration (MBC) values against several strains (including clinical isolates) of methicillin-sensitive *Staphylococcus aureus* (MSSA), methicillin-resistant *S. aureus* (MRSA), mupirocin-resistant MRSA, aminoglycoside-resistant *Enterococcus faecalis* and aminoglycoside-resistant *E. faecium* were 31–125, 31–250, 31–125, 125–500 and 250–500 mg/L, respectively.

Chelerythrine and the quaternary benzophenanthridine alkaloid fraction (containing chelerythrine and sanguinarine 7 : 3 with traces of chelirubine) isolated from *C. majus* root were ineffective *in vitro* against several Gram-negative bacterial strains, including *Escherichia coli*, *Pseudomonas aeruginosa* and *Klebsiella pneumoniae*.[40] In contrast, substantial activity was observed *in vitro* for the alkaloid fraction against Gram-positive bacteria, including *Staphylococcus aureus*, beta-haemolytic streptococci and alpha-haemolytic streptococci, and against *Candida albicans* (minimum inhibitory concentration (MIC) values: 5, 10, 20 and 5 μg/mL, respectively). MBC values for the alkaloid fraction against these species were 40, 10, 40 and >160 μg/mL, respectively.

These findings are supported to some extent by those of other studies. In tests using the liquid dilution method, crude ethanolic extracts of the aerial parts of *C. majus* were inactive against *E. coli*, *P. aeruginosa*, *Bacillus cereus*, *Salmonella enteritidis* and *Candida albicans*.[42] In contrast, an ethanolic extract of *C. majus* roots had MIC values of 15.63, 62.50 and 62.50 mg dry plant material/mL for *B. cereus*, *S. enteritidis* and *C. albicans*, but was inactive against *E. coli* and *P. aeruginosa*.

Berberine chloride and chelerythrine chloride, isolated from another plant species (*Fagara zanthoxyloides*, Rutaceae), have activity against *S. aureus*, *Bacillus subtilis*, *Streptococcus pneumoniae*, *E. coli*, *Klebsiella pneumoniae*, *P. aeruginosa*, *Proteus* sp. and *C. albicans*.[43]

Antifungal activity *in vitro* has also been documented for *C. majus* extracts against *Fusarium* strains. In liquid medium assays, a methanolic extract of the whole plant harvested at the flowering stage appeared to display the greatest antifungal activity: five days after inoculation, growth of two *Fusarium* strains tested was reduced to less than 40% of that seen with control, whereas this was achieved for only one strain with an ethanolic extract and not at all with an aqueous extract.[44] *F. oxysporum* f. sp. *cubense* was the strain most sensitive to the methanolic extract, and *F. solani* was the most sensitive strain to all three extracts. In contrast, *F. culmorum* was insensitive to all three extracts. Methanolic extracts of *C. majus* roots achieved greater inhibition of fungal growth than did methanolic extracts of *C. majus* shoots: growth of *F. oxysporum* f. sp. *cubense*, *F. oxysporum* f. sp. *melonis* and *F. solani* was reduced to less than 30% of that seen with control, although growth of *F. culmorum* was unaffected.

Further experiments used alkaloids isolated from *C. majus* roots and shoots: chelerythrine and sanguinarine were reported to be active against both *F. solani* and *F. culmorum*, berberine was active against *F. solani*, and chelidonine was inactive against both strains.[44] However, data supporting these statements were not provided in the published report.

Antifungal activity against *Cladosporium herbarum* has been described for the alkaloids chelidonine, dihydrochelerythrine and dihydrosanguinarine isolated from a methanolic extract of *C. majus* fresh root: minimum quantities of these compounds for inhibition of growth of *C. herbarum* on thin-layer chromatography (TLC) plates were 10, 6 and 4 μg, respectively.[45]

Other work has shown little variation in the antimycotic activity of *C. majus* plant material collected during different months. Ethanolic extracts of *C. majus* plants collected in late July or early September were active against *Candida pseudotropicalis*, *M. gypseum*, *T. mentagrophytes*, *M. canis* and *E. floccosum* (zone of inhibition from 21 to 30 or more millimetres in diameter). Ethanolic extracts of *C. majus* plants collected in early September were also active against *C. albicans*.[46]

Antiviral activity *In vitro* activity against adenoviruses and herpes simplex virus type I (HSV-1) has been documented for the squeezed sap and a sodium chloride extract of the aerial parts of *C. majus*.[47] Subsequent bioassay-guided fractionation of extracts of the aerial parts and the root of the plant produced several fractions of which one in particular at a concentration of 35 μg/mL showed antiviral activity when incubated with cells infected with adenovirus type 12. This fraction also showed virucidal action against HSV-1, achieving 100% loss of virus infectivity after 90 minutes' incubation, although adenoviruses types 5 and 12 were less sensitive, retaining 50% infectivity after 120 minutes' incubation with the fraction.

An extract obtained from the 'green' parts of mature *C. majus* plants was found to have inhibitory activity against cysteine, but not serine, proteinases. The phytocystatin chelidocystatin, isolated from the extract, inhibited the activity of the cysteine proteinases cathepsin L, papain and cathepsin H (inhibition constant, K_i values: 5.6×10^{-11} mol/L, 1.1×10^{-10} mol/L and 7.5×10^{-9} mol/L, respectively).[4]

The pure compound chelidonine has weak inhibitory activity (IC_{50} around 200 μg/mL) against human immunodeficiency virus type-1 reverse transcriptase (HIV-1 RT), whereas berberine chloride has moderate inhibitory activity against this enzyme (IC_{50} = 100 μg/mL).[48]

Other activities A liquid alcoholic extract of *C. majus* herb, containing 0.64 mg/mL total alkaloids, calculated as chelidonine, protected against indometacin-induced (10 mg/kg body weight) gastric damage in a dose-dependent manner (2.5–10 mL/kg) when administered orally one hour before indometacin to rats.[49] Doses of *C. majus* herb extract of 5 and 10 mL/kg body weight afforded over 50% protection against the development of ulcers, compared with control.

Antioxidant activity, determined using the FRAP (ferric reducing and antioxidant power) method, has been reported for 20% and 40% alcohol–water (type not stated) extracts of the fresh aerial parts of *C. majus* collected in Hungary.[50]

C

Clinical studies

Pharmacokinetics No information relating to the clinical pharmacokinetics of *C. majus* preparations was found.

Therapeutics Clinical investigation of *C. majus* preparations is limited. The few clinical trials available have investigated the effects of proprietary products containing *C. majus*, often in combination with other herbal ingredients, in patients with functional epigastric disorders. Further investigation of the efficacy and effectiveness of *C. majus* preparations is required.

In a randomised, double-blind, placebo-controlled trial, 60 patients with functional epigastric complaints, including cramp-like pains in the biliary and gastrointestinal tracts, received tablets containing *C. majus* extract (comprising 66.0 to 167.2 mg native dry extract, equivalent to 4 mg total alkaloids, calculated as chelidonine), or placebo, at a dosage of two tablets three times daily for six weeks.[14] At the end of the study, the reduction in symptom score (one of the primary outcome variables), assessed using the Zerssen list, was significantly greater in the *C. majus* group, compared with the placebo group ($p = 0.003$). Also, the physician's assessment of efficacy was that 18/30 patients in the treatment group were improved or symptom-free, compared with 8/30 in the placebo group ($p = 0.0038$).[14]

The effects of a combination preparation (Iberogast) containing extract of *C. majus* herb (as well as extracts of bitter candy tuft, chamomile flower, peppermint leaves, caraway fruit, liquorice root, lemon balm leaves, angelica root and milk thistle fruit) were investigated in a randomised, double-blind, placebo-controlled trial involving 60 patients with functional dyspepsia.[51] Participants received Iberogast, a preparation similar to Iberogast but lacking bitter candy tuft extract, or placebo, 20 drops three times daily for four weeks. At the end of the study, participants who received one of the two combination preparations, compared with those in the placebo group, had a significant improvement in gastrointestinal symptom scores, one of the primary outcome variables ($p < 0.001$).

Another double-blind, placebo-controlled trial assessed the effects of a combination preparation (Cholagogum F Nattermann) containing dry extracts of *C. majus* and *Curcuma longa* in patients with upper abdominal pain due to biliary system dysfunction.[52] Participants received the herbal preparation ($n = 39$), or placebo ($n = 37$), one capsule three times daily for three weeks. Capsules of the herbal preparation were standardised to contain 4 mg total alkaloids calculated as chelidonine. During the first week of treatment, reductions in the frequency of cramp-like pain were reported for both the treatment and placebo groups, although the difference between the groups was not statistically significant ($p = 0.069$). There was, however, a statistically significant difference in the frequency of episodes of dull/hollow pain between the treatment and placebo groups ($p = 0.009$).[52]

A small number of other clinical investigations has explored the effects of a preparation (Ukrain) comprising a semi-synthetic thiophosphoric (triaziridide) derivative of the purified alkaloid chelidonine isolated from *C. majus* (*see* Pharmacological Actions). Most of these investigations, typically case series and small studies of varying methodological quality, have involved patients with different types of cancer, including lung cancer,[53,54] Kaposi's sarcoma,[55] rectal or ovarian cancer,[56] breast cancer,[54] and children from areas contaminated with radioactive material after the Chernobyl accident with recurrent bronchopulmonary pathology.[57]

A systematic review of seven randomised controlled trials of Ukrain in patients with different types of cancer found that all included trials reported beneficial effects for Ukrain, but that as most of the trials had methodological limitations, their results were not definitive and further investigation in the form of well-designed randomised controlled trials is required.[58]

In one study, a randomised, controlled trial involving 90 patients with pancreatic cancer, participants received gemcitabine alone, Ukrain (NSC-631570) alone, or gemcitabine followed by Ukrain.[59] Survival rates after six months were reported to be 26, 65 and 74% for the gemcitabine, Ukrain, and gemcitabine plus Ukrain groups, respectively ($p < 0.01$ for gemcitabine plus Ukrain versus gemcitabine alone). A further study has assessed the effects of Ukrain in patients with hepatitis C virus infection.[60]

Side-effects, Toxicity

There is a limited amount of information relating to the safety and toxicity of preparations of *C. majus*.

Clinical data

Only limited data relating to safety aspects of *C. majus* are available from clinical trials. Such studies in any case are not designed primarily to assess safety, and generally have the statistical power only to detect common, acute adverse events.

A randomised, double-blind, placebo-controlled trial involving 60 patients with functional epigastric complaints who received tablets containing *C. majus* extract (comprising 66.0 to 167.2 mg native dry extract, equivalent to 4 mg total alkaloids, calculated as chelidonine), or placebo, at a dosage of two tablets three times daily for six weeks reported a similar number of adverse events for both groups (three and five for the *C. majus* preparation and placebo, respectively).[14] In another double-blind, placebo-controlled trial, no adverse events occurred in patients ($n = 39$) with upper abdominal pain due to biliary system dysfunction who received a preparation (Cholagogum F Nattermann) containing dry extracts of *C. majus* and *Curcuma longa* one capsule (standardised to contain 4 mg total alkaloids calculated as chelidonine) three times daily for three weeks.[52]

Hepatotoxicity Several case reports have described hepatotoxic effects, including severe hepatitis, severe cholestasis and fibrosis, associated with the use of preparations of *C. majus*.[61] One report describes ten cases of acute hepatitis in women who had ingested preparations containing *C. majus* extract for one to nine months before the onset of symptoms of hepatotoxicity.[62] In all ten cases, other common causes for hepatitis were excluded, and liver function test values before intake of *C. majus* were normal for the seven patients for whom these data were available. The ten cases concerned use of five different German manufacturers' preparations of *C. majus*, three of which formulations include only *C. majus* extract as the active component; such preparations are usually standardised for content of chelidonine. A mechanism for *C. majus* induced hepatotoxicity has not been established, although because of the apparent lack of a dose-dependent effect and variable latent period in the reported cases, an idiosyncratic reaction may be the most plausible explanation.[62]

Two further cases describe a 39-year-old woman and a 69-year-old man who both presented with symptoms of acute hepatitis, including dark brown urine and jaundice; laboratory tests revealed that both patients had highly elevated liver function test values.[63] The woman had been taking a preparation containing *C. majus* for four weeks before the onset of symptoms, and the man had taken capsules containing C. *majus* (each capsule standardised for 4 mg chelidonine) and *Curcuma longa* for six weeks before symptom onset; other possible causes of hepatotoxicity were excluded. Both patients recovered after stopping treatment with C. *majus*.

The World Health Organization's Uppsala Monitoring Centre (WHO-UMC; Collaborating Centre for International Drug Monitoring) receives summary reports of suspected adverse drug reactions from national pharmacovigilance centres of over 70 countries worldwide, including the UK. At the end of June 2005, the WHO-UMC's Vigisearch database contained a total of 47 reports, describing a total of 147 adverse reactions, for products containing C. *majus* only as the active ingredient (*see* Table 1). All but one (Belgium) of these reports originated from Germany.[64]

The specific products (manufacturer) associated with the reactions were: Ardeycholan N (Ardeypharm), two reports; Chol 4000 (Lichtenstein), six reports; Chol Sabona (Sabona), two reports; Cholarist (Steiner), ten reports; Gallopas (Pascoe), four reports; Panchelidon (Kanoldt), eight reports; Panchelidon N (Boots Pharmaceuticals), ten reports; Siosol Febna (one report); celandine/chelidonium extract (specific product not stated), four reports. In seven cases, the patient concerned was taking other medicines, although C. *majus* extract was the sole suspected drug in five of these seven reports.

Six of the total number of reports provided information on dechallenge; in all six cases, the reaction(s) had abated on stopping C. *majus* extract. The outcomes for the 47 reports were stated as: died (one report); not recovered (six reports); recovered (ten reports); unknown (30 reports). (These data were obtained from the Vigisearch database held by the WHO Collaborating Centre for International Drug Monitoring, Uppsala, Sweden. The information is not homogeneous at least with respect to origin or likelihood that the pharmaceutical product caused the adverse reaction. Any information included in this report does not represent the opinion of the World Health Organization.)

In May 2003, the Complementary Medicines Evaluation Committee, which advises the Australian Government's Therapeutic Goods Administration, recommended that preparations of C. *majus* for oral administration should include on their label statements advising consumers to use such products only under the supervision of a healthcare professional, to seek advice from a healthcare professional before using the product if the potential user has a history of liver disease, and to stop using C. *majus* preparations if symptoms associated with liver disease occur.[65] Healthcare professionals who identify suspected adverse drug reactions associated with C. *majus* preparations should report these using the appropriate spontaneous reporting form.

Other reactions Contact dermatitis has been reported in a 64-year-old woman who had used C. *majus* juice externally to treat warts.[66] Within a few hours of applying the preparation, the woman experienced severe itching and erythema, with papules, at the application site. Six weeks later, the woman experienced the same symptoms after applying the juice to a facial wart. In both instances, the reaction resolved within a few days without treatment. Subsequently, the woman displayed positive reactions to patch testing with C. *majus* juice and to extracts of C. *majus* branch, stem and root at concentrations of 0.1, 1 and 10 mg/mL.[66] A case report describing this reaction does not state the source of the plant material and authentication and phytochemical analysis of the materials do not appear to have been undertaken.

Preclinical data

In vitro inhibition of rat liver alanine aminotransferase (ALT) has been described for the benzophenanthridine alkaloids sanguinarine and chelerythrine. Sanguinarine was a more powerful inhibitor than was chelerythrine (ID_{50} values: 3.4×10^{-6} mol/L and 4.0×10^{-6} mol/L, respectively).[67] In other experiments, sanguinarine, chelerythrine, berberine and coptisine inhibited oxygen uptake by

Table 1 Summary of spontaneous reports ($n = 47$) of adverse drug reactions associated with single-ingredient *Chelidonium majus* preparations held in the Vigisearch database of the World Health Organization's Uppsala Monitoring Centre for the period up to end of June 2005.[a, 64]

System organ class. **Adverse drug reaction name (number)**	**Total**
Central nervous system. Paraesthesia (1)	1
Foetal. Biliary atresia (1)	1
General. Asthenia (3); death (1); fatigue (2); malaise (1); necrosis ischaemic (1)	8
Gastrointestinal. Abdominal pain (4); diarrhoea (2); faeces, discoloured (3); mouth dry (1); nausea (6); pancreatitis (1); tongue oedema (1); vomiting (3)	21
Liver-biliary. Bilirubinaemia (11); cholelithiasis (1); gamma-GT increased (6); hepatic enzymes increased (13); hepatic failure (1); hepatic function abnormal (1); hepatitis (19); hepatitis, cholestatic (8); hepatitis, viral (1); hepatocellular damage (4); jaundice (16); SGOT increased (7); SGPT increased (7)	95
Metabolic. Cholinesterase decreased (1); LDH increased (2); phosphatase alkaline, increased (5)	8
Psychiatric. Anorexia (1); insomnia (1); nervousness (2)	4
Respiratory. Dyspnoea (1); larynx oedema (1)	2
Skin. Pruritus (3); skin discoloration (1)	4
Urinary. Urine abnormal (3)	3
Total number of adverse drug reactions	**147**

Key: GT = glutamyl transferase; LDH = lactate dehydrogenase; SGOT = serum glutamic-oxaloacetic transaminase (= aspartate transaminase/aspartate aminotransferase); SGPT = serum glutamate pyruvate transaminase (= alanine transaminase/alanine aminotransferase)

[a]Caveat statement. These data were obtained from the Vigisearch database held by the WHO Collaborating Centre for International Drug Monitoring, Uppsala, Sweden. The information is not homogeneous at least with respect to origin or likelihood that the pharmaceutical product caused the adverse reaction. Any information included in this report does not represent the opinion of the World Health Organization

C

mitochondria obtained from mouse liver, whereas chelidonine had virtually no effect.[68]

In a randomised controlled experiment, swine were fed sanguinarine and chelerythrine (isolated from *Macleya cordata* (Wild.), Papaveraceae) in their feed (mean daily intake 0.1 or 5 mg/kg body weight), or a standard diet, for 90 days (n = 3 per group).[15] At the 30-, 60- and 90-day assessments, there were no statistically significant differences between the alkaloid-fed groups and the control group with respect to the following haematological and biochemical parameters: haemoglobin, haematocrit, erythrocyte and leukocyte counts, total protein, albumin, glucose, cholesterol, triacylglycerols, creatinine, urea, total bilirubin and alkaline phosphatase (ALP). However, at day 90, statistically significant differences were observed for ALT, aspartate aminotransferase (AST) and gamma-glutamyl transferase (GGT) for the higher alkaloid intake group, compared with control and, for GGT, for the lower alkaloid intake group ($p <$ 0.05 for all).[15]

There are conflicting results regarding possible cytotoxicity of *C. majus* preparations (*see* Pharmacological Actions, *In-vitro* and animal studies, Anticancer activity). Sanguinarine–intercalates with DNA.[26]

Contra-indications, Warnings

Greater celandine is contraindicated in patients with biliary obstructions, existing or previous liver disease.[G76] In view of the evidence of hepatotoxicity, use of *C. majus* extracts at dosages higher than those recommended (*see* Dosage) and/or for longer periods should be avoided. Monitoring of liver enzyme activity is recommended for patients using *C. majus* preparations for longer than four weeks.[G76]

Drug interactions No interactions have been documented for *C. majus*. However, in view of the documented pharmacological effects, whether or not there is potential for clinically important interactions with other medicines with similar or opposing effects and used concurrently should be considered.

Pregnancy and lactation The safety of *C. majus* has not been established. In view of the lack of information on the use of *C. majus* during pregnancy and lactation, its use should be avoided during these periods.

References

1 Medicines Act 1968, Statutory Instrument 1977 No. 2130 (Retail Sale or Supply of Herbal Remedies) Order, 1977.
2 Hahn R, Nahrstedt A. Hydroxycinnamic acid derivatives, caffeoylmalic and new caffeoylaldonic acid esters, from *Chelidonium majus*. *Planta Med* 1993; 59: 71–75.
3 De Rosa S, Di Vincenzo G. Isochelidonine, a benzophenanthridine alkaloid from *Chelidonium majus*. *Phytochemistry* 1992; 31: 1085–1086.
4 Rogelj B *et al*. Chelidocystatin, a novel phytocystatin from *Chelidonium majus*. *Phytochemistry* 1998; 49: 1645–1649.
5 Kim HK *et al*. Biological and phytochemical evaluation of plants. V: isolation of two cytotoxic alkaloids from *Chelidonium majus*. *J Pharm Sci* 1969; 58: 372–374.
6 Chang H-M, But PP-H (eds). Pharmacology and applications of Chinese materia medica. Volume 1. Singapore: World Scientific Publishing Co, 1986.
7 Fik E *et al*. New plant glycoprotein against methicillin resistant Staphylococci and Enterococci. *Acta Microbiologica Polonica* 1997; 46: 325–327.
8 Fik E *et al*. Isolation and characterisation of glycoproteins from milky juice levaes [sic] and roots of *Chelidonium maius* [sic] L. *Herba Pol* 1995; 41: 84–95.
9 Fik E *et al*. Comparative biochemical analysis of lectin and nuclease from *Chelidonium majus* L. *Acta Biochim Pol* 2000; 47: 413–420.
10 Kadan G *et al*. (−)-Turkiyenine, a new alkaloid from *Chelidonium majus*. *J Nat Prod* 1990; 53: 531–532.
11 Kadan G *et al*. (+)-Norchelidonine from *Chelidonium majus*. *Planta Med* 1992; 58: 477.
12 Colombo ML, Bosisio E. Pharmacological activities of *Chelidonium majus* L. (Papaveraceae). *Pharm Res* 1996; 33: 127–134.
13 Tome F, Colombo ML. Distribution of alkaloids in *Chelidonium majus* and factors affecting their accumulation. *Phytochemistry* 1995; 40: 37–39.
14 Ritter R *et al*. Clinical trial on standardised celandine extract in patients with functional epigastric complaints: results of a placebo-controlled double-blind trial. *Complement Ther Med* 1993; 1: 189–193.
15 Kosina P *et al*. Sanguinarine and chelerythrine: assessment of safety on pigs in ninety days feeding experiment. *Food Chem Tox* 2004; 42: 85–91.
16 Boegge S *et al*. Reduction of ACh-induced contraction of rat isolated ileum by coptisine, (+)-caffeoylmalic acid, *Chelidonium majus*, and *Corydalis lutea* extracts. *Planta Med* 1996; 62: 173–174.
17 Hiller K-O *et al*. Antispasmodic and relaxant activity of chelidonine, protopine, coptisine, and *Chelidonium majus* extracts on isolated guinea-pig ileum. *Planta Med* 1998; 64: 758–760.
18 Häberlein H *et al*. *Chelidonium majus* L.: components with *in vitro* affinity for the $GABA_A$ receptor. Positive cooperation of alkaloids. *Planta Med* 1996; 62: 227–231.
19 Kardos J *et al*. Enhancement of γ-aminobutyric acid receptor binding by protopine-type alkaloids. *Arzneim Forsch/Drug Res* 1986; 36(I): 939–940.
20 Kim Y *et al*. Modulation of *Chelidonii herba* on GABA activated chloride current in rat PAG neurons. *Am J Chin Med* 2001; 29: 265–279.
21 Shin M-C *et al*. Modulation of *Chelidonii herba* on glycine-activated and glutamate-activated ion currents in rat periaqueductal gray neurons. *Clin Chim Acta* 2002; 337: 93–101.
22 Vahlensieck U *et al*. The effect of *Chelidonium majus* herb extract on choleresis in the isolated perfused rat liver. *Planta Med* 1995; 61: 267–271.
23 Kim DJ *et al*. Potential preventive effects of *Chelidonium majis* [sic] L. (Papaveraceae) herb extract on glandular stomach tumor development in rats treated with *N*-methyl-*N*'-nitro-*N*-nitrosoguanidine (MNNG) and hypertonic sodium chloride. *Cancer Lett* 1997; 112: 203–208.
24 Kim HK *et al*. Biological and phytochemical evaluation of plants V: isolation of two cytotoxic alkaloids from *Chelidonium majus*. *J Pharm Sci* 1969; 58: 372–374.
25 Song J-Y *et al*. Immunomodulatory activity of protein-bound polysaccharide extracted from *Chelidonium majus*. *Arch Pharm Res* 2002; 25: 158–164.
26 Smékal E *et al*. Interaction of benzophenanthridine alkaloid sanguinarine with DNA. *Stud Biophys* 1984; 101: 125–132.
27 Smékal E, Kubova N. Alkaloids of protoberberine and benzophenanthridine groups as intercalating drugs with DNA. *Stud Biophys* 1984; 101: 121–123.
28 Vavrečková C *et al*. Benzophenanthridine alkaloids of *Chelidonium majus*: II. Potent inhibitory action against the growth of human keratinocytes. *Planta Med* 1996; 62: 491–494.
29 Bruller W. Studies concerning the effect of Ukrain in vivo and in vitro. *Drugs Exp Clin Res* 1992; 18 (Suppl. Suppl.): 13–16.
30 Panzer A *et al*. Chemical analyses of Ukrain™, a semi-synthetic *Chelidonium majus* alkaloid derivative, fail to confirm its trimeric structure. *Cancer Lett* 2000; 160: 237–241.
31 Jagiello-Wójtowicz E *et al*. Ukrain (NSC-631570) in experimental and clinical studies: a review. *Drugs Exp Clin Res* 1998; 14: 213–219.
32 Roublevskaia IN *et al*. Induced G2/M arrest and apoptosis in human epidermoid carcinoma cell lines by semisynthetic drug Ukrain. *Anticancer Res* 2000; 20: 3163–3168.
33 Cordes N *et al*. Ukrain®, an alkaloid thiophosphoric acid derivative of *Chelidonium majus* L. protects human fibroblasts but not human tumour cells in vitro against ionizing radiation. *Int J Radiat Biol* 2002; 78: 17–27.

C

34 Boyko VN *et al.* Action of Ukrain, a cytostatic and immunomodulating drug, on effects of irradiation. *Drugs Exp Clin Res* 1996; 22: 167–171.
35 Jabłoński M. Ukrain (NSC-631570) influences on bone status: a review. *Drugs Exp Clin Res* 2000; 26: 317–320.
36 Panzer A *et al.* Ukrain™, a semisynthetic *Chelidonium majus* alkaloid derivative, acts by inhibition of tubulin polymerization in normal and malignant cells. *Cancer Lett* 2000; 160: 149–157.
37 Panzer A *et al.* The antimitotic effects of Ukrain™, A *Chelidonium majus* alkaloid derivative, are reversible in vitro. *Cancer Lett* 2000; 150: 85–92.
38 Song J-Y *et al.* Radiation protective effect of an extract from *Chelidonium majus. Int J Hematol* 2003; 78: 226–232.
39 Chung H-S *et al.* Water extract isolated from *Chelidonium majus* enhances nitric oxide and tumour necrosis factor-α production via nuclear factor-κB activation in mouse peritoneal macrophages. *J Pharm Pharmacol* 2004; 56: 129–134.
40 Lenfeld J *et al.* Antiinflammatory activity of quaternary benzophenanthridine alkaloids from *Chelidonium majus. Planta Med* 1981; 43: 161–165.
41 Vavrečková C *et al.* Benzophenanthridine alkaloids of *Chelidonium majus*: I. Inhibition of 5- and 12-lipoxygenase by a non-redox mechanism. *Planta Med* 1996; 62: 397–401.
42 Kokoska L *et al.* Screening of some Siberian medicinal plants for antimicrobial activity. *J Ethnopharmacol* 2002; 82: 51–53.
43 Odebiyi OO, Sofowara EA. Antimicrobial alkaloids from a Nigerian chewing stick (*Fagara zanthoxyloides*). *Planta Med* 1979; 36: 204–207.
44 Matos OC *et al.* Sensitivity of *Fusarium* strains to *Chelidonium majus* L. extracts. *J Ethnopharmacol* 1999; 66: 151–158.
45 Ma WG *et al.* Fungitoxic alkaloids from Hokkaido Papaveraceae. *Fitoterapia* 2000; 71: 527–534.
46 Vukušić I *et al.* Investigation of the antimycotic activities of *Chelidonium majus* extract. *Planta Med* 1991; 57 (Suppl. Suppl.2): 1459.
47 Kéry A *et al.* Antiviral alkaloid in *Chelidonium majus* L. *Acta Pharm Hung* 1987; 57: 19–25.
48 Tan GT *et al.* Evaluation of natural products as inhibitors of human immunodeficiency virus type 1 (HIV-1) reverse transcriptase. *J Nat Prod* 1991; 54: 143–154.
49 Khayyal MT *et al.* Antiulcerogenic effect of some gastrointestinally acting plant extracts and their combination. *Arzneim-Forsch/Drug Res* 2001; 51: 545–553.
50 Then M *et al.* Examination on antioxidant activity in the greater celandine (*Chelidonium majus* L.) extracts by FRAP method. *Acta Biol Szegediensis* 2003; 47: 115–117.
51 Madisch A *et al.* Ein Phytotherapeutikum und seine modifizierte Rezeptur bei funktioneller Dyspepsie. Ergebnisse einer doppelblinden plazebokontrollierten Vergleichstudie. *Z Gastroenterol* 2001; 39: 511–517.
52 Niederau C, Göpfert E. Die Wirkung von Schöllkraut- und Curcumawurzelstock-Extrakt auf Oberbauch-beschwerden infolge funktioneller Störungen des ableitenden Gallensystems. Ergebnisse einer plazebokontrollierten Doppelblindstudie. *Med Klinik* 1999; 94: 425–430.
53 Staniszewski A *et al.* Lymphocyte subsets in patient with lung cancer treated with thiophosphoric acid alkaloid derivatives from *Chelidonium majus* L. (Ukrain). *Drugs Exptl Clin Res* 1992; 18 (Suppl. Suppl.): 63–67.
54 Nowicky JW *et al.* Evaluation of thiophosphoric acid alkaloid derivatives from *Chelidonium majus* L. ("Ukrain") an an immunostimulant in patients with various carcinomas. *Drugs Exptl Clin Res* 1991; 17: 139–143.
55 Voltchek IV *et al.* Potential therapeutic efficacy of Ukrain (NSC 631570) in AIDS patients with Kaposi's sarcoma. *Drugs Exptl Clin Res* 1996; 22: 283–286.
56 Nowicky JW *et al.* Ukrain both as an anticancer and immunoregulatory agent. *Drugs Exptl Clin Res* 1992; 18 (Suppl. Suppl.): 51–54.
57 Zahriychuk O. Ukrain, a thiophosphoric acid derivative of alkaloids of *Chelidonium majus* L., is effective in the treatment of recurrent bronchopulmonary pathology in children from areas contaminated after the Chernobyl accident. *Int J Immunotherapy* 2003; 19: 47–53.
58 Ernst E, Schmidt K. Ukrain – a new cancer cure? A systematic review of randomised clinical trials. *BMC Cancer* 2005; 5: 69.
59 Gansuage F *et al.* NSC-631570 (Ukrain) in the palliative treatment of pancreatic cancer. Results of a phase II trial. *Langenbeck's Arch Surg* 2002; 386: 570–574.
60 Sologub TV *et al.* Efficacy and safety of the drug Ukrain in chronic hepatits C patients. *Int J Immunother* 2003; 19: 55–59.
61 De Smet PAGM. Safety concerns about kava not unique. *Lancet* 2002; 360: 1336.
62 Benninger J *et al.* Acute hepatitis induced by Greater Celandine (*Chelidonium majus*). *Gastroenterology* 1999; 117: 1234–1237.
63 Stickel F *et al.* Acute hepatitis induced by Greater Celandine (*Chelidonium majus*). *Scand J Gastroenterol* 2003; 5: 565–568.
64 Vigibase, WHO Adverse Reactions database, Uppsala Monitoring Centre (accessed June 27, 2005).
65 Therapeutic Goods Administration. Greater celandine (*Chelidonium majus*). Proposed labelling advisory statement for the herb greater celandine (*Chelidonium majus*). http://www.tga.gov.au/docs/html/celandine.htm (accessed 29 June 2005).
66 Etxenagusia MA *et al.* Contact dermatitis from *Chelidonium majus* (greater celandine). *Contact Dermatitis* 2000; 43: 47.
67 Walterová D *et al.* Inhibition of liver alanine aminotransferase activity by some benzophenanthridine alkaloids. *J Med Chem* 1981; 24: 1100–1103.
68 Barreto MC *et al.* Inhibition of mouse liver respiration by *Chelidonium majus* isoquinoline alkaloids. *Tox Lett* 2003; 146: 37–47.

Celery

Summary and Pharmaceutical Comment

Celery fruit should not be confused with the commercial celery stem, which is commonly eaten as a food. The chemistry of celery fruit is well studied and the phototoxic furanocoumarin constituents are well documented. Phototoxicity appears to be associated with the handling of the celery stems, especially diseased plant material. Limited scientific evidence is available to justify the herbal uses of celery, although bacteriostatic activity has been documented for the oil. Celery fruit should be used cautiously in view of the documented allergic reactions.

Species (Family)

Apium graveolens L. (Apiaceae/Umbelliferae)

Synonym(s)

Apii Fructus, Celery Fruit, Celery Seed, Smallage, Wild Celery

Part(s) Used

Fruit

Pharmacopoeial and Other Monographs

BHC 1992[G6]
BHP 1996[G9]
Martindale 35th edition[G85]

Legal Category (Licensed Products)

GSL[G37]

Constituents

The following is compiled from several sources, including General References G2, G6, G48 and G58.

Flavonoids Apigenin, apiin, isoquercitrin and others.[1]

Coumarins Apigravin, apiumetin, apiumoside, bergapten, celerin, celereoside, isoimperatorin, isopimpinellin, osthenol, rutaretin, seselin, umbelliferone and 8-hydroxy-5-methoxypsoralen.[1–9]

Low concentrations (not exceeding 1.3 ppm) of furanocoumarins have been identified in commercial celery,[10] although concentrations are reported to rise considerably in diseased stems.[11]

Volatile oils 2–3%. Many components including limonene (60%) and selenine (10–15%), and various sesquiterpene alcohols (1–3%), e.g. α-eudesmol and β-eudesmol, santalol.[12,13] Phthalide compounds, 3-*n*-butyl phthalide and sedanenolide, provide the characteristic odour of the oil (presence of sedanolide and sedanonic anhydride disputed).[14,15]

Other constituents Choline ascorbate,[16] fatty acids (e.g linoleic, myristic, myristicic, myristoleic, oleic, palmitic, palmitoleic, petroselinic and stearic acids).

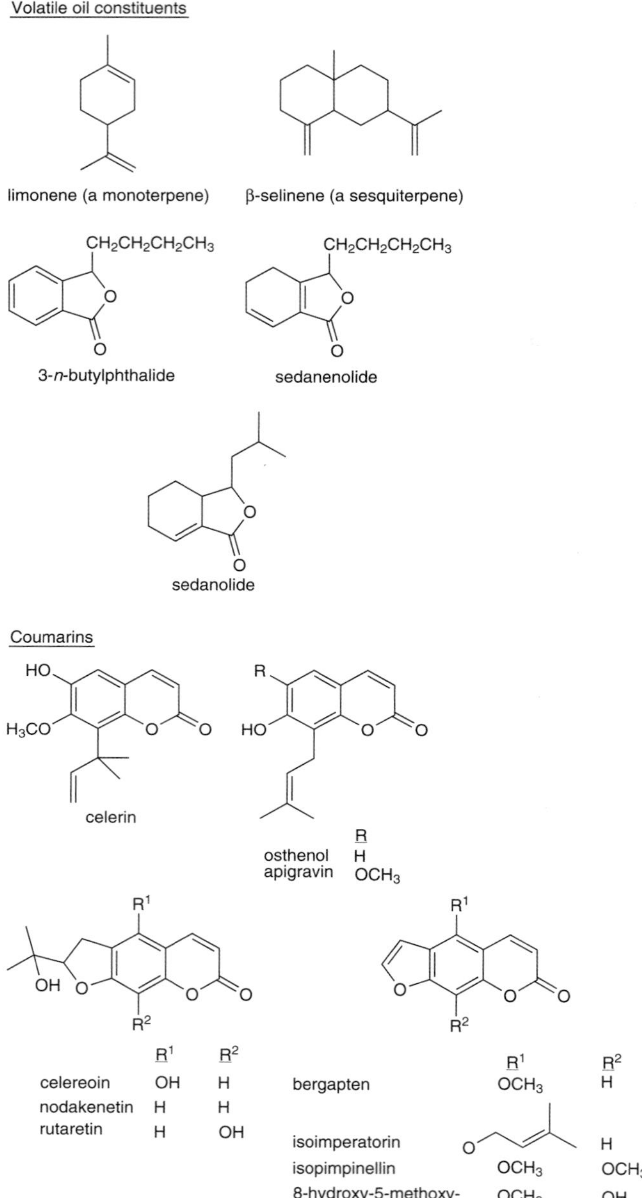

Figure 1 Selected constituents of celery.

Food Use

Celery is listed by the Council of Europe as a natural source of food flavouring (category N2). This category indicates that celery can be added to foodstuffs in small quantities, with a possible limitation of an active principle (as yet unspecified) in the final product.[G16] Celery stem (not the fruit) is commonly used in foods. Previously, celery seed has been listed as GRAS (Generally Recognised As Safe).[G41]

Herbal Use

Celery is stated to possess antirheumatic, sedative, mild diuretic and urinary antiseptic properties. It has been used for arthritis, rheumatism, gout, urinary tract inflammation, and specifically for rheumatoid arthritis with mental depression.[G2, G6, G7, G8, G64]

Dosage

Dosages for oral administration (adults) for traditional uses recommended in older standard herbal reference texts are given below.

Dried fruits 0.5–2.0 g as a decoction 1 : 5 three times daily.[G7]

Liquid extract 0.3–1.2 mL (1 : 1 in 60% alcohol) three times daily.[G7]

Liquid Extract of Celery (BPC 1934) 0.3–1.2 mL.

Pharmacological Actions

In vitro and animal studies

In mice, sedative and antispasmodic activities have been documented for the phthalide constituents.[17, G22] Celery seed oil has been reported to exhibit bacteriostatic activity against *Bacillus subtilis*, *Vibrio cholerae*, *Staphylococcus aureus*, *Staphylococcus albus*, *Shigella dysenteriae*, *Corynebacterium diphtheriae*, *Salmonella typhi*, *Streptococcus faecalis*, *Bacillus pumilus*, *Streptococcus pyogenes* and *Pseudomonas solanacearum*.[9] No activity was observed against *Escherichia coli*, *Sarcina lutea* or *Pseudomonas aeruginosa*.

Apigenin has exhibited potent antiplatelet activity *in vitro*, inhibiting the aggregation of rabbit platelets induced by collagen, ADP, arachidonic acid and platelet-activating factor (PAF), but not that induced by thrombin or ionophore A23187.[18]

Studies with celery plant extracts have demonstrated anti-inflammatory activity in the mouse ear test and against carrageenan-induced rat paw oedema,[19] and a hypotensive effect in rabbits and dogs after intravenous administration.[G41] In addition, hypoglycaemic activity has been documented.[G22]

Celery juice has been reported to exhibit choleretic activity and the phthalide constituents are stated to possess diuretic activity.[13]

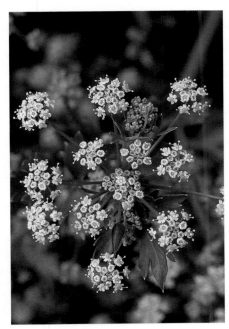

Figure 2 Celery (*Apium graveolens*).

Clinical studies

There is a lack of clinical research assessing the effects of celery fruit and rigorous randomised controlled clinical trials are required.

Side-effects, Toxicity

None documented. However, there is a lack of clinical safety and toxicity data for celery fruit and further investigation of these aspects is required.

Photosensitivity reactions have been reported as a result of external contact with celery stems.[20, 21, G51] These reactions have been attributed to the furanocoumarin constituents which are known to possess photosensitising properties.[11, 22] The concentrations of these compounds are reported to increase considerably in diseased celery stems.[11, 22] It is thought that psoralen, the most potent phototoxic furanocoumarin, acts as a transient precursor for other furanocoumarins and does not accumulate in celery.[5, 11]

Instances of allergic and anaphylactic reactions to celery have also been documented[23] following oral ingestion of the stems.[24] Celery allergy is reported to be mediated by IgE antibodies and an association between pollen and celery allergy has been postulated,

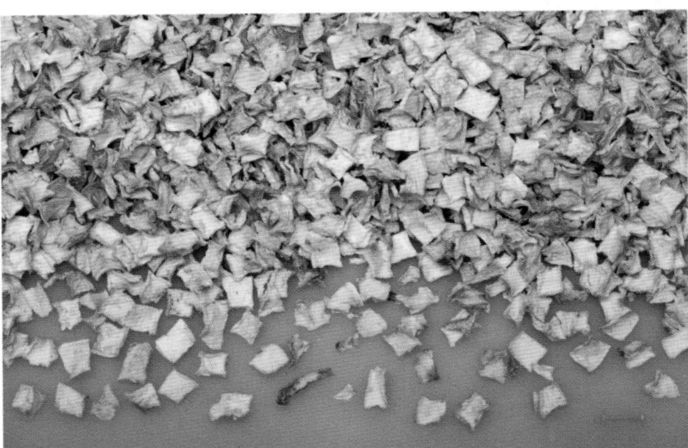

Figure 3 Celery – dried drug substance (root).

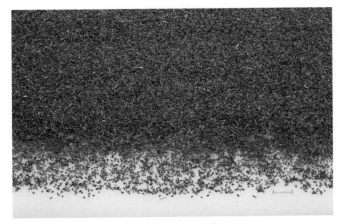

Figure 4 Celery – dried drug substance (fruit).

C

C

although the common antigen has not been determined.[25] Cross-sensitivities to celery have been documented in patients with existing allergies to dandelion and wild carrot.[G51]

Acute LD_{50} values (rats, by mouth; rabbits, dermal) have been reported as greater than 5 g/kg body weight.[26] Celery seed oil is stated to be non-irritant, non-phototoxic and non-sensitising in humans.[26, G58]

Contra-indications, Warnings

Celery fruit contains phototoxic compounds, furanocoumarins, which may cause photosensitive reactions. Celery fruit may precipitate allergic reactions, particularly in individuals with existing plant, pollen or food allergies. Diseased celery stems (indicated by a browning of the stem) should not be ingested.

Drug interactions None documented. However, the potential for preparations of celery to interact with other medicines administered concurrently, particularly those with similar or opposing effects, should be considered.

Pregnancy and lactation Celery fruit is reputed to affect the menstrual cycle and to be abortifacient.[G30] Uterine stimulant activity has been documented for the oil,[G22, G30] and the use of celery fruits is contra-indicated during pregnancy.[G49] This does not refer to celery stems that are commonly ingested as a food, although excessive consumption should be avoided. It is not known whether constituents of celery fruit appear in breast milk.

Preparations

Proprietary multi-ingredient preparations

Australia: Arthritic Pain Herbal Formula 1; Boswellia Complex; Devils Claw Plus; Fluid Loss; Guaiacum Complex; Lifesystem Herbal Formula 1 Arthritic Aid. *Canada:* Herbal Diuretic. *India:* Flexi-muv. *Malaysia:* Celery Plus. *UK:* Mixed Vegetable Tablets; Modern Herbals Rheumatic Pain; Napiers Backache Tea; Rheumatic Pain; Rheumatic Pain Tablets; Sciatica Tablets; Vegetex.

References

1 Garg SK *et al.* Glucosides of *Apium graveolens. Planta Med* 1980; 38: 363–365.

2 Garg SK *et al.* Apiumetin – a new furanocoumarin from the seeds of *Apium graveolens. Phytochemistry* 1978; 17: 2135–2136.

3 Garg SK *et al.* Celerin, a new coumarin from *Apium graveolens. Planta Med* 1980; 38: 186–188.

4 Garg SK *et al.* Minor phenolics of *Apium graveolens* seeds. *Phytochemistry* 1979; 18: 352.

5 Dall'Acqua *et al.* Biosynthesis of O-alkylfurocoumarins. *Planta Med* 1975; 27: 343–348.

6 Garg SK *et al.* Apiumoside, a new furanocoumarin glucoside from the seeds of *Apium graveolens. Phytochemistry* 1979; 18: 1764–1765.

7 Garg SK *et al.* Coumarins from *Apium graveolens* seeds. *Phytochemistry* 1979; 18: 1580–1581.

8 Innocenti G *et al.* Investigations of the content of furocoumarins in *Apium graveolens* and in *Petroselinum sativum. Planta Med* 1976; 29: 165–170.

9 Kar A, Jain SR. Investigations on the antibacterial activity of some Indian indigenous aromatic plants. *Flavour Industry* 1971; February.

10 Beier RC *et al.* Hplc analysis of linear furocoumarins (psoralens) in healthy celery (*Apium graveolens*). *Food Chem Toxicol* 1983; 21: 163–165.

11 Chaudhary SK *et al.* Increased furocoumarin content of celery during storage. *J Agric Food Chem* 1985; 33: 1153–1157.

12 Fehr D. Untersuchung über aromastoffe von sellerie (*Apium graveolens* L.). *Pharmazie* 1979; 34: 658–662.

13 Stahl E. *Drug Analysis by Chromatography and Microscopy.* Ann Arbor, Michigan: Ann Arbor Science, 1973.

14 Bjeldanes LF, Kim I-S. Phthalide components of celery essential oil. *J Org Chem* 1977; 42: 2333–2335.

15 Bos R *et al.* Composition of the volatile oils from the roots, leaves and fruits of different taxa of *Apium graveolens. Planta Med* 1986; 52: 531.

16 Kavalali G, Akcasu A. Isolation of choline ascorbate from *Apium graveolens. J Nat Prod* 1985; 48: 495.

17 Gijbels MJM *et al.* Phthalides in roots of *Apium graveolens, A. graveolens* var. *rapaceum.* Bifora testiculata and *Petroselinum crispum* var. *tuberosum. Fitoterapia* 1985; 56: 17–23.

18 Teng CM *et al.* Inhibition of platelet aggregation by apigenin from *Apium graveolens. Asia Pac J Pharmacol* 1988; 1: 85–89.

19 Lewis DA *et al.* The anti-inflammatory activity of celery *Apium graveolens* L. (Fam. Umbelliferae). *Int J Crude Drug Res* 1985; 23: 27–32.

20 Berkley SF *et al.* Dermatitis in grocery workers associated with high natural concentrations of furanocoumarins in celery. *Ann Intern Med* 1986; 105; 351–355.

21 Austad J, Kavli G. Phototoxic dermatitis caused by celery infected by *Sclerotinia sclerotiorum. Contact Dermatitis* 1983; 9: 448–451.

22 Ashwood-Smith MJ *et al.* Mechanisms of photosensitivity reactions to diseased celery. *BMJ* 1985; 290: 1249.

23 Déchamp C *et al.* Choc anaphylactique au céleri et sensibilisation à l'ambroisie et à l'armoise. Allergie croisée ou allergie concomitante? *Presse Med* 1984; 13: 871–874.

24 Forsbeck M, Ros A-M. Anaphylactoid reaction to celery. *Contact Dermatitis* 1979; 5: 191.

25 Pauli G *et al.* Celery sensitivity: clinical and immunological correlations with pollen allergy. *Clin Allergy* 1985; 15: 273–279.

26 Opdyke DLJ. Celery seed oil. *Food Cosmet Toxicol* 1974; 12: 849–850.

Centaury

Summary and Pharmaceutical Comment

There is little published information specifically concerning *Centaurium erythraea*. Bitter components support the traditional use of centaury as an appetite stimulant, although it is said to be less active than comparable bitter herbs, such as gentian. In view of the lack of pharmacological and toxicological data, excessive use should be avoided.

Species (Family)

Centaurium erythraea Rafn. (Gentianaceae)

Synonym(s)

Centaurium minus auct., *C. minus* auct. subsp. *minus*, *C. umbellatum* Gilib., Common Centaury, *Erythraea centaurium* (L.) Pers. subsp. *centaurium*

Part(s) Used

Herb

Pharmacopoeial and Other Monographs

BHP 1996[G9]
BP 2007[G84]
Complete German Commission E[G3]
ESCOP 2003[G76]
Martindale 35th edition[G85]
Ph Eur 2007[G81]

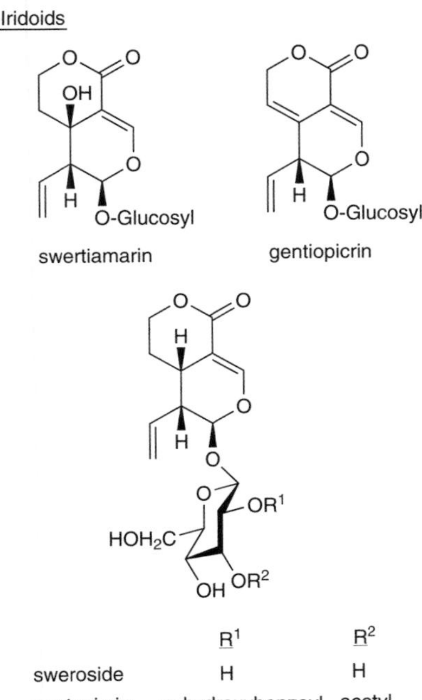

Figure 1 Selected constituents of centaury.

Legal Category (Licensed Products)

GSL[G37]

Constituents

The following is compiled from several sources, including General Reference G2.

Acids Phenolic. Protocatechuic, *m*- and *p*-hydroxybenzoic, vanillic, syringic, *p*-coumaric, ferulic, sinapic and caffeic, hydroxyterephthalic and 2,5-dihydroxyterephthalic acids among others.

Alkaloids Pyridine-type. Traces of gentianine, gentianidine, gentioflavine and others.

Monoterpenoids Iridoids (bitters).[1,2] Gentiopicroside (about 2%) as major, others include centapicrin, gentioflavoside, sweroside and swertiamarin; intensely bitter *m*-hydroxybenzoylesters of sweroside and catapicrin.

Triterpenoids Includes α- and β-amyrin, erythrodiol, crataegolic acid, oleanolic acid and sitosterol.

Xanthones Highly methylated xanthones, including eustomin and 8-demethyleustomin.

Other constituents Flavonoids, fatty acids, alkanes and waxes.

Food Use

Centaury is listed by the Council of Europe as a natural source of food flavouring (category N2). This category indicates that centaury can be added to foodstuffs in small quantities, with a possible limitation of an active principle (as yet unspecified) in the final product.[G16] Previously, the bitter properties of centaury were utilised in alcoholic and non-alcoholic beverages with maximum permitted doses between 0.0002% and 0.0008%.[G41]

Herbal Use

Centaury is reputed to act as a bitter, aromatic and stomachic. Traditionally, it has been used for anorexia and dyspepsia.[G2, G7, G52]

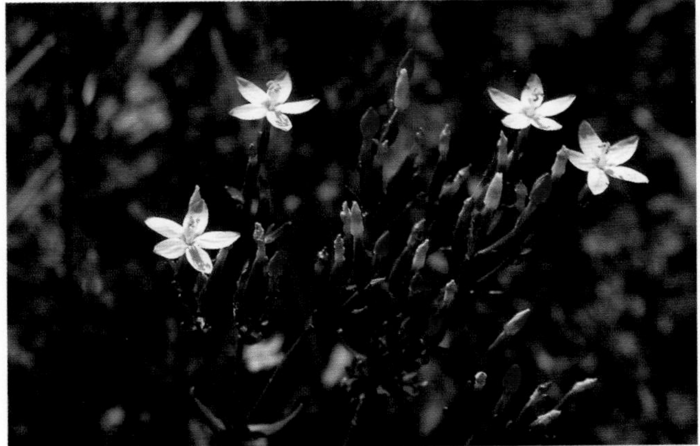

Figure 2 Centaury (*Centaurium erythraea*).

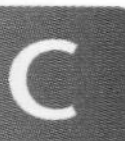

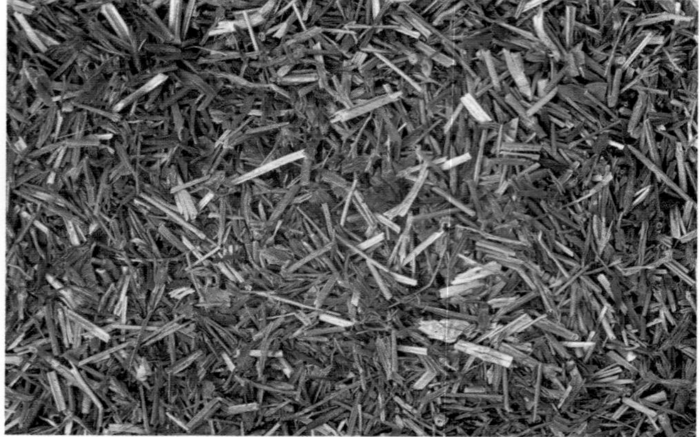

Figure 3 Centaury – dried drug substance (herb).

Dosage

Dosages for oral administration (adults) for traditional uses recommended in standard herbal reference texts are given below.

Herb 2–4 g as an infusion three times daily.(G7)

Liquid extract 2–4 mL (1 : 1 in 25% alcohol) three times daily.(G7)

Pharmacological Actions

In vitro and animal studies

Anti-inflammatory activity has been documented in two rat models; subchronic inflammation (air pouch granuloma and polyarthritis) test,[3] and the carrageenan rat paw oedema test (19% compared to 45% with indometacin).[4] Antipyretic activity has also been exhibited by a centaury extract against experimentally induced hyperthermia in rats, although pretreatment with the extract did not prevent hyperthermia;[3] antipyretic activity is stated to be due to the phenolic acid constituents.(G45) In the same study, no analgesic activity could be demonstrated in mice (writhing syndrome and hotplate models).[3] Gentiopicroside (30 mg/kg/day intraperitoneally) inhibited tumour necrosis factor (TNF) production in carbon tetrachloride-induced and bacillus Calmette–Guérin/lipopolysaccharide-induced models of hepatic injury in mice.(G52)

In rats, anticholinesterase activity has been demonstrated for swertiamarin in a dose-dependent manner following oral administration, demonstrated by inhibition of carbachol-induced contraction of proximal colon.(G52) In mice, gentianine has central nervous system (CNS)-depressant activity at oral doses of 30 mg/kg, demonstrated by inhibition of spontaneous movement and prolonged hexobarbital-induced sleeping time.(G52) Anti-ulcerogenic and inhibitory gastric secretion in rats (100 mg/kg) have been shown for gentianine.(G52)

Clinical studies

There is a lack of clinical research assessing the effects of centaury and rigorous randomised controlled clinical trials are required.

Side-effects, Toxicity

There is a lack of clinical safety and toxicity data for centaury and further investigation of these aspects is required.

An alcoholic extract of centaury (200 mL/plate) was antimutagenic in *Salmonella typhimurium* strains TA8 and TA100.(G52)

Contra-indications, Warnings

Centaury is contra-indicated for individuals with peptic ulcers.(G52)

Drug interactions None documented. However, the potential for preparations of centaury to interact with other medicines administered concurrently, particularly those with similar or opposing effects, should be considered.

Pregnancy and lactation The safety of centaury taken during pregnancy has not been established. In view of the lack of toxicity data, use of centaury during pregnancy and lactation should be avoided.

Preparations

Proprietary single-ingredient preparations

Czech Republic: Nat Zemezluce.

Proprietary multi-ingredient preparations

Austria: Montana N; China-Eisenwein; Eryval; Magentee St Severin; Mariazeller. *Czech Republic:* Naturland Grosser Swedenbitter; Stomaran. *France:* Diacure; Tisane Hepatique de Hoerdt. *Germany:* Amara-Tropfen; Canephron; Stullmaton. *Russia:* Canephron N (*Канефрон Н*); Herbion Drops for the Stomach (*Гербион Желудочные Капли*); Original Grosser Bittner Balsam (*Оригинальный Большой Бальзам Биттнера*). *South Africa:* Amara; Clairo. *Spain:* Natusor Hepavesical; Odisor. *Switzerland:* Gastrosan; Tisane pour l'estomac.

References

1 Van der Sluis WG, Labadie RP. Onderzok naar en van secoiridoid glucosiden en zanthonen in het gescglacht *Centaurium*. *Pharm Weekbl* 1978; 113: 21–32.

2 Van der Sluis WG, Labadie RP. Secoiridoids and xanthones in the genus *Centaurium*. Part 3. Decentapicrins A, B and C, new *m*-hydroxybenzoyl esters of sweroside from *Centaurium littorale*. *Planta Med* 1981; 41: 150–160.

3 Berkan T *et al*. Antiinflammatory, analgesic, and antipyretic effects of an aqueous extract of *Erythraea centaurium*. *Planta Med* 1991; 57: 34–37.

4 Mascolo N *et al*. Biological screening of Italian medicinal plants for anti-inflammatory activity. *Phytother Res* 1987; 1: 28–31.

Cereus

C

Summary and Pharmaceutical Comment

Little phytochemical or pharmacological information has been documented for cereus, although the presence of tyramine, a cardiotonic amine, may support the traditional use of cereus as a cardiac stimulant. Cardiac complaints are not considered to be suitable for self-medication.

Species (Family)

Selenicereus grandiflorus (L.) Britt. & Rose (Cactaceae)

Synonym(s)

Cactus grandiflorus L., *Cereus grandiflorus* (L.) Mill., Night Blooming Cereus

Part(s) Used

Stem

Pharmacopoeial and Other Monographs

Martindale 35th edition[G85]

Legal Category (Licensed Products)

Cereus is not included in the GSL.[G37]

Constituents

The following is compiled from several sources, including General References G22 and G40.

Alkaloids Isoquinoline-type. Unidentified alkaloids.[1]

Amines Tyramine[2], hordenine,[3] previously referred to as cactine.

Flavonoids Rutin, kaempferitrin, hyperoside, isorhamnetin-3-β-(galactosyl)-rutinoside.

Other constituents Resin

Food Use

Cereus is not used in foods.

Herbal Use

Cereus is reputed to act as a cardiac stimulant and as a partial substitute for digitalis, although there is no proof of its therapeutic value. Cereus has been used in cases of dropsy and various cardiac disorders.[G10, G64]

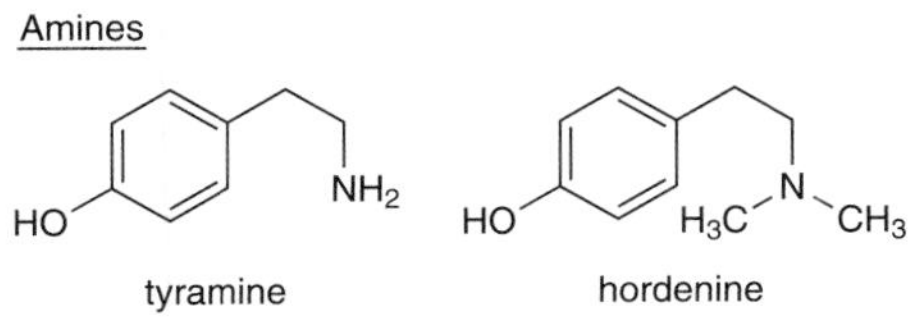

Amines

tyramine

hordenine

Figure 1 Selected constituents of cereus.

Dosage

Dosages for oral administration (adults) for traditional uses recommended in older standard reference texts are given below.

Liquid extract of cereus (BPC 1934) 0.06–0.6 mL.

Tincture of cereus (BPC 1934) 0.12–2.0 mL.

Pharmacological Actions

In vitro and animal studies

None documented for cereus. Cereus is reported to contain a cardiotonic amine, tyramine, which has positive inotropic activity.

Clinical studies

There is a lack of clinical research assessing the effects of cereus and rigorous randomised controlled clinical trials are required.

Side-effects, Toxicity

There is a lack of clinical safety data and toxicity data for cereus and further investigation of these aspects is required.

The fresh juice of cereus is irritant to the oral mucosa, causing a burning sensation, nausea and vomiting. Diarrhoea has also been reported following cereus consumption.[G22]

Contra-indications, Warnings

Cereus is stated to contain tyramine;[2] on this basis, whether or not it is appropriate for use by patients with cardiac disorders should be considered.

Drug interactions None documented. However, the potential for preparations of cereus to interact with other medicines administered concurrently, particularly those with similar or opposing effects, should be considered. Cereus is stated to contain tyramine;[2] until further information is available, its use in patients receiving monoamine oxidase inhibitors should be avoided.

Pregnancy and lactation The safety of cereus has not been established. In view of the limited information available on cereus, its use during pregnancy and lactation should be avoided.

References

1. Brown SD *et al*. Cactus alkaloids. *Phytochemistry* 1968; 7: 2031–2036.
2. Wagner H, Grevel J. Neue herzwirksame drogen II, nachweis und isolierung herzwirksamer amine durch ionenpaar-HPLC. *Planta Med* 1982; 44: 36–40.
3. Petershofer-Halbmayer H *et al*. Isolierung von Hordenin (Cactin) aus *Selenicereus grandiflorus* (L.) Britt. & Rose und *Selenicereus pteranthus* (Link & Otto) Britt. & Rose. *Sci Pharm* 1982; 50: 29–34.

Chamomile, German

Summary and Pharmaceutical Comment

The chemistry of German chamomile, especially of the volatile oil component, is well documented and is similar to that of Roman chamomile. Pharmacological activity is associated with the flavonoid and volatile oil fractions. A range of pharmacological actions has been documented (e.g. anti-inflammatory and antispasmodic activities) and many of these support the reputed herbal uses. Rigorous clinical research assessing the effects of German chamomile is limited, and randomised controlled clinical trials are required to establish the reported anti-inflammatory, wound-healing and sedative effects. Toxicity studies to date have indicated chamomile to be of low toxicity, although allergic reactions are documented.

Species (Family)

Matricaria recutita L. (Asteraceae/Compositae)

Synonym(s)

Chamomilla recutita (L.) Rauschert, Hungarian Chamomile, Matricaria Flowers, Scented Mayweed, Sweet False Chamomile, Wild Chamomile

Part(s) Used

Flowerhead

Pharmacopoeial and Other Monographs

BHC 1992[G6]
BHP 1996[G9]
BP 2007 (Matricaria Flower)[G84]
Complete German Commission E [G3]
ESCOP 2003[G76]
Martindale 35th edition[G85]
Ph Eur 2007 (Matricaria Flower)[G81]
USP29/NF24[G86]
WHO volume 1 1999[G63]

Legal Category (Licensed Products)

GSL[G37]

Constituents

The following is compiled from several sources, including General References G2, G6 and G52.

Coumarins Umbelliferone and its methyl ether, heniarin.

Flavonoids Apigenin, apigetrin, apiin, luteolin, quercetin, quercimeritrin and rutin.

Volatile oils 0.24–1.9%. Pharmacopoeial standard not less than 4 mg/kg blue oil.[G84] Main components are (−)-α-bisabolol (up to 50%)[1] and chamazulene (1–15%).[2] Others include (−)-α-bisabolol oxide A and B, (−)-α-bisabolone oxide A, spiroethers (e.g. *cis*- and *trans*-en-yn-dicycloether), sesquiterpenes (e.g. anthecotulid), cadinene, farnesene, furfural, spathulenol and proazulenes (e.g. matricarin and matricin).

Chamazulene is formed from matricin during steam distillation of the oil. It varies in yield depending on the origin and age of the flowers.[2]

Other constituents Amino acids, anthemic acid (bitter), choline, polysaccharide, plant and fatty acids, tannin and triterpene hydrocarbons (e.g. triacontane).

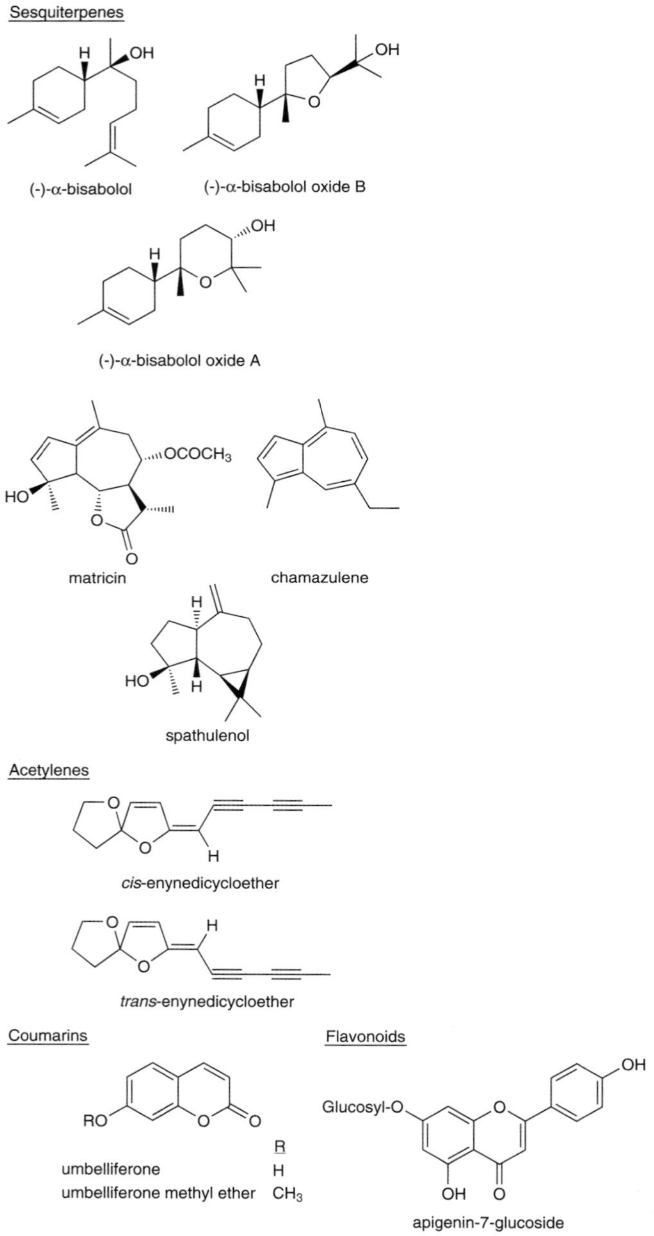

Sesquiterpenes

(-)-α-bisabolol

(-)-α-bisabolol oxide B

(-)-α-bisabolol oxide A

matricin

chamazulene

spathulenol

Acetylenes

cis-enynedicycloether

trans-enynedicycloether

Coumarins

	R
umbelliferone	H
umbelliferone methyl ether	CH_3

Flavonoids

apigenin-7-glucoside

Figure 1 Selected constituents of German chamomile.

Food Use

German chamomile is listed by the Council of Europe as a natural source of food flavouring (category N2). This category indicates that chamomile can be added to foodstuffs in small quantities, with a possible limitation of an active principle (as yet unspecified) in the final product.[G16] German chamomile is commonly used in herbal teas. Previously, German chamomile has been listed as GRAS (Generally Recognised As Safe).[G41]

Herbal Use

German chamomile is stated to possess carminative, antispasmodic, mild sedative, anti-inflammatory, antiseptic and anticatarrhal properties.[G2, G4, G6, G7, G8, G43, G52, G64] It has been used for flatulent nervous dyspepsia, travel sickness, nasal catarrh, nervous diarrhoea, restlessness and specifically for gastrointestinal disturbance with associated nervous irritability in children. It has been used topically for haemorrhoids, mastitis and leg ulcers. German Commission E approved use for gastrointestinal spasms and inflammatory diseases of the gastrointestinal tract and externally for skin and mucous membrane inflammation and bacterial skin diseases including oral cavity and gums. It is also approved for inflammations and irritations of the respiratory tract (by inhalation) and ano-genital inflammation (baths and irrigation).[G3]

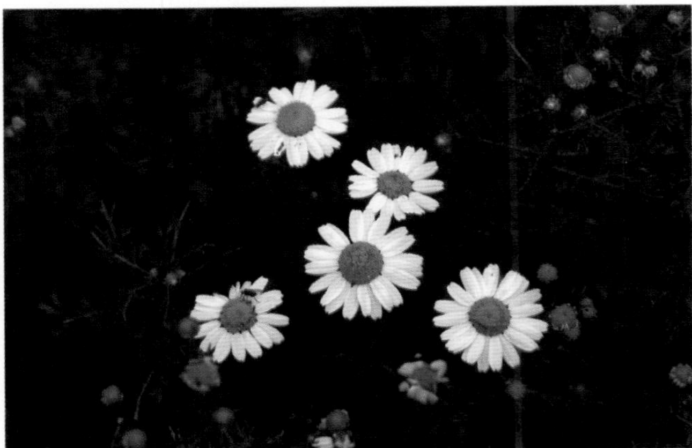

Figure 2 German chamomile (*Matricaria recutita*).

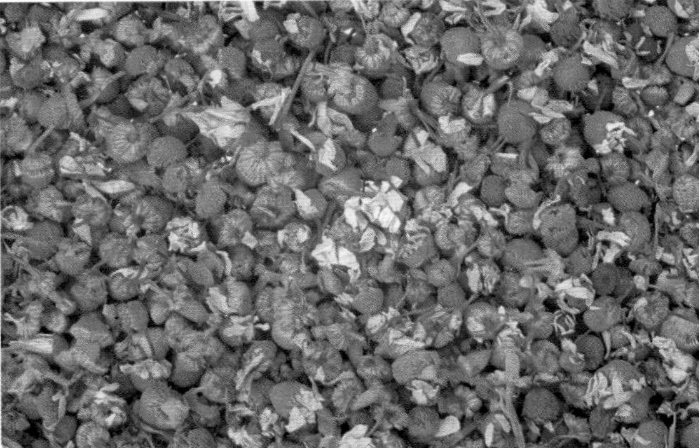

Figure 3 German chamomile – dried drug substance (flowerhead).

Dosage

Dosages for oral administration (adults) for traditional uses recommended in standard herbal reference texts are given below.

Dried flowerheads 2–8 g as an infusion three times daily.[G7]

Liquid extract 1–4 mL (1 : 1 in 45% alcohol) three times daily.[G7]

Pharmacological Actions

In vitro and animal studies

A wide range of pharmacological activities has been documented for German chamomile, including antibacterial, anti-inflammatory, antispasmodic, anti-ulcer, antiviral and hypo-uraemic activities.

Anti-inflammatory and anti-allergic activity Anti-allergic and anti-inflammatory activities[2, 3] are well documented for German chamomile. The azulene components of the volatile oil are thought to contribute by inhibiting histamine release and they have been reported to prevent allergic seizures in guinea-pigs.[2] Aqueous alcoholic extracts inhibited 5-lipoxygenase and cyclooxygenase activity, and oxidation of arachidonic acid, and a supercritical carbon dioxide extract had IC_{50} values of 6–25 μg/mL for these three activities.[G52] The active compounds identified included apigenin, chamazulene, *cis*-en-yn spiroether and (−)-α-bisabolol.[G52] Matricin, the precursor to chamazulene, is reported to be a more effective anti-inflammatory agent than chamazulene.[2, 4] Anti-inflammatory activity has also been documented for the sesquiterpene bisabolol compounds, with greatest activity reported for (−)-α-bisabolol,[2, 5] and for *cis*-spiroether.[2] Anti-inflammatory activity (rat paw carrageenan test) has also been documented for a *cis*-spiroether against dextran induced oedema; no activity was observed against oedema induced by serotonin, histamine or bradykinin.[6] In addition, flavonoids are known to possess anti-inflammatory activity.

Sedative activity Apigenin competitively inhibited binding of flunitrazepam to the central benzodiazepine receptor, but lacked activity at other receptors, including muscarinic, α_1-adrenoreceptor and $GABA_A$.[G52] High-performance liquid chromatography (HPLC) fractions of a methanol extract displaced flunitrazepam from its receptors in rat cerebellum membranes and muscimol from GABA receptors in rat cortical membranes, due to the presence of GABA in the fractions. Prolongation of hexobarbital-induced sleeping time and reduction in activity of mice have been documented.[G52]

Anti-ulcerogenic activity Anti-ulcerogenic activity in rats has been reported for (−)-α-bisabolol; the development of ulcers induced by indometacin, stress or ethanol was inhibited.[2, 7]

Antimicrobial and antiviral activities German chamomile oil has been reported to have antifungal activity and antibacterial activity against Gram-positive bacteria.[G52] The coumarin herniarin has antibacterial and antifungal activities in the presence of UV light. Antibacterial activity has been documented for the coumarin constituents.[2] An ethanolic extract of the entire plant has been reported to inhibit the growth of poliovirus and herpesvirus.[8]

Antispasmodic activity Antispasmodic activity on the isolated guinea-pig ileum has been documented for the flavonoid and bisabolol constituents.[2, 9] Greatest activity was exhibited by the flavonoids, especially apigenin which was found to be more than

C

three times as potent as papaverine.[2] (−)-α-Bisabolol activity was found to be comparable to that of papaverine, while the total volatile oil was considerably less active.[2] Smooth muscle relaxant properties have also been documented for a *cis*-spiroether.[2,6,10]

Enhancement of uterine tone in the guinea-pig and rabbit has been reported for an aqueous extract at a concentration of 1–2 mg extract/cm^3.[11]

Other activities High molecular weight polysaccharides with immunostimulating activity have been isolated from German chamomile.[12] The oil has been reported to increase bile secretion and concentration of cholesterol in the bile, following the administration of 0.1 mL/kg by mouth to cats and dogs.[13] A dose of 0.2 mL/kg was stated to exhibit hypotensive, and cardiac and respiratory depressant properties.[13]

The ability of the volatile oil to regenerate liver tissue in partially hepatectomised rats has been attributed to the azulene constituents.[2]

The volatile oil has been documented to reduce the serum concentration of urea in rabbits with experimentally induced uraemic conditions.[14]

Clinical studies

Rigorous clinical research assessing the effects of German chamomile is limited and large randomised controlled clinical trials are required.

Anti-inflammatory and wound-healing effects Clinical studies investigating the anti-inflammatory effects and wound-healing properties of German chamomile preparations have been reviewed.[G52] A summary of this information is given below. Many of the studies and reports mentioned below have important methodological limitations (e.g. no control group, small numbers of participants) and this should be considered when interpreting the results.

A cream containing German chamomile extract was reported to have effects equivalent to 0.25% hydrocortisone, and superior effects to 0.1% diflucortolone and 5% bufexamax in inflammatory dermatoses, as assessed in 161 patients. Studies involving healthy volunteers who received German chamomile preparations have reported that German chamomile ointment was superior to 0.1% hydrocortisone acetate in dermatitis, and German chamomile cream (20 mg/g) reduced visual sores and redness of skin in an adhesive-tape stripping test. A randomised, double-blind trial involving 25 participants indicated that a cream containing an aqueous alcoholic extract of German chamomile was more effective than hydrocortisone against UVB-induced erythema.

In an open study involving 98 patients with cancer, an extract preparation (containing 50 mg α-bisabolol and 150–300 mg apigenin-7-glucoside/100 g) used three times daily was reported to reduce oral mucositis caused either by irradiation or chemotherapy. However, a double-blind, placebo-controlled trial involving 164 patients showed that a mouthwash containing German chamomile did not decrease 5-fluorouracil-induced stomatitis.

The healing effects of German chamomile ointment and dexapanthenol 5% cream administered for six days were reported to have comparable effects in a study involving 147 female patients who underwent episiotomy during childbirth. A standardised extract (50 mg α-bisabolol and 3 mg chamazulene/100 g) significantly decreased weeping wound area and drying of wound in 14 patients following removal of tattoos. An ointment preparation improved haemorrhage, itching, burning and oozing due to haemorrhoids in a study involving 120 patients.

Sedative effects Oral administration of a German chamomile extract was reported to induce a deep sleep in 10 of 12 patients undergoing cardiac catheterisation.[2]

Side-effects, Toxicity

There is a lack of clinical safety data and toxicity data for German chamomile and further investigation of these aspects is required.

Reports of allergic reactions to chamomile are common, although in the majority of cases the plant species is not specified.[15] Patients with an existing hypersensitivity to German chamomile have demonstrated cross-sensitivities to other members of the family Asteraceae/Compositae[16,G51] and also to celery (family Umbelliferae).[G51] There are reports of anaphylactic reactions to chamomile (species unspecified)[17,18] and in both cases the individuals concerned had an existing hypersensitivity to ragweed (member of Asteraceae/Compositae). The symptoms they experienced included abdominal cramps, thickness of the tongue and a tight sensation in the throat,[18] angioedema of the lips and eyes, diffuse pruritus, a full sensation of the ears, generalised urticaria, upper airway obstruction, and pharyngeal oedema.[17] Both patients made a full recovery following medical treatment.

Allergic skin reactions have been documented following external contact with German chamomile.[2,19,G51] Consumption of chamomile tea may exacerbate existing allergic conditions and the use of a chamomile enema has been documented to cause asthma and urticaria.[G51]

The allergenic properties documented for chamomile have been attributed to anthecotulid, a sesquiterpene lactone present in low concentrations,[15] and to matricarin, a proazulene which has produced positive patch tests in patients with an existing sesquiterpene lactone hypersensitivity.[G51] Sesquiterpene lactones have been implicated in the allergenic activity of many plants, especially those belonging to the Asteraceae/Compositae family (*see* Feverfew). The prerequisite for allergenic activity is thought to be an exocyclic α-methylene group.[20]

The flowerheads contain anthemic acid, which is reported to act as an emetic in large doses.[G22]

The acute toxicity of chamomile oil (German and Roman) is reported to be low.[21] Oral and dermal LD_{50} values in rabbits have been documented as greater than 5 g/kg,[21] and the application of undiluted oil to the hairless backs of mice, to rabbit skin, and to human skin was not found to produce any observable irritation.[21] An LD_{50} value (mouse, by mouth) for German chamomile oil has been documented as 2.5 mL/kg.[13] The acute oral toxicity of (−)-α-bisabolol in mice and rats is reported to be low at approximately 15 mL/kg.[22] The subacute oral toxicity of (−)-α-bisabolol has been estimated to be between 1.0 and 2.0 mL/kg in rats and dogs.[22] An LD_{50} value (mouse, intraperitoneal injection) for *cis*-spiroether has been stated as 670 mg/kg.[6]

Contra-indications, Warnings

In view of the documented allergic reactions and cross-sensitivities, German chamomile should be avoided by individuals with a known hypersensitivity to any members of the Asteraceae/Compositae family. In addition, German chamomile may precipitate an allergic reaction or exacerbate existing symptoms in susceptible individuals (e.g. asthmatics).

The use of chamomile preparations for teething babies is not recommended.

Drug interactions None documented. However the potential for preparations of German chamomile to interact with other medicines administered concurrently, particularly those with similar or opposing effects, should be considered (particularly where oral preparations of German chamomile are used).

Coumarin compounds detected so far in German chamomile do not possess the minimum structural requirements (a C-4 hydroxyl substituent and a C-3 non-polar carbon substituent)[G87] for anticoagulant activity.

Pregnancy and lactation German chamomile is reputed to affect the menstrual cycle[G30] and extracts are reported to be uterotonic.[2, 11] Teratogenicity studies in rats, rabbits and dogs have been documented for (−)-α-bisabolol, with the oral toxic dose stated as 1–3 mL/kg.[22] A dose of 3 mL/kg was found to increase the number of fetuses reabsorbed and reduce the body weight of live offspring.[22] (−)-α-Bisabolol administered orally (250 and 500 mg/kg) to pregnant rats has been reported to have no effect on the fetus.[1] There are insufficient data on the use of German chamomile preparations during pregnancy and breast-feasting, and excessive use (particularly oral preparations) should be avoided during these periods.

Preparations

Proprietary multi-ingredient preparations

UK: Culpeper After Dinner Tea; Napiers Monthly Calm Tea. *USA:* Hot Flashex; Kavatrol; Laci Throat Care Soothing Citrus; MSM with Glucosamine Creme.

References

1 Isaac O. Pharmacological investigations with compounds of chamomile I. On the pharmacology of (−)-α-bisabolol and bisabolol oxides (review). *Planta Med* 1979; 35: 118–124.

2 Mann C, Staba EJ. The chemistry, pharmacology, and commercial formulations of chamomile. In: Craker LE, Simon JE, eds. *Herbs, Spices, and Medicinal Plants: Recent Advances in Botany, Horticulture, and Pharmacology*, vol 1. Arizona: Oryx Press, 1986: 235–280.

3 Tubaro A *et al*. Evaluation of antiinflammatory activity of a chamomile extract after topical application. *Planta Med* 1984; 50: 359.

4 Jakovlev V *et al*. Pharmacological investigations with compounds of chamomile VI. Investigations on the antiphlogistic effects of chamazulene and matricine. *Planta Med* 1983; 49: 67–73.

5 Jacovlev V *et al*. Pharmacological investigations with compounds of chamomile II. New investigations on the antiphlogistic effects of (−)-α-bisabolol and bisabolol oxides. *Planta Med* 1979; 35: 125–140.

6 Breinlich VJ, Scharnagel K. Pharmakologische Eigenschaften des EN-IN-dicycloäthers aus *Matricaria chamomilla. Arzneimittelforschung* 1968; 18: 429–431.

7 Szelenyi I *et al*. Pharmacological experiments with compounds of chamomile III. Experimental studies of the ulcerprotective effect of chamomile. *Planta Med* 1979; 35: 218–227.

8 Suganda AG *et al*. Effets inhibiteurs de quelques extraits bruts et semi purifiés de plantes indigènes françaises sur la multiplication de l'herpesvirus humain 1 et du poliovirus humain 2 en culture cellulaire. *J Nat Prod* 1983; 46: 626–632.

9 Achterrath-Tuckermann U *et al*. Pharmacological investigations with compounds of chamomile. V. Investigations on the spasmolytic effect of compounds of chamomile and Kamillosan on the isolated guinea pig ileum. *Planta Med* 1980; 39: 38–50.

10 Hölzl J *et al*. Preparation of ^{14}C-spiro ethers by chamomile and their use by an investigation of absorption. *Planta Med* 1986; 52: 533.

11 Shipochliev T. Extracts from a group of medicinal plants enhancing the uterine tonus. *Vet Med Nauki* 1981; 18: 94–98.

12 Wagner VH *et al*. Immunstimulierend wirkende polysaccharide (heteroglykane) aus höheren pflanzen. *Arzneimittelforschung* 1985; 35: 1069.

13 Ikram M. Medicinal plants as hypocholesterolemic agents. *JPMA* 1980; 30: 278–282.

14 Grochulski VA, Borkowski B. Influence of chamomile oil on experimental glomerulonephritis in rabbits. *Planta Med* 1972; 21: 289–292.

15 Hausen BM *et al*. The sensitizing capacity of Compositae plants. *Planta Med* 1984; 50: 229–234.

16 Hausen BM. The sensitising capacity of Compositae plants. III. Test results and cross-reactions in Compositae-sensitive patients. *Dermatologica* 1979; 159: 1–11.

17 Casterline CL. Allergy to chamomile tea. *JAMA* 1980; 4: 330–331.

18 Benner MH, Lee HJ. Anaphylactic reaction to chamomile tea. *J Allergy Clin Immunol* 1973; 52: 307–308.

19 Kettel WG. Allergy to *Matricaria chamomilla. Contact Dermatitis* 1987; 16: 50–51.

20 Mitchell JC, Dupuis G. Allergic contact dermatitis from sesquiterpenoids of the Compositae family of plants. *Br J Derm* 1971; 84: 139–150.

21 Opdyke DLJ. Chamomile oil German. *Food Cosmet Toxicol* 1974; 12: 851–852.

22 Habersang S *et al*. Pharmacological studies with compounds of chamomile IV. Studies on toxicity of (−)-α-bisabolol. *Planta Med* 1979; 37: 115–123.

Chamomile, Roman

C

Summary and Pharmaceutical Comment

The chemistry of Roman chamomile, particularly of the volatile oil, is well documented and is similar to that of German chamomile. Limited pharmacological data are available for Roman chamomile, although many actions have been reported for German chamomile. In view of the similar chemical compositions, many of the activities described for German chamomile are thought to be applicable to Roman chamomile and thus support the traditional herbal uses. However, rigorous clinical research assessing the efficacy and safety of preparations of Roman chamomile is required. Roman chamomile is stated to be of low toxicity, although allergic reactions (mainly contact dermatitis) have been reported.

Species (Family)

Chamaemelum nobile (L.) All. (Asteraceae/Compositae)

Synonym(s)

Anthemis nobilis L., Chamomile, *ormenis nobilis* (L.) J. Gay ex Coss. & Germ.

Part(s) Used

Flowerhead

Pharmacopoeial and Other Monographs

BHC 1992[G6]
BHP 1996[G9]
BP 2007[G84]
Martindale 35th edition[G85]
Ph Eur 2007[G81]
USP29/NF24[G86]

Legal Category (Licensed Products)

GSL[G37]

Constituents

The following is compiled from several sources, including General References G2 and G6.

Coumarins Scopoletin-7-glucoside.

Flavonoids Apigenin, luteolin, quercetin and their glycosides (e.g. apiin, luteolin-7-glucoside and rutin).

Volatile oils 0.4–1.75%. Angelic and tiglic acid esters (85%);[1] others include 1,8-cineole, *l-trans*-pinocarveol, *l-trans*-pinocarvone, chamazulene, farnesol, nerolidol; germacranolide-type sesquiterpene lactones (0.6%),[2] including nobilin, 3-epinobilin, 1,10-epoxynobilin, 3-dehydronobilin; various alcohols including amyl and isobutyl alcohols, anthemol.[1–4] Chamazulene is formed from a natural precursor during steam distillation of the oil, and varies in yield depending on the origin and the age of flowers.[1]

Other constituents Anthemic acid (bitter), phenolic and fatty acids, phytosterol, choline and inositol.

Food Use

Roman chamomile is listed by the Council of Europe as a natural source of food flavouring (category N2). This category indicates that Roman chamomile can be added to foodstuffs in small quantities, with a possible limitation of an active principle (as yet unspecified) in the final product.[G16] Chamomile is commonly used as an ingredient of herbal teas. Previously, Roman chamomile has been listed as GRAS (Generally Recognised As Safe).[G41]

Herbal Use

Roman chamomile is stated to possess carminative, anti-emetic, antispasmodic, and sedative properties. It has been used for dyspepsia, nausea and vomiting, anorexia, vomiting of pregnancy, dysmenorrhoea, and specifically for flatulent dyspepsia associated with mental stress.[G2, G6, G7, G8, G64]

Dosage

Dosages for oral administration (adults) for traditional uses recommended in standard herbal reference texts are given below.

Dried flowerheads 1–4 g as an infusion three times daily.[G7]

Liquid extract 1–4 mL (1 : 1 in 70% alcohol) three times daily.[G7]

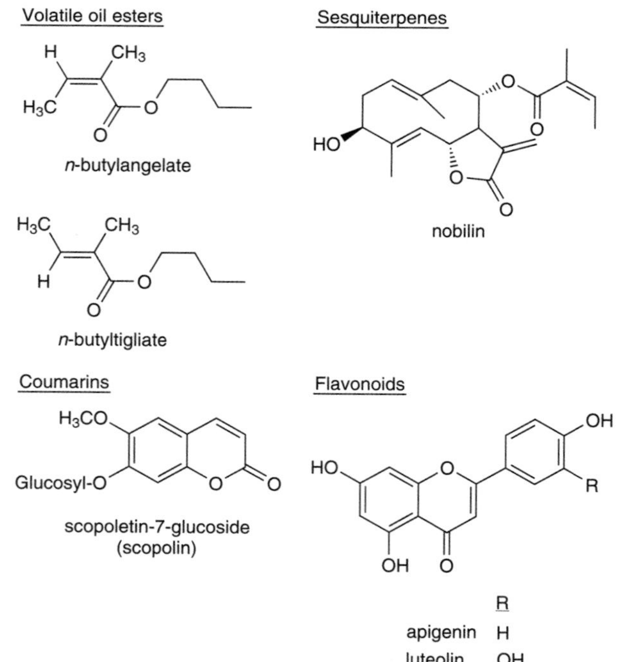

Figure 1 Selected constituents of Roman chamomile.

C

Pharmacological Actions

German and Roman chamomile possess similar pharmacological activities (*see* Chamomile, German for a fuller description of documented pharmacological actions).

In vitro and animal studies

Few studies have been documented specifically for Roman chamomile. The azulene compounds are reported to possess anti-allergic and anti-inflammatory properties; their mechanism of action is thought to involve inhibition of histamine release (*see* Chamomile, German). The volatile oil has been documented as having anti-inflammatory activity (carrageenan rat paw oedema test), and antidiuretic and sedative effects following intraperitoneal administration of doses up to 350 mg/kg body weight to rats.[5]

The azulenes have been reported to stimulate liver regeneration following oral, but not subcutaneous, administration.

The sesquiterpenoids nobilin, 1,10-epoxynobilin and 3-dehydronobilin have demonstrated *in vitro* antitumour activity against human cells.[1] The concentration of hydroxyisonobilin required for cytotoxic activity is reported to be low enough to warrant further investigations (ED_{50} 0.56 µg/mL versus HeLa; ED_{50} 1.23 µg/mL versus KB; arbitrary acceptable test level 4 µg/mL).

Clinical studies

Clinical research assessing the effects of Roman chamomile is limited, and rigorous randomised controlled clinical trials are required.

Side-effects, Toxicity

There is a lack of clinical safety data and toxicity data for Roman chamomile and further investigation of these aspects is required.

Instances of allergic and anaphylactic reactions to chamomile have been documented (*see* Chamomile, German) The allergenic principles in chamomile are thought to be the sesquiterpene lactones.[1] Roman chamomile yields nobilin, a sesquiterpene lactone that is reported to be potentially allergenic.[1] However, Roman chamomile oil has also been reported to be non-irritant and non-sensitising to human skin.[2] Animal studies have indicated the oil to be either mildly or non-irritant, and to lack any phototoxic effects.[2]

Large doses of Roman chamomile are stated to act as an emetic[G44] and this has been attributed to the anthemic acid content.[6]

The acute toxicity of Roman chamomile in animals is reported to be relatively low.[1] Acute LD_{50} values in rabbits (dermal) and rats (by mouth) have been stated to exceed 5 g/kg.[2]

Contra-indications, Warnings

In view of the documented allergic reactions and cross-sensitivities (*see* Chamomile, German), Roman chamomile should be avoided by individuals with a known hypersensitivity to any members of the Asteraceae/Compositae family. In addition, Roman chamomile may precipitate an allergic reaction or exacerbate existing symptoms in susceptible individuals (e.g. asthmatics).

The use of chamomile preparations in teething babies is not recommended.

Drug interactions None documented. However the potential for preparations of Roman chamomile to interact with other medicines administered concurrently, particularly those with similar or opposing effects, should be considered (particularly where oral preparations of Roman chamomile are used). Coumarin compounds detected so far in Roman chamomile do not possess the minimum structural requirements (a C-4 hydroxyl substituent and a C-3 non-polar carbon substituent) for anticoagulant activity.

Pregnancy and lactation Roman chamomile is reputed to be an abortifacient and to affect the menstrual cycle.[G30] In view of this and the potential for allergic reactions, the excessive use of Roman chamomile during pregnancy and lactation should be avoided.

Preparations

Proprietary multi-ingredient preparations

UK: Summertime Tea Blend.

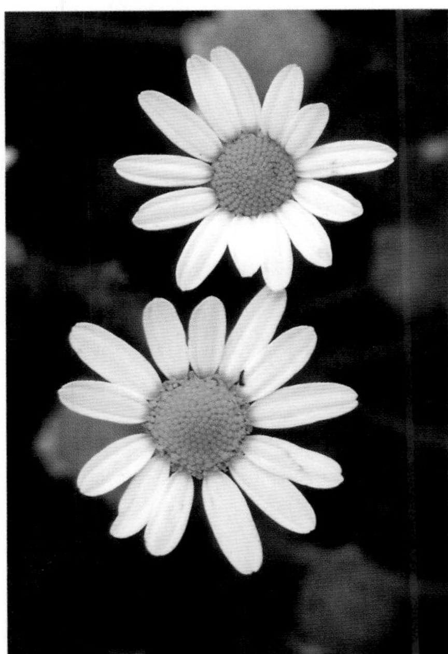

Figure 2 Roman chamomile (*Chamaemelum nobile*).

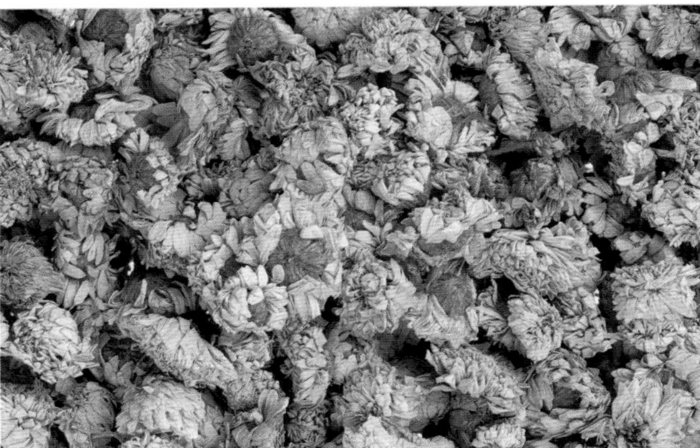

Figure 3 Roman chamomile – dried drug substance (flowerhead).

References

1 Mann C, Staba EJ. The chemistry, pharmacology, and commercial formulations of chamomile. In: Craker LE, Simon JE, eds. *Herbs, Spices, and Medicinal Plants: Recent Advances in Botany, Horticulture, and Pharmacology*, vol 1. Arizona: Oryx Press, 1986: 235–280.

2 Opdyke DLJ. Chamomile oil roman. *Food Cosmet Toxicol* 1974: 12: 853.

3 Casterline CL. Allergy to chamomile tea. *JAMA* 1980; 4: 330–331.

4 Hausen BM *et al*. The sensitizing capacity of Compositae plants. *Planta Med* 1984; 50: 229–234.

5 Melegari M *et al*. Chemical characteristics and pharmacological properties of the essential oils of *Anthemis nobilis*. *Fitoterapia* 1988; 59: 449–455.

6 Achterrath-Tuckermann U *et al*. Pharmacologisch Untersuchungen von Kamillen-Inhaltestoffen. *Planta Med* 1980; 39: 38–50.

Chaparral

Summary and Pharmaceutical Comment

The chemistry of chaparral is well studied and extensive literature has been published on the principal lignan component nordihydroguaiaretic acid (NDGA). However, little documented evidence is available to justify the herbal uses of chaparral. In view of the concerns over the hepatic toxicity, the use of chaparral as a herbal remedy cannot be recommended.

Species (Family)

Larrea tridentata Cov. var. *glutinosa* Jepson (Zygophyllaceae)

Synonym(s)

Creosote Bush. *L. tridentata* (south-western USA and northern Mexico) is now regarded as a separate species to *Larrea divaricata* Gav. (north-western Argentina).[1]

Part(s) Used

Herb

Pharmacopoeial and Other Monographs

Martindale 35th edition[G85]

Legal Category (Licensed Products)

Chaparral is not included in the GSL.[G37]

Constituents

The following is compiled from several sources, including General Reference G22.

Amino acids Arginine, aspartine, cystine, glutamic acid, glycine, isoleucine, leucine, phenylalanine, tryptophan, tyrosine and valine.

Flavonoids More than 20 different compounds reported, including isorhamnetin, kaempferol and quercetin and their glycosidic and ether derivatives; gossypetin, herbacetin, and their acetate derivatives;[1–7] two *C*-glucosyl flavones.

Lignans Major constituent nordihydroguaiaretic acid (NDGA) (up to 1.84%), norisoguaiacin, dihydroguaiaretic acid, partially demethylated dihydroguaiaretic acid, 3′-demethoxyisoguaiacin.[8–10]

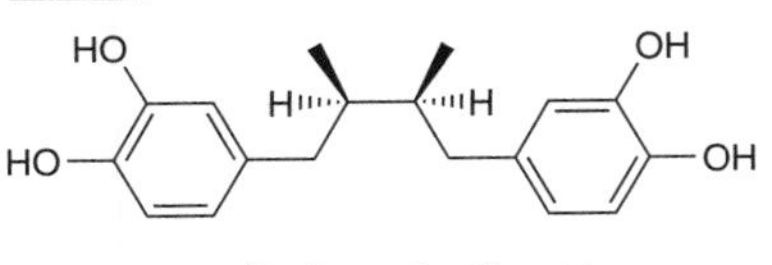

Lignans

HO HO H H OH OH

nordihydroguaiaretic acid

Figure 1 Selected constituents of chaparral.

Resins 20%. Phenolic constituents on external leaf surfaces of *L. divaricata* and *L. tridentata* are reported to be identical, containing a number of flavone and flavonol glycosides, and two lignans (including NDGA).[5]

Volatile oils Many identified terpene components include calamene, eudesmol, limonene, α- and β-pinene, and 2-rossalene.[11]

Other constituents Two pentacyclic triterpenes,[12] saponins.

Other plant parts A cytotoxic naphthoquinone derivative, larreantin, has been isolated from the roots.[13]

Food Use

Chaparral is not used in foods, although a related species, *Larrea mexicana* Moric., also termed creosote bush, is listed by the Council of Europe as a natural source of food flavouring (category N2). This category indicates that creosote bush can be added to foodstuffs in small quantities, with a possible limitation of an active principle (as yet unspecified) in the final product.[G16] In the USA, NDGA is no longer permitted to be used as an antioxidant in foods following the results of toxicity studies in animals (*see* Side-effects, Toxicity).

Herbal Use

Chaparral has been used for the treatment of arthritis, cancer, venereal disease, tuberculosis, bowel cramps, rheumatism and colds.[G60]

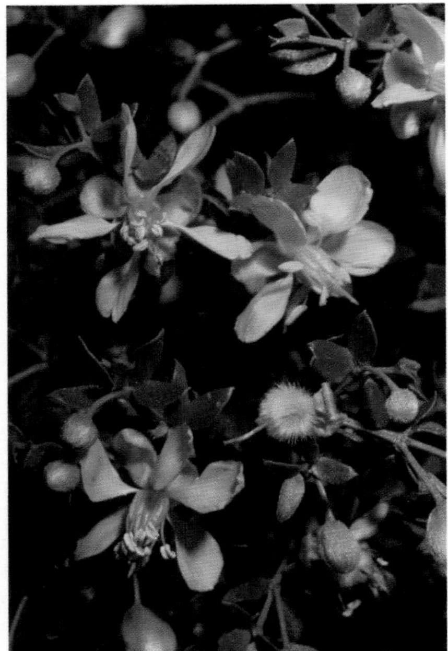

Figure 2 Chaparral (*Larrea tridentata*).

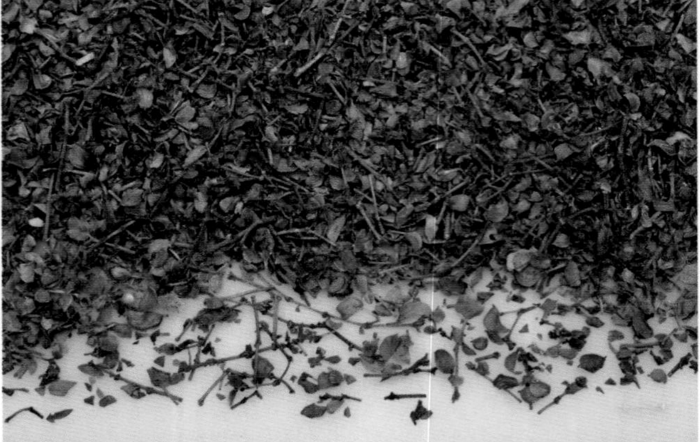

Figure 3 Chaparral – dried drug substance (herb).

Dosage

None documented.

Pharmacological Actions

In vitro and animal studies

Amoebicidal action against *Entamoeba histolytica* has been reported for a chaparral extract (0.01%).[14] This action may be attributable to the lignan constituents, which are documented as both amoebicidal and fungicidal.[9] NDGA has been reported to have antimicrobial activity against a number of organisms including *Penicillium* spp., *Salmonella* spp., *Streptococcus* spp., *Staphylococcus aureus*, *Bacillus subtilis*, *Pseudomonas aeruginosa* and various other pathogens and moulds.[8, 15]

NDGA is an antioxidant, and has been documented to cause inhibition of hepatic microsomal enzyme function.[15–17]

Clinical studies

Medical interest in chaparral increased following claims that ingestion of an aqueous infusion of the herb was associated with regression of a malignant melanoma in the cheek of an 85-year-old man.[18] However, an isolated care report is not adequate scientific evidence, results of a subsequent study that investigated the antitumour action of chaparral, as a tea, were inconclusive.[G60]

Side-effects, Toxicity

There is a lack of clinical safety data and toxicity data for chaparral and further investigation of these aspects is required.

Acute hepatitis has been associated with chaparral ingestion.[19–21] Contact dermatitis to chaparral has been reported.[22, 23] Chaparral-induced toxic hepatitis has been reported for two patients in different parts of the USA. The adverse effects were attributed to ingestion of a herbal nutritional supplement derived from the leaves of chaparral. Five cases of serious poisoning in the USA and another three in Canada have been linked to chaparral-containing products.[20, 24] Some patients have developed irreversible reno-hepatic failure. Initially, NDGA was thought to have low toxicity: doses of up to 400 mg/kg body weight by intramuscular injection had been administered to humans for 5–6 months, with little or no toxicity reported.[15] Documented oral LD_{50} values for NDGA include 4 g/kg (mouse), 5.5 g/kg (rat) and 830 mg/kg (guinea-pig).[15] Results of chronic feeding studies (two years, 0.25–1.0% of diet) in rats and mice reported no abnormalities in histological tests of the liver, spleen and kidney. Inflammatory caecal lesions and slight cystic enlargement of lymph nodes near the caecum were observed in rats at the 0.5% feeding level. At this point NDGA was considered to be safe for food use. However, two later studies in rats (using NDGA at up to 3% of the diet) reported the development of cortical and medullary cysts in the kidney.[15] On the basis of these findings, NDGA was removed from GRAS (Generally Recognised As Safe) status in the USA and is no longer permitted to be used as an antioxidant in foods.[15]

Contra-indications, Warnings

In view of the reports of acute hepatitis associated with chaparral ingestion, and the uncertainty regarding NDGA toxicity, consumption should be avoided.

Drug interactions None documented. However the potential for preparations of chaparral to interact with other medicines administered concurrently, particularly those with similar or opposing effects, should be considered. Chaparral has amino acid constituents and, therefore, may not be suitable for use by patients receiving treatments with monoamine oxidase inhibitors.

Pregnancy and lactation *In vitro* utero activity has been documented for chaparral.[G30] In view of the concerns regarding toxicity, chaparral should not be ingested during pregnancy or lactation.

Preparations

Proprietary multi-ingredient preparations

Australia: Proyeast.

References

1 Bernhard HO, Thiele K. Additional flavonoids from the leaves of *Larrea tridentata. Planta Med* 1981; 41: 100–103.

2 Sakakibara M *et al.* 6,8-Di-C-glucosylflavones from *Larrea tridentata* (Zygophyllaceae). *Phytochemistry* 1977; 16: 1113–1114.

3 Sakakibara M *et al.* A new 8-hydroxyflavonol from *Larrea tridentata. Phytochemistry* 1975; 14: 2097–2098.

4 Sakakibara M *et al.* New 8-hydroxyflavonols from *Larrea tridenta. Phytochemistry* 1975; 14: 849–851.

5 Sakakibara M *et al.* Flavonoid methyl ethers on the external leaf surface of *Larrea tridentata* and *L. divaricata. Phytochemistry* 1976; 15: 727–731.

6 Chirikdjian JJ. Isolation of kumatakenin and 4′,5-dihydroxy-3,3′,7-trimethoxyflavone from *Larrea tridentata. Pharmazie* 1974; 29: 292–293.

7 Chirikdjian JJ. Flavonoids of *Larrea tridentata. Z Naturforsch* 1973; 28: 32–35.

8 Gisvold O, Thaker E. Lignans from *Larrea divaricata. J Pharm Sci* 1974; 63: 1905–1907.

9 Fronczek FR *et al.* The molecular structure of 3′-demethoxynorisoguaiacin triacetate from creosote bush (*Larrea tridentata*). *J Nat Prod* 1987; 50: 497–499.

10 Page JO. Determination of nordihydroguaiaretic acid in creosote bush. *Anal Chem* 1955; 27: 1266–1268.

11 Bohnstedt CF, Mabry TJ. The volatile constituents of the genus *Larrea* (Zygophyllaceae). *Rev Latinoam Quim* 1979; 10: 128–131.

12 Xue H-Z *et al.* 3-β-(3,4-Dihydroxycinnamoyl)-erythrodiol and 3β-(4-hydroxycinnamoyl)-erythrodiol from *Larrea tridentata. Phytochemistry* 1988; 27: 233–235.

13 Luo Z *et al.* Larreatin, a novel, cytotoxic naphthoquinone from *Larrea tridentata. J Org Chem* 1988; 53: 2183–2185.

14 Segura JJ *et al.* In-vitro amebicidal activity of *Larrea tridentata. Bol Estud Med Biol* 1979; 30: 267–268.

15 Oliveto EP. Nordihydroguaiaretic acid. A naturally occurring antioxidant. *Chem Ind* 1972: 677–679.
16 Burk D, Woods M. Hydrogen peroxide, catalase, glutathione peroxidasequinones, nordihydroguaiaretic acid, and phosphopyridine in relation to X-ray action on cancer cells. *Radiation Res Suppl* 1963; 3: 212–246.
17 Pardini RS *et al*. Inhibition of mitochondrial electron transport by nor-dihydroguaiaretic acid (NDGA). *Biochem Pharmacol* 1970; 19: 2695–2699.
18 Smart CR *et al*. An interesting observation on nordihydroguaiaretic acid (NSC-4291; NDGA) and a patient with malignant melanoma—a preliminary report. *Cancer Chemother Rep Part 1* 1969; 53: 147.
19 Katz M, Saibil F. Herbal hepatitis: subacute hepatic necrosis secondary to chaparral leaf. *J Clin Gastroenterol* 1990; 12: 203–206.
20 Clark F, Reed R. Chaparral-induced toxic hepatitis – California and Texas, 1992. *Morb Mortal Wkly Rep* 1992; 41: 812–814.
21 Gordon DW *et al*. Chaparral ingestion – the broadening spectrum of liver injury caused by herbal medicines. *JAMA* 1995; 273: 489–490.
22 Leonforte JF. Contact dermatitis from *Larrea* (creosote bush). *J Am Acad Dermatol* 1986; 14: 202–207.
23 Shasky DR. Contact dermatitis from *Larrea tridentata* (creosote bush). *J Am Acad Dermatol* 1986; 15: 302.
24 Anon. Toxic tea. *Pharm J* 1993; 250: 366.

Cinnamon

C

Summary and Pharmaceutical Comment

The reputed antimicrobial, antiseptic, anthelmintic, carminative and antispasmodic properties of cinnamon are probably attributable to the volatile oil. The astringent properties of tannins may account for the claimed antidiarrhoeal action. However, rigorous clinical research assessing the efficacy and safety of cinnamon preparations is required. Cinnamon should not be used in amounts greatly exceeding those used in foods.

Species (Family)

**Cinnamomum zeylanicum* Bl. (Lauraceae)
†*Cinnamomum loureirii* Nees
‡*Cinnamomum burmanii* (Nees) Bl.

Synonym(s)

*Ceylon Cinnamon, *Cinnamomum verum* J.S. Presl., True Cinnamon
†*Cinnamomum obtusifolium* Nees var. *loureirii* Perr. & Eb., Saigon Cassia, Saigon Cinnamon
‡Batavia Cassia, Batavia Cinnamon, Padang-Cassia, Panang Cinnamon

Part(s) Used

Inner bark

Pharmacopoeial and Other Monographs

BHP 1996[G9]
BP 2007[G84]
Complete German Commission E[G3]
Martindale 35th edition[G85]
Ph Eur 2007[G81]
WHO volume 1 1999[G63]

Legal Category (Licensed Products)

GSL[G37]

Constituents

The following is compiled from several sources, including General References G2, G58, G59 and G62.

Tannins Condensed.

Volatile oils Up to 4%. Cinnamaldehyde (60–75%), benzaldehyde and cuminaldehyde; phenols (4–10%) including eugenol, and methyleugenol, pinene, phellandrene, cymeme and caryophyllene (hydrocarbons), eugenol acetate, cinnamyl acetate and benzyl benzoate (esters), linalool (an alcohol). Of the various types of cinnamon bark the oil of *C. zeylanicum* is stated to contain the highest amount of eugenol. Cinnamon oil differs from the closely related cassia oil in that the latter is reported to be devoid of eugenol, monoterpenoids and sesquiterpenoids (*see* Cassia).

Other constituents Calcium oxalate, cinnzeylanin, cinnzeylanol, coumarin, gum, mucilage, resins and sugars.

Other plant parts Cinnamon leaf oil contains much higher concentrations of eugenol, from 80 to 96% depending on the species. A cinnamon leaf oil of Chinese origin, *Cinnamomum japonicum* Sieb., contains a high concentration of safrole (60%) and only about 3% eugenol.

Food Use

Cinnamon is listed by the Council of Europe as a natural source of food flavouring (category N2). This category indicates that cinnamon can be added to foodstuffs in small quantities, with a possible limitation of an active principle (as yet unspecified) in the final product.[G16] It is commonly used as a spice in cooking, although at levels much less than the stated therapeutic doses. The acceptable daily intake of cinnamaldehyde has been temporarily estimated as 700 μg/kg body weight.[G45] Previously, cinnamon has been listed as GRAS (Generally Recognised As Safe).[G41]

Herbal Use

Cinnamon is stated to possess antispasmodic, carminative, orexigenic, antidiarrhoeal, antimicrobial, refrigerant and anthelmintic properties. It has been used for anorexia, intestinal colic, infantile diarrhoea, common cold, influenza, and specifically for flatulent colic, and dyspepsia with nausea.[G7] Cinnamon bark is also stated to be astringent, and cinnamon oil is reported to possess carminative and antiseptic properties.[G2, G41, G64]

Dosage

Dosages for oral administration (adults) for traditional uses recommended in older standard herbal and pharmaceutical reference texts are given below.

Dried bark 0.5–1.0 g as an infusion three times daily.[G7]

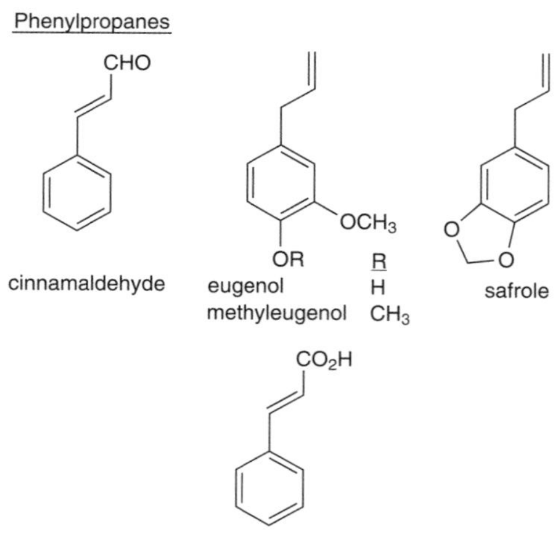

Figure 1 Selected constituents of cinnamon.

Liquid extract 0.5–1.0 mL (1 : 1 in 70% alcohol) three times daily.[(G7)]

Tincture of Cinnamon (BPC 1949) 2–4 mL.

Pharmacological Actions

In vitro and animal studies

Cinnamon oil has antifungal, antiviral, bactericidal and larvicidal properties.[(G41)] A carbon dioxide extract of cinnamon bark (0.1%) has been documented to suppress completely the growth of numerous microorganisms including *Escherichia coli*, *Staphylococcus aureus* and *Candida albicans*.[(G41)] (*See* Cassia for details of the many pharmacological actions documented for cinnamaldehyde and cinnamomi cortex (cinnamon bark).)

Antiseptic and anaesthetic properties have been documented for eugenol[(1)] and two insecticidal compounds, cinnzeylanin and cinnzeylanol, have been isolated.[(G41)] Tannins are known to possess astringent properties.

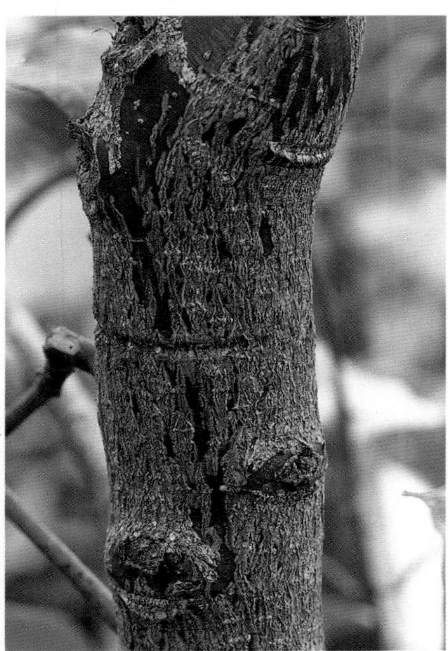

Figure 2 Cinnamon (*Cinnamomum zeylanicum*).

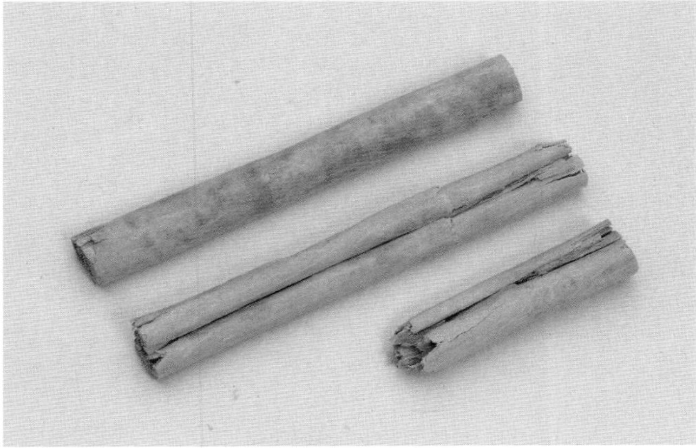

Figure 3 Cinnamon – dried drug substance (inner bark).

Weak tumour-promoting activity on the mouse skin and weak cytotoxic activity against HeLa cells has been documented for eugenol.[(G41)]

Clinical studies

There is a lack of clinical research assessing the effects of cinnamon and rigorous randomised controlled clinical trials are required.

Side-effects, Toxicity

None documented for cinnamon bark. However, clinical safety data and toxicity data for cinnamom are limited and further investigation of these aspects is required. Cinnamon oil contains cinnamaldehyde, an irritant and sensitising principle.[(G58)] The dermal LD_{50} of the oil is reported to be 690 mg/kg body weight (*see* Cassia). The accepted daily intake of eugenol is up to 2.5 mg/kg.[(G45)]

Contra-indications, Warnings

Contact with cinnamon bark or oil may cause an allergic reaction.[(G51)] Cinnamon oil is stated to be a dermal and mucous membrane irritant, and a dermal sensitiser.[(G58)] It is a hazardous oil and should not be used on the skin.[(G58)] The oil should not be taken internally.

Drug interactions None documented.

Pregnancy and lactation There are no known problems with the use of cinnamon during pregnancy and lactation, provided that doses do not greatly exceed the amounts used in foods.

Preparations

Proprietary single-ingredient preparations

USA: Cinnamon Extract.

Proprietary multi-ingredient preparations

Austria: Brady's-Magentropfen; China-Eisenwein; Mariazeller; Montana; Montana N; Passedan. *Brazil:* Balsamo Branco; Paratonico. *Czech Republic:* Blahungstee N; Dr Theiss Rheuma Creme; Dr Theiss Schwedenbitter; Magen- und Darmtee N. *France:* Elixir Grez; Quintonine. *Germany:* Amara-Pascoe; Gastrosecur; Klosterfrau Melisana; Melissengeist; Schwedentrunk Elixier; Sedovent. *India:* Carmicide. *Israel:* Davilla. *Italy:* Biophase Shampoo; Dam. *Russia:* Doppelherz Melissa (Доппельгерц Мелисса); Himcolin (Химколин). *South Africa:* Melissengeist; Rooilavental; Spiritus Contra Tussim Drops. *Spain:* Agua del Carmen; Vigortonic. *Switzerland:* Odontal; Tisane pour les problemes de prostate. *Thailand:* Meloids. *UK:* Melissa Comp.. *Venezuela:* Aftil.

Reference

1 Wagner H, Wolff P (eds). *New Natural Products and Plant Drugs with Pharmacological, Biological or Therapeutical Activity.* Berlin: Springer Verlag, 1977.

Clivers

Summary and Pharmaceutical Comment

Limited chemical information is available for clivers. No scientific evidence was found to support the herbal uses, although documented tannin constituents may account for the reputed mild astringent action. In view of the paucity of toxicity data, excessive use of clivers should be avoided.

Species (Family)

Galium aparine L. (Rubiaceae)

Synonym(s)

Cleavers, Galium, Goosegrass

Part(s) Used

Herb

Pharmacopoeial and Other Monographs

BHC 1992[G6]
BHP 1996[G9]
Martindale 35th edition[G85]

Legal Category (Licensed Products)

GSL[G37]

Constituents

The following is compiled from several sources, including General Reference G6.

Acids Caffeic acid, *p*-coumaric acid, gallic acid, *p*-hydroxybenzoic acid, salicylic acid and citric acid.[1]

Coumarins Unspecified. Scopoletin and umbelliferone reported for related species *Galium cruciata* and *Galium tauricum*.[2]

Iridoids Asperuloside (rubichloric acid), monotropein.[3,4]

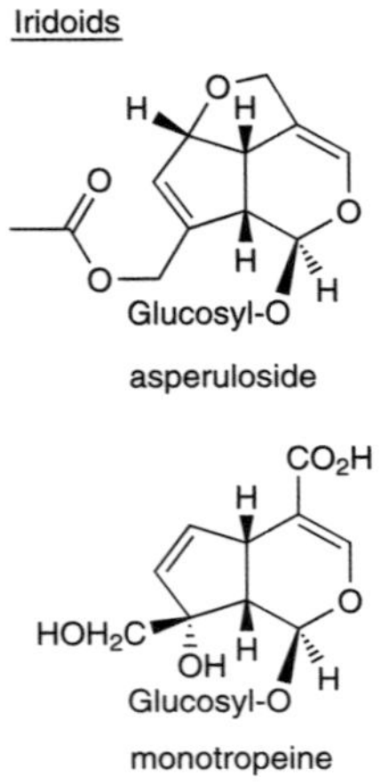

Iridoids

asperuloside

monotropeine

Figure 1 Selected constituents of clivers.

Tannins Unspecified;[5] gallic acid is usually associated with hydrolysable tannins.

Other constituents Alkanes (C_{19}–C_{31}),[4] flavonoids.

Other plant parts Anthraquinones have been documented for the roots, but not for the aerial parts.[1]

Food Use

Clivers is not used in foods.

Herbal Use

Clivers is stated to possess diuretic and mild astringent properties. It has been used for dysuria, lymphadenitis, psoriasis, and specifically for enlarged lymph nodes.[G6, G7, G8, G64]

Dosage

Dosages for oral administration (adults) for traditional uses recommended in standard herbal reference texts are given below.

Dried herb 2–4 g as an infusion three times daily.[G6, G7]

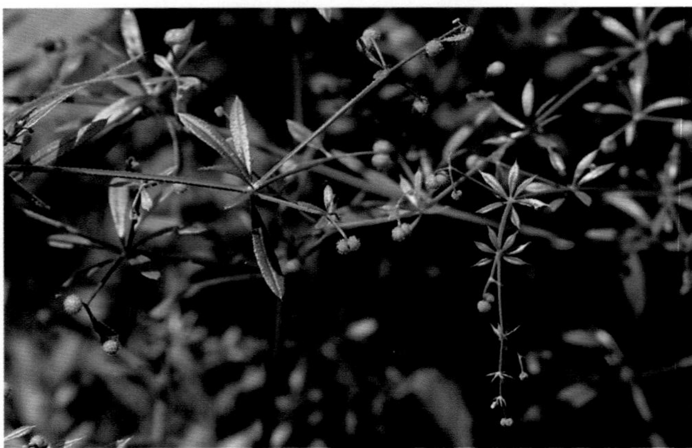

Figure 2 Clivers (*Galium aparine*).

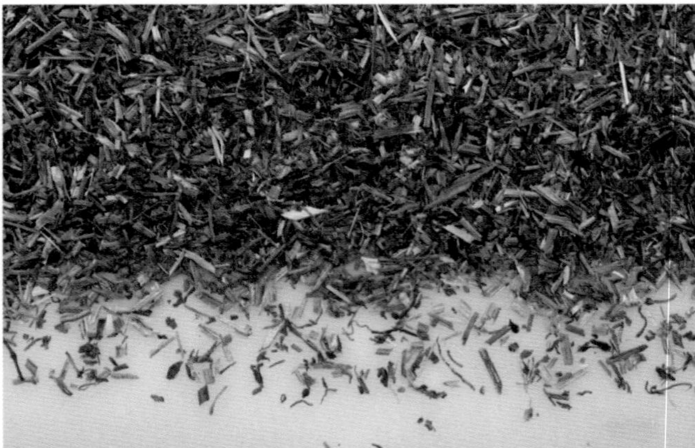

Figure 3 Clivers – dried drug substance (herb).

Liquid extract 2–4 mL (1 : 1 in 25% alcohol) three times daily.(G6, G7)

Expressed juice 3–15 mL three times daily.(G6, G7)

Pharmacological Actions

In vitro and animal studies

None documented for clivers. Asperuloside and monotropein have been reported to elicit a mild laxative action in mice.[6] The action was stated to be approximately 15 times less potent than that of senna, and of shorter duration.

Clinical studies

None documented. Tannins are known to possess astringent activities.

Side-effects, Toxicity

None documented.

Contra-indications, Warnings

It has been stated that diabetics should only use the expressed juice with caution(G34) although no pharmacological data were located to support this statement.

Drug interactions None documented. However the potential for preparations of clivers to interact with other medicines administered concurrently, particularly those with similar or opposing effects, should be considered.

Pregnancy and lactation In view of the lack of pharmacological and toxicological information, the use of clivers during pregnancy and lactation should be avoided.

Preparations

Proprietary multi-ingredient preparations

Australia: Dermaco; Galium Complex; Herbal Cleanse; Uva-Ursi Complex. *UK:* Antitis; Aqua Ban Herbal; Athera; Backache; Cascade; Fenneherb Cystaid; Gerard House Water Relief Tablets; HealthAid Boldo-Plus; Kas-Bah; Modern Herbals Menopause; Modern Herbals Water Retention; Napiers Breathe Easy Tea; Psorasolv; Sciargo; Skin Cleansing; Tabritis; Tabritis Tablets; Water Naturtabs; Watershed.

References

1 Hegnauer R. *Chemotaxonomie der Pflanzen*, vol 6. Basel and Stuttgart: Birhauser Verlag, 1973: 158–159.

2 Borisov MI. Coumarins of the genus Asperula and Galium. *Khim Prir Soedin* 1974; 10: 82.

3 Grimshaw J. Structure of asperuloside. *Chem Ind* 1961: 403–404.

4 Corrigan D *et al*. Iridoids and alkanes in twelve species of *Galium* and *Asperula*. *Phytochemistry* 1978; 17: 1131–1133.

5 Buckova A *et al*. Contents of tannins in some species of the Asperula and Galium genera. *Acta Fac Pharm Univ Comeniana* 1970; 19: 7–28.

6 Inouye H *et al*. Purgative activities of iridoid glucosides. *Planta Med* 1974; 25: 285–288.

Clove

C

Summary and Pharmaceutical Comment

The pharmacological properties documented for cloves are associated with the volatile oil, in particular with eugenol which has local anaesthetic action. However, rigorous clinical research assessing the efficacy and safety of clove preparations is required. Cloves should not be taken in doses greatly exceeding those used in foods and caution should be exerted in patients taking anticoagulant or antiplatelet therapy.

Species (Family)

Syzygium aromaticum (L.) Merr. & Perry (Myrtaceae)

Synonym(s)

Caryophyllus aromaticus L., *Eugenia aromatica* (L.) Baill., *Eugenia caryophyllata* Thunb., *Eugenia caryophyllus* (Spreng.) Bull. & Harr.

Part(s) Used

Clove (dried flowerbud), leaf, stem

Pharmacopoeial and Other Monographs

BHP 1996[(G9)]
BP 2007[(G84)]
Complete German Commission E[(G3)]
Martindale 35th edition[(G85)]
Ph Eur 2007[(G81)]

Legal Category (Licensed Products)

GSL[(G37)]

Constituents

The following is compiled from several sources, including General References G2 and G58.

Volatile oils Clove bud oil (15–18%) containing eugenol (80–90%), eugenyl acetate (2–27%), β-caryophyllene (5–12%). Others include methylsalicylate, methyleugenol, benzaldehyde, methylamyl ketone and α-ylangene.

Leaf oil (2%) containing eugenol 82–88%.

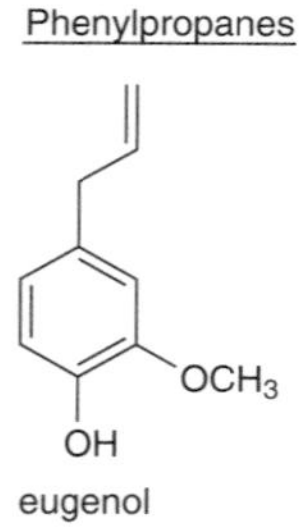

Phenylpropanes

OCH_3

OH

eugenol

Figure 1 Selected constituents of clove.

Stem oil (4–6%) with eugenol 90–95%. A more comprehensive listing is provided elsewhere.[(G22)]

Other constituents Campesterol, carbohydrates, kaempferol, lipids, oleanolic acid, rhamnetin, sitosterol, stigmasterol and vitamins.

Food Use

Clove is listed by the Council of Europe as a natural source of food flavouring (category N2). This category indicates that clove can be added to foodstuffs in small quantities, with a possible limitation of an active principle (as yet unspecified) in the final product.[(G16)] Clove is commonly used in cooking, and as a flavouring agent in food products. Previously, clove has been listed as GRAS (Generally Recognised As Safe).[(G41)]

Herbal Use

Clove has been traditionally used as a carminative, anti-emetic, toothache remedy and counter-irritant.[(G2, G41, G64)]

Clove oil is stated to be a carminative, occasionally used in the treatment of flatulent colic[(G54)] and is commonly used topically for symptomatic relief of toothache.[(G45)]

Dosage

Dosages for oral administration (adults) for traditional uses recommended in older standard pharmaceutical reference texts are given below. In dentistry, clove oil is applied undiluted using a plug of cottonwool soaked in the oil and applied to the cavity of the tooth (*see* Contra-indications, Warnings).

Clove 120–300 mg.[(G44)]

Clove oil 0.05–0.2 mL.[(G44)]

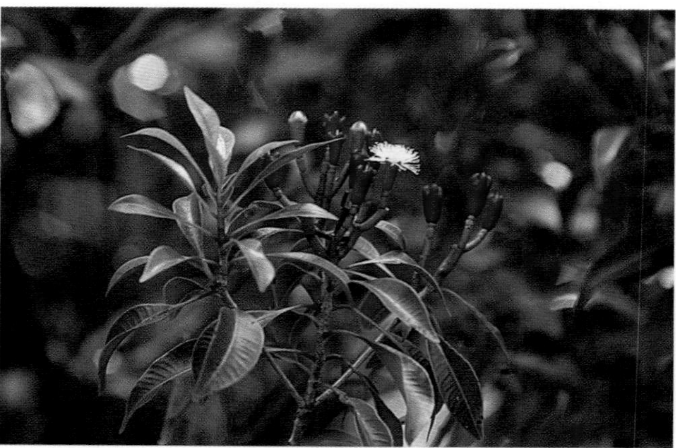

Figure 2 Clove (*Syzygium aromaticum*).

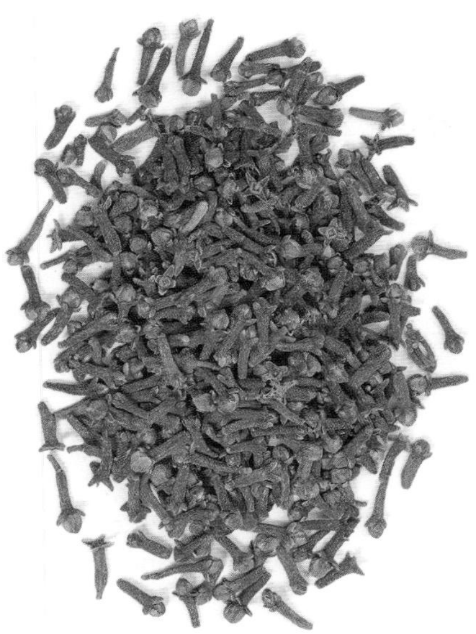

Figure 3 Clove – dried drug substance (flowerbud).

Pharmacological Actions

In vitro and animal studies

The anodyne and mild antiseptic properties documented for clove oil have been attributed to eugenol.[G41] Clove oil is stated to possess antihistaminic and antispasmodic properties.[G41] Eugenol, eugenol acetate and methyl acetate are reported to exhibit trypsin-potentiating activity.[G41]

Antibacterial, hypoglycaemic and potent CNS-depressant activities have been documented for *Syzygium cuminii* L., a related species cultivated in India.[1]

Clinical studies

There is a lack of clinical research assessing the effects of cloves and rigorous randomised controlled clinical trials are required.

Side-effects, Toxicity

There is a lack of clinical safety data and toxicity data for clove oil and further investigation of these aspects is required. Clove oil is stated to be a dermal and mucous membrane irritant;[G58] contact dermatitis, cheilitis, and stomatitis have been reported for clove oil.[G51] The irritant nature of the oil can be attributed to the eugenol content. Eugenol is also stated to have sensitising properties.[G51] An LD_{50} (rat, by mouth) value for clove oil is stated as 2.65 g/kg body weight.[G22]

Contra-indications, Warnings

None documented for the bud, leaf or stem. It is recommended that clove oil should be used with caution orally and should not be used on the skin.[G58] Repeated application of clove oil as a toothache remedy may result in damage to the gingival tissue.[G45] In view of the irritant nature of the volatile oil, concentrated clove oil is not suitable for internal use in doses larger than those recommended.

There is limited evidence from *in vitro* investigations that eugenol inhibits prostaglandin synthesis,[2] and coagulation disorders have been reported following childhood ingestion of clove oil.[3,4]

Drug interactions None documented. However, the potential for preparations of clove oil to interact with other medicines administered concurrently, particularly those with similar or opposing effects, should be considered. Eugenol, a major consituent of clove oil, inhibits prostaglandin synthesis, although the clinical relevance of this, if any, is unclear.

Pregnancy and lactation There are no known problems with the use of clove during pregnancy or lactation, provided that doses taken do not greatly exceed the amounts used in foods.

Preparations

Proprietary multi-ingredient preparations

Austria: Mariazeller. *Brazil:* Balsamo Branco. *Czech Republic:* Naturland Grosser Swedenbitter; Stomatosan. *Germany:* Inconturina; Klosterfrau Melisana; Melissengeist. *Italy:* Biophase Shampoo; Saugella Uomo. *Portugal:* Midro. *Russia:* Doppelherz Melissa (Доппельгерц Мелисса); Maraslavin (Мараславин); Original Grosser Bittner Balsam (Оригинальный Большой Бальзам Биттнера). *South Africa:* Clairo; Melissengeist; Spiritus Contra Tussim Drops. *Switzerland:* Odontal; Tisane pour les problemes de prostate. *UK:* Melissa Comp.; Revitonil.

References

1 Chakraborty D *et al*. A new neuropsychopharmacological study of *Syzygium cuminii*. *Planta Med* 1986; 52: 139–143.

2 Rasheed A *et al*. Eugenol and prostaglandin biosynthesis. *New Eng J Med* 1984; 310(1): 50–51.

3 Brown SA *et al*. Disseminated intravascular coagulation and hepatocellular necrosis due to clove oil. *Blood Coag Fibrinol* 1992; 3 (5): 665–668.

4 Hartnoll G *et al*. Near fatal ingestion of oil of cloves. *Arch Dis Childhood* 1993; 69(3): 392–393.

Cohosh, Black

C

Summary and Pharmaceutical Comment

The chemistry of black cohosh is well-documented. The triterpene glycosides and flavonoids are considered to be important for activity, although as a mechanism of action for black cohosh has not been established, whether or not other known or as yet undocumented constituents contribute to the observed effects is unclear. Most of the reputed traditional uses of black cohosh are not supported by data from preclinical or clinical studies. One exception is the use of black cohosh in rheumatism and rheumatoid arthritis – there are data from *in vitro* and *in vivo* studies in rodents that indicate that black cohosh extracts have anti-inflammatory activity.

Evidence from rigorous randomised controlled clinical trials to support the efficacy of extracts of black cohosh rhizome in relieving menopausal symptoms is lacking; two recent studies have reported a lack of effect for black cohosh preparations on certain primary outcome variables (*see* Pharmacological Actions; Clinical studies). Further investigation to assess the effects of well-characterised black cohosh preparations in well-designed randomised controlled trials involving sufficient numbers of participants is required. Two such studies are in progress in the USA.

Preclinical research has provided conflicting data on the oestrogenic activity of preparations of black cohosh. On balance, recent findings indicate that extracts of black cohosh root/rhizome do not have oestrogenic effects, but further study is required to confirm this and to elucidate the mechanism(s) of action of black cohosh constituents. Evidence from clinical studies on this point is also unclear. Until further information is available, black cohosh preparations should not be taken by individuals with oestrogen-sensitive tumours, such as certain breast cancers. There are only limited data on other safety aspects of black cohosh preparations.

There are now several case reports of hepatotoxic reactions associated with the use of black cohosh preparations. Individuals taking black cohosh preparations and who feel unwell or experience new symptoms, particularly those associated with liver disease, should be advised to stop taking black cohosh and to consult their doctor. Patients with previous or existing liver disorders should be advised not to take black cohosh without first consulting their doctor. In view of the lack of conclusive evidence for the efficacy of black cohosh, and the serious nature of the potential harm, it is extremely unlikely that the benefit–harm balance would be in favour of such patients using black cohosh.

Use of black cohosh preparations at doses higher than those recommended for therapeutic effects and/or for excessive periods (exceeding three months)[G56] should be avoided until further information is available on the safety of black cohosh with long-term use. In view of the documented pharmacological actions of black cohosh preparations, the potential for interactions with other medicines administered concurrently, particularly those with similar or opposing effects, should be considered.

Species (Family)

Cimicifuga racemosa (L.) Nutt. (Ranunculaceae)

Synonym(s)

Actaea racemosa L., *A. monogyna* Walter, Black Snakeroot, Cimicifuga, Macrotys Actaea

Part(s) Used

Rhizome, root

Pharmacopoeial and Other Monographs

AHP 2002[G1]
BHC 1992[G6]
BHP 1996[G9]
BHMA 2003[G66]
BPC 1934[G10]
Complete German Commission E[G3]
ESCOP 2003[G76]
Martindale 35th edition[G85]
WHO volume 1 (1999)[G63]

Legal Category (Licensed Products)

GSL[G37]

Constituents

The following is compiled from several sources, including General References G1 and G75.

Alkaloids Quinolizidine-type, including cytisine, *N*-methylcytisine and other unidentified compounds.[G75]

Flavonoids Formononetin (isoflavonoid),[1,2] although it was not detected in 13 samples analysed.[3]

Phenylpropanoids Phenylpropanoid esters cimiracemates A-D, isoferulic and ferulic acids, methylcaffeate.[4]

Terpenoids [16] Complex mixture of 9,19-cycloartenol-type triterpene glycosides with either xylose or arabinose. The isolated compounds include actein[1,5–11,G6] and related compounds cimicifugoside (cimigoside), 26-deoxycimicifugoside, cimiacerooside A, cimiracemosides A-H,[12–14] cimicifugosides H-3, H-4 and H-6,[15] cimigenol,[G63] 26-deoxyactein, 23-epi-26-deoxyactein (revised structure proposed for 27-deoxyactein),[11–13] cimiracemosides I-P and thirteen other cimiracemosides: 25-anhydrocimigenol-3-O-β-D-xyloside, 25-anhydrocimigenol-3-O-α-L-arabinoside, cimigenol-3-O-β-D-xyloside, cimigenol-3-O-α-L-arabinoside, 25-O-acetylcimigenin-3-O-β-D-xyloside, 25-O-acetylcimigenol-3-O-α-L-arabinoside, 23-O-acetylshengmanol-3-O-α-L-arabinoside, cimifugosides H-1 and H-2, 24-O-acetylshengmanol-α-arabinoside, 26-deoxycimicifugoside,[16,17] and actaeaepoxide-3-O-β-D-xylopyranoside.[18] Daucosterol-6′-lineolate.The major triterpene glycosides of this complex mixture appear to be cimicifugoside, actein, 23-epi-26-deoxyactein and cimiracemosides A, C and F.[G76]

Other constituents Acetic acid, butyric acid, formic, palmitic and salicylic acids, hydroxycinnamic acid esters of fukiic and piscidic acids (e.g. fukinolic acid, cimicifugic acids A, B, E, F),[19] glyceryl-L-palmitate.[16]

Related species 23-epi-26-deoxyactein (formerly 27-deoxyactein) is present in *C. dahurica* and *C. foetida*. The triterpenoid pattern differs in seven species.[20]

Quality of plant material and commercial products

As with other herbal medicinal products, there is variation in the qualitative and quantitative composition of black cohosh crude plant material and commercial black cohosh root/rhizome preparations.

Analysis of methanol extracts of black cohosh rhizomes using thin-layer chromatography and fluorometry found the content of formononetin to be in the range 3.1–3.5 μg/g dry weight (detection limit 0.08 parts per million).[2] Contents of isoferulic acid and total triterpene glycosides, analysed using other techniques, were within the range 1.22–1.35 and 20.1–22.1 mg/g dry weight, respectively. By contrast, formononetin was not detected in any of 13 samples of black cohosh root and rhizome collected in the year 2000 from various locations in the Eastern United States of America and extracted with 80% methanol, according to thin-layer chromatographic and high-performance liquid chromatographic techniques.[3] Similarly, formononetin and ononin (formononetin-7-glucoside) were not detected in two commercial products (Remifemin and CimiPure) available in the USA. However, the method for determination of the limits of detection used in this study, and the reliability of the results, have been questioned.[2] Another analytical study of commercial preparations of black cohosh also did not detect formononetin in the products tested, although other flavonoids were present.[21]

In another analytical study, a sample of black cohosh plant material and six commercial products purchased from shops in North Carolina, USA, and labelled as containing black cohosh, were examined for content of 23-epi-26-deoxyactein and other triterpene glycosides using LC/TIS-MS (liquid chromatography/turbo-ion spray-mass spectrometry). The crude plant material, extracted with chloroform–methanol (1 : 1, v/v), contained 0.8 mg/g 23-epi-26-deoxyactein (10.6% of total triterpene glycosides) and had a total triterpene glycoside content of 7.2 mg/g.[20] The 23-epi-26-deoxyactein and total triterpene glycoside contents of commercial products varied, ranging from 0.1–0.4 mg/capsule and 1.3–3.0 mg/capsule, respectively, for the three products formulated as capsules, and were 0.3 mg/mL and 3.6 mg/mL, respectively, for a liquid extract, 0.1 mg/tablet and 0.4 mg/tablet, respectively, for a tablet product, and 0.1 mg/tablet and 0.5 mg/tablet, respectively, for a sublingual tablet product. The actual total triterpene glycoside content also varied from that stated on the product labels for the five products providing this information; in three cases, the actual content was substantially higher than the quantity stated on the labels (3.0, 1.6 mg/capsule and 3.6 mg/mL versus 1.0, 1.0 mg/capsule and 2.0 mg/mL), and for the two other products, was substantially lower than that stated on the labels (0.38 and 0.45 versus one mg/tablet for both).

Contamination of *C. racemosa* products with other species, such as *C. foetida*, *C. dahurica* and *C. heracleifolia*, has occurred.[22] While some of these other species do contain 23-epi-26-deoxyactein and certain other constituents of *C. racemosa*, the phytochemical profile of different *Cimicifuga* species differs qualitatively and quantitatively.[3]

Detailed descriptions of *C. racemosa* rhizome for use in botanical, microscopic and macroscopic identification have been published, along with qualitative and quantitative methods for the assessment of *C. racemosa* rhizome raw material.[G1]

Food Use

Black cohosh is not used in foods.

Herbal Use

Black cohosh is stated to possess antirheumatic, antitussive, sedative and emmenagogue properties. It has been used for intercostal myalgia, sciatica, whooping cough, chorea, tinnitus, dysmenorrhoea, uterine colic, and specifically for muscular rheumatism and rheumatoid arthritis.[G6, G7, G8, G32, G64] Modern use of black cohosh is focused on its use in treating peri- and postmenopausal symptoms.

Dosage

Dosages for oral administration (adults) for traditional uses recommended in older and contemporary standard herbal reference texts are given below.

Dried rhizome/root 40–200 mg daily.[G6]

Liquid extract Ethanolic extracts equivalent to 40 mg dried rhizome/root daily.[G3, G50]

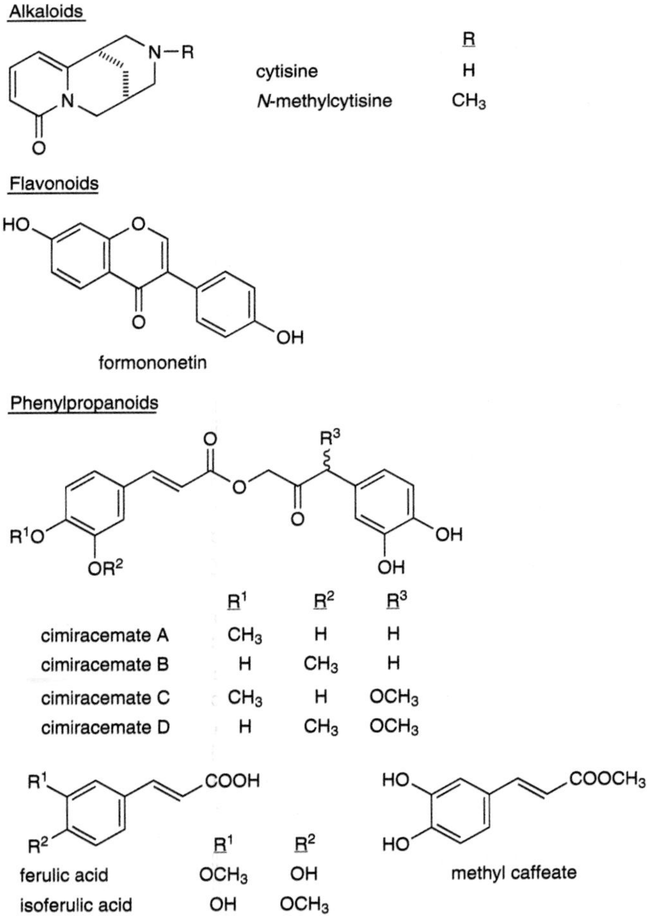

Alkaloids

	R
cytisine	H
N-methylcytisine	CH_3

Flavonoids

formononetin

Phenylpropanoids

	R^1	R^2	R^3
cimiracemate A	CH_3	H	H
cimiracemate B	H	CH_3	H
cimiracemate C	CH_3	H	OCH_3
cimiracemate D	H	CH_3	OCH_3

	R^1	R^2
ferulic acid	OCH_3	OH
isoferulic acid	OH	OCH_3

methyl caffeate

Figure 1 Selected constituents of black cohosh.

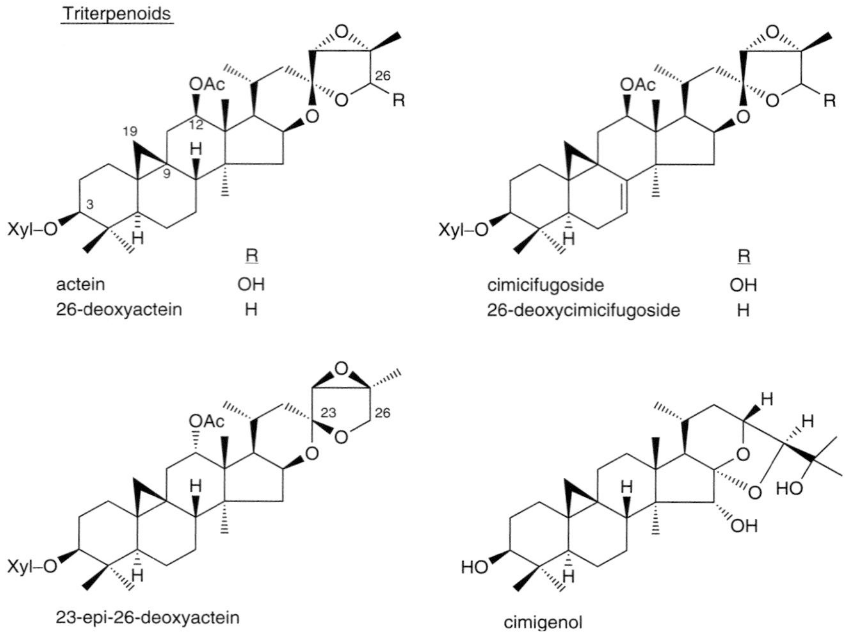

Triterpenoids

	R
actein	OH
26-deoxyactein	H

	R
cimicifugoside	OH
26-deoxycimicifugoside	H

23-epi-26-deoxyactein

cimigenol

Figure 2 Selected constituents of black cohosh.

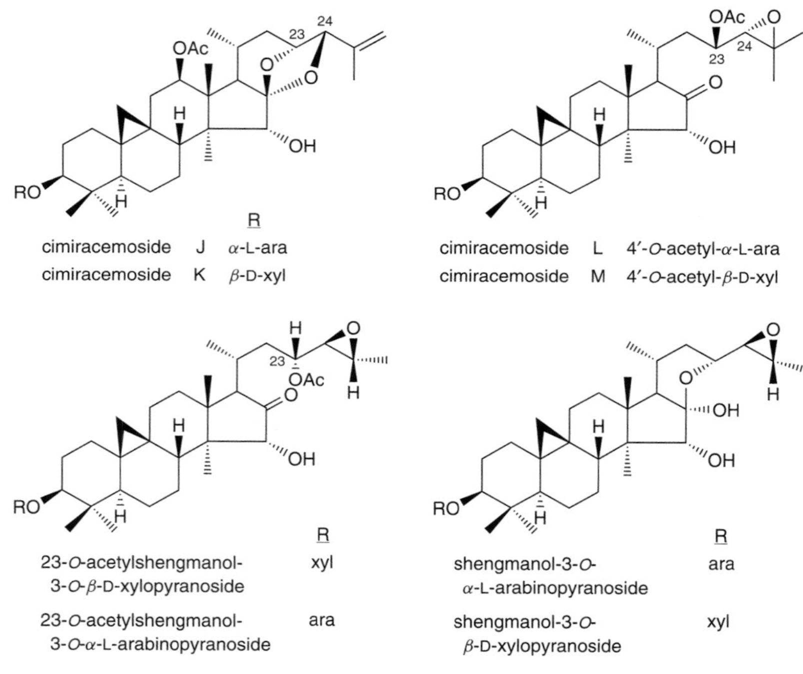

Figure 3 Selected constituents of black cohosh.

Tincture 0.4–2 mL (1 : 10 in 60% ethanol) daily.[G6]

Controlled clinical trials assessing black cohosh preparations for the treatment of menopausal symptoms typically have used an aqueous-isopropanolic standardised extract of black cohosh rhizome (Remifemin; each 20 mg tablet contains 1 mg triterpene glycosides, calculated as 27-deoxyactein (now known as 23-epi-26-deoxyactein)) 40 mg twice daily for up to 24 weeks, or an aqueous-ethanolic extract of black cohosh rhizome (Klimadynon/Menofem/BNO-1055; not further specified) at doses equivalent to 40 mg crude drug daily; treatment in clinical trials typically has been for 12 weeks.

Pharmacological Actions

In vitro and animal studies

Preclinical research with black cohosh preparations has focused on exploring hormonal activity, and there are conflicting results on this. Several other pharmacological activities, including anti-inflammatory and analgesic activities, have been documented for black cohosh extracts and/or their constituents. The triterpene glycosides and flavonoids are considered to be important for activity, although as a mechanism of action for black cohosh has not been established, whether or not other known or as yet undocumented constituents contribute to the observed effects is unclear.

Hormonal activity There are conflicting results regarding oestrogenic activity of black cohosh root/rhizome preparations. There is evidence from older *in vitro* and *in vivo* studies that black cohosh preparations have oestrogenic activity, although more recent research has indicated a lack of oestrogenic activity, antioestrogenic activity and, in some studies, antioestrogenic activity and selective oestrogen receptor activity. A review of 15 *in vitro* and 15 *in vivo* (animals) experiments assessing the effects of different extracts and fractions of black cohosh material concluded that *C. racemosa* does not have hormonal effects and that it may act by a central mechanism,[23] although data to support the latter are limited at present. Further research using well-characterised extracts is required to determine the precise mechanism(s) of action of black cohosh rhizome. The following is a summary of some of the preclinical research on the pharmacological effects of black cohosh extracts and their constituent compounds.

A methanolic extract of the rhizome of black cohosh reduced the serum concentration of luteinising hormone (LH) in ovariectomised rats, and exhibited a binding affinity to oestrogen receptors in isolated rat uterus.[5] *In vivo*, the activity of the methanolic extract was significantly reduced following enzymatic hydrolysis of glucosides present. Subsequent *in vitro* studies isolated three compounds with endocrine activity, including an isoflavone, formononetin. Formononetin was found to exhibit competitive oestrogen receptor activity, but did not cause a reduction in serum concentrations of LH.[5]

In ovariectomised rats, administration of a lipophilic extract of black cohosh (140 mg by intraperitoneal injection for three days) led to a significant reduction in serum LH concentrations, compared with control ($p < 0.01$), whereas no effect was observed with a hydrophilic extract (216 mg intraperitoneally for three days).[24] Subsequent studies using fractions of the lipophilic extract demonstrated that constituents inhibited LH secretion and/or exhibited activity in an oestrogen receptor-binding assay.

Oestrogenic activity has been documented *in vitro* for fukinolic acid, a hydroxycinnamic acid ester of fukiic acid, in oestrogen-dependent MCF-7 cells (a breast cancer cell line).[19] Fukinolic acid at concentrations of 5×10^{-7} mol/L and 5×10^{-8} mol/L led to significantly increased cell proliferation (mean (standard deviation): +120 (6%) and +126 (5%), respectively), compared with control. These effects were reported to be equivalent to those of estradiol at 10^{-10} mol/L.

By contrast, in animal models of cancer, black cohosh extracts have not demonstrated oestrogenic activity. An isopropanolic extract of black cohosh rhizome administered by gavage at doses of 0.71, 7.1 and 71.4 mg/kg body weight daily (estimated to be 1-, 10- and 100-fold times the therapeutic dose used in humans) for six weeks did not stimulate growth of chemically induced breast tumours in ovariectomised rats (tumours were induced five to nine weeks before ovariectomy), whereas rats treated with mestranol 450 μg/kg/day for six weeks had a significantly higher number of tumours, compared with control ($p < 0.01$).[25] Similarly, in an animal model of endometrial cancer, an isopropanolic extract of black cohosh rhizome administered via animals' drinking water to achieve a dose of 60 mg herbal drug/kg body weight daily and initiated on the same day as inoculation of animals with RUCA-I rat endometrial adenocarcinoma cells,[26] mean tumour mass after five weeks was reported to be similar in black cohosh treated animals and control animals, although no statistical tests were reported to support this.

Several *in vitro* studies using black cohosh preparations have also described a lack of oestrogenic activity and inhibition, or lack of promotion, of proliferation of breast cancer cells. A methanol extract of black cohosh rhizomes and roots did not demonstrate oestrogenic activity in several assays, including binding affinity for oestrogen receptors α and β, stimulation of pS2 mRNA expression in S30 cells (S30 is a subclone of an oestrogen receptor-negative

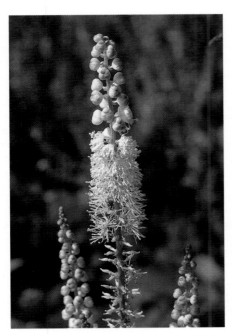

Figure 4 Black cohosh (*Cimicifuga racemosa*).

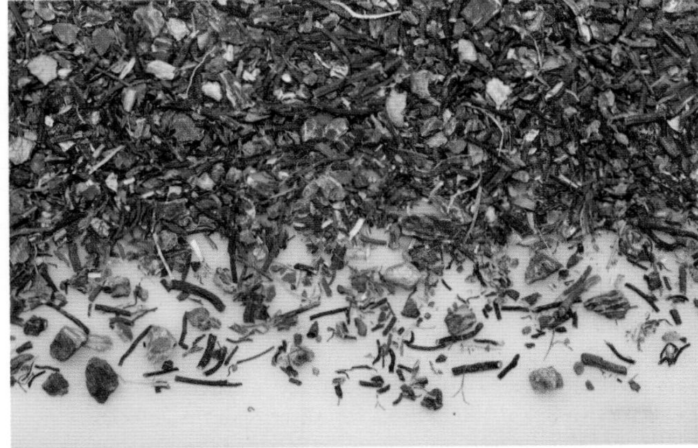

Figure 5 Black cohosh – dried drug substance (root).

C

breast cancer cell line), and induction of alkaline phosphatase in an oestrogen receptor-positive endometrial adenocarcinoma cell line.[27]

In studies using the oestrogen receptor-positive breast cancer cell lines MCF-7 and T47D, hexane, ethyl acetate and aqueous extracts of black cohosh dried roots and rhizomes (obtained from crude plant material initially extracted with 80% methanol which was then fractionated),[28] and phenolic esters from a 50% ethanolic extract of black cohosh rhizomes[29] did not have oestrogenic activity and did not lead to proliferation effects in these cell lines. An ethyl acetate extract was found to be more potent than hexane and water extracts in inhibiting growth of MCF-7 cells and oestrogen receptor-negative MDA-MB-453 cells, with IC_{50} values of 20 and 10 µg/mL, respectively.[30]

In another *in vitro* study using oestrogen receptor-positive breast cancer cells, black cohosh extract did not stimulate cancer cell growth and, at a concentration of 2.5 µg/mL, led to a marked inhibition of breast cancer cell proliferation.[31] Inhibition of MCF-7 cell proliferation has also been described for an isopropanolic extract of black cohosh rhizome *in vitro*, and further experiments indicated that the black cohosh extract at certain dilutions enhanced the proliferation-inhibiting effect of tamoxifen in the same system.[32] Further work has suggested that extracts of black cohosh root and rhizome activate caspase enzymes and induce apoptosis in both MCF-7 oestrogen receptor-positive breast cancer cells and MDA-MB-231 oestrogen receptor-negative breast cancer cells.[33] Triterpene glycoside and cinnamic acid ester fractions inhibited growth of MCF-7 cells with IC_{50} values of 59.3 and 26.1 µg/mL, respectively, and induced apoptosis at concentrations of 25 and 5 µg/mL, respectively.[34] An ethyl acetate fraction of black cohosh rhizome extract induced cell-cycle arrest at the G1 and G2/M phases at concentrations of 30 and 60 µg/mL, respectively, in MCF-7 cells.[30]

Anti-oestrogenic activity and a lack of oestrogenic activity have been described for ethanolic and isopropanolic extracts of black cohosh rhizome (not further specified) in three experimental systems. Oestradiol-induced stimulation of proliferation of MCF-7 cells was inhibited by black cohosh extract at a concentration of 1 µg/mL and, in two assays based on oestradiol-induced gene expression, black cohosh extract at concentrations ranging from 100–1000 µg/mL suppressed gene expression.[35] An anti-oestrogenic effect would require binding of constituents of black cohosh to oestrogen receptors, yet previous research has found that a methanol extract of black cohosh rhizomes and roots did not display binding affinity for either α or β oestrogen receptors.[27]

Other *in vitro* experiments have shown that an aqueous-ethanol extract of black cohosh rhizomes inhibited the proliferation of LNCaP (androgen-sensitive human prostate carcinoma) cells in a concentration-dependent manner. A significant reduction in cell growth was observed with the extract at concentrations over the range 0.05–10 µg/mL, when compared with control ($p < 0.05$ for all).[36] An isopropanolic extract of black cohosh rhizome activated caspase enzymes and induced apoptosis in both androgen-sensitive LNCaP cells and androgen-insensitive PC-3 and DU-145 prostate cancer cells.[37] IC_{50} values for the extract were 37.1, 53.2 and 62.7 µg/mL for LNCaP, DU-145 and PC-3 cells, respectively.

Further work has suggested that black cohosh extract has selective oestrogen receptor modifying effects. In ovariectomised rats given an aqueous-ethanolic extract of black cohosh rhizome or 17β-estradiol in their food for three months, uterine weight increased significantly in the 17β-estradiol group, but not in animals given black cohosh extract, compared with control ($p < 0.05$).[38] Black cohosh extract and 17β-estradiol reduced the extent of loss of bone mass from the metaphysis of the tibia, compared with control, three months after ovariectomy ($p < 0.05$ for both versus control). Similar results were obtained from another experiment in ovariectomised rats given a black cohosh rhizome extract (Remifemin) in their diet (equivalent to 4500 µg/kg body weight triterpene glycosides daily, calculated as 27-deoxyactein (now known as 26-deoxyactein)) for 12 weeks. At the end of the study, bone mineral density and a score for bone quality were significantly greater in the black cohosh and raloxifene (a selective oestrogen receptor modulator; positive control) groups, compared with those for the control group ($p < 0.05$ for both).[39] Bone-sparing effects have also been described for an aqueous-ethanolic extract of black cohosh rhizome in orchidectomised rats when given in the diet at a dose of around 133 mg extract daily for three months.[40]

An alternative mechanism for the activity of black cohosh extract, which does not involve oestrogenic pathways, has been proposed (*see* Pharmacological Actions, Other Activities).

Anti-inflammatory and analgesic activities Anti-inflammatory and analgesic activities have been described for constituents of black cohosh following *in vitro* and *in vivo* studies (mice and rats).

In vitro, caffeic acid, fukinolic acid and cimicifugic acids A, B, E and F inhibited the activity of neutrophil elastase in a concentration-dependent manner.[41] (Raised plasma concentrations of neutrophil elastase are a typical feature of active inflammation. Neutrophil elastase contributes to the destruction of basement membranes during inflammation.) Caffeic acid inhibited the enzyme with an IC_{50} of 16 µg/mL (93 µmol/L), whereas fukinolic acid had an IC_{50} of 0.1 µg/mL (0.23 µmol/L), relative to controls. Of the cimicifugic acids, A and B were the strongest inhibitors of the enzyme, with IC_{50} values of 2.2 µmol/L and 11.4 µmol/L, respectively.

Compared with controls, a methanol extract, a butanol-soluble fraction and a water-soluble fraction obtained from *Cimicifuga* rhizome inhibited carrageenan-induced rat paw oedema by 73–76%, 80–84% and 46–54%, respectively, compared with controls, 30–120 minutes after injection of 0.1 mL carrageenan 1%.[42] The same fractions (100 mg/kg by intraperitoneal injection), compared with controls, demonstrated analgesic activity determined by significant reductions in acetic acid-induced writhing in mice, and the methanol extract and butanol-soluble fraction also displayed analgesic activity in a tail-flick test (demonstrated by increased latency time upon infrared light exposure). All three fractions (40 µg/mL) inhibited bradykinin and histamine receptor-mediated contractions of guinea-pig ileum, and all inhibited lipopolysaccharide-induced 6-keto prostaglandin $F_{1\alpha}$ ($PGF_{1\alpha}$) formation in macrophages. Incubation of macrophages with lipopolysaccharide and the water-soluble fraction 10 µg/mL almost completely blocked (99% inhibition) lipopolysaccharide-induced 6-keto-$PGF_{1\alpha}$ formation. Lipopolysaccharide-induced 6-keto-$PGF_{1\alpha}$ formation in macrophages is related to selective expression of cyclooxygenase 2 (COX-2). The inhibitory effects of fractions of *Cimicifuga* rhizome in this model, and their inhibitory effects on bradykinin and histamine receptor-mediated reactions are possible mechanisms for the observed anti-inflammatory and analgesic activities.

Other activities A mechanism for the activity of black cohosh extract that does not involve oestrogenic pathways has been described following *in vitro* experiments. In radioligand binding studies, constituents of a 40% isopropanol extract of black cohosh roots/rhizomes were found to bind to serotonin receptors, particularly those of the 5-HT_{1A}, 5-HT_{1D} and 5-HT_7 subtypes.[43] Subsequent experiments showed that the isopropanol extract inhibited the binding of [^{3}H]-lysergic acid diethylamide to the human 5-HT_7 receptor with an IC_{50} value of 2.4 µg/mL, but inhibited the binding of a ligand to the 5-HT_{1A} receptor with less affinity (IC_{50} 13.9 µg/mL). A methanol extract inhibited the binding of ligands to these receptor subtypes with equal affinities (IC_{50} values: 2.5 and 2.2 µg/mL for the 5-HT_{1A} and 5-HT_7 subtypes, respectively). Further work indicated that a constituent (s) of the methanol extract was a mixed competitive ligand for the 5-HT_7 receptor and behaved as a partial agonist.[43]

In vitro studies using rat aortic strips have investigated the vasoactive effects of constituents of *Cimicifuga* species.[44] Cimicifugic acid D and fukinolic acid (3×10^{-4} mol/L) caused a sustained relaxation of aortic strips precontracted with noradrenaline (norepinephrine) in preparations with or without endothelium. By contrast, cimicifugic acid C inversely caused a weak contraction, and fukiic acid and cimicifugic acids A, B and E showed no vasoactivity at the concentration tested.

Triterpene compounds in black cohosh have been shown to possess hypocholesterolaemic activity *in vivo*, and an inhibitory effect on phytohaemagglutin-induced proliferative response *in vitro*. These activities were thought to be linked to molecular characteristics between the identified triterpenes and intermediates in cholesterol biosynthesis.[45]

Triterpenoid constituents from several *Cimicifuga* species, including actein from *C. racemosa*, have been investigated for antimalarial activity using *Plasmodium falciparum in vitro*.[46] Cimicifugoside (isolated from *C. simplex*) and actein were among the compounds with potent antiplasmodial activity (EC_{50} 5.0 µmol/L and 10.0 µmol/L, respectively), although activity was two- to three-fold less than that of positive controls (quinine, chloroquine and pyrimethamine).

Actein, isolated from black cohosh rhizome, has been reported to exhibit anti-HIV activity *in vitro* (EC_{50} = 0.375 µg/mL).[47]

The root of a related species, *Cimicifuga dahurica*, has been reported to exhibit antibacterial activity towards Gram-positive (*Bacillus subtilis*, *Mycobacterium smegmatis*, *Staphylococcus aureus*), and Gram-negative (*Escherichia coli*, *Shigella flexneri*, *Shigella sonnei*) organisms.[48]

In ovariectomised rats, ethyl acetate-soluble fractions from the rhizome of the related species *Cimicifuga heracleifolia* and *C. foetida* administered orally at doses of 100 mg/kg/day for 42 days led to a significant increase in bone mineral density of the lumbar spine, compared with that in untreated ovariectomised control rats.[49]

Clinical studies

Clinical trials of extracts of black cohosh preparations mainly have investigated effects in women with peri- and/or postmenopausal symptoms.

Pharmacokinetics Pharmacokinetic data for preparations of black cohosh are extremely limited. In a phase I study involving six perimenopausal women who ingested single doses (32, 64 or 128 mg) of a 70% ethanol extract of black cohosh (not further specified), mercapturate conjugates of certain constituents of black cohosh (fukinolic acid, fukiic acid, caffeic acid and cimiracemate B) were not detected in urine samples collected from participants over the following 24 hours (*see also* Side Effects, Toxicity, Preclinical data).[50]

Menopausal symptoms In a randomised (2 : 1 to the active treatment group), double-blind, controlled trial, 127 women aged 45–60 years who were in the peri or early menopausal period and were experiencing climacteric disorders, including at least three hot flushes per day during the six weeks prior to commencement of the study, received capsules containing a 60% ethanol extract of black cohosh rhizome (Cr-99, each capsule contained 6.5 mg extract; drug to extract ratio, 4.5–8.5 : 1, equivalent to 29–55 mg crude drug) one daily, or placebo, for 12 weeks.[51] At the end of the study, data from 122 participants were available for an intention-to-treat analysis (n = 81 and 41 for the black cohosh and placebo groups, respectively). There were no statistically significant differences between the two groups with respect to the two primary outcome variables (weekly weighted score for hot flushes, and the change in the Kupperman Menopausal Index score, a tool which measures major menopausal symptoms). Subgroup analysis of participants with a Kupperman Index score of at least 20 at baseline showed that the Kupperman Index score and the Menopause Rating Scale score were significantly improved in black cohosh recipients, compared with placebo recipients (p = 0.018 and 0.009, respectively). However, as the study was not designed primarily to assess the effects of black cohosh in women with moderate to severe (rather than mild) symptoms, the hypothesis that black cohosh is effective in women with moderate or severe menopausal symptoms requires testing in further randomised controlled trials involving sufficient numbers of participants.

In a randomised, double-blind, placebo-controlled trial, 80 women (mean (standard deviation) age: 51.2 (3.1) years) with menopausal symptoms received standardised black cohosh extract (Remifemin; each 20-mg tablet contained 1 mg triterpene glycosides, calculated as 27-deoxyactein) 40 mg twice daily, conjugated oestrogens 0.625 mg daily, or placebo, for 12 weeks.[52] At the end of the study, somatic and psychological symptoms, measured by the Kupperman Menopausal Index and the Hamilton Anxiety Scale, had improved significantly only in women who received black cohosh, compared with those who received oestrogen or placebo. Similarly, a significant increase in proliferation of vaginal epithelium was noted only in the black cohosh group. However, there is a view that the dose of oestrogen used in the study was too low to provide a useful comparison.

Another randomised, double-blind, placebo-controlled trial compared the effects of an aqueous-ethanolic extract of black cohosh rhizome (Klimadynon/Menofem/BNO-1055), corresponding to 40 mg herbal drug daily for three months, with those of conjugated oestrogens 0.6 mg daily for three months, in postmenopausal women (last menstrual bleed at least six months ago) aged 40–60 years with serum FSH concentrations at least 25 mU/mL and experiencing at least three hot flushes daily. Initially, 97 women were randomised to one of the three study groups, although the analysis included only 62 participants as two women withdrew before any post-baseline data were collected and data for 33 women were excluded as it was subsequently found that they did not meet the inclusion criteria with respect to having masked ovulatory or anovulatory cycles and oestrogen production in fatty tissue.[53]

The results of the study showed that Menopause Rating Scale scores (the primary outcome variable) were reduced in both the black cohosh extract and conjugated oestrogen groups, compared with baseline values, although neither of these reductions was statistically significant when compared with the reduction observed in the placebo group (p = 0.051 for both).[53] It was also reported that the black cohosh extract had no effect on endometrial thickness, whereas endometrial thickness was significantly increased, compared with placebo, in the conjugated oestrogens group ($p < 0.05$). Black cohosh extract did have beneficial effects on parameters relating to bone metabolism: serum concentrations of bone-specific alkaline phosphatase (indicating increased activity of osteoblast cells, which are responsible for bone formation) were significantly increased in the black cohosh group, but not in the conjugated oestrogens group, compared with placebo. These findings were interpreted as being indicative of selective oestrogen receptor modulatory effects for black cohosh extract,[53] although this hypothesis requires testing in further clinical studies.

A randomised, double-blind, placebo-controlled trial involving 85 women with a history of breast cancer assessed the effects of black cohosh (no details of extract provided) one tablet twice daily for 60 days on the frequency and intensity of hot flushes.[54] Participants were stratified according to whether or not they were using tamoxifen. Both treatment and placebo groups reported decreases in the number and intensity of hot flushes, compared with baseline values. There were no statistically significant differences between the two groups, and subgroup analysis of tamoxifen users and non-users did not reveal any statistically significant differences. Changes in other parameters measured during the study (other menopausal symptoms, serum concentrations of follicle-stimulating hormone (FSH) and luteinising hormone (LH)) were also not statistically significant between groups.

Another study specifically assessed the effects of black cohosh extract on gonadotrophin secretion. In a placebo-controlled trial involving 110 women with menopausal symptoms, black cohosh extract (Remifemin) two tablets daily for two months significantly reduced serum LH concentrations, compared with placebo ($p < 0.05$).[24] There was no significant difference between the two groups with respect to serum FSH concentrations.

The effects of an aqueous-isopropanolic extract of black cohosh rhizome (Remifemin) on menopausal symptoms were compared with those of low-dose transdermal estradiol treatment in a randomised controlled trial. In the study, 64 women with menopausal status for at least six months, serum FSH concentrations of > 30 mIU/L and experiencing at least five hot flushes per day received the black cohosh extract 40 mg daily for three months, or transdermal estradiol patches 25 μg every seven days for three months plus dihydrogesterone 10 mg daily for the last 12 days of the 3-month period of estradiol treatment.[55] At the end of the study, the number of hot flushes experienced by women was significantly reduced for both groups, compared with baseline values ($p < 0.001$ for both) and there was no statistically significant difference between groups, although details of statistical tests for the latter were not provided in a report of the study. There were no statistically significant changes in serum FSH and LH concentrations in either group at the end of the study ($p > 0.05$). The study has several methodological limitations, such as lack of a placebo arm, and apparent lack of blinding (the use of dummy patches and tablets was not mentioned), and the equivalence of black cohosh extract with standard treatment for menopausal symptoms requires further investigation.

In an open study, 60 women with at least one intact ovary who had undergone hysterectomy and who were experiencing menopausal symptoms were randomised to receive estriol (1 mg daily), conjugated oestrogens (1.25 mg daily), oestrogen–progestagen sequential therapy (dose not specified), or black cohosh extract (Remifemin) 40 mg twice daily, for 24 weeks.[56] At the end of the study, improvements in Kupperman Index scores were significantly lower, compared with baseline values, in all groups. There were no statistically significant differences between groups.

Another open, controlled study involving women with menopausal symptoms ($n = 60$) assessed the effects of black cohosh extract administered as a tincture (80 drops daily), compared with oestrogen (0.625 mg daily) or diazepam (2 mg daily), over a 12-week period.[57] Cytological responses (proliferation and maturation of vaginal epithelial cells) were observed for participants in the black cohosh and oestrogen groups, but not in the diazepam group. For all three groups, improvements in neurovegetative and psychological symptoms (e.g. self-assessed depression) were reported.

Other studies of black cohosh extracts involving women with menopausal symptoms lack control groups and, therefore, do not provide an unbiased assessment of effects. Generally, these studies report significant improvements in menopausal symptoms, compared with baseline values, after at least four weeks' treatment; some studies involved administration of black cohosh extract for up to 24 weeks.[58]

In a randomised, double-blind trial, 152 peri- and postmenopausal women received an isopropanolic extract of black cohosh rhizome (Remifemin) at a dose equivalent to 39 or 127 mg crude drug daily for 24 weeks.[59] At the 12-week and 24-week endpoints, data from 149 and 116 participants, respectively, were available for intention-to-treat analyses. Kupperman Index scores decreased significantly in both the low- and high-dose groups, compared with baseline values, and there was no statistically significant difference between groups ($p = 0.73$). No statistically significant differences were observed for either group in the degree of vaginal cell proliferation, and serum concentrations of FSH, LH, prolactin and 17β-oestradiol, compared with baseline values. The results of this study provide some supporting clinical evidence for a lack of oestrogenic activity of black cohosh extract, and raise the possibility of tissue-selective effects,[59] although the design of this study (no placebo or oestrogen control groups) precludes definitive conclusions.

Other conditions In an open trial, 136 women who had undergone segmental or total mastectomy, radiation therapy and/or adjuvant cancer chemotherapy were randomised to receive tamoxifen 20 mg orally daily for five years with ($n = 90$) or without ($n = 46$) an aqueous-ethanolic extract of black cohosh rhizome (BNO-1055), corresponding to 20 mg herbal drug daily for 12 months, to assess the effects of treatment with black cohosh on hot flushes caused by tamoxifen.[60] At the end of the study, significantly fewer women in the tamoxifen plus black cohosh extract group were experiencing severe hot flushes than were women in the tamoxifen alone group (25% versus 74%) and more women in the tamoxifen plus black cohosh extract group were not experiencing hot flushes at all (47% versus 0%); proportions of women experiencing hot flushes of moderate severity were similar (29% versus 26%). The difference in outcome between the two groups was reported to be statistically significant ($p < 0.01$),[60] although as baseline values for the proportions of women in each group experiencing hot flushes of different severities were not reported, and as the study used an open-label design, it is not possible to draw firm conclusions from this finding.

A randomised, double-blind, placebo-controlled trial assessed the prophylactic effects of a combination preparation (tablets containing 75 mg soy extract, standardised for 40% isoflavones, 50 mg dong quai extract, standardised for 1% ligustilide, and 25 mg black cohosh extract, standardised for 8% triterpenes; not further specified) in 49 women who experienced migraine attacks associated with menstruation.[61] Participants took one tablet twice daily, or placebo, for 24 weeks. At the end of the study, the mean number of menstrual migraine attacks was significantly lower in the treatment group, compared with the placebo group ($p < 0.01$). The contribution of black cohosh to the observed effect is unclear in view of recent studies that have described a lack of oestrogenic activity for black cohosh extracts. (There is evidence of an association between oestrogen concentrations and menstrual migraine attacks).[61]

In a randomised, double-blind, controlled trial, 82 patients with osteoarthritis or rheumatoid arthritis received a proprietary combination herbal preparation containing black cohosh 35 mg (other ingredients: white willow bark, guaiacum resin, sarsaparilla and poplar bark; Reumalex), or placebo, two tablets daily for two months.[62] At the end of the study, there was a small, but statistically significant improvement in pain symptoms (as assessed by the Arthritis Pain Scale) in the treatment group, compared with the placebo group ($p < 0.05$).

Side-effects, Toxicity

Clinical data

There are only limited clinical data on safety aspects of black cohosh preparations from clinical trials and post-marketing surveillance-type studies.

Randomised, double-blind, placebo-controlled trials of black cohosh preparations in women with menopausal symptoms have reported that the frequency of adverse events was similar for the black cohosh and placebo groups. Clinical trials, however, are designed primarily to assess efficacy, not safety, and have the statistical power only to detect common, acute adverse effects. In a randomised, double-blind, controlled trial in which 127 women aged 45–60 years in the peri- or early menopausal period received capsules containing a 60% ethanol extract of black cohosh rhizome (Cr-99, each capsule contained 6.5 mg extract; drug to extract ratio, 4.5-8.5 : 1, equivalent to 29–55 mg crude drug) one daily, or placebo, for 12 weeks, 20 and 23% of participants in the black cohosh and placebo groups, respectively, reported adverse events.[51] In another randomised, double-blind, placebo-controlled trial in which postmenopausal women received an aqueous-ethanolic extract of black cohosh rhizome (BNO-1055), corresponding to 40 mg herbal drug daily, conjugated oestrogens 0.6 mg daily, or placebo, for three months, no serious adverse events occurred and the frequency of mild or moderate non-serious adverse events was stated to be similar in all three groups.[53] Another randomised, double-blind, placebo-controlled trial involving women with menopausal symptoms ($n = 80$) who received standardised black cohosh extract (Remifemin) 40 mg twice daily, conjugated oestrogens, or placebo, for 12 weeks reported that non-specific adverse events, such as headaches, not considered to be treatment-related, occurred in all three groups.[52]

In a further randomised, double-blind, placebo-controlled trial, which involved 85 women with a history of breast cancer who received black cohosh (no details of extract provided) one tablet twice daily, or placebo, for 60 days, ten adverse events occurred in the treatment group, compared with three in the placebo group.[54] Three events were considered serious (treatment group: hysterectomy, recurrence of breast cancer; placebo group: appendectomy) all of which occurred in women who were also receiving tamoxifen. Minor adverse events (including constipation, weight gain, cramping, indigestion, vaginal bleeding) were not thought to be treatment related.

Post-marketing surveillance studies involving over 2500 women with menopausal symptoms have reported few serious adverse events for black cohosh extracts, although these studies have been of relatively short duration (up to 12 weeks) and have monitored the effects of different black cohosh preparations. In view of this, further, large, long-term drug monitoring studies of well-characterised black cohosh extracts are required to provide data on the safety of these preparations. In a post marketing surveillance study involving 629 women with menopausal symptoms who received standardised black cohosh extract as a tincture (40 drops twice daily for 6–8 weeks, tolerability was rated as 'good' in 93% of patients; mild, transient adverse events, such as nausea, vomiting, headache and dizziness, were noted in 7% of patients.[63] In a post-marketing surveillance study involving 2016 Hungarian women with menopausal symptoms who received an isopropanolic extract of black cohosh rhizome (Remifemin) for up to 12 weeks, 24% of participants found the treatment to be ineffective, 16% did not attend a final assessment, and 12% reported 'unexpected adverse effects'.[64] Overall, 35 participants reported specific adverse effects, most commonly stiffening of the extremeties ($n = 8$), gastric pain (7) and allergic reactions (6). Other adverse effects reported included breast tenderness, bleeding disturbances (not further specified) and gastrointestinal complaints. A report of the study indicates that these data were collected using postal questionnaires, although it is not clear how questions regarding safety aspects were phrased, including whether participants were asked to report adverse effects or adverse events.

Systematic reviews, conducted during 2001 and 2002,[65, 66] of information concerning safety aspects of black cohosh preparations have concluded that on the basis of the available limited evidence, certain black cohosh preparations (i.e. those that have been the subject of clinical investigations and/or have otherwise been subject to safety monitoring) are well-tolerated when used according to recommended dosage regimens.

Hepatotoxicity Several case reports describe hepatoxic reactions associated with the use of preparations containing black cohosh. One report describes a 47-year-old woman who developed jaundice and raised liver function test values one week after beginning treatment with a product stated to contain black cohosh for menopausal symptoms.[67] Biopsy confirmed severe hepatitis and the woman underwent liver transplantation. In a second case, a 43-year-old woman was reported to have taken a combination herbal preparation containing black cohosh as well as skullcap, valerian and five other herbal ingredients. The woman developed jaundice and raised liver function test values.[67] For both of these cases, descriptions of the products taken lack important details, and it appears that samples of the products were not available, therefore, analysis of the preparations implicated was not undertaken. Causality in these cases has not been established.

In a randomised controlled trial in which 64 menopausal women received an aqueous-isopropanolic extract of black cohosh rhizome (Remifemin) 40 mg daily for three months, or low-dose estradiol treatment (transdermal patches delivering 25 µg every seven days for three months plus dihydrogesterone 10 mg daily for the last 12 days of the 3-month period of estradiol treatment), there were no statistically significant differences in liver function test values (aspartate transaminase and alanine transaminase concentrations) in the black cohosh group at the end of the study, compared with baseline values.[55]

The World Health Organization's Uppsala Monitoring Centre (WHO-UMC; Collaborating Centre for International Drug Monitoring) receives summary reports of suspected adverse drug reactions from national pharmacovigilance centres of over 70 countries worldwide. To the end of the year 2005, the WHO-UMC's Vigisearch database contained a total of 143 reports, describing a total of 328 adverse reactions, for products reported to contain *C. racemosa* only as the active ingredient (*see* Table 1).[68] This number may include the case reports described above. Reports originated from several 13 different countries. The total number of reports included 31 reports, originating from five countries (18 reports originated from the UK), describing a total of 46 reactions associated with liver and biliary system disorders (*see* Table 1), including two cases of hepatic failure. Where the age and gender of the cases were known (n = 30 reports), all were female and aged between 38 and 66 years. Where the outcome of the case was documented (n = 24 reports), ten cases recovered and 14 had not recovered. Causality had been assessed for seven cases; for these, a causal association with black cohosh use was determined to be 'possible' in five cases and 'certain' in two cases. (These data were obtained from the Vigisearch database held by the WHO Collaborating Centre for International Drug Monitoring, Uppsala, Sweden. The information is not homogeneous at least with respect to origin or likelihood that the pharmaceutical product caused the adverse reaction. Any information included in this report does not represent the opinion of the World Health Organization).

By March 2006, the UK's spontaneous reporting scheme for suspected adverse drug reactions (ADRs) had received 21 reports of suspected ADRs describing reactions in the liver associated with the use of preparations containing black cohosh rhizome/root; the total number of reports received in the UK for all

Table 1 Summary of spontaneous reports (n = 143) of suspected adverse drug reactions associated with single-ingredient *Cimicifuga racemosa* preparations held in the Vigisearch database of the World Health Organization's Uppsala Monitoring Centre for the period up to end of 2005.[a, b, 68]

System organ class. **Adverse drug reaction name (number)**	**Total**
Body as a whole – general disorders. Including back pain (5); chest pain (3); malaise (3); pain (7)	40
Cardiovascular disorders, general. Including hypertension (5)	6
Central and peripheral nervous system disorders. Including convulsions (5); dizziness (3); headache (6)	17
Collagen disorders.	2
Endocrine disorders.	1
Gastrointestinal system disorders. Including abdominal pain (8); diarrhoea (5); dyspepsia (3); nausea (10)	44
Hearing and vestibular disorders.	1
Heart rate and rhythm disorders. Including tachycardia (3)	9
Liver and biliary system disorders. Including hepatic function abnormal (13); hepatitis (12); jaundice (3); hepatic enzymes increased (4); SGPT increased (4)	46
Metabolic and nutritional disorders. Including diabetes mellitus (3)	8
Musculo-skeletal system disorders.	4
Myo-endopericardial and valve disorders.	1
Neoplasm. Including breast, neoplasm benign female (3)	7
Platelet, bleeding and clotting disorders.	7
Psychiatric disorders.	15
Red blood cell disorders.	1
Reproductive disorders, female and male. Including menstrual disorder (3); breast enlargement (5); breast pain (4); breast pain, female (6); post-menstrual bleeding (5)	40
Resistance mechanism disorders.	1
Respiratory system disorders. Including dyspnoea (5)	8
Skin and appendages disorders. Including angioedema (4); pruritus (7); rash (7); rash, erythematous (5)	35
Special senses other, disorders.	1
Urinary system disorders. Including face oedema (4); urinary tract infection (3)	15
Vascular (extracardiac) disorders.	5
Vision disorders.	2
White cell and res. disorders. Including granulocytopenia (3)	1
Other reactions described using terms not included in database	11
Total number of suspected adverse drug reactions	**328**

[a]Specific reactions described where n = 3 or more
[b]Caveat statement. These data were obtained from the Vigisearch database held by the WHO Collaborating Centre for International Drug Monitoring, Uppsala, Sweden. The information is not homogeneous at least with respect to origin or likelihood that the pharmaceutical product caused the adverse reaction. Any information included in this report does not represent the opinion of the World Health Organization

reactions associated with black cohosh was 31.[69] After assessment, 14 reports were considered to support a relationship between use of black cohosh rhizome and liver damage: hepatitis ($n = 4$); abnormal liver function test values (9); jaundice (1). For ten of these cases, black cohosh use was considered to have 'probably' led to liver damage. For a further six cases, the relationship could not be assessed because of limited available information.[69]

On the basis of these data, in July 2006, the UK Medicines and Healthcare products Regulatory Agency (MHRA) issued recommendations that warnings should be added to preparations containing black cohosh rhizome/root regarding the association between such products and liver ADRs,[69] and advised that patients taking black cohosh preparations and who feel unwell and/or experience new symptoms (particularly those indicative of liver disease) should consult their doctor.[70] Individuals who have previously experienced liver complaints or other serious health conditions should not use black cohosh preparations without first consulting their doctor.

The European Medicines Agency undertook a similar assessment of reports originating within the European Union, and issued the following advice:

- patients should stop taking preparations containing black cohosh rhizome/root and consult their doctor immediately if they experience signs and/or symptoms indicative of liver injury, such as tiredness, loss of appetite, yellowing of the skin, and eyes, severe upper stomach pain with nausea and vomiting, dark urine
- healthcare professionals should ask patients about use of preparations containing black cohosh rhizome/root.[71]

Preclinical data

In an *in vitro* study in which a 70% ethanol extract of black cohosh (not further specified) was incubated with GSH (glutathione), NADPH and a preparation of rat liver microsomes, the formation of eight electrophilic metabolites, including quinoid metabolites of fukinolic acid, fukiic acid, caffeic acid and cimiracemate B, was described.[50]

In mice, LD_{50} values for a black cohosh extract following intragastric and intravenous administration have been found to be 7.7 and 1.1 g/kg body weight, respectively.[72]

Contra-indications, Warnings

There are reports of hepatotoxic reactions associated with the use of black cohosh rhizome/root preparations. Patients should be advised to stop taking black cohosh preparations, and to consult their doctor if they experience symptoms that may indicate liver injury.

Until further information is available, it is appropriate to advise that black cohosh preparations should not be taken by individuals with oestrogen-sensitive tumours, such as breast cancer. The scientific basis for this statement is that there are conflicting results from preclinical studies regarding oestrogenic activity of black cohosh preparations. There is evidence from older *in vitro* and *in vivo* studies that black cohosh preparations have oestrogenic activity, although more recent research has indicated a lack of oestrogenic activity and a small number of studies has described selective oestrogen receptor activity or anti-oestrogenic activity. On balance, preclinical research seems to indicate that extracts of black cohosh root/rhizome do not have hormonal effects, but further study is required to confirm this and to elucidate the mechanism(s) of action of black cohosh constituents. Evidence from clinical studies is also unclear: some studies have described effects for black cohosh preparations indicative of oestrogenic activity, whereas in other studies such effects have not been observed, or selective effects (e.g. effects on bone but not uterine tissue) have been described.

There is concern that the use of herbal medicines with oestrogenic activity by women with breast cancer might stimulate the growth of breast cancer cells and interfere with the effects of competitive oestrogen receptor antagonists such as tamoxifen[73] (although, in general, preclinical studies have not observed breast cancer cell proliferation and one *in vitro* study found that black cohosh extract enhanced the proliferation inhibiting effect of tamoxifen on breast cancer cells.[32]) In a randomised, double-blind, placebo-controlled trial involving 85 women with a history of breast cancer, one woman receiving both black cohosh and tamoxifen experienced a recurrence of breast cancer, although it was reported that the woman had an increase in carcinoembryonic antigen concentration when she entered the trial (this had not been reported to the referring physician).[54]

Drug interactions In view of the documented pharmacological actions of black cohosh the potential for preparations of black cohosh to interfere with other medicines administered concurrently, particularly those with similar or opposing effects, should be considered.

In a randomised, crossover study, 12 healthy volunteers received a black cohosh root extract (stated to be standardised for 0.2% triterpene glycosides; not further specified) 1090 mg twice daily for 28 days to assess effects on cytochrome P450 enzyme activity. Presence of 27-deoxyactein (now known as 23-epi-26-deoxyactein), actein and cimiracemoside was confirmed using reversed-phase HPLC with light scattering detection. It was reported that black cohosh extract significantly inhibited CYP2D6 activity, but the extent of inhibition may not be clinically relevant.[74]

In vitro experiments using EMT6 mouse mammary tumour cells have shown that black cohosh extracts at concentrations equivalent to 2.5 times recommended therapeutic doses increased the cytotoxicity of doxorubicin when the two substances were added to the cell system.[75] In similar experiments, black cohosh extracts also increased the cytotoxicity of docetaxel and decreased the cytotoxicity of cisplatin. The clinical relevance of these findings, particularly with respect to the effects of increased doxorubicin sensitivity in bone marrow and myocardial cells, is unknown.

Pregnancy and lactation There are insufficient data on the use of black cohosh preparations during pregnancy and breastfeeding, and the use of such preparations is contraindicated during these periods.

There are conflicting data on oestrogenic activity of black cohosh, including the effects of black cohosh preparations on uterine tissue (*see* Pharmacological Actions).

There is an isolated report of a child born with no spontaneous breathing and who subsequently experienced brain hypoxia and seizures following the oral administration of black cohosh and blue cohosh by a midwife in an attempt to induce labour in a woman who had had an uneventful pregnancy.[76] The report has been criticised as it did not provide any further details of the dose or formulation of the herbs, and as the authors of the report make several assumptions about the clinical activity of the herbs on the basis of studies in animals.[77]

C

Preparations

Proprietary single-ingredient preparations

Argentina: Menofem. *Austria:* Agnukliman; Jinda; Klimadynon. *Brazil:* Aplause; Clifemin; Mencirax; Menoliv; Tensiane. *Chile:* Ginemaxim; Mensifem. *Czech Republic:* Menofem. *France:* Cimipax. *Germany:* Cefakliman mono; Cimisan; Femi; Femikliman uno; Femilla N; Feminon C; Femisana gyn; Jinda; Klimadynon; Natu-fem; Remifemin; Sinei; Solcosplen C. *Hong Kong:* Klimadynon. *Hungary:* Cefakliman mono; Remifemin. *Russia:* Klimadynon (Климадинон). *Singapore:* Klimadynon; Remifemin. *Spain:* Avala; Remifemin. *Switzerland:* Cimifemine; Climavita; Femicine; Maxifem. *Thailand:* Remifemin.

Proprietary multi-ingredient preparations

Australia: Cimicifuga Compound; Dong Quai Complex; Dyzco; Extralife Meno-Care; Extralife PMS-Care; Herbal PMS Formula; Lifesystem Herbal Formula 4 Women's Formula; Medinat Esten; PMT Complex; Proesten; Soy Forte with Black Cohosh; Women's Formula Herbal Formula 3. *Austria:* Remifemin plus. *Canada:* Natural HRT. *Czech Republic:* Dr Theiss Rheuma Creme; Dr Theiss Schwedenbitter. *Germany:* Remifemin plus. *Italy:* Climil Complex; Climil-80; Hiperogyn. *Singapore:* Phytoestrin. *UK:* Gerard House Reumalex; Modern Herbals Rheumatic Pain; St Johnswort Compound; Vegetable Cough Remover; Vegetex. *USA:* Black Cohosh; Estrocare; Hot Flashex; Menopause Relief; Menopause Support; Natrol Complete Balance for Menopause AM/PM Formula; Women's Menopause Formula.

References

1 Jarry H *et al.* Untersuchungen zur endokrinen wirksamkeit von inhaltsstoffen aus *Cimicifuga racemosa* 2. In vitro-bindung von inhaltsstoffen an östrogenrezeptoren. *Planta Med* 1985; 51: 316–319.

2 Panossian A *et al.* Methods of phytochemical standardisation of rhizoma *Cimicifugae racemosae. Phytochemical Anal* 2004; 15: 100–108.

3 Kennelly EJ *et al.* Analysis of thirteen populations of black cohosh for formononetin. *Phytomedicine* 2002; 9: 461–467.

4 Chen S-N *et al.* Cimiracemates A-D, phenylpropanoid esters from the rhizomes of *Cimicifuga racemosa. Phytochemistry* 2002; 61: 409–413.

5 Jarry H, Harnischfeger G. Untersuchungen zur endokrinen wirksamkeit von inhaltsstoffen aus *Cimicifuga racemosa* 1. Einfluss auf die serum spiegel von hypophysenhormonen ovariektomierter ratten. *Planta Med* 1985; 51: 46–49.

6 Linde H. Die inhaltsstoffe von Cimicifuga racemosa 2. Mitt.: zur struktur des acteins. *Arch Pharm* 1967; 300: 885–892.

7 Linde H. Die inhaltsstoffe von Cimicifuga racemosa 3. Mitt.: über die konstitution der ringe A, B and C des acteins. *Arch Pharm* 1967; 300: 982–992.

8 Linde H. Die inhaltsstoffe von Cimicifuga racemosa 4. Mitt.: actein: der ring D und seitenkette. *Arch Pharm* 1968; 301: 120–138.

9 Linde H. Die inhaltsstoffe von Cimicifuga racemosa 5. Mitt.: 27-desoxyacetylacteol. *Arch Pharm* 1968; 301: 335–341.

10 Radics L *et al.* Carbon-13 NMR spectra of some polycyclic triterpenoids. *Tetrahedron Lett* 1975; 48: 4287–4290.

11 Chen S-N *et al.* Isolation, structure elucidation, and absolute configuration of 26-deoxyactein from *Cimicifuga racemosa* and clarification of nomenclature associated with 27-deoxyactein. *J Nat Prod* 2002; 65: 601–605.

12 Bedir E, Khan IA. Cimiracemoside A: a new cyclolanostanol xyloside from the rhizome of *Cimicifuga racemosa. Chem Pharm Bull* 2000; 48: 425–427.

13 Shao Y *et al.* Triterpene glycosides from *Cimicifuga racemosa. J Nat Prod* 2000; 63: 905–910.

14 Bedir E, Khan IA. A new cyclolanostanol arabinoside from the rhizome of *Cimicifuga racemosa. Pharmazie* 2001; 56: 268–269.

15 Sakurai N *et al.* Studies on the Chinese crude drug 'Shoma.' X. Three new trinor-9,19-cyclolanostanol xylosides, cimicifugosides H-3, H-4 and H-6, from Cimicifuga rhizome and transformation of cimicifugoside H-1 into cimicifugosides H-2, H-3 and H-4. *Chem Pharm Bull* 1995; 43: 1475–1482.

16 Chen S-N *et al.* Cimiracemosides I-P, new 9,19-cycloanostane triterpene glycosides from *Cimicifuga racemosa. J Nat Prod* 2002; 65: 1391–1397.

17 Hamburger M *et al.* Cycloartane glycosides from *Cimicifuga racemosa. Pharm Pharmacol Lett* 2001; 2: 98–100.

18 Wende K *et al.* Actaeaepoxide 3-O-β-D-xylopyranoside, a new cycloartane glycoside from the rhizomes of *Actaea racemosa* (*Cimicifuga racemosa*). *J Nat Prod* 2001; 64: 986–989.

19 Kruse SO *et al.* Fukiic and piscidic acid esters from the rhizome of *Cimicifuga racemosa* and the in vitro estrogenic activity of fukinolic acid. *Planta Med* 1999; 65: 763–764.

20 Wang H-K *et al.* LC/TIS-MS fingerprint profiling of *Cimicifuga* species and analysis of 23-epi-26-deoxyactein in *Cimicifuga racemosa* commercial products. *J Agric Food Chem* 2005; 53: 1379–1386.

21 Struck D *et al.* Flavones in extracts of *Cimicifuga racemosa. Planta Med* 1997; 63: 289.

22 Halliday J. AHPA urges black cohosh, caffeine action. USA NutraIngredients.com. http://www.nutraingredients-usa.com/news/ (accessed August 22, 2005).

23 Borrelli F *et al.* Pharmacological effects of *Cimicifuga racemosa. Life Sci* 2003; 73: 1215–1229.

24 Düker E-M *et al.* Effects of extracts from *Cimicifuga racemosa* on gonadotropin release in menopausal women and ovariectomized rats. *Planta Med* 1991; 57: 420–424.

25 Freudenstein J *et al.* Lack of promotion of estrogen-dependent mammary gland tumors *in vivo* by an isopropanolic *Cimicifuga racemosa* extract. *Cancer Res* 2002; 62: 3448–3452.

26 Nißlein T, Freudenstein J. Concomitant administration of an isopropanolic extract of black cohosh and tamoxifen in the *in vivo* tumor model of implanted RUCA-I rat endometrial adenocarcinoma cells. *Toxicol Lett* 2004; 150: 271–275.

27 Liu J *et al.* Evaluation of estrogenic activity of plant extracts for the potential treatment of menopausal symptoms. *J Agric Food Chem* 2001; 49: 2472–2479.

28 Lupu R *et al.* Black cohosh, a menopausal remedy, does not have estrogenic activity and does not promote breast cancer cell growth. *Int J Oncology* 2003; 23: 1407–1412.

29 Stromeier S *et al.* Phenolic esters from the rhizomes of *Cimicifuga racemosa* do not cause proliferation effects in MCF-7 cells. *Planta Med* 2005; 71: 495–500.

30 Einbond LS *et al.* Growth inhibitory activity of extracts and purified components of black cohosh on human breast cancer cells. *Breast Cancer Res Treat* 2004; 83: 221–231.

31 Nesselhut T *et al.* Untersuchungen zur proliferativen Potenz von Phytopharmaka mit östrogenähnlicher Wirkung bei Mammakarzinomzellen. *Arch Gynecol Obstet* 1993; 254: 817–818.

32 Bodinet C, Freudenstein J. Influence of *Cimicifuga racemosa* on the proliferation of estrogen receptor-positive human breast cancer cells. *Breast Cancer Res Treat* 2002; 76: 1–10.

33 Hostanska K *et al. Cimicifuga racemosa* extract inhibits proliferation of estrogen receptor-positive and negative breast carcinoma cell lines by induction of apoptosis. *Breast Cancer Res Treat* 2004; 84: 151–160.

34 Hostanska K *et al.* Evaluation of cell death caused by triterpene glycosides and phenolic substances from *Cimicifuga racemosa* extract in human MCF-7 breast cancer cells. *Biol Pharm Bull* 2004; 27: 1970–1975.

35 Zierau O *et al.* Antiestrogenic activities of *Cimicifuga racemosa* extracts. *J Steroid Biochem Mol Biol* 2002; 80: 125–130.

36 Jarry H *et al. Cimicifuga racemosa* extract BNO 1055 inhibits proliferation of the human prostate cancer cell line LNCaP. *Phytomedicine* 2005; 12: 178–182.

37 Hostanska K *et al.* Apoptosis of human prostate androgen-dependent and -independent carcinoma cells induced by an isopropanolic extract of black cohosh involves degradation of cytokeratin (CK) 18. *Anticancer Res* 2005; 25: 139–148.

38 Seidlová-Wuttke D *et al*. Evidence for selective estrogen receptor modulator activity in a black cohosh (*Cimicifuga racemosa*) extract: comparison with estradiol-17β. *Eur J Endocrinol* 2003; 149: 351–362.
39 Nißlein T, Freudenstein J. Effects of an isopropanolic extract of *Cimicifuga racemosa* on urinary crosslinks and other parameters of bone quality in an ovariectomized rat model of osteoporosis. *J Bone Miner Metab* 2003; 21: 370–376.
40 Seidlová-Wuttke D *et al*. Effects of estradiol-17β, testosterone and a black cohosh preparation on bone and prostate in orchidectomized rats. *Maturitas* 2005; 51: 177–186.
41 Löser B *et al*. Inhibition of neutrophil elastase activity by cinnamic acid derivatives from *Cimicifuga racemosa*. *Planta Med* 2000; 66: 751–753.
42 Kim S-J, Kim M-S. Inhibitory effects of Cimicifugae rhizoma extracts on histamine, bradykinin and COX-2 mediated inflammatory actions. *Phytother Res* 2000; 14: 596–600.
43 Burdette JE *et al*. Black cohosh acts as a mixed competitive ligand and partial agonist of the serotonin receptor. *J Agric Food Chem* 2003; 51: 5661–5670.
44 Noguchi M *et al*. Vasoactive effects of cimicifugic acids C and D, and fukinolic acid in Cimicifuga rhizome. *Biol Pharm Bull* 1998; 21: 1163–1168.
45 Resing K, Fitzgerald A. Crystal data for 15-*o*-acetylacerinol and two related triterpenes isolated from Japanese *Cimicifuga* plants. *J Appl Crystallogr* 1978; 11: 58.
46 Takahara M *et al*. Antimalarial activity and nucleoside transport inhibitory activity of the triterpenic constituents of *Cimicifuga* spp. *Biol Pharm Bull* 1998; 21: 823–828.
47 Sakurai N *et al*. Anti-AIDS agents. Part 57: actein, an anti-HIV principle from the rhizome of *Cimicifuga racemosa* (black cohosh), and the anti-HIV activity of related saponins. *Bioorganic Med Chem Lett* 2004; 14: 1329–1332.
48 Moskalenko SA. Preliminary screening of Far-Eastern ethnomedicinal plants for antibacterial activity. *J Ethnopharmacol* 1986; 15: 231–259.
49 Li JX *et al*. Effects of Cimicifugae rhizoma on serum calcium and phosphate levels in low calcium dietary rats and on bone mineral density in ovariectomized rats. *Phytomedicine* 1996/97; 3: 379–385.
50 Johnson BM, van Breemen RB. In vitro formation of quinoid metabolites of the dietary supplement *Cimicifuga racemosa* (black cohosh). *Chem Res Toxicol* 2003; 16: 838–846.
51 Frei-Kleiner S *et al*. *Cimicifuga racemosa* dried ethanolic extract in menopausal disorders: a double-blind placebo-controlled clinical trial. *Maturitas* 2005; 51: 397–404.
52 Stoll W. (Phytopharmacon influences atrophic vaginal epithelium: double-blind study, *Cimicifuga* vs estrogenic substances). *Therapeuticon* 1987; 1: 23–31.
53 Wuttke W *et al*. The Cimicifuga preparation BNO 1055 vs conjugated estrogens in a double-blind placebo-controlled study: effects on menopause symptoms and bone markers. *Maturitas* 2003; 44 (Suppl. Suppl.1): S67–S77.
54 Jacobson JS *et al*. Randomized trial of black cohosh for the treatment of hot flashes among women with a history of breast cancer. *J Clin Oncol* 2001; 19: 2739–2745.
55 Nappi RE *et al*. Efficacy of *Cimicifuga racemosa* on climacteric complaints: a randomized study versus low-dose transdermal estradiol. *Gynecol Endocrinol* 2005; 20: 30–35.
56 Lehman-Willenbrock E, Riedel H-H. Klinische und endokrinologische Untersuchungen zur Therapie ovarieller Ausfallserscheinungen nach Hysterektomie unter Belassung der Adnexe. *Z Gynäkol* 1988; 110: 611–618.
57 Warnecke G. Beeinflussung klimakterischer Beschwerden durch ein Phytotherapeutikum. Erfolgreiche Therapie mit Cimicifuga-Mono extrakt. *Med Welt* 1985; 36: 871–874.
58 Mahady G. Black cohosh (*Actaea/Cimicifuga racemosa*). Review of the clinical data for safety and efficacy in menopausal symptoms. *Treat Endocrinol* 2005; 4: 177–184.
59 Liske E *et al*. Physiological investigation of a unique extract of black cohosh (*Cimicifugae racemosae* rhizoma): a 6-month clinical study demonstrates no systemic estrogenic effect. *J Women's Health Gender-Based Med* 2002; 11: 163–174.
60 Hernández Muñoz G, Pluchino S. *Cimicifuga racemosa* for the treatment of hot flushes in women surviving breast cancer. *Maturitas* 2003; 44 (Suppl. Suppl.1): S59–S65.
61 Burke BE *et al*. Randomized, controlled trial of phytoestrogen in the prophylactic treatment of menstrual migraine. *Biomed Pharmacother* 2002; 56: 283–288.
62 Mills SY *et al*. Effect of a proprietary herbal medicine on the relief of chronic arthritic pain: a double-blind study. *Br J Rheumatol* 1996; 35: 874–878.
63 Stolze H. Der andere Weg, klimakterische Beschwerden zu behandeln. *Gyne* 1982; 3: 14–16.
64 Vermes G *et al*. The effects of Remifemin® on subjective symptoms of menopause. *Adv Ther* 2005; 22: 148–154.
65 Huntley A, Ernst E. A systematic review of the safety of black cohosh. *Menopause* 2003; 10: 58–64.
66 Low Dog T *et al*. Critical evaluation of the safety of *Cimicifuga racemosa* in menopause symptom relief. *Menopause* 2003;10: 299–313.
67 Whiting PW *et al*. Black cohosh and other herbal remedies associated with acute hepatitis. *Med J Aust* 2002; 177: 440–443.
68 Vigibase. WHO Adverse Reactions database, Uppsala Monitoring Centre (accessed January 20, 2006).
69 Black Cohosh. UK Public Assessment Report. Medicines and Healthcare products Regulatory Agency, July 2006. Available at http://www.mhra.gov.uk (accessed September 25, 2006).
70 Black cohosh (Cimicifuga racemosa) – risk of liver problems. Medicines and Healthcare products Regulatory Agency, July 2006. Available at http://www.mhra.gov.uk (accessed September 25, 2006).
71 *EMEA public statement on herbal medicinal products containing Cimicifugae racemosae rhizome (black cohosh, root) – serious hepatic reactions*. European Medicines Agency, 18 July 2006. Doc. Ref.: EMEA/269259/2006.
72 Beuscher N. *Cimicifuga racemosa* L. Black cohosh. *Z Phytother* 1995; 16: 310–310.
73 Boyle FM. Adverse interaction of herbal medicine with breast cancer treatment. *Med J Aust* 1997; 167: 286.
74 Gurley BJ *et al*. In vivo effects of goldenseal, kava kava, black cohosh, and valerian on human cytochrome P450 1A2, 2D6, 2E1, and 3A4/5 phenotypes. *Clin Pharmacol Ther* 2005; 77: 415–426.
75 Rockwell S *et al*. Alteration of the effects of cancer therapy agents on breast cancer cells by the herbal medicine black cohosh. *Breast Cancer Res Treat* 2005; 90: 233–239.
76 Gunn TR, Wright IMR. The use of black and blue cohosh in labour. *N Z Med J* 1996; 109: 410–411.
77 Baillie N, Rasmussen P. Black and blue cohosh in labour. *N Z Med J* 1997; 110: 20–21.

Cohosh, Blue

C

Summary and Pharmaceutical Comment

Limited data are available on the chemistry of blue cohosh. Documented pharmacological actions support some of the reputed traditional uses, although many of these are not suitable indications for self-medication. No evidence regarding antirheumatic properties was located, although anti-inflammatory action has been documented for the aerial plant parts. In view of the potential toxicity associated with blue cohosh, it should be used with caution. The potential for preparations of blue cohosh to interfere with other medicines administered concurrently, particularly those with similar or opposing effects, should be considered. The use of blue cohosh preparations during pregnancy and breastfeeding should be avoided.

Species (Family)

Caulophyllum thalictroides (L.) Mich. (Berberidaceae)

Synonym(s)

Caulophyllum, *Leontice thalictroides* L., Papoose Root, Squaw Root

Part(s) Used

Rhizome, root

Pharmacopoeial and Other Monographs

BHP 1983[G7]
Martindale 35th edition[G85]

Legal Category (Licensed Products)

GSL[G37]

Constituents

The following is compiled from several sources, including General References G22, G41 and G48.

Alkaloids Quinolizidine and isoquinoline-types. Anagyrine, baptifoline, magnoflorine, methylcytisine (caulophylline). Other unidentified minor tertiary alkaloids.[1]

Saponins Caulosaponin and cauloside D yielding hederagenin on hydrolysis.[2]

Other constituents Citrullol, gum, resins, phosphoric acid, phytosterol and starch.

Other Caulophyllum species A related species, *C. robustum* Maxim., is rich in triterpene glycosides (caulosides A–G), most of which possess hederagenin as their aglycone.

Food Use

Blue cohosh is not used in foods.

Herbal Use

Blue cohosh is stated to possess antispasmodic, emmenagogue, uterine tonic and antirheumatic properties. Traditionally, it has been used for amenorrhoea, threatened miscarriage, false labour pains, dysmenorrhoea, rheumatic pains, and specifically for conditions associated with uterine atony.[G7, G64]

Dosage

Dosages for oral administration (adults) for traditional uses recommended in standard herbal reference texts are given below.

Dried rhizome/root 0.3–1.0 g as a decoction three times daily.[G7]

Liquid extract 0.5–1.0 mL (1 : 1 in 70% alcohol) three times daily.[G7]

Pharmacological Actions

In vitro and animal studies

A blue cohosh extract exhibited stimulant properties on the isolated guinea-pig uterus, although subsequent *in vivo* studies in cats, dogs and rabbits demonstrated no uterine activity.[3]

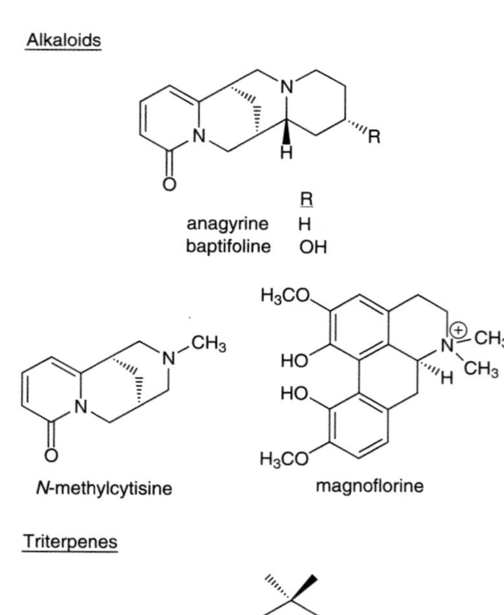

Figure 1 Selected constituents of blue cohosh.

Antifertility actions documented in rats were reported to be caused by inhibition of ovulation[4] and by interruption of implantation.[5]

Smooth muscle stimulation has been documented for a crystalline glycoside constituent on the uterus (*in vitro*), the small intestine (*in vitro*), and the coronary blood vessels (*in vivo*) of various small mammals.[6] The glycoside was also reported to cause erythrolysis and to be of an irritant nature. An earlier study that used a crystalline glycoside identified as caulosaponin, reported a variety of actions including an oxytocic effect on the isolated rat uterus, constriction of coronary and carotid blood vessels, a toxic action on cardiac muscle, and a spasmogenic action on the isolated intestine.[6]

Methylcytisine is stated to have a nicotinic-like action, causing an elevation in blood pressure and stimulating both respiration and intestinal motility.[G60]

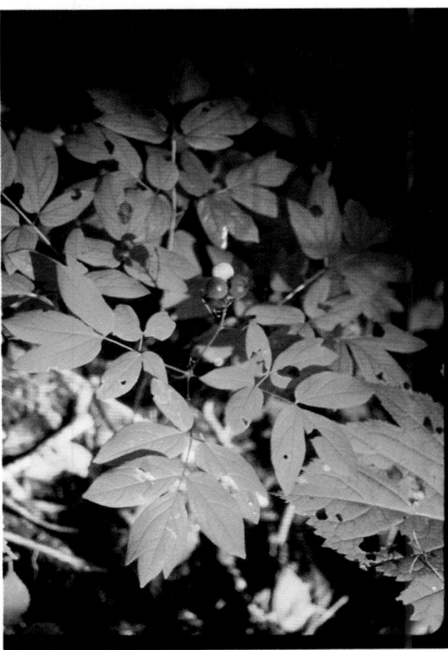

Figure 2 Blue cohosh (*Caulophyllum thalictroides*).

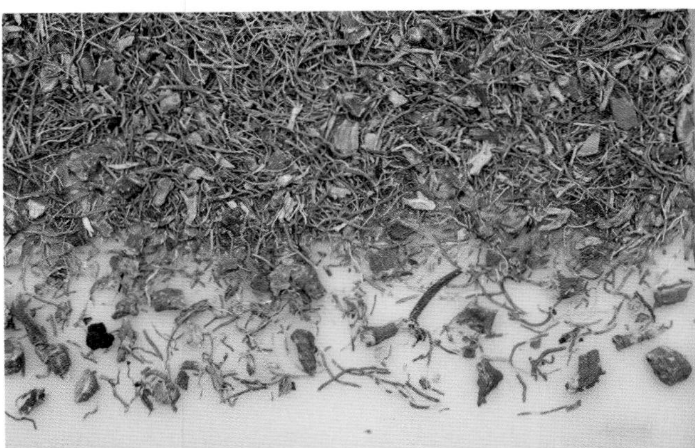

Figure 3 Blue cohosh – dried drug substance (root).

An alcoholic extract of the aerial parts of blue cohosh produced up to 55% inhibition of inflammation in the carrageenan rat paw test.[7]

Clinical studies

There is a lack of clinical research assessing the effects of blue cohosh and rigorous randomised controlled clinical trials are required.

C

Side-effects, Toxicity

Clinical data

There is a lack of clinical safety and toxicity data for blue cohosh and further investigation of these aspects is required.

Powdered blue cohosh is stated to be irritant, especially to mucous membranes.[G51] The leaves and seeds are reported to contain methylcytisine and some glycosides that can cause severe stomach pains. Children have been poisoned by eating the bright blue bitter-tasting seeds.[G22] Caulosaponin is reported to be cardiotoxic, causing constriction of coronary blood vessels, to produce intestinal spasms, and to possess oxytocic properties.[G60]

There is an isolated report of tachycardia, diaphoresis, muscle weakness and fasciculations in a 21-year-old woman who ingested blue cohosh tincture in an attempt to induce an abortion. The woman's symptoms, which resolved over the following 24 hours, were considered to be consistent with those of nicotine toxicity.[8]

Preclinical data

N-methylcytisine isolated from blue cohosh root material demonstrated teratogenic activity in rat embryo culture, an *in-vitro* system used to detect potential teratogens.[9] The clinical significance of this finding has not been established.

Contra-indications, Warnings

Blue cohosh may irritate gastrointestinal conditions. It is not known whether excessive doses of blue cohosh may cause a rise in blood pressure, because of the methylcytisine content.

Drug interactions None documented. However, in view of the limited information on the chemistry of blue cohosh, and documented pharmacological actions, the potential for preparations of blue cohosh to interfere with other medicines administered concurrently, particularly those with similar or opposing effects, should be considered.

Pregnancy and lactation There are insufficient data on the use of blue cohosh preparations during pregnancy and breastfeeding, and the use of blue cohosh should be avoided during these periods.

Blue cohosh is reputed to be an abortifacient and to affect the menstrual cycle.[G30]

Preparations

Proprietary multi-ingredient preparations

Australia: Dyzco; Lifesystem Herbal Formula 4 Women's Formula; Women's Formula Herbal Formula 3.

C

References

1 Flom MS *et al*. Isolation and characterization of alkaloids from *Caulophyllum thalictroides*. *J Pharm Sci* 1967; 56: 1515–1517.
2 Strigina LI *et al*. Cauloside D a new triterpenoid glycoside from *Caulophyllum robustum*. Maxim. Identification of cauloside A. *Phytochemistry* 1976; 15: 1583–1586.
3 Pilcher JD *et al*. The action of various female remedies on the excised uterus of the guinea-pig. *Arch Intern Med* 1916; 18: 557–583.
4 Chaudrasekhar K, Sarma GHR. Observations on the effect of low and high doses of Caulophyllum on the ovaries and the consequential changes in the uterus and thyroid in rats. *J Reprod Fertil* 1974; 38: 236–237.
5 Chaudrasekhar K, Raa Vishwanath C. Studies on the effect of Caulophyllum on implantation in rats. *J Reprod Fertil* 1974; 38: 245–246.
6 Ferguson HC, Edwards LD. A pharmacological study of a crystalline glycoside of *Caulophyllum thalictroides*. *J Am Pharm Assoc* 1954; 43: 16–21.
7 Benoit PS *et al*. Biological and phytochemical evaluation of plants XIV. Anti-inflammatory evaluation of 163 species of plants. *Lloydia* 1976; 393: 160–171.
8 Rao RB, Hoffman RS. Nicotinic toxicity from tincture of blue cohosh (Caulophyllum thalictroides) used as an abortifacient. *Vet Hum Toxicol* 2002; 44: 221–222.
9 Kennelly EJ *et al*. Detecting potential teratogenic alkaloids from blue cohosh rhizomes using an in vitro rat embryo culture. *J Nat Prod* 1999; 62: 1385–1389.

Cola

Summary and Pharmaceutical Comment

The principal active constituent in cola is caffeine. The reputed herbal uses of cola can be attributed to the actions of caffeine, and precautions associated with other xanthine-containing beverages are applicable to cola.

Species (Family)

Cola nitida (Vent.) Schott & Endl. (Sterculiaceae)
**Cola acuminata* (P. Beauv.) Schott & Endl.

Synonym(s)

Cola Seed, Guru Nut, Kola Nut
**Sterculia acuminata* Beauv.

Part(s) Used

Cotyledon

Pharmacopoeial and Other Monographs

BHC 1992[G6]
BHP 1996[G9]
BP 2007[G84]
Complete German Commission E[G3]
Martindale 35th edition[G85]
Ph Eur 2007[G81]

Legal Category (Licensed Products)

GSL[G37]

Constituents

The following is compiled from several sources, including General References G6 and G62.

Alkaloids Xanthine-types. Caffeine (0.6–3.0%), theobromine (up to 0.1%).

Tannins Condensed type, catechins.

Other constituents Betaine, cellulose, enzyme, fats, a glucoside, protein, red pigment and sugars.

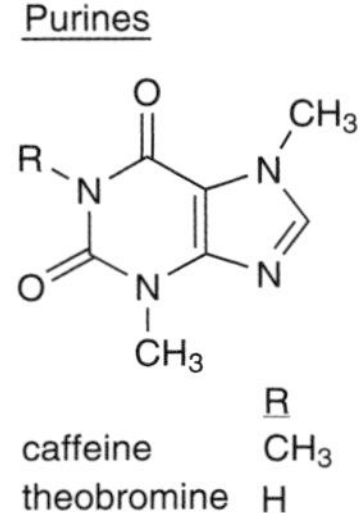

Figure 1 Selected constituents of cola.

Food Use

Cola is listed by the Council of Europe as a natural source of food flavouring (cola and cola nut extract: category N4, with limits on caffeine) (*see* Appendix 3).[G17] Cola is commonly used in foods. Previously, cola has been listed as GRAS (Generally Recognised As Safe).[G41]

Herbal Use

Cola is stated to possess CNS stimulant, thymoleptic, antidepressant, diuretic, cardioactive and antidiarrhoeal properties. It has been used for depressive states, melancholy, atony, exhaustion, dysentery, atonic diarrhoea, anorexia, migraine and specifically for depressive states associated with general muscular weakness.[G6, G7, G8, G64]

Dosage

Dosages for oral administration (adults) for traditional uses recommended in older standard herbal and pharmaceutical reference texts are given below.

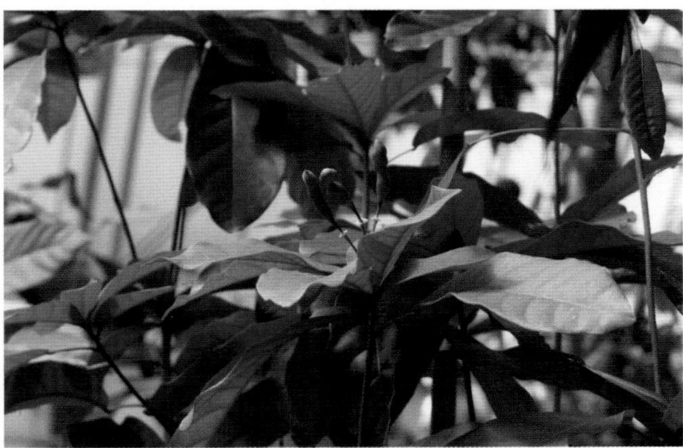

Figure 2 Cola (*Cola nitida*).

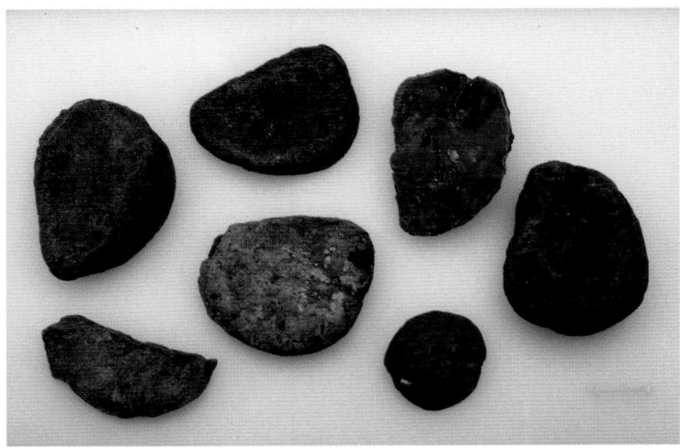

Figure 3 Cola – dried drug substance (cotyledon).

Powdered cotyledons 1–3 g as a decoction three times daily.[G6, G7]

Liquid Extract of cola (BPC 1949) 0.6–1.2 mL (1 : 1 in 60% alcohol).

Tincture of cola (BPC 1934) 1–4 mL (1 : 5 in 60% alcohol).

Pharmacological Actions

The xanthine constituents, caffeine and theobromine, are the active principles in cola. The pharmacological properties of caffeine are well documented and include stimulation of the CNS, respiratory system and skeletal muscle, cardiac stimulation, coronary dilatation, smooth muscle relaxation and diuresis.[G41] Cola-containing beverages are stated to provide active doses of caffeine.[G45]

Side-effects, Toxicity

Side-effects commonly associated with xanthine-containing beverages include sleeplessness, anxiety, tremor, palpitations and withdrawal headache.[G54]

Contra-indications, Warnings

Consumption of cola should be restricted in individuals with hypertension or cardiac disorders, because of the caffeine content.

Drug interactions None documented. However, the potential for preparations of cola to interact with other medicines administered concurrently, particularly those with similar or opposing effects, should be considered.

Pregnancy and lactation It is generally recommended that caffeine consumption should be restricted during pregnancy, although conflicting reports have been documented regarding the association between birth defects and caffeine consumption. In view of this, excessive consumption of cola during pregnancy should be avoided. Caffeine is excreted in breast milk, but at concentrations considered too low to represent a hazard to breastfed infants.[G45] However, as with all xanthine-containing beverages, excessive consumption of cola by lactating mothers should be avoided.

Coltsfoot

Summary and Pharmaceutical Comment

The majority of the traditional uses associated with coltsfoot can be attributed to the mucilage content. However, coltsfoot also contains toxic pyrrolizidine alkaloids albeit at a low concentration. The risk of exposure to low concentrations of unsaturated pyrrolizidine alkaloids is unclear although hepatotoxicity following prolonged exposure has been documented (*see* Comfrey). The regular or excessive consumption of coltsfoot, especially in the form of herbal teas, should therefore be avoided.

Species (Family)

Tussilago farfara L. (Asteraceae/Compositae)

Synonym(s)

Farfara

Part(s) Used

Flower, leaf

Pharmacopoeial and Other Monographs

BHC 1992[G6]
BHP 1983[G7]
Complete German Commission E[G3]
Martindale 35th edition[G85]

Legal Category (Licensed Products)

GSL[G37]

Constituents

The following is compiled from several sources, including General Reference G2.

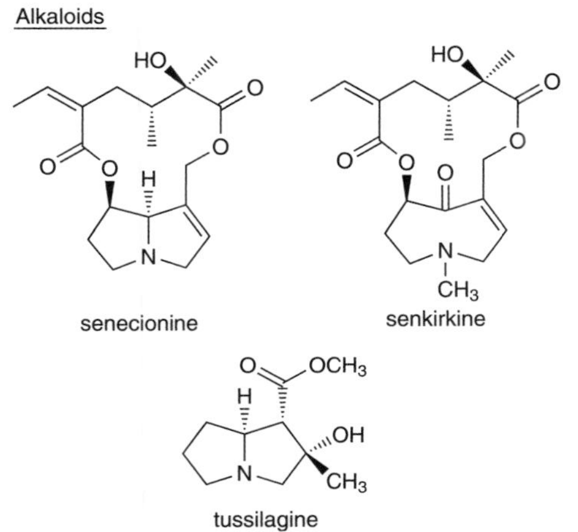

Figure 1 Selected constituents of coltsfoot.

Acids Caffeic acid, caffeoyltartaric acid, ferulic acid, gallic acid, *p*-hydroxybenzoic acid, and tannic acid (phenolic); malic acid and tartaric acid (aliphatic).[1]

Alkaloids Pyrrolizidine-type. Senkirkine 0.015% and senecionine (minor) (unsaturated)[2,3] and tussilagine (saturated).[4]

Carbohydrates Mucilage (water-soluble polysaccharides) 7–8% yielding various sugars following hydrolysis (e.g. arabinose, fructose, galactose, glucose, uronic acid and xylose); inulin (polysaccharide).[5]

Flavonoids Flavonols (e.g. kaempferol, quercetin) and their glycosides.[1]

Tannins Up to 17% (type unspecified).

Other constituents Bitter (glycoside), choline, paraffin (fatty acid), phytosterols (sitosterol, stigmasterol, taraxasterol), triterpene (amyrin), tussilagone (sesquiterpene)[6] and volatile oil.

Food Use

Coltsfoot is not commonly used as a food but it is listed by the Council of Europe as a source of natural food flavouring (category N4). This category indicates that although coltsfoot is permitted for use as a food flavouring, there are insufficient data available for an assessment of toxicity to be made.[G16]

Herbal Use

Coltsfoot is stated to possess expectorant, antitussive, demulcent and anticatarrhal properties. It has been used for asthma, bronchitis, laryngitis and pertussis.[G2, G7, G49, G64]

Dosage

Dosages for oral administration (adults) for traditional uses recommended in standard herbal reference texts are given below.

Dried herb 0.6–2.0 g by decoction three times daily.[G6]

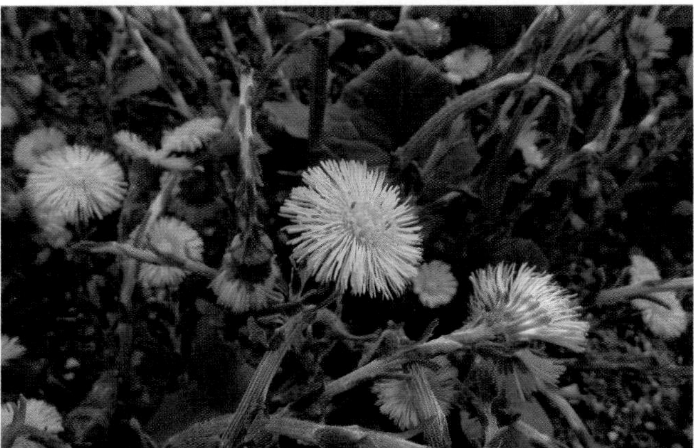

Figure 2 Coltsfoot (*Tussilago farfara*).

C

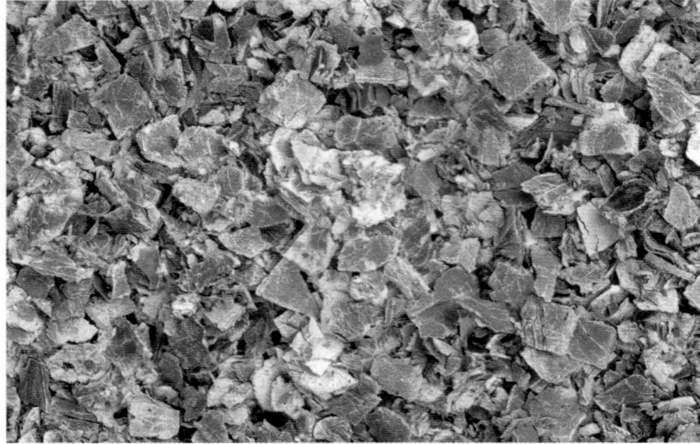

Figure 3 Coltsfoot – dried drug substance (leaf).

Liquid extract 0.6–2.0 mL (1 : 1 in 25% alcohol) three times daily.[G7]

Tincture 2–8 mL (1 : 5 in 45% alcohol) three times daily.[G7]

Syrup 2–8 mL (liquid extract 1 : 4 in syrup) three times daily.[G7]

Pharmacological Actions

In vitro and animal studies

Antibacterial activity has been documented for coltsfoot against various Gram-negative bacteria including *Staphylococcus aureus*, *Proteus hauseri*, *Bordetella pertussis*, *Pseudomonas aeruginosa* and *Proteus vulgaris*.[7–9]

Anti-inflammatory activity comparable to that of indometacin, determined in Selye's experimental chronic inflammation test, has been attributed to water-soluble polysaccharides in coltsfoot.[10] Weak acute anti-inflammatory activity has been reported for coltsfoot when tested against carrageenan-induced rat paw oedema.[11, 12]

Platelet-activating factor (PAF) is known to be involved in various inflammatory, respiratory and cardiovascular disorders. The aggregating action of PAF is known to be weaker if intracellular concentrations of calcium are low. A sesquiterpene, L-652469, isolated from coltsfoot buds has been reported to be a weak inhibitor of both PAF receptor binding and calcium channel blocker binding to membrane vesicles.[13] This combination of actions was found to effectively block PAF-induced platelet aggregation. L-652469 was also found to be active orally, inhibiting PAF-induced rat paw oedema.[13] Interestingly, L-652469 was reported to interact with the cardiac calcium channel blocker receptor complex (dihydropyridine receptor), but was also found to be a calcium channel blocker.[13]

Tussilagine has been reported to be a potent cardiovascular and respiratory stimulant.[6, 14] Dose-dependent pressor activity following intravenous injection has been observed in the cat, rat and dog.[14] The pressor effect is stated to be similar to that of dopamine, but without tachyphylaxis. A significant stimulation of respiration was also observed.[6] Cardiovascular and respiratory effects are thought to be mediated by peripheral and central mechanisms, respectively.[6]

Clinical studies

There is a lack of clinical research assessing the effects of coltsfoot and rigorous randomised controlled clinical trials are required.

Side-effects, Toxicity

There is a lack of clinical safety and toxicity data for coltsfoot and further investigation of these aspects is required.

Coltsfoot has been reported to be phototoxic in guinea-pig skin.[15]

Pyrrolizidine alkaloids with an unsaturated pyrrolizidine nucleus are known to be hepatotoxic in both animals and humans (*see* Comfrey). Of the pyrrolizidine alkaloids documented for coltsfoot, senecionine and senkirkine are unsaturated. Chronic hepatotoxicity has been described in rats following the incorporation of coltsfoot into their diet at concentrations ranging from 4–33%.[16] After 600 days, it was found that rats fed more than 4% coltsfoot had developed hepatic tumours (haemangioendothelial sarcoma) while none were observed in the control group. Furthermore, histological changes associated with pyrrolizidine alkaloid toxicity, such as centrilobular necrosis of the liver and cirrhosis, were observed in many of the rats who had ingested coltsfoot but who had not developed tumours.[16] The hepatotoxicity of coltsfoot was attributed to senkirkine, which is present at a concentration of only 0.015%, thus highlighting the dangers associated with chronic exposure to low concentrations of pyrrolizidine alkaloids.

Newborn rats have been found to be more susceptible than weanlings to the hepatotoxic effects of senkirkine despite lacking the hepatic microsomal enzymes required for the formation of the toxic pyrrolic metabolites.[17] Fatal hepatic veno-occlusive disease has been documented in a newborn infant whose mother had regularly consumed a herbal tea during pregnancy.[18] Analysis of the herbal tea revealed the presence of 10 different plants including coltsfoot and a *Senecio* species (known source of pyrrolizidine alkaloids, *see* Liferoot). The mother exhibited no signs of hepatic damage, suggesting an increased sensitivity of the fetal liver to pyrrolizidine alkaloid toxicity.

Pre-blooming coltsfoot flowers are reported to contain the highest concentration of alkaloids.[3] Considerable loss of both senkirkine and senecionine has been observed upon prolonged storage of the dried plant material.[3] Senkirkine and senecionine are both easily extracted into hot water and, therefore, would presumably be ingested in a herbal tea prepared from the fresh plant.[3] A cup of tea prepared from 10 g pre-blooming flowers has been estimated to contain a maximum of 70 µg senecionine and 1.4 mg senkirkine. Tea from the young leaves or mature plant would presumably contain considerably lower concentrations of alkaloids.[3] These concentrations are not considered to represent a health hazard compared to the known hepatotoxicity of senecionine (intravenous LD_{50} 64 mg/kg body weight, mice).[3] However, prolonged exposure to low concentrations of pyrrolizidine alkaloids has resulted in hepatotoxicity (*see* Comfrey).

Tussilagine LD_{50} (mice, intravenous injection) has been determined as 28.9 mg/kg.[14]

Contra-indications, Warnings

In view of the known pyrrolizidine alkaloid content, excessive or prolonged ingestion should be avoided. In particular, herbal teas containing coltsfoot should be avoided.

Drug interactions None documented. However, the potential for preparations of coltsfoot to interact with other medicines administered concurrently, particularly those with similar or opposing effects, should be considered. There is limited evidence from preclinical studies that tussilagine, a constituent of coltsfoot, has pressor activity. However, the clinical significance of this, if any, is not known.

Pregnancy and lactation Coltsfoot should not be taken during pregnancy or lactation in view of the toxicity associated with the pyrrolizidine alkaloid constituents. Coltsfoot is reputed to be an abortifacient.[G30]

Preparations

Proprietary multi-ingredient preparations

Argentina: Arceligasol; Negacne. *Czech Republic:* Perospir; Species Pectorales Planta. *Italy:* Lozione Same Urto. *Spain:* Llantusil. *UK:* Antibron; Chesty Cough Relief.

References

1 Didry N *et al*. Phenolic compounds from *Tussilago farfara*. *Ann Pharm Fr* 1980; 38: 237–241.
2 Culvenor CCJ *et al*. The occurrence of senkirkine in *Tussilago farfara*. *Aust J Chem* 1976; 29: 229–230.
3 Rosberger DF *et al*. The occurrence of senecione in *Tussilago farfara*. *Mitt Geb Lebensm Hyg* 1981; 72: 432–436.
4 Röder E *et al*. Tussilagine – a new pyrrolizidine alkaloid from *Tussilago farfara*. *Planta Med* 1981; 41: 99–102.
5 Haaland E. Water-soluble polysaccharides from the leaves of *Tussilago farfara* L. *Acta Chem Scand* 1969; 23: 2546–2548.
6 Yi-Ping L, Wang Y-M. Evaluation of tussilagone: a cardiovascular-respiratory stimulant isolated from Chinese herbal medicine. *Gen Pharmacol* 1988; 19: 261–263.
7 Didry N *et al*. Components and activity of *Tussilago farfara*. *Ann Pharm Fr* 1982; 40: 75–80.
8 Didry N, Pinkas M. Antibacterial activity of fresh leaves of *Tussilago* spp. *Bull Soc Pharm (Lille)* 1982; 38: 51–52.
9 Ieven M *et al*. Screening of higher plants for biological activities I. Antimicrobial activity. *Planta Med* 1979; 36: 311–321.
10 Engalycheva E-I *et al*. Anti-inflammatory activity of polysaccharides obtained from *Tussilago farfara* L. *Farmatsiya* 1982; 31: 37–40.
11 Benoit PS *et al*. Biological and phytochemical evaluation of plants. XIV. Antiinflammatory evaluation of 163 species of plants. *Lloydia* 1976; 39: 160–171.
12 Mascolo N *et al*. Biological screening of Italian medicinal plants for anti-inflammatory activity. *Phytother Res* 1987; 1: 28–31.
13 Hwang S-B *et al*. L-652,469 – a dual receptor antagonist of platelet activating factor and dihydropyridines from *Tussilago farfara* L. *Eur J Pharmacol* 1987; 141: 269–281.
14 Wang Y-M. Pharmacological studies of extracts of *Tussilago farfara* L. II Effects on the cardiovascular system. *Acta Pharm Sin* 1979; 5: 268–276.
15 Masaki H *et al*. Primary skin irritation and phototoxicity of plants extracts for cosmetic ingredients. *J Soc Cosmet Chem Jpn* 1984; 18: 47–49.
16 Hirono I *et al*. Carcinogenic activity of coltsfoot, *Tussilago farfara* L. *Gann* 1976; 67: 125–129.
17 Schoental R. Hepatotoxic activity of retrorsine, senkirkine and hydroxysenkirkine in newborn rats, and the role of epoxides in carcinogenesis by pyrrolizidine alkaloids and aflatoxins. *Nature* 1970; 227: 401–402.
18 Roulet M *et al* Hepatic veno-occlusive disease in newborn infant of a woman drinking herbal tea. *J Pediatr* 1988; 112: 433–436.

Comfrey

Summary and Pharmaceutical Comment

Comfrey is characterised by its pyrrolizidine alkaloid constituents. The hepatotoxicity of these compounds is well known, and cases of human poisoning involving comfrey have been documented. Human hepatotoxicity with pyrrolizidine-containing plants is well documented, particularly following the ingestion of *Crotalaria*, *Heliotropium* and *Senecio* species. Comfrey has traditionally been used topically for treating wounds. Percutaneous absorption of pyrrolizidine alkaloids present in comfrey is reported to be low, although application of comfrey preparations to the broken skin should be avoided.

Licensed herbal products intended for internal use are not permitted to contain comfrey. The inclusion of comfrey in products intended for topical application is permitted, provided the preparation is only applied to the unbroken skin and that its use is restricted to ten days or less at any one time.

As a result of a 1993 report by the Committee on Toxicity of Chemicals in Food to the Food Advisory Committee and the Ministry of Agriculture, Fisheries and Food (UK), the health food trade voluntarily withdrew all products, such as tablets and capsules, and advice was issued that the root and leaves should be labelled with warnings against ingestion. It was considered that comfrey teas contained relatively low concentrations of pyrrolizidine alkaloids and did not need any warning labels.

Species (Family)

Symphytum officinale L. (Boraginaceae)

Synonym(s)

Symphytum Radix

Related species include Prickly Comfrey (*Symphytum asperum*), Quaker and Russian Comfrey (*Symphytum uplandicum*, hybrid of *S. officinale* × *S. asperum*)

Part(s) Used

Leaf, rhizome, root

Pharmacopoeial and Other Monographs

BHC 1992[G6]
BHP 1996[G9]
Complete German Commission E[G3]
Martindale 35th edition[G85]

Legal Category (Licensed Products)

GSL (external use only)[G37]

Constituents

The following is compiled from several sources, including General References G2 and G6.

Alkaloids Pyrrolizidine-type. 0.3%. Symphytine, symlandine, echimidine, intermidine, lycopsamine, myoscorpine, acetyllycopsamine, acetylintermidine, lasiocarpine, heliosupine, viridiflorine and echiumine.[1–5]

Carbohydrates Gum (arabinose, glucuronic acid, mannose, rhamnose, xylose); mucilage (glucose, fructose).

Tannins Pyrocatechol-type. 2.4%.

Triterpenes Sitosterol and stigmasterol (phytosterols), steroidal saponins and isobauerenol.

Other constituents Allantoin 0.75–2.55%, caffeic acid, carotene 0.63%, chlorogenic acid, choline, lithospermic acid, rosmarinic acid and silicic acid.

Food Use

Comfrey is occasionally used as an ingredient of soups and salads. It is listed by the Council of Europe as natural source of food flavouring (category N4). This category indicates that although comfrey is permitted for use as a food flavouring, insufficient data are available to assess toxicity.[G16]

Herbal Use

Comfrey is stated to possess vulnerary, cell-proliferant, astringent, antihaemorrhagic and demulcent properties. It has been used for colitis, gastric and duodenal ulcers, haematemesis, and has been applied topically for ulcers, wounds and fractures.[G2, G6, G7, G8, G49, G64]

Dosage

Dosages for oral (unless otherwise stated) administration (adults) for traditional uses recommended in standard herbal reference texts are given below. Note: internal use is no longer advised.

Alkaloids

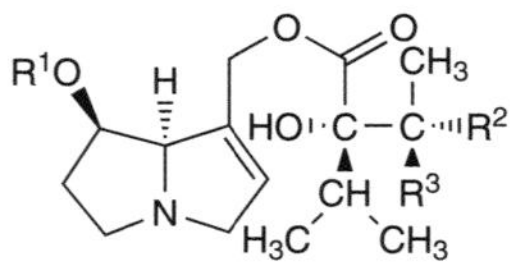

	R^1	R^2	R^3
intermedine	H	H	OH
echimidine	angelyl	H	OH
acetylechimidine	acetyl	H	OH
lycopsamine	H	OH	H
symphytine	tiglyl	OH	H
acetylsymphytine	acetyl	OH	H

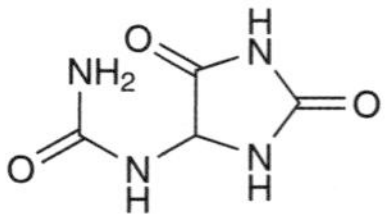

allantoin

Figure 1 Selected constituents of comfrey.

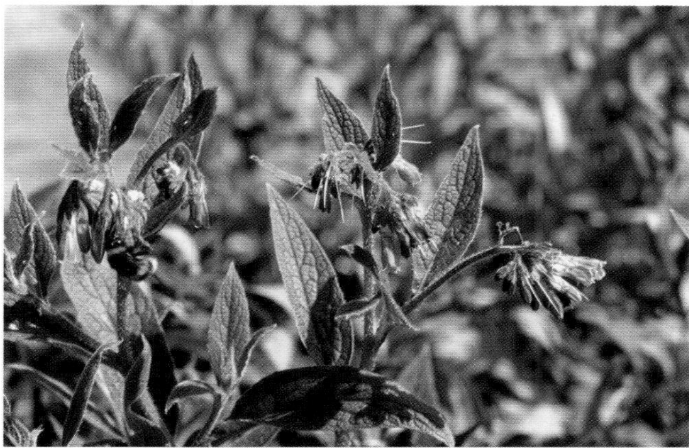

Figure 2 Comfrey (*Symphytum officinale*).

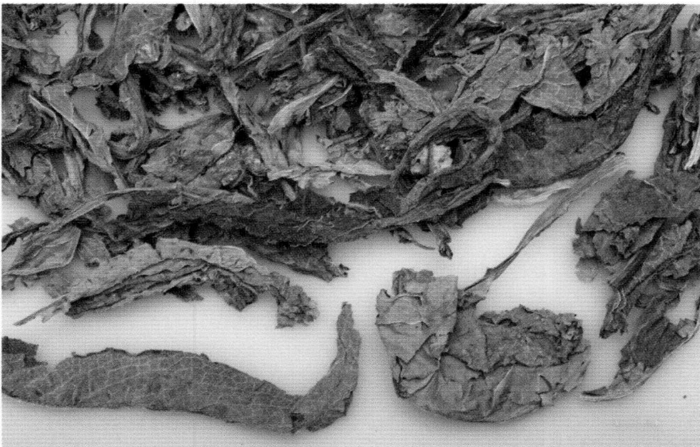

Figure 3 Comfrey – dried drug substance (leaf).

Dried root/rhizome 2–4 g as a decoction three times daily.[G7]

Root, liquid extract 2–4 mL (1 : 1 in 25% alcohol) three times daily.[G7]

Ointment symphytum root 10–15% root extractive in usual type ointment basis applied topically three times daily.[G7]

Dried leaf 2–8 g or by infusion three times daily.[G7]

Leaf, liquid extract 2–8 mL (1 : 1 in 25% alcohol) three times daily.[G7]

Pharmacological Actions

The classical pharmacology of pyrrolizidine alkaloids is overshadowed by the well-recognised toxicity of this class of compounds. Consequently, the majority of data documented for comfrey involve toxicity. Many useful reviews have been published on the toxicity of pyrrolizidine alkaloids in humans (*see below*).[5–11]

In vitro and animal studies

Wound-healing and analgesic activities have been documented in rats administered comfrey extract orally.[12] Percutaneous absorption of pyrrolizidine alkaloids obtained from comfrey is reported to be low in rats, with minimal conversion of the pyrrolizidine alkaloid *N*-oxides to the free pyrrolizidine alkaloids in the urine (reduction of the *N*-oxides is required before they can be metabolised into the reactive pyrrolic esters).[13, 14]

Rosmarinic acid has been isolated from comfrey (*S. officinale*) as the main constituent with *in vitro* anti-inflammatory activity.[15] Biological activity was determined by inhibition of malonic dialdehyde formation in human platelets. Minor components, chlorogenic and caffeic acids, were not found to exhibit any significant activity. The pyrrolic esters have been reported to possess mild antimuscarinic activity, which is more pronounced in the non-hepatotoxic esters of saturated amino alcohols.[16] Conversely, the free amino alcohols are reported to exert indirect cholinomimetic action involving the release of acetylcholine from postganglionic sites in the guinea-pig ileum.[16]

Comfrey has been reported to stimulate the activity of the hepatic drug-metabolising enzyme aminopyrine *N*-demethylase in rats.[17]

A comfrey extract has been reported to enhance uterine tone *in vitro*.[18] The action of comfrey was reported to be weaker than that exhibited by German chamomile, calendula and plantain, but stronger than that shown by shepherd's purse, St. John's wort and uva-ursi.

Clinical studies

There is a lack of clinical research assessing the effects of comfrey and rigorous randomised controlled clinical trials are required.

The antimuscarinic properties of certain pyrrolic esters have been utilised. Two non-hepatotoxic pyrrolizidine alkaloids, sarracine and platyphylline, have been used for the treatment of gastrointestinal hypermotility and peptic ulceration.[16]

Side-effects, Toxicity

Two reports of human hepatotoxicity associated with the ingestion of comfrey have been documented.[19, 20] One case involved a 13-year-old boy who had been given a comfrey root preparation in conjunction with acupuncture to treat Crohn's disease.[19] The boy was diagnosed with veno-occlusive disease of the liver and the authors concluded comfrey to be the only possible causal factor of the liver disease. The second case involved a 49-year-old woman diagnosed with veno-occlusive disease.[20] She had been taking various food supplements including a herbal tea and comfrey-pepsin pills. Pyrrolizidine alkaloids were identified in both the tea (stated to contain ginseng) and the comfrey-pepsin pills. The authors estimated that over a period of six months the woman had ingested 85 mg of pyrrolizidine alkaloids, equivalent to 15 μg/kg body weight per day. This report highlighted the potential toxicity associated with chronic ingestion of relatively small amounts of pyrrolizidine alkaloids.

The toxicity of pyrrolizidine alkaloids is well recognised. Pyrrolizidine alkaloids with an unsaturated pyrrolizidine nucleus are metabolised in the liver to toxic pyrrole metabolites.[8] Acute toxicity results in hepatic necrosis, whereas chronic toxicity typically results in veno-occlusive disease characterised by the presence of greatly enlarged liver cells.[8, 10]

Reports of human hepatotoxicity associated with pyrrolizidine alkaloid ingestion have been documented.[5, 8–10, 21–30] Many of these reports have resulted from crop (and subsequently flour and bread) contamination with *Crotalaria*, *Heliotropium* and *Senecio* species and from the use of pyrrolizidine-containing plants in medicinal 'bush' teas. In addition, pyrrolizidine alkaloid poisoning has been associated with the use of herbal teas in Europe and the United States.[20, 25–27] The diagnosis of veno-occlusive disease in a newborn infant who subsequently died highlights the susceptibility of the fetus to pyrrolizidine alkaloid toxicity.[30] In this case, the mother had consumed a herbal tea as an expectorant during pregnancy. The tea, which was purchased from a pharmacy in Switzerland, was analysed and found to contain pyrrolizidine alkaloids. The mother did not exhibit any signs of hepatotoxicity.

Interestingly, liver function tests in 29 chronic comfrey users have been reported to show no abnormalities.[31]

The hepatotoxicity of pyrrolizidine alkaloids is well documented in animals.[5] In addition, carcinogenicity has been described in rats fed a diet supplemented with comfrey.[32] The mutagenicity of comfrey has been attributed to lasiocarpine,[23] which is known to be mutagenic and carcinogenic. However, other workers have reported a lack of mutagenic activity for comfrey following assessment using direct bacterial test systems (Ames), host mediated assay (Legator), liver microsomal assay and the micronucleus technique.[33,34]

Contra-indications, Warnings

In view of the hepatotoxic properties documented for the pyrrolizidine alkaloid constituents, comfrey should not be taken internally. The topical application of comfrey-containing preparations to broken skin should be avoided.

Drug interactions None documented. However, the potential for preparations of comfrey to interact with other medicines administered concurrently, particularly those with similar or opposing effects, should be considered.

Pregnancy and lactation The safety of comfrey has not been established. In view of the toxicity associated with the alkaloid constituents, comfrey should not be taken during pregnancy or lactation.

Preparations

Proprietary single-ingredient preparations

Austria: Traumaplant. *Czech Republic:* Traumaplant. *Germany:* Kytta-Plasma f; Kytta-Salbe f; Traumaplant. *Switzerland:* Kytta Pommade. *Venezuela:* Traumaplant.

Proprietary multi-ingredient preparations

Czech Republic: Dr Theiss Beinwell Salbe; Stomatosan. *Germany:* Kytta-Balsam f; Rhus-Rheuma-Gel N. *Israel:* Comfrey Plus. *Switzerland:* Gel a la consoude; Keppur; Keppur; Kytta Baume. *USA:* MSM with Glucosamine Creme.

References

1 Culvenor CCJ *et al*. Structure and toxicity of the alkaloids of Russian comfrey (*Symphytum* × *uplandicum* Nyman), a medicinal herb and item of human diet. *Experientia* 1980; 36: 377–379.
2 Smith LW, Culvenor CCJ. Hepatotoxic pyrrolizidine alkaloids. *J Nat Prod* 1981; 44: 129–152.
3 Huizing HJ. Phytochemistry, systematics and biogenesis of pyrrolizidine alkaloids of *Symphytum* taxa. *Pharm Weekbl (Sci)* 1987; 9: 185–187.
4 Mattocks AR. Toxic pyrrolizidine alkaloids in comfrey. *Lancet* 1980; ii: 1136–1137.
5 *Pyrrolizidine alkaloids. Environmental Health Criteria 80*. Geneva: WHO, 1988.
6 Abbott PJ. Comfrey: assessing the low-dose health risk. *Med J Aust* 1988; 149: 678–682.
7 Awang DVC. Comfrey. *Can Pharm J* 1987; 120: 101–104.
8 McLean EK. The toxic actions of pyrrolizidine (Senecio) alkaloids. *Pharmacol Rev* 1970; 22: 429–483.
9 Huxtable RJ. Herbal teas and toxins: novel aspects of pyrrolizidine poisoning in the United States. *Perspect Biol Med* 1980; 24: 1–14.
10 Mattocks AR. *Chemistry and Toxicology of Pyrrolizidine Alkaloids*. London: Academic Press, 1986.
11 Jadhav SJ *et al*. Pyrrolizidine alkaloids: A review. *J Food Sci Technol* 1982; 19: 87–93.
12 Goldman RS *et al*. Wound healing and analgesic effect of crude extracts of *Symphytum officinale*. *Fitoterapia* 1985; 6: 323–329.
13 Brauchli J *et al*. Pyrrolizidine alkaloids from *Symphytum offinale* L. and their percutaneous absorption in rats. *Experientia* 1982; 38: 1085–1087.
14 Brauchli J *et al*. Pyrrolizidine alkaloids in *Symphytum officinale* L. and their dermal absorption in rats. *Experientia* 1981; 37: 667.
15 Gracza L *et al*. Biochemical-pharmacological investigations of medicinal agents of plant origin, I: Isolation of rosmarinic acid from *Symphytum officinale* L. and its anti-inflammatory activity in an *in-vitro* model. *Arch Pharm (Weinheim)* 1985; 318: 1090–1095.
16 Culvenor CCJ. Pyrrolizidine alkaloids: some aspects of the Australian involvement. *Trends Pharmacol Sci* 1985; 6: 18–22.
17 Garrett BJ *et al*. Consumption of poisonous plants (*Senecio jacobaea*, *Symphytum officinale*, *Pteridium aquilinum*, *Hypericum perforatum*) by rats: Chronic toxicity, mineral metabolism, and hepatic drug-metabolizing enzymes. *Toxicol Lett* 1982; 10: 183–188.
18 Shipochliev T. Extracts from a group of medicinal plants enhancing the uterine tonus. *Vet Med Nauki* 1981; 18: 94–98.
19 Weston CFM *et al*. Veno-occlusive disease of the liver secondary to ingestion of comfrey. *Br Med J* 1987; 295: 183.
20 Ridker PM *et al*. Hepatic venocclusive disease associated with the consumption of pyrrolizidine-containing dietary supplements. *Gastroenterology* 1985; 88: 1050–1054.
21 Anderson C. Comfrey toxicity in perspective. *Lancet* 1981; i: 944.
22 Huxtable RJ *et al*. Toxicity of comfrey-pepsin preparations. *N Engl J Med* 1986; 315: 1095.
23 Furmanowa M *et al*. Mutagenic effects of aqueous extracts of *Symphytum officinale* L. and of its alkaloidal fractions. *J Appl Toxicol* 1983; 3: 127–130.
24 Ridker PM, McDermott WV. Comfrey herb tea and hepatic veno-occlusive disease. *Lancet* 1989; i: 657–658.
25 Lyford CL *et al*. Hepatic veno-occlusive disease originating in Ecuador. *Gastroenterology* 1976; 70: 105–108.
26 Kumana CR *et al*. Herbal tea induced hepatic veno-occlusive disease: quantification of toxic alkaloid exposure in adults. *Gut* 1985; 26: 101–104.
27 Stillman AE *et al*. Hepatic veno-occlusive disease due to pyrrolizidine (Senecio) poisoning in Arizona. *Gastroenterology* 1977; 73: 349–352.
28 McGee JO'D *et al*. A case of veno-occlusive disease of the liver in Britain associated with herbal tea consumption. *J Clin Pathol* 1976; 29: 788–794.
29 Datta DV *et al*. Herbal medicines and veno-occlusive disease in India. *Postgrad Med J* 1978; 54: 511–515.
30 Roulet M *et al*. Hepatic veno-occlusive disease in newborn infant of a woman drinking herbal tea. *J Pediatr* 1988; 112: 433–436.
31 Anderson PC, McLean AEM. Comfrey and liver damage. *Hum Toxicol* 1989; 8: 55–74.
32 Hirono I *et al*. Carcinogenic activity of *Symphytum officinale*. *J Natl Cancer Inst* 1978; 61: 865–869.
33 Lim-Sylianco CY *et al*. Mutagenicity studies of aqueous extracts from leaves of comfrey (*Symphytum officinale* Linn). *NRCP Res Bull* 1977; 32: 178–191.
34 White RD *et al*. An evaluation of acetone extracts from six plants in the Ames mutagenicity test. *Toxicol Lett* 1983; 15: 23–31.

Corn Silk

Summary and Pharmaceutical Comment

Limited information is available on the constituents of corn silk. Extracts have been reported to exhibit diuretic actions in both humans and animals, thus justifying the reputed herbal uses. However, no additional data were located to support these reported actions. In view of the lack of toxicity data, excessive use of corn silk should be avoided.

Species (Family)

Zea mays L. (Gramineae)

Synonym(s)

Stigma Maydis, Maize, Zea

Part(s) Used

Stigma, style

Pharmacopoeial and Other Monographs

BHC 1992[G6]
BHP 1996[G9]
Martindale 35th edition[G85]

Legal Category (Licensed Products)

Corn silk is not included in the GSL.[G37]

Constituents

The following is compiled from several sources, including General References G2 and G6.

Amines 0.05%. Type not specified, although hordenine is listed for the genus *Zea*.

Fixed oils 1.85–2.25%. Contain glycerides of linoleic, oleic, palmitic and stearic acids.

Saponins 3% (unspecified).

Tannins Up to 11.5–13% (unspecified).

Other constituents Allantoin, bitter glycosides (1%), cryptoxanthin, cyanogenetic compound (unidentified),[1] flavone (maysin), gum, phytosterols (e.g. sitosterol, stigmasterol), pigments, resin, vitamins (C and K).

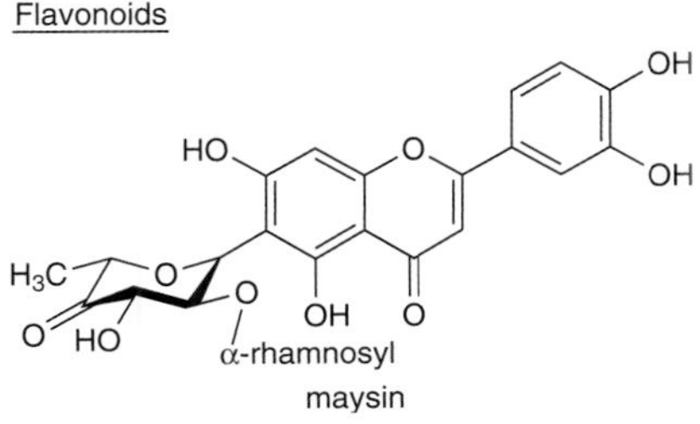

Figure 1 Selected constituents of corn silk.

Food Use

Corn silk is listed as a natural source of food flavouring (category N2). This category indicates that corn silk can be added to foodstuffs in small quantities, with a possible limitation of an active principle (as yet unspecified) in the final product. Previously, corn silk has been listed as GRAS (Generally Recognised As Safe).[G41] The fruits are classified as category N1 with no restriction on their use.[G16] Corn (maize) oil and flour are commonly used in cooking.

Herbal Use

Corn silk is stated to possess diuretic and stone-reducing properties. It has been used for cystitis, urethritis, nocturnal enuresis, prostatitis, and specifically for acute or chronic inflammation of the urinary system.[G2, G6, G7, G8, G64]

Dosage

Dosages for oral administration (adults) for traditional uses recommended in standard herbal reference texts are given below.

Dried style/stigma 4–8 g as an infusion three times daily.[G6, G7]

Liquid Extract of Maize Stigmas (BPC 1923) 4–8 mL.

Tincture 5–15 mL (1 : 5 in 25% alcohol) three times daily.[G6, G7]

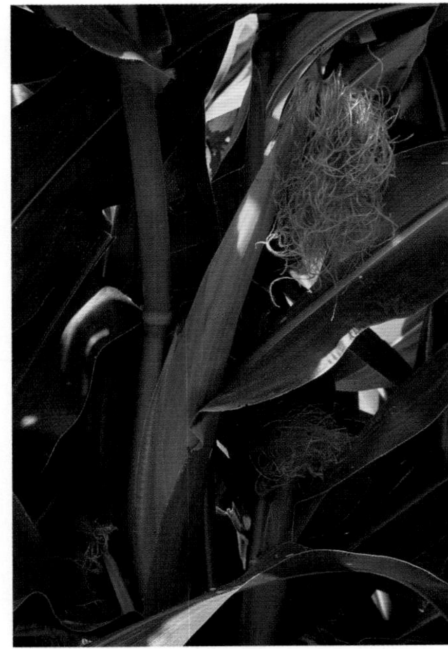

Figure 2 Corn silk (*Zea mays*).

C

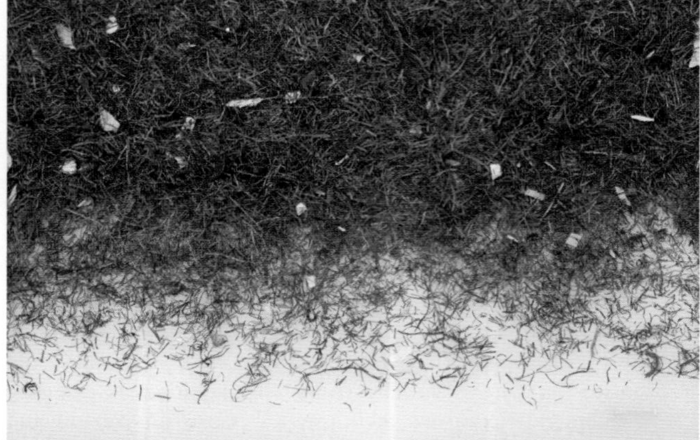

Figure 3 Corn silk – dried drug substance (stigma).

Pharmacological Actions

In vitro and animal studies

Corn silk is stated to possess cholagogue, diuretic, hypoglycaemic, and hypotensive activities in laboratory animals.[2, G41] Utilising aqueous extracts, a methanol-insoluble fraction has been reported to exhibit diuretic activity in rabbits,[G41] and an isolated crystalline component has been documented to have a hypotensive action and to stimulate uterine contraction in rabbits.[3] The latter two actions were thought to involve a cholinergic mechanism. The action of corn silk extract on experimental periodontolysis in hamsters has been documented.[4]

Cryptoxanthin is stated to possess vitamin A activity,[G48] and tannins are known to possess astringent properties.

Clinical studies

There is a lack of clinical research assessing the effects of corn silk and rigorous randomised controlled clinical trials are required.

It has been stated that an aqueous extract is strongly diuretic in humans,[G41] and that clinical studies have indicated corn silk to be effective in kidney and other diseases.[G41] No further information on human studies was located to support these statements.

Side-effects, Toxicity

There is a lack of clinical safety and toxicity data for corn silk and further investigation of these aspects is required.

Allergic reactions including contact dermatitis and urticaria have been documented for corn silk, its pollen and for starch derived from corn silk.[G51] Cornstarch is considered to be a known allergen.[G51] The toxicity of a methanol-insoluble fraction of an aqueous corn silk extract has been reported to be low in rabbits. The effective intravenous dose for a diuretic action was documented as 1.5 mg/kg body weight compared to the lethal intravenous dose of 250 mg/kg.[G41] Corn silk contains an unidentified toxic principle,[1, 2] and is listed as being capable of producing a cyanogenetic compound.[1]

Contra-indications, Warnings

Corn silk may cause an allergic reaction in susceptible individuals.

Drug interactions None documented. However, the potential for preparations of corn silk to interact with other medicines administered concurrently, particularly those with similar or opposing effects, should be considered. There is limited evidence from preclinical studies that corn silk has hypoglycaemic and hypotensive activity.

Pregnancy and lactation Corn silk has been documented to stimulate uterine contractions in rabbits. In view of this, doses of corn silk greatly exceeding amounts used in foods should not be taken during pregnancy or lactation.

Preparations

Proprietary single-ingredient preparations

UK: Protat.

Proprietary multi-ingredient preparations

Spain: Diurinat; Renusor. *UK:* Elixir Damiana and Saw Palmetto; Napiers Uva Ursi Tea; Roberts Black Willow Compound Tablets. *USA:* Cran Support.

References

1 Seigler DS. Plants of the northeastern United States that produce cyanogenic compounds. *Economic Bot* 1976; 30: 395–407.

2 Bever BO, Zahnd GR. Plants with oral hypoglycaemic action. *Q J Crude Drug Res* 1979; 17: 139–196.

3 Hahn SJ. Pharmacological action of Maydis stigma. *K'at'ollik Taehak Uihakpu Nonmunjip* 1973; 25: 127–141.

4 Chaput A *et al*. Action of *Zea mays* L. unsaponifiable titre extract on experimental periodontolysis in hamsters. *Med Hyg (Geneve)* 1972; 30: 1470–1471.

Couchgrass

Summary and Pharmaceutical Comment

Limited chemical data are available for couchgrass and little scientific evidence was located to justify the traditional herbal uses. Agropyrene is regarded as the main active principle in couchgrass on account of its antibiotic effect, although the presence of agropyrene in the volatile oil has been disputed. In view of the lack of toxicity data, excessive ingestion should be avoided.

Species (Family)

Elymus repens (L.) Gould [*Elytrigia repens* (L.) Desv. Ex Nevski] (Gramineae)

Synonym(s)

Agropyron, *Agropyron repens* Beauv., Dogs Grass, Quackgrass, Triticum, *Triticum repens* L., Twitch, Twitchgrass

Part(s) Used

Rhizome

Pharmacopoeial and Other Monographs

BHP 1996[G9]
BP 2007[G84]
Complete German Commission E[G3]
Martindale 35th edition[G85]
Ph Eur 2007[G81]
WHO volume 1 1999[G63]

Legal Category (Licensed Products)

GSL (Agropyron)[G37]

Constituents

The following is compiled from several sources, including General References G2 and G7.

Carbohydrates Fructose, glucose, inositol, mannitol, mucilaginous substances (10%), pectin, triticin.

Cyanogenetic glycosides Unspecified.

Flavonoids Tricin and other unidentified flavonoids.

Saponins No details documented.

Volatile oils 0.05%. Agropyrene (95%). Presence of agropyrene has been disputed,[1] with the oil reported to consist mainly of the monoterpenes carvacrol, *trans*-anethole, carvone, thymol, menthol, menthone and *p*-cymene and three sesquiterpenes.

Other constituents Fixed oil, vanillin glucoside.

Food Use

Couchgrass is listed by the Council of Europe as a natural source of food flavouring (category N2). This category indicates that couchgrass can be added to foodstuffs in small quantities, with a possible limitation of an active principle (as yet unspecified) in the final product.[G16] Previously, couchgrass has been listed as GRAS (Generally Recognised As Safe).[G41]

Herbal Use

Couchgrass is stated to possess diuretic properties. It has been used for cystitis, urethritis, prostatitis, benign prostatic hypertrophy, renal calculus, lithuria, and specifically for cystitis with irritation or inflammation of the urinary tract.[G2, G7, G64]

Dosage

Dosages for oral administration (adults) for traditional uses recommended in older and contemporary standard herbal reference texts are given below.

Dried rhizome 4–8 g as an decoction three times daily.[G7]

Liquid extract 4–8 mL (1 : 1 in 25% alcohol) three times daily.[G7]

Tincture 5–15 mL (1 : 5 in 40% alcohol) three times daily.[G7]

Pharmacological Actions

In vitro and animal studies

Couchgrass is stated to exhibit diuretic and sedative activities in rats and mice, respectively.[G41] Broad antibiotic activity has been documented for agropyrene and its oxidation product.[G41] An ethanolic extract was found to exhibit only weak inhibition (14%) of carrageenan-induced inflammation in the rat paw.[2]

Couchgrass has been reported to be phytotoxic with flavonoid components implicated as the active constituents.[3]

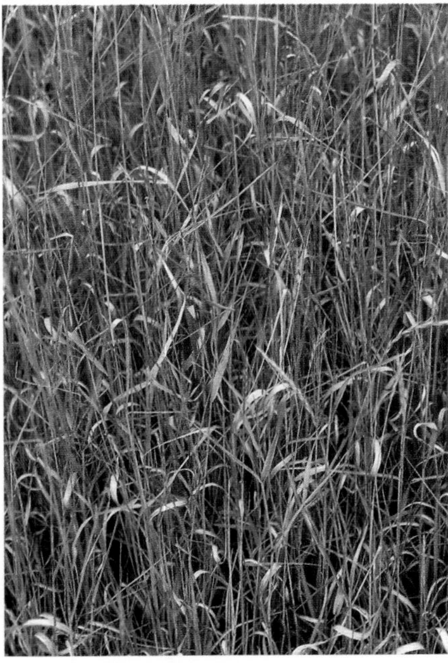

Figure 1 Couchgrass (*Elymus repens*).

C

Clinical studies

There is a lack of clinical research assessing the effects of couchgrass and rigorous randomised controlled clinical trials are required.

Side-effects, Toxicity

None documented. However, there is a lack of clinical safety and toxicity data for couchgrass and further investigation of these aspects is required. An unspecified cyanogenetic glycoside has been reported as a constituent of couchgrass, although no further details were located.(G7)

Contra-indications, Warnings

Drug interactions None documented. However, the potential for preparations of couchgrass to interact with other medicines administered concurrently, particularly those with similar or opposing effects, should be considered. The clinical relevance of the reputed diuretic action is unclear.

Pregnancy and lactation In view of the limited pharmacological and toxicological data, the use of couchgrass during pregnancy and lactation should be avoided.

Preparations

Proprietary single-ingredient preparations

Germany: Acorus.

Proprietary multi-ingredient preparations

France: Herbesan; Mediflor Tisane Antirhumatismale No 2; Mediflor Tisane No 4 Diuretique; Obeflorine; Tisane Hepatique de Hoerdt. *Germany:* Hevert-Blasen-Nieren-Tee N; Renob Blasen- und Nierentee. *Italy:* Emmenoiasi; Tisana Kelemata. *Spain:* Diurinat; Renusor. *UK:* Antitis; Fenneherb Cystaid; Kas-Bah; Napiers Uva Ursi Tea. *USA:* Natural Herbal Water Tablets.

References

1 Boesel R, Schilcher H. Composition of the essential oil of *Agropyrum repens* rhizome. *Planta Med* 1989; 55: 399–400.
2 Mascolo N. Biological screening of Italian medicinal plants for anti-inflammatory activity. *Phytother Res* 1987; 1: 28–29.
3 Weston LA *et al*. Isolation, characterization and activity of phytotoxic compounds from quackgrass [*Agropyron repens* (L.) Beauv.]. *J Chem Ecol* 1987; 13: 403–421.

Cowslip

Summary and Pharmaceutical Comment

The chemistry of cowslip is not well-documented and it is unclear whether saponins reported as constituents of the underground plant parts are also present in the flowers. Little pharmacological information has been documented to justify the herbal uses of cowslip. In view of the lack of toxicity data, excessive use of cowslip should be avoided.

Species (Family)

Primula veris L. (Primulaceae)

Synonym(s)

Paigle, Peagle, Primula, *Primula officinalis* (L.) Hill.

Part(s) Used

Flower

Pharmacopoeial and Other Monographs

BHP 1983[G7]
Complete German Commission E (Primrose flower)[G3]
ESCOP 1997[G52]
Martindale 35th edition[G85]

Legal Category (Licensed Products)

GSL[G37]

Constituents

The following is compiled from several sources, including General References G2 and G59.

Carbohydrates Arabinose, galactose, galacturonic acid, glucose, rhamnose, xylose and water-soluble polysaccharide (6.2–6.6%).

Flavonoids Apigenin, gossypetin, isorhamnetin, kaempferol, luteolin and quercetin.[1]

Phenols Glycosides primulaveroside (primulaverin) and primveroside.

Quinones Primin and other quinone compounds.

Saponins Primula acid in sepals but saponins absent from other parts of the flower.

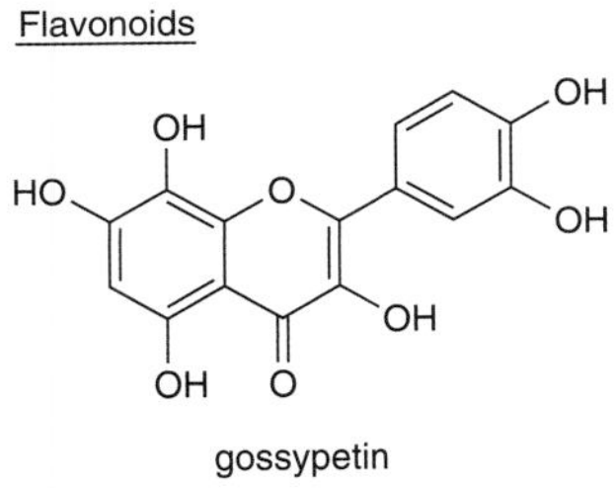

Flavonoids

gossypetin

Figure 1 Selected constituents of cowslip.

Tannins Condensed (e.g. proanthocyanidin B2), pseudotannins (e.g. epicatechin, epigallocatechin).[1]

Other constituents Silicic acid and volatile oil (0.1–0.25%).

Other plant parts Saponins have been documented for the underground parts.[1] 'Primulic acid' is a collective term for the saponin mixture.[2] Primulic acid A glycoside (5–10%) yields primulagenin A as aglycone together with arabinose, galactose, glucose, glucuronic acid, rhamnose and xylose.[3,4] The saponin content of the roots is stated to peak at two years.[5] After five years of storage the saponin content was reported to have decreased by 45%.

Food Use

Cowslip is not commonly used in foods. A related species, *Primula eliator*, is listed by the Council of Europe as a natural source of food flavouring (category N2). This category indicates that *Primula eliator* can be added to foodstuffs, provided that the concentration of coumarin does not exceed 2 mg/kg.[G16] Coumarins, however, are not documented as constituents of *Primula veris*, the subject of this monograph.

Herbal Use

Cowslip is stated to possess sedative, antispasmodic, hypnotic, mild diuretic, expectorant and mild aperient properties. It has been used for insomnia, nervous excitability, hysteria and specifically for anxiety states associated with restlessness and irritability.[G2, G7, G64]

Dosage

Dosages for oral administration (adults) for traditional uses recommended in standard herbal reference texts are given below.

Dried flowers 1–2 g as an infusion three times daily.[G7]

Liquid extract 1–2 mL (1 : 1 in 25% alcohol) three times daily.[G7]

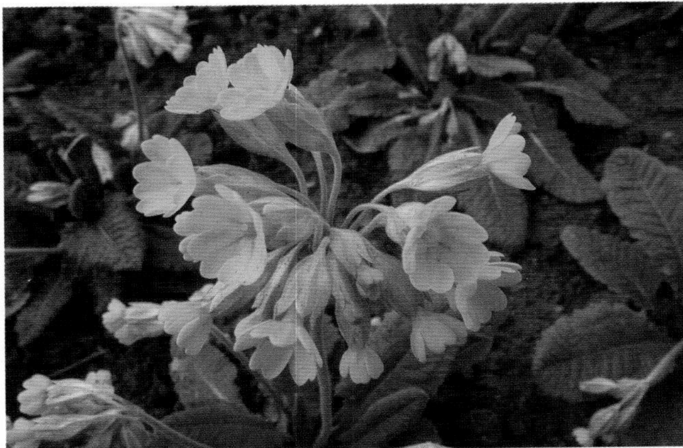

Figure 2 Cowslip (*Primula veris*).

C

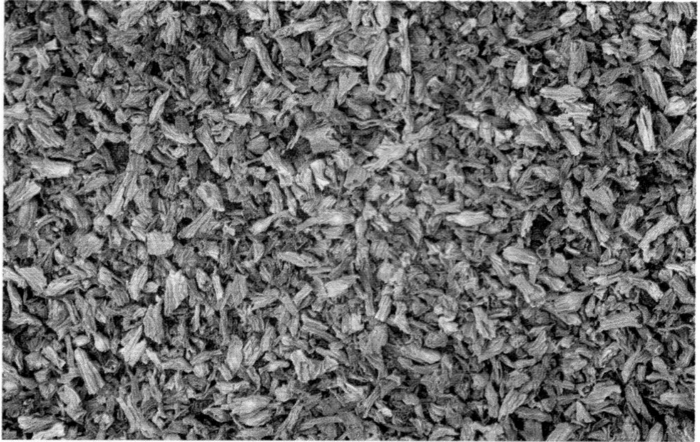

Figure 3 Cowslip – dried drug substance (flowerhead).

Pharmacological Actions

In vitro and animal studies

The saponin fraction has been reported to cause an initial hypotension followed by a long-lasting hypertension in anaesthetised animals.[(6)]

In vitro, the saponins have been documented to inhibit prostaglandin (PG) synthetase, but to a lesser extent than aspirin because of insignificant protein binding; to exhibit a slight anti-inflammatory effect against carrageenan rat paw oedema; to contract isolated rabbit ileum; and to possess analgesic and antigranulation activity.[(6)]

Flavonoid and tannin constituents have been documented for cowslip. A variety of activities has been reported for flavonoids including anti-inflammatory and antispasmodic effects. The tannins are known to be astringent.

Clinical studies

There is a lack of clinical research assessing the effects of cowslip and rigorous randomised controlled clinical trials are required.

Side-effects, Toxicity

There is a lack of clinical safety and toxicity data for cowslip and further investigation of these aspects is required.

Allergic contact reactions to related *Primula* species have been documented; quinone compounds are stated to be the allergenic principles with primin described as a strong contact allergen.[(7)] Two positive patch test reactions to cowslip have been recorded, although allergenicity was not proven.[(G51)] An LD_{50} value (mice, intraperitoneal injection) for the saponin fraction is documented as 24.5 mg/kg body weight compared to a value of 9.5 mg/kg for reparil (aescin). Haemolytic activity has been reported for the saponins, and an aqueous extract of cowslip is stated to contain saponins that are toxic to fish. Saponins are stated to be irritant to the gastrointestinal tract.

The toxicity of cowslip seems to be associated with the saponin constituents. However, these compounds have only been documented for the underground plant parts, and not for the flowers which are the main plant parts used in the UK.

Contra-indications, Warnings

Cowslip may cause an allergic reaction in sensitive individuals.

Drug interactions None documented. However, the potential for preparations of cowslip to interact with other medicines administered concurrently, particularly those with similar or opposing effects, should be considered. There is limited evidence from preclinical studies that cowslip has hypo- and hypertensive activity.

Pregnancy and lactation The safety of cowslip has not been established. In view of the lack of toxicity data, use of cowslip during pregnancy and lactation should be avoided.

Preparations

Proprietary multi-ingredient preparations

Argentina: Expectosan Hierbas y Miel. *Austria:* Bronchithym; Cardiodoron; Heumann's Bronchialtee; Krauter Hustensaft; Sinupret; Thymoval. *Canada:* Original Herb Cough Drops. *Czech Republic:* Biotussil; Bronchialtee N; Bronchicum Elixir; Bronchicum Hustensirup; Bronchicum Sekret-Loser; Sinupret. *Germany:* Bronchicum Elixir S; Bronchicum; Bronchipret; Brust- und Hustentee; Cardiodoron; Drosithym-N; Equisil N; Expectysat N; Harzer Hustenloser; Heumann Bronchialtee Solubifix T; Kinder Em-eukal Hustensaft; Phytobronchin; Sinuforton; Sinuforton; Sinupret; Solvopret; Tussiflorin Hustensaft; Tussiflorin Hustentropfen; TUSSinfant N. *Hong Kong:* Sinupret. *Hungary:* Sinupret. *Netherlands:* Bronchicum. *Russia:* Bronchicum (Бронхикум); Bronchicum Husten (Бронхикум Сироп от Кашля); Sinupret (Синупрет). *South Africa:* Cardiodoron. *Singapore:* Sinupret. *Switzerland:* Demo-Pectol; Kernosan Elixir; Pectoral N; Sinupret; Sirop pectoral contre la toux S; Sirop S contre la toux et la bronchite; Strath Gouttes contre la toux; Strath Gouttes pour les veines; Strath Gouttes Rhumatisme; Tisane pectorale pour les enfants. *Thailand:* Sinupret; Solvopret TP. *UK:* Bio-Strath Willow Formula; Onopordon Comp B.

References

1 Karl C *et al*. Die flavonoide in den blüten von Primula officinalis. *Planta Med* 1981; 41: 96–99.
2 Grecu L, Cucu V. Saponine aus *Primula officinalis* und *Primula elatior*. *Planta Med* 1975; 27: 247–253.
3 Kartnig T, Ri CY. Dünnschichtchromatographische untersuchungen an den zuckerkomponenten der saponine aus den wurzeln von *Primula veris* und *P. elatior*. *Planta Med* 1973; 23: 379–380.
4 Grecu L, Cucu V. Primulic acid aglycone from the roots of *Primula officinalis*. *Farmacia (Bucharest)* 1975; 23: 167–170.
5 Jentzsch K *et al*. Saponin level in the radix of *Primula veris*. *Sci Pharm* 1973; 41: 162–165.
6 Cebo B *et al*. Pharmacological properties of saponin fractions from Polish crude drugs. *Herb Pol* 1976; 22: 154–162.
7 Hausen BM. On the occurrence of the contact allergen primin and other quinoid compounds in species of the family of Primulaceae. *Arch Dermatol Res* 1978; 261: 311–321.

Cranberry

Summary and Pharmaceutical Comment

Limited chemical information is available for cranberry. Documented *in vitro* and animal studies provide supporting evidence for a mechanism of action for cranberry in preventing urinary tract infections. However, little is known about the specific active constituent(s); proanthocyanidins have been reported to be important.

A Cochrane systematic review of cranberry for the prevention of urinary tract infections found that there is some evidence to support the efficacy of cranberry juice for the prevention of urinary tract infections in women with symptomatic urinary tract infections. However, there is no clear evidence as to the quantity and concentration of cranberry juice that should be consumed, or as to the duration of treatment. Rigorous randomised controlled trials using appropriate outcome measures are required to determine the efficacy of cranberry juice in other populations, including children and older men and women. Prevention trials should be of at least six-months' duration in order to take into account the natural course of the illness. Another Cochrane systematic review found that there is no reliable evidence to support the efficacy of cranberry juice in the treatment of urinary tract infections.

Patients wishing to use cranberry for urinary tract infections should be advised to consult a pharmacist, doctor or other suitably trained health care professional for advice.

There are several reports of an interaction between cranberry juice and warfarin. Most reports have involved increases in patients' international normalised ratios (INR) and/or bleeding episodes. It is not possible to indicate a safe quantity or preparation of cranberry juice, and it is not known whether or not other cranberry products might also interact with warfarin. Patients taking warfarin should be advised to avoid taking cranberry juice and other cranberry products unless the health benefits are considered to outweigh the risks. In view of the lack of conclusive evidence for the efficacy of cranberry, and the serious nature of the potential harm, it is extremely unlikely that the benefit–harm balance would be in favour of such patients using cranberry.

Doses of cranberry greatly exceeding the amounts used in foods should not be taken during pregnancy and lactation.

Species (Family)

**Vaccinium macrocarpon* Aiton (Ericaceae)
†*Vaccinium oxycoccus* L.

Synonym(s)

*Large Cranberry *Oxycoccus macrocarpus* (Aiton) Pursh. is the species grown for commercial purposes.[1]
†European Cranberry, Mossberry, *Oxycoccus palustris* Pursh.

Part(s) Used

Fruit (whole berries)

Pharmacopoeial and Other Monographs

AHP[G1]
Martindale 35th edition[G85]
USP29/NF24[G86]

Legal Category (Licensed Products)

Cranberry is not included in the GSL.[G37]

Constituents

Acids Citric, malic, quinic and benzoic acids are present.[2]

Carbohydrates Fructose and oligosaccharides.

Phenolics Anthocyanins and proanthocyanidins.

Other constituents Trace glycoside has been isolated from *V. oxycoccus*.[3] Cranberries are also a good source of fibre. Cranberry juice cocktail contains more carbohydrate than do products (i.e. soft or hard gelatin capsules) based on cranberry powder (prepared from rapidly dried fruits), whereas the latter contain more fibre.[2] Alkaloids (*N*-methylazatricyclo type) have been isolated from the leaves.[4]

Food Use

Cranberries are commonly used in foods;[5] cranberry juice cocktail (containing approximately 25% cranberry juice) is widely available.[2, 5] Cranberry is listed by the Council of Europe as a natural source of food flavouring (fruit: category N1) (*see* Appendix 3).[G17]

Herbal Use

Cranberry juice and crushed cranberries have a long history of use in the treatment and prevention of urinary tract infections.[1] Traditionally, cranberries have also been used for blood disorders, stomach ailments, liver problems, vomiting, loss of appetite, scurvy and in the preparation of wound dressings.[5]

Dosage

The doses used in clinical trials of cranberry for prevention of urinary tract infections have been variable. One study used 300 mL cranberry juice cocktail (containing 30% cranberry concentrate) daily for six months.[6]

Pharmacological Actions

Documented activity for cranberry is mainly of its use in the prevention and treatment of urinary tract infections.[1]

Initially it was thought that the antibacterial effect of cranberry juice was due to its ability to acidify urine and, therefore, to inhibit bacterial growth. However, recent work has focused on the effects of cranberry in inhibiting bacterial adherence and on determining anti-adhesion agents in cranberry juice. Bacterial adherence to mucosal surfaces is considered to be an important step in the development of urinary tract infections;[7] it is facilitated by fimbriae (proteinaceous fibres on the bacterial cell wall) which produce adhesins that attach to specific receptors on uroepithelial cells.[8]

In vitro and animal studies

C

In *in vitro* studies using human urinary tract isolates of *Escherichia coli*, cranberry cocktail (which contains fructose and vitamin C in addition to cranberry juice) inhibited bacterial adherence to uroepithelial cells by 75% or more in over 60% of the clinical isolates.[9] In addition, urine from mice fed cranberry juice significantly inhibited *E. coli* adherence to uroepithelial cells when compared with urine from control mice.[9] However, these studies did not define the bacteria tested in terms of the type of fimbriae they might have expressed (specific fimbriae mediate bacterial adherence to cells).

Irreversible inhibition of adherence of urinary isolates of *E. coli* expressing type 1 and type P fimbriae has been demonstrated with cranberry juice cocktail.[10] It was thought that fructose might be responsible for the inhibition of type 1 fimbriae[10] and an unidentified high molecular weight substance responsible for type P fimbriae inhibition.[11] Further *in vitro* studies in which cranberry juice was added to the growth medium of P-fimbriated *E. coli* duplicated immediate inhibition of adherence, but also showed the loss of fimbriae with cellular elongation after long-term exposure; such changed bacteria are unable to adhere to urothelium.[12]

Proanthocyanidins extracted from cranberries have been shown to inhibit the adherence of P-fimbriated *E. coli* to uroepithelial cell surfaces at concentrations of 10–50 μg/mL, suggesting that proanthocyanidins may be important for the stated effects of cranberry in urinary tract infections.[13]

The effects of a high molecular weight constituent of cranberry juice on adhesion of bacterial strains found in the human gingival crevice have also been investigated.[14] A non-dialysable material derived from cranberry juice concentrate used at concentrations of 0.6–2.5 mg/mL reversed the interspecies adhesion of 58% of 84 bacterial pairs. Gram- negative dental plaque bacteria appeared to be more sensitive to the inhibitory effects of the cranberry constituent on adhesion.[14]

Crude extracts of cranberry have been reported to exhibit potential anticarcinogenic activity *in vitro* as demonstrated by inhibition of the induction of ornithine decarboxylase (ODC) by the tumour promoter phorbol 12-myristate 13-acetate (TPA).[15] The greatest activity appeared to be in the polymeric proanthocyanidin fraction which had an IC_{50} for ODC activity of 6.0 μg. The anthocyanidin fraction and the ethyl acetate extract were either inactive or relatively weak inhibitors of ODC activity.

A cranberry extract with a polyphenolic content of 1548 mg gallic acid equivalents per litre inhibited low-density lipoprotein (LDL) oxidation *in vitro*.[16]

Cranberry juice has demonstrated marked *in vitro* antifungal activity against *Epidermophyton floccosum* and against several *Microsporum* and *Trichophyton* species, but had no effect against *Candida albicans*.[17] Benzoic acid and/or other low molecular weight constituents of cranberry juice were reported to be responsible for the fungistatic action.

Clinical studies

Clinical trials investigating the use of cranberries for the prevention and treatment of urinary tract infections have been subject to Cochrane systematic reviews; both of these systematic reviews sought to include all randomised or quasi-randomised controlled trials.[18, 19]

Prevention of urinary tract infections Seven trials were included in a Cochrane systematic review of cranberries for prevention of urinary tract infections; six trials compared the effectiveness of cranberry juice (or cranberry–lingonberry juice) versus placebo or water and two trials compared cranberry tablets or capsules with placebo.[18] Studies differed in the formulations of cranberry, doses and treatment periods used.

In the two trials assessed as being of good methodological quality, use of cranberry was associated with a statistically significant reduction in the incidence of urinary tract infections after 12 months (relative risk (95% confidence interval): 0.61 (0.40–0.91)). One of these trials involved the administration of cranberry concentrate 7.5 g daily (in 50 mL) and the other assessed the effects of cranberry concentrate (1 : 30) in tablet form or in 250 mL juice. Apart from these two trials, the methodological quality of the trials was found to be poor and the reliability of their results questionable. The conclusions of the review were that there was some evidence to support the efficacy of cranberry juice for the prevention of urinary tract infections in women with symptomatic urinary tract infections. However, there was no clear evidence as to the quantity and concentration of cranberry juice that should be consumed, or as to the duration of treatment.[18] In addition, rigorous randomised controlled trials are required to determine the efficacy of cranberry juice in other populations, including children and older men and women.

The largest study of cranberry juice for the prevention of urinary tract infections was a double-blind, placebo-controlled trial involving 153 women (mean age 78.5 years) randomised to receive 300 mL cranberry juice cocktail (n = 72) or an indistinguishable placebo (n = 81) daily for six months.[6] The odds of experiencing bacteriuria with pyuria were significantly lower in cranberry-treated subjects than in those who received a placebo beverage (p = 0.004). The validity of the results of this trial have been questioned because of methodological shortcomings in the study design, particularly the method of randomisation.[20, 21]

Several of the other studies included in the review are summarised below. These also have methodological limitations, for example, several controlled studies claiming to involve random assignment to treatment[22–24] either did not employ true randomisation[23] or the method of randomisation was not stated.[22, 24]

A randomised, controlled, crossover study was conducted involving 38 persons (mean age 81 years) who had had hospital treatment and were waiting to be transferred to a nursing home.[23] Subjects received cranberry juice (15 mL) mixed with water or water alone twice daily for four weeks before crossing over to the alternative regimen. Seventeen participants completed the study and, of the seven from whom data were suitable for comparison, there were fewer occurrences of bacteriuria during the period of treatment with cranberry juice.[23]

The role of cranberry in the prevention of urinary tract infections in younger women has been explored in a randomised, double-blind, placebo-controlled, crossover trial involving 19 non-pregnant, sexually active women aged 18–45 years.[24] Participants received capsules containing 400 mg cranberry solids daily (exact dose not stated) or placebo for three months before crossing over to the alternative regimen. Ten subjects completed the six-month study period. Of the 21 incidents of urinary tract infection recorded among these participants, significantly fewer occurred during periods of treatment with cranberry than with placebo ($p < 0.005$).[24]

A randomised, physician-blind, crossover study investigated the efficacy of cranberry cocktail (30% cranberry concentrate) (15 mL/kg/day) for six months in 40 children (age range 1.4–18 years, mean age 9.35 years) with neuropathic bladder and managed by clean intermittent catheterisation; water was used as a control.[22] No benefit was reported for cranberry compared with control.

A randomised, double-blind, placebo-controlled, crossover trial of the effects of consumption of cranberry concentrate on the prevention of bacteriuria and symptomatic urinary tract infection has been carried out in children (n = 15) with neurogenic bladder receiving clean intermittent catheterisation.[25] Children drank 2 oz of cranberry concentrate or placebo daily for three months before changing to the alternative regimen. At the end of the study, the number of urinary tract infections occurring under each regimen was identical (n = 3). There was no significant difference between cranberry treatment and placebo with regard to the number of collected urine samples testing positively for a pathogen (75% of samples for both cranberry and placebo) (p = 0.97). It was concluded that cranberry concentrate had no effect on the prevention of bacteriuria in the population studied.[25]

Treatment of urinary tract infections Although several trials investigating the effectiveness of cranberry juice and cranberry products for treating urinary tract infections were found, none of these trials met all the inclusion criteria for systematic review.[19] Two of the studies identified[26,27] did report a beneficial effect with cranberry products, although both contained methodological flaws and no firm conclusions can be drawn from these studies.[19] Thus, it was stated that there was no evidence to suggest that cranberry juice or other cranberry products are effective in treating urinary tract infections.[19]

Other studies Early studies involving the administration of large amounts of cranberry juice to human subjects reported reductions in mean urinary pH values.[28,29] A crossover study involving eight subjects with multiple sclerosis reported that administration of cranberry juice and ascorbic acid was more effective than orange juice and ascorbic acid in acidifying the urine. However, neither treatment consistently maintained a urinary pH lower than 5.5, the pH previously determined as necessary for maintaining bacteriostatic urine.[30] Inhibition of bacterial adherence (*see* Pharmacological Actions, *In vitro* and animal studies) has been observed with urine from 22 human subjects who had ingested cranberry cocktail 1–3 hours previously.[9] Protection against bacterial adhesion has also been reported in a study involving urine collected from ten healthy male volunteers who had ingested water, ascorbic acid (500 mg twice daily for 2.5 days) or cranberry (400 mg three times daily for 2.5 days) supplements.[31] Urine samples were used to determine uropathogen adhesion to silicone rubber in a parallel plate flow chamber; urine obtained after ascorbic acid or cranberry supplementation reduced the initial deposition rates and numbers of adherent *E. coli* and *Enterococcus faecalis*, but not *Pseudomonas aeruginosa*, *Staphylococcus epidermidis* or *C. albicans*.

Other preliminary studies have explored the use of cranberry juice in reducing urine odours,[32] in improving peristomal skin conditions in urostomy patients[33] and in reducing mucus production in patients who have undergone entero-uroplasty.[34]

The ingestion of cranberry juice by subjects with hypochlorhydria due to omeprazole treatment or atrophic gastritis has been shown to result in increased protein-bound vitamin B_{12} absorption, although the clinical benefit of ingesting cranberry juice along with a meal (i.e. with the buffering action of food) remains to be determined.[35] Possible mechanisms by which the ingestion of an acidic drink such as cranberry juice could result in improved protein-bound vitamin B_{12} absorption include increased release of vitamin B_{12} from protein by direct action of acid on the vitamin B_{12}–protein bond and a pH-sensitive bacterial binding activity of vitamin B_{12} that is altered in an acidic environment.[35]

C

Side-effects, Toxicity

Clinical data

A Cochrane systematic review of cranberry products for the prevention of urinary tract infections reported that the drop-out rates in the seven studies included were high (20–55%).[18] In one of these studies, of 17 withdrawals during cranberry treatment (a further two occurred during the control period), nine participants gave the taste of cranberry as the reason for withdrawal.[22]

It has been claimed that ingesting large amounts of cranberry juice may result in the formation of uric acid or oxalate stones secondary to a constantly acidic urine and because of the high oxalate content of cranberry juice.[1] However, it has also been stated that the role of cranberry juice as a urinary acidifier has not been well established.[36] The use of cranberry juice in preventing the formation of stones which develop in alkaline urine, such as those comprising magnesium ammonium phosphate and calcium carbonate, has been described.[28]

Contra-indications, Warnings

The calorific content of cranberry juice should be borne in mind. Patients with diabetes who wish to use cranberry juice should be advised to use sugar-free preparations. Patients using cranberry juice should be advised to drink sufficient fluids in order to ensure adequate urine flow.[G31] Although a constituent of cranberry juice has been reported to have potential for altering the subgingival microbiota, some commercially available cranberry juice cocktails may not be suitable for oral hygiene purposes because of their high dextrose and fructose content.[14]

Drug interactions There are several reports of an interaction between cranberry juice and warfarin. By October 2004, the UK Committee on Safety of Medicines had received 12 such reports, of which eight involved increases in patients' international normalised ratios (INR) and/or bleeding episodes, three involved unstable INR and one a decrease in INR.[37] These reports include a death in a man whose INR rose to over 50 six weeks after starting to drink cranberry juice. The man experienced gastrointestinal and pericardial haemorrhage and died.[38] It is not possible to indicate a safe quantity or preparation of cranberry juice, and it is not known whether or not other cranberry products might also interact with warfarin.

Against this background, patients taking warfarin should be advised to avoid taking cranberry juice and other cranberry products unless the health benefits are considered to outweigh the risks.[39] In view of the lack of conclusive evidence for the efficacy of cranberry, and the serious nature of the potential harm, it is extremely unlikely that the benefit–harm balance would be in favour of such patients using cranberry.

The mechanism for the interaction between cranberry constituents and warfarin is not known. The suggestion that it may involve inhibition of the cytochrome P450 enzyme CYP2C9 (by which warfarin is predominantly metabolised),[38] requires investigation.

While not a drug interaction, it is reasonable to provide the following information here. Interference with dipstick tests for glucose and haemoglobin in urine has been reported in a study involving 28 patients who had drunk 100 or 150 mL of low-sugar or regular cranberry juice daily for seven weeks;[40] ascorbic acid in cranberry juice was reported to be the component responsible for interference resulting in negative test results.

Pregnancy and lactation There are no known problems with the use of cranberry during pregnancy. Doses of cranberry greatly exceeding the amounts used in foods should not be taken during pregnancy and lactation.

Preparations

Proprietary single-ingredient preparations

Australia: Uricleanse. *Canada:* Cran Max. *France:* Gyndelta. *UK:* Seven Seas Cranberry Forte.

Proprietary multi-ingredient preparations

Australia: Bioglan Cranbiotic Super; Cranberry Complex; Cranberry Complex; Extralife Uri-Care. *Canada:* Cran-C; Prostease. *Hong Kong:* Prostease. *USA:* CranAssure; Cranberry; Cran Support; Calcium with Magnesium; My Defense.

References

1 Kingwatanakul P, Alon US. Cranberries and urinary tract infection. *Child Hosp Q* 1996; 8: 69–72.
2 Hughes BG, Lawson LD. Nutritional content of cranberry products. *Am J Hosp Pharm* 1989; 46: 1129.
3 Jankowski K, Paré JRJ. Trace glycoside from cranberries (*Vaccinium oxycoccus*). *J Nat Prod* 1983; 46: 190–193.
4 Jankowski K. Alkaloids of cranberries V. *Experientia* 1973; 29: 1334–1335.
5 Siciliano AA. Cranberry. *Herbalgram* 1996; 38: 51–54.
6 Avorn J *et al.* Reduction of bacteriuria and pyuria after ingestion of cranberry juice. *JAMA* 1994; 271: 751–754.
7 Reid G, Sobel JD. Bacterial adherence in the pathogenesis of urinary tract infection: a review. *Rev Infect Dis* 1987; 9: 470–487.
8 Beachey EH. Bacterial adherence: adhesin–receptor interactions mediating the attachment of bacteria to mucosal surface. *J Infect Dis* 1981; 143: 325–345.
9 Sobota AE. Inhibition of bacterial adherence by cranberry juice: potential use for the treatment of urinary tract infections. *J Urol* 1984; 131: 1013–1016.
10 Zafiri D *et al.* Inhibitory activity of cranberry juice on adherence of type 1 and type P fimbriated *Escherichia coli* to eucaryotic cells. *Antimicrob Agents Chemother* 1989; 33: 92–98.
11 Ofek I *et al.* Anti-*Escherichia coli* adhesin activity of cranberry and blueberry juices. *Adv Exp Med Biol* 1996; 408: 179–183.
12 Ahuja S *et al.* Loss of fimbrial adhesion with the addition of *Vaccinium macrocarpon* to the growth medium of P-fimbriated *Escherichia coli*. *J Urol* 1998; 159: 559–562.
13 Howell AB *et al.* Inhibition of the adherence of P fimbriated *Escherichia coli* to uroepithelial-cell surfaces by proanthocyanidin extracts from cranberries. *N Engl J Med* 1998; 339: 1085–1086.
14 Weiss EI *et al.* Inhibiting interspecies coaggregation of plaque bacteria with a cranberry juice constituent. *J Am Dent Assoc* 1998; 129: 1719–1723.
15 Bomser J *et al.* *In vitro* anticancer activity of fruit extracts from *Vaccinium* species. *Planta Med* 1996; 62: 212–216.
16 Wilson T *et al.* Cranberry extract inhibits low density lipoprotein oxidation. *Life Sci* 1998; 62: 381–386.
17 Swartz JH, Medrek TF. Antifungal properties of cranberry juice. *Appl Microbiol* 1968; 16: 1524–1527.
18 Jepson RG *et al.* Cranberries for preventing urinary tract infections (Cochrane Review). The Cochrane Database of Systematic Reviews 2004, Issue 2. Art. No.: CD001321.pub3.
19 Jepson RG *et al.* Cranberries for treating urinary tract infections (Cochrane Review). The Cochrane Database of Systematic Reviews 1998, Issue 4. Art. No.: CD001322.
20 Hopkins WJ *et al.* Reduction of bacteriuria and pyuria using cranberry juice (letter). *JAMA* 1994; 272: 589.
21 Katz LM. Reduction of bacteriuria and pyuria using cranberry juice (letter). *JAMA* 1994; 272: 589.
22 Foda MM *et al.* Efficacy of cranberry in prevention of urinary tract infection in a susceptible pediatric population. *Can J Urol* 1995; 2: 98–102.
23 Haverkorn MJ, Mandigers J. Reduction of bacteriuria and pyuria using cranberry juice (letter). *JAMA* 1994; 272: 590.
24 Walker EB *et al.* Cranberry concentrate: UTI prophylaxis. *J Family Pract* 1997; 45: 167–168.
25 Schlager TA *et al.* Effect of cranberry juice on bacteriuria in children with neurogenic bladder receiving intermittent catheterization. *J Pediatr* 1999; 135: 698–702.
26 Papas PN *et al.* Cranberry juice in the treatment of urinary tract infections. *Southwest Med* 1966; 47: 17–20.
27 Rogers J. Pass the cranberry juice. *Nurs Times* 1991; 87: 36–37.
28 Kahn HD *et al.* Effect of cranberry juice on urine. *J Am Diet Assoc* 1967; 51: 251–254.
29 Kinney AB, Blount M. Effect of cranberry juice on urinary pH. *Nurs Res* 1979; 28: 287–290.
30 Schultz A. Efficacy of cranberry juice and ascorbic acid in acidifying the urine in multiple sclerosis subjects. *J Commun Health Nurs* 1984; 1: 159–169.
31 Habash MB *et al.* The effect of water, ascorbic acid, and cranberry derived supplementation on human urine and uropathogen adhesion to silicone rubber. *Can J Microbiol* 1999; 45: 691–694.
32 DuGan CR, Cardaciotto PS. Reduction of ammoniacal urine odors by sustained feeding of cranberry juice. *J Psych Nurs* 1966; 8: 467–470.
33 Tsukada K *et al.* Cranberry juice and its impact on peri-stomal skin conditions for urostomy patients. *Ostomy/Wound Manage* 1994; 40: 60–67.
34 Rosenbaum TP *et al.* Cranberry juice helps the problem of mucus production in entero-uroplasties. *Neurol Urodynamics* 1989; 8: 344–345.
35 Saltzman JR *et al.* Effect of hypochlorhydria due to omeprazole treatment or atrophic gastritis on protein-bound vitamin B_{12} absorption. *J Am Coll Nutr* 1994; 13: 584–591.
36 Soloway MS, Smith RA. Cranberry juice as a urine acidifier. *JAMA* 1988; 260: 1465.
37 Anon. Interaction between warfarin and cranberry juice: new advice. *Curr Prob Pharmacovigilance* 2004; 30: 10.
38 Anon. Possible interaction between warfarin and cranberry juice. *Curr Prob Pharmacovigilance* 2003; 29: 8.
39 Medicines and Healthcare products Regulatory Agency. Herbal Safety News. Cranberry. http://www.mhra.gov.uk (accessed January 9, 2006).
40 Kilbourn JP. Interference with dipstick tests for glucose and hemoglobin in urine by ascorbic acid in cranberry juice. *Clin Chem* 1987; 33: 1297.

Damiana

Summary and Pharmaceutical Comment

There is limited chemical information available on damiana. There has been little documented evidence to justify the herbal uses, and the reputation of damiana as an aphrodisiac is unproven. In view of the lack of toxicity data and reported cyanogenetic and arbutin constituents, excessive use of damiana should be avoided.

Species (Family)

Turnera diffusa Willd. ex Schult. (Turneraceae)

Synonym(s)

Turnera aphrodisiaca Ward, *T. diffusa* var. *aphrodisiaca* (Ward) Urb.

Part(s) Used

Leaf, stem

Pharmacopoeial and Other Monographs

BHC 1992[G6]
BHP 1996[G9]
Martindale 35th edition[G85]

Legal Category (Licensed Products)

GSL[G37]

Constituents

The following is compiled from several sources, including General Reference G6.

Carbohydrates Gum 13.5%, starch 6%, sugars.

Cyanogenetic glycosides Tetraphyllin B.[1]

Phenolic glycoside Arbutin (up to 0.7%).[2]

Tannins 3.5%. Type unspecified.

Volatile oils 0.5–1.0%. At least 20 components including 1,8-cineole (11%), *p*-cymene (2%), α- and β-pinene (2%), thymol, α-copaene, δ-cadinene and calamene. The presence of 1,8-cineole and *p*-cymene has been disputed.[2]

Other constituents Acids (fatty, plant), alkanes (e.g. hexacosanol-1 and triacontane), damianin (7%) (a bitter principle), flavone (gonzalitosin-1), β-sitosterol, resin (6.5%).[3]

Food Use

Damiana is used in foods and is listed by the Council of Europe as a natural source of food flavouring (category N2). This category indicates that damiana can be added to foodstuffs in small quantities with a possible limitation of an active principle (as yet unspecified) in the final product.[G16] Previously in the USA, damiana has been approved for food use.[G41]

Herbal Use

Damiana is stated to possess antidepressant, thymoleptic, mild purgative, stomachic and reputedly aphrodisiac properties.[4] It

Phenolic glycosides

arbutin

Monoterpenes

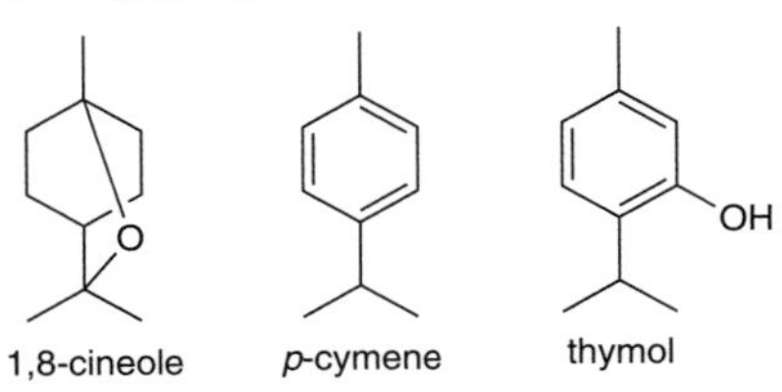

Sesquiterpenes

δ-cadine

α-copaene

calamene

Cyanogenic glycoside

tetraphyllin B

Flavonoids

gonzalitosin 1

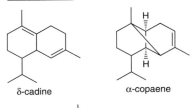

Figure 1 Selected constituents of damiana.

has been used for depression, nervous dyspepsia, atonic constipation, coital inadequacy, and specifically for anxiety neurosis with a predominant sexual factor.[G6, G7, G8, G64]

Dosage

Dosages for oral administration (adults) for traditional uses recommended in older and contemporary standard reference texts are given below.

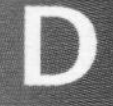

Dried leaf 2–4 g as an infusion three times daily.[G6, G7]

Liquid Extract of Damiana (BPC 1934) 2–4 mL.

Pharmacological Actions

In vitro and animal studies

Hypoglycaemic activity has been reported in mice following both oral and intraperitoneal administration of damiana.[5] An ethanolic extract was stated to exhibit CNS-depressant activity although no other experimental details were available.[6]

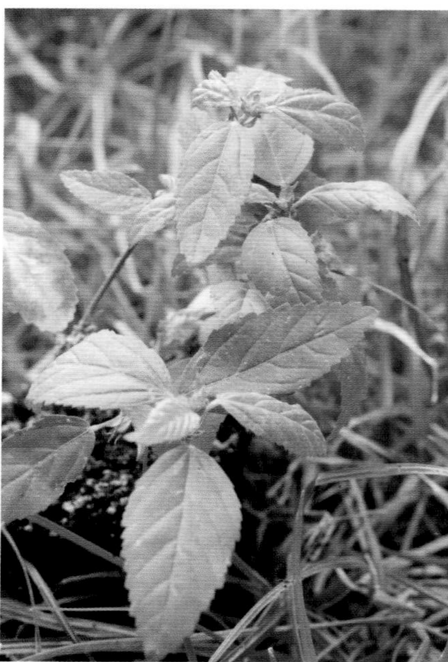

Figure 2 Damiana (*Turnera diffusa*).

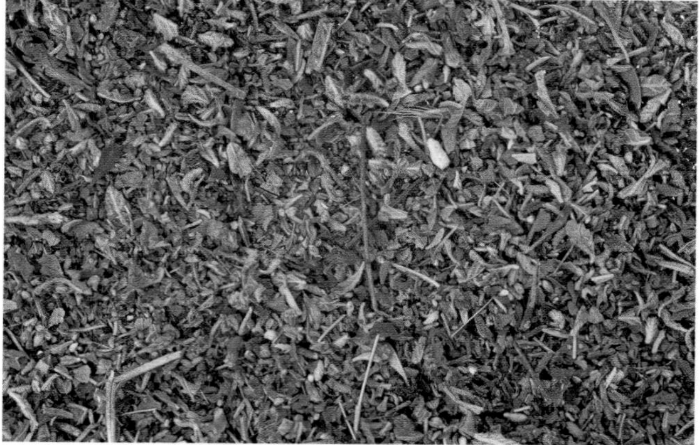

Figure 3 Damiana – dried drug substance.

Antibacterial activity against *Escherichia coli*, *Proteus mirabilis*, *Pseudomonas aeruginosa* and *Staphylococcus aureus* has been documented for a mixed herbal preparation, with some of the activity attributed to damiana.[7] The same herbal preparation was also reported to inhibit acetylcholine-induced spasm of the isolated guinea-pig ileum, although none of the antispasmodic activity was attributed to damiana.[7]

Arbutin is stated to be responsible for the urinary antiseptic properties (*see* Uva-Ursi). However, the arbutin content of damiana is much less than that quoted for uva-ursi (0.7% and 5 to 18%, respectively).

Clinical studies

There is a lack of clinical research assessing the effects of damiana and rigorous randomised controlled clinical trials are required.

A herbal preparation containing damiana as one of the ingredients was reported to have a favourable effect on the symptoms of irritable bladder associated with functional and neurohormonal disorders, and on bacterial bladder infections.[7] However, because of the methodological limitations of this study, these effects cannot be attributed to damiana.

Side-effects, Toxicity

There is a lack of clinical safety and toxicity data for damiana and further investigation of these aspects is required.

Tetanus-like convulsions and paroxysms resulting in symptoms similar to those of rabies or strychnine poisoning have been described in one individual following the ingestion of approximately 200 g damiana extract; cyanide poisoning was considered to be a possible cause. No other reported side-effects for damiana were located.

High doses of arbutin (e.g. 1 g) are considered to be toxic, although the concentration of arbutin documented for damiana (1 g arbutin is equivalent to more than 100 g plant material) is probably too low to warrant concerns over safety.

Contra-indications, Warnings

Excessive use should be avoided because of the presence of cyanogenetic glycosides and arbutin.

Drug interactions None documented. However, the potential for preparations of damiana to interact with other medicines administered concurrently, particularly those with similar or opposing effects, should be considered. There is limited evidence from preclinical studies that damiana has hypoglycaemic activity.

Pregnancy and lactation The safety of damiana has not been established. In view of the lack of toxicity data and possible cyanogenetic constituents, doses greatly exceeding amounts used in foods should not be taken during pregnancy or lactation.

Preparations

Proprietary multi-ingredient preparations

Australia: Bioglan Mens Super Soy/Clover; Bioglan The Blue One; Medinat Esten; Nevaton. *Canada:* Damiana-Sarsaparilla Formula. *Italy:* Dam; Four-Ton. *Malaysia:* Total Man. *Spain:* Energysor. *UK:* Daily Fatigue Relief; Damiana and Kola Tablets; Elixir Damiana and Saw Palmetto; Regina Royal Concorde; Strength; Strength Tablets; Supa-Tonic Tablets; VitAmour; Zotrim. *USA:* Women's Menopause Formula.

References

1 Spencer KC, Siegler DS. Tetraphyllin B from *Turnera diffusa*. *Planta Med* 1981; 43: 175–178.

2 Auterhoff H, Häufel H-P. Inhaltsstoffe der damiana-droge. *Arch Pharm* 1968; 301: 537–544.

3 Domínguez XA, Hinojosa M. Mexican medicinal plants. XXVIII Isolation of 5-hydroxy-7,3′,4′-trimethoxy-flavone from *Turnera diffusa*. *Planta Med* 1976; 30: 68–71.

4 Braun JK, Malone MH. Legal highs. *Clin Toxicol* 1978; 12: 1–31.

5 Pérez RM *et al*. A study of the hypoglycemic effect of some Mexican plants. *J Ethnopharmacol* 1984; 12: 253–262.

6 Jiu J. A survey of some medical plants of Mexico for selected biological activity. *Lloydia* 1966; 29: 250–259.

7 Westendorf J. Carito-In-vitro-Untersuchungen zum Nachweis spasmolytischer und kontraktiler Einflüsse. *Therapiewoche* 1982; 32: 6291–6297.

Dandelion

Summary and Pharmaceutical Comment

Dandelion is a well-known traditional herbal remedy, although limited scientific information, particularly clinical research, is available to justify the reputed uses. Several investigations have failed to demonstrate significant diuretic effects in laboratory animals and have proposed that any diuretic activity is due to the high potassium content of the leaf and root. Dandelion has also been used in foods for many years. Animal studies indicate dandelion to be of low toxicity. However, excessive ingestion of dandelion, particularly in amounts exceeding those normally consumed in foods, should be avoided.

Species (Family)

Taraxacum officinale Weber (Asteraceae/Compositae)

Synonym(s)

Lion's Tooth, *Taraxacum palustre* (Lyons) Lam & DC., *Leontodon taraxacum* L., Taraxacum

Part(s) Used

Leaf, root

Pharmacopoeial and Other Monographs

BHC 1992[(G6)]
BHP 1996[(G9)]
Complete German Commission E[(G3)]
ESCOP 2003[(G76)]
Martindale 35th edition[(G85)]

Legal Category (Licensed Products)

GSL[(G37)]

Constituents

The following is compiled from several sources, including General References G2, G6 and G64.

Acids and phenols Caffeic acid, *p*-hydroxyphenylacetic acid, chlorogenic acid,[(1)] cichoric acid, monocaffeoyl tartaric acids,[(2)] taraxacoside, linoleic acid, linolenic acid, oleic acid and palmitic acid.

Coumarins Cichoriin and aesculin.[(2)]

Flavonoids Luteolin-7-glucoside and luteolin-7-diglucosides.[(2)]

Minerals Potassium 4.5% in leaf, 2.45% in root.[(3)]

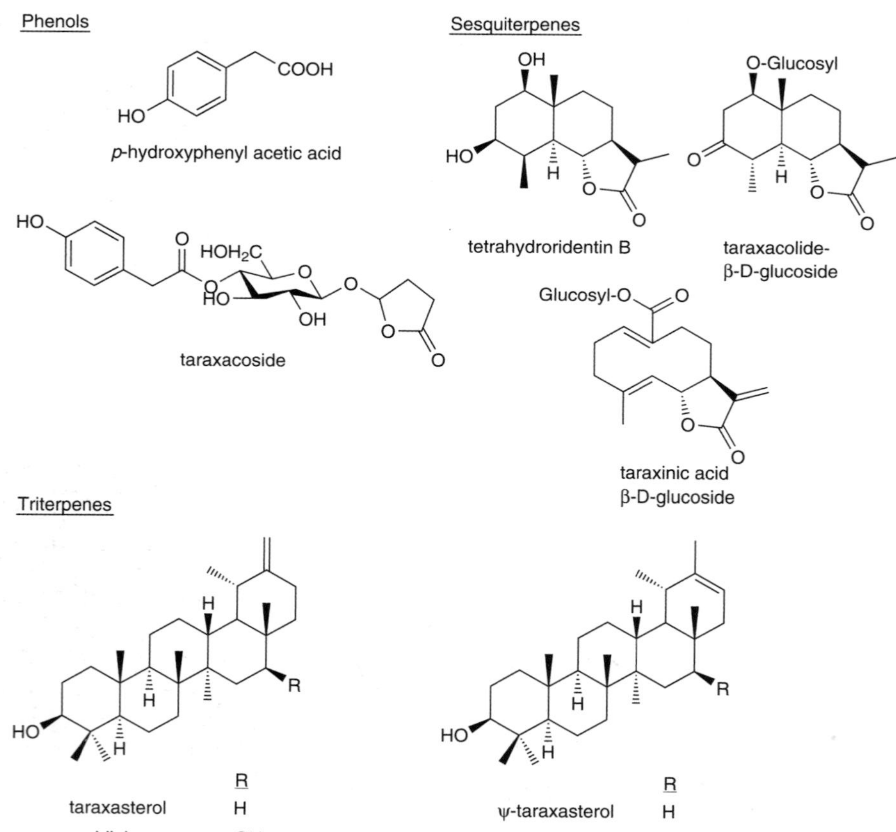

Figure 1 Selected constituents of dandelion.

Resin Undefined bitter complex (taraxacin).

Terpenoids Sesquiterpene lactones taraxinic acid (germacranolide) esterified with glucose,[4] and eudesmanolides.[5]

Vitamins Vitamin A 14 000 iu/100 g leaf (compared with 11 000 iu/100 g carrots).

Other constituents Carotenoids, choline, inulin, pectin, phytosterols (e.g. sitosterol, stigmasterol, taraxasterol, homotaraxasterol), sugars (e.g. fructose, glucose, sucrose), triterpenes (e.g. β-amyrin, taraxol, taraxerol).

Food Use

Dandelion is used as a food, mainly in salads and soups. The roasted root and its extract have been used as a coffee substitute.[G41] Dandelion is listed by the Council of Europe as a natural source of food flavouring (category N2). This category indicates that dandelion can be added to foodstuffs in small quantities, with a possible limitation of an active principle (as yet unspecified) in the final product.[G16] Previously in the USA, dandelion has been listed as GRAS (Generally Recognised As Safe).[G41]

Herbal Use

Dandelion is stated to possess diuretic, laxative, cholagogue and antirheumatic properties. It has been used for cholecystitis, gallstones, jaundice, atonic dyspepsia with constipation, muscular rheumatism, oliguria, and specifically for cholecystitis and dyspepsia. The German Commission E approved use of root and herb for disturbance of bile flow, stimulation of diuresis, loss of appetite and dyspepsia.[G3] Root is used in combination with celandine herb and artichoke for epigastric discomfort due to functional disorders of the biliary system.[G3]

Dosage

Dosages for oral administration (adults) for traditional uses recommended in older and contemporary standard herbal reference texts are given below.

Dried leaf 4–10 g as an infusion three times daily.[G6, G7]

Leaf, liquid extract 4–10 mL (1 : 1 in 25% alcohol) three times daily.[G6, G7]

Leaf tincture 2–5 mL.[G3]

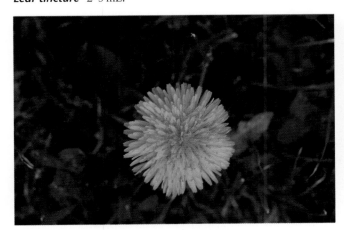

Figure 2 Dandelion (*Taraxacum officinale*).

Leaf, fresh juice 5–10 mL.[G52]

Dried root 2–8 g or by infusion or decoction three times daily.[G6, G7]

Root, tincture 5–10 mL (1 : 5 in 45% alcohol) three times daily.[G6, G7]

Liquid Extract of Taraxacum (BPC 1949) 2–8 mL.

Juice of Taraxacum (BPC 1949) 4–8 mL.

Pharmacological Actions

In vitro and animal studies

A diuretic effect in rats and mice has been documented for dandelion extracts, following oral administration.[6] Herb extracts were found to produce greater diuresis than root extracts; a dose of 50 mL (equivalent to 2 g dried herb/kg body weight) produced an effect comparable to that of furosemide 80 mg/kg. By contrast, no significant increases in urine volume or sodium excretion were observed in mice following oral administration of either leaf or root extracts, or of purified fractions.[3] Similarly, oral and intravenous administration of an ethanolic extract of dandelion root failed to produce a diuretic effect in laboratory animals.[7]

Moderate anti-inflammatory activity against carrageenan-induced rat paw oedema has been documented for a dandelion root extract.[8] An 80% ethanol extract of root (100 mg/kg orally)

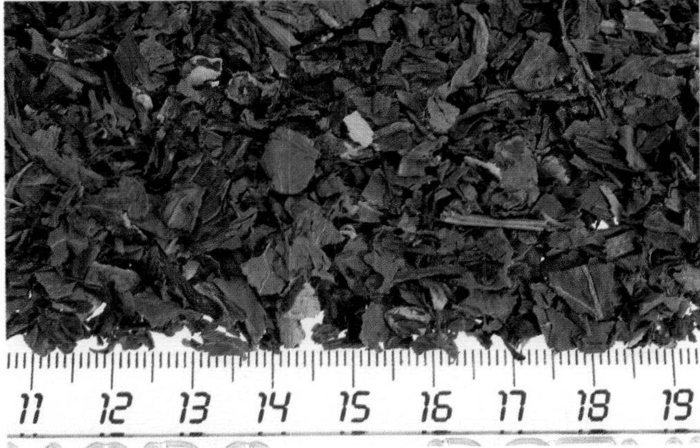

Figure 3 Dandelion – dried drug substance (leaf).

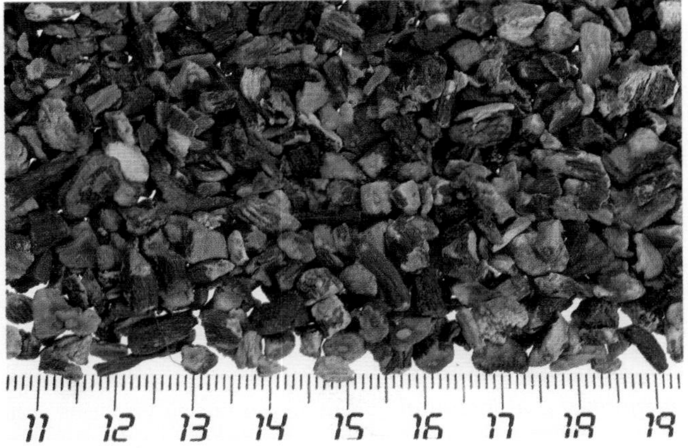

Figure 4 Dandelion – dried drug substance (root).

inhibited oedema by 43% in the carrageenan-induced rat paw oedema test at 3 hours.[7]

Bile secretion was doubled in dogs by a decoction of fresh root (equivalent to 5 g dried plant); similar activity has been observed for rats.[G52]

Hypoglycaemic activity has been described in normal, but not in diabetic rabbits, following oesophageal administration of dandelion.[9] Doses greater than 500 mg/kg produced a significant blood glucose concentration which had returned to normal after 24 hours. The maximum decrease produced by a dose of 2 g/kg was reported to be 65% of the effect produced by tolbutamide 500 mg/kg. Sulfonylureas (e.g. tolbutamide) act by stimulating pancreatic beta-cells and a similar mechanism was proposed for dandelion.

In vitro antitumour activity has been documented for an aqueous extract of dandelion, given by intraperitoneal injection, in the tumour systems ddY-Ehrlich and C3H/He-MM46.[10] The mechanism of action was thought to be similar to that of tumour polysaccharides such as lentinan.

Clinical studies

There is a lack of clinical research assessing the effects of dandelion and rigorous randomised controlled clinical trials are required.

Side-effects, Toxicity

There is a lack of clinical safety and toxicity data for dandelion and further investigation of these aspects is required.

Contact allergic reactions to dandelion have been documented[11, G51] and animal studies have reported dandelion to have a weak sensitising capacity.[12] Sesquiterpene lactones are thought to be the allergenic principles in dandelion.[4] These compounds contain an exocyclic α-methylene β-lactone moiety, which is thought to be a prerequisite for allergenic activity of sesquiterpene lactones.

The acute toxicity of dandelion appears to be low, with LD_{50} values (mice, intraperitoneal injection) estimated at 36.8 g/kg and 28.8 g/kg for the root and herb, respectively.[6] No visible signs of toxicity were observed in rabbits administered dandelion 3, 4, 5 and 6 g/kg body weight by mouth for up to seven days.[9] In addition, no behavioural changes were recorded.

Contra-indications, Warnings

Treatment with dandelion is contraindicated for patients with occlusion of bile duct, gall bladder empyema and obstructive ileus.[G3, G52] Dandelion may precipitate an allergic reaction in susceptible individuals, although no reports following the ingestion of dandelion have been documented.

Drug interactions None documented. However, the potential for preparations of dandelion to interact with other medicines administered concurrently, particularly those with similar or opposing effects, should be considered. There is limited evidence from preclinical studies that dandelion has diuretic and hypoglycaemic activities.

Pregnancy and lactation There are no known problems with the use of dandelion during pregnancy, provided that doses do not greatly exceed the amounts used in foods.

Preparations

Proprietary single-ingredient preparations

Czech Republic: Gallentee. *Germany:* Carvicum.

Proprietary multi-ingredient preparations

Argentina: Quelodin F. *Australia:* Berberis Complex; Bioglan Cranbiotic Super; Colax; Colax; Digest; Extralife Fluid-Care; Extralife Liva-Care; Feminine Herbal Complex; Fluid Loss; Glycoplex; Herbal Cleanse; Herbal Diuretic Formula; Lifesystem Herbal Formula 7 Liver Tonic; Liver Tonic Herbal Formula 6; Livstim; Livton Complex; Profluid; Silybum Complex; St Mary's Thistle Plus; Trifolium Complex; Uva-Ursi Complex; Uva-Ursi Plus. *Austria:* Gallen- und Lebertee St Severin; Magentee St Severin; Montana; Original Schwedenbitter; Urelium Neu. *Canada:* Milk Thistle Extract Formula. *Czech Republic:* Cynarosan; Diabetan; Diabeticka Cajova Smes-Megadiabetin; The Salvat; Ungolen. *France:* Diacure; Hydracur; Romarene. *Germany:* Alasenn; Amara-Tropfen; Carmol Magen-Galle-Darm; Cholosom SL; Cholosom-Tee; Gallemolan forte; Gallexier; Gallexier; Tonsilgon. *Hong Kong:* Hepatofalk. *Italy:* Varicofit. *Malaysia:* Dandelion Complex. *Russia:* Tonsilgon N (Тонзилгон Н). *South Africa:* Amara. *Spain:* Diurette. *Switzerland:* Boldocynara; Demonatur Gouttes pour le foie et la bile; Gastrosan; Heparfelien; Strath Gouttes pour les reins et la vessie; Tisane hepatique et biliaire. *UK:* Adios; Aqualette; Aqualette; Backache; Boldex; Culpeper DeTox Tea; Fenneherb Slim Aid; HealthAid Boldo-Plus; Herbulax; HRI Water Balance; Napiers Slimming Tablets; Natravene; Natural Herb Tablets; Nervous Dyspepsia Tablets; Out-of-Sorts; Reducing (Slimming) Tablets; Rheumatic Pain; Stomach Mixture; Uvacin; Uvacin; Weight Loss Aid; Wind & Dyspepsia Relief. *USA:* Liver Formula Herbal Blend.

References

1 Clifford MN *et al.* The chlorogenic acids content of coffee substitutes. *Food Chem* 1987; 24: 99–107.

2 Williams CA *et al.* Flavonoids, cinnamic acids and coumarins from the different tissues and medicinal preparations of *Taraxacum officinale*. *Phytochem* 1996; 42: 121–127.

3 Hook I *et al.* Evaluation of dandelion for diuretic activity and variation in potassium content. *Int J Pharmacog* 1993; 31: 29–34.

4 Hausen BM. Taraxinsäure-1′-O-β-D-glucopyranosid, das kontaktallergen des löwenzahns (*Taraxacum officinale* Wiggers). *Dermatosen* 1982; 30: 51–53.

5 Hänsel R *et al.* Sequiterpenlacton-β-D-glucopyranoside sowie ein neues eudesmanolid aus *Taraxacum officinale*. *Phytochem* 1980; 19: 857–861.

6 Rácz-Kotilla *et al.* The action of *Taraxacum officinale* extracts on the body weight and diuresis of laboratory animals. *Planta Med* 1974; 26: 212–217.

7 Tita B *et al.* *Taraxacum officinale* W.: Pharmacological effect of ethanol extract. *Pharmacol Res* 1993; 27: 23–24.

8 Mascolo N *et al.* Biological screening of Italian medicinal plants for anti-inflammatory activity. *Phytother Res* 1987; 1: 28–29.

9 Akhtar MS *et al.* Effects of *Portulaca oleracae* (kulfa) and *Taraxacum officinale* (dhudhal) in normoglycaemic and alloxan-treated hyperglycaemic rabbits. *J Pak Med Assoc* 1985; 35: 207–210.

10 Baba K *et al.* Antitumor activity of hot water extract of dandelion, *Taraxacum officinale* – correlation between antitumor activity and timing of administration. *Yagugaku Zasshi* 1981; 101: 538–543.

11 Hausen BM, Schulz KH. Allergische kontaktdermatitis durch löwenzahn (*Taraxacum officinale* Wiggers). *Dermatosen* 1978; 26: 198.

12 Davies MG, Kersey PJW. Contact allergy to yarrow and dandelion. *Contact Dermatitis* 1986; 14: 256–257.

Devil's Claw

Summary and Pharmaceutical Comment

The chemistry of devil's claw has been well documented. The iridoid constituents are thought to be responsible for the reputed anti-inflammatory activity of devil's claw, although it is not known precisely which of these are the most important for pharmacological activity, and the importance of other compounds. There is conflicting evidence from *in vitro*, animal and human studies regarding the anti-inflammatory activity of devil's claw and possible mechanisms of action. Several randomised trials using devil's claw extracts standardised on harpagoside content have reported superiority over placebo for some aspects of low back pain and rheumatic complaints. However, some studies used non-standard outcome measures and carried out several post-hoc analyses. Further studies have used recognised, predefined outcome measures to establish the therapeutic value of standardised devil's claw extracts in patients with arthritic and rheumatic conditions.

On the basis of randomised controlled trials involving patients with arthritic and rheumatic disorders, devil's claw extracts appear to have a favourable short-term adverse effect profile when taken in recommended doses. Mild, transient gastrointestinal effects, such as diarrhoea and flatulence, may occur. Chronic toxicity studies and clinical experience with prolonged use are lacking, so the effects of long-term use are not known. On this basis, and in view of the possible cardioactivity of devil's claw, devil's claw should not be used for long periods of time at doses higher than recommended. Further studies involving large numbers of patients are required.

Species (Family)

Harpagophytum procumbens (Burch.) DC. ex Meissn. (Pedaliaceae)

Synonym(s)

Harpagophytum, *Harpagophytum burchelii* Decne, Grapple Plant, Wood Spider

Part(s) Used

Secondary root tuber

Pharmacopoeial and Other Monographs

BHC 1992[G6]
BHMA 2003[G66]
BHP 1996[G9]
BP 2007[G84]
Complete German Commission E[G3]
ESCOP 2003[G76]
Martindale 35th edition[G85]
Ph Eur 2007[G81]

Legal Category (Licensed Products)

Devil's claw is not included in the GSL.[G37]

Constituents

See also General Reference G2.

Carbohydrates Fructose, galactose, glucose and *myo*-inositol (monosaccharides), raffinose, stachyose (46%) and sucrose (oligosaccharides).[1]

Diterpenes (+)-8,11,13-totaratriene-12,13-diol and (+)-8,11,13-abietatrien-12-ol.[2]

Iridoids Harpagoside (1–3%), harpagide, 8-*p*-coumaroylharpagide, 8-feruloylharpagide, 8-cinnamylmyoporoside, 6′-*O*-*p*-coumaroylharpagide, 6′-*p*-coumaroylprocumbide, and pagoside.[3–5] *p*-Coumaroyl esters occur as E and Z isomers.[5]

Phenylpropanoids Acteoside and isoacteoside, 6-O-acetylacteoside,[4–6] 2,6-*O*-diacetylacteoside.[7]

Other constituents Amino acids, flavonoids (e.g. kaempferol, luteolin), triterpenoids, sterols.[4, G75]

Other plant parts The flower, stem and ripe fruit are reported to be devoid of harpagoside; the leaf contains traces of iridoids.[8]

Quality of plant material and commercial products

According to the British and European Pharmacopoeias, devil's claw root consists of the cut and dried tuberous secondary roots of *H. procumbens* DC. It contains not less than 1.2% of harpagoside, calculated with reference to the dried drug.[G81, G84] As with other herbal medicinal products, there is variation in the qualitative and quantitative composition of commercial devil's claw root preparations.

Some commercial extracts of devil's claw root may have been prepared not only from the roots of *H. procumbens*, but also from the roots of *H. zeyheri*, which are similar macroscopically.[9] However, the two species differ in the concentration of the constituents harpagoside and 8-*p*-coumaroylharpagide. On this basis it has been stated that the species can be distinguished chemically by determining the ratio harpagoside : 8-*p*-coumaroylharpagide. The ratio is stated to be near one for *H. zeyheri* and between 20 and 38 for *H. procumbens* which has a low 8-*p*-coumaroylharpagide content.[9] While this ratio may be sufficient for chemotaxonomic differentiation, it may not be adequate for quality control.[10]

Other studies have demonstrated that the harpagoside content of several powdered dry extracts of devil's claw from different manufacturers varies, and that each extract has a unique profile of other constituents.[11] The harpagoside content of commercial extracts of *H. procumbens* has been reported to range from 0.8–2.3%.[12]

Food Use

Devil's claw is not used in foods.

Herbal Use

Devil's claw is stated to possess anti-inflammatory, antirheumatic, analgesic, sedative and diuretic properties. Traditionally, it has been used as a stomachic and a bitter tonic, and for arthritis, gout, myalgia, fibrositis, lumbago, pleurodynia and rheumatic disease.[G2, G6–G8, G32, G64] Modern use of devil's claw is focused on its use in the treatment of rheumatic and arthritic conditions, and low back pain.

Dosage

Dosages for oral administration (adults) recommended in older and more contemporary standard herbal reference texts are given below.

Painful arthrosis and tendonitis

1.5–3 g dried tuber as a decoction, three times daily; 1–3 g drug or equivalent aqueous or hydroalcoholic extracts;[G76] liquid extract 1–3 mL (1 : 1, 25% ethanol) three times daily.[G6]

Diterpenes

	R^1	R^2
(+)-8,11,13-totaratriene-12,13-diol	OH	isopropyl
(+)-8,11,13-abietatrien-12-ol	isopropyl	H

Iridoids

	R
harpagoside	*trans*-cinnamoyl
harpagide	H

procumbide

	R^1	R^2	R^3	R^4	R^5	R^6
8-*p*-coumaroylharpagide	OH	OH	H	OH	H	H
8-feruloylharpagide	OH	OH	OCH_3	OH	H	H
8-cinnamoylmyoporoside	H	H	H	H	OH	H
6′-*p*-coumaroylharpagide	OH	OH	H	OH	H	*p*-coumaroyl

pagoside

Figure 1 Selected constituents of devil's claw.

Phenylpropanoids

	R^1	R^2	R^3
acteoside	H	caffeoyl	H
isoacteoside	H	H	caffeoyl
6-*O*-acetyl-acteoside	H	caffeoyl	acetyl
2,6-di-*O*-acetyl-acteoside	acetyl	caffeoyl	acetyl

Figure 2 Selected constituents of devil's claw.

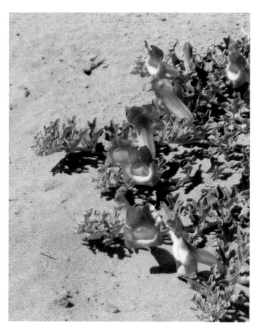

Figure 3 Devil's claw (*Harpagophytum procumbens*).

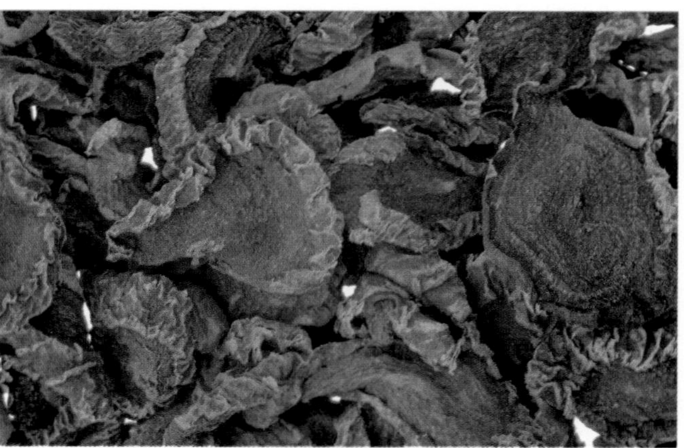

Figure 4 Devil's claw – dried drug substance (root).

Loss of appetite or dyspepsia

Dried tuber 0.5 g as a decoction, three times daily.[G6]

Tincture 1 mL (1 : 5, 25% ethanol) three times daily.[G6]

Clinical trials of devil's claw root extracts for the treatment of low back pain typically have tested oral doses ranging from 2000–4500 mg daily, in two or three divided doses (equivalent to less than 30 mg up to 100 mg harpagoside daily, depending on the particular extract), for four to 20 weeks.[13] In a clinical trial in osteoarthritis, participants received capsules containing powdered cryoground devil's claw root 2610 mg daily for four months.[14]

Pharmacological Actions

The active constituents of devil's claw are widely held to be the iridoid glucosides although, of these, it has not been definitively established whether harpagoside is the most important pharmacologically active constituent of the whole extract. Other compounds present in the root may contribute to the pharmacological activities of devil's claw.[15,16] It has also been suggested that harpagogenin, formed by *in vivo* acid hydrolysis of harpagoside, may have biological activity.[17]

In vitro and animal studies

Pharmacokinetics Transformation of the iridoids harpagide, harpagoside and 8-*O*-(*p*-coumaroyl)-harpagide into the pyridine monoterpene alkaloid aucubinine B, chemically or by human intestinal bacteria *in vitro*, has been documented.[18,19] However, it is not known if aucubinine B is formed *in vivo* by intestinal bacteria and, therefore, whether it contributes to the pharmacological activity of devil's claw.[19]

Anti-inflammatory and analgesic activities Animal studies of the anti-inflammatory and analgesic activities of devil's claw have reported conflicting results. Activity appears to differ depending on the route of administration of devil's claw, and the model of inflammation, whether acute or subacute. Also, studies have assessed the effects of different preparations of *H. procumbens* (e.g. aqueous extracts and ethanolic extracts) and it is important to consider this when interpreting the results.

In controlled experiments in rats, a 60% ethanol extract of *H. procumbens* roots injected (compartment and site not specified) at doses of 25, 50 and 100 mg/kg body weight daily for four days beginning five days after sub-plantar injection of Freund's adjuvant produced a significantly greater antinociceptive response in the hot-plate test and significantly reduced paw oedema than did control (distilled water) on days 6–8 after induction of experimental arthritis ($p < 0.01$ for all).[20] Similar results were obtained when administration of *H. procumbens* extract was initiated 20 days after sub-plantar injection of Freund's adjuvant and continued for 20 days, with tests for antinociceptive and anti-inflammatory activity performed on four occasions during this period.

Pretreatment with a dried aqueous extract of devil's claw root at doses of 100 mg/kg and above, administered intraperitoneally, resulted in peripheral analgesic activity demonstrated by a significant reduction in the number of writhings induced by acetic acid in mice.[16] However, no effect was observed in the hot-plate test, indicating a lack of central analgesic activity with devil's claw extract.

The peripheral analgesic properties of intraperitoneal dried aqueous extract of devil's claw have been confirmed in other studies for doses of 400 mg/kg and above.[9] A subsequent series of experiments found that administration of an aqueous extract of *H. procumbens* root at doses of 200–800 mg/kg body weight intraperitoneally resulted in significantly greater antinociceptive effects than did control in both the hot-plate and acetic-acid induced writhings tests in mice ($p < 0.05$ versus control) and, at a dose of 400 or 800 mg/kg body weight, in a significant reduction in egg-albumin induced hind-paw inflammation in rats, compared with control ($p < 0.05$).[21]

In contrast, other studies have reported that dried aqueous extract of devil's claw administered orally had no effect on carrageenan- or *Mycobacterium butyricum*- (Freund's adjuvant) induced oedema in rat paw, whereas both indometacin and aspirin displayed significant anti-inflammatory activity.[22,23] However, dried aqueous extract of devil's claw administered by intraperitoneal injection demonstrated significant activity in the carrageenan-induced oedema test in rats, an acute model of inflammation.[16] The effect on oedema was dose-dependent for doses of devil's claw extract 100–400 mg/kg, and reached a maximum three hours after carrageenan injection. Other studies in rats have reported significant reductions in oedema using the same model following pretreatment with intraperitoneal[9,24] and intraduodenal, but not oral, dried aqueous extract of devil's claw.[24]

Anti-inflammatory activity of harpagoside has been demonstrated in experimental models, including the croton oil-induced granuloma pouch test, and for harpagogenin, the aglucone of harpagoside, in the croton oil-induced granuloma pouch test and in formalin-induced arthritis in rats.[25]

Studies have also reported peripheral analgesic and anti-inflammatory properties for the related species *Harpogophytum zeyheri*.[9] Animal studies using aqueous extracts of devil's claw have suggested that the extract may be inactivated by passage through the acid environment of the stomach.[16,24] One study compared the anti-inflammatory activities of aqueous devil's claw extract administered by different routes. Intraperitoneal and intraduodenal administration led to a significant reduction in the carrageenan-induced rat paw oedema test, but there was no effect following oral administration.[24] In another study, aqueous devil's claw extract pretreated with hydrochloric acid to mimic acid conditions in the stomach showed no activity in pharmacological models of pain and inflammation.[16]

A clear mechanism of action for the purported anti-inflammatory effects of devil's claw has yet to be established. *In vitro*, devil's claw (100 mg/mL) had no significant effect on prostaglandin (PG) synthetase activity, whereas indometacin (316 μg/mL) and aspirin (437 μg/mL) caused 50% inhibition of this enzyme.[23] In other *in vitro* studies in human whole blood samples, devil's claw extracts and fractions of extracts were tested for their effects on thromboxane B2 (TXB_2) and leukotriene (LT) biosynthesis.[26] TXB_2 is an end-product of arachidonic acid metabolism by the cyclooxygenase 1 (COX-1) pathway. Inhibition appeared to be dependent on the harpagoside content of the extracts or fractions.[26] An aqueous extract of *H. procumbens* inhibited lipopolysaccharide-induced enhancement of cyclooxygenase-2 activity, resulting in suppression of PGE_2 synthesis in *in-vitro* experiments using the mouse fibroblast cell line L929.[27] In the same system, the extract inhibited inducible nitric oxide synthase (iNOS) mRNA expression, resulting in suppression of nitric oxide production. Inhibition of iNOS expression by an aqueous extract of *H. procumbens* roots, resulting in suppression of nitrite production, has also been described following experiments in rat renal mesangial cells. The effect was observed with a harpagoside-free extract and with an extract containing a high concentration (27%) of harpagoside, but not with extracts containing around 2% harpagoside, indicating that high concentrations of harpagoside as well as other concentrations are necessary to bring about the effect.[28]

Harpagoside (100 µmol/L), but not harpagide (100 µmol/L), inhibited calcium ionophore A23187-stimulated release of TXB_2 from human platelets.[29] However, harpagoside and harpagide had no significant inhibitory effect on calcium ionophore A23187-stimulated release of PGE_2 and LTC_4 from mouse peritoneal macrophages.[29]

Other preclinical studies have described effects for devil's claw extracts and/or isolated constituents on other pathways involved in inflammatory processes. *In vitro* inhibition of tumour-necrosis-factor-α (TNF-α) synthesis in lipopolysaccharide-stimulated human monocytes by a hydroalcoholic extract of devil's claw (SteiHap 69) has also been documented.[30] Inhibitory activity against human leukocyte elastase (a serine proteinase involved in inflammatory processes) has been reported for an aqueous extract of *H. procumbens* roots (drug to extract ratio 1.5-2.5 : 1) and the isolated constituents 6′-*O*-acetylacteoside, isoacteoside, 8-*p*-coumaroylharpagide, pagoside and caffeic acid, with IC_{50} values of 542, 47, 179, 179, 154 and 86 µg/mL, respectively. The IC_{50} values for several other constituents, including acteoside and harpagoside were higher than 300 µg/mL (4). An ethanol extract of *H. procumbens* significantly reduced IL-1β-induced production of several matrix metalloproteinase enzymes (MMPs) in human chondrocytes.[31] (In inflammatory diseases, there is increased production of cytokines such as IL-1β and TNF-α, which results in an increased production of MMPs which breakdown the extracellular cartilage matrix.)

Other activities Crude methanolic extracts of devil's claw have been shown to be cardioactive *in vitro* and *in vivo* in animals. A protective action against ventricular arrhythmias induced by aconitine, calcium chloride and epinephrine (adrenaline)/chloroform has been reported for devil's claw given intraperitoneally or added to the reperfusion medium.[32,33] The crude extract was found to exhibit greater activity than pure harpagoside.[33] In isolated rabbit heart, low concentrations of a crude methanolic extract had mild negative chronotropic and positive inotropic effects,[32] whereas high concentrations caused a marked negative inotropic effect with reduction in coronary blood flow.[32] In anaesthetised dogs, harpagoside administered orally by gavage caused a decrease in mean aortic pressure and arterial and pulmonary capillary pressure.[34]

In vitro, harpagoside has been shown to decrease the contractile response of smooth muscle to acetylcholine and barium chloride on guinea-pig ileum and rabbit jejunum. Harpagide was found to increase this response at lower concentrations, but antagonised it at higher concentrations.[35] On the basis of these studies in isolated smooth muscle, it was suggested that the constituents of devil's claw may influence mechanisms regulating calcium influx.[35]

Methanolic extracts have also exhibited hypotensive properties in normotensive rats, causing a decrease in arterial blood pressure following oral doses of 300 mg/kg and 400 mg/kg body weight.[32]

Aqueous fractions derived from an extract of devil's claw root (drug to extract ratio 2 : 1 containing 2.6% harpagoside) showed antioxidant activity in an *in-vitro* assay based on ability to scavenge 2,2′-azino-bis(3-ethylbenzthiazoline-6-sulfonic acid)-derived radicals.[36] However, harpagoside showed only weak antioxidant activity. In mice, a methanol extract of *H. procumbens* root tubers applied topically to shaven skin 30 minutes before application of 12-*O*-tetradecanoylphorbol-13-acetate (TPA), a stimulator of COX-2 expression, led to a significant reduction in COX-2 protein when assessed four hours after TPA administration.[37] The extract did not have any effect on TPA-induced activation of nuclear factor-κB, but inhibited TPA-induced activation of activator protein-1, which is involved in the regulation of COX-2 in mouse skin. Overexpression of COX-2 is thought to be involved in tumour promotion.

Antidiabetic activity has been described for an aqueous extract of *H. procumbens* root in *in vivo* experiments in rats with streptozotocin-induced diabetes mellitus.[21] The extract significantly reduced blood glucose concentrations in both fasted normoglycaemic rats and fasted diabetic rats when administered intraperitoneally at doses of 800 mg/kg body weight.

Two diterpene constituents ((+)-8,11,13-totaratriene-12,13-diol and (+)-8,11,13-abietatrien-12-ol) isolated using bioassay-guided fractionation from a petroleum ether extract of *H. procumbens* root were found to be active against a chloroquine-sensitive (D10) and a chloroquine-resistant (K1) strain of *Plasmodium falciparum in vitro* ($IC_{50} < 1$ µg/mL).[2]

Devil's claw extracts possess weak antifungal activity against *Penicillium digitatum* and *Botrytis cinerea*.[38]

Clinical studies

Pharmacokinetics There is little published information on the pharmacokinetics of devil's claw extracts in humans. A pharmacokinetic study involving a small number of healthy male volunteers ($n = 3$) measured plasma harpagoside concentrations after oral administration of devil's claw extract (WS1531 containing 9% harpagoside) 600, 1200 and 1800 mg as film-coated tablets.[26] Maximal plasma concentrations of harpagoside were reached after 1.3–1.8 hours, and were 8.2 ng/mL and 27.8 ng/mL for doses of harpagoside of 108 and 162 mg, respectively (corresponding to 1200 and 1800 mg devil's claw extract, respectively). Other studies involving small numbers of healthy male volunteers indicated that the half-life ranged between 3.7 and 6.4 hours. Other results suggested that there may be low oral absorption or a considerable first-pass effect with devil's claw extract, although this needs further investigation.[26]

Pharmacodynamics A study involving healthy volunteers investigated the effects on eicosanoid production of orally administered devil's claw (four 500-mg capsules of powder, containing 3% glucoiridoids, daily for 21 days).[39] No statistically significant differences on PGE_2, TXB_2, 6-keto-$PGF_{1\alpha}$ and LTB_4 were observed following the period of devil's claw administration, compared with baseline values. By contrast, in a subsequent study involving whole blood samples taken from healthy male volunteers, a biphasic decrease in basal cysteinyl-leukotriene (Cys-LT) biosynthesis, compared with baseline values, was observed following oral administration of devil's claw extract (WS1531 containing 9% harpagoside) 600, 1200 and 1800 mg as film-coated tablets.[26]

Therapeutic activity The efficacy and effectiveness of devil's claw have been investigated in around 20 clinical studies involving patients with rheumatic and arthritic conditions, and low back pain.[15,40] These studies have involved different methodological designs, including several uncontrolled studies, and different preparations of devil's claw, including crude drug and aqueous extracts. Evaluating the evidence is further complicated as preparations tested in clinical trials typically have been standardised for their harpagoside content and, although harpagoside is believed to contribute to activity, it is not yet clear to what extent and which other constituents are important. Therefore, at present, there is insufficient evidence to draw definitive conclusions regarding the efficacy of specific devil's claw preparations, and because of the differences in the pharmaceutical quality of individual preparations, general conclusions on efficacy cannot be drawn.[41]

A systematic review of the quality of clinical trials involving devil's claw found that although the results of some studies have provided evidence for the effectiveness of certain devil's claw preparations, the quality of evidence was not sufficient to support the use of any of the available products.[42]

A systematic review of 12 controlled, randomised or quasi-randomised trials of *H. procumbens* preparations in patients with osteoarthritis (5 trials), low back pain (4 trials) and mixed pain conditions (3 trials) found differing levels of evidence for the different *H. procumbens* preparations assessed. There was evidence (from two trials involving a total of 325 participants) that an aqueous extract of *H. procumbens* administered orally at a dose equivalent to harpagoside 50 mg daily for four weeks was superior to placebo in reducing pain in patients with acute episodes of chronic non-specific low-back pain.[13] There was also evidence (from one trial for each) that the same extract administered orally at a dose equivalent to harpagoside 100 mg daily for four weeks was superior to placebo, and at a dose equivalent to harpagoside 60 mg daily for six weeks was not inferior to rofecoxib 12.5 mg daily, in reducing pain in patients with acute episodes of chronic non-specific low-back pain. There was evidence that powdered *H. procumbens* plant material at a dose equivalent to 57 mg harpagoside daily for 16 weeks was not inferior to diacerhein. Overall, however, the limited amount of data and heterogeneous nature of the available studies, indicate that further randomised controlled trials assessing well-characterised *H. procumbens* preparations and involving sufficient numbers of patients are required.

Several of the trials mentioned above are discussed in more detail below.

A randomised, double-blind, placebo-controlled study involving 118 patients with acute exacerbations of chronic low back pain investigated the effects of devil's claw extract 800 mg three times daily (equivalent to 50 mg harpagoside daily) for four weeks.[43] There was no statistically significant difference between the devil's claw and placebo groups in the primary outcome measure – consumption of the opioid analgesic tramadol over weeks 2–4 of the study – among the 109 patients who completed the study. This was an unusual choice of primary outcome measure as it gives no direct indication of the degree of pain experienced by participants. There was a trend towards improvement in a modified version of the Arhus Low Back Pain Index (a measure of pain, disability and physical impairment) for devil's claw recipients compared with placebo recipients, although this did not reach statistical significance. A greater proportion of patients in the devil's claw group were pain-free at the end of the study, although this was only a secondary outcome measure.

On the basis of these findings, a subsequent randomised, double-blind, placebo-controlled trial involving 197 patients with exacerbations of low back pain tested the effects of two doses of devil's claw (WS1531) extract against placebo.[44] Participants received devil's claw extract 600 mg or 1200 mg daily (equivalent to 50 mg and 100 mg harpagoside daily, respectively), or placebo, for four weeks. There was a statistically significant difference (p = 0.027) between devil's claw and placebo with respect to the primary outcome measure – the number of patients who were pain-free without tramadol for at least five days during the last week of the study. However, numbers of patients who were pain-free were low (3, 6 and 10 for placebo, devil's claw 600 mg daily and devil's claw 1200 mg daily, respectively). Furthermore, this is a non-standard outcome measure. Arhus Low Back Pain Index scores improved significantly in all three groups, compared with baseline values, although there was no statistically significant difference between groups.

In a randomised, double-blind, placebo-controlled study involving patients with non-specific low back pain, 65 participants received devil's claw extract (LI-174, Rivoltan), or placebo, 480 mg twice daily (equivalent to 24 mg harpagoside daily) for four weeks.[45] There was a significant improvement ($p < 0.001$) in visual analogue scale (VAS) scores for muscle pain in the devil's claw group, but not the placebo group, compared with baseline values, after two and four weeks' treatment. Differences in VAS scores between the two groups were statistically significant after four weeks' treatment ($p < 0.001$). Significant differences between the two groups in favour of devil's claw after four weeks' treatment were also observed with several other parameters, including muscle stiffness and muscular ischaemic pain.

A small number of studies has compared the efficacy of devil's claw with that of conventional pharmaceutical agents in the treatment of low back pain. In a randomised, double-blind, pilot trial, 88 participants with acute exacerbations of low back pain received an aqueous extract of devil's claw (Doloteffin; drug to extract ratio 1.5-2.5:1) 2400 mg daily in three divided doses (equivalent to 60 mg harpagoside daily), or rofecoxib (Vioxx) 12.5 mg daily for six weeks.[46] At the end of this period, compared with baseline values, there were improvements in Arhus Low Back Pain Index scores, health assessment questionnaire scores, and increases in the numbers of pain-free patients for both groups. There were no statistically significant differences between groups for any of the outcome measures but, because the study did not include sufficient numbers of patients, these findings do not demonstrate clinical equivalence between the two treatments.[46]

A randomised, double-blind, pilot trial in which 88 participants with acute exacerbations of low back pain received an aqueous extract of devil's claw (Doloteffin), or rofecoxib (Vioxx) for six weeks offered participants continuing treatment with devil's claw aqueous extract two tablets three times daily for up to one year after the six-week pilot study. Participants were not aware of their initial study group (i.e. devil's claw extract or rofecoxib) until towards the end of the one-year follow-up study.[47] In total, 38 and 35 participants who had previously received devil's claw and rofecoxib, respectively, participated in the follow-up study, and underwent assessment every six weeks. After 24 and 54 weeks, 53 and 43 participants, respectively, remained in the study. There were no convincing differences between the two groups (i.e. those who previously received devil's claw and those who received rofecoxib) with respect to pain scores, use of additional analgesic medication, Arhus Index scores and health assessment questionnaire scores.

Furthermore, the uncontrolled design of the follow-up study would have precluded any definitive conclusions regarding differences between the two groups.

A randomised, double-blind trial compared the efficacy of devil's claw extract with that of diacerein in 122 patients with osteoarthritis of the knee and hip.[14] Participants received powdered cryoground devil's claw (Harpadol) 2.61 g daily, or diacerein 100 mg daily, for four months.

VAS scores for spontaneous pains improved significantly in both groups, compared with baseline values, and there were no differences between devil's claw and diacerein with respect to VAS scores. In a placebo-controlled study involving 89 patients with rheumatic complaints, devil's claw recipients (who received powdered crude drug 2 g daily for two months) showed significant improvements in sensitivity to pain and in motility (as measured by the finger-to-floor distance), compared with placebo recipients.[48]

Several, open, uncontrolled, post-marketing surveillance studies[49–53] have assessed the effects of devil's claw preparations in patients with rheumatic and arthritic disorders, and back pain. These studies typically have reported improvements in pain scores at the end of the treatment period, compared with baseline values. However, the design of these studies (i.e. no control group) does not allow any conclusions to be drawn on the effects of devil's claw in these conditions as there are alternative explanations for the observed effects.

Another study involved 45 patients with osteo- or rheumatoid arthritis who received devil's claw root extract 2.46 g daily for two weeks in addition to non-steroidal anti-inflammatory drug (NSAID) treatment, followed by devil's claw extract alone, for four weeks.[54] It was reported that there were no statistically significant changes in pain intensity and duration of morning stiffness during the period of treatment with devil's claw extract alone. In subgroups of patients with rheumatoid arthritis and those with osteoarthritis, small decreases were observed in concentrations of C-reactive protein and creatinine, respectively. The design of this study in terms of the treatment regimen (NSAID followed by devil's claw extract without a wash-out period), also precludes definitive conclusions about the effects of devil's claw preparations.

Side-effects, Toxicity

The mechanism of action of devil's claw remains unclear, in particular, whether it has significant effects on the mediators of acute inflammation. Data from *in vitro* and clinical studies in this regard do not yet give a clear picture (*see* Pharmacological Actions, *In vitro* and animal studies and Clinical studies, Pharmacodynamics). It has been stated that adverse effects associated with the use of NSAIDs are unlikely to occur with devil's claw, even during long-term treatment.[G50, G76] While there are no documented reports of gastrointestinal bleeding or peptic ulcer associated with the use of devil's claw, the latter statement requires confirmation. Use of devil's claw in gastric and duodenal ulcer is contraindicated, although this appears to be because of the drug's bitter properties.[G50]

Clinical data

Randomised, placebo-controlled trials involving patients with rheumatic and arthritic conditions who have received devil's claw extracts or powdered drug at approximately recommended doses for four weeks have reported mild, transient gastrointestinal symptoms (such as diarrhoea, flatulence) in a small proportion (less than 10%) of devil's claw recipients.[43–45] No serious adverse events were reported, although one patient withdrew from one study because of tachycardia.[43]

A small number of reports of randomised trials comparing the effects of devil's claw preparations with those of standard pharmaceutical agents has included data on adverse events. In a randomised, double-blind, pilot trial, 88 participants with acute exacerbations of low back pain received an aqueous extract of devil's claw (Doloteffin; drug to extract ratio 1.5-2.5:1) 2400 mg daily in three divided doses (equivalent to 60 mg harpagoside daily), or rofecoxib (Vioxx) 12.5 mg daily for six weeks.[46] In total, 28 (32%) participants (14 in each group) experienced adverse events, most commonly gastrointestinal complaints (9 in each group).

In a follow-up study, participants in the six-week pilot study were offered continuing treatment with devil's claw aqueous extract two tablets three times daily for up to one year. Participants were not aware of their initial study group (i.e. devil's claw extract or rofecoxib) until towards the end of the one-year follow-up study.[47] In total, 38 and 35 participants who had previously received devil's claw and rofecoxib, respectively, participated in the follow-up study and, after 24 and 54 weeks, a total of 53 and 43 participants, respectively, remained in the study. Overall, 17 (23%) of the 73 participants in the follow-up study experienced a total of 21 adverse events. Of these, the causality for three events was classified (by a physician not involved in the study) as 'likely' (one allergic skin reaction) or 'possible' (diarrhoea, acid 'hiccup') with respect to devil's claw treatment. Five participants (7%) withdrew from the study because of adverse events.

In a randomised, controlled trial comparing devil's claw extract with diacerein in patients with osteoarthritis, numbers of patients ending the study prematurely because of suspected adverse drug reactions were 8 and 14 for devil's claw and diacerein recipients, respectively.[14] In total, 26 diacerein recipients and 16 devil's claw recipients reported one or more adverse events ($p = 0.042$). The numbers of adverse events attributed to the treatment was significantly lower for devil's claw than for diacerein (10 versus 21; $p = 0.017$). The most frequently reported adverse event, diarrhoea, occurred in 8.1% and 26.7% of devil's claw and diacerein recipients, respectively.

Several, open, uncontrolled studies,[51–53] which have assessed the effects of devil's claw preparations in patients with arthritic disorders and back pain, have reported data on adverse events. In an open, uncontrolled, multicentre, surveillance study involving patients with arthrosis of the hip or knee, 75 participants received tablets containing an aqueous extract of the secondary tubers of devil's claw (Doloteffin; drug extract ratio = 1.5-2.5 : 1) at a dosage of two 400 mg tablets three times daily (equivalent to 50 mg iridoidglycosides, calculated as harpagoside) for 12 weeks.[51] During the study, four (5%) participants experienced adverse events (dyspeptic complaints, 2; sensation of fullness, 1; panic attack, 1), although none stopped treatment with devil's claw. Causality was assessed as 'possible' for two of these events. In a similar open, uncontrolled, multicentre study, 130 participants with chronic non-radicular back pain received tablets containing 480 mg devil's claw extract (LI-174; drug extract ratio = 4.4-5 : 1) at a dosage of one tablet twice daily for eight weeks.[52] Overall, 13 (10%) participants withdrew from the study for various reasons, including no apparent improvement in their condition. No serious adverse events were reported, but three partipants reported minor adverse events (bloating, insomnia and outbreaks of sweating). In a post-marketing surveillance study, 250 patients with non-specific low back pain or osteoarthritic pain of the knee or hip received an aqueous extract of *H. procumbens* (Doloteffin) at an oral dose equivalent to harpagoside 60 mg daily in three divided doses for eight weeks in addition to any existing treatment and/or additional analgesic medicines as required. Fifty participants experienced adverse events; most commonly gastrointestinal complaints ($n = 22$); two participants experienced allergic skin reactions.[53] In 27 participants, the adverse event was considered by an independent investigator to be possibly (n = 11), likely (15) or certainly (1) related to ingestion of devil's claw.

In another open, uncontrolled study, one patient withdrew after four days' treatment with devil's claw aqueous extract 1.23 g daily because of several symptoms, including frontal headache, tinnitus, anorexia and loss of taste.[(55)]

There is an isolated report of conjunctivitis, rhinitis and respiratory symptoms in a 50-year-old woman who had experienced chronic occupational exposure to devil's claw.[(56)]

Preclinical data

Acute and subacute toxicity tests in rodents have demonstrated low toxicity of devil's claw extracts. In a study in mice, the acute oral lethal dose (LD) LD_0 and LD_{50} were greater than 13.5 g/kg body weight.[(23)] In rats, clinical, haematological and gross pathological findings were unremarkable following administration of devil's claw extract 7.5 g/kg by mouth for seven days. Hepatic effects (liver weight, and concentrations of microsomal protein and several liver enzymes) were not observed following oral treatment with devil's claw extract 2 g/kg for seven days.[(23)] Other studies in mice have reported acute oral acute intravenous LD_0 values of greater than 4.64 g/kg and greater than 1 g/kg, respectively.[(57)] For an extract containing harpagoside 85%, acute oral LD_0, acute intravenous LD_0 and acute intravenous LD_{50} values were greater than 4.64 g/kg, 395 mg/kg and 511 mg/kg, respectively.[(57)]

Contra-indications, Warnings

Devil's claw is stated to be contra-indicated in gastric and duodenal ulcers,[(G3, G76)] and in gallstones should be used only after consultation with a physician.[(G3)]

Drug interactions None have been described for devil's claw preparations. However, on the basis of pharmacological evidence of devil's claw's cardioactivity, the possibility of excessive doses interfering with existing treatment for cardiac disorders or with hypo/hypertensive therapy should be considered. Inhibitory effects on certain cytochrome P450 (CYP) drug metabolising enzymes have been documented for a devil's claw root extract (Bioforce) *in vitro* using a technique involving liquid chromatography-mass spectrometry and automated online extraction.[(58)] Mean (standard deviation) IC_{50} values for the devil's claw extract when tested in assays with individual CYP enzymes were 997 (23), 254 (17), 121 (8), 155 (9), 1044 (80) and 335 (14) for the CYPs 1A2, 2C8, 2C9, 2C19, 2D6 and 3A4, respectively.

Pregnancy and lactation It has been stated that devil's claw has oxytocic properties,[(59)] although the reference gives no further details and the basis for this statement is not known. In addition, there is no further evidence to substantiate the statement. However, given the lack of data on the effects of devil's claw taken during pregnancy and lactation, its use should be avoided during these periods.

Preparations

Proprietary single-ingredient preparations

France: Harpadol; Harpagocid. *Germany:* Ajuta; Allya; Arthrosetten H; Arthrotabs; Bomarthros; Cefatec; Dolo-Arthrodynat; Dolo-Arthrosetten H; Doloteffin; flexi-loges; Harpagoforte Asmedic; HarpagoMega; Harpagosan; Jucurba; Matai; Pargo; Rheuferm Phyto; Rheuma-Sern; Rivoltan; Sogoon; Teltonal; Teufelskralle. *Spain:* Fitokey Harpagophytum; Harpagofito Orto.

Proprietary multi-ingredient preparations

Australia: Arthriforte; Arthritic Pain Herbal Formula 1; Bioglan Arthri Plus; Boswellia Compound; Devils Claw Plus; Extralife Arthri-Care; Guaiacum Complex; Herbal Arthritis Formula; Lifesystem Herbal Formula 1 Arthritic Aid; Prost-1. *Czech Republic:* Antirevmaticky Caj. *France:* Arkophytum. *Germany:* Dr Wiemanns Rheumatonikum. *Italy:* Bodyguard; Nevril; Pik Gel. *Malaysia:* Celery Plus. *Spain:* Dolosul; Natusor Harpagosinol.

References

1 Ziller KH, Franz G. Analysis of the water-soluble fraction from the roots of *Harpagophytum procumbens*. *Planta Med* 1979; 37: 340–348.

2 Clarkson C *et al*. *In vitro* antiplasmodial activity of abietana and totarane diterpenes isolated from *Harpagophytum procumbens* (Devil's claw). *Planta Med* 2003; 69: 720–724.

3 Kikuchi T *et al*. New iridoid glucosides from *Harpagophytum procumbens* DC. *Chem Pharm Bull* 1983; 31: 2296–2301.

4 Boje K *et al*. New and known iridoid- and phenylethanoid glycosides from *Harpagophytum procumbens* and their in vitro inhibition of human leukocyte elastase. *Planta Med* 2003; 69: 820–825.

5 Seger C *et al*. LC-DAD-MS/SPE-NMR hyphenation. A tool for the analysis of pharmaceutically used plant extracts: identification of isobaric iridoid glycoside regioisomers from *Harpagophytum procumbens*. *Anal Chem* 2005; 77: 878–885.15679357

6 Burger JFW *et al*. Iridoid and phenolic glycosides from *Harpagophytum procumbens*. *Phytochemistry* 1987; 26: 1453–1457.

7 Munkombwe NM. Acetylated phenolic glycosides from *Harpagophytum procumbens*. *Phytochemistry* 2003; 62: 1231–1234.12648542

8 Czygan FC, Krueger A. Pharmaceutical biological studies of the genus *Harpagophytum*. Part 3 Distribution of the iridoid glycoside harpagoside in the different organs of *Harpagophytum procumbens* and *Harpagophytum zeyheri*. *Planta Med* 1977; 31: 305–307.

9 Baghdikian B *et al*. An analytical study, anti-inflammatory and analgesic effects of *Harpagophytum procumbens* and *Harpagophytum zeyheri*. *Planta Med* 1997; 63: 171–176.

10 Eich J *et al*. HPLC analysis of iridoid compounds of *Harpagophytum* taxa: quality control of pharmaceutical drug material. *Pharmac Pharmacol Lett* 1998; 8: 75–78.

11 Chrubasik S *et al*. Zum Harpagosidehalt verschiedener Trockenextraktpulver aus *Harpagophytum procumbens*. *Forsch Komplementärmed* 1996; 3: 6–11.

12 Chrubasik S *et al*. Zum Wirkstoffgehalt in Arzneimitteln *Harpagophytum procumbens*. 1996, 3: 57–63.

13 Gagnier JJ *et al*. *Harpagophytum procumbens* for osteoarthritis and low back pain: a systematic review. *BMC Complementary and Alternative Medicine* 2004; 4: 13.

14 Chantre P *et al*. Efficacy and tolerance of *Harpagophytum procumbens* versus diacerhein in treatment of osteoarthritis. *Phytomedicine* 2000; 7: 177–183.

15 Wegener T. Devil's claw: from African traditional remedy to modern analgesic and antiinflammatory. *Herbalgram* 2000; 50: 47–54.

16 Lanhers M-C *et al*. Anti-inflammatory and analgesic effects of an aqueous extract of *Harpagophytum procumbens*. *Planta Med* 1992; 58: 117–123.

17 Vanhaelen M *et al*. Biological activity of *Harpagophytum procumbens*. 1. Preparation and structure of Harpagogenin. *J Pharm Belg* 1981 36: 38–42.

18 Baghdikian B *et al*. Two new pyridine monoterpene alkaloids by chemical conversion of a commercial extract of *Harpagophytum procumbens*. *J Nat Prod* 1999; 62: 211–213.

19 Baghdikian B *et al*. Formation of nitrogen-containing metabolites from the main iridoids of *Harpagophytum procumbens* and *H. zeyheri* by human intestinal bacteria. *Planta Med* 1999; 65: 164–166.

D

20 Andersen ML. Evaluation of acute and chronic treatments with *Harpagophytum procumbens* on Freund's adjuvant-induced arthritis in rats. *J Ethnopharmacol* 2004; 91: 325–330.
21 Mahomed IM Analgesic, antiinflammatory and antidiabetic properties of *Harpagophytum procumbens* DC (Pedaliaceae) secondary root aqueous extract. *Phytotherapy Res* 2004; 18: 982–989.
22 McLeod DW *et al.* Investigations of *Harpagophytum procumbens* (devil's claw) in the treatment of experimental inflammation and arthritis in the rat. *Br J Pharmacol* 1979; 66: P140.
23 Whitehouse LW *et al.* Devil's claw (*Harpagophytum procumbens*): no evidence for anti-inflammatory activity in the treatment of arthritic disease. *Can Med Assoc J* 1983; 129: 249–251.
24 Soulimani R *et al.* The role of stomachal digestion on the pharmacological activity of plant extracts, using as an example extracts of *Harpagophytum procumbens*. *Can J Physiol Pharmacol* 1994; 72: 1532–1536.
25 Sticher O. Plant mono-, di- and sesquiterpenoids with pharmacological and therapeutical activity. In: Wagner H, Wolff P, eds. *New Natural Products with Pharmacological, Biological or Therapeutical Activity.* Berlin: Springer Verlag, 1977: 137–176.
26 Loew D *et al.* Investigations on the pharmacokinetic properties of *Harpagophytum* extracts and their effects on eicosanoid biosynthesis in vitro and ex vivo. *Clin Pharmacol Ther* 2001; 69: 356–364.
27 Jang MH. *Harpagophytum procumbens* suppresses lipopolysaccharide-stimulated expressions of cyclooxygenase-2 and inducible nitric oxide synthase in fibroblast cell line L929. *J Pharmacol Sci* 2003; 93: 367–371.
28 Kaszkin M. Downregulation of iNOS expression in rat mesangial cells by special extracts of *Harpagophytum procumbens* derives from harpagoside-dependent and independent effects. *Phytomedicine* 2004; 11: 585–595.
29 Benito PB *et al.* Effects of some iridoids from plant origin on arachidonic acid metabolism in cellular systems. *Planta Med* 2000; 66: 324–328.
30 Fiebich BL *et al.* Inhibition of TNF-α synthesis in LPS-stimulated primary human monocytes by *Harpagophytum* extract SteiHap 69. *Phytomedicine* 2001; 8: 28–30.
31 Schulze-Tanzil G, Wirkung des Extraktes aus *Harpagophytum procumbens* DC auf Matrix-Metalloproteinasen in menschlichen Knorpelzellen in vitro. *Arzneim Forsch* 2004; 54: 213–220.
32 Circosta C *et al.* A drug used in traditional medicine: *Harpagophytum procumbens* DC. II. Cardiovascular activity. *J Ethnopharmacol* 1984; 11: 259–274.
33 Costa de Pasquale R *et al.* A drug used in traditional medicine: *Harpagophytum procumbens* DC. III. Effects on hyperkinetic ventricular arrhythmias by reperfusion. *J Ethnopharmacol* 1985; 13: 193–199.
34 Occhiuto F, De Pasquale A. Electrophysiological and haemodynamic effects of some active principles of *Harpagophytum procumbens* DC in the dog. *Pharmacological Res* 1990; 22: 72–73.
35 Occhiuto F *et al.* A drug used in traditional medicine: *Harpagophytum procumbens* DC. IV. Effects on some isolated muscle preparations. *J Ethnopharmacol* 1985; 13: 201–208.
36 Betancor-Fernández A, Screening pharmaceutical preparations containing extracts of turmeric rhizome, artichoke leaf, devil's claw root and garlic or salmon oil for antioxidant capacity. *J Pharm Pharmacol* 2003; 55: 981–986.
37 Kundu JK Inhibitory effects of the extracts of *Sutherlandia frutescens* (L.) R. Br. and *Harpagophytum procumbens* DC. on phorbol ester-induced COX-2 expression in mouse skin: AP-1 and CREB as potential upstream targets. *Cancer Lett* 2005; 218: 21–31.
38 Guérin J-C, Réveillère H-P. Activité antifongique d'extraits végétaux à usage thérapeutique. II. Étude de 40 extraits sur 9 souches fongiques. *Ann Pharmaceut Fr* 1985; 43: 77–81.
39 Moussard C *et al.* A drug used in traditional medicine, *Harpagophytum procumbens*: no evidence for NSAID-like effect on whole blood eicosanoid production in human. *Prostaglandins Leukot Essent Fatty Acids* 1992; 46: 283–286.
40 Wegener T, Wiedenbrück R. Die Teufelskralle (*Harpagophytum procumbens* DC.)in der Therapie rheumatischer Erkrankungen. *Z Phytother* 1998; 19: 284–294.
41 Chrubasik S. Effectiveness of devil's claw for osteoarthritis. *Rheumatology* 2002; 41: 1332–1333.
42 Chrubasik S. The quality of clinical trials with *Harpagophytum procumbens. Phytomedicine* 2003; 10 :613–623.
43 Chrubasik S *et al.* Effectiveness of *Harpagophytum procumbens* in treatment of acute low back pain. *Phytomedicine* 1996; 3: 1–10.
44 Chrubasik S *et al.* Effectiveness of *Harpagophytum* extract WS 1531 in the treatment of exacerbation of low back pain: a randomized, placebo-controlled, double-blind study. *Eur J Anaesthesiol* 1999; 16: 118–129.
45 Göbel H *et al. Harpagophytum* extract LI 174 (Devil's claw) for treating non-specific back pain. Effects on sensory, motor and vascular muscle response. *Schmerz* 2001; 15: 10–18.
46 Chrubasik S. A randomized double-blind pilot study comparing Doloteffin and Vioxx in the treatment of low back pain. *Rheumatology* 2003; 42: 141–148.
47 Chrubasik S. A 1-year follow-up after a pilot study with Doloteffin for low back pain. *Phytomedicine* 2005; 12: 1–9.
48 Lecomte A, Costa JP. Harpagophytum dans l'arthrose: étude en double insu contre placebo. *Le Magazine* 1992; 27–30.
49 Pinget M, Lecomte A. Die Wirkung der 'Harpagophytum Arkocaps' bei degenerativem Rheuma. *Naturheilpraxis* 1992; 50: 267–269.
50 Bélaiche P. Étude clinique de 630 cas d'arthrose traités par le nébulisat aqueux d'*Harpagophytum procumbens* (Radix). *Phytothérapy* 1982; 1: 22–28.
51 Wegener T, Lüpke NP. Treatment of patients with arthrosis of hip or knee with an aqueous extract of devil's claw (*Harpagophytum procumbens* DC.). *Phytotherapy Res* 2003; 17: 1165–1172.
52 Laudahn D, Walper A. Efficacy and tolerance of *Harpagophytum* extract LI 174 in patients with chronic non-radicular back pain. *Phytotherapy Res* 2001; 15: 621–624.
53 Chrubasik S Comparison of outcome measures during treatment with the proprietary *Harpagophytum* extract Doloteffin in patients with pain in the lower back, knee or hip. *Phytomedicine* 2002; 9: 181–194.
54 Szczepański L. (Efficacy and tolerability of 'Pagosid' (*Harpagophytum procumbens* root extract) in the treatment of rheumatoid arthritis and osteoarthritis). *Reumatologia* 2000; 38: 67–73.
55 Grahame R, Robinson BV. Devil's claw (*Harpagophytum procumbens*): pharmacological and clinical studies. *Ann Rheum Dis* 1981; 40: 632.
56 Altmeyer N *et al.* Conjonctivite, rhinite et asthme rythmés par l'exposition professionelle à l'*Harpagophytum. Arch Mal Prof Med Trav Soc* 1992; 53: 289–291.
57 Erdös A *et al.* Beitrag zur pharmakologie und toxikologie verschiedener extrakte, sowie des harpagosids aus *Harpagophytum procumbens* DC. *Planta Med* 1978; 34: 97–108.
58 Unger M, Frank A. Simultaneous determination of the inhibitory potency of herbal extracts on the activity of six major cytochrome P450 enzymes using liquid chromatography/mass spectrometry and automated online extraction. *Rapid Comm Mass Spectrometry* 2004; 18: 2273–2281.
59 Abramowitz M. Toxic reactions to plant products sold in health food stores. *Med Lett Drugs Ther* 1979; 21: 29–30.

Drosera

Summary and Pharmaceutical Comment

Limited chemical information is available for drosera. Documented animal studies support some of the herbal uses. Reported immunostimulant and immunosuppressant activities may warrant further research into the pharmacological activities of drosera. In view of the lack of chemical and toxicity data, excessive use of drosera should be avoided.

Species (Family)

Drosera rotundifolia L. (Droserceae)

Synonym(s)

Round-leaved Sundew, Sundew

Part(s) Used

Herb

Pharmacopoeial and Other Monographs

BHP 1983[G7]
Complete German Commission E (Sundew)[G3]
Martindale 35th edition[G85]

Legal Category (Licensed Products)

Drosera is not included in the GSL.[G37]

Constituents

The following is compiled from several sources, including General Reference G2.

Flavonoids Kaempferol, myricetin, quercetin and hyperoside.[1]

Quinones Plumbagin,[2] hydroplumbagin glucoside[3] and rossoliside (7-methyl-hydrojuglone-4-glucoside).[4]

Other constituents Carotenoids, plant acids (e.g. butyric acid, citric acid, formic acid, gallic acid, malic acid, propionic acid), resin, tannins (unspecified) and ascorbic acid (vitamin C).

Food Use

Drosera is not used in foods.

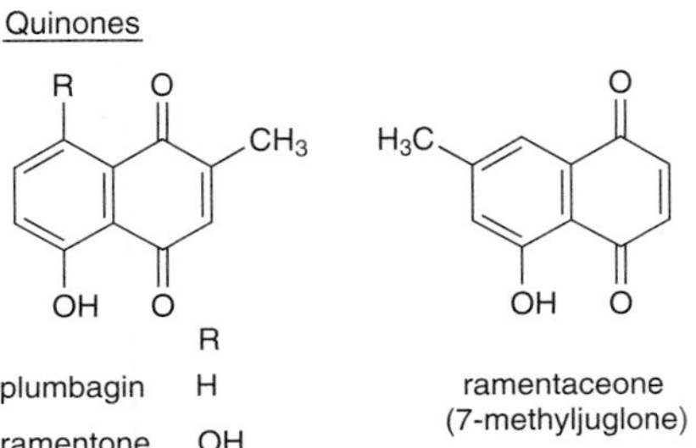

Figure 1 Selected constituents of drosera.

Herbal Use

Drosera is stated to possess antispasmodic, demulcent and expectorant properties. It has been used for bronchitis, asthma, pertussis, tracheitis, gastric ulceration and specifically for asthma and chronic bronchitis with peptic ulceration or gastritis.[G2, G7, G64]

Dosage

Dosages for oral administration (adults) for traditional uses recommended in older and contemporary standard herbal reference texts are given below.

Dried plant 1–2 g as an infusion three times daily.[G7]

Liquid extract 0.5–2.0 mL (1 : 1 in 25% alcohol) three times daily.[G7]

Tincture 0.5–1.0 mL (1 : 5 in 60% alcohol) three times daily.[G7]

Pharmacological Actions

In vitro and animal studies

Drosera is reported to prevent acetylcholine- or histamine-induced bronchospasm, and to relax acetylcholine- or barium chloride-induced spasm of the isolated intestine.[5] Drosera is stated to possess antitussive properties and has been reported to prevent coughing induced by excitation of the larynx nerve in the rabbit.[5] These antispasmodic actions have been attributed to the naphthoquinone constituents.[G53]

Antimicrobial properties have also been documented for the naphthoquinones.[6] *In vivo*, plumbagin is reported to exert a broad spectrum of activity against Gram-positive and Gram-negative bacteria, influenza viruses, pathogenic fungi, and parasitic protozoa. *In vitro*, a plumbagin solution (1 : 50 000) was reported to exhibit activity against staphylococci, streptococci and pneumococci (Gram-positive bacteria), but to lack activity against *Haemophilus pertussis* (Gram-negative bacteria).[5] Plumbagin administered orally to mice for five days, was found to be ineffective against *Lamblia muris* and tuberculosis infection.

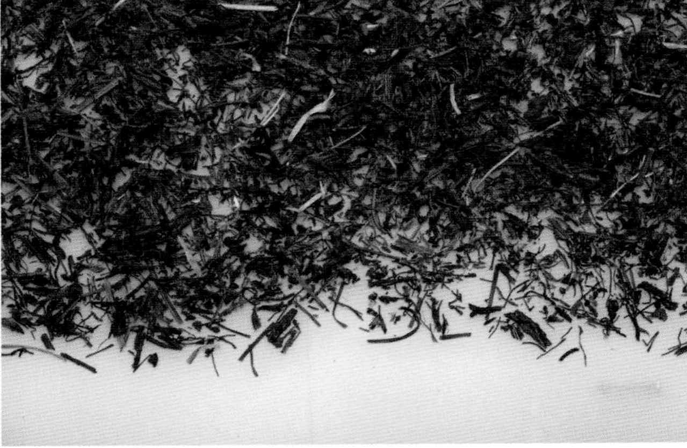

Figure 2 Drosera – dried drug substance (herb).

Microsporum infections in guinea-pigs were treated successfully by local applications of 0.25–0.5% solutions (in 40% alcohol) or of 1% emulsions.(6)

An aqueous drosera extract was reported to possess pepsin-like activity.(G53)

In vitro, drosera extracts and plumbagin, in concentrations of 0.01–1.0 mg/mL, have been documented to exert a cytotoxic or immunosuppressive effect in human granulocytes and lymphocytes.(2) Lower concentrations were reported to exhibit immunostimulating properties. Plumbagin possesses chemotherapeutic properties, but is irritant when administered at therapeutic doses.(6)

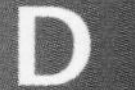

Clinical studies

There is a lack of clinical research assessing the effects of drosera and rigorous randomised controlled clinical trials are required.

Side-effects, Toxicity

None documented. However, there is a lack of clinical safety and toxicity data for drosera and further investigation of these aspects is required. Plumbagin is stated to be an irritant principle(G51) and an LD_{50} (mice, intraperitoneal injection) has been reported to be 15 mg/kg body weight.(G48)

Cytotoxic properties have been documented for drosera and plumbagin (*see* Pharmacological Actions, *In vitro* and animal studies).

Contra-indications, Warnings

Drug interactions None documented. However, the potential for preparations of drosera to interact with other medicines administered concurrently, particularly those with similar or opposing effects, should be considered.

Pregnancy and lactation The safety of drosera has not been established. In view of the lack of toxicity data, the use of drosera during pregnancy and lactation should be avoided.

Preparations

Proprietary single-ingredient preparations

Germany: Makatussin Saft Drosera; Makatussin Tropfen Drosera.

Proprietary multi-ingredient preparations

Australia: Asa Tones. *Austria:* Pilka Forte; Pilka. *Chile:* Fitotos; Gotas Nican; Notosil; Pectoral Pasteur; Pulmagol; Ramistos; Sedotus. *Czech Republic:* Bronchicum Pflanzlicher Hustenstiller; Stodal; Tussilen. *France:* Pastilles Monleon; Tussidoron. *Germany:* Drosithym-N; Lomal; Makatussin Tropfen forte. *Israel:* Pilka. *Mexico:* Citos; Fen-y-Tos. *Portugal:* Pilka F. *South Africa:* Cough Elixir. *Spain:* Broncovital; Pazbronquial; Pilka. *Switzerland:* Bromocod N; Demo Elixir pectoral N; DemoTussil; Escotussin; Famel; Gouttes contre la toux "S"; Makaphyt Gouttes antitussives; Makaphyt Sirop; Nican; Pastilles bronchiques S nouvelle formule; Pastilles pectorales Demo N; Sirop pectoral contre la toux S; Sirop S contre la toux et la bronchite. *Venezuela:* Codebromil; Pi-Fedrin.

References

1 Ayuga C *et al*. Contribución al estudio de flavonoides en *D. rotundifolia* L. *An R Acad Farm* 1985; 51: 321–326.
2 Wagner H *et al*. Immunological investigations of naphthoquinone-containing plant extracts, isolated quinones and other cytostatic compounds in cellular immunosystems. *Phytochem Soc Eur Symp* 1986; 43.
3 Vinkenborg J *et al*. De aanwezigheid van hydroplumbagin-glucoside in *Drosera rotundifolia*. *Pharm Weekbl* 1969; 104: 45–49.
4 Sampara-Rumantir N. Rossoliside. *Pharm Weekbl* 1971; 106: 653–664.
5 Oliver-Bever B. *Plants in Tropical West Africa*. Cambridge University Press: Cambridge, 1986: 129.
6 Vichkanova SA *et al*. Chemotherapeutic properties of plumbagin. In: Aizenman BE, ed. *Fitontsidy Mater Soveshch, 6th 1969*. Kiev: Naukova Dumka, 1972: 183–185.

Echinacea

Summary and Pharmaceutical Comment

The chemistry of echinacea is well documented (*see* Constituents). The three species are chemically dissimilar. *Echinacea purpurea* and *E. angustifolia* both contain alkamides as their major lipophilic constituents, but of differing structural types. By contrast, the lipophilic fraction of *E. pallida* is characterised by polyacetylenes and contains only very low concentrations, if any, of alkamides. The alkene constituents are stated to be susceptible to auto-oxidation, resulting in the formation of artefacts during storage.[G2]

Commercial echinacea samples and marketed echinacea products may contain one or more of the three echinacea species mentioned above. Analysis of commercial samples of raw echinacea material and marketed echinacea products has shown that in some cases the echinacea species assigned to the sample or product was incorrect, and that the pharmaceutical quality and labelling of some finished products was inadequate (*see* Constituents, Quality of plant material and commercial products). Users and potential users of echinacea products should be made aware of the possible differences between products and the implications of this for efficacy and safety.

Evidence from *in vitro* and animal studies supports some of the uses for echinacea, particularly the reputed immunostimulant properties, although immunostimulant activity has been disputed following one series of studies (*see* Pharmacological Actions, *In vitro* and animal studies, Immunomodulatory activity). Reported pharmacological activities have been documented for the polyene and high molecular weight polysaccharide constituents, as well as the alkamides and caffeic acid derivatives.

Several, but not all, clinical trials of echinacea preparations have reported effects superior to those of placebo in the prevention and treatment of upper respiratory tract infections (URTIs). However, evidence of efficacy is not definitive as studies have included different patient groups and tested various different preparations and dosage regimens of echinacea. As such, there is insufficient evidence to recommend any specific echinacea products, or to advise on optimal dose and treatment duration (*see* Clinical studies). Further well-designed clinical trials using well-defined, standardised preparations are necessary in order to establish efficacy.

There is a lack of clinical research on the anti-inflammatory and wound-healing properties of echinacea preparations documented *in vitro* and in animal studies. Several other areas of interest, related to the immunostimulant effects of echinacea, such as prevention of recurrence of genital herpes and other infections, and reduction of adverse effects associated with antineoplastic treatment, also require further clinical investigation.

Another area that requires further study is whether certain groups of constituents, such as the polysaccharides, are active after oral administration and, if so, what is the mechanism of action since polysaccharides usually would be broken down into simple inactive sugars. There is a lack of data on the pharmacokinetics of echinacea preparations, although very preliminary studies have reported transportation of isobutylamides across Caco-2 cells, an *in vitro* model of intestinal absorption, and detection of alkamides in blood taken from healthy volunteers who ingested echinacea preparations (*see* Clinical studies, Pharmacokinetics).

On the basis of the available (limited) safety data, which come mostly from short-term clinical trials of echinacea preparations for the prevention and treatment of URTIs in otherwise generally healthy individuals, echinacea appears to be well-tolerated. However, firm conclusions cannot be drawn from these limited data, and further investigation is required to establish the safety profile of different echinacea preparations. At present, the main safety issues are the possibility of allergic reactions, and concern about the use of echinacea by patients with progressive systemic diseases, such as tuberculosis, leukaemia, collagen disorders, multiple sclerosis and other autoimmune diseases (*see* Side-effects, Toxicity and Contra-indications, Warnings). In view of the lack of toxicity data, excessive use of echinacea should be avoided. In placebo-controlled trials of echinacea preparations for the prophylaxis of URTIs, treatment was taken typically for 8–12 weeks.

As with other herbal medicines, the potential for echinacea preparations to interact with conventional medicines should be considered. As *E. purpurea* root can inhibit CYP1A2 and selectively modulate CYP3A, echinacea should be used with caution in patients receiving therapeutic agents with a narrow therapeutic range and which are substrates for these CYP enzymes.

Species (Family)

**Echinacea angustifolia* DC. (Asteraceae/Compositae)
†*Echinacea pallida* (Nutt.) Nutt.
‡*Echinacea purpurea* (L.) Moench

Synonym(s)

Black Sampson, Coneflower
**E. angustifolia* var. *strigosa*
†*Rudbeckia pallida* Nutt., *Brauneria pallida* (Nutt.) Britton, *E. angustifolia* Hook. f.
‡*Rudbeckia purpurea* L., sp., *R. serotina* (Nutt.) Sweet, *R. hispida* Hoffm., *E. intermedia* Lindl., *E. purpurea* (L.) Moench var. *arkansana* Stey., *E. purpurea* var. *purpurea* f. liggettii

Part(s) Used

Rhizome, root. *E. purpurea* herb (aerial parts) is also used

Pharmacopoeial and Other Monographs

AHP (*E. purpurea* root)[G1]
BHC 1992[G6]
BHMA 2003[G66]
BHP 1996[G9]

E

BP 2007[G84]
Complete German Commission E 1998[G3]
ESCOP 2003[G76]
Expanded German Commission E 2000[G4]
Martindale 35th edition[G85]
Ph Eur 2007[G81]
USP29/NF24[G86]
WHO volume 1 1999[G63]

E

Legal Category (Licensed Products)

GSL[G37]

Constituents

Alkamides At least 20, mainly isobutylamides of straight-chain fatty acids with olefinic and/or acetylenic bonds,[1–5] e.g. isomeric dodeca-2*E*,4*E*,8*Z*,10*E*/*Z*-tetraenoic isobutylamide,[6] present in the roots and aerial parts of *Echinacea angustifolia* and *Echinacea purpurea*, but mainly absent from *Echinacea pallida*. Isobutylamides from the roots of *E. purpurea* contain mainly 2,4-dienoic units whilst those of *E. angustifolia* contain mainly 2-monoene units.[4] The synthesis of the acetylenic amide *N*-(2-methylpropyl)-2*E*-undecene-8,10-diynamide, a constituent of *E. angustifolia* root, has been reported.[7] *E. purpurea* root reportedly contains 0.01–0.04% alkamides.[G52]

Phenylpropanoids Caffeic acid glycosides (e.g. echinacoside,[8] verbascoside, caffeoylechinacoside), caffeic acid esters of quinic acid (e.g. chlorogenic acid = 5-caffeoylquinic acid, isochlorogenic acid = 3,4- and 3,5-dicaffeoylquinic acid, cynarin = 1,3-dicaffeoylquinic acid) and of tartaric acid (e.g. caftaric acid = 2-caffeoyltartaric acid, cichoric acid = 2,3-dicaffeoyltartaric acid).[9] Varying mixtures of caffeic acid derivatives are present in the three species, with echinacoside being the major component of the roots of *E. angustifolia* and *E. pallida*[9] (0.5–1.0%),[G52] and cichoric acid being a major component of *E. purpurea* roots (0.14–2.05%),[10] and aerial parts (1.2–3.1%).[11, G52] Cynarin is reportedly present in *E. angustifolia* root,[6, 9] but not in the roots of the other two species.

Polysaccharides Polysaccharides PS1 (a methylglucuronoarabinoxylan, mol. wt 35 kDa),[12] PS2 (an acidic rhamnoarabinogalactan, mol. wt 450 kDa) and a xyloglucan (mol. wt 79 kDa) have been isolated from *E. purpurea* herb.[13, 14, G52] Polysaccharides and glycoproteins are present in *E. purpurea* herb and *E. pallida* root.[G52] The pressed juice from the aerial parts of *E. purpurea* (and the herbal medicinal product Echinacin prepared from the juice) contain heterogeneous polysaccharides (mol. wt <10 kDa), inulin-type fractions (mol. wt 6 kDa) and an acidic highly branched arabinogalactan polysaccharide (mol. wt 70 kDa).[15] The pressed juice of *E. purpurea* aerial parts has yielded an arabinogalactan-protein (AGP) comprising 83% polysaccharide (galactose–arabinose 1.8 : 1), uronic acids (4–5%) and protein (7%) with high concentrations of serine, alanine and hydroxyproline.[16] The AGP (mol. wt 1.2×10^6 Da) has a highly branched polysaccharide core of 3-, 6-, and 3,6-linked galactose residues with terminal arabinose and glucuronic acid units.[16]

Volatile oils *E. pallida* root (0.2–2.0%)[G52] mainly contains polyenes and polyacetylenes including pentadeca-1,8*Z*-diene and a range of ketoalkenes and ketoalkenynes (ketopolyacetylenes), principally pentadeca-8*Z*-ene-2-one, pentadeca-8*Z*,11*Z*-diene-2-one, pentadeca-8*Z*,13*Z*-diene-11-yne-2-one, tetradeca-8*Z*-ene-11,13-diyne-2-one and others.[17, G52] These alkenes are unstable and readily oxidise to 8-hydroxy derivatives.[G52] The alkenes of *E. pallida* and *E. purpurea* root are distinctly different from those of *E. angustifolia* which are mainly alkylketones.[5] The volatile oil from the aerial parts of the three species contains borneol, bornyl acetate, germacrene D, caryophyllene and other components.[G2, G52]

Other constituents A series of other constituents has been reported including the saturated pyrrolizidine-type alkaloids tussilagine and isotussilagine (0.006%) from *E. angustifolia* and *E. purpurea*.[18] Flavonoids, including quercetin, kaempferol, isorhamnetin and their glycosides[G52] and also anthocyanins, are present in the aerial parts of *E. purpurea* (0.48%).[G2] The major flavonoid of the aerial parts of *E. angustifolia* has been identified as patuletin-3-rutinoside,[19] and not rutin as previously reported.[20] Free phenolic acids, including *p*-coumaric, *p*-hydroxybenzoic and protocatechuic acids, have been isolated from the aerial parts of *E. angustifolia* and *E. purpurea*.[21] Other miscellaneous compounds reported include betaine, fatty acids, simple sugars, sterols and vanillin. The presence of 'melanin' in material from cultured *E. angustifolia* plants has been reported.[22] Phytomelanin deposits are stated to be present in the roots of *E. pallida* and *E. angustifolia*, but absent from *E. purpurea* roots.[G75]

Quality of plant material and commercial products

Alkamide concentrations vary between species and between different parts of the plant.[23] Commercial root samples of *E. purpurea* have been shown to vary in their alkamide content (0.12–1.2%).[11] In Germany, 25 commercial echinacea preparations were assayed for their alkamide (dodeca-2*E*,4*E*,8*Z*,10*E*/*Z*-tetraenoic acid isobutylamide) and cichoric acid contents.[24] Some products were highly concentrated, whereas others had no detectable concentrations of alkamide or cichoric acid. Large differences were observed between comparable products from different manufacturers.

Several commercial echinacea products have performed poorly in examinations of their quality. Of 25 commercial echinacea products purchased in the USA only 14 (56%) passed assessments for their quality.[25] Six were inadequately labelled, three of them not stating the species used, one not stating the plant part and two liquid preparations had no concentrations given for their echinacea content. The remaining 19 products were assessed for their stated content of particular species and for claimed concentrations of phenols. Twelve of these products were labelled as containing only *E. purpurea* and two of them failed, as one contained only 54% of the expected concentration of phenols and the other had three times the accepted concentration of microbes as set out in World Health Organization (WHO) guidelines. Two products were allegedly prepared from *E. angustifolia* and both failed, one having only one-third of the stated phenolic content and the other having no detectable echinacoside. Five further products allegedly containing a mixture of species were also assessed and one failed because echinacoside could not be detected. Analysis of 59 commercial products available in the US revealed that 10% had no measurable echinacea content, 48% were not consistent with their labels in respect of the species present, and of 21 standardised preparations, 57% did not meet the standards stated on their labels; often products did not contain the species stated.[26]

A fresh plant product of echinacea herb has been shown to possess three times the amount of alkamide than a product prepared from dried plants and this has been attributed to loss on drying.(27) The alkamide and cichoric acid contents of six commercial preparations of *E. purpurea* expressed juice have been shown to be variable (0.1–1.8 mg/mL and 0.0–0.4%, respectively).(28) Ten commercial preparations of echinacea were analysed for their betaine content and concentrations ranged from 0.04–0.64%.(29)

The concentrations of some constituents may be affected during growing, drying or storage of the plant material. The yields of some constituents are affected when plants are grown under conditions of drought stress.(30) Analysis of roots of *E. angustifolia* dried at a range of temperatures between 23°C and 60°C indicated that there were no significant changes in the alkamide content, whereas 25% and 45% of the echinacoside content was lost at 30°C and 60°C, respectively.(31) By contrast, roots of *E. purpurea* at −18°C in deep-freeze for 64 weeks were found to have lost 40% of their alkamide content.(32) An aqueous–alcoholic extract of *E. purpurea* and its dried extract were stored at different temperatures for seven months and then assayed for their alkamide and phenylpropanoid content.(33) The amount of the major alkamide (dodeca-2*E*,4*E*,8*Z*,10*E*/*Z*-tetraenoic acid isobutylamide) in the liquid preparation was not significantly affected by storage at 25°C and 40°C, whereas the cichoric acid content declined. However, the reverse occurred for the dried extract when there was a significant loss of alkamide at storage temperatures of 25°C and 40°C but no significant loss of cichoric acid content.

The effects of drying temperatures on the constituents of all three echinacea species have been investigated.(34) The results showed that there was an increase in cichoric acid for *E. purpurea* and *E. pallida*. Furthermore, increased moisture content resulted in higher concentrations of echinacoside for *E. angustifolia* and *E. pallida* and of chlorogenic acid in *E. angustifolia*. The polysaccharide contents were significantly decreased by raised moisture levels in the roots of *E. angustifolia* and *E. pallida*.

The presence of colchicine in commercial echinacea products in the USA has been reported,(35) although subsequent analysis of 17 commercial echinacea products purchased in pharmacies in Chicago, USA, did not detect colchicine in any of the samples.(36)

Detailed descriptions of *E. purpurea* root for use in botanical, microscopic and macroscopic identification have been published, along with qualitative and quantitative methods for the assessment of *E. purpurea* root raw material.(37)

Phenylpropanoids

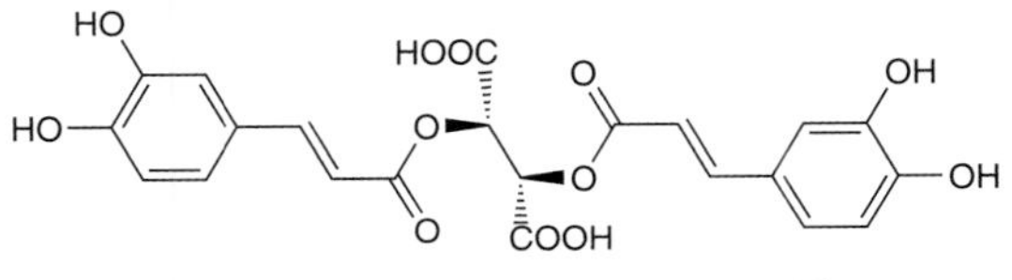

cichoric acid (2,3-dicaffeoyltartaric acid)
(cafartic acid = 2-caffeoyltartaric acid)

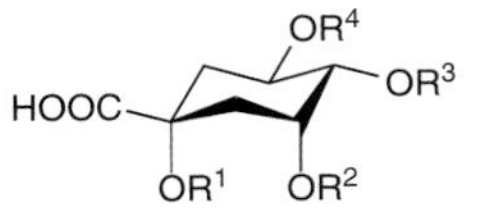

	R^1	R^2	R^3	R^4
chlorogenic acid (5-caffeoylquinic acid)	H	H	H	caffeoyl
isochlorogenic acid (3,4-dicaffeoylquinic acid)	H	caffeoyl	caffeoyl	H
isochlorogenic acid (3,5-dicaffeoylquinic acid)	H	caffeoyl	H	caffeoyl
cynarin	caffeoyl	caffeoyl	H	H

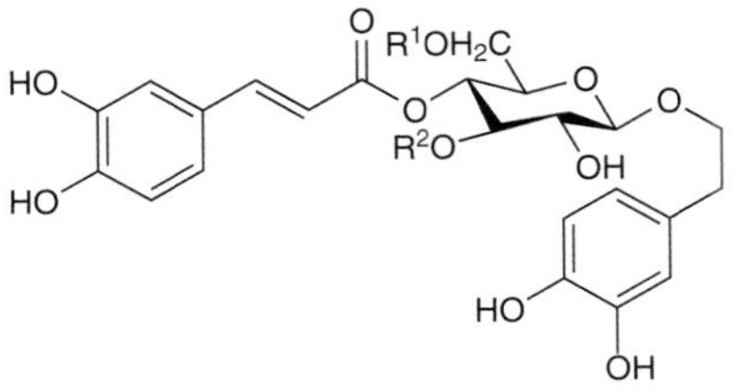

	R^1	R^2
echinacoside	glucose (1→6)	rhamnosyl (1→3)
verbascoside	H	rhamnosyl (1→3)
caffeoyl-echinacoside	6-caffeoylglucosyl (1→6)	rhamnosyl (1→3)

Figure 1 Selected constituents of echinacea.

Herbal Use

Echinacea has a long history of medicinal use for a wide variety of conditions, mainly infections, such as syphilis and septic wounds, but also as an 'anti-toxin' for snakebites and blood poisoning.(38, G50) Traditionally, echinacea was known as an 'anti-infective' agent, and was indicated in bacterial and viral infections, mild septicaemia, furunculosis (persistent recurring episodes of painful nodules in the skin) and other skin conditions, including boils, carbuncles and abscesses.(G6, G7, G60, G69) Other traditional uses listed include naso-pharangeal catarrh, pyorrhoea (periodontitis) and tonsillitis, and as supportive treatment for influenza-like infections and recurrent infections of the respiratory tract and lower urinary tract and, externally, for poorly healing superficial wounds.(G66)

Current interest in the medicinal use of echinacea is focused on its immunostimulant (increasingly described as immunomodulatory) effects, particularly in the treatment and prevention of the common cold, influenza and other upper respiratory tract infections (*see* Pharmacological Actions; Clinical studies).

Dosage

In standard herbal reference texts

Dosages for oral administration (adults) recommended in older standard herbal reference texts(G6, G7) are the same for several indications; examples are given below.

E. angustifolia *root and/or* E. pallida *root* For various indications, including chronic viral and bacterial infections, skin complaints, prophylaxis of colds and influenza, mild septicaemia, furunculosis, naso-pharyngeal catarrh, pyorrhoea and tonsillitis.

Dried root/rhizome 1 g by infusion or decoction three times daily.(G6, G7)

Liquid extract 0.5–1.0 mL (1 : 5 in 45% alcohol) three times daily,(G6) or 0.25–1.0 mL (1 : 1 in 45% alcohol) three times daily.(G7)

Tincture 2–5 mL (1 : 5 in 45% alcohol) three times daily,(G6) or 1–2 mL (1 : 5 in 45% alcohol) three times daily.(G7)

In more recent texts

Dosages for oral administration (adults) described in more recent texts are provided for more specific indications.

As adjuvant therapy and for prophylaxis of recurrent infections of the upper respiratory tract (common colds); treatment should not exceed eight weeks' duration.[G3, G52]

E. pallida *root* Hydroethanolic extract corresponding to 900 mg crude drug daily,[G52] e.g. tincture (1 : 5 in 50% ethanol by volume) from dry extract (7–11 : 1 in 50% ethanol).[G3]

E. purpurea *herb* 6–9 mL expressed juice daily.[G3, G52]

E. purpurea *root* 3 × 60 drops of tincture (1 : 5 in 55% ethanol), equivalent to 3 × 300 mg crude drug daily.[G52]

E. angustifolia *root* 1–3 g daily

Echinacea preparations (i.e. containing different echinacea species and plant parts) and, therefore, dosage regimens tested in clinical trials have varied widely (*see* Pharmacological Actions, Clinical studies). Trials of echinacea preparations for the prevention of upper respiratory tract infections have typically involved an 8- or 12-week duration of treatment; trials of echinacea preparations for the treatment of upper respiratory tract infections typically involve administration of the study medication for 6–10 days.

Pharmacological Actions

There is a vast scientific literature on the pharmacological activities of *Echinacea* species based on *in vitro* and *in vivo* (animal) studies. Research has focused on investigating the immunomodulatory activity of echinacea preparations, although other activities, such as antiviral, antifungal, anti-inflammatory and antioxidant properties have also been explored. Effects on the immune system may play a role in some of these other activities.

The pharmacological activities of echinacea preparations cannot be attributed to a single constituent or group of constituents. Rather, several groups of constituents – the alkamides, caffeic acid derivatives, polysaccharides and alkenes – appear to contribute to activity.

However, it has been reported that following oral administration in man, alkamides are bioavailable, whereas caffeic acid derivatives are not and, therefore, cannot contribute to activity (*see* Clinical studies, Pharmacokinetics).[39]

In vitro and animal studies

Immunomodulatory activity Currently, there is a view that immunomodulatory, rather than immunostimulatory, is the most appropriate term to describe the immunological effects of echinacea,[40] although 'immunostimulatory' is still used and is ubiquitous in the earlier scientific literature on echinacea. It has

Alkamides

dodeca-2*E*,4*E*,8*Z*,10*Z*-tetraenoic acid isobutylamide

undeca-2*E*-enoic-8,10-diyne acid isobutylamide

Polyenes

pentadeca-1,8*Z*-diene

pentadeca-8*Z*-ene-2-one

pentadeca-8*Z*,11*Z*-diene-2-one

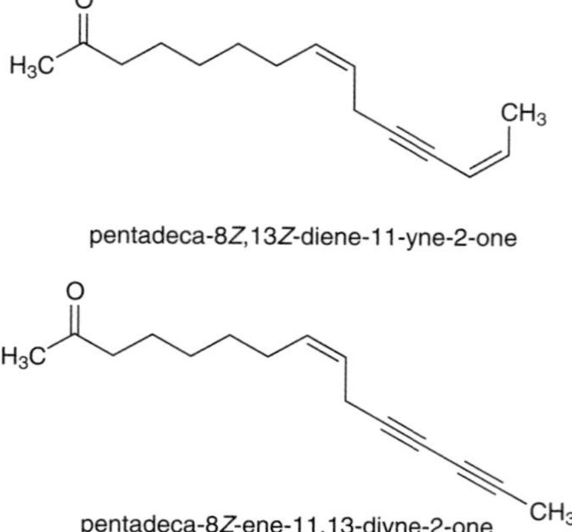

Figure 2 Selected constituents of echinacea.

been suggested that broad stimulation of the various highly complex components of the immune system is unlikely to be beneficial, since some immune responses are harmful.[40]

The immunological effects of a wide range of echinacea preparations comprising different species, plant parts and types of extract, have been investigated extensively *in vitro* and *in vivo*. Collectively, the data indicate that echinacea preparations do have effects on certain indices of immune function,[40,41] although at present there is no clear picture as to which specific preparations have the greatest activity. A summary of some of the scientific literature on the immunological effects of echinacea is given below.

Enhancement of macrophage function has been documented for various preparations of echinacea *in vitro* and *in vivo* in studies using a range of methods, such as the carbon clearance test and measurement of cytokine production, as indicators of macrophage activity.[42–44] *In vitro* experiments with human macrophages found that fresh pressed juice and dried juice from the aerial parts of *E. purpurea* stimulated production of cytokines, including interleukin 1 (IL-1), IL-10, and tumour necrosis factor α (TNFα).[45]

Other studies have reported that purified polysaccharides from *E. purpurea* induced macrophage production of IL-1,[46] and that a polysaccharide arabinogalactan isolated from plant cell cultures of *E. purpurea* induced TNFα and interferon β2 production by murine macrophages.[47] Polysaccharides obtained from plant cell cultures of *E. purpurea* have also been shown previously to have immunological activity *in vitro*.[48] In another series of *in vitro* experiments, *E. purpurea* induced macrophage activation (as assessed by TNFα production) following simulated digestion (incubation of echinacea with gastric fluid) in an attempt to mimic effects following oral administration.[49] Other work has demonstrated that *E. purpurea* dry root powder (containing 1.5% total polyphenols, calculated as chlorogenic acid) increased the resistance of splenic lymphocytes to apoptosis; splenic lymphocytes were obtained from mice administered the echinacea preparation orally at dosages of 30 or 100 mg/kg daily for 14 days.[50]

In an *in vitro* study, peripheral blood mononuclear cells (PBMCs) from healthy individuals and from patients with chronic fatigue syndrome and acquired immune deficiency syndrome (AIDS) incubated with increasing concentrations of extracts of *E. purpurea* led to enhanced natural killer function of PBMCs.[51] *In vivo*, oral administration of *E. purpurea* root extract has been reported to increase numbers of natural killer cells in normal,[52] leukaemic,[53] and ageing mice.[54]

A subsequent *in vivo* study, conducted using a rigorous randomised, double-blind design, assessed the effects of an echinacea product (Nature's Resource, CVS Pharmacy, USA; capsules containing echinacea aerial parts 1.05 g and cichoric acid 10.5 mg) in 16 ageing male rats.[55] Animals received echinacea (species and method of preparation were not stated although, as aerial parts were used, the species may have been *E. purpurea*) 50 mg/kg body weight (equivalent to cichoric acid 0.5 mg/kg), or placebo, orally as a bolus dose in peanut butter each morning for eight weeks. Mean circulating total white cell counts were significantly higher in echinacea-treated rats than in the control group for the first two weeks ($p < 0.05$), although baseline counts for the two groups and a precise p value or confidence intervals were not given in a report of the study, and concentrations of IL-2 were significantly higher in echinacea-treated rats, compared with the control group, for the last five weeks of the study ($p < 0.05$). Differential white cell counts were significantly altered throughout the 8-week study period in the echinacea group, compared with the control group: proportions of lymphocytes and monocytes increased while those of neutrophils and eosinophils decreased with echinacea, compared with placebo.[55] There were no changes in the phagocytic activity of circulating leukocytes, as assessed by ability to ingest latex particles, in either group during the study.

Other *in vivo* studies (rats) have shown that administration of water–ethanol extracts (100 μL twice daily by oral gavage for four days) of *E. purpurea* roots and aerial parts containing defined concentrations of cichoric acid, polysaccharides and alkamides stimulated phagocytic activity of macrophages; activity was increased with increasing concentrations of the three components.[56] Subsequently, an increase in lipopolysaccharide-stimulated nitric oxide release was observed by macrophages obtained from the spleens of rats previously treated with the echinacea extracts. A similar set of experiments demonstrated stimulation of alveolar macrophage function by alkamides administered to healthy rats.[57]

A proprietary preparation containing *E. purpurea* root extract and liquorice (*Glycyrrhiza glabra*) root extract stimulated phagocytosis *in vitro* and *in vivo*, as demonstrated by the carbon clearance test, following oral administration to mice.[58] The combination product produced a greater immunostimulatory effect in this test than did either extract tested alone. Another combination preparation, comprising aqueous–ethanol extracts of *E. purpurea* and *E. pallida* root, *Baptisia tinctoria* root and *Thuja occidentalis* herb, administered orally via the diet or drinking water to mice for seven days enhanced the antibody response to sheep red blood cells.[59]

In contrast with the extensive body of research supporting the immunostimulatory effects of echinacea preparations, some recent work has reported a lack of effect. No evidence of natural killer cell activity or antibody formation was found in studies involving rats fed various preparations of echinacea, including an alcoholic extract of *E. purpurea* root and an alcoholic extract of the roots of *E. angustifolia*, *E. purpurea* and *E. pallida*, in their diet.[60]

A concentration-dependent and cell-type specific *de novo* synthesis of TNF-α mRNA in primary human CD14+ monocytes/macrophages *in vitro* has been described for an *E. purpurea* extract (Echinaforce, Bioforce).[61] The alkamide constituents appeared to be responsible for this effect, at least in part, mediated via the cyclic AMP and other pathways and involving activation of NF-κB. Further experiments using these cells and an anti-cannabinnoid-2 (CB2) polyclonal antibody and the CB2 antagonist SR-144528 resulted in inhibition of the induction of TNF-α mRNA.

Antiviral activity Antiviral activity has been described for various different preparations of echinacea following *in vitro* studies. An 'indirect' antiviral effect was documented in experiments involving addition of glycoprotein-containing fractions obtained from *E. purpurea* root to mouse spleen cell cultures.[62] Interferon-α and -β produced by the cells were then tested for activity against vesicular stomatitis virus. These glycoprotein-containing fractions were also tested directly against herpes simplex virus (HSV) and were reported to reduce the number of plaques by up to 80%, although raw data were lacking and statistical tests do not appear to have been carried out.

In other *in vitro* studies, the antiviral activity of an aqueous solution of *E. purpurea* herb was tested against aciclovir-susceptible and aciclovir-resistant strains of HSV-1 and HSV-2.[63] In aciclovir-susceptible strains of HSV-1 and HSV-2, median ED_{50} (effective dose) values for the echinacea preparation were 1 : 100 (range 1 : 25 to 1 : 400) and 1 : 200 (range 1 : 50 to 1 : 1600), respectively. Similarly, for aciclovir-resistant HSV-1 and HSV-2, median ED_{50} values (range) were 1 : 100 (1 : 50 to 1 : 400) and 1 : 200 (1 : 50 to 1 : 3200), respectively.

An *n*-hexane extract of *E. purpurea* root, an ethanolic extract of *E. pallida* var. *sanguinea* herb and the isolated constituent cichoric acid were the most potent inhibitors of HSV-1 in *in vitro* studies designed to assess light-activated antiviral activity.[64] The minimum inhibitory concentrations (MIC) for these preparations were 0.12, 0.026 and 0.045 mg/mL, respectively.

Other *in vitro* studies using mouse fibroblasts found that preincubation with *E. purpurea* herb juice and methanolic and aqueous extracts of *E. purpurea* root resulted in resistance to influenza A2, herpes, and vesicular stomatitis virus infection for 24 hours.[65]

Antifungal and antibacterial activities Activity against several yeast strains, including *Saccharomyces cerevisiae* and *Candida albicans*, has been described for *n*-hexane extracts of *E. purpurea* roots.[66] Antifungal activity was observed under near ultraviolet light irradiation and, in some cases, was also light independent. The pure polyacetylenic compound trideca-1-ene-3,5,7,9,10-pentayne, isolated from *E. purpurea* root extracts, demonstrated marked light-mediated inhibition of growth of *S. cerevisiae*.[66] Anti-*Candida* activity for *E. purpurea* extracts has also been described previously.[40]

In contrast, *n*-hexane extracts of the fresh roots of *E. pallida* var. *pallida* and *E. pallida* var. *angustifolia* (identified according to a revised taxonomy[67] showed no measurable inhibition of *C. albicans*, but an amphotericin-B-resistant strain (D10) of *C. albicans* and *Tricophyton mentagrophytes* were susceptible to *E. pallida* var. *pallida* root extract in the presence of UV light.[68]

Studies in mice have described a dose-dependent protective effect for polysaccharide fractions from *E. purpurea* plant cell cultures against lethal-dose infection with *C. albicans* and *Listeria monocytogenes* when administered intravenously within less than 18 hours of the infection dose.[69] A similar finding was reported when such polysaccharide fractions were administered to immunosuppressed mice both before and after lethal dose infection with *C. albicans* and *L. monocytogenes*.[70]

Antibacterial activity against *Escherichia coli*, *Proteus mirabilis*, *Pseudomonas aeruginosa* and *Staphylococcus aureus* has been demonstrated for a multi-herbal preparation containing *E. purpurea* root extract, although it was stated that the observed antibacterial effects were most likely attributable to one of the other ingredients, extract of onion.[71]

Anti-inflammatory activity *In vivo* anti-inflammatory activity has been reported for a polysaccharide fraction (PSF) obtained from *E. angustifolia* roots in the carrageenan-induced rat paw oedema test and in the croton oil mouse ear test, with the PSF administered intravenously and topically, respectively.[72] The isolated PSF was twice as active as the total aqueous extract in the carrageenan-induced oedema test, and about half as active as indometacin in the croton oil test. An aqueous extract of *E. angustifolia* roots was also reported to be more effective than benzydamine (a topical non-steroid anti-inflammatory drug (NSAID)) in the croton oil test.[73] Further work using fractions of an aqueous extract of *E. angustifolia* roots administered topically to mice in the croton oil test attributed the observed anti-inflammatory activity mainly to intermediate and high molecular weight fractions.[74]

Oral administration of higher (100 mg/kg) but not lower (30 mg/kg) doses of *E. purpurea* dry root powder (containing 1.5% total polyphenols, calculated as chlorogenic acid) inhibited carrageenan-induced paw oedema in mice; the effect was stated to be similar to that of indometacin 0.25 mg/kg, although this was not tested statistically.[75] Further exploration suggested that the observed effect may be due to downregulation of cyclooxygenase 2 (COX-2) expression by the echinacea preparation. *In vitro* inhibition of cyclooxygenase 1 (COX-1) and, to a lesser extent, COX-2 has been described for alkamides isolated from *E. purpurea* roots,[76] and *in vitro* inhibition of 5-lipoxygenase (5-LO) and cyclooxygenase (from sheep seminal microsomes) has been reported for polyunsaturated alkamides from *E. angustifolia* roots.[77]

Inhibition of 5-LO has also been described for extracts of roots of *E. purpurea*, *E. pallida* var. *pallida* and *E. pallida* var. *angustifolia* (identified according to a revised taxonomy).[67] IC_{50} values (μg root/mL assay volume) were 0.642, 1.08 and 0.444, respectively, and corresponding alkamide concentrations in the root of each species were 0.05%, trace, and 0.2%, respectively.[68]

Anti-inflammatory and cicatrising activities have been reported for gel preparations containing echinacoside 0.4 mg and *E. pallida* root extract 100 mg following studies in rats with experimental skin abrasions and excision wounds.[78] These effects were observed 48 and 72 hours after topical administration, and were stated to be greater than those observed for *E. purpurea* root extract and control. However, no statistical analysis was reported.

The wound-healing properties documented for echinacea have been attributed in part to a polysaccharide fraction, which is thought to inhibit the action of hyaluronidase.[79] Ethanol extracts of *E. purpurea* roots and aerial parts have been reported to inhibit fibroblast-induced collagen contraction, although the significance of this activity for wound healing needs to be investigated.[80] Other studies have documented a protective effect for echinacoside, isolated from *E. angustifolia* root, and other caffeoyl esters against free radical-induced degradation of collagen, an experimental model for skin damage caused by exposure to ultraviolet light.[81]

Other activities A long-chain alkene from *E. angustifolia* is stated to possess antitumour activity *in vivo*, inhibiting the growth of Walker tumours in rats and lymphocytic leukaemia (P388) in mice.[82]

In an assay of the mosquitocidal activity of alkamides isolated from dried *E. purpurea* roots, a mixture of dodeca-2*E*,4*E*,8*Z*,10*E*-tetraenoic acid isobutylamide and dodeca-2*E*,4*Z*,8*Z*,10*Z*-tetraenoic acid isobutylamide at a concentration of 100 μg/mL achieved 87.5% mortality of *Aedes aegyptii* L. mosquito larvae within 15 minutes. Several other alkamides assayed also demonstrated mosquitocidal activity, but required longer incubation periods and were less effective.[76]

Free radical-scavenging activity has been documented for alcoholic extracts of the roots and leaves of *E. purpurea*, *E. angustifolia* and *E. pallida in vitro*.[7]

Dodeca-2*E*,4*E*,8*Z*,10*E*/*Z*-tetraenoic isobutylamides found in *Echinacea* species (but isolated in this experiment from *Echinacea atrorubens* root) were transported across Caco-2 monolayers, an *in vitro* model for intestinal absorption, over a 6-hour period.[83] Transport kinetics did not differ significantly following modification of the model (by preincubation of Caco-2 cells with lipopolysaccharide and phorbol 12-myristate-13-acetate) to mimic inflammation.

A similar study explored the transport of 12 alkamides and 5 caffeic acid conjugates from a proprietary preparation of echinacea (Echinacea Premium Liquid; MediHerb, Australia), which contains a 60% ethanol/water extract of *E. angustifolia* root (200 mg/mL) and *E. purpurea* root (300 mg/mL).[84] Almost all of the caffeic acid conjugates permeated poorly through the Caco-2 monolayers: their uptake was no better than that of control (mannitol, which is poorly absorbed); only cinnamic acid diffused readily (apparent permeability coefficient, P_{app}, = 1 × 10^{-4} cm/second). By contrast, both 2,4-diene and 2-ene alkamides readily diffused through the monolayers, although P_{app} values varied (range: 3 × 10^{-6} to 3 × 10^{-4} cm/second), depending on structure. Saturated compounds and those with N-terminal methylation had lower permeability coefficients. These findings suggest that alkamides, but not caffeic acid conjugates, are likely to cross the intestinal barrier and thus be bioavailable following oral administration.[84]

Clinical studies

Pharmacokinetics There are only limited data on the clinical pharmacokinetics of echinacea preparations (*see also* Pharmacological Actions, *In vitro* and animal studies, Other activities). One study reported that dodeca-2*E*,4*E*,8*Z*,10*E*/*Z*-tetraenoic acid isobutylamide (alkamide) was detectable in blood one hour after oral administration of 65 mL of a concentrated ethanolic extract of *E. purpurea* herb (containing 4.3 mg isobutylamides) on an empty stomach to a single healthy volunteer.[85]

In a study involving nine healthy volunteers who ingested four Echinacea Premium tablets (MediHerb, Australia; each tablet contains *E. angustifolia* root extract 150 mg, containing 2.0 mg alkamides, and *E. purpurea* root extract 112.5 mg, containing 2.1 mg alkamides) after a high-fat breakfast, alkamides were detected in plasma obtained from blood samples taken 20 minutes after ingestion and some alkamides were detectable for 12 hours post echinacea ingestion.[86] The mean (standard error of mean) maximum plasma concentration (C_{max}) for total alkamides was 336 (131), time to C_{max} was 2.3 (0.5) hours and the area under the plasma concentration time curve (AUC_t) was 714 (181) μg equivalent/h/L. Most alkamides found in echinacea were detected in plasma. In contrast, caffeic acid conjugates could not be detected and therefore were reported not to be bioavailable.[86]

In a randomised, open, crossover study, in which 11 healthy volunteers received a single oral dose of 2.5 mL of a 60% ethanolic extract of *E. angustifolia* roots (containing 2.0 mg tetraene per 2.5 mL) in the morning following an overnight fast, C_{max} for tetraene (a polyene) was reported to be around 11 ng/mL.[87]

Therapeutic effects Clinical trials of preparations containing echinacea have focused on testing effects in preventing and treating the common cold and other upper respiratory tract infections (URTIs); some preliminary studies have explored the effects of echinacea in other infections, such as genital herpes, and as an adjunctive treatment in cancer chemotherapy. The rationale for the use of echinacea in these conditions is for its immunomodulatory activity. Collectively, the findings of studies of echinacea are difficult to interpret as studies have assessed preparations containing different species of echinacea and/or different plant parts of echinacea, administered as monopreparations or in combination with other herbal ingredients, and products manufactured by different processes and with different dosage forms. Hence, the different preparations tested will vary quantitatively and qualitatively in their chemical composition (i.e. will contain different profiles and concentrations of chemical constituents).

Immunomodulatory activity One of the first systematic reviews of studies of echinacea-containing preparations assessed evidence of their immunomodulatory effects.[88] The review included 26 controlled clinical trials, of which six investigated the treatment of URTIs and influenza-like syndromes, seven explored the treatment of other infections, such as sinusitis, bronchitis and candida, six studied the prophylaxis of URTIs and influenza-like syndromes, four tested the reduction by echinacea of adverse effects of antineoplastic treatment and three explored the effects on immunological parameters in patients with infections or malignancies.[88]

Most studies reported that echinacea-containing preparations were superior to placebo in the indications tested. However, trials included in the review tested different species, parts and preparations (e.g. pressed juice, extract) of echinacea administered via different routes (including oral and parenteral) and with different dosage regimens. In addition, many studies were of poor methodological quality (only eight achieved more than 50% of the maximum score in an assessment of quality), several preparations tested included other herbs in addition to echinacea, and the review included trials involving patients with a range of conditions, so evidence for the immunomodulatory activity of echinacea from this review can only be considered tentative at best.

The same research group carried out another systematic review of five of their randomised, placebo-controlled studies (four were also conducted double-blind) which investigated the immunomodulatory activity of preparations of echinacea in healthy volunteers. Again, there were marked differences between the preparations tested in the studies included in the review: combination homeopathic preparations containing *E. angustifolia* at potencies of D1 and D4 (which can be considered to contain reasonable quantities of starting material) for intravenous administration; ethanolic extracts of *E. purpurea* root and *E. pallida* root for oral administration; ethanolic extract of 95% *E. purpurea* herb and 5% *E. purpurea* root. In two of the five studies, phagocytic activity of polymorphonuclear neutrophil granulocytes (the primary outcome measure) was significantly increased in the echinacea groups, compared with the placebo groups, although no such effects were noted in the other studies.[89]

Recent studies investigating the immunomodulatory activity of echinacea species administered to healthy volunteers have reported different findings. In a randomised, double-blind, placebo-controlled trial, compared with a placebo group, volunteers who received extracts of *E. purpurea* and *E. angustifolia* with or without the addition of an arabinogalactan extracted from *Larix occidentalis* (larch) for four weeks were found to have increased concentrations of complement properdin (thought to be an indication of immune system stimulation).[90] Other small placebo-controlled studies have reported stimulatory effects following 28 days' oral pretreatment with pressed juice of *E. purpurea* on the exercise-induced immune response in athletes,[91] and of administration of purified polysaccharides from cell cultures of *E. purpurea* to healthy volunteers.[92] By contrast, a double-blind, placebo-controlled, crossover study involving 40 healthy volunteers found that oral administration of freshly expressed juice of *E. purpurea* herb, or placebo, for two weeks did not enhance phagocytic activity of polymorphonuclear leukocytes or monocytes, or affect TNFα and IL-1 production.[93]

Preliminary studies have assessed the effects of a combination preparation containing extracts of *E. angustifolia*, *Eupatorium perfoliatum* (boneset) and *Thuja occidentalis* (thuja) on cytokine production in patients who have undergone curative surgery for various solid malignant tumours,[94] and the immunostimulatory effects of a regimen comprising intramuscular *E. purpurea* extract, low-dose intramuscular cyclophosphamide and intravenous thymostimulin in patients with advanced colorectal cancer.[95] In another study, the effects of a polysaccharide fraction of *E. purpurea* herb obtained from cell cultures in reducing the adverse effects of cancer chemotherapy were explored in patients with advanced gastric cancer receiving palliative therapy with etoposide, leucovorin and 5-fluorouracil.[96] Although these studies reported some positive findings with echinacea, no firm conclusions can be drawn because of the nature of the study designs, therefore further research in this area is required.

Upper respiratory tract infections (URTIs) Numerous studies have explored the effects of echinacea preparations in preventing or treating the common cold and other URTIs. Overall, several, but not all, studies have reported beneficial effects for certain echinacea preparations, compared with placebo, for the prevention and treatment of URTIs. However, for the reasons given (*see* Pharmacological Actions, Therapeutic effects), current consensus is that there is insufficient evidence to recommend any specific echinacea preparations, or to advise on optimal dose and treatment duration.

Prophylaxis A Cochrane systematic review included 16 randomised and quasi-randomised controlled trials – involving a total of almost 3400 participants – of extracts of echinacea for preventing (n = 8) or treating (n = 8) URTIs.[97] The eight 'prevention' trials comprised five which were placebo-controlled (n = 1272 participants), and which largely were considered to be of adequate methodological quality, and three (n = 1139 participants) in which the control group received no treatment. The five placebo-controlled trials tested combination echinacea preparations (n = 2) or monopreparations of *E. purpurea* herb or root, or *E. angustifolia* root (n = 3), administered orally typically for 8–12 weeks. Two of these studies reported a statistically significant reduction in the incidence of URTIs in echinacea recipients, compared with placebo recipients (odds ratios, 95% confidence interval (CI): 0.45, 0.22–0.92 and 0.27, 0.11–0.66). One of these studies also found that in participants who did acquire infections, the duration was significantly shorter in those who had received echinacea compared with placebo recipients, although two other studies reported no difference in this outcome.

The three other 'prevention' trials all involved children and compared a combination preparation containing extracts of *E. angustifolia* and *E. pallida* root, *Baptisia tinctoria* root and *Thuja occidentalis* herb, as well as several homeopathic dilutions, with no treatment. All three studies reported that the frequency of infection was significantly lower in the treatment compared with no treatment group (pooled odds ratio 0.36; 95% CI 0.28–0.46), although the methodological quality of all three studies was considered inadequate.[97]

An updated Cochrane review used more restrictive inclusion criteria for trials (e.g. randomised controlled trials only, trials assessing multi-herb products excluded), such that the revised review included only five trials that had been included in the earlier review, and 11 new trials.[98] Two of the 16 included trials involving children, and the others, adults; 15 trials used a placebo control design, one compared an echinacea preparation with another herbal product and no treatment, three trials involved two echinacea arms, and one involved comparisons with both placebo and no treatment, thus the total number of comparisons in the review was 22.

In contrast with the earlier review, only three comparisons (from two trials[99, 100]) investigated echinacea preparations for the prevention of colds, and none of these found statistically significant differences between the echinacea and placebo groups with respect to proportion of participants experiencing one or more colds.[98] Details of the two prevention trials included in the review,[99, 100] as well as those of several excluded trials, are given below. These trials did not show beneficial effects for echinacea preparations, compared with placebo, on main outcome measures.[101–104]

A randomised, double-blind, placebo-controlled trial involved 302 healthy volunteers recruited from military institutions and an industrial plant who received an ethanolic extract of *E. purpurea* root or *E. angustifolia* root (drug : extract ratio, 1 : 11 in 30% alcohol), or placebo, 50 drops twice daily on five days per week (Monday to Friday) for 12 weeks.[99] In an intention-to-treat analysis (n = 289), the proportion of participants who experienced at least one URTI was 32% (95% CI: 23–41%) for *E. angustifolia* recipients, 29% (95% CI: 20–38%) for *E. purpurea* recipients, and 37% (95% CI: 27–47%) for placebo recipients; these differences were not statistically significant (p = 0.55). Similarly, there were no statistically significant differences between groups in time to occurrence of the first URTI (p = 0.49), or in the duration of infections (p = 0.29), although it is possible that the study was not large enough to detect differences. However, a greater proportion of echinacea recipients believed they had benefited from the study medication than did placebo recipients (78%, 70% and 56% for *E. angustifolia*, *E. purpurea* and placebo, respectively; p = 0.04).[99]

In another randomised, double-blind, placebo-controlled trial, involving 109 individuals who had experienced more than three colds or respiratory infections in the previous year, a fluid extract of *E. purpurea* prepared from the aerial parts of fresh flowering plants, administered at a dose of 4 mL twice daily for eight weeks, had no statistically significant effect compared with placebo on the incidence of colds and URTIs (rate ratio for number of participants in each group with at least one cold or URTI = 0.88, 95% CI: 0.60–1.22).[100] Likewise, there was no statistically significant difference between groups in the duration and severity of occurring colds or URTIs.

Three further studies[101–103] tested the effects of echinacea for the prevention of colds due to experimental rhinovirus infection. In one study, adult volunteers (n = 117 enrolled) with a serum titre of neutralising antibody to rhinovirus of $\leqslant$1 : 4 received echinacea (300 mg) or placebo three times daily for 14 days prior to and for five days after challenge with rhinovirus (n = 92 challenged due to study withdrawals). It is not stated in a report of the study[101] whether random allocation to study group was undertaken, or whether participants were masked (blind) to treatment allocation, although a blinding check before virus challenge found that 30 (60%) of the 50 echinacea recipients and 19 (45%) of the 42 placebo recipients thought they were receiving the 'active' treatment (p = 0.21).

The study did not provide evidence to suggest that echinacea had effects over those of placebo: rhinovirus infection occurred in 22 (44%) of echinacea recipients and in 24 (57%) of placebo recipients (rate ratio = 0.77; p = 0.3), 'clinical' colds developed in 50% and 59% of echinacea and placebo recipients, respectively (p = 0.77), and there was no difference in mean total symptom scores (11.4, 95% CI 3.9–18.9 and 13.6, 95% CI 7.5–19.7 for echinacea and placebo, respectively). However, the study involved small numbers of participants and a sample size calculation was not reported, hence it is possible that the study was not large enough to be able to detect a difference if one existed. Additionally, information on the species of echinacea, plant part used, type of preparation (e.g. extract) and route of administration used was not provided in a report of this study.[101] It was stated that the preparation contained cichoric acid 0.16% and almost no echinacosides or alkamides, but with this limited information, it is not possible to say with certainty which species is likely to have been used, although it may have been *E. purpurea*.

In a subsequent study[102] a randomised, double-blind trial, 48 healthy adults received a preparation containing the pressed juice of the aerial parts of *E. purpurea* in a 22% alcohol base (EchinaGuard) 2.5 mL three times daily, or placebo, for seven days before and after inoculation with rhinovirus (RV-39) by intranasal administration in two inocula about 30 minutes apart (total dose: 0.25 mL per nostril). The proportions (95% confidence intervals (CI)) of participants with laboratory evidence of infection (at least a fourfold increase in RV-39 neutralising antibody titre and/or recovery of rhinovirus on viral culture), the primary outcome measure, were 92% (95% CI: 73–99) and 96% (95% CI: 77–100) for echinacea recipients and placebo recipients, respectively, and with clinical illness (presence of a cold defined as a five-day total symptom score of five or more and three successive days of rhinorrhea or participant's positive self-report of a cold) 58% (95% CI: 37-78) and 82% (95% CI: 60-94) for the echinacea and placebo groups, respectively (p = 0.114). Thus, the results indicate that, in this study, echinacea was no more effective than placebo in preventing rhinovirus infection. However, it is possible that the study did not have sufficient statistical power to detect a difference between the two groups.[102]

The lack of effect observed in these two studies raises the question whether or not the durations of administration (14 and seven days in the respective studies[101, 102]) of echinacea prior to experimental rhinovirus infection were sufficient. On the other hand, the observed lack of effect may simply be because the studies were not large enough to be able to detect a difference between the treatment and placebo groups.

The effects of three different extracts of *E. angustifolia* root on the prevention and treatment of experimental rhinovirus infections were assessed in a randomised, double-blind, placebo controlled trial involving 437 young healthy volunteers.[103] In the 'prevention' phase of the study, volunteers received one of the three echinacea extracts 1.5 mL three times daily, or placebo, for 7 days before challenge with 100 50% tissue culture infectious doses of rhinovirus type 39 (asymptomatic participants only). The chemical profile of the extracts was reported to be: supercritical carbon dioxide extract, alkamides 74%, polysaccharides not present; 60% ethanol extract, polysaccharides 49%, alkamides 2.3%, cynarin 0.16 mg/mL; 20% ethanol extract, polysaccharides 42%, alkamides 0.1%; echinacoside was not detected in any of the extracts. At the end of the seven-day period, there were no statistically significant differences between the echinacea and placebo groups with respect to the proportion of participants in each group who developed an infection following rhinovirus challenge ($p > 0.05$ for all comparisons). Participants who were challenged with rhinovirus remained in the study for a 'treatment' phase (*see* Clinical studies, Treatment).

E

A further 'prevention' trial assessed the effects of a combination preparation containing extracts of aerial parts of *E. purpurea* and roots of *E. angustifolia* (Chizukit, Hadas Corporation Limited, Israel) 50 mg/mL, propolis 50 mg/mL and vitamin C 10 mg/mL in children.[104] In this randomised, double-blind study, 430 children aged one to five years received 5 mL of the preparation (7.5 mL for children aged four to five years), or placebo, twice daily for 12 weeks over a winter period. If a respiratory tract infection (RTI) occurred, the dosage was increased to four times daily for the duration of the episode. In total, 328 children completed the study. According to an efficacy analysis, the total number of episodes of illness, the mean number of episodes per child and the proportion of children with one or more episodes of illness were all significantly lower in the echinacea group, compared with the placebo group (reductions of 55%, 50% and 43%, respectively; $p <$ 0.001 for each).[104]

The authors' justification for not carrying out an intention-to-treat analysis was that all dropouts occurred in the first week of the trial; however, this decision should have been made *a priori* and not because of high dropout rates.[105] Other methodological limitations of the study are that baseline data, other than mean age, for the two groups are lacking, so it is not possible to assess the success of randomisation, and several, rather than one, primary outcomes were assessed.[105] Additionally, there is a lack of detail regarding the preparation studied (e.g. types of extracts, content of active constituents).

Treatment The earlier Cochrane systematic review described above (*see* Clinical studies, Prophylaxis) included eight randomised, placebo-controlled trials of echinacea preparations for the treatment of URTIs.[97] These trials tested three different combinations of echinacea extracts and two monopreparations, taken orally typically for 6–10 days. Six studies reported statistically significant beneficial effects for echinacea recipients, compared with placebo recipients, on outcome measures such as duration of illness or symptoms (e.g. 'running nose'). However, heterogeneity of the studies precluded any further summary of the results. In addition, several of the studies had methodological flaws or their methodological quality could not be determined due to a lack of detail about the study designs in published reports. For these reasons, although the majority of the studies described reported positive results for echinacea preparations, it was not possible to recommend any specific product for the treatment of the common cold and further research was considered necessary.[97]

An updated Cochrane review used more restrictive inclusion criteria for trials (*see* Clinical studies, Prophylaxis), as well as new trials, and included 14 trials (involving

Table 1 Summary of recent trials of echinacea preparations in the prevention and treatment of the common cold and other URTIs

Ref	Study design	Participants; *n*	Treatment group(s) regimen; *n* (ITT analysis)	Control group; *n* (ITT analysis)	Primary outcome measure(s)	Results (primary outcome measure)
Prevention trials						
99	R, DB, PC	Healthy adults from military/ industrial organisations in Germany; *n* = 302 enrolled, *n* = 289 ITT analysis	Ethanolic extract (DER 1:11 in 30% alcohol) of: (*a*) Ep root (*n* = 99) or (*b*) Ea root (*n* = 100); 50 drops bd on 5 days/ week for 12 weeks	Placebo (coloured ethanolic solution); *n* = 90	Time to first URTI	No statistically significant difference between groups: mean time (95% CI) in days to first URTI 69 (64–74), 66 (61–72) and 65 (59–70) for Ep, Ea and placebo, respectively; *p* = 0.49
100	R, DB, PC	Adults from a large general practice in Germany who had >3 colds/URTIs in the previous year; *n* = 109 enrolled, *n* = 108 treated, ITT analysis	Fluid extract of Ep herb 4 mL bd for 8 weeks; *n* = 55	Placebo (coloured ethanolic solution); *n* = 54	Investigator-assessed incidence, severity of colds/URTI	No statistically significant differences between groups: mean number colds/URTI per subject 0.78 and 0.93 for Ep and placebo, respectively (difference = 0.15; 95% CI –0.12, 0.41, *p* = 0.33); severity of infections (*p* = 0.15)
101	DB, PC	Healthy adults from university community in USA; *n* = 117 enrolled, *n* = 92 treated, analysed	Echinacea (0.16% cichoric acid; species, plant part not stated) 300 mg tds for 14 days before rhinovirus challenge and for 5 days after; *n* = 50	Placebo; *n* = 42	Incidence of colds	No statistically significant differences between groups: proportions with rhinovirus infection = 44 and 57% for echinacea and placebo, respectively (*p* = 0.3); proportions with clinical colds = 50 and 59% for echinacea and placebo, respectively (*p* = 0.77)
102	R, DB, PC	Healthy adults; *n* = 48 enrolled	Pressed juice of aerial parts of Ep in 22% alcohol, 2.5 mL tds for 7 days before rhinovirus inoculation and for 7 days afterwards; *n* = 24	Placebo; *n* = 24	Frequency of rhinovirus infection as assessed by laboratory evidence; incidence of colds	No statistically significant differences between groups: proportions (95% CI) with laboratory evidence of rhinovirus infection = 92% (73–99) and 96% (77–100) for Ep and placebo, respectively (*p* value not reported); proportions (95% CI) with clinical colds = 58 (37–78) and 82 (60–94) for Ep and placebo, respectively (*p* = 0.114)
103	R, DB, PC	Healthy young adults from university community in USA; *n* = 437 enrolled, *n* = 419 treated, *n* = 399 analysed; this study included both a prevention and a treatment phase	(*a*) Carbon dioxide Ea root extract; (*b*) 60% ethanol Ea root extract; or (*c*) 20% ethanol Ea root extract; 1.5 mL three times daily for each, for 7 days before virus challenge and for 5 days after; *n* = 163 randomised for prevention phase; *n* = 328 for treatment phase	Placebo; *n* = 274 for prevention phase; *n* = 109 for treatment phase	Proportions of participants who developed clinical colds (prevention phase) and total symptom scores (treatment phase)	No statistically significant differences between echinacea and placebo groups: difference with respect to proportions of participants who developed clinical colds (prevention phase) and total symptom scores (treatment phase) (*p* > 0.05 for both)
104	R, DB, PC	Children aged 1–5 years; *n* = 430 enrolled, *n* = 328 efficacy analysis	Combination preparation containing extracts of aerial parts of Ep and roots of Ea, 5 mL (7.5 mL for 4–5 year-olds) bd for 12 weeks; *n* = 160	Placebo; *n* = 168	Several stated, including total number of episodes of illness, mean number of episodes per child, proportion of children with one or more episodes of illness	Total number of episodes of illness, mean number of episodes per child, proportion of children with one or more episodes of illness were significantly lower (reductions of 55, 50 and 43%, respectively) in the Ep/ Ea group compared with the placebo group (*p* < 0.001)

table continues

Table 1 *continued*

Ref	Study design	Participants; *n*	Treatment group(s) regimen; *n* (ITT analysis)	Control group; *n* (ITT analysis)	Primary outcome measure(s)	Results (primary outcome measure)
Treatment trials						
106	R, DB, PC	University students in USA with colds of recent onset; *n* = 148 enrolled, *n* = 142 analysed (no post-enrolment data available for 6 participants)	Capsules containing dried Ea root 123 mg, Ep root 62 mg and Ep herb 62 mg plus flavourings, 4 capsules 6 times during first 24 hours of cold onset, then 4 capsules tds until symptoms resolved (max 10 days); *n* = 69	Placebo (alfalfa 333 mg); *n* = 73	Self-reported duration, severity of colds	No statistically significant differences between groups: difference (95% CI) in duration = –0.52 days (–1.09 to 0.22); global severity (numerical data not shown)
107	R, DB, PC	Healthy adults 'prone' to common cold in Sweden; *n* = 559 enrolled, *n* = 246 who took study medication ITT analysis	Tablets containing crude extract of:(*a*) Ep 6.78 mg herb (95%), root (5%), *n* = 55; (*b*) Ep 48.27 mg herb (95%), root (5%), *n* = 64; (*c*) Ep 29.6 mg root (100%), *n* = 63; 2 tablets tds at cold onset until symptoms resolved (max 7 days)	Placebo; *n* = 64	Physician-assessed reduction in symptom index	Treatments *a* and *b*, but not treatment *c*, significantly more effective than placebo: mean (95% CI) relative reduction in symptoms = 58.7% (48.7, 68.7), 58.1% (47.7, 69.7), 46.1% (30.1, 62.1) and 33.6% (16.6, 50.6), for *a*, *b*, *c* and placebo, respectively (p = 0.045, 0.027 and 0.133 for *a*, *b* and *c* versus placebo, respectively)
108	R, DB, PC	Adults with symptoms of a cold in Germany; *n* = 80 enrolled and analysed	EC31J0 (pressed juice of Ep herb) 5 mL bd for 10 days; *n* = 41	Placebo; *n* = 39	Duration of illness (full picture of common cold based on self-reported symptoms)	Duration significantly shorter in echinacea group compared with placebo group (6 and 9 days, respectively; p = 0.0112)
109	QR, DB, PC	Adults with cold onset employed at nursing home in USA; *n* = 95	Tea comprising Ep and Ea herb and extract of Ep root (equivalent to 1275 mg dried herb and root per tea bag); 5–6 cups of tea on day 1, titrating down to 1 cup per day over next 5 days; *n* = 48	Placebo – herbal tea containing 7 herbal ingredients, including peppermint leaf and ginger rhizome; *n* = 47	No primary outcome stated; measures included self-reported symptoms and duration	Self-reported mean (SD) 'effectiveness score' significantly higher for echinacea compared with placebo (4.125 (0.959) and 2.787 (0.954), respectively; $p < 0.001$) but self-reported mean duration of symptoms significantly longer (4.33 (0.930) and 2.34 (1.09), respectively; $p < 0.001$)
110	R, DB, PC	Adults within 24 hours of first symptoms of a cold in USA; *n* = 128	Capsules containing 100 mg freeze-dried pressed juice of Ep; one tds until symptoms resolved or max imum of 14 days)	Placebo	Modified Jackson method for severity of symptoms; time to resolution of symptoms	No statistically significant differences between groups for total symptom scores, mean individual symptom scores and duration of symptoms (p range = 0.29–0.90, p range = 0.09–0.93, p = 0.73, respectively)
111	R, DB, PC	Adults with history of colds in Canada; *n* = 282, of whom 128 contracted a cold	Echinilin (standardised Ep extract) 10 × 4 mL on day 1 then 4 × 4 mL for next 6 days; *n* = 59	Placebo; *n* = 69	Change in total daily symptom scores (TDSS) for 7-day treatment period, duration of symptoms	Mean TDSS were significantly lower for E recipients, compared with placebo recipients ($p < 0.05$), but there was no statistically significant difference in duration of symptoms, according to ITT analysis (*n* = 128) ($p > 0.05$ for all symptoms)
112	R, DB, PC	Children aged 2–11 years; *n* = 524 enrolled	Dried pressed juice of aerial parts of Ep in syrup; *n* = 263	Placebo; *n* = 261	Duration and severity of symptoms	No statistically significant differences between groups for duration and severity of symptoms (p = 0.89 and 0.69, respectively)

bd = twice daily; DB = double-blind; DER = drug:extract ratio; E = Echinacea; Ea = *E. angustifolia*; Ep = *Echinacea purpurea*; ITT = intention-to-treat; PC = placebo-controlled; QR = quasi-randomised; R = randomised; tds = three times daily; URTIs = upper respiratory tract infections

E

19 comparisons) investigating echinacea preparations for the treatment of colds.[98] Most of the included trials were considered to be of 'reasonable to good quality'. However, trials assessed a variety of different preparations of echinacea, administered according to different dosage regimens, and more than one trial was available only for preparations of pressed juice obtained from the aerial parts of *E. purpurea*. In these two placebo-controlled trials, treatment was taken at the first signs of a cold; the number of participants developing a full cold was significantly lower in the echinacea group, whereas in the other trial, the difference did not reach statistical significance.[98] Details of eight trials included in the review (all are new trials published since the earlier Cochrane review) are summarised below. Collectively, the findings of available trials are difficult to interpret because of the wide variations in preparations tested; many marketed preparations of echinacea have not been tested at all in clinical trials.[98] Future trials should report the chemical composition of the echinacea material tested, and ideally assess the effects of standardised preparations.

Several new trials of echinacea preparations in the treatment of URTIs have been completed since the Cochrane review (Table 1) and have reported conflicting results.[106–113]

The effects of capsules containing 100 mg freeze-dried pressed juice of the aerial parts of *E. purpurea*, standardised for 2.4% β-1,2-D-fructofuranosides, were explored in a randomised, double-blind, placebo-controlled trial involving 128 adults enrolled into the study within 24 hours of their first symptoms of a cold.[110] Participants ingested one capsule three times daily until symptoms resolved, or for a maximum of 14 days. At the end of the study, there were no statistically significant differences between groups with respect to time to resolution of symptoms, daily self-recorded symptom scores, and frequency of adverse events. It is unclear why the preparation was standardised for content of β-1,2-D-fructofuranosides rather than, for example, alkamides, and why content of other constituents was not reported. Thus, it is difficult to interpret these results in the context of the findings of other studies.

In a larger randomised, double-blind, placebo-controlled trial, 282 adults with a history of two or more colds in the previous year received a standardised preparation of echinacea (Echinilin), or placebo, taken at the start of a cold (ten 4-mL doses over day 1, then four 4-mL doses daily for the next six days).[111] The echinacea preparation contained concentrated water–ethanol extracts of alkamides, cichoric acid and polysaccharides, obtained from various parts (no further details provided) of freshly harvested *E. purpurea* plants, and combined in 40% ethanol to provide concentrations of 0.25, 2.5 and 25.5 mg/mL, respectively. At the end of the study, according to an intention-to-treat analysis for the 128 participants who contracted a cold, self-assessed mean total daily symptom scores (TDSS; the primary efficacy parameter) were significantly lower for echinacea recipients than for placebo recipients (mean TDSS (95% CI) were 16.3 (13.6–19.0) and 19.9 (17.5–22.5), respectively for the echinacea and placebo groups; $p < 0.05$).

A report of this study lacks several important details. Numbers of participants initially randomised to the echinacea and placebo groups, and demographic data (e.g. mean age, gender etc) are not provided for the 282 participants who entered the study, so it is not possible to judge whether or not the randomisation process was successful in balancing the two groups with respect to these variables. These data are reported for the intention-to-treat analysis, and the placebo group has a markedly higher proportion of females than does the echinacea group (75% versus 54%, respectively). However, it is not possible to establish whether the placebo group originally comprised a greater proportion of females simply by chance through randomisation, or whether a markedly greater proportion of women in the placebo group perceived that they contracted a cold. This imbalance, and the implications it may have for the results, has not been considered adequately in the analysis.

A randomised, double-blind, placebo-controlled, community-based trial involving 148 students with common colds of recent onset, assessed the effects of capsules containing unrefined *E. purpurea* herb (62 mg), root (62 mg) and *E. angustifolia* root (123 mg).[106] Analysis of samples of the preparation by independent laboratories found that they contained cichoric acid and alkamides (0.5% to <1.0%), and echinoside, chlorogenic acid and caffeoyltartaric acid (all >0.1% to <0.5%). Participants took four capsules six times during the first 24 hours of the onset of a cold, followed by four capsules three times daily until symptoms resolved, or for up to 10 days. Among the 142 participants who completed the study, there was no difference in the mean duration of cold symptoms (6.27 and 5.75 days for the echinacea and placebo groups, respectively; difference: −0.52 days, 95% CI −1.09 to 0.22 days), even though the study had an adequate sample size: with a sample size of 150 participants, the study would have had 80% power to detect a benefit of two days' duration.

Three different preparations and doses of *E. purpurea* were tested in a randomised, double-blind, placebo-controlled trial in healthy adults.[107] The four arms of the study were: 6.78 mg *E. purpurea* crude extract, based on 95% herb and 5% root (Echinaforce); 48.27 mg *E. purpurea* crude extract, based on 95% herb and 5% root; 29.60 mg *E. purpurea* crude extract, based on root only; and placebo. In total, 246 participants experienced symptoms typical of the onset of a common cold and took their allocated study medication two tablets three times daily until they felt better, or for up to seven days. According to an intention-to-treat analysis, the two echinacea extracts prepared from both *E. purpurea* herb and root were significantly more effective than *E. purpurea* root extract and placebo in reducing symptoms as assessed by the investigator (the primary outcome measure): the relative reductions in the mean complaint index for these preparations were 58.7% (95% CI 48.7–68.7; $p = 0.045$ versus placebo) and 58.1% (95% CI 47.7–69.7; $p = 0.027$ versus placebo).[107]

Statistically significant effects for an extract of *E. purpurea* herb (Echinacin) on median duration of illness were reported in another randomised, double-blind, placebo-controlled trial involving 80 adults who experienced onset of a cold (median duration six and nine days for echinacea and placebo, respectively; $p = 0.0112$).[108] Participants started taking their allocated medication on first experiencing symptoms, and continued treatment (5 mL twice daily) until symptoms resolved.

A further placebo-controlled study involving adults with early symptoms of a cold ($n = 95$) explored the effects of a combination preparation containing *E. purpurea* and *E. angustifolia* herb and extract of *E. purpurea* root, as well as lemongrass leaf and spearmint leaf as flavourings, formulated as a tea.[109] When prepared as directed, tea prepared from one bag was stated to provide 31.5 mg of phenolic compounds, calculated as caftaric acid, cichoric acid, chlorogenic acid and echinacoside. The results suggested a statistically significant difference between the treatment and placebo groups in self-rated effectiveness – mean (standard deviation, SD) effectiveness score 4.13 (0.96) and 2.78 (0.95) for echinacea tea and placebo, respectively ($p < 0.001$) – although the mean (SD) duration of symptoms was significantly longer in the echinacea group, compared with the placebo group (4.33 (0.93) and 2.34 (1.09) for echinacea tea and placebo, respectively; $p < 0.001$). In addition, the study had several methodological limitations. For example, although stated to be randomised, the study did not involve true randomisation (participants were allocated to groups alternately), the 'placebo' tea contained low doses of several herbs (peppermint leaf, sweet fennel seed, ginger rhizome, papaya leaf, alfalfa leaf and cinnamon bark), and outcomes were self-assessed only.

The effects of three different extracts of *E. angustifolia* root on the prevention and treatment of experimental rhinovirus infections were assessed in a randomised, double-blind, placebo controlled trial involving 437 young healthy volunteers.[103] In the 'prevention' phase of the study (*see* Clinical studies, Prophylaxis), volunteers received one of the three echinacea extracts 1.5 mL three times daily, or placebo, for 7 days before challenge with 100 50% tissue culture infectious doses of rhinovirus type 39 (asymptomatic participants only). Participants who were challenged with rhinovirus remained in the study for a 'treatment' phase during which they continued with their initial treatment allocation (i.e. one of the three echinacea extracts or placebo) or, having received placebo during the 'prevention' phase, received one of the three echinacea extracts during the treatment phase. Treatment was given according to the same dosage regimen for five days after virus challenge.

At the end of the study, there were no statistically significant differences between the echinacea and placebo groups with respect to total symptom scores and proportions of participants who developed clinical colds.

The chemical profile of the extracts was reported to be: supercritical carbon dioxide extract, alkamides 74%, polysaccharides not present; 60% ethanol extract, polysaccharides 49%, alkamides 2.3%, cynarin 0.16 mg/mL; 20% ethanol extract, polysaccharides 42%, alkamides 0.1%; echinacoside was not detected in any of the extracts. It remains possible that other constituents or combinations of constituents have pharmacological effects,[103] although bioavailability would need to be demonstrated. The alkamide constituents of *E. angustifolia* root and *E. purpurea* root have been detected in plasma following administration of an echinacea product to healthy volunteers.[86]

Two other studies have assessed the effects of echinacea preparations in the treatment of URTIs in children. In a randomised, double-blind, placebo-controlled trial, 524 children aged two to eleven years received dried pressed juice of the aerial parts of *E. purpurea* (harvested at flowering) combined with syrup, or placebo (syrup only) 3.75 mL (5 mL for 6 to 11 year olds) twice daily during a URTI and until all symptoms had resolved up to a maximum of 10 days.[112] Data were available for 707 of 759 (94%) URTIs that occurred during the study period; 370 and 337 of these occurred in the placebo and echinacea groups, respectively. A significantly greater proportion of children in the placebo group had more than one URTI, when compared with the echinacea group (64.4% vs 52.3% for placebo and echinacea, respectively; $p = 0.015$). There were no statistically significant differences between groups for the primary outcome measures duration ($p = 0.89$) and severity of symptoms ($P = 0.69$) or for secondary outcome measures, including peak severity of symptoms, number of days of peak symptoms and number of days with fever ($p > 0.08$ for all). This study has been criticised, in particular, because the preparation tested was not analysed to determine its chemical composition;[114] in response, the authors stated that the constituent(s) responsible for the putative clinical effects have not been definitively established.[115] While this is indeed the case, it is nevertheless important to describe the chemical composition of the product tested (e.g. its alkamide and polysaccharide content) so that the findings of the study can be considered in the context of other research.

The effects of a preparation containing expressed juice (80 mL/100 mL preparation) from freshly collected flowering *E. purpurea* plants (Immunal, SIA International, Volgograd, Russia) were compared with those of a preparation (SHA-10, Swedish Herbal Institutue, Gothenburg, Sweden) containing a standardised extract of *Andrographis paniculata* (5.25 mg andrographolide and deoxyandrographolide per tablet) and extract of *Eleutherococcus senticosus* (9.7 mg per tablet) in a randomised, double-blind, placebo-controlled trial involving 133 children aged four to eleven years with uncomplicated URTI for whom treatment could begin within 24 hours of the onset of symptoms.[113] The dosage regimens were 10 drops three times daily for the echinacea preparation, and two tablets three times daily for the *A. paniculata* preparation; the duration of treatment was 10 days for both. The interventions were given in addition to standard treatment (warm drinks, throat gargles, nose drops and paracetamol 500 mg three times daily if required), and a control group received standard treatment alone.

At the end of the study, *A. paniculata* recipients had recovered more quickly than had participants in the other two groups ($p < 0.002$), and the amount of nasal secretion was significantly lower in the *A. paniculata* group, compared with the echinacea group, from day five of the study ($p < 0.01$).[113] This study, however, has several methodological flaws: there was no pre-specified primary outcome measure, and a sample size calculation does not appear to have been carried out; the study was reported to be double-blind, although it is not stated that placebo drops and tablets were used; a doctor helped the children with their self-assessment of symptoms, and it is not clear if and how blinding was maintained throughout these interactions; the study was focused on *A. paniculata* and analyses comparing the echinacea and placebo groups were not carried out.

Several trials of echinacea preparations in the prevention of URTIs provide data on duration and severity of infections occurring in participants (*see* Clinical studies, Prophylaxis). While these data have some relevance to treatment, they should not be grouped together, since the dosage regimens are entirely different – in 'prevention' trials, participants may have received study medication for several weeks or more before experiencing an infection, whereas in 'treatment' trials, participants usually start study medication immediately after the onset of symptoms.

Other infections A randomised, double-blind, placebo-controlled, crossover trial assessed the effects of an extract of *E. purpurea* herb (95%) and root (5%) (Echinaforce) on the incidence and severity of recurrent genital herpes in 50 patients who had not been exposed to aciclovir or similar medicines within 14 days of enrollment into the study and who had had at least four recurrences of genital herpes within the previous 12 months.[116] Study medication, or placebo, was taken orally 800 mg twice daily for six months. The study did not show any significant difference between the two groups on the outcomes measured (frequency and duration of recurrences, pain score, CD4 cell count, neutrophil count), although there was a high drop-out rate during the study.

A systematic review of studies exploring the immunomodulatory effects of echinacea-containing preparations included seven controlled clinical trials in infections such as sinusitis, bronchitis and candida (*see* Clinical studies, Immunomodulatory activity).[88]

Side-effects, Toxicity

Frequency and type of adverse events Data on numbers of participants experiencing adverse events were provided by several studies included in a Cochrane systematic review of 16 randomised and quasi-randomised controlled trials of extracts of echinacea for preventing or treating URTIs (*see* Clinical studies, Prophylaxis, and Treatment).[97] Four placebo-controlled 'prevention' trials of echinacea reported these data: in three trials, involving a total of around 1000 participants, the frequency of adverse events in the echinacea group was similar to that in the corresponding placebo group; in one trial, adverse events did not occur in either the echinacea or placebo groups. Three 'treatment' trials provided adverse event data: in two studies, adverse events were not observed in either the echinacea or the placebo groups, and in one, numbers of patients experiencing adverse events in the echinacea and placebo groups were similar (four and five, respectively).[97]

New clinical trials published since the Cochrane review also report that there was no statistically significant difference in the frequency of adverse events noted for echinacea preparations and placebo.[99–112] with the exception of one study which reported a significantly higher frequency of rash in the echinacea group, compared with the placebo group (7.1% vs 2.7% for echinacea and placebo, respectively; $p = 0.008$).[112] The updated Cochrane review drew similar conclusions that data from the available randomised controlled trials indicated that adverse effects or events associated with the use of the echinacea preparations assessed were infrequent, minor and similar to those noted for placebo.[99]

Where adverse events were reported, most commonly these were mild gastrointestinal symptoms.[100, 104, 106, 107, 111, 112] Another review of clinical data, mostly from clinical trials, concluded that oral administration of the expressed juice of *E. purpurea* herb is well-tolerated.[117] The review included data from an unpublished post-marketing surveillance study involving over 1200 individuals aged 2–20 years who used oral *E. purpurea* lozenges for 4–6 weeks for URTIs, and which indicated that unpleasant taste was the most frequently reported adverse event.

On the basis of these limited data, it seems that the risk of acute adverse effects with echinacea is very small. However, it is not possible to draw firm conclusions from these data for several reasons – different echinacea preparations and regimens were tested, different patient populations (adults, children) were involved, and echinacea preparations were administered for only a short time period, particularly in the 'treatment' trials.[118] In addition, since clinical trials usually have the statistical power only to detect common, acute adverse effects and, as there is a lack of data on the safety of the longer term use of echinacea preparations, there is a need for further evaluation of the safety of different echinacea preparations.

The low number of reports of suspected adverse reactions associated with echinacea preparations set against estimates of the high frequency of use of echinacea has been used as an argument for the safety of echinacea.[40] However, this argument is flawed since it fails to consider that under-reporting of suspected adverse reactions associated with herbal medicines is likely at several levels,[119, G21] and that in general reporting systems for herbal medicines are not well-established. The use of sales data to estimate the frequency of an adverse reaction can be misleading at best and, in addition, the argument takes no account of the differences in preparations of echinacea.

The UK Committee on Safety of Medicines (CSM) and Medicines and Healthcare products Regulatory Agency (MHRA) spontaneous reporting scheme (the 'yellow card' scheme) for suspected adverse drug reactions (ADR) reporting received 34 reports describing 64 suspected ADRs associated with echinacea preparations for the period 1 July 1963 to 1 June 2004 (*see* Table 2).[120] For the majority of these cases, echinacea had been administered orally; details of specific products, species of echinacea, type of extract and other details are not available.

The World Health Organization's Uppsala Monitoring Centre (WHO-UMC; Collaborating Centre for International Drug Monitoring) receives summary reports of suspected adverse drug reactions from national pharmacovigilance centres of over 70 countries worldwide, including the UK. To the end of the year 2004, the WHO-UMC had received a total of 259 reports, describing a total of 537 adverse reactions, for products containing a single species of *Echinacea*.[121] The vast majority of these reports describes reactions associated with *E. purpurea*, most commonly (reaction listed 10 times or more): abdominal pain ($n = 10$); angioedema (10); dyspnoea (18); nausea (14); pruritus (17); rash (18); rash, erythematous (23); urticaria (23). (These data were obtained from the Vigisearch database held by the WHO Collaborating Centre for International Drug Monitoring, Uppsala, Sweden. The information is not homogeneous at least with respect to origin or likelihood that the pharmaceutical product caused the adverse reaction. Any information included in this report does not represent the opinion of the World Health Organization.)

Allergic reactions

Echinacea species belong to the Asteraceae (Compositae, daisy) family, members of which are known to cause allergic reactions. Individuals with allergic tendencies, particularly those with

Table 2 Spontaneous reports of suspected adverse drug reactions associated with echinacea preparations submitted to the UK Committee on Safety of Medicines/Medicines and Healthcare products Regulatory Agency for the period 01/07/1963 to 01/06/2004 (Adverse Drug Reactions On-line Information Tracking 2004).[120]

System organ class. **Reaction names**	**Total**
Blood and lymphatic system disorders. Aplastic anaemia (1), coagulopathy (1), idiopathic thrombocytic purpura (1)	3
Cardiac disorders. Supraventricular tachycardia (1), ventricular arrhythmia NOS (1), palpitations (1)	3
Central and peripheral nervous system disorders. Including convulsions (5); dizziness (3); headache (6)	17
Endocrine disorders. Basedow's disease (1)	1
Eye disorders. Blurred vision (1)	1
Gastrointestinal disorders. Faecal incontinence (1), irritable bowel syndrome (1), dysphagia (1), nausea (1), tongue oedema (1)	5
General disorders and administration site conditions. Rigors (1), drug interaction NOS (3), drug interaction potentiation (1), fatigue (1), malaise (1), feeling abnormal (1)	8
Hepatobiliary disorders. Sclerosing cholangitis (1)	1
Infections and infestations. Parotitis (1)	1
Investigations. Blood pressure increased (1), INR increased (2), liver function test abnormal (1), weight increased (1)	5
Metabolism and nutrition disorders. Hyponatraemia (1)	1
Musculoskeletal and connective tissue disorders. Arthralgia (2), myalgia (1), muscle twitching (1)	4
Nervous system disorders. Central pontine myelinolysis (1), memory impairment (1), ataxia (1), abnormal co-ordination NOS (1), loss of consciousness (1), burning sensation NOS (1), dysarthria (1), epilepsy NOS (1)	8
Psychiatric disorders. Agitation (1), panic reaction (1), confusional state (2), insomnia (1), sleep disorder NOS (1)	6
Renal and urinary disorders. Pollakiuria (1), urinary incontinence (1), haematuria (1)	3
Respiratory , thoracic and mediastinal disorders. Asthma NOS (1), dyspnoea (1), dry throat (1), pharyngolaryngeal pain (1)	4
Skin and subcutaneous tissue disorders. Face oedema (1), urticaria NOS (3), erythema multiforme (1), erythema (1), pruritus (1), rash NOS (1)	8
Vascular disorders. Flushing (1), hypertension NOS (1)	2
Total number of reactions	**64**

INR = international normalised ratio; NOS = not otherwise stated

known allergy to other members of the Asteraceae family (e.g. chamomile) should be advised to avoid echinacea preparations containing aerial parts.[G50]

Isolated spontaneous reports of suspected ADRs associated with the use of echinacea preparations include allergic skin reactions (*see also* Side-effects, Toxicity, Frequency and type of adverse events).[117] In Australia, detailed assessment of five cases of allergic reactions temporally associated with echinacea (anaphylaxis, 2; acute asthma attack in an echinacea-naive individual, 1; recurrent mild asthma, 1; macropapular rash, 1), three of which reported positive rechallenge, revealed that three patients had positive skin-prick test results for echinacea.[122] One case report described a 37-year-old woman with atopy who experienced anaphylaxis 30 minutes after ingesting several dietary supplements (vitamins B_{12} and E, an iron preparation, 'folate', vitamin B complex, a multivitamin preparation, zinc, antioxidants, a garlic and onion preparation, evening primrose oil) and 15 minutes after taking 5 mL of an echinacea preparation, stated to be equivalent to *E. angustifolia* whole plant extract 3825 mg and *E. purpurea* dried root 150 mg.[123] The woman took promethazine and was observed in an emergency department for 2 hours, and her symptoms resolved without further treatment. Two weeks later she gave a positive skin-prick test to the echinacea product, but not to 'crude' extracts of the other supplements she had taken. She had been taking echinacea for 2–3 years and had previously taken the same product without experiencing any adverse effects. A causal association in this case has been questioned.[124]

Positive skin-prick test results for echinacea were also reported for 20% of 100 echinacea-naive atopic individuals, and over 50% of 26 Australian suspected ADR reports of hypersensitivity associated with echinacea involved individuals with atopy.[122] Echinacea has previously been reported to have produced positive patch test reactions in four individuals with a previous history of plant dermatitis.[G51] These reports raise hypotheses that require testing in formal studies.

An isolated report describes a 41-year-old man who experienced four episodes of erythema nodosum after using an echinacea preparation at each onset of an influenza-like illness.[125] The man had been using echinacea intermittently for 18 months, as well as loratadine on an as required basis and St John's wort for the previous six months. Each episode of erythema nodosum responded to conventional treatment including prednisone. The man was advised to discontinue treatment with echinacea and, after one year, had not experienced any further recurrences. However, the report does not provide any details (species, plant part, formulation, dosage regimen) of the echinacea preparation involved and therefore is difficult to interpret. Causality has not been established.

Other reactions

A case of hypokalaemic renal tubular acidosis due to Sjögren's syndrome (a symptom complex of unknown aetiology, marked by keratoconjunctivitis sicca, xerostamia, with or without lachrymal and salivary gland enlargement, respectively, and presence of connective tissue disease, usually rheumatoid arthritis, but sometime systemic lupus erythematosus, scleroderma or polymyositis) has been reported in a 36-year-old woman.[126] She was stated to have begun taking echinacea, St. John's wort and kava two weeks before becoming ill, but the report does not provide any further details of the echinacea species contained in the product(s), nor of the types of preparations, formulations, dosages and routes of administration of any of the herbal medicines listed. The woman was hospitalised with severe generalised muscle weakness and tests revealed she had a serum potassium ion concentration of 1.3 mEq/L. She was given electrolyte replacement for four days, after which the muscle weakness resolved, and was started on hydroxychloroquine 200 mg daily for 'probable' Sjögren's syndrome. The authors suggested that ingestion of echinacea may have aggravated an autoimmune disorder, although rechallenge with echinacea was not undertaken, and causality has not been established.[126]

Another report describes a 49-year-old woman who presented with a five-day history of numbness and weakness in her right arm.[127] For the previous seven weeks she had received echinacea comp 2 mL mixed with 5 mL of her venous blood intramuscularly twice weekly to prevent infections and 'boost' her immune system. The injection was stated to contain *E. angustifolia* D2 1.1 mL, Aconitum D4 0.3 mL and Lachesis (bushmaster snake venom) D8 0.3 mL. (D nomenclature relates to a homeopathic dilution step; D2 is equivalent to a 1 in 100 dilution, whereas D8 is equivalent to a 1 in 100 000 000 dilution.)[128] The woman was admitted to hospital with mild spastic paresis and fluctuating numbness of the right arm and was described as having acute disseminated encephalomyelitis; symptoms resolved after treatment with methylprednisolone 500 mg daily by intravenous infusion. Causality has not been established.

There is an isolated report of exacerbation of pre-existing pemphigus vulgaris (a chronic, serious skin disorder characterized by the development of easily ruptured blisters on skin and mucous membranes) in a 55-year-old man who began taking an echinacea product orally after developing an upper respiratory tract infection.[129] Within a week, he developed blisters on his trunk, head and oral mucosa; partial disease control was achieved after discontinuing the product. It is possible that this exacerbation was part of the natural course of disease, and causality in this case has not been established. Furthermore, no further details of the product, including species of echinacea, plant part, type of preparation, and dosage were provided, and it is not stated whether or not a sample of the product was retained. Without verification that the product implicated did contain echinacea material and was free of other ingredients or adulterants, this report adds little to the debate on the safety of use of echinacea by individuals with autoimmune disorders.

Toxicology

In general, animal studies with different preparations and fractions of echinacea species have indicated low toxicity.[40] In acute toxicity studies involving polysaccharide fractions from *E. purpurea* administered by intraperitoneal injection to small numbers of mice, the LD_{50} (lethal dose) for female mice was 2500 mg/kg.[130] Other acute toxicity studies using a preparation comprising pressed juice from *E. purpurea* herb have provided LD_{50} values in mice of >30 000 mg/kg and >10 000 mg/kg for oral and intravenous administration, respectively, and in rats of >15 000 mg/kg and >5000 mg/kg or oral and intravenous administration, respectively.[131, 132] Further experiments showed no evidence of mutagenic activity in bacteria and mammalian cells *in vitro* and *in vivo* in mice.[132]

High concentrations of *E. purpurea* (8 mg/mL) have been reported to reduce sperm motility, sperm penetration of hamster oocytes and to be associated with sperm DNA denaturation *in vitro*; no such effects were observed with low concentrations.[133, 134] These findings are difficult to interpret since there is a lack of detail regarding the preparation of *E. purpurea*, and their clinical relevance is questionable.

The pyrrolizidine alkaloids isotussilagine and tussilagine have been documented for echinacea, although they possess a saturated pyrrolizidine nucleus and are not thought to be toxic.

In vivo antitumour activity and *in vitro* stimulation of TNFα secretion have been reported for echinacea. In addition to its antitumour effects, TNF is stated to be a mediator of cachexia and the manifestations of endotoxic shock.

Contra-indications, Warnings

It has been stated that echinacea is contra-indicated in patients with progressive systemic diseases, such as tuberculosis, leukaemia and leukaemia-like diseases, collagen disorders, multiple sclerosis and other autoimmune diseases.[G56] In the UK, some products also advise against use in AIDS and HIV infections. The basis for these statements appears to be a theoretical one, based on evidence that echinacea preparations have immunomodulatory activity; there is an opposing view that echinacea is not harmful in autoimmune diseases.[G50] At present, there is a lack of reliable clinical evidence to support these views, although in view of the seriousness of the conditions listed, it is appropriate to avoid use in these disorders until further information is available.

Interactions There are no reported drug interactions for echinacea, although on the basis of its documented immunomodulatory activity, as a general precaution, echinacea should only be used with caution in patients taking immunosuppressant drugs.

A study involving 12 healthy non-smoking volunteers assessed the effects of *E. purpurea* root (Nature's Bounty, Bohemia, New York, USA) on the activity of the cytochrome P450 enzymes CYP1A2, CYP2C9 and CYP2D6 and CYP3A using caffeine, tolbutamide, dextromethorphan and midazolam, respectively, as probe drugs (i.e. substrates for the respective CYP enzymes).[135] After a control phase in which volunteers received all of the probe drugs orally (with the exception of midazolam which was given intravenously and, later, orally), participants took *E. purpurea* root 400 mg four times daily for eight days; the product was stated to contain more than 1% phenols (caftaric acid, chlorogenic acid, echinacoside and cichoric acid). On the sixth day, the probe drugs were administered and blood and urine samples were collected as during the control phase.

The clearance of caffeine after oral administration was reduced significantly during echinacea administration compared with values obtained during the control phase (mean (SD): 6.6 (3.8) L/hour and 4.9 (2.3) L/hour for echinacea and control periods, respectively; $p = 0.049$), although the half-life ($t_{½}$) of caffeine, area under the curve (AUC) and maximum concentration (C_{max}) were not significantly altered. Time to maximum concentration (t_{max}) was significantly increased for both caffeine and tolbutamide during echinacea administration, compared with baseline values ($p = 0.015$ and 0.004, respectively). Dextromethorphan pharmacokinetics were unaltered during echinacea administration in the 11 participants who were extensive metabolisers. The clearance of midazolam following intravenous, but not oral, administration was significantly increased during echinacea administration, compared with baseline values (mean (SD): 43 (16) L/hour and 32 (7) L/hour, respectively; $p = 0.003$).

These findings suggest that *E. purpurea* root inhibits CYP1A2, but not CYP2C9 and CYP2D6, and that CYP3A activity is selectively modulated: intestinal CYP3A activity is inhibited and hepatic CYP3A activity is induced. There are several possible explanations for the selective effects of *E. purpurea* root on CYP3A activity: the constituent(s) of echinacea responsible for CYP3A inhibition may not be systemically available, thus avoiding hepatic CYP3A inhibition; the constituent(s) of echinacea responsible for CYP3A induction may be rapidly absorbed, thus intestinal CYP3A induction is avoided; hepatic CYP3A may be induced by a systemically formed metabolite of a constituent of echinacea; CYP3A induction may involve tissue-specific activators which are differentially influenced by constituents of echinacea.[135]

In a subsequent, similar study, 12 healthy volunteers received capsules containing a whole plant extract of *E. purpurea* (containing cichoric acid 13.7 mg; chlorogenic acid and echinacoside were not detected by HPLC analysis) 800 mg twice daily for 28 days. Participants also received three other herbal products (*Citrus aurantium*, *Serenoa serrulata* and *Silybum marianum*), each administered separately for 28 days; the four herbal products were administered in random sequence, with a 30-day wash-out period between each, until each participant had received all four herbal products. It was stated that there were no statistically significant differences between serum ratios of probe drugs and their respective metabolites obtained before and after administration of *E. purpurea* extract and, therefore, that the extract had no significant effect on CYP1A2, CYP2D6, CYP2E1 or CYP3A4 activities. The authors' conclusions, however, included the caveat that the effects of *E. purpurea* extract on CYP enzyme activity, particularly that of CYP1A2 and CYP3A4, merit further study.[136]

The effects of echinacea products available in Canada on inhibition of the human cytochrome P450 drug metabolising enzyme CYP3A4 have been tested *in vitro* using a fluorometric mitrotitre plate assay.[137] In the study, 10 mL samples of preparations of *E. angustifolia* roots, *E. purpurea* roots and herb, and a 1 : 1 blend of *E. angustifolia* and *E. purpurea* (plant parts not specified) were standardised to contain ethanol 55% and used as stock solutions. Samples of serial dilutions of these preparations, as well as different concentrations of the pure compounds echinacoside and cichoric acid, were assayed. The blend of *E. angustifolia* and *E. purpurea*, and *E. purpurea* herb showed 'moderate' inhibition of CYP3A4: median (95% CI) inhibitory concentration (IC_{50}) values (% of full strength preparation) were 6.73 (4.75, 10.09) and 8.56 (5.95, 13.05), respectively. Echinacoside also showed moderate inhibitory activity (median IC_{50} values (95% CI) 6.29 (2.07, 71.56)), whereas cichoric acid showed low inhibitory activity.[137]

A study in mice fed both melatonin and an extract of *E. purpurea* root in their diet reported reduced numbers of proliferating myeloid cells in the spleen and bone marrow.[138]

Further research is needed to determine whether these findings are clinically important.

Pregnancy and lactation There is a lack of data on the safety of echinacea preparations taken during pregnancy and lactation and, given that the benefits of specific echinacea preparations have not been established definitively, excessive use during these periods should be avoided as a general precaution.

A cohort study compared numbers of live births, and spontaneous and therapeutic abortions occurring among women who had taken echinacea preparations during pregnancy ($n = 206$, 112 of whom took echinacea during the first trimester) with those occurring among a control group of 206 women matched for disease (URTI), maternal age and alcohol and cigarette use.[139] The exposed group of women had telephoned a hospital teratogen information service regarding the use of echinacea during pregnancy; the unexposed group had also telephoned the service for this reason, but subsequently did not use echinacea or used a non-teratogenic antibiotic instead.

There were no statistically significant differences between the two groups in assessed outcomes including number of live births, spontaneous and therapeutic abortions, gestational age, birth weight and rates of malformations. In the exposed group there were six major and six minor malformations, compared with seven major and seven minor malformations in the control group.[139] The study has several limitations, particularly the small sample size, meaning that the study would have the statistical power only to detect common malformations, and self-report of exposure, since it is possible that misclassification could have occurred (e.g. exposed women reported as unexposed). In addition, participants used a range of different preparations of echinacea at different dosage regimens, so the study does not provide adequate evidence for any specific preparation. Further study is required to establish the safety profile of echinacea during pregnancy.

Preparations

Proprietary single-ingredient preparations

Australia: Echinacin. *Austria:* Echinacin; Echinaforce; Sanvita Immun. *Belgium:* Echinacin. *Brazil:* Enax; Equinacea; Imunnal; Imunocel; Imunogreen. *Canada:* Citranacea; Triple Blend Echinacea. *Czech Republic:* Immunal. *Germany:* aar vir; Cefasept; Echan; Echifit; Echiherb; Echinacin; Echinacin; Echinaforce; Echinapur; Echinatur; Episcorit; Esberitox mono; Lymphozil; Pascotox forte-Injektopas; Pascotox mono; Resistan mono; Resplant; Wiedimmun. *Greece:* Echinacin. *Hungary:* Echinacin. *Italy:* EuMunil. *Mexico:* Inmune Booster; Regripax. *Russia:* Immunal (Иммунал); Immunorm (Иммунорм). *Spain:* Echinacin; Ekian. *Switzerland:* Echinacin; Echinaforce; EchinaMed. *UK:* Echinacea; Echinaforce; Phytocold; Skin Clear. *USA:* Echinacea; Laci Echinacea with Hint of Mint.

Proprietary multi-ingredient preparations

Argentina: Parodontax Fluor; SX-22. *Australia:* Andrographis Complex; Andrographis Compound; Astragalus Complex; Broncafect; Cats Claw Complex; Cold and Flu Relief; Cough Relief; Digest; Echinacea 4000; Echinacea ACE + Zinc; Echinacea Complex; Echinacea Lozenge; Euphrasia Complex; Flavons; Galium Complex; Gartech; Herbal Cleanse; Herbal Cold & Flu Relief; Lifesystem Herbal Plus Formula 8 Echinacea; Logicin Natural Lozenges; Odourless Garlic; Proyeast; Sambucus Complex; Urgenin; Urinase. *Austria:* Parodontax; Parodontax; Spasmo-Urgenin; Urgenin. *Belgium:* Urgenin. *Brazil:* Malvatricin Natural Organic; Malvatricin Natural; Parodontax. *Canada:* Bentasil Licorice with Echinacea; Benylin First Defense; Echinacea Goldenseal Formula. *Chile:* Citro-C; Paltomiel Plus. *Germany:* Esberitox; Esberitox N; Hewenephron duo. *Hong Kong:* Urgenin. *Israel:* Urgenin. *Italy:* Bodyguard; Dermilia Flebozin; Golatux; Immumil; Influ-Zinc; Probigol; Ribovir; Sclerovis H. *Malaysia:* Echinacea Plus; Total Man. *Mexico:* Gripaleta. *New Zealand:* Lice Blaster; Strepsils Echinacea Defence. *Portugal:* Spasmo-Urgenin; Vitace. *Russia:* Prostanorm (Простанорм). *South Africa:* Wecesin. *Spain:* Neo Urgenin; Spasmo-Urgenin; Urgenin. *Switzerland:* Demonatur Capsules contre les refroidissements; Demonatur Dragees pour les reins et la vessie; Drosana Resiston avec vitamine C; Esberitop; Gel a la consoude; Prosta-Caps Chassot N; Spagymun; Spagyrom; Wala Echinacea. *Thailand:* Spasmo-Urgenin. *UK:* AllerClear; Antifect; Catarrh Tablets; Echinaboost; Echinacea; Goodypops; Hay Fever & Sinus Relief; Hayfever & Sinus Relief; Höfels Echinacea and Rosehip; Immune Insurance; Modern Herbals Cold & Catarrh; Napiers Echinacea Tea; Revitonil; Sinotar; Sinus and Hay Fever Tablets. *USA:* Echinacea Golden Seal; Laci Throat Care Soothing Citrus; Laci Supplement Power Time; Immune Support; TriMune.

References

1 Bauer R *et al*. Alkamides from the roots of *Echinacea angustifolia*. *Phytochemistry* 1989; 28: 505–508.

2 Bauer R, Wagner H. Echinacea. In: *Ein Handbuch für Ärzte, Apotheker und andere Naturwissenschaftler*. Stuttgart: Wissenschaftliche Verlagsgesellschaft, 1990: 182.

3 Bauer R, Wagner H. Echinacea – Der Sonnenhut – Stand der Forschung. *Z Phytother* 1988; 9: 151–159.

4 Bauer R, Remiger P. TLC and HPLC analysis of alkamides in *Echinacea* drugs. *Planta Med* 1989; 55: 367–371.

5 Lienert D *et al*. Gas chromatography-mass spectral analysis of roots of *Echinacea* species and classification by multivariate data analysis. *Phytochem Anal* 1998; 9: 88–89.

6 Sloley BD *et al*. Comparison of chemical components and antioxidant capacity of different *Echinacea* species. *J Pharm Pharmacol* 2001; 53: 849–857.

7 Kraus GA, Bae J. Synthesis of *N*-(2-methylpropyl)-2*E*-undecene-8,10-diynamide, a novel constituent of *Echinacea angustifolia*. *Tetrahedron Lett* 2003; 44: 5505–5506.

8 Becker H *et al*. Structure of echinoside. *Z Naturforsch* 1982; 37c: 351–353.

9 Pietta P, Mauri P, Bauer R. MEKC analysis of different species. *Planta Med* 1998; 64: 649–652.

10 Wills RBH, Stuart DL. Alkylamide and cichoric acid levels in *Echinacea purpurea* grown in Australia. *Food Chem* 1999; 67: 385–388.

11 Nüsslein B *et al*. Enzymatic degradation of cichoric acid in *Echinacea purpurea* preparations. *J Nat Prod* 2000; 63: 1615–1618.

12 Proksch A, Wagner H. Structural analysis of a 4-O-methylgluconoarabinoxylan with immunostimulating activity from *Echinacea purpurea*. *Phytochemistry* 1987; 26: 1989–1993.

13 Wagner H *et al*. Immunostimulating action of polysaccharides (heteroglycans) from higher plants. *Arzneimittelforschung* 1985; 35: 1069–1075.

14 Bauer R. Echinacea – Pharmazeutische qualität und therapeutischer wert. *Z Phytother* 1997; 18: 207–214.

15 Blaschek W *et al*. Echinacea – Polysaccharide. *Z Phytother* 1998; 19: 255–262.

16 Classen B *et al*. Characterisation of an arabinogalactan-protein isolated from pressed juice of *Echinacea purpurea* by precipitation with the β-glucosyl Yariv reagent. *Carbohydrate Res* 2000; 327: 497–504.

17 Bauer R *et al*. TLC and HPLC analysis of *Echinacea pallida* and *E. angustifolia* root. *Planta Med* 1988; 54: 426–430.

18 Röder E *et al*. Pyrrolizidine in *Echinacea angustifolia* DC und *Echinacea purpurea* M. *Arzneimittelforschung* 1984; 124: 2316–2317.

19 Lin L *et al*. Patuetin-3-O-Rutinoside from the aerial parts of *Echinacea angustifolia*. *Pharm Biol* 2002; 40: 92–95.

20 Bauer R *et al*. New alkamides from *Echinacea angustifolia* and *E. purpurea* roots. *Planta Med* 1988; 563–564.

21 Glowniak K *et al*. Solid phase extraction and reversed-phase high-performance liquid chromatography of free phenolic acids in some *Echinacea* species. *J Chromatogr A* 1996; 730: 25–29.

22 Pugh N *et al*. Elusive immunostimulatory compound discovered in *Echinacea* and other immune enhancing botanicals. *International Congress on Natural Product Research*. Phoenix, Arizona, 2004: 44 [abstract].

23 Perry NB *et al*. Alkamide levels in *Echinacea purpurea*: a rapid analytical method revealing differences among roots, rhizomes, stems, leaves and flowers. *Planta Med* 1997; 63: 8–62.

24 Osowski S *et al*. Zur pharmazeutischen Vergleichbarkeit von therapeutisch verwendeten Echinacea-Präparaten. *Forsch Komplementärmed Klass Naturheilk* 2000; 7: 294–300.

25 ConsumerLab. Product review: Echinacea. [accessed September 23, 2003]

26 Gilroy CM *et al*. Echinacea and truth in labeling. *Arch Intern Med* 2003; 163: 699–704.

27 Tobler M *et al*. Characteristics of whole fresh plant extracts. *Schweiz Zschr GanzheitsMedizin* 1994; 6: 257–266.

28 Bauer R. Standardization of *Echinacea purpurea* expressed juice with reference to cichoric acid and alkalamides. *J Herbs Spices Med Plants* 1999; 6: 51–62.

29 Ganzera M *et al*. An improved method for the determination of betaine in *Echinacea* products. *Pharmazie* 2001; 56: 552–553.

30 Gray DE *et al*. Acute drought stress and plant age effects on alkalamide and phenolic acid content in purple coneflower roots. *Planta Med* 2003; 69: 50–55.

31 Kabganian R *et al*. Drying of *Echinacea angustifolia* roots. *J Herbs Spices Med Plants* 2002; 10: 11–19.

32 Perry NB *et al*. Alkamide levels in *Echinacea purpurea*: effects of processing, drying and storage. *Planta Med* 2000; 66: 54–56.

33 Livesey J *et al*. Effect of temperature on stability of marker constituents in *Echinacea purpurea* root formulations. *Phytomedicine* 1999; 6: 347–349.

34 Li TS, Wardle DA. Effects of root drying temperature and moisture content on the levels of active ingredients in *Echinacea* roots. *J Herbs Spices Med Plants* 2001; 8: 15–22.

35 Petty HR *et al*. Identification of colchicine in placental blood from patients using herbal medicines. *Chem Res Toxicol* 2001; 14: 1254–1258.

36 Li W *et al*. Evaluation of commercial ginkgo and echinacea dietary supplements for colchicine using liquid chromatography-tandem mass spectrometry. *Chem Res Toxicol* 2002; 15: 1174–1178.

37 Upton R (ed). *Echinacea purpurea* root. *Echinacea purpurea* (L.) Moench. Standards of analysis, quality control, and therapeutics. Scotts Valley: *American Herbal Pharmacopoeia and Therapeutic Compendium*, 2004.

38 Hobbs C. Echinacea. A literature review. *HerbalGram* 1994; 30 (Suppl): 33–47.

39 Matthias A *et al*. Echinacea – what constituents are therapeutically important? *International Congress on Natural Product Research*. Phoenix, Arizona, 2004: 43 [abstract].

40 Barrett B. Medicinal properties of *Echinacea*: a critical review. *Phytomedicine* 2003; 10: 66–86.

41 Bauer R *et al*. [Pressaft aus dem Kraut von *Echinacea purpurea*: ein allopathisches Phytoimmunstimulans]. *Wien med Wschr* 1999; 149: 185–189.

42 Schulte KE *et al*. Das Vorkommen von Polyacetylen-Verbindungen in *Echinacea purpurea* Mnch. und *Echinacea angustifolia* DC. *Arzneimittelforschung* 1967; 17: 825–829.

43 Bauer R *et al*. Immunologische *in-vivo* und *in-vitro* Untersuchungen mit Echinacea Extracten. *Arzneimittelforschung* 1988; 38: 276–281.

44 Vömel T. Der einfluss eines pflanzelischen Immunostimulans auf die Phagozytose von Erythozyten durch das retikulohistozytäre System der isoliert perfundierten Rattenleber. *Arzneimittelforschung* 1985; 35: 1437–1439.

45 Burger A *et al*. Echinacea-induced cytokine production by human macrophages. *Int J Immunopharmacol* 1997; 19: 371–379.

46 Stimpel M *et al.* Macrophage activation and induction of macrophage cytotoxicity by purified polysaccharide fractions from the plant *Echinacea purpurea*. *Infect Immun* 1984; 46: 845–849.
47 Luettig B *et al.* Macrophage activation by the polysaccharide arabinogalactan isolated from plant cell cultures of *Echinacea purpurea*. *J Natl Cancer Inst* 1989; 81: 669–675.
48 Wagner H *et al.* Immunologically active polysaccharides of *Echinacea purpurea* cell cultures. *Phytochemistry* 1988; 27: 119–126.
49 Rininger JA *et al.* Immunopharmacological activity of *Echinacea* preparations following simulated digestion on murine macrophages and human peripheral blood mononuclear cells. *J Leukoc Biol* 2000; 68: 503–510.
50 Di Carlo G *et al.* Modulation of apoptosis in mice treated with *Echinacea* and St John's wort. *Pharmacol Res* 2003; 48: 273–277.
51 See DM *et al. In vitro* effects of echinacea and ginseng on natural killer and antibody-dependent cell cytotoxicity in healthy subjects and chronic fatigue syndrome or acquired immunodeficiency syndrome patients. *Immunopharmacology* 1997; 35: 229–235.
52 Sun LZ-Y *et al.* The American coneflower: a prophylactic role involving nonspecific immunity. *J Altern Complement Med* 1999; 5: 437–446.
53 Currier NL, Miller SC. *Echinacea purpurea* and melatonin augment natural-killer cells in leukemic mice and prolong life span. *J Altern Complement Med* 2001; 7: 241–251.
54 Currier NL, Miller SC. Natural killer cells from aging mice treated with extracts from *Echinacea purpurea* are quantitatively and functionally rejuvenated. *Exp Gerontol* 2000; 35: 627–639.
55 Cundell DR *et al.* The effect of aerial parts of Echinacea on the circulating white cell levels and selected immune functions of the aging male Sprague-Dawley rat. *International Immunopharmacol* 2003; 3: 1041–1048.
56 Goel V *et al.* Echinacea stimulates macrophage function in the lung and spleen of normal rats. *J Nutr Biochem* 2002; 13: 487–492.
57 Goel V *et al.* Alkylamides of *Echinacea purpurea* stimulate alveolar macrophage function in normal rats. *Int Immunopharmacol* 2002; 2: 381–387.
58 Wagner H, Jurcic K. Immunological studies of Revitonil®, a phytopharmaceutical containing *Echinacea purpurea* and *Glycyrrhiza glabra* root extract. *Phytomedicine* 2002; 9: 390–397.
59 Bodinet C, Freudenstein J. Effects of an orally applied aqueous-ethanolic extract of a mixture of *Thujae occidentalis* herba, *Baptisiae tinctoriae* radix, *Echinaceae purpureae* radix and *Echinaceae pallidae* radix on antibody response against sheep red blood cells in mice. *Planta Med* 1999; 65: 695–699.
60 South EH, Exon JH. Multiple immune functions in rats fed echinacea extracts. *Immunopharmacol Immunotoxicol* 2001; 23: 411–421.
61 Gertsch J *et al.* Echinacea alkylamides modulate TNF-alpha gene expression via cannabinoid receptor CB2 and multiple signal transduction pathways. *FEBS Lett* 2004; 577: 563–569.
62 Bodinet C, Beuscher N. Antiviral and immunological activity of glycoproteins from *Echinacea purpurea* radix. *Planta Med* 1991; 57 (Suppl 2): A33–34.
63 Thompson KD. Antiviral activity of Viracea® against acyclovir susceptible and acyclovir resistant strains of herpes simplex virus. *Antiviral Res* 1998; 39: 55–61.
64 Binns SE *et al.* Antiviral activity of characterized extracts from *Echinacea* spp. (Heliantheae: Asteraceae) against herpes simplex virus (HSV-1). *Planta Med* 2002; 68: 780–783.
65 Wacker A, Hilbig W. Virus inhibition by *Echinacea purpurea*. *Planta Med* 1978; 33: 89–102.
66 Binns SE *et al.* Light-mediated antifungal activity of *Echinacea* extracts. *Planta Med* 2000; 66: 241–244.
67 Binns SE *et al.* A taxonomic revision of the genus Echinacea (Helianthae; Asteraceae). *Systematic Bot* 2002; 27: 610–632.
68 Merali S *et al.* Antifungal and anti-inflammatory activity of the genus *Echinacea*. *Pharmaceutical Biol* 2003; 41: 412–420.
69 Roesler J *et al.* Application of purified polysaccharides from cell cultures of the plant *Echinacea purpurea* to mice mediates protection against systemic infection with *Listeria monocytogenes* and *Candida albicans*. *Int J Immunopharmacol* 1991; 13: 27–37.
70 Steinmüller C *et al.* Polysaccharides isolated from plant cell cultures of *Echinacea purpurea* enhance the resistance of immunosuppressed mice against systemic infection with *Candida albicans* and *Listeria monocytogenes*. *Int J Immunopharmacol* 1993; 15: 605–614.
71 Westendorf J. Carito® – *in-vitro* Untersuchungen zum Nachweiss spasmolytischer und kontraktiler Einflüsse. *Therapiewoche* 1982; 32: 6291–6297.
72 Tubaro A *et al.* Anti-inflammatory activity of a polysaccharidic fraction of *Echinacea angustifolia*. *J Pharm Pharmacol* 1987; 39: 567–569.
73 Tragni E *et al.* Evidence from two classical irritation tests for an anti-inflammatory action of a natural extract, echinacea B. *Food Chem Toxicol* 1985; 23: 317–319.
74 Tragni E *et al.* Anti-inflammatory activity of *Echinacea angustifolia* fractions separated on the basis of molecular weight. *Pharmacol Res Commun* 1988; 20(Suppl V): 87–90.
75 Mattace Raso G *et al.* In-vivo and in-vitro anti-inflammatory effect of *Echinacea purpurea* and *Hypericum perforatum*. *J Pharm Pharmacol* 2002; 54: 1379–1383.
76 Clifford LJ *et al.* Bioactivity of alkamides isolated from *Echinacea purpurea* (L.) Moench. *Phytomedicine* 2002; 9: 249–253.
77 Müller-Jakic B *et al. In vitro* inhibition of cyclooxygenase and 5-lipoxygenase by alkamides from *Echinacea* and *Achillea* species. *Planta Med* 1994; 60: 37–40.
78 Speroni E *et al.* Anti-inflammatory activity and cicatrizing activity of *Echinacea pallida* Nutt. root extract. *J Ethnopharmacol* 2002; 79: 265–272.
79 Busing K. Hyaluronidasehemmung durch echinacin. *Arzneimittelforschung* 1952; 2: 467–469.
80 Zoutewelle G, van Wijk R. Effects of *Echinacea purpurea* extracts on fibroblast populated collagen lattice contraction. *Phytother Res* 1990; 4: 77–81.
81 Facino RM *et al.* Echinacoside and caffeoyl conjugates protect collagen from free radical-induced degradation: a potential use of *Echinacea* extracts in the prevention of skin photodamage. *Planta Med* 1995; 61: 510–514.
82 Voaden DJ, Jacobson M. Tumour inhibitors. 3. Identification and synthesis of an oncolytic hydrocarbon from American coneflower roots. *J Med Chem* 1972; 15: 619–623.
83 Jager H *et al.* Transport of alkamides from *Echinacea* species through Caco-2 monolayers. *Planta Med* 2002; 68: 469–471.
84 Matthias A *et al.* Permeability studies of alkylamides and caffeic acid conjugates from Echinacea using a Caco-2 cell monolayer model. *J Clin Pharm Ther* 2004; 29: 7–13.
85 Dietz B *et al.* Absorption of dodeca-2E,4E,8Z,10E/Z-tetraenoic acid isobutylamides after oral application of *Echinacea purpurea* tincture. *Planta Med* 2001; 67: 863–864.
86 Matthias A *et al.* Bioavailability and pharmacokinetics of alkylamides from Echinacea. *International Congress on Natural Product Research*. Phoenix, Arizona, 2004: p57, p133 [abstract].
87 Wölkart K *et al.* Pharmacokinetics and bioavailability of alkamides from the roots of *Echinacea angustifolia* in humans after oral application. *International Congress on Natural Product Research*. Phoenix, Arizona, 2004: 44 [abstract].
88 Melchart D *et al.* Immunomodulation with *Echinacea* – a systematic review of controlled clinical trials. *Phytomedicine* 1994; 1: 245–254.
89 Melchart D *et al.* Results of five randomized studies on the immunomodulatory activity of preparations of echinacea. *J Altern Complement Med* 1995; 1: 145–160.
90 Kim LS *et al.* Immunological activity of larch arabinogalactan and *Echinacea*: a preliminary, randomized, double-blind, placebo-controlled trial. *Altern Med Rev* 2002; 7: 138–149.
91 Berg A *et al.* Influence of Echinacin (EC31) treatment on the exercise-induced immune response in athletes. *J Drug Assessment* 1998; 1: 625–638.
92 Roesler J *et al.* Application of purified polysaccharides from cell cultures of the plant *Echinacea purpurea* to test subjects mediates activation of the phagocyte system. *Int J Immunopharmacol* 1991; 13: 931–941.
93 Schwarz E *et al.* Oral administration of freshly expressed juice of *Echinacea purpurea* herb fail to stimulate the nonspecific immune response in healthy young men: results of a double-blind, placebo-controlled crossover study. *J Immunother* 2002; 25: 413–420.

E

94 Elsässer-Beile U *et al*. Cytokine production in leukocyte cultures during therapy with echinacea extract. *J Clin Lab Anal* 1996; 10: 441–445.
95 Lersch C *et al*. Nonspecific immunostimulation with low doses of cyclophosphamide (LDCY), thymostimulin, and *Echinacea purpurea* extracts (Echinacin) in patients with far advanced colorectal cancers: preliminary results. *Cancer Invest* 1992; 10: 343–348.
96 Melchart D *et al*. Polysaccharides isolated from *Echinacea purpurea* herba cell cultures to counteract undesired effects of chemotherapy – a pilot study. *Phytother Res* 2002; 16: 138–142.
97 Melchart D *et al*. Echinacea for preventing and treating the common cold (Cochrane review). In: *The Cochrane Library*, Issue 3, 2003. Oxford: Update Software.
98 Linde K *et al*. Echinacea for preventing and treating the common cold (Review). Cochrane Database of Systematic Reviews 2006, Issue 1. Art. No.: CD000530.
99 Melchart D *et al*. Echinacea root extracts for the prevention of upper respiratory tract infections. A double-blind, placebo-controlled, randomized trial. *Arch Fam Med* 1998; 7: 541–545.
100 Grimm W, Müller H-H. A randomized controlled trial of the effect of fluid extract of *Echinacea purpurea* on the incidence and severity of colds and respiratory infections. *Am J Med* 1999; 106: 138–143.
101 Turner RB *et al*. Ineffectiveness of echinacea for prevention of experimental rhinovirus colds. *Antimicrob Agents Chemother* 2000; 44: 1708–1709.
102 Sperber SJ *et al*. *Echinacea purpurea* for prevention of experimental rhinovirus colds. *Clin Infect Dis* 2004; 38: 1367–1371.
103 Turner RB *et al*. An evaluation of *Echinacea angustifolia* in experimental rhinovirus infection. *N Engl J Med* 2005; 353: 341–348.
104 Cohen HA *et al*. Effectiveness of an herbal preparation containing Echinacea, propolis, and vitamin C in preventing respiratory tract infections in children. A randomized, double-blind, placebo-controlled, multicenter study. *Arch Pediatr Adolesc Med* 2004; 158: 217–221.
105 Christakis DA, Lehmann HP. Can an herbal preparation of echinacea, propolis, and vitamin C reduce respiratory illnesses in children? *Arch Pediatr Adolesc Med* 2004; 158: 222–224.
106 Barrett BP *et al*. Treatment of the common cold with unrefined echinacea. A randomized, double-blind, placebo-controlled trial. *Ann Intern Med* 2002; 137: 939–946.
107 Brinkeborn RM *et al*. Echinaforce® and other *Echinacea* fresh plant preparations in the treatment of the common cold. A randomized, placebo-controlled, double-blind clinical trial. *Phytomedicine* 1999; 6: 1–5.
108 Schulten B *et al*. Efficacy of *Echinacea purpurea* in patients with a common cold. A placebo-controlled, randomised, double-blind clinical trial. *Arzneimittelforschung* 2001; 51: 563–568.
109 Lindenmuth GF, Lindenmuth EB. The efficacy of echinacea compound herbal tea preparation on the severity and duration of upper respiratory and flu symptoms: a randomized, double-blind, placebo-controlled study. *J Altern Complement Med* 2000; 6: 327–334.
110 Yale SH, Liu K. Echinacea purpurea therapy for the treatment of the common cold: a randomized, double-blind, placebo-controlled clinical trial. *Arch Intern Med* 2004; 164: 1237–1241.
111 Goel V *et al*. Efficacy of a standardized echinacea preparation (Echinilin) for the treatment of the common cold: a randomized, double-blind, placebo-controlled trial. *J Clin Pharm Ther* 2004; 29: 75–83.
112 Taylor JA *et al*. Efficacy and safety of Echinacea in treating upper respiratory tract infections in children. A randomized controlled trial. *JAMA* 2003; 290: 2824–2830.
113 Spasov AA *et al*. Comparative controlled study of Andrographis paniculata fixed combination, Kan Jang® and an Echinacea preparation as adjuvant in the treatment of uncomplicated respiratory disease in children. *Phytother Res* 2004; 18: 47–53.
114 Firenzuoli F, Gori L. Echinacea for treating colds in children [letter]. *JAMA* 2004; 291: 1323–1324.
115 Taylor JA *et al*. Echinacea for treating colds in children [letter]. *JAMA* 2004; 291: 1324.
116 Vonau B *et al*. Does the extract of the plant *Echinacea purpurea* influence the clinical course of recurrent genital herpes? *Int J STD AIDS* 2001; 12: 154–158.
117 Parnham MJ. Benefit-risk assessment of the squeezed sap of the purple coneflower (*Echinacea purpurea*) for long-term oral immunostimulation. *Phytomedicine* 1996; 3: 95–102.
118 Barnes J. Herbal therapeutics (7). Colds. *Pharm J* 2002; 269: 716–718.
119 Barnes J *et al*. Different standards for reporting ADRs to herbal remedies and conventional OTC medicines: face-to-face interviews with 515 users of herbal remedies. *Br J Clin Pharmacol* 1998; 45: 496–500.
120 Barnes J *et al*. Echinacea species (*Echinacea angustifolia* (DC.) Hell., *Echinacea pallida* (Nutt.) Nutt., *Echinacea purpurea* (L.) Moench): a review of their chemistry, pharmacology and clinical properties. *J Pharm Pharmacol* 2005; 57: 929–954.
121 Vigibase, WHO Adverse Reactions database, Uppsala Monitoring Centre [accessed 3 February 2005].
122 Mullins RJ, Heddle R. Adverse reactions associated with echinacea: the Australian experience. *Ann Allergy Asthma Immunol* 2002; 88: 42–51.
123 Mullins RJ. Echinacea-associated anaphylaxis. *Med J Aust* 1998; 168: 170–171.
124 Myers SP, Wohlmuth H. Echinacea-associated anaphylaxis. *Med J Aust* 1998; 168: 583.
125 Soon SL, Crawford RI. Recurrent erythema nodosum associated with echinacea herbal therapy. *J Am Acad Dermatol* 2001; 44: 298–299.
126 Logan JL, Ahmed J. Critical hypokalemic renal tubular acidosis due to Sjögren's syndrome: association with the purported immune stimulant echinacea. *Clin Rheumatol* 2003; 22: 158–159.
127 Schwarz S *et al*. Acute disseminated encephalomyelitis after parenteral therapy with herbal extracts: a report of two cases. *J Neurol Neurosurg Psychiatry* 2000; 69: 516–518.
128 Kayne SB. *Homoeopathic Pharmacy. An Introduction and Handbook*. Edinburgh: Churchill Livingstone, 1997.
129 Lee AN, Werth VP. Activation of autoimmunity following use of immunostimulatory herbal supplements. *Arch Dermatol* 2004; 140: 723–727.
130 Lenk M. Akute Toxizität von verschieden Polysacchariden aus *Echinacea purpurea* an der Maus. *Z Phytother* 1989; 10: 49–51.
131 Mengs U *et al*. Toxicity studies with Echinacin [abstract presented at Third International Conference on Phytomedicine, Munich Germany, October 2000]. *Phytomedicine* 2000; 2(Suppl): 32.
132 Mengs U *et al*. Toxicity of *Echinacea purpurea*. Acute, subacute and genotoxicity studies. *Arzneimittel Forschung* 1991; 41: 1076–1081.
133 Ondrizek RR *et al*. An alternative medicine study of herbal effects on the penetration of zona-free hamster oocytes and the integrity of sperm deoxyribonucleic acid. *Fertil Steril* 1999; 71: 517–522.
134 Ondrizek RR *et al*. Inhibition of human sperm motility by specific herbs used in alternative medicine. *J Assist Reprod Genet* 1999; 16: 87–91.
135 Gorski JC *et al*. The effect of Echinacea (*Echinacea purpurea* root) on cytochrome P450 activity in vivo. *Clin Pharmacol Ther* 2004; 75: 89–100.
136 Gurley BJ *et al*. In vivo assessment of botanical supplementation on human cytochrome P450 phenotypes: *Citrus aurantium*, *Echinacea purpurea*, milk thistle, and saw palmetto. *Clin Pharmacol Ther* 2004; 76: 428–440.
137 Budzinski JW *et al*. An *in vitro* evaluation of human cytochrome P450 3A4 inhibition by selected commercial herbal extracts and tinctures. *Phytomedicine* 2000; 7: 273–282.
138 Currier NL *et al*. Deleterious effects of *Echinacea purpurea* and melatonin on myeloid cells in mouse spleen and bone marrow. *J Leukoc Biol* 2001; 70: 274–276.
139 Gallo M *et al*. Pregnancy outcome following gestational exposure to echinacea: a prospective controlled study. *Arch Intern Med* 2000; 160: 3141–3143.

Elder

Summary and Pharmaceutical Comment

Phytochemical details have been documented for elder, with flavonoids and triterpenes representing the main biologically active constituents. Anti-inflammatory, antiviral and diuretic effects have been observed in *in vivo* studies, thus supporting the herbal uses of elder. No documented studies in humans were found. Potentially toxic compounds have been reported for the bark (lectins) and the leaves (cyanogenetic glycosides); the flowers are suitable for use as a herbal remedy.

Species (Family)

Sambucus nigra L. (Caprifoliaceae)

Synonym(s)

Black Elder, European Elder, Sambucus
Sambucus canadensis L. refers to American Elder

Part(s) Used

Flower

Pharmacopoeial and Other Monographs

BHC 1992[(G6)]
BHP 1996[(G9)]
BP 2007[(G84)]
Complete German Commission E[(G3)]
Martindale 35th edition[(G85)]
Ph Eur 2007[(G81)]

Legal Category (Licensed Products)

GSL[(G37)]

Constituents

The following is compiled from several sources, including General References G6, G41, G62 and G75.

Flavonoids Flavonols (kaempferol, quercetin), quercetin glycosides (1.5–3.0%) including hyperoside, isoquercitrin and rutin.

Triterpenes α- and β-amyrin, oleanolic and ursolic acids.

Volatile oils 0.3%. 66% fatty acids (primarily linoleic, linolenic and palmitic) and 7% alkanes (C_{19}, C_{21}, C_{23} and C_{25}). Numerous other constituent types have been identified including ethers and oxides, ketones, aldehydes, alcohols and esters.[(1)]

Other constituents Chlorogenic acid, tannin, mucilage, plastocynin (protein),[(2)] pectin and sugar.

Other plant parts Leaf Sambunigrin (0.042%), prunasin, zierin and holocalin (cyanogenetic glycosides),[(3)] choline, flavonoids (rutin, quercetin), sterols (sitosterol, stigmasterol, campesterol), triterpenes (α- and β-amyrin palmitates, oleanolic and ursolic acids), alkanes, fatty acids, tannins and others.[(G41)]

Bark Lectin (mol. wt 140 000) rich in asparagine/aspartic acid, glutamine/glutamic acid, valine and leucine,[(4)] phytohaemagglutinin,[(5)] triterpenoids (α-amyrenone, α-amyrin, betulin, oleanolic acid, β-sito sterol).[(6)]

Food Use

Elder is listed by the Council of Europe as a source of natural food flavouring (categories N1 and N2). Category N1 refers to the fruit and indicates that there are no restrictions on quantities used. Category N2 refers to the restrictions on the concentrations of hydrocyanic acid that are permitted, namely 1 mg/kg in beverages and foods, 1 mg/kg for every per cent proof of alcoholic beverages, 5 mg/kg in stone fruit juices, 25 mg/kg in confectionery and 50 mg/kg in marzipan.[(G16)] Previously, the flowers have had a regulatory status of GRAS (Generally Recognised As Safe).[(G41)]

Herbal Use

Elder is stated to possess diaphoretic and anticatarrhal properties. Traditionally, it has been used for influenza, colds, chronic nasal catarrh with deafness and sinusitis.[(G8)] Elder is also stated to act as a diuretic, laxative and local anti-inflammatory agent.[(G2, G6–8, G41, G49, G64)]

Dosage

Dosages for oral administration (adults) for traditional uses recommended in standard herbal reference texts are given below.

Dried flower 2–4 g by infusion three times daily.[(G6, G7)]

Liquid extract 2–4 mL (1 : 1 in 25% alcohol) three times daily.[(G6, G7)]

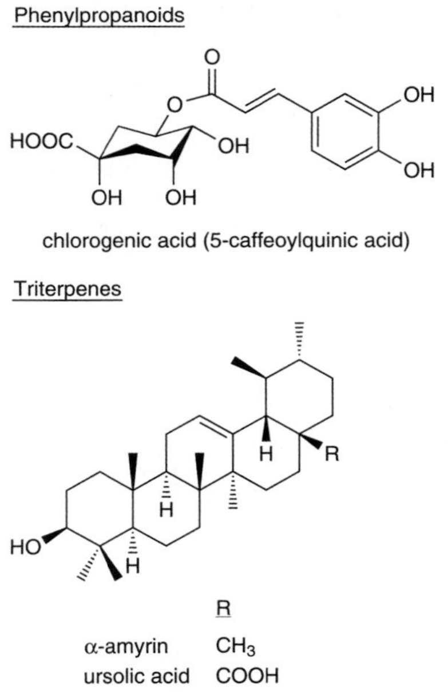

Phenylpropanoids

HOOC, O, OH, OH, OH, OH

chlorogenic acid (5-caffeoylquinic acid)

Triterpenes

	R
α-amyrin	CH_3
ursolic acid	COOH

Figure 1 Selected constituents of elder.

E

Pharmacological Actions

In vitro and animal studies

Elder is stated to possess diuretic and laxative properties.[G41]

Moderate (27%) anti-inflammatory action in carrageenan-induced rat paw oedema has been documented for an elder preparation given one hour before carrageenan (100 mg/kg, by mouth).[7] Indometacin as a control exhibited 45% inhibition at a dose of 5 mg/kg.[7]

An infusion made from the flowers of elder, St John's wort herb and root of soapwort (*Saponaria officinalis*) has exhibited antiviral activity against influenza types A and B (*in vivo* and *in vitro*) and herpes simplex virus type 1 (*in vitro*).[8]

A diuretic effect in rats exceeding that exerted by theophylline has been reported for elder.[9] An infusion and extracts rich in potassium and in flavonoids all caused diuresis. Greatest activity was exerted by the combined potassium- and flavonoid-rich extracts.

In vitro antispasmodic activity (rat ileum, rabbit/guinea-pig intestine) and spasmogenic activity (rat uterus) have been reported for lectins isolated from elder.[10]

A lectin isolated from elder bark was found to be a lactose-specific haemagglutinin with a slightly higher affinity for erythrocytes from blood group A.[4] Unlike many other plant lectins, the lectin did not inhibit protein synthesis.[4] The carbohydrate-binding properties of a lectin isolated from elder bark have been studied.[11]

Phytohaemagglutinins are biologically active extracts isolated from various plants and represent a class of lectin. They are associated with haemagglutination and mitogenic, antigenic and immunosuppressant properties.[5] *In vitro*, phytohaemagglutinin has been found to stimulate production of an interferon-like substance in human leukocytes.[G45]

Hepatoprotective activity against carbon tetrachloride-induced toxicity has been reported for triterpenes isolated from *Sambucus formosana* Nakai.[12]

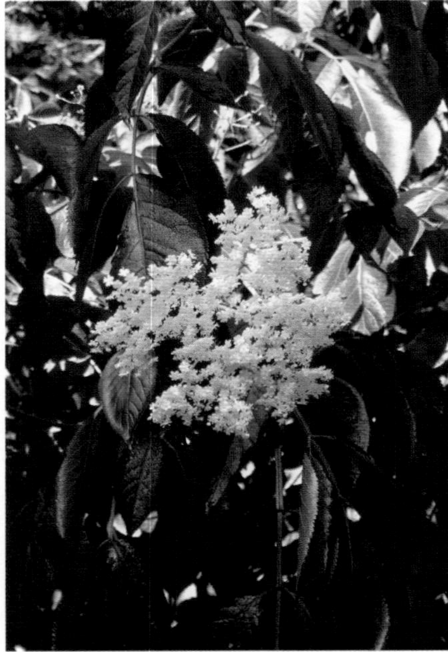

Figure 2 Elder (*Sambucus nigra*).

Clinical studies

There is a lack of clinical research assessing the effects of elder and rigorous randomised controlled clinical trials are required. Phytohaemagglutinin extracts have been used clinically to treat drug-induced leucopenia and some types of anaemia.[5] The blastogenic response of lymphocytes to phytohaemagglutinin has been used extensively as a measure of immunocompetence.[G45]

Side-effects, Toxicity

No reported side-effects specifically for elder were located. However, there is a lack of clinical safety and toxicity data for elder and further investigation of these aspects is required. Human poisoning has occurred with *Sambucus* species.[13] The roots, stems and leaves and, much less so, the flowers and unripe berries, are stated to contain a poisonous alkaloid and cyanogenic glycoside causing nausea, vomiting and diarrhoea.[13] The flowers and ripe fruit are stated to be edible without harm.[13]

The effects of a lectin isolated from elder bark on mammalian embryonic and fetal development has been studied.[5] The lectin exerted mainly a toxic effect and, to a lesser degree, a teratogenic effect when administered subcutaneously to pregnant mice. In view of the high doses administered, the authors stated that the results did not indicate a potential hazard to human fetuses exposed to lectins.[5]

Contra-indications, Warnings

Plant parts other than the flowers are reported to be poisonous and should not be ingested. There is limited evidence from preclinical studies that elder has a diuretic effect; the clinical relevance of this, if any, is unclear.

Drug interactions None documented. However, the potential for preparations of elder to interact with other medicines administered concurrently, particularly those with similar or opposing effects, should be considered.

Pregnancy and lactation The safety of elder taken during pregnancy has not been established. In view of the lack of toxicity data, the use of elder during pregnancy and lactation should be avoided.

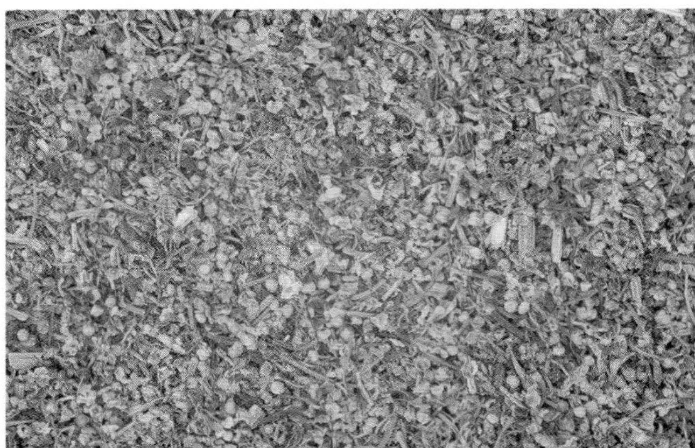

Figure 3 Elder – dried drug substance (flower).

Preparations

Proprietary single-ingredient preparations

Czech Republic: Caj z Kvetu Bezu Cerneho; Kvet Bazy Ciernej. *Russia:* Novo-Passit (Ново-Пассит).

Proprietary multi-ingredient preparations

Australia: Sambucus Complex. *Austria:* Entschlackender Abfuhrtee EF-EM-ES; Grippetee St Severin; Krauter Hustensaft; Laxalpin; Sinupret; Tuscalman. *Canada:* Original Herb Cough Drops. *Czech Republic:* Biotussil; Cajova Smes pri Nachlazeni; Detsky Caj s Hermankem; Erkaltungstee; Novo-Passit; Perospir; Pulmoran; Reduktan; Sinupret; Species Urologicae Planta; Urcyston Planta. *Germany:* Sinupret; Solvopret. *Hong Kong:* Sinupret. *Hungary:* Sinupret. *Russia:* Sinupret (Синупрет). *Singapore:* Sinupret. *Spain:* Natusor Gripotul; Natusor Sinulan. *Switzerland:* Sinupret; Tisane contre les refroidissements. *Thailand:* Sinupret. *UK:* Cleansing Herbs; EP&C Essence; Hay Fever & Sinus Relief; Hayfever & Sinus Relief; Herb and Honey Cough Elixir; Life Drops; Lion Cleansing Herbs; Lustys Herbalene; Modern Herbals Cold & Catarrh; Sinotar; Summertime Tea Blend; Tabritis; Tabritis Tablets. *USA:* Liquid Elderberry with Ester-C.

References

1 Toulemonde B, Richard HMJ. Volatile constituents of dry elder (*Sambucus nigra* L.) flowers. *J Agric Food Chem* 1983; 31: 365–370.

2 Scawen MD *et al.* The amino-acid sequence of plastocyanin from *Sambucus nigra* L. (elder). *Eur J Biochem* 1974; 44: 299–303.

3 Jensen SR, Nielsen BJ. Cyanogenic glucosides in *Sambucus nigra* L. *Acta Chem Scand* 1973; 27: 2661–2685.

4 Broekaert WF *et al.* A lectin from elder (*Sambucus nigra* L.) bark. *Biochem J* 1984; 221: 163–169.

5 Paulo E. Effect of phytohaemagglutinin (PHA) from the bark of *Sambucus nigra* on embryonic and foetal development in mice. *Folia Biol (Kraków)* 1976; 24: 213–222.

6 Lawrie W *et al.* Triterpenoids in the bark of elder (*Sambucus nigra*). *Phytochemistry* 1964; 3: 267–268.

7 Mascolo N *et al.* Biological screening of Italian medicinal plants for anti-inflammatory activity. *Phytother Res* 1987; 1: 28.

8 Serkedjieva J *et al.* Antiviral activity of the infusion (SHS-174) from flowers of *Sambucus nigra* L., aerial parts of *Hypericum perforatum* L., and roots of *Saponaria officinalis* L. against influenza and herpes simplex viruses. *Phytother Res* 1990; 4: 97.

9 Rebuelta M *et al.* Étude de l'effet diurétique de différentes préparations des fleurs du *Sambucus nigra* L. *Plant Méd Phytothér* 1983; 17: 173–181.

10 Richter A. Changes in the motor activity of smooth muscles of the rat uterus *in vitro* as the effect of phytohaemagglutinins from *Sambucus nigra*. *Folia Biol* 1973; 21: 33–48.

11 Shibuya N *et al.* The elderberry (*Sambucus nigra* L.) bark lectin recognizes the Neu5Ac(α2–6)Gal/GalNAc sequence. *J Biol Chem* 1987; 262: 1596–1601.

12 Lin C-N, Tome W-P. Antihepatotoxic principles of *Sambucus formosana*. *Planta Med* 1988; 54: 223–224.

13 Hardin JW, Arena JM, eds. *Human Poisoning from Native and Cultivated Plants*, 2nd edn. North Carolina: Duke University Press, 1974.

Elecampane

Summary and Pharmaceutical Comment

The pharmacological actions documented for elecampane seem to be attributable to the sesquiterpene lactone constituents, in particular alantolactone and isoalantolactone. The demulcent action of mucilage and reported *in vivo* antispasmodic activity of the volatile oil support the traditional uses of this remedy in coughs. In addition, alantolactone has been utilised as an anthelmintic. A number of interesting cardiovascular activities have been documented for a related species, *I. racemosa*. Whether the constituents responsible for these actions are also present in elecampane is unclear. In view of the paucity of toxicity data for elecampane, excessive or prolonged use should be avoided.

Species (Family)

Inula helenium L. (Asteraceae/Compositae)

Synonym(s)

Alant, Horseheal, Inula, Scabwort, Tu Mu Xiang, Yellow Starwort

An elecampane extract has been referred to as helenin. Alantolactone is also known as elecampane camphor, alant camphor, helenin and inula camphor.[G45]

Part(s) Used

Rhizome, root

Pharmacopoeial and Other Monographs

BHC 1992[G6]
BHP 1996[G9]
Martindale 35th edition[G85]

Legal Category (Licensed Products)

GSL[G37]

Constituents

The following is compiled from several sources, including General References G2, G6 and G75.

Carbohydrates Inulin (up to 44%), mucilage.

Terpenoids β- and γ-sitosterols, stigmasterol and damaradienol (sterols), friedelin.

Volatile oils 1–4%. Mainly contains sesquiterpene lactones including alantolactone, isoalantolactone and dihydroalantolactone (eudesmanolides), alantic acid and azulene.

Other constituents Resin.

Food Use

Elecampane is listed by the Council of Europe as a natural source of food flavouring (category N2). This category indicates that elecampane can be added to foodstuffs in small quantities, with a possible limitation of an active principle (as yet unspecified) in the final product.[G16]

Previously in the USA, elecampane was only approved for use in alcoholic beverages.[G41]

Herbal Use

Elecampane is stated to possess expectorant, antitussive, diaphoretic and bactericidal properties. Traditionally, it has been used for bronchial/tracheal catarrh, cough associated with pulmonary tuberculosis and dry irritating cough in children.[G2, G6, G7, G8, G64]

Alantolactone has been used as an anthelmintic in the treatment of roundworm, threadworm, hookworm and whipworm infection.[G44, G45]

Dosage

Dosages for oral administration (adults) for traditional uses recommended in standard herbal reference texts are given below.

Rhizome/root 1.5–4.0 g as a decoction three times daily.[G6, G7]

Liquid extract 1.5–4.0 mL (1 : 1 in 25% alcohol) three times daily.[G6, G7]

Pharmacological Actions

In vitro and animal studies

Elecampane infusion has exhibited a pronounced sedative effect in mice.[G41] Alantolactone has been reported to exhibit hypotensive, hyperglycaemic (large doses) and hypoglycaemic (smaller doses) actions in animals.[G41] Antibacterial properties have also been documented. Alantolactone and isoalantolactone have been reported to exhibit high bactericidal and fungicidal properties *in vitro*.[G41]

The volatile oil has been reported to exert a potent smooth muscle relaxant effect *in vitro* on guinea-pig ileal and tracheal muscle.[1]

Various activities have been documented for *Inula racemosa*: an extract lowered plasma insulin and glucose concentrations in rats 75 minutes after oral administration,[2] counteracted adrenaline-induced hyperglycaemia in rats,[2] exhibited negative inotropic and chronotropic effects on the frog heart,[2] and provided a preventative and curative action against experimentally induced myocardial infarction in rats.[3] Pretreatment was found to be most effective.[3]

Sesquiterpene lactones with antitumour activity have been isolated from *Helenium microcephalum*.[4, 5]

Clinical studies

There is a lack of rigorous clinical research assessing the effects of elecampane and rigorous randomised controlled clinical trials are required.

Alantolactone has been used as an anthelmintic in the treatment of roundworm, threadworm, hookworm and whipworm infection.[G44, G45]

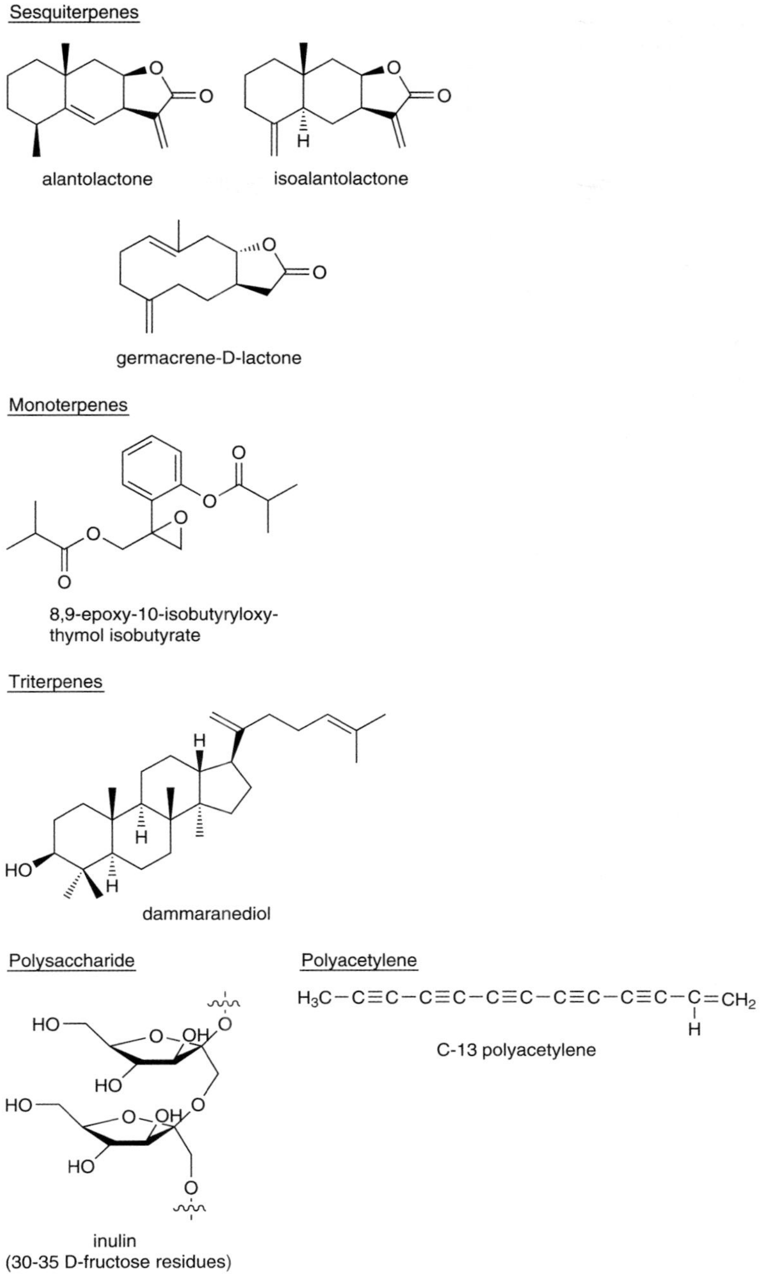

Sesquiterpenes

alantolactone

isoalantolactone

germacrene-D-lactone

Monoterpenes

8,9-epoxy-10-isobutyryloxy-thymol isobutyrate

Triterpenes

dammaranediol

Polysaccharide

inulin (30-35 D-fructose residues)

Polyacetylene

$H_3C-C\equiv C-C\equiv C-C\equiv C-C\equiv C-C\equiv C-CH=CH_2$

C-13 polyacetylene

Figure 1 Selected constituents of elecampane.

Inula racemosa has been reported to prevent ST-segment depression and T-wave inversion in patients with proven ischaemic heart disease,[(2)] and to have a beneficial effect on angina pectoris.[(6)]

Side-effects, Toxicity

There is a lack of clinical safety and toxicity data for elecampane and further investigation of these aspects is required.

Elecampane has been reported to cause allergic contact dermatitis.[(G51)] Sensitising properties have been documented for the volatile oil,[(G51, G58)] and for alantolactone and isoalantolactone.[(7)] *In vitro* cytotoxicty has been reported for alantolactone and isoalantolactone.[(8)]

Contraindications, Warnings

Elecampane may cause an allergic reaction, particularly in individuals with an existing allergy or sensitivity to other plants in the Asteraceae family.

Drug interactions None documented. However, the potential for preparations of elecampane to interact with other medicines administered concurrently, particularly those with similar or opposing effects, should be considered. There is limited evidence from preclinical studies that alantolactone, a constituent of elecampane, has hypotensive and hypo- and hyperglycaemic activities.

E

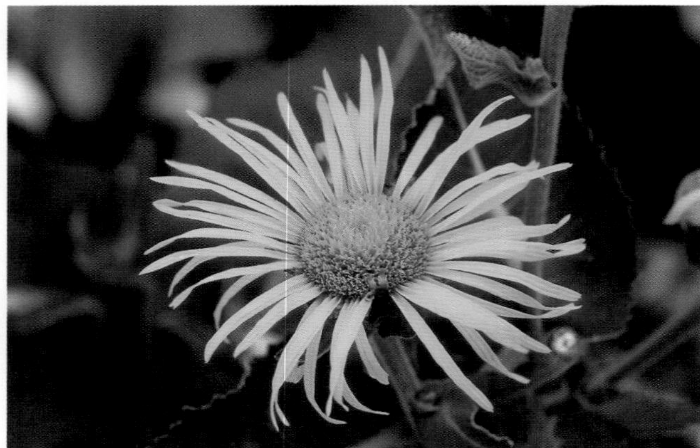

Figure 2 Elecampane (*Inula helenium*).

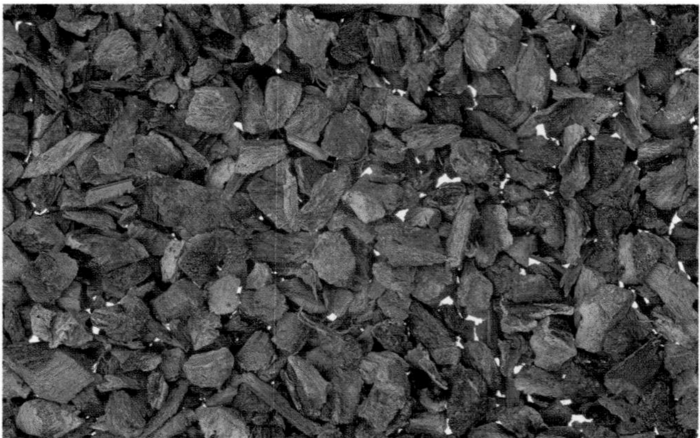

Figure 3 Elecampane – dried drug substance (rhizome).

Pregnancy and lactation The safety of elecampane taken during pregnancy has not been established. In view of the lack of toxicity data, the use of elecampane during pregnancy and lactation should be avoided.

Preparations

Proprietary multi-ingredient preparations

Austria: Brust- und Hustentee St Severin. *Czech Republic:* Species Cholagogae Planta. *France:* Mediflor Tisane Digestive No 3; Mediflor Tisane Hepatique No 5. *Germany:* Klosterfrau Melisana. *Russia:* Original Grosser Bittner Balsam (Оригинальный Большой Бальзам Биттнера). *South Africa:* Wonderkroonessens. *Spain:* Bronpul; Natusor Asmaten; Natusor Broncopul. *Switzerland:* Hederix; Padmed Laxan. *UK:* Catarrh-eeze; Cough-eeze; Horehound and Aniseed Cough Mixture; Vegetable Cough Remover.

References

1 Reiter M, Brandt W. Relaxant effects on tracheal and ileal smooth muscles of the guinea pig. *Arzneimittelforschung* 1985; 35: 408–414.
2 Tripathi YB *et al*. Assessment of the adrenergic beta-blocking activity of *Inula racemosa*. *J Ethno pharmacol* 1988; 23: 3–9.
3 Patel V *et al*. Effect of indigenous drug (puskarmula) on experimentally induced myocardial infarction in rats. *Act Nerv Super (Praha)* 1982; (Suppl 3): 387–394.
4 Sims D *et al*. Antitumor agents 37. The isolation and structural elucidation of isohelenol, a new antileukemic sesquiterpene lactone, and isohelenalin from *Helenium microcephalum*. *J Nat Prod* 1979; 42: 282–286.
5 Imakura Y *et al*. Antitumor agents XXXVI: Structural elucidation of sesquiterpene lactones microhelenins-A, B, and C, microlenin acetate, and plenolin from *Helenium microcephalum*. *J Pharm Sci* 1980; 69: 1044–1049.
6 Tripathi SN *et al*. Beneficial effect of *Inula racemosa* (pushkarmoola) in angina pectoris: a preliminary report. *Indian J Physiol Pharmacol* 1984; 28: 73–75.
7 Stampf JL *et al*. The sensitising capacity of helenin and two of its main constituents the sesquiterpene lactones alantolactone and isoalantolactone: a comparison of epicutaneous and intradermal sensitising methods in different strains of guinea pig. *Contact Dermatitis* 1982; 8: 16–24.
8 Woerdenbag HJ. In vitro cytotoxicity of sesquiterpene lactones from *Eupatorium cannabinum* L. and semi-synthetic derivatives from eupatoriopicrin. *Phytother Res* 1988; 2: 109–114.

Ephedra

Summary and Pharmaceutical Comment

The activities of ephedra are due to the presence of the ephedra alkaloids; of these, the pharmacological effects of ephedrine and pseudoephedrine are most well-documented and support their modern uses. There is less information on the pharmacological effects of ephedra extracts and clinical trials, in particular, are generally lacking.

In view of the safety concerns regarding the use of ephedra products, individuals wishing to use these products should be advised to consult an appropriately trained health care professional. Pharmacists and other health care professionals should be aware that ephedra may be included in unlicensed herbal products and food supplements under the name Ma Huang. Such products will not include reference to ephedra in the labelling.

Species (Family)

**Ephedra sinica* Stapf (Ephedraceae)
†*E. equisetina* Bunge
‡*E. intermedia* Shrenk ex Meyer
§*E. gerardiana* Wallich ex Meyer
||*E. major* Host

Synonym(s)

*Cao Ma Huang, *E. mahuang* Liu
†*E. shennungiana* Tang
‡Zhong Ma Huang
§*E. gerardiana* var. *congesta* C.Y. Cheng, Shan Ling Ma Huang
||*E. scoparia* Lange, *E. nebrodensis* Tineo ex Guss

Ephedra (and some other herbs) has also been referred to as 'herbal ecstasy'.

Part(s) Used

Aerial parts

Pharmacopoeial and Other Monographs

Complete German Commission E[G3]
Martindale 35th edition[G85]
WHO volume 1 1999[G63]

Legal Category (Licensed Products)

Ephedra is not included in the GSL.[G37]

Ephedra is included in Parts II and III of SI 2130.[1] This allows supply of ephedra (maximum dose of 600 mg and a maximum daily dose of 1800 mg) following a one-to-one consultation with a practitioner.

Ephedrine and pseudoephedrine are not included on the GSL. Both are prescription-only medicines (POM), but can be supplied through pharmacies at certain permitted doses, as follows. Ephedrine for internal preparations: maximum dose 30 mg, maximum daily dose 60 mg; nasal preparations, ephedrine 2%. Pseudoephedrine hydrochloride for internal preparations: maximum dose 60 mg, maximum daily dose 240 mg; prolonged-release preparations: maximum dose 120 mg, maximum daily dose 240 mg. Pseudoephredine sulfate for internal preparations: maximum dose 60 mg, maximum daily dose 180 mg.

E

Constituents

Alkaloids 0.5–2.0%. Mainly (−)-ephedrine (30–90% in most species, except *E. intermedia*) and (+)-pseudoephedrine, also (−)-norephedrine, (+)-nor pseudoephedrine, (−)-methylephedrine and (+)-methylpseudoephedrine.[2, G63]

Volatile oil Mainly terpenoids (e.g. α-terpineol, limonene, tetramethylpyrazine, terpinen-4-ol, linalol).[3]

Other constituents Tannins (catechin, gallic acid), ephedrans (glycans) and acids (citric, malic, oxalic).

Roots

Alkaloids Ephedroxane, ephedradines A to D, feruloylhistamine and maokonine.[4]

Flavonoids A flavonoflavonol (ephedrannin A), bisflavonols (mahuannins A to D).[4]

Food Use

Ephedra is not used in foods.

Herbal Use

Ephedra has traditionally been used for the treatment of bronchial asthma, hayfever, coughs and colds, fever, urticaria, enuresis, narcolepsy, myasthenia gravis, chronic postural hypotension and rheumatism.[G32, G34, G36, G49, G54, G63, G64]

It is stated to have vasoconstricting, bronchodilating and central stimulating properties.[G56] Modern interest in ephedra is focused on its use in cough and bronchitis,[G56] and in nasal congestion due to hayfever, allergic rhinitis, common cold and

Alkaloids

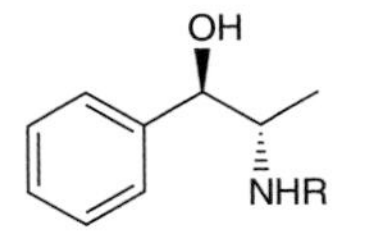

	R
(-)-norephedrine	H
(-)-ephedrine	CH_3

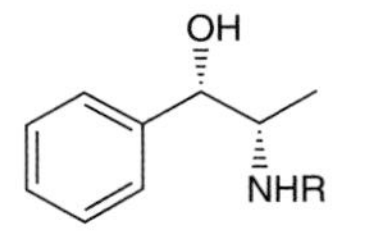

	R
(+)-norpseudoephedrine	H
(+)-pseudoephedrine	CH_3

Figure 1 Selected constituents of ephedra.

sinusitis.[G63] There is also interest in the potential of ephedra as an appetite suppressant.

Dosage

Dosages for oral administration (adults) for traditional uses recommended in standard herbal reference texts are given below.

Herb 1.2–2.3 g cut herbs containing approximately 1.3% (13 mg/g) total alkaloids.[G4]

Extract Adults: 15–30 mg alkaloids (maximum daily dose 300 mg), calculated as ephedrine.[G56]

Tincture 6–8 mL (1 : 4) three times daily.[G36]

In 1997, the US Food and Drugs Administration (FDA) proposed restrictions on the use of ephedra. The FDA proposals included a restriction on the maximum dose of ephedrine: 8 mg taken every six hours to a maximum daily dose of 24 mg for no more than seven days.[5, G56]

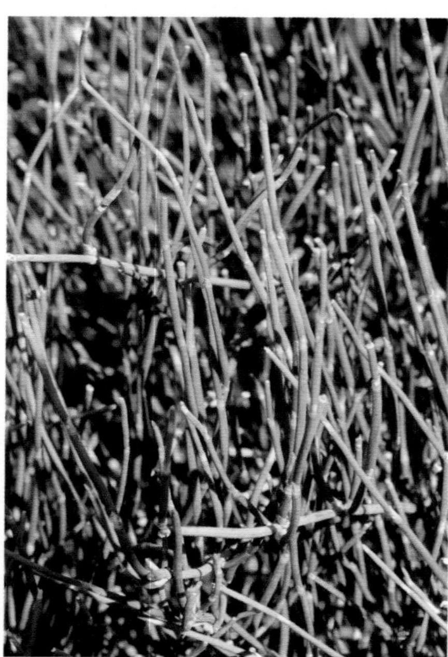

Figure 2 Ephedra (*Ephedra sinica*).

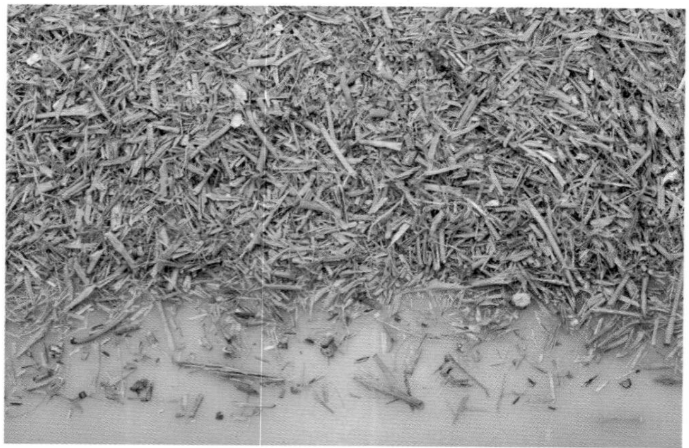

Figure 3 Ephedra – dried drug substance (herb).

E

Pharmacological Actions

The pharmacological properties of ephedra are due to the presence of ephedrine, pseudoephedrine and other ephedra alkaloids (*see* Constituents). Ephedrine and pseudoephedrine are sympathomimetic agents that have direct and indirect effects on both α- and β-adrenoceptors, as well as stimulating the central nervous system (CNS).[G43, G63] Pseudoephedrine is stated to have less pressor activity and fewer CNS effects than ephedrine.[G43]

In vitro and animal studies

Pharmacological activities documented for ephedrine and/or pseudoephedrine *in vitro* or *in vivo* (animals) include smooth muscle relaxant, cardiovascular, anti-inflammatory, immunomodulatory, CNS stimulatory and antimicrobial effects. The pharmacology of ephedra and its constituent alkaloids has been reviewed.[4, 6–8]

Ephedrine and pseudoephedrine have been stated to have a relaxant effect on bronchial smooth muscle in isolated rabbit lung and bronchi.[6] Relaxant effects on gastrointestinal smooth muscle have also been noted.[4, 6]

Ephedrine has been shown to cause vasoconstriction and to have hypertensive effects in several animal models.[4, 6] Maokonine, a constituent of ephedra root, has been reported to have hypertensive effects in anaesthetised rats.[9] By contrast, other constituents of ephedra roots, such as ephedrannin A and feruloylhistamine, have been reported to have hypotensive activity.[10, 11] An aqueous extract of ephedra and its alkaloid fraction increased blood pressure, heart rate and blood glucose concentration in anaesthetised dogs following intravenous administration.[12]

Anti-inflammatory activity has been documented for ephedrine and pseudoephedrine in carrageenan-induced hind-paw oedema in mice.[13] Oral administration of ephedrine and pseudoephedrine also inhibited hind-paw oedema induced by histamine, serotonin, bradykinin and prostaglandin E_1. Crude extracts of ephedra have been reported to inhibit complement *in vitro*.[14] Further investigation, using an aqueous extract of *E. sinica* leaves, showed that the complement-inhibiting component of ephedra inhibited the classical complement pathway in sera from several species, including human, pig, guinea-pig, rat and rabbit.[14]

In vitro antibacterial activity against several species, including *Staphylococcus aureus*, has been reported.[6]

In vitro studies have assessed the cytotoxicity of extracts of ephedra prepared under various conditions (e.g. using ground or unground material boiled for 0.5 or 2 hours) against a range of cell lines, including a human hepatoblastoma cell line (HepG2), a mouse neuroblastoma cell line (Neuro-2a) and a mouse fibroblastoma cell line.[15] Ephedrine and ephedra extracts prepared from ground material appeared to be significantly more cytotoxic in these cell lines than did preparations from unground material. Also, Neuro-2a cells were more sensitive to ephedra extracts than were the other cell lines tested. Findings of this *in vitro* work also indicated that ephedra contains toxins other than ephedrine, as IC_{50} values were lower (i.e. indicating greater cytotoxicity) for ephedra extracts than for ephedrine alone.

Clinical studies

Pharmacokinetics Ephedrine and pseudoephedrine are readily absorbed from the gastrointestinal tract and are excreted, largely unchanged, in the urine.[G43] Small amounts of metabolites following hepatic metabolism may be produced. The half-lives of ephedrine and pseudoephedrine range from 3–6 hours and from 5–8 hours, respectively, depending on urinary pH.[G43]

In a study involving 12 healthy volunteers aged 23–40 years, four capsules of an ephedra product were administered twice, nine hours apart. Each capsule contained ephedra 375 mg (*E. sinica*), with a mean (standard deviation (SD)) ephedrine content of 4.84 (0.45) mg.[16] The half-life was reported to be 5.2 hours, maximum plasma concentration (C_{max}) was 81.0 ng/mL, the time to reach C_{max} (t_{max}) was 3.9 hours, and clearance was 24.3 L/hour.

In a randomised, crossover study, 10 healthy volunteers received ephedrine 25 mg or one of three ephedrine-containing nutritional supplements on one day during different phases of the study, each with a one-week wash-out period.[17] Following single-dose administration of ephedrine 25 mg, mean (SD) half-life, C_{max}, t_{max} and clearance were found to be 5.37 (1.67) hours, 86.5 (15.4) ng/mL, 2.81 (1.35) hours and 28.5 (5.92) L/hour, respectively.

Therapeutic effects The pharmacological properties of ephedrine and pseudoephedrine in humans have been documented and include cardiovascular, bronchodilator and CNS stimulant effects.[G43, G63]

Ephedrine is stated to raise blood pressure by increasing cardiac output and also by peripheral vasoconstriction. Ephedrine relaxes bronchial smooth muscle, reduces intestinal tone and motility, relaxes the bladder wall and reduces the activity of the uterus. Ephedrine is a CNS stimulant; this has led to its investigation for use in assisting weight loss.

There is a lack of clinical research assessing the effects of ephedra and rigorous randomised controlled clinical trials are required.

A randomised, double-blind, placebo-controlled trial assessed the effects of a herbal combination preparation which included ephedra and other herbal ingredients.[18] In the study, 67 overweight to obese individuals (body mass index 29–35 kg/m^2) received the ephedra-containing preparation, or placebo, for eight weeks. Among the 48 participants who completed the study (24 in each group), a greater mean (SD) weight loss was noted for the treatment group, compared with the placebo group (4.0 (3.4) kg versus 0.8 (2.4) kg, respectively; $p < 0.006$).

Side-effects, Toxicity

The most common adverse effects of ephedrine and pseudoephedrine are tachycardia, anxiety, restlessness and insomnia.[G43] Tremor, dry mouth, impaired circulation to the extremities, hypertension and cardiac arrhythmias may also occur with ephedrine, and skin rashes and urinary retention have been reported for pseudoephedrine.[G43] There are isolated reports of hallucinations in children following use of pseudoephedrine.[G43]

There is a lack of clinical safety and toxicity data for ephedra and further investigation of these aspects is required.

In the US, adverse effects have been reported following self-treatment with products containing ephedra alkaloids marketed for several uses, including as an aid to weight loss, to increase athletic performance, and as an alternative to illegal drugs of abuse.[19, G43]

A review assessed 140 reports of adverse events related to the use of products containing ephedra alkaloids, usually combined with caffeine, submitted to the US FDA between June 1997 and March 1999.[19] The main reasons for use of these products were weight loss (59%) and to increase athletic performance (16%); the reason for use was unknown in 17% of cases. Thirty-one per cent of cases (n = 43) were considered to be 'definitely' or 'probably' related to the use of products containing ephedra alkaloids, and a further 31% (n = 44) were judged to be 'possibly' related; for 29 cases, insufficient information was available to assess causation, and 24 cases were deemed to be 'unrelated' to use of these products. In several cases, individuals were thought to be ingesting up to 60 mg ephedra alkaloids daily. Of the 87 cases where causality was assessed, cardiovascular symptoms (mainly hypertension, palpitations, tachycardia) were the most common adverse events (47%). The most common CNS events were stroke (n = 10) and seizures (n = 7). Where events were 'definitely' or 'probably' related (n = 43), clinical outcomes were death (three cases), permanent impairment (seven) and ongoing treatment (four); a full recovery occurred in 29 cases.[19]

In a randomised, double-blind, placebo-controlled trial of a herbal supplement containing ephedra (72 mg/day) and guarana (240 mg/day), as well as other herbal ingredients, 23% (n = 8) of participants in the treatment group withdrew from the study because of adverse events (e.g. dry mouth, insomnia, headache) that may have been treatment-related; there were no withdrawals among placebo recipients.[18]

There are isolated reports of myocarditis,[20] exacerbation of autoimmune hepatitis,[21] acute hepatitis,[22] nephrolithiasis[23] and psychiatric complications[24] associated with the use of ephedra-containing products. There is a report of sudden death associated with ephedrine toxicity in a 23-year-old man.[25] Several other reports also document psychosis and renal calculi following chronic use or misuse of ephedrine.[G18]

In a study involving 12 normotensive adults who ingested four capsules each containing 375 mg powdered ephedra, followed by four more capsules nine hours later, a statistically significant increase in heart rate, compared with baseline values, was noted in six participants, although effects on blood pressure were variable.[16]

Preclinical data

A study involving 47 dogs who were considered to have accidentally ingested herbal products containing ephedra and guarana reported that most dogs (80%) developed clinical signs of toxicosis, within eight hours of ingestion, which persisted for up to 48 hours.[26] Hyperactivity, tremors, seizures and behaviour changes were reported in 83% of dogs; other signs and symptoms included vomiting, tachycardia and hyperthermia.

Contra-indications, Warnings

Ephedra is stated to be contra-indicated in coronary thrombosis, diabetes, glaucoma, heart disease, hypertension, thyroid disease, phaeochromocytoma and enlarged prostate.[G63] Another source states that ephedrine (and, therefore, ephedrine-containing products) should be used with caution in patients with diabetes, ischaemic heart disease, hypertension, hyperthyoidism, renal impairment and angle-closure glaucoma, and that in patients with prostate enlargement, ephedrine may increase difficulty with micturition.[G43] It has been recommended to reduce the dose or discontinue treatment if nervousness, tremor, sleeplessness, loss of appetite or nausea occur with use of ephedra preparations.[G63]

There is a report of a professional sportsman who tested positive for norpseudoephedrine after having consumed a liquid herbal product listing ephedra as one of the 15 ingredients.[27]

Drug interactions Warnings documented for ephedrine are applicable.

Ephedrine-containing products should be avoided in patients receiving monoamine oxidase inhibitors as concomitant treatment may lead to a hypertensive crisis.[G43] Ephedrine should also be avoided or used with caution in patients undergoing anaesthesia with cyclopropane, halothane or other volatile anaesthetics. There may be an increased risk of arrhythmias in patients receiving ephedrine together with cardiac glycosides, quinidine or tricyclic antidepressants, and there is an increased risk of vasoconstrictor or pressor effects in patients receiving ergot alkaloids or oxytocin.[G43]

E

Pregnancy and lactation There are no reliable data on the use of ephedra during pregnancy and lactation. The safety of ephedra during pregnancy and lactation has not been established and its use should be avoided.

Preparations

Proprietary multi-ingredient preparations

Canada: Herbal Cold Relief. *Germany:* Cefadrin.

References

1 Medicines Act 1968, Statutory Instrument 1977 No. 2130 (Retail Sale of Supply of Herbal Remedies) Order, 1977.
2 Dewick P. *Medicinal Natural Products. A Biosynthetic Approach.* Wiley: Chichester, 1997.
3 Miyazawa M *et al.* Volatile components of *Ephedra sinica* Stapf. *Flavour Fragrance J* 1997; 12: 15–17.
4 Tang W, Eisenbrand G. *Chinese Drugs of Plant Origin. Chemistry, Pharmacology and Use in Traditional and Modern Medicine.* Berlin: Springer-Verlag, 1992: 481–490.
5 Blumenthal M. Ephedra update: industry coalition asks FDA to adopt national labeling guidelines on ephedra; offers co-operative research with NIH. *Herbal Gram* 2000; 50: 64–65.
6 Chang H-M, But PP-H, eds. *Pharmacology and Applications of Chinese Materia Medica*, vol 2. Singapore: World Scientific Publishing, 1987: 1119–1124.
7 Kalix P. The pharmacology of psychoactive alkaloids from Ephedra and Catha. *J Ethnopharmacol* 1991; 32: 201–208.
8 Bowman WC, Rand MJ. *Textbook of Pharmacology*, 2nd edn. Oxford: Blackwell, 1980.
9 Tamada M *et al.* Maokonine, hypertensive principle of *Ephedra* roots. *Planta Med* 1978; 34: 291–293.
10 Hikino H *et al.* Structure of feruloylhistamine, a hypotensive principle of *Ephedra* roots. *Planta Med* 1983; 48: 108–110.
11 Hikino H *et al.* Structure of ephedrannin A, a hypotensive principle of *Ephedra* roots. *Tetrahedron Lett* 1982; 23: 673–676.
12 Harada M, Nichimura M. Contribution of alkaloid fraction to pressor and hyperglycemic effect of crude ephedra extract in dogs. *J Pharm Dyn* 1981; 4: 691–699.
13 Kasahara Y *et al.* Antiinflammatory actions of ephedrines in acute inflammations. *Planta Med* 1985; 51: 325–331.
14 Ling M *et al.* A component of the medicinal herb ephedra blocks activation in the classical and alternative pathways of complement. *Clin Exp Immunol* 1995; 102: 582–588.
15 Lee MK *et al.* Cytotoxicity assessment of Ma-huang (Ephedra) under different conditions of preparation. *Toxicol Sci* 2000; 56: 424–430.
16 White LM *et al.* Pharmacokinetics and cardiovascular effects of ma-huang (*Ephedra sinica*) in normotensive adults. *J Clin Pharmacol* 1997; 37: 116–122.
17 Gurley BJ *et al.* Ephedrine pharmacokinetics after the ingestion of nutritional supplements containing *Ephedra sinica* (ma huang). *Ther Drug Monitoring* 1998; 20: 439–445.
18 Boozer CN *et al.* An herbal supplement containing Ma-Huang-Guarana for weight loss: a randomised, double-blind trial. *Int J Obesity* 2001; 25: 316–324.
19 Haller CA, Benowitz NL. Adverse cardiovascular and central nervous system events associated with dietary supplements containing ephedra alkaloids. *N Engl J Med* 2000; 343: 1833–1838.
20 Zaacks SM *et al.* Hypersensitivity myocarditis associated with ephedra use. *J Toxicol Clin Toxicol* 1999; 37: 485–489.
21 Borum ML. Fulminant exacerbation of autoimmune hepatitis after the use of Ma Huang. *Am J Gastroenterol* 2001; 96: 1654–1655.
22 Nadir A *et al.* Acute hepatitis associated with the use of a Chinese herbal product, ma-huang. *Am J Gastroenterol* 1996; 91: 1436–1438.
23 Powell T *et al.* Ma-Huang strikes again: ephedrine nephrolithiasis. *Am J Kidney Dis* 1998; 32: 153–159.
24 Jacobs KM, Hirsch KA. Psychiatric complications of Ma-huang. *Psychosomatics* 2000; 41: 58–62.
25 Theoharides TC. Sudden death of a healthy college student related to ephedrine toxicity from a ma huang-containing drink. *J Clin Psychopharmacol* 1997; 17: 437–439.
26 Ooms TG *et al.* Suspected caffeine and ephedrine toxicosis resulting from ingestion of an herbal supplement containing guarana and ma huang in dogs: 47 cases (1997–1999). *J Am Vet Med Assoc* 2001; 218: 225–229.
27 Ros JJW *et al.* A case of positive doping associated with a botanical food supplement. *Pharm World Sci* 1999; 21: 44.

Eucalyptus

Summary and Pharmaceutical Comment

Eucalyptus is characterised by its volatile oil components. Antiseptic and expectorant properties have been attributed to the oil, in particular to the principal component eucalyptol. The undiluted oil is toxic if taken internally. Essential oils should not be applied to the skin unless they are diluted with a carrier vegetable oil.

Species (Family)

Eucalyptus globulus Labill. (Myrtaceae)

Synonym(s)

E. maidenii subsp. *globulus* (Labill.) Kirkp., Fevertree, Gum Tree, Tasmanian Bluegum

Part(s) Used

Leaf

Pharmacopoeial and Other Monographs

BHP 1996[(G9)]
BP 2007[(G84)]
Complete German Commission E[(G3)]
Martindale 35th edition[(G85)]
Ph Eur 2007[(G81)]

Legal Category (Licensed Products)

GSL[(G37)]

Constituents

The following is compiled from several sources, including General References G2 and G75.

Flavonoids Eucalyptrin, hyperoside, quercetin, quercitrin and rutin.

Volatile oils 0.5–3.5%. Eucalyptol (cineole) 70–85%. Others include monoterpenes (e.g. α-pinene, β-pinene, *d*-limonene, *p*-cymene, α-phellandrene, camphene, γ-terpinene) and sesquiterpenes (e.g. aromadendrene, alloaromadendrene, globulol, epiglobulol, ledol, viridiflorol), aldehydes (e.g. myrtenal) and ketones (e.g. carvone, pinocarvone).

Monoterpenes

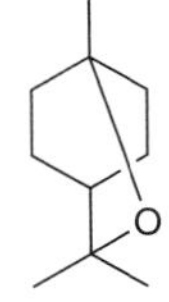

1,8-cineole
(eucalyptol)

Figure 1 Selected constituents of eucalyptus.

Other constituents Tannins and associated acids (e.g. gallic acid, protocatechuic acid), caffeic acid, ferulic acids, gentisic acid, resins and waxes.

Food Use

Eucalyptus is listed by the Council of Europe as a natural source of food flavouring (leaves, flowers and preparations: category N4, with limits on eucalyptol) (*see* Appendix 3).[(G17)] Both eucalyptus and eucalyptol (cineole) are used as flavouring agents in many food products.[(G41)] Previously in the USA, eucalyptus was approved for food use and eucalyptol was listed as a synthetic flavouring agent.[(G41)]

Herbal Use

Eucalyptus leaves and oil have been used as an antiseptic, febrifuge and expectorant.[(G2, G41, G64)]

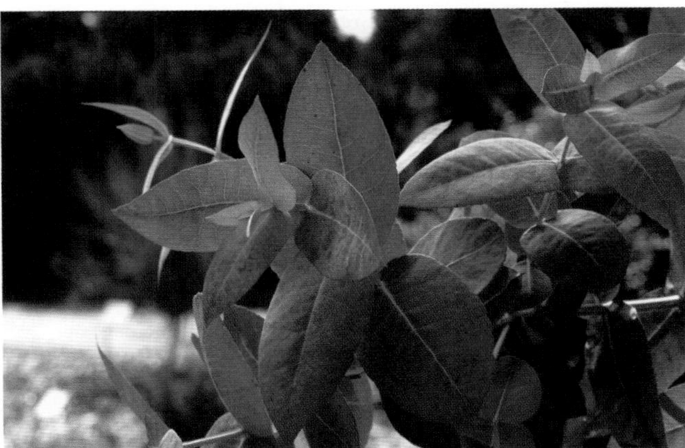

Figure 2 Eucalyptus (*Eucalyptus globulus*).

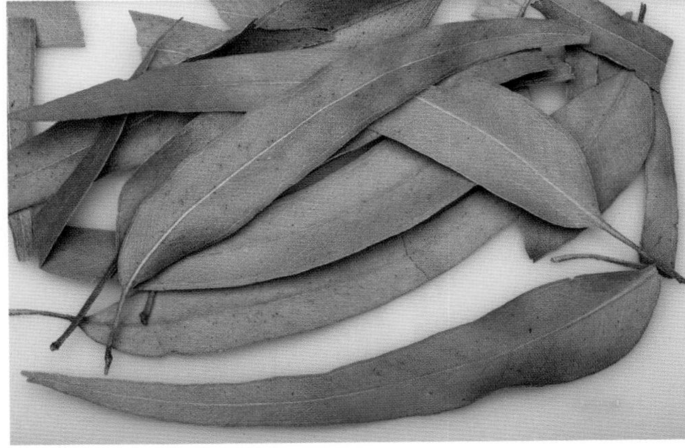

Figure 3 Eucalyptus – dried drug substance (leaf).

E

Dosage

Dosages for oral (unless otherwise stated) administration (adults) for traditional uses recommended in older standard reference texts are given below.

Eucalyptol (cineole BPC 1973) 0.05–0.2 mL.

Eucalyptus Oil (BPC 1973) 0.05–0.2 mL.

Fluid extract 2–4 g.

Oil for local application 30 mL oil to 500 mL lukewarm water.

Pharmacological Actions

In vitro and animal studies

Hypoglycaemic activity in rabbits has been documented for a crude leaf extract rich in phenolic glycosides. Purification of the extract resulted in a loss of activity.[G41] Expectorant and antibacterial activities have been reported for eucalyptus oil and for eucalyptol.[G41] Various *Eucalyptus* species have been shown to possess antibacterial activity against both Gram-positive and Gram-negative organisms. Gram-positive organisms were found to be the most sensitive, particularly *Bacillus subtilis* and *Micrococcus glutamious.*[1]

In vitro antiviral activity against influenza type A has been documented for quercitrin and hyperoside.[G41]

Clinical studies

There is a lack of clinical research assessing the effects of eucalyptus and rigorous randomised controlled clinical trials are required.

Eucalyptus oil has been taken orally for catarrh, used as an inhalation and applied as a rubefacient.[G45] A plant preparation containing tinctures of various herbs including eucalyptus has been used in the treatment of chronic suppurative otitis.[2]

Side-effects, Toxicity

Externally, eucalyptus oil is stated to be generally non-toxic, non-sensitising and non-phototoxic.[G58] Undiluted eucalyptus oil is toxic and should not be taken internally. A dose of 3.5 mL has proved fatal.[G45] Symptoms of poisoning with eucalyptus oil include epigastric burning, nausea and vomiting, dizziness, muscular weakness, miosis, a feeling of suffocation, cyanosis, delirium and convulsions.

Contra-indications, Warnings

Eucalyptus oil should be diluted before internal or external use.

Drug interactions None documented. However, the potential for preparations of eucalyptus to interact with other medicines administered concurrently, particularly those with similar or opposing effects, should be considered. There is limited evidence from preclinical studies that constituents of eucalyptus have hypoglycaemic activity.

Pregnancy and lactation Eucalyptus oil should not be taken internally during pregnancy or lactation.

References

1 Kumar A *et al.* Antibacterial properties of some *Eucalpytus* oils. *Fitoterapia* 1988; 59: 141–144.

2 Shaparenko BA *et al.* On use of medicinal plants for treatment of patients with chronic suppurative otitis. *Zh Ushn Gorl Bolezn* 1979; 39: 48–51.

Euphorbia

Summary and Pharmaceutical Comment

There is little published information concerning euphorbia, although documented actions observed in animals support the traditional herbal uses. There is a lack of information concerning toxicity and excessive or prolonged ingestion should be avoided.

Species (Family)

Chamaesyce hirta (L.) Millsp. (Euphorbiaceae)

Synonym(s)

Euphorbia capitata Lam., *E. hirta* L., Pillbearing Spurge, Snakeweed

Part(s) Used

Herb

Pharmacopoeial and Other Monographs

BHP 1983[G7]
Martindale 35th edition[G85]

Legal Category (Licensed Products)

GSL[G37]

Constituents

The following is compiled from several sources, including General References G41 and G48.

Flavonoids Leucocyanidin, quercetin, quercitrin and xanthorhamnin.

Terpenoids α- and β-Amyrin, taraxerol and esters, friedelin; campesterol, sitosterol and stigmasterol (sterols).

Other constituents Choline, alkanes, inositol, phenolic acids (e.g. ellagic, gallic, shikimic), sugars and resins.

Food Use

Euphorbia is not used in foods.

Herbal Use

Euphorbia is stated to be used for respiratory disorders, such as asthma, bronchitis, catarrh and laryngeal spasm. It has also been used for intestinal amoebiasis.[G7, G64]

Dosage

Dosages for oral administration (adults) for traditional uses recommended in older standard reference texts are given below.

Herb 120–300 mg as an infusion.[G7]

Liquid Extract of Euphorbia (BPC 1949) 0.12–0.3 mL.

Euphorbia Tincture (BPC 1923) 0.6–2.0 mL.

Pharmacological Actions

In vitro and animal studies

Euphorbia has been reported to have antispasmodic and histamine-potentiating properties.[G41] Smooth muscle relaxing

Triterpenes

HO
H
H
H

α-amyrin

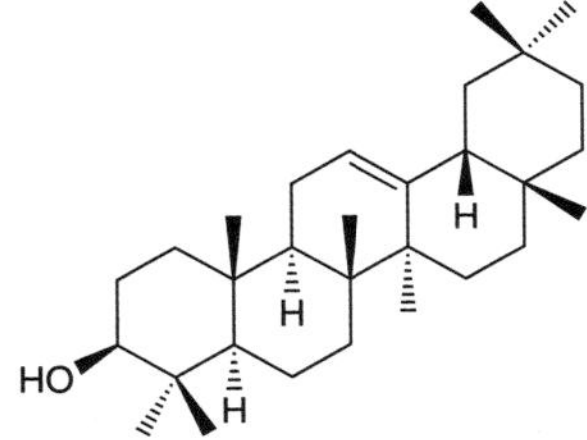

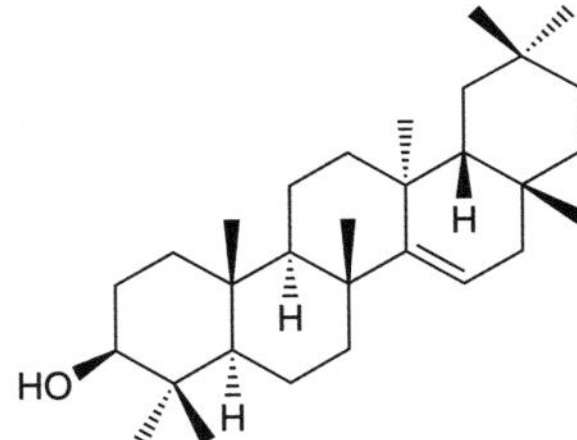

Figure 1 Selected constituents of euphorbia.

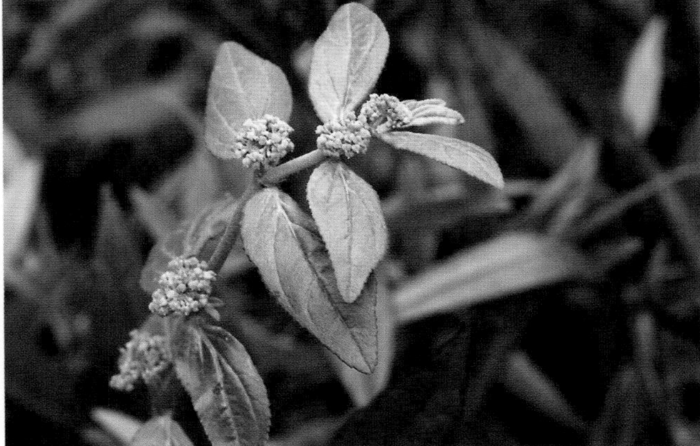

Figure 2 Euphorbia (*Chamaesyce hirta*).

E

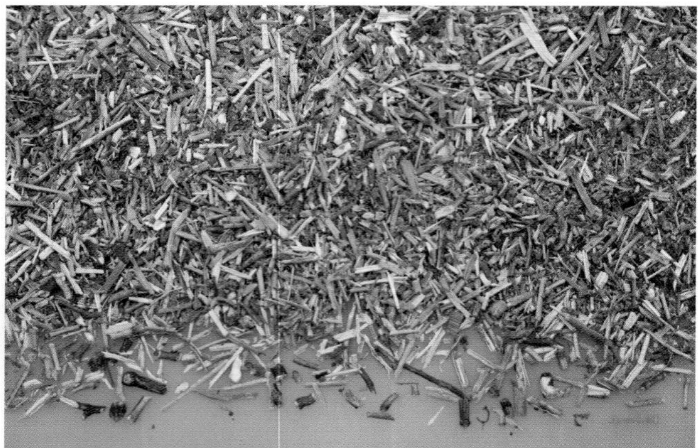

Figure 3 Euphorbia – dried drug substance (herb).

and contracting activities have been exhibited by euphorbia *in vitro* (guinea-pig ileum) and have been attributed to shikimic acid and to choline, respectively.[1]

In vivo antitumour activities have been documented for euphorbia.[G41]

Antibacterial activity *in vitro* versus both Gram-positive and Gram-negative bacteria has been documented for euphorbia.[2] Stem extracts were slightly more active than leaf extracts. *In vitro* amoebicidal activity versus *Entamoeba histolytica* has been reported for a euphorbia decoction.[3]

Clinical studies

There is a lack of clinical research assessing the effects of euphorbia and rigorous randomised controlled clinical trials are required.

Side-effects, Toxicity

None documented. However, there is a lack of clinical safety and toxicity data for euphorbia and further investigation of these aspects is required. Carcinogenic properties in mice have been reported for shikimic acid, although no mutagenic activity was observed in the Ames assay.[G41]

Contra-indications, Warnings

None documented.

Drug interactions None documented. However, the potential for preparations of euphorbia to interact with other medicines administered concurrently, particularly those with similar or opposing effects, should be considered.

Pregnancy and lactation The safety of euphorbia has not been established. Euphorbia has been reported to cause both contraction and relaxation of smooth muscle. In view of the lack of pharmacological and toxicity data, the use of euphorbia during pregnancy and lactation should be avoided.

Preparations

Proprietary single-ingredient preparations

India: Thankgod.

Proprietary multi-ingredient preparations

Australia: Asa Tones; Euphorbia Complex; Procold; Sambucus Complex. *Canada:* Sirop Cocillana Codeine. *Hong Kong:* Cocillana Christo; Cocillana Compound; Cocillana Compound; Cocillana Compound; Mefedra-N. *UK:* Antibron.

References

1 El-Naggar L *et al.* A note on the isolation and identification of two pharmacologically active constituents of *Euphorbia pilulifera*. *Lloydia* 1978; 41: 73–75.

2 Ajao AO *et al.* Antibacterial activity of *Euphorbia hirta*. *Fitoterapia* 1985; 56: 165–167.

3 Basit N *et al.* In vitro effect of extracts of *Euphorbia hirta* Linn. on *Entamoeba histolytica*. *Riv Parasitol* 1977; 38: 259–262.

Evening Primrose

Summary and Pharmaceutical Comment

Interest in the seed oil of the evening primrose plant lies in its essential fatty acid content, in particular in the linoleic acid (LA) and gamolenic acid (GLA) content. Both of these compounds are prostaglandin precursors and dietary gamolenic acid supplementation has been shown to increase the ratio of non-inflammatory to inflammatory prostaglandin compounds.

The use of evening primrose oil in various disease states associated with low gamolenic acid concentrations has been extensively investigated and a vast body of published literature is available. However, while some clinical studies have reported benefits following administration of evening primrose oil, for the most part, the available data are inconclusive, and/or arise from studies with methodological limitations. The efficacy of evening primrose oil in the various conditions for which it has been investigated, therefore, has not been established and further, rigorous research is required. In particular, authoritative reviews of studies assessing the effects of evening primrose oil preparations concluded that there are no reliable data on their efficacy in atopic eczema and in relieving symptoms of premenstrual syndrome, including mastalgia, and product licences for evening primrose preparations (Epogam, Efamast) licensed in the UK for these indications were withdrawn in 2002. Unlicensed preparations of evening primrose oil (which cannot make efficacy claims in the UK) remain available.

Evening primrose oil is well-tolerated when uesd at recommended dosages; minor adverse effects, such as headache, nausea, diarrhoea, have occasionally been associated with its use. Evening primrose oil may have the potential to make manifest undiagnosed temporal lobe epilepsy, especially in schizophrenic patients and/or those who are already receiving known epileptogenic drugs, such as phenothiazines (*see* Contra-indications, Warnings). Evening primrose oil should be used with caution by such patients and those with a history of epilepsy. In view of the lack of safety data, evening primrose oil should not be taken during pregnancy. As LA and gamolenic acid occur naturally in breast milk, it is reasonable to expect that evening primrose oil can be taken during breastfeeding, although whether or not concentrations of LA and gamolenic acid in breast milk of mothers ingesting high doses of evening primrose oil can reach levels that may be harmful to the neonate should be considered.

Species (Family)

Oenothera biennis L. (Onagraceae)

Synonym(s)

Common Evening Primrose, King's Cureall, *Onagra biennis* (L.) Scop.

Part(s) Used

Seed oil

Pharmacopoeial and Other Monographs

BP 2007[G84]
Martindale 35th edition[G85]
Ph Eur 2007[G81]

Legal Category (Licensed Products)

Evening primrose is not included in the GSL.[G37] Gamolenic acid is a prescription-only medicine. Product licences for the products Epogam and Efamast (which contain gamolenic acid derived from evening primrose oil) were withdrawn in the UK on 7 October, 2002.[1,2]

Constituents

Fixed oils 14%. cis-Linoleic acid (LA) 72% (65–80%), cis-gammalinolenic acid (gamolenic acid, GLA) 2–16%, oleic acid 9%, palmitic acid 7% and stearic acid (3%).[3–7]

Food Use

Evening primrose root has been used as a vegetable with a peppery flavour.[7] The seed oil has been used as a food supplement for many years. LA and gamolenic acid are both essential fatty acids (EFAs), with LA representing the main EFA in the diet, whilst gamolenic acid is found in human milk, in oats and barley, and in small amounts in a wide variety of common foods.[6,7]

Herbal Use

An infusion of the whole plant is reputed to have sedative and astringent properties, and has traditionally been used for asthmatic coughs, gastrointestinal disorders, whooping cough and as a sedative painkiller.[7] Externally, poultices were reputed to ease bruises and to speed wound-healing.[7]

Evening primrose oil (EPO) was licensed in the UK for the treatment of atopic eczema, and cyclical and non-cyclical

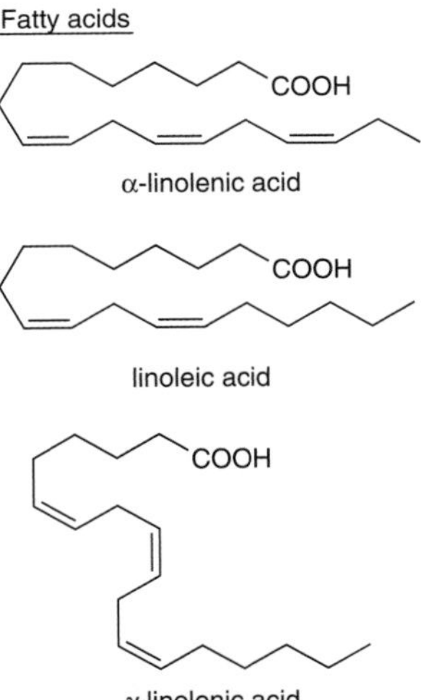

Figure 1 Selected constituents of evening primrose.

mastalgia, but product licences for two products were withdrawn in 2002 due to a lack of data sufficient to support efficacy in these conditions.[1,2,8] Other conditions in which evening primrose oil has been used include premenstrual syndrome, psoriasis, multiple sclerosis, hypercholesterolaemia, rheumatoid arthritis, Raynaud's phenomenon, Sjögren's syndrome, postviral fatigue syndrome, asthma and diabetic neuropathy.[3–5,7]

Dosage

Dosages recommended for previously licensed evening primrose oil products in the UK are given below; doses were based on a standardised gamolenic acid content of 8%. However, evening primrose oil products licensed in the UK had their product licences withdrawn in 2002 due to a lack of data sufficient to support efficacy.[8] Thus, there is no evidence that the dosages described below are efficacious in the conditions stated.

Atopic eczema: 6–8 g daily (adults); 2–4 g daily (children); cyclical and non-cyclical mastalgia: 3–4 g daily. The manufacturer advised that treatment for three months may be necessary before a clinical response is observed.[9]

Pharmacological Actions

The actions of evening primrose oil are attributable to the essential fatty acid content of the oil and to the involvement of these compounds in prostaglandin biosynthetic pathways.[3–5,7]

In vitro and animal studies

Gamolenic acid and its metabolite dihomogamma-linolenic acid (DGLA) are precursors of both the inflammatory prostaglandin E_2 (PGE_2) series via arachidonic acid (AA), and of the less inflammatory prostaglandin E_1 (PGE_1) series. Actions attributed to PGE_1 include anti-inflammatory, immunoregulatory and vasodilatory properties, inhibition of platelet aggregation and cholesterol biosynthesis, hypotension and elevation of cyclic AMP (inhibits phospholipase A_2, see below).[3–5]

Dietary supplementation with gamolenic acid has been noted to have a favourable effect on the DGLA : AA ratio. Although an increase in arachidonic acid concentrations is also seen, this is much smaller and less consistent compared with the increase seen for DGLA.[5] Contributory factors to this negative effect on arachidonic acid are PGE_1 and 15-hydroxy-DGLA. The latter inhibits conversion of arachidonic acid to inflammatory lipoxygenase metabolites including leukotrienes, whilst PGE_1 inhibits the enzyme phospholipase A_2 which is required for the mobilisation of arachidonic acid from phospholipid membrane stores.[5] In addition, DGLA desaturation to arachidonic acid is a rate-limiting step in humans and proceeds very slowly.[5]

Gamolenic acid is not normally obtained directly from dietary sources and the body relies on metabolic conversion from dietary LA. This conversion is readily saturable and is considered to be the rate-limiting step in the production of gamolenic acid. A reduced rate of LA conversion to gamolenic acid has been observed in a number of clinical situations including ageing, diabetes, cardiovascular disorders and high cholesterol concentrations, high alcohol intake, viral infections, cancer, nutritional deficits, atopic eczema and premenstrual syndrome.[3–5] Direct dietary supplementation with gamolenic acid effectively bypasses this rate-limiting conversion step and has a beneficial effect on the ratio of inflammatory : non-inflammatory prostaglandin compounds.

Gamolenic acid, administered as evening primrose oil, can prevent or reverse diabetic neuropathy in animal models.

Administration of gamolenic acid to animals has been reported to prevent or attenuate renal damage. Gamolenic acid decreases blood pressure and platelet aggregation in animals.[5] *In vitro* studies have observed that malignant cells die following exposure to gamolenic acid and related fatty acids at concentrations that are non-lethal to normal cells. *In vitro* studies have shown gamolenic acid to inhibit the growth of various human cancer cell lines, and *in vivo* studies have described an inhibitory effect of gamolenic acid on tumour growth.[5]

Evening primrose oil represents a good source of both LA and, more importantly, of gamolenic acid. There is a large body of literature on the biochemical rationale for the therapeutic uses of evening primrose oil.[5] Alternative natural oil sources such as blackcurrant or borage that offer a higher gamolenic acid yield compared with that of evening primrose oil have been identified, although these oils have not been found to exhibit the same biological effects as those observed for evening primrose oil.[5]

Clinical studies

There is a large body of literature on the effects of evening primrose oil and gamolenic acid in various disease states associated with low concentrations of gamolenic acid. For the most part, the available data are inconclusive, and/or arise from studies with methodological limitations. The efficacy of evening primrose oil in these conditions, therefore, has not been

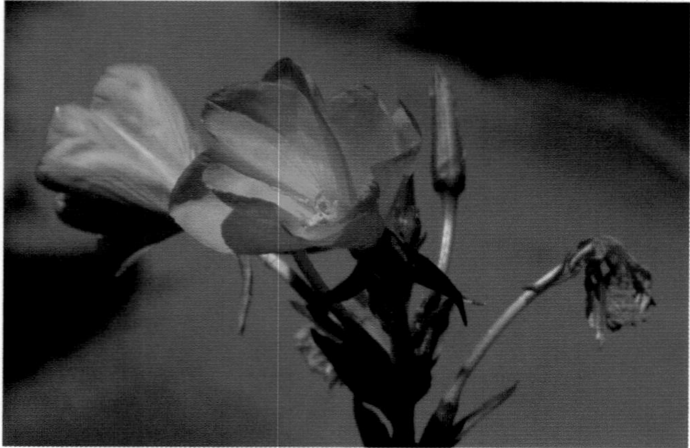

Figure 2 Evening primrose (*Oenothera biennis*).

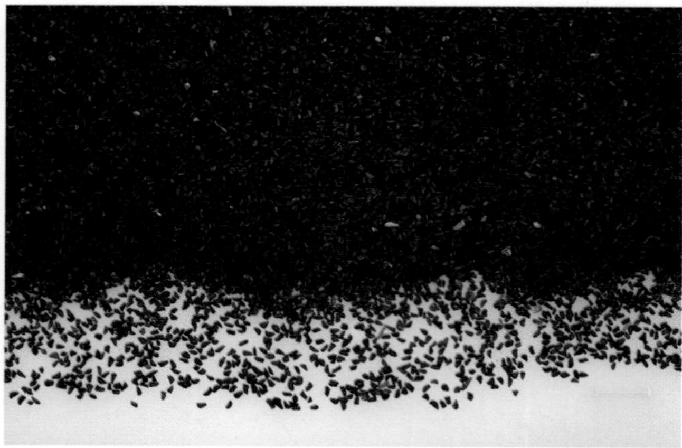

Figure 3 Evening primrose – dried drug substance (seed).

established and further, rigorous research is required. The following is a summary of some of the clinical studies of evening primrose oil and gamolenic acid.

Atopic eczema An inherited slow rate of 6-desaturation (LA to gamolenic acid conversion) has been documented in this condition. Normal or elevated concentrations of LA are associated with reduced concentrations of their metabolites. Some randomised, double-blind, placebo-controlled trials have suggested gamolenic acid improves features of atopic eczema, especially in itch.[3–5, 10–13] However, two large trials have not shown evidence of benefit.[14, 15] A review of the available evidence to support the efficacy of evening primrose oil preparations in atopic eczema concluded that there were insufficient data, and product licences for evening primrose preparations licensed in the UK for atopic eczema were withdrawn in 2002.[2, 8]

Cyclical/non-cyclical mastalgia and premenstrual syndrome PGE_1 is thought to modulate the action of prolactin. Abnormal concentrations may result in an excessive peripheral action of prolactin.[5] The use of evening primrose oil for the treatment of premenstrual syndrome has been rationalised on the grounds that hypersensitivity to prolactin is due to low levels of PGE_1.[16] High levels of linoleic acid and low levels of gamma-linolenic acid have been observed for patients with premenstrual syndrome.

Several placebo-controlled studies in the older literature have reported that gamolenic acid is better than placebo in the treatment of premenstrual syndrome and/or breast pain.[3–5, 17] However, conflicting results have been obtained from other clinical studies. Authoritative reviews of studies assessing the effects of evening primrose oil preparations have concluded that there are no reliable data on their efficacy in relieving symptoms of premenstrual syndrome, including mastalgia,[18] and product licences for evening primrose preparations licensed in the UK for the treatement of mastalgia were withdrawn in 2002.[2, 8]

Diabetic neuropathy Diabetes has been associated with reduced ability to desaturate essential fatty acids, with deficits resulting in abnormal neuronal membrane structure. A double-blind, placebo-controlled trial has described reversal of diabetic neuropathy by gamolenic acid.[19]

Multiple sclerosis The results of clinical trials on the use of evening primrose oil for the treatment of multiple sclerosis are contradictory.[3, 4] Patients with recent onset or less severe forms of the disease are more likely to respond. Linoleic acid may have a beneficial effect on the severity and duration of relapses and on the progression of the disease.[3] It is suggested that linoleic acid is involved in the immunosuppressive effect at the cellular level and may be of use when combined with a low animal fat/high polyunsaturated fat diet.[4]

Rheumatoid arthritis A randomised, double-blind trial has demonstrated a significant improvement in subjective symptoms of rheumatoid arthritis (RA) (indicated by a reduction in required non-steroidal anti-inflammatory drug treatment) in the active group receiving evening primrose oil compared with the placebo group. However, no objective changes were observed in any of the biochemical indicators of RA.[3–5]

Sjögren's syndrome This disease is associated with the loss of secretions from exocrine glands throughout the body, but especially from the salivary and lacrimal glands. One of the features of EFA deficiency is exocrine gland atrophy. Placebo-controlled trials have shown a modest improvement in tear flow together with relief of lethargy, a prominent feature of the syndrome.[3, 5]

Coronary heart disease Abnormal intake and metabolism of EFAs (both *n*-3 and *n*-6) are thought to be important risk factors for coronary heart disease (CHD), resulting in enhanced cholesterol and triglyceride biosynthesis, enhanced platelet aggregation and elevated blood pressure. Dietary supplementation with foods or oils rich in LA (*n*-6) or in marine (*n*-3) EFAs have been found to decrease significantly the risk of CHD, although it is considered that an optimum balance between *n*-3 and *n*-6 EFAs may well be important.[3–5, 20] gamolenic acid has been reported to decrease blood pressure and platelet aggregation in humans.[5]

Renal disease Renal tissue is especially rich in EFAs, and prostaglandins of the E series are believed to be important in maintaining adequate renal blood flow. A single placebo-controlled trial involving postrenal transplant patients demonstrated better graft survival rate for the group receiving evening primrose oil (45 patients) compared with the placebo group (44 patients).[5]

Gastrointestinal disorders A double-blind placebo-controlled crossover trial has indicated a beneficial effect of evening primrose oil on irritable bowel syndrome exacerbated by premenstrual syndrome. A beneficial effect superior to that of fish oil or placebo has been reported for evening primrose oil in ulcerative colitis.

Viral infections/postviral fatigue A single placebo-controlled study has demonstrated significant beneficial effects in patients with well-defined postviral fatigue (PVF) receiving evening primrose oil compared with those receiving placebo. Symptoms arrested were muscle weakness, aches and pains, lack of concentration, exhaustion, memory loss, depression, dizziness and vertigo.[3, 5]

Endometriosis A placebo-controlled trial has shown that gamolenic acid in combination with eicosapentaenoic acid (*n*-3 EFA metabolite) reduced symptoms of endometriosis in 90% women, whereas 90% of the placebo group reported no relief from symptoms.[5]

Schizophrenia It is believed that EFAs, in particular PGE_1, antagonise the excessive central dopaminergic activity that is thought to be a possible cause of schizophrenia. Low concentrations of LA in plasma phospholipids have been observed in populations of schizophrenics from Ireland, England, Scotland, Japan and the USA. It is thought that a poor recovery rate from the disease is associated with the presence of saturated fats in the diet, but not with unsaturated fats. Various open and placebo-controlled trials of gamolenic acid and DGLA supplementation have reportedly produced mixed results. Administration of evening primrose oil with co-factors known to be important in EFA metabolism (zinc, pyridoxine, niacin and vitamin C) enhanced the improvements in memory loss, schizophrenic symptoms and tardive dyskinesia that were observed in evening primrose oil-treated compared with placebo-treated patients.[3–5]

Alcoholism Evening primrose oil has been documented to reduce symptoms in the first three weeks of withdrawal, indicated by a reduced requirement for tranquillisers, and to significantly improve the rate of return to normal liver function. However, in the longer term, evening primrose did not affect the relapse rate.[5]

Dementia Alzheimer's disease and other forms of dementia are associated with low serum concentrations of EFAs. A single

E

Table 1 Summary of spontaneous reports (n = 187) of suspected adverse drug reactions associated with single-ingredient *Oenothera biennis* preparations held in the Vigisearch database of the World Health Organization's Uppsala Monitoring Centre for the period up to end of 2005.[21]

System organ class. **Adverse drug reaction name (number)**[a, b]	**Total**
Body as a whole – general disorders. Including allergic reaction (4); therapeutic response decreased (5); condition aggravated (5); fatigue (4); fever (6); malaise (7); pain (7); withdrawal syndrome (3)	65
Cardiovascular disorders, general. Including hypertension (3)	5
Central and peripheral nervous system disorders. Including convulsions (16); convulsions, aggravated (8); dizziness (5); headache (27); paraesthesia (9)	84
Endocrine disorders.	2
Foetal disorders.	1
Gastrointestinal system disorders. Including abdominal pain (18); constipation (3); diarrhoea (12); dyspepsia (7); eructation (3); flatulence (5); nausea (19); vomiting (5)	74
Heart rate and rhythm disorders.	2
Liver and biliary system disorders. Including hepatic function abnormal (4); hepatitis (3)	11
Metabolic and nutritional disorders. Including thirst (3); weight decrease (3)	15
Musculo-skeletal system disorders. Including arthralgia (3); myalgia (3)	8
Neoplasm.	2
Platelet, bleeding and clotting disorders. Including purpura (3)	13
Psychiatric disorders. Including nervousness (4); aggressive reaction (3); confusion (3)	38
Red blood cell disorders.	1
Reproductive disorders, female and male. Including menorrhagia (4); menstrual disorder (3)	17
Resistance mechanism disorders.	1
Respiratory system disorders. Including bronchospasm, aggravated (4); dyspnoea (4)	18
Skin and appendages disorders. Including acne (4); alopecia (3); eczema (5); pruritus (11); skin exfoliation (4); sweating increased (4); rash (9); rash, erythematous (11); rash, macropapular (5); urticaria (16)	96
Urinary system disorders. Including face oedema (5)	13
Vascular (extracardiac) disorders. Including flushing (4)	6
Vision disorders. Including abnormal vision (4)	12
White cell and res. disorders.	1
Other reactions described using terms not included in database	4
Total number of suspected adverse drug reactions	**489**

[a]Specific reactions described where n = 3 or more
[b]Caveat statement. These data were obtained from the Vigisearch database held by the WHO Collaborating Centre for International Drug Monitoring, Uppsala, Sweden. The information is not homogeneous at least with respect to origin or likelihood that the pharmaceutical product caused the adverse reaction. Any information included in this report does not represent the opinion of the World Health Organization

placebo-controlled trial in patients with Alzheimer's disease reported improvements in cerebral function in the evening primrose oil group compared with the placebo group.

Hyperactivity in children Hyperactive children tend to have abnormal levels of essential fatty acids. No improvements in behavioural patterns and no changes in blood fatty acids were observed in one trial with evening primrose oil.[4]

Side-effects, Toxicity

Clinical data

There is a lack of clinical safety and toxicity data for evening primrose and further investigation of these aspects is required. Limited clinical data on safety aspects of evening primrose oil preparations are available from clinical trials.

Evening primrose oil appears to be well tolerated when taken at recommended dosages.[5] Mild gastrointestinal effects, indigestion, nausea and softening of stools and headache have occasionally occurred.[5,7] It has been noted that there may be an increased risk of temporal lobe epilepsy in schizophrenic patients being treated with epileptogenic drugs such as phenothiazines.[9] In cases of overdosage, symptoms of loose stools and abdominal pain have been noted; no special treatment is required.[9] The two principal components in evening primrose oil are LA and gamolenic acid. LA is commonly ingested as part of the diet. It has been estimated that the concentration of gamolenic acid provided by evening primrose oil is comparable to that metabolised in the body from normal dietary LA.[6]

The World Health Organization's Uppsala Monitoring Centre (WHO-UMC; Collaborating Centre for International Drug Monitoring) receives summary reports of suspected adverse drug reactions from national pharmacovigilance centres of over 70 countries worldwide. To the end of the year 2005, the WHO-UMC's Vigisearch database contained a total of 291 reports, describing a total of 489 adverse reactions, for products reported to contain *Oenothera biennis* only as the active ingredient (*see* Table 1).[21] Reports originated from 12 different countries. (These data were obtained from the Vigisearch database held by the WHO Collaborating Centre for International Drug Monitoring, Uppsala, Sweden. The information is not homogeneous at least with respect to origin or likelihood that the pharmaceutical product caused the adverse reaction. Any information included in this report does not represent the opinion of the World Health Organization.)

Preclinical data

Toxicity studies have indicated evening primrose oil to be non-toxic.[5]

Contra-indications, Warnings

Evening primrose oil may have the potential to make manifest undiagnosed temporal lobe epilepsy, especially in schizophrenic patients and/or those who are already receiving known epileptogenic drugs such as phenothiazines.[9] Evening primrose oil should be used with caution by such patients and those with a history of epilepsy.

Drug interactions In view of the documented pharmacological actions of evening primrose oil, the potential for preparations of evening primrose oil to interfere with other medicines administered concurrently, particularly those with similar or opposing effects, should be considered. Evening primrose oil may increase the risk of seizure in patients receiving phenothiazines.

Pregnancy and lactation Animal studies have indicated evening primrose oil to be non-teratogenic.[9] However, data on the safety of evening primrose oil during human pregnancy are not available and therefore patients should be advised not to take evening primrose oil during pregnancy unless the potential benefits outweigh the potential harms. In view of the lack of conclusive evidence for the efficacy of evening primrose oil, it is unlikely that the benefit–harm balance would be in favour of patients using evening primrose oil.

Both LA and gamolenic acid are normally present in breast milk (*see* Side-effects, Toxicity) and it has been calculated that a breastfed infant receives a higher proportion (mg/kg) of LA and gamolenic acid from human milk than from evening primrose oil ingested by the breastfeeding mother.[6] It is reasonable to assume, therefore, that evening primrose oil may be taken while breastfeeding, although whether or not concentrations of LA and gamolenic acid in breast milk of mothers ingesting high doses of evening primrose oil can reach levels that may be harmful to the neonate should be considered.

Preparations

Proprietary multi-ingredient preparations

Italy: Sclerovis H. *UK:* Boots Alternatives Premenstrual; Seven Seas Evening Primrose Oil and Starflower Oil. *USA:* Evening Primrose Oil; PMS Control.

References

1 Anon. Withdrawal of Epogam and Efamast. *Curr Prob Pharmacovigilance* 2002; 28: 12.

2 Anon. What's new. Epogam and Efamast (gamolenic acid) – withdrawal of marketing authorisations. www.mca.gov.uk/whatsnew/epogam.html [accessed November 19, 2002]

3 Li Wan Po A. Evening primrose oil. *Pharm J* 1991; 246: 670–676.

4 Barber HJ. Evening primrose oil: a panacea? *Pharm J* 1988; 240: 723–725.

5 Horrobin DF. Gammalinolenic acid: an intermediate in essential fatty acid metabolism with potential as an ethical pharmaceutical and as a food. *Rev Contemp Pharmacother* 1990; 1: 1–45.

6 Carter JP. Gamma-linolenic acid as a nutrient. *Food Technol* 1988; 72.

7 Briggs CJ. Evening primrose. *Rev Pharm Can* 1986; 119: 249–254.

8 Barnes J. Herbal therapeutics (9). Women's health. *Pharm J* 2003; 270: 16–18.

9 Anon. *Data Sheet Compendium 1994–95*, 1520-1. Efamast, Epogam, Epogam Paediatric (Searle).

10 Lovell CR *et al.* Treatment of atopic eczema with evening primrose oil. *Lancet* 1981; 1: 278.

11 Schalin-Karrila M *et al.* Evening primrose oil in the treatment of atopic eczema: effect on clinical status, plasma phospholipid fatty acids and circulating blood prostaglandins. *Br J Dermatol* 1987; 117: 11–19.

12 Wright S, Burton JL. Oral evening primrose seed oil improves atopic eczema. *Lancet* 1982; ii: 1120–1122.

13 Stewart JCM *et al.* Treatment of severe and moderately severe atopic dermatitis with evening primrose oil (Epogam); a multicentre study. *J Nutr Med* 1991; 2: 9–15.

14 Bamford JTM *et al.* Atopic eczema unresponsive to evening primrose oil (linolenic and gamma-linolenic acids). *J Am Acad Dermatol* 1985; 13: 959–965.

15 Berth-Jones J, Graham-Brown RAC. Placebo-controlled trial of essential fatty acid supplementation in atopic dermatitis. *Lancet* 1993; 341: 1557–1560.

16 Brush MG. Efamol (evening primrose oil) in the treatment of the premenstrual syndrome. In: Horrobin DF, ed. *Clinical Uses for Essential Fatty Acids.* Buffalo, New York: Eden Press, 1982: 155.

17 Pye JK *et al.* Clinical experience of drug treatments for mastalgia. *Lancet* 1985; ii: 373–377.

18 Bandolier. Evening primrose oil for premenstrual syndrome. www.jr2.ox.ac.uk/bandolier/booth/alternat/AT058.html [accessed November 19, 2002]

19 Jamal GA *et al.* Gamma-linolenic acid in diabetic neuropathy. *Lancet* 1986; i: 1098.

20 Horrobin DF, Manku MS. How do polyunsaturated fatty acids lower plasma cholesterol levels?. *Lipids* 1983; 18: 558–562.

21 Vigibase, WHO Adverse Reactions database, Uppsala Monitoring Centre [accessed January 20, 2006]

Eyebright

Summary and Pharmaceutical Comment

Limited information is available regarding the constituents of eyebright and it is unclear which *Euphrasia* species is most commonly utilised. In addition, eyebright is also used as a common name for plants other than *Euphrasia* species. Little scientific information was found to justify the reputed herbal uses, although tannin constituents would provide an astringent effect. The use of home-made preparations for ophthalmic purposes should be avoided. Little is known regarding the toxicity of eyebright and, in view of the reported presence of unidentified alkaloids, it should be used with caution and excessive doses and prolonged treatment should be avoided.

Species (Family)

Euphrasia officinalis L. (Scrophulariaceae)

Other *Euphrasia* species, including *E. rostkoviana* Hayne, are used and these may differ in their chemical constituents. The genus *Euphrasia* consists of around 450 *Euphrasia* species and their wild hybrids and these are difficult to identify botanically.

Synonym(s)

Euphrasia

Part(s) Used

Herb

Pharmacopoeial and Other Monographs

BHP 1983[G7]
Martindale 35th edition[G85]

Legal Category (Licensed Products)

Eyebright is not included in the GSL.[G37]

Constituents

The following is compiled from several sources, including General References G2, G40 and G75.

Unless otherwise stated, constituents listed are for *E. officinalis*.

Acids Caffeic acid, ferulic acid.[1]

Alkaloids Unidentified tertiary alkaloids, choline, steam volatile bases.[1]

Amino acids Glycine, leucine and valine.

Flavonoids Four compounds (unidentified). Quercetin and rutin stated to be absent.[1] Quercetin, quercitrin and rutin have been documented for *E. rostkoviana*.

Iridoids Aucubin 0.05%. Additional glycosides have been reported for related *Euphrasia* species including catalpol, euphroside, eurostoside, geniposide, ixoroside and mussaenoside for *E. rostkoviana*.[2–5]

Phenethyl glycosides Dehydroconiferyl alcohol-4-β-D-glucoside[3] and eukovoside (3,4-dihydroxy-4-phenethyl-O-α-L-rhamnoside(13)-4-O-isoferuoyl-β-D- glucoside)[4] from *E. rostkoviana*.

Tannins About 12%. Condensed and hydrolysable; gallic acid is among the hydrolysis products.[1]

Volatile oils About 0.2%. Seven major and numerous minor components, mainly unidentified; four of the major compounds are thought to be aldehydes or ketones.[1]

Other constituents Bitter principle, β-carotene, phytosterols (e.g. β-sitosterol, stigmasterol),[1] resin, carbohydrates (e.g. arabinose, glucose, galactose) and vitamin C.

Food Use

Eyebright is listed by the Council of Europe as a natural source of food flavouring (category N3). This category indicates that eyebright can be added to foodstuffs in the traditionally accepted manner, although there is insufficient information available for an adequate assessment of potential toxicity.[G16]

Herbal Use

Eyebright is stated to possess anticatarrhal, astringent and anti-inflammatory properties. Traditionally it has been used for nasal catarrh, sinusitis and specifically for conjunctivitis when applied locally as an eye lotion.[G2, G7, G64]

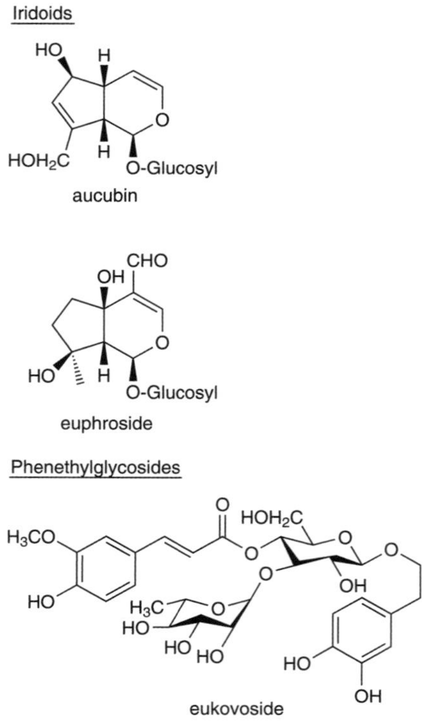

Figure 1 Selected constituents of eyebright.

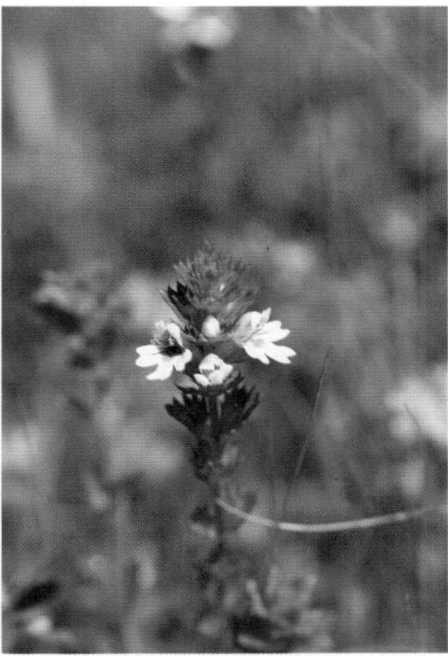

Figure 2 Eyebright (*Euphrasia officinalis*).

Dosage

Dosages for oral administration (adults) for traditional uses recommended in standard herbal reference texts are given below.

Dried herb 2–4 g as an infusion three times daily.(G7)

Liquid extract 2–4 mL (1 : 1 in 25% alcohol) three times daily.(G7)

Tincture 2–6 mL (1 : 5 in 45% alcohol) three times daily.(G7)

Pharmacological Actions

In vitro and animal studies

None documented for eyebright. Caffeic acid is bacteriostatic,(1) and a purgative action in mice has been documented for iridoid glycosides.(6) The purgative action of aucubin is approximately 0.05 times the potency of sennosides, with onset of diarrhoea stated to occur more than six hours after aucubin administration.(6) Tannins are known to possess astringent properties.

Clinical studies

There is a lack of clinical research assessing the effects of eyebright and rigorous randomised controlled clinical trials are required.

Side-effects, Toxicity

There is a lack of clinical safety and toxicity data for eyebright and further investigation of these aspects is required. Information in older literature states that doses of as little as 10–60 drops of eyebright tincture could lead to adverse effects, including mental confusion,(G22) although this requires confirmation.

Contra-indications, Warnings

The use of eyebright for ophthalmic application has been discouraged.(G60)

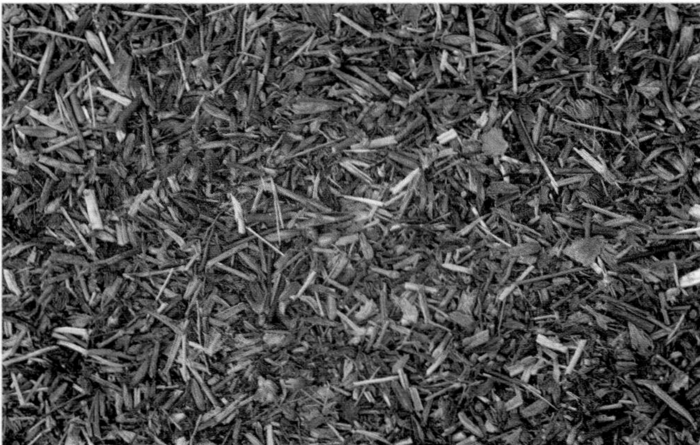

Figure 3 Eyebright – dried drug substance (herb).

Drug interactions None documented. However, the potential for preparations of eyebright to interact with other medicines administered concurrently, particularly those with similar or opposing effects, should be considered.

Pregnancy and lactation The safety of eyebright has not been established. In view of the lack of pharmacological and toxicity data, the use of eyebright during pregnancy and lactation should be avoided.

Preparations

Proprietary single-ingredient preparations

UK: Snore Calm.

Proprietary multi-ingredient preparations

Australia: Euphrasia Complex; Euphrasia Compound; Eye Health Herbal Plus Formula 4; Lifesystem Herbal Plus Formula 5 Eye Relief; Sambucus Complex. *Italy:* Eulux; Iridil. *Malaysia:* Eyebright Plus. *Switzerland:* Collypan; Oculosan; Tendro. *UK:* Se-Power; Summertime Tea Blend; Vital Eyes. *USA:* Eye Support Formula Herbal Blend.

References

1 Harkiss KJ, Timmins P. Studies in the Scrophulariaceae Part VIII. Phytochemical investigation of *Euphrasia officinalis*. *Planta Med* 1973; 23: 342–347.

2 Sticher O, Salama O. Iridoid glucosides from *Euphrasia rostkoviana*. *Planta Med* 1981; 42: 122–123.

3 Salama O *et al*. A lignan glucoside from *Euphrasia rostkoviana*. *Phytochemistry* 1981; 20: 2003–2004.

4 Sticher O *et al*. Structure analysis of eukovoside, a new phenylpropanoid glycoside from *Euphrasia rostkoviana*. *Planta Med* 1982; 45: 159.

5 Salama O, Sticher O. Iridoidglucoside von *Euphrasia rostkoviana* 4. Mitteilung über Euphrasia-Glykoside. *Planta Med* 1983; 47: 90–94.

6 Inouye H *et al*. Purgative activities of iridoid glycosides. *Planta Med* 1974; 25: 285–288.

False Unicorn

Summary and Pharmaceutical Comment

The chemistry of false unicorn is poorly documented and no scientific evidence was located to justify the herbal uses. In view of this and the lack of toxicity data, the use of false unicorn should be avoided.

F

Species (Family)

Chamaelirium luteum (L.) A. Gray (Melanthiaceae)

Synonym(s)

Blazing Star, *Chamaelirium carolianum* Wild., Devil's-bit, Helonias, *Helonias dioica* (Walter) Pursh., *Helonias lutea* (L.) Ker Gawl., Starwort, *Veratrum luteum* L.

Part(s) Used

Rhizome, root

Pharmacopoeial and Other Monographs

BHP 1996[G9]
Martindale 35th edition[G85]

Legal Category (Licensed Products)

GSL[G37]

Constituents

The following is compiled from several sources, including General References G40 and G48.

Limited chemical information is available on false unicorn. It is stated to contain a steroidal saponin glycoside, chamaelirin, and another glycoside helonin.

Food Use

False unicorn is not used in foods.

Herbal Use

False unicorn is stated to possess an action on the uterus. Traditionally it has been used for ovarian dysmenorrhoea, leucorrhoea and specifically for amenorrhoea. It is reported to be useful for vomiting of pregnancy and threatened miscarriage.[G7, G8, G64]

Dosage

Dosages for oral administration (adults) for traditional uses recommended in standard herbal reference texts are given below.

Dried rhizome/root 1–2 g as an infusion three times daily.[G7]

Liquid extract 1–2 mL (1 : 1 in 45% alcohol) three times daily.[G7]

Tincture 2–5 mL (1 : 5 in 45% alcohol) three times daily.[G7]

Pharmacological Actions

None documented.

Clinical studies

There is a lack of clinical research assessing the effects of centaury and rigorous randomised controlled clinical trials are required.

Side-effects, Toxicity

There is a lack of clinical safety and toxicity data for false unicorn and further investigation of these aspects is required. It is stated

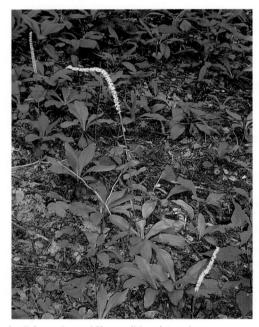

Figure 1 False unicorn (*Chamaelirium luteum*).

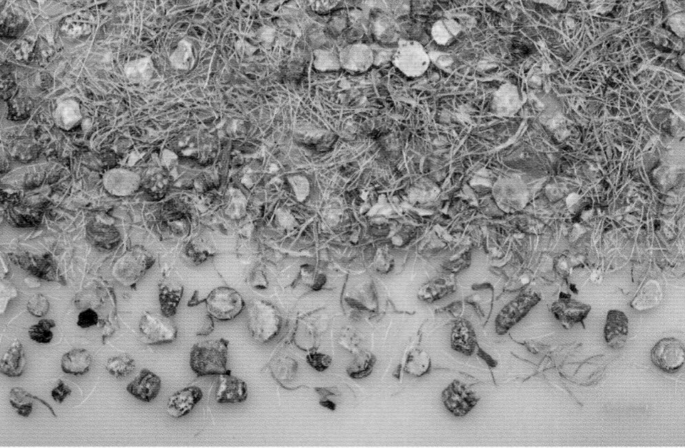

Figure 2 False unicorn – dried drug substance (root).

that large doses of false unicorn may cause nausea and vomiting.[G7]

Contra-indications, Warnings

None documented.

Drug interactions None documented. However, in view of the lack of phytochemical and pharmacological information for false unicorn, the potential for preparations of false unicorn to interact with other medicines administered concurrently, particularly those with similar or opposing effects, should still be considered.

Pregnancy and lactation The safety of false unicorn has not been established. In view of the lack of phytochemical, pharmacological and toxicity data, and its reputed action as a uterine tonic, the use of false unicorn during pregnancy and lactation should be avoided.

Preparations

Proprietary multi-ingredient preparations

Australia: Nervatona Plus. *UK:* Period Pain Relief.

Fenugreek

Summary and Pharmaceutical Comment

Fenugreek seeds contain a high proportion of mucilaginous fibre, together with various other pharmacologically active compounds including steroidal and amine components. The majority of the traditional uses of fenugreek are probably attributable to the mucilage content. In addition, hypocholesterolaemic and hypoglycaemic actions have been documented for fenugreek in both laboratory animals and humans. The mechanism by which fenugreek exerts these actions is unclear. Proposed theories include a reduction in carbohydrate absorption by the mucilaginous fibre, and an effect on cholesterol metabolism, cholesterol absorption and bile acid excretion by the saponin components. Toxicity studies indicate fenugreek seeds to be relatively non-toxic, although the presence of pharmacologically active constituents would suggest that excessive ingestion is inadvisable.

Species (Family)

Trigonella foenum-graecum L. (Leguminosae)

Synonym(s)

Bockshornsame

Part(s) Used

Seed

Pharmacopoeial and Other Monographs

BHP 1996(G9)
BP 2007(G84)
Complete German Commission E(G3)
Martindale 35th edition(G85)
Ph Eur 2007(G81)

Legal Category (Licensed Products)

GSL(G37)

Constituents

The following is compiled from several sources, including General Reference G2.

Alkaloids Pyridine-type. Gentianine, trigonelline (up to 0.13%), choline (0.05%).

Proteins and amino acids Protein (23–25%) containing high quantities of lysine and tryptophan. Free amino acids include 4-hydroxyisoleucine (0.09%), histidine, lysine and arginine.

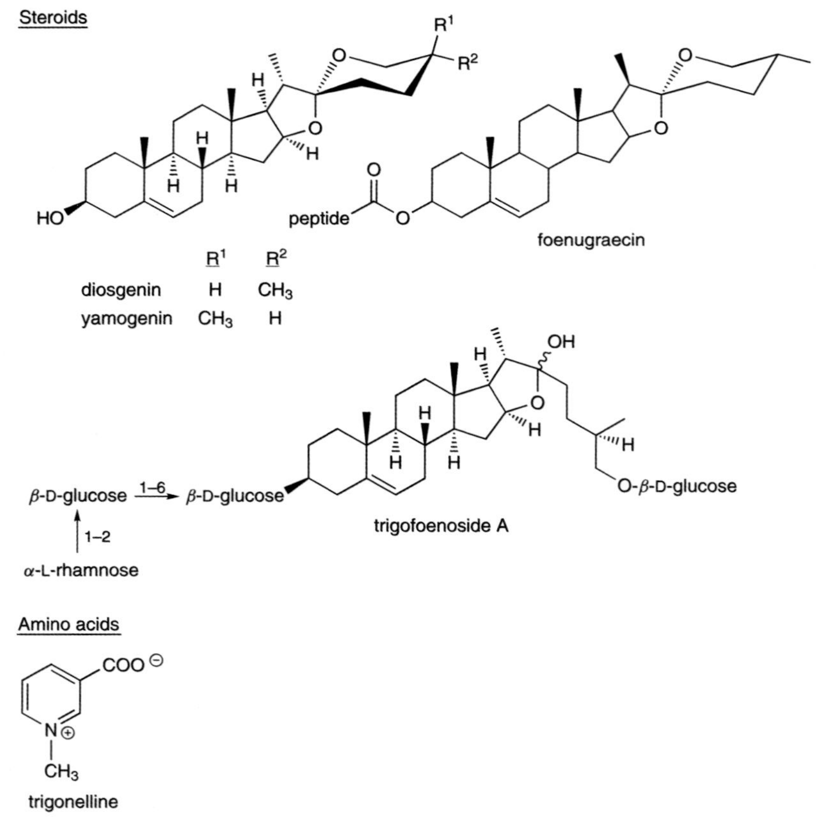

Steroids

	R^1	R^2
diosgenin	H	CH_3
yamogenin	CH_3	H

foenugraecin

trigofoenoside A

β-D-glucose →(1–6) β-D-glucose; α-L-rhamnose →(1–2) β-D-glucose; O-β-D-glucose

Amino acids

trigonelline

Figure 1 Selected constituents of fenugreek.

Flavonoids Flavone (apigenin, luteolin) glycosides including orientin and vitexin, quercetin (flavonol).

Saponins 0.6–1.7%. Glycosides yielding steroidal sapogenins diosgenin and yamogenin (major), with tigogenin, neotigogenin, gitogenin, neogitogenin, smilagenin, sarsasapogenin, yuccagenin;[1] fenugreekine, a sapogenin-peptide ester involving diosgenin and yamogenin;[2] trigofoenosides A–G (furostanol glycosides).[3–6]

Other constituents Coumarin,[7] lipids (5–8%),[8] mucilaginous fibre (50%),[8] vitamins (including nicotinic acid) and minerals.

Food Use

Fenugreek is listed by the Council of Europe as a natural source of food flavouring (category N2). This category indicates that fenugreek can be added to foodstuffs in small quantities, with a possible limitation of an active principle (as yet unspecified) in the final product.[G16] Previously fenugreek extracts have been permitted in foods at concentrations usually below 0.05%. In addition, fenugreek has been listed as GRAS (Generally Recognised As Safe).

Herbal Use

Fenugreek is stated to possess mucilaginous demulcent, laxative, nutritive, expectorant and orexigenic properties, and has been used topically as an emollient and vulnerary. Traditionally, it has been used in the treatment of anorexia, dyspepsia, gastritis and convalescence, and topically for furunculosis, myalgia, lymphadenitis, gout, wounds and leg ulcers.[G2, G7, G22, G64]

Dosage

Dosages for oral administration (adults) for traditional uses recommended in older standard herbal reference texts are given below.

Seed 1–6 g or equivalent three times daily.[G49]

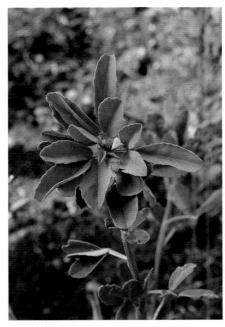

Figure 2 Fenugreek (*Trigonella foenum-graecum*).

Figure 3 Fenugreek – dried drug substance (seed).

Pharmacological Actions

In vitro and animal studies

Hypocholesterolaemic activity has been reported for fenugreek in rats[9, G41] and alloxan-diabetic dogs.[10] Activity has been attributed to the fibre and saponin fractions, and not to lipid or amino acid fractions.[9, 10] Studies have reported a reduction in cholesterol but not triglyceride concentrations,[9] or in both cholesterol and triglyceride concentrations, but without significant alterations in high-density lipoprotein (HDL) and low-density lipoprotein (LDL) concentrations.[10]

Hypoglycaemic activity has been observed in rabbits, rats and dogs, and attributed to the defatted seed fraction (DSF),[8] trigonelline, nicotinic acid and coumarin.[7, 11] Oral administration of DSF reduced hyperglycaemia in four alloxan-diabetic dogs, and reduced the response to an oral glucose tolerance test in eight normal dogs, whereas the lipid fraction had no effect on serum glucose and insulin concentrations.[8] The high fibre content (50%) of DSF was thought to contribute to its antidiabetic effect although the initial rate of glucose absorption was not affected.[8] Nicotinic acid and coumarin were reported to be the major hypoglycaemic components of fenugreek seeds, following administration to normal and alloxan-diabetic rats.[7] The hypoglycaemic action exhibited by coumarin was still significant 24 hours post administration.[7] In addition, a slight antidiuretic action was noted for coumarin.[7] Trigonelline inhibited cortisone-induced hyperglycaemia in rabbits if administered (250 mg/kg) concomitantly or two hours before, but not two hours after, cortisone.[11] In addition, trigonelline exhibited significant hypoglycaemic activity in alloxan-diabetic rats (50 mg/kg), lasting 24 hours.[11]

A stimulant action on the isolated uterus (guinea-pig), especially during late pregnancy, has been noted for both aqueous and alcoholic extracts.[G41] An aqueous extract is stated to increase the number of heart beats in the isolated mammalian heart.[G41]

In vitro antiviral activity against vaccinia virus has been reported for fenugreekine, which also possesses cardiotonic, hypoglycaemic, diuretic, antiphlogistic and antihypertensive properties.[2]

Clinical studies

There is a lack of clinical research assessing the effects of fenugreek and rigorous randomised controlled clinical trials are required.

A transient hypoglycaemic effect was observed in 5 of 10 diabetic patients who received 500 mg oral trigonelline whilst fasting.[11] Increasing the dose did not increase this effect, and 500 mg ingested three times a day for five days did not alter the diurnal blood glucose concentration.[11] Hypoglycaemic activity in healthy individuals has been reported for whole seed extracts, with slightly lesser activity exhibited by gum isolate, extracted seeds and cooked seeds.[12] The addition of fenugreek to an oral glucose tolerance test reduced serum glucose and insulin concentrations. Chronic ingestion (21 days) of extracted seeds (25 g seeds daily incorporated into two meals) by non-insulin-dependent diabetics improved plasma glucose and insulin responses (no control group), and reduced 24-hour urinary glucose concentrations.[12] Furthermore, in two diabetic insulin-dependent subjects, daily administration of 25 g fenugreek seed powder reduced fasting plasma-glucose profile, glycosuria and daily insulin requirements (56–20 units) after eight weeks. A significant reduction in serum cholesterol concentrations in diabetic patients was also noted.[12]

F

Side-effects, Toxicity

None documented. However, there is a lack of clinical safety and toxicity data for fenugreek and further investigation of these aspects is required. Acute toxicity values (LD_{50}) documented for fenugreek alcoholic seed extract are 5 g/kg (rat, oral) and 2 g/kg (rabbit, dermal).[13] The alcoholic seed extract is reported to be non-irritating and non-sensitising to human skin and non-phototoxic (mice, pigs).[13] Coumarin is a toxic seed component.[7] Acute LD_{50} (rat, oral) values per kilogram documented for various seed constituents are 5 g (trigonelline), 8.8 g (nicotinic acid), 7.4 g (nicotinamide) and 0.72 g (coumarin).[7]

Contra-indications, Warnings

Drug interactions None documented. However, the potential for preparations of fenugreek to interact with other medicines administered concurrently, particularly those with similar or opposing effects, should be considered. There is limited evidence from preclinical and preliminary clinical studies that fenugreek has hypoglycaemic activity. Caution may be advisable in patients receiving monoamine oxidase inhibitor (MAOI), hormonal or anticoagulant therapies in view of amine, steroidal saponin and coumarin constituents, respectively, although their clinical significance is unclear. Cardioactivity has been documented *in vitro*. The absorption of drugs taken concomitantly with fenugreek may be affected (high mucilaginous fibre content).

Pregnancy and lactation Fenugreek is reputed to be oxytocic[G22] and *in vitro* uterine stimulant activity has been documented. In view of this, and the documented pharmacologically active components, the use of fenugreek during pregnancy and lactation in doses greatly exceeding those normally encountered in foods is not advisable.

Preparations

Proprietary single-ingredient preparations

France: Fenugrene; Sthenorex.

Proprietary multi-ingredient preparations

Australia: Garlic and Horseradish + C Complex; Panax Complex. *India:* Happy'tizer. *Malaysia:* Horseradish Plus.

References

1 Gupta RK *et al.* Minor steroidal sapogenins from fenugreek seeds, *Trigonella foenum-graecum*. *J Nat Prod* 1986; 49: 1153.
2 Ghosal S *et al.* Fenugreekine, a new steroidal sapogenin-peptide ester of *Trigonella foenum-graecum*. *Phytochemistry* 1974; 13: 2247–2251.
3 Gupta RK *et al.* Two furostanol saponins from *Trigonella feonum-graecum*. *Phytochemistry* 1986; 25: 2205–2207.
4 Varshney IP *et al.* Saponins from *Trigonella foenum-graecum* leaves. *J Nat Prod* 1984; 47: 44–46.
5 Gupta RK *et al.* Furostanol glycosides from *Trigonella foenum-graecum* seeds. *Phytochemistry* 1984; 23: 2605–2607.
6 Gupta RK *et al.* Furostanol glycosides from *Trigonella foenum-graecum* seeds. *Phytochemistry* 1985; 24: 2399–2401.
7 Shani J *et al.* Hypoglycaemic effect of *Trigonella foenum graecum* and *Lupinus termis* (Leguminosae) seeds and their major alkaloids in alloxan-diabetic and normal rats. *Arch Int Pharmacodyn Ther* 1974; 210: 27–37.
8 Ribes G *et al.* Hypocholesterolaemic and hypotriglyceridaemic effects of subfractions from fenugreek seeds in alloxan diabetic dogs. *Phytother Res* 1987; 1: 38–42.
9 Ribes G *et al.* Effects of fenugreek seeds on endocrine pancreatic secretions in dogs. *Ann Nutr Metab* 1984; 28: 37–43.
10 Sharma RD. An evaluation of hypocholesterolemic factor of fenugreek seeds (*T. foenum graecum*) in rats. *Nutr Rep Int* 1986; 33: 669–677.
11 Mishkinsky J *et al.* Hypoglycaemic effect of trigonelline. *Lancet* 1967; 2: 1311–1312.
12 Sharma RD. Effect of fenugreek seeds and leaves on blood glucose and serum insulin responses in human subjects. *Nutr Res* 1986; 6: 1353–1364.
13 Opdyke DLJ. Fenugreek absolute. *Food Cosmet Toxicol* 1978; 16 (Suppl. Suppl.): 755–756.

Feverfew

Summary and Pharmaceutical Comment

Feverfew is characterised by the sesquiterpene lactone constituents, in particular by parthenolide which is thought to be the main active component. *In vitro* studies provide some evidence to support the reputation of feverfew as a herb used to treat migraine and arthritis. Some clinical studies have suggested that feverfew leaf preparations may be a useful prophylactic remedy against migraine, although further research is deemed necessary to establish the benefits. It has been recommended that feverfew should only be used by sufferers who have proved unresponsive to conventional forms of migraine treatment. Those using feverfew as a remedy for migraine should preferably do so under medical supervision.

Results of a study that investigated the usefulness of feverfew in treating rheumatoid arthritis were less encouraging: feverfew provided no additional benefit when added to existing non-steroidal anti-inflammatory treatment. Feverfew products currently available are unlicensed and vary in their recommended daily doses. Furthermore, variation between the stated and actual amount of feverfew in commercial products (based on their ability to inhibit platelet secretion) has been reported.

Species (Family)

Tanacetum parthenium (L.) Schultz Bip. (Asteraceae/Compositae)

Synonym(s)

Altamisa, *Chrysanthemum parthenium* (L.) Bernh., non (Lam.) Gaterau, *Leucanthemum parthenium* (L.) Gren & Godron, *Pyrethrum parthenium* (L.) Sm.

Part(s) Used

Leaf, aerial parts

Pharmacopoeial and Other Monographs

BHC 1992[G6]
BHP 1996[G9]
BP 2007[G84]
ESCOP 2003[G76]
Martindale 35th edition[G85]
Ph Eur 2007[G81]
USP29/NF24[G86]

Legal Category (Licensed Products)

Feverfew is not included in the GSL.[G37]

Constituents

The following is compiled from several sources, including General Reference G6.

Terpenoids Sesquiterpene lactones: germacranolides (GE), guaianolides (GU) and eudesmanolides (EU). The structural feature common to all three types is an α-unsaturated γ-lactone moiety, and examples of each type include parthenolide, 3-β-hydroxy-parthenolide, costunolide, 3-β-hydroxycostunolide, artemorin, 8-α-hydroxyestafiatin and chrysanthemonin (novel dimeric nucleus) (GE); artecanin, chrysanthemin A (canin) and B (stereoisomers), chrysanthemolide, partholide, two chlorine-containing sesquiterpene lactones (GU); magnolialide, reynosin, santamarine, 1-β-hydroxyarbusculin and 5-β-hydroxyreynosin (EU).[1–5]

Volatile oils (0.02–0.07%). Various monoterpene and sesquiterpene components (e.g. camphor, borneol, α-pinene derivatives, germacrene, farnesene and their esters).

Other constituents Pyrethrin, flavonoids, tannins (type unspecified) and melatonin.[6]

Food Use

Feverfew is not generally used in foods.

Herbal Use

Feverfew has traditionally been used in the treatment of migraine, tinnitus, vertigo, arthritis, fever, menstrual disorders, difficulty during labour, stomach ache, toothache and insect bites. Modern use of feverfew is focused on its effects in the prevention and treatment of migraine.[7, 8]

Feverfew products currently available are unlicensed adn vary in their recommended daily doses.[9]

Dosage

Limited information is available regarding the traditional dose of feverfew. The doses (oral administration, adults) that have been recommended for migraine prophylaxis are as follows.

Leaf (fresh) 2.5 leaves daily with or after food.

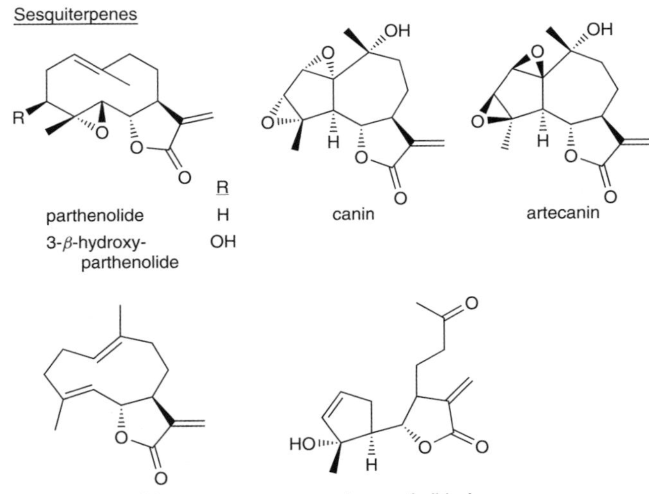

Figure 1 Selected constituents of feverfew.

Leaf (freeze-dried) 50 mg daily with or after food.

Aerial parts (dried) 50–200 mg daily; equivalent to 0.2–0.6 mg parthenolide daily.[G6, G52]

Clinical trials of feverfew for the prevention of migraine have assessed the effects of, for example, 143 mg of a dried alcoholic extract of feverfew daily (equivalent to 0.5 mg parthenolide),[10] and capsules containing powdered feverfew leaf 50 mg daily,[11, 12] for one to six months.

Pharmacological Actions

In vitro and animal studies

Feverfew extracts have been documented to inhibit platelet aggregation and prostaglandin, thromboxane and leukotriene production, although feverfew has also been reported to have no effect on cyclooxygenase (the mechanism by which non-steroidal anti-inflammatory drugs inhibit prostaglandin production).[13–15] Instead, feverfew is thought to act by inhibiting the enzyme phospholipase A_2, which facilitates the release of arachidonic acid from the phospholipid cellular membrane.[14–16] The clinical significance of this action has been questioned.[17] In addition, *in vitro* experiments have shown that feverfew extracts inhibit the interaction of human platelets with collagen substrates.[18, 19] Feverfew has been shown to inhibit granule secretion in blood platelets and neutrophils, which has been associated with the aetiology of migraine and rheumatoid arthritis, respectively.[20] Feverfew was also found to inhibit the release of vitamin B_{12}-binding protein from polymorphonuclear leukocytes, but to be ineffective against platelet and polymorphonucleocyte secretion induced by calcium ionophore A2318.[20] Sesquiterpene lactone constituents of feverfew containing an α-methylene butyrolactone unit are thought to be responsible for the antisecretory activity.[21] Their inhibitory effect on platelet aggregation is thought to involve neutralisation of sulfhydryl groups on specific enzymes of proteins that are necessary for platelet aggregation and secretion.[22] A similar mode of action has been proposed for the inhibitory action of feverfew on polymorphonuclocyte secretion.[23] In addition, feverfew extracts have been reported to produce a concentration-dependent inhibition of anti-IgE-induced histamine release from mast cells.[24] The authors concluded that the mechanism of action of the feverfew extract was different to that of both cromoglycate and quercetin.

Parthenolide markedly interfered with contractile and relaxant mechanisms in blood vessels.[G52] An aqueous extract of feverfew administered intravenously significantly inhibited collagen-induced bronchoconstriction in guinea-pigs.[G52]

The presence of large numbers of lymphocytes and monocytes in the synovium is considered to be of significance in rheumatoid arthritis.[25] Feverfew extract and parthenolide have been documented to inhibit mitogen-induced proliferation of human peripheral blood mononuclear cells and mitogen-induced prostaglandin E_2 (PGE_2) production by synovial cells.[25] The feverfew extract and parthenolide also proved to be cytotoxic to mitogen-treated peripheral blood mononuclear cells and the authors considered that this cytotoxicity was responsible for the actions observed.[25] *In vitro* studies using crude feverfew extracts and parthenolide have documented other activities that may contribute to the reported anti-inflammatory effects of feverfew. Pretreatment of human synovial fibroblasts with feverfew extract and with purified parthenolide inhibited cytokine-induced expression of intercellular adhesion molecule 1 (ICAM-1) expression.[26] A reduction in T cell adhesion to the treated fibroblasts also occurred. In other *in vitro* studies, parthenolide inhibited lipopolysaccharide-induced interleukin-12 (IL-12) production by mouse macrophages in a concentration-dependent manner.[27] Parthenolide has also been shown to inhibit promoter activity of the inducible nitric oxide synthase gene in a human monocyte cell line, THP-1, in a concentration-dependent manner.[28] (Excessive nitric oxide production in inflammatory cells is thought to be a causative factor in cellular injury in inflammatory disease.) Anti-inflammatory activity of feverfew has also been attributed to the presence of flavonoids, e.g. santonin.[29]

Anti-inflammatory properties have also been documented for feverfew extract and parthenolide *in vivo*. Oral administration of feverfew extract (10, 20 and 40 mg/kg) reduced carrageenan-induced oedema in rat paw in a dose-dependent manner.[30] Intraperitoneal parthenolide (1 and 2 mg/kg) also demonstrated anti-inflammatory effects in this model.

Parthenolide has been documented to have cytotoxic activity in Eagle's 9KB carcinoma of the nasopharynx cell culture system, the activity being associated with the presence of an α-methylene-γ-lactone moiety in the molecule.[31] *In vitro*, parthenolide has been shown to inhibit growth of mouse fibrosarcoma (MN-11) and human lymphoma (TK6) cell lines.[32] The effect appeared to be reversible.

Antinociceptive properties have been reported for feverfew and parthenolide *in vivo*. Oral administration of feverfew extract (10, 20 and 40 mg/kg) and intraperitoneal administration of parthe-

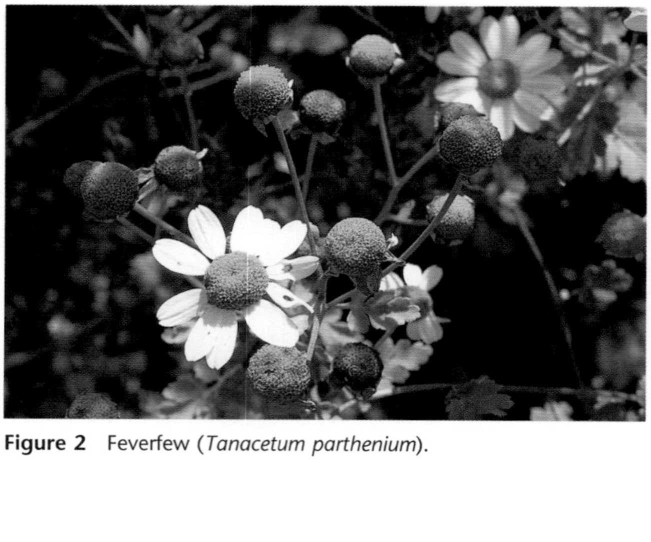

Figure 2 Feverfew (*Tanacetum parthenium*).

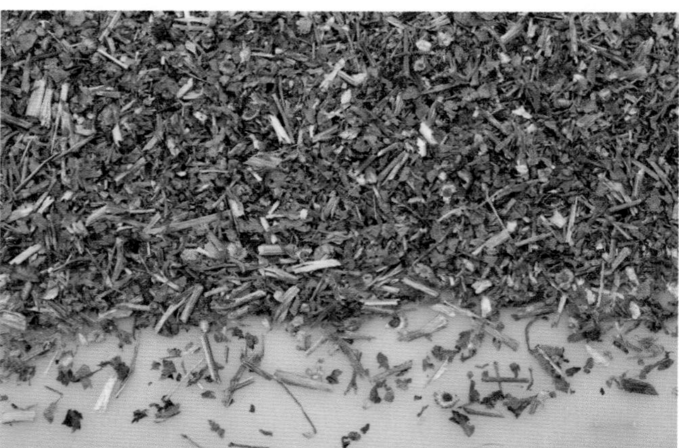

Figure 3 Feverfew – dried drug substance (herb).

nolide (1 and 2 mg/kg) led to reductions in acetic acid-induced writhing in mice.[30]

Antimicrobial properties against Gram-positive bacteria, yeasts and filamentous fungi *in vitro* have been documented for parthenolide.[33] Gram-negative bacteria were not affected.

Clinical studies

Migraine Several placebo-controlled clinical trials have assessed the effects of preparations of feverfew in the prevention of migraine.[10–12, 34]

A randomised, double-blind, placebo-controlled trial involved 17 patients who had been successfully controlling their migraine by eating raw feverfew leaves for at least three months.[11] Patients either continued to receive feverfew (50 mg daily) or were given placebo for six periods of four weeks. The authors reported that the placebo group experienced a significant increase in the frequency and severity of headache. Those given feverfew showed no change. It was suggested that the placebo group was in fact suffering withdrawal symptoms from feverfew and a 'post-feverfew syndrome' was described (*see* Side-effects, Toxicity).

Another study, a randomised double-blind, placebo-controlled, crossover trial involved 72 adults who had experienced migraine for more than two years and who had at least one attack per month.[34] The only concurrent medication allowed was the oral contraceptive pill. Patients completed a one-month, single-blind, placebo run-in phase, followed by four months' administration of placebo/active and four months' crossover. It was reported that patients experienced a 24% reduction in the number of attacks during feverfew treatment (one capsule daily; 70–114 mg feverfew equivalent to 2.19 μg parthenolide) although the duration of each individual attack was not significantly affected. Patients allocated to the active and then placebo group did not experience the withdrawal symptoms documented in another study,[11] although patients involved in the previous study had used feverfew over a longer period of time.

In a randomised, double-blind, placebo-controlled trial, 57 patients received capsules of dried, powdered feverfew leaves (parthenolide 0.2%) 100 mg daily for 60 days (open-label phase), followed by randomisation to feverfew or placebo (ground parsley) for 30 days then crossover to the other arm for 30 days.[12] There was no wash-out between crossover. At the end of the open-label phase (i.e. during which all participants received feverfew), there was a significant reduction in pain intensity and symptoms, such as vomiting and sensitivity to light, compared with baseline values ($p < 0.001$). At the end of the double-blind, crossover phase, it was reported that pain intensity was significantly lower during feverfew administration, compared with placebo administration ($p < 0.01$).

Thus, these three studies reported beneficial effects for feverfew, as demonstrated by fewer and/or less severe migraine episodes and/or reductions in pain intensity, compared with placebo.[11, 12, 34] However, one double-blind, placebo-controlled trial involving 50 feverfew-naïve patients who experienced migraine attacks at least once a month reported no difference in the number of migraine attacks between placebo recipients and participants who received capsules containing a dried alcoholic extract of feverfew equivalent to 0.5 mg parthenolide daily for nine months.[10] Another randomised, double-blind, placebo-controlled, crossover trial involving 20 patients with migraine assessed the effects of feverfew 100 mg daily for two months on serotonin uptake and platelet activity.[35] This trial found no effect for feverfew in the prevention of migraine attacks and also reported that feverfew administration had no effect on the uptake of serotonin by platelets.

The authors of a Cochrane systematic review of five randomised, double-blind, placebo-controlled trials (four studies mentioned above,[10–12, 34] plus one another) concluded that although some trials suggest that feverfew preparations are superior to placebo in preventing migraine, further well-designed clinical trials are required to establish the beneficial effects of feverfew for migraine prophylaxis.[36] Furthermore, the trials included in the review assessed the effects of different feverfew preparations (e.g. fresh or dried leaves), administered according to different dosage regimens (e.g. approximately 50–143 mg powdered feverfew leaf daily for one to six months). Many other marketed preparations of feverfew leaf have not been assessed at all in controlled clinical trials.

F

Rheumatoid arthritis A double-blind, placebo-controlled, non-crossover trial studying the use of feverfew in rheumatoid arthritis has also been documented.[37] Forty-one female patients with inflammatory joint symptoms inadequately controlled by non-steroidal anti-inflammatory drugs were given either one feverfew capsule (70–86 mg equivalent to 2–3 μmol parthenolide) daily, or one placebo capsule, for six weeks. Current non-steroidal therapy was maintained. It was concluded that patients in the trial had experienced no additional benefit from feverfew.[37] The authors commented that while concomitant non-steroidal anti-inflammatory drug therapy has been stated to reduce the effectiveness of feverfew, the majority of rheumatoid arthritis sufferers will use feverfew to supplement existing therapy.

Side-effects, Toxicity

Clinical safety and toxicity data for feverfew is limited, and further investigation of these aspects is required.

Randomised, double-blind, placebo-controlled trials have documented the following adverse effects during feverfew administration, although most effects were also reported (sometimes more frequently) during placebo administration: mouth ulcers (reported more frequently during placebo administration in one study[34]), sore mouth, abdominal pain and indigestion, diarrhoea, flatulence, nausea, dizziness and skin rash.[10, 11, 34] On balance, adverse effects reported for feverfew are mild and transient, are similar to those reported during placebo administration and occur with a similar frequency.

A 'post-feverfew syndrome' has been described on stopping feverfew administration[11] (*see* Pharmacological Action, Clinical studies) with symptoms such as nervousness, tension headaches, insomnia, stiffness/pain in joints and tiredness.

The onset of side-effects with feverfew is reported to vary, with symptoms becoming apparent within the first week of treatment, or appearing gradually over the first two months.

Sesquiterpene lactones that contain an α-methylene butyrolactone ring are known to cause allergic reactions.[38, G51] Compounds with this structure are present in feverfew and reports of contact dermatitis have been documented.[39–42] No documented allergic reactions following oral ingestion were located.

No chronic toxicity studies have been reported. However, detailed haematological analysis of 60 feverfew users, some of whom had used feverfew for more than one year, did not show any significant differences when compared with analysis of controls.[43] A human toxicity study has investigated whether the sesquiterpene lactones in feverfew induce chromosomal or other changes in normal human cells of individuals who have taken the herb.[44] The study compared 30 chronic female feverfew users (leaves, tablets or capsules taken daily for more than 11 consecutive months) with matched non-users. The results of lymphocyte cultures established from blood samples taken over a period of several months were stated to indicate that feverfew affects neither the frequency of chromosomal aberrations nor the frequency of sister chromatid exchanges in the circulating peripheral lymphocytes.

Preclinical data

An LD_{50} value for feverfew has not been estimated. No adverse effects were reported for rats and guinea-pigs receiving feverfew at doses 100 and 150 times the human daily dose, respectively.[43]

Contra-indications, Warnings

Feverfew is contra-indicated in individuals with a known hypersensitivity to other members of the family Compositae (Asteraceae), such as chamomile, ragweed and yarrow. Feverfew should not be ingested by individuals who develop a rash on contact with the plant.

Feverfew should only be considered as a treatment for migraine that has proved unresponsive to conventional forms of medication. Although traditionally recommended as a remedy for rheumatic conditions, self-medication with feverfew should not be undertaken without first consulting a doctor.

Drug interactions None documented. However, in view of the documented pharmacological actions of feverfew, the potential for preparations of feverfew to interact with other medicines administered concurrently, particularly those with similar or opposing effects, should be considered.

Pregnancy and lactation Feverfew is contra-indicated during pregnancy. It is reputed to be an abortifacient and to affect the menstrual cycle. It is documented to modify menstrual flow, cause abortion in cattle and induce uterine contraction in full-term women.[G30]

Preparations

Proprietary single-ingredient preparations

Australia: Herbal Headache Relief. *Brazil:* Tanaceto; Tenliv. *Canada:* Tanacet. *UK:* Tanacet.

Proprietary multi-ingredient preparations

Australia: Albizia Complex; Extralife Arthri-Care; Extralife Migrai-Care; Guaiacum Complex.

References

1 Stefanovic M *et al*. Sesquiterpene lactones from the domestic plant species *Tanacetum parthenium* L. (Compositae). *J Serb Chem Soc* 1985; 50: 435–441.
2 Bohlmann F, Zdero C. Sesquiterpene lactones and other constituents from *Tanacetum parthenium*. *Phytochemistry* 1982: 21: 2543–2549.
3 Osawa T, Taylor D. Revised structure and stereochemistry of chrysartemin B. *Tetrahedron Lett* 1977; 13: 1169–1172.
4 Hylands DM, Hylands PJ. New sesquiterpene lactones from feverfew. *Phytochem Soc Eur Symp* 1986: 17.
5 Wagner H *et al*. New chlorine-containing sesquiterpene lactones from *Chrysanthemum parthenium*. *Planta Med* 1988; 54: 171–172.
6 Murch SJ *et al*. Melatonin in feverfew and other medicinal plants. *Lancet* 1997; 350: 1598–1599.
7 Awang DVC. Feverfew fever – a headache for the consumer. *Herbalgram* 1993; 29: 34–36.
8 Berry M. Feverfew. *Pharm J* 1994; 253: 806–808.
9 Baldwin CA *et al*. What pharmacists should know about feverfew. *Pharm J* 1987; 239: 237–238.
10 De Weerdt CJ, Bootsma HPR, Hendriks H. Herbal medicines in migraine prevention. Randomized double-blind placebo-controlled crossover trial of a feverfew preparation. *Phytomedicine* 1996; 3: 225–230.
11 Johnson ES *et al*. Efficacy of feverfew as prophylactic treatment of migraine. *BMJ* 1985; 291: 569–573.
12 Palevitch D *et al*. Feverfew (*Tanacetum parthenium*) as a prophylactic treatment for migraine: a double-blind placebo-controlled study. *Phytother Res* 1997; 11: 508–511.
13 Collier HOJ *et al*. Extract of feverfew inhibits prostaglandin biosynthesis. *Lancet* 1980; ii: 922–973.
14 Makheja AM, Bailey JM. The active principle in feverfew. *Lancet* 1981; ii, 1054.
15 Capasso F. The effect of an aqueous extract of *Tanacetum parthenium* L. on arachidonic acid metabolism by rat peritoneal leucocytes. *J Pharm Pharmacol* 1986; 38: 71–72.
16 Makheja AM, Bailey JM. A platelet phospholipase inhibitor from the medicinal herb feverfew (*Tanacetum parthenium*). *Prostaglandins Leukot Med* 1982: 8: 653–660.
17 Biggs MJ *et al*. Platelet aggregation in patients using feverfew for migraine. *Lancet* 1982; ii: 776.
18 Loesche W *et al*. Feverfew – an antithrombotic drug? *Folia Haematol* 1988; 115: 181–184.
19 Groenewegen WA, Heptinstall S. Amounts of feverfew in commercial preparations of the herb. *Lancet* 1986; i: 44–45.
20 Heptinstall S *et al*. Extracts of feverfew inhibit granule secretion in blood platelets and polymorphonuclear leucocytes. *Lancet* 1985; i: 1071–1073.
21 Groenewegen WA *et al*. Compounds extracted from feverfew that have anti-secretory activity contain an α-methylene butyrolactone unit. *J Pharm Pharmacol* 1986; 38: 709–712.
22 Heptinstall S *et al*. Extracts of feverfew may inhibit platelet behaviour via neutralization of sulphydryl groups. *J Pharm Pharmacol* 1987; 39: 459–465.
23 Lösche W *et al*. Inhibition of the behaviour of human polynuclear leukocytes by an extract of *Chrysanthemum parthenium*. *Planta Med* 1988; 54: 381–384.
24 Hayes NA, Foreman JC. The activity of compounds extracted from feverfew on histamine release from rat mast cells. *J Pharm Pharmacol* 1987; 39: 466–470.
25 O'Neill LAJ *et al*. Extracts of feverfew inhibit mitogen-induced human peripheral blood mononuclear cell proliferation and cytokine mediated responses: a cytotoxic effect. *Br J Clin Pharmac* 1987; 23: 81–83.
26 Piela-Smith TH, Liu X. Feverfew extracts and the sesquiterpene lactone partenolide inhibit intercellular adhesion molecule-1 expression in human synovial fibroblasts. *Cell Immunol* 2001; 209: 89–96.
27 Kang BY *et al*. Inhibition of interleukin-12 production in lipopolysaccharide-activated mouse macrophages by parthenolide, a predominant sesquiterpene lactone in *Tanacetum parthenium*: involvement of nuclear factor-kappa-B. *Immunol Lett* 2001; 77: 159–163.
28 Fukuda K *et al*. Inhibition by parthenolide of phorbol ester-induced transcriptional activation of inducible nitric oxide synthase gene in a human monocyte cell line THP-1. *Biochem Pharmacol* 2000; 60: 595–600.
29 Williams CA *et al*. A biologically active lipophilic flavonol from *Tanacetum parthenium*. *Phytochemistry* 1995; 38: 267–270.
30 Jain NK, Kulkarni SK. Antinociceptive and anti-inflammatory effects of *Tanacetum parthenium* L. extract in mice and rats. *J Ethnopharmacol* 1999; 68: 251–259.
31 Berry MI. Feverfew faces the future. *Pharm J* 1984; 232: 611–614.
32 Ross JJ *et al*. Low concentrations of the feverfew component parthenolide inhibit in vitro growth of tumor lines in a cytostatic fashion. *Planta Med* 1999; 65: 126–129.
33 Blakeman JP, Atkinson P. Antimicrobial properties and possible role in host–pathogen interactions of parthenolide, a sesquiterpene lactone

isolated from glands of *Chrysanthemum parthenium*. *Physiol Plant Pathol* 1979; 15: 183–192.

34 Murphy JJ *et al*. Randomised double-blind, placebo-controlled trial of feverfew in migraine prevention. *Lancet* 1988; ii: 189–192.

35 Kuritzky A *et al*. Feverfew in the treatment of migraine: its effects on serotonin uptake and platelet activity. *Neurology* 1994; 44(Suppl 2): A201.

36 Pittler MH, Ernst E. Feverfew for preventing migraine (Review). Cochrane Database of Systematic Reviews 2004, Issue 1. Art. No. CD002286

37 Pattrick M *et al*. Feverfew in rheumatoid arthritis: a double blind, placebo controlled study. *Ann Rheum Dis* 1989; 48: 547–549.

38 Rodríguez E *et al*. The role of sesquiterpene lactones in contact hypersensitivity to some North and South American species of feverfew (*Parthenium* – Compositae). *Contact Dermatitis* 1977; 3: 155–162.

39 Burry J. Compositae dermatitis in South Australia: Contact dermatitis from *Chrysanthemum parthenium*. *Contact Dermatitis* 1980; 6: 445.

40 Mitchell JC *et al*. Allergic contact dermatitis caused by *Artemisia* and *Chrysanthemum* species. The role of sesquiterpene lactones. *J Invest Dermatol* 1971; 56: 98–101.

41 Schmidt RJ, Kingston T. Chrysanethemum dermatitis in South Wales; diagnosis by patch testing with feverfew (*Tanacetum parthenium*) extract. *Contact Dermatitis* 1985; 13: 120–127.

42 Mensing H *et al*. Airborne contact dermatitis. *Der Hautarzt* 1985; 36: 398–402.

43 Johnson S. *Feverfew.* London: Sheldon Press, 1984.

44 Johnson ES *et al*. Investigation of possible genetoxic effects of feverfew in migraine patients. *Hum Toxicol* 1987; 6: 533–534.

Figwort

Summary and Pharmaceutical Comment

The chemistry of figwort is well studied. Little scientific evidence was located to justify the herbal uses. In view of the lack of toxicity data and possible cardioactive properties, excessive use of figwort should be avoided.

Species (Family)

Scrophularia nodosa L. (Scrophulariaceae)

Synonym(s)

Common Figwort, Scrophularia

Part(s) Used

Herb

Pharmacopoeial and Other Monographs

BHP 1983[(G7)]

Legal Category (Licensed Products)

Figwort is not included in the GSL.[(G37)]

Constituents

The following is compiled from several sources, including General Reference G62.

Amino acids Alanine, isoleucine, leucine, lysine, phenylalanine, threonine, tyrosine and valine.[(1)]

Flavonoids Diosmetin, diosmin and acacetin rhamnoside.[(2)]

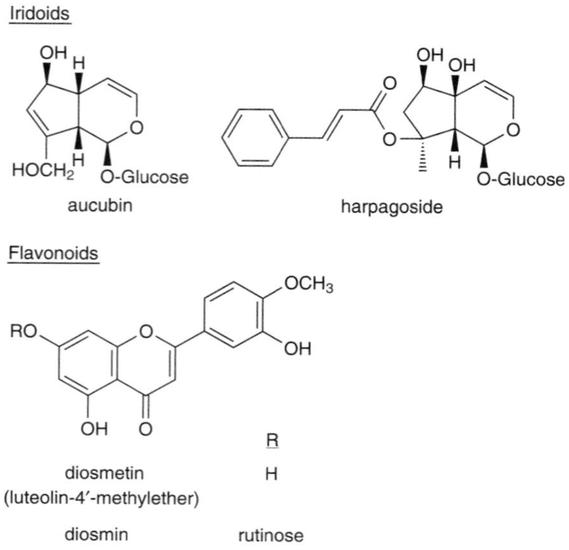

Iridoids

aucubin

harpagoside

Flavonoids

	R
diosmetin (luteolin-4′-methylether)	H
diosmin	rutinose

Figure 1 Selected constituents of figwort.

Iridoids Aucubin, acetylharpagide, harpagide, harpagoside, isoharpagoside, procumbid and a catalpol glycoside.[(3–5)] Figwort is stated to have the same qualitative iridoid composition as devil's claw, but about half the content of harpagoside.

Acids Various acids, including caffeic acid, cinnamic acid, ferulic acid, sinapic acid and vanillic acid, present as both esters and glycosides.[(6, 7)]

Food Use

Figwort is not used in foods.

Herbal Use

Figwort is stated to act as a dermatological agent and a mild diuretic, and to increase myocardial contraction. Traditionally, it has been used for chronic skin disease, and specifically for eczema, psoriasis and pruritus.[(G7, G64)]

Dosage

Dosages for oral administration (adults) for traditional uses recommended in standard herbal reference texts are given below.

Dried herb 2–8 g by infusion.[(G7)]

Liquid extract 2–8 mL (1 : 1 in 25% alcohol).[(G7)]

Tincture 2–4 mL (1 : 10 in 45% alcohol).[(G7)]

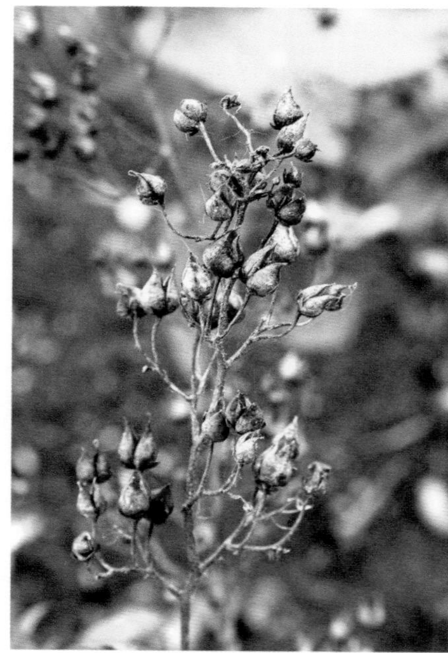

Figure 2 Figwort (*Scrophularia nodosa*).

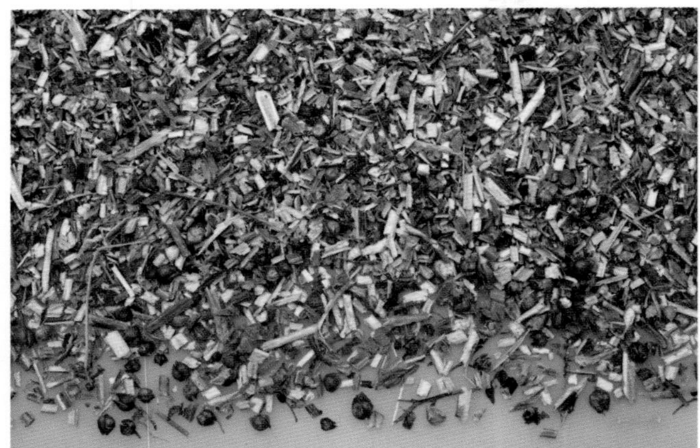

Figure 3 Figwort – dried drug substance (herb).

Pharmacological Actions

In vitro and animal studies

The iridoid glycosides aucubin and catalpol have been documented to exert a purgative action in mice.(8) Cardioactive properties and anti-inflammatory activity have been claimed for harpagide and the other iridoid constituents (*see* Devil's Claw).(G62)

Clinical studies

There is a lack of clinical research assessing the effects of figwort and rigorous randomised clinical trials are required. The iridoids are stated to be bitter principles.(G62)

Side-effects, Toxicity

None documented. However, there is a lack of clinical safety and toxicity data for figwort and further investigation of these aspects is required.

Contra-indications, Warnings

Figwort should be avoided in ventricular tachycardia.(G7)

Drug interactions None documented. However, the potential for preparations of figwort to interact with other medicines administered concurrently, particularly those with similar or opposing effects, should be considered.

Pregnancy and lactation The safety of figwort has not been established. In view of the lack of pharmacological and toxicity data, use of figwort during pregnancy and lactation should be avoided.

F

References

1 Toth L *et al*. Amino acids in Scrophulariaceae species. *Bot Kozl* 1977; 64: 43–52.
2 Marczal G *et al*. Flavonoids as biologically active agents and their occurrence in the Scrophulariaceae family. *Acta Pharm Hung* 1974: 44 (Suppl. Suppl.): 83–90.
3 Swann K, Melville C. Iridoid content of some *Scrophularia* species. *J Pharm Pharmacol* 1972; 24: 170P.
4 Swiatek L. Iridoid glycosides in the Scrophulariaceae family. *Acta Pol Pharm* 1973; 30: 203–212.
5 Weinges K, Von der Eltz H. Natural products from medicinal plants. XXIII. Iridoid glycosides from *Scrophularia nodosa* L. *Justus Liebigs Ann Chem* 1978; 12: 1968–1973.
6 Swiatek L. Phenolic acids of underground parts of *Scrophularia nodosa*. *Pol J Pharmacol Pharm* 1973; 25: 461–464.
7 Swiatek L. Pharmacobotanical investigations of some Scrophulariaceae species. *Diss Pharm Pharmacol* 1970; 22: 321–328.
8 Inouye H *et al*. Purgative activities of iridoid glucosides. *Planta Med* 1974; 25:285– 288.

Frangula

Summary and Pharmaceutical Comment

The chemistry of frangula is characterised by the anthraquinone glycoside constituents. The laxative action of these compounds is well recognised and supports the herbal use of frangula as a laxative. The use of non-standardised anthraquinone-containing preparations should be avoided, since their pharmacological effect will be variable and unpredictable. In particular, the use of products containing combinations of anthraquinone laxatives should be avoided.

Species (Family)

Frangula alnus Mill. (Rhamnaceae)

Synonym(s)

Alder Buckthorn, *Rhamnus frangula* L., *Frangula nigra* Samp.

Part(s) Used

Bark

Pharmacopoeial and Other Monographs

BHC 1992[G6]
BHP 1996[G9]
BP 2007[G84]
Complete German Commission E (Buckthorn)[G3]
ESCOP 2003[G76]
EMEA HMPC Community Herbal Monograph[1]
Martindale 35th edition[G85]
Ph Eur 2007[G81]

Anthraquinones

R^2O O OH (8, 1); R^1O (6); 3 CH_3; O

	R^1	R^2
frangulin A	α-L-rhamnose	H
frangulin B	β-D-apiose	H
glucofrangulin A	α-L-rhamnose	β-D-glucose
glucofrangulin B	β-D-apiose	β-D-glucose
frangula emodin	H	H
physcion	CH_3	H
chrysophanol	(unsubstituted)	H

Dihydroanthracenes

OH O OH; H H; CH_3

frangula emodin anthrone

Figure 1 Selected constituents of frangula.

Legal Category (Licensed Products)

GSL[G37]

Constituents

The following is compiled from several sources, including General References G2, G6, G59 and G62.

Anthraquinones 3–7%. Frangulosides as major components including frangulin A and B (emodin glycosides) and glucofrangulin A and B (emodin diglycosides); emodin derivatives including emodin dianthrone and its monorhamnoside, palmidin C (*see* Rhubarb) and its monorhamnoside, emodin glycoside; also glycosides of chrysophanol and physcion, and various free aglycones.

Other constituents Flavonoids and tannins.

Food Use

Frangula is listed by the Council of Europe as a natural source of food flavouring (category N4). While this category recognises the use of frangula as a flavouring agent, it indicates that there is insufficient information available to classify it further into categories N1, N2, or N3.[G16]

Herbal Use

Frangula is stated to possess mild purgative properties and has been used traditionally for constipation.[G2, G6, G7, G8, G64]

The European Medicines Agency Committee on Herbal Medicinal Products (HMPC) has adopted a Community Herbal monograph for frangula. The monograph includes indications for short-term use of frangula in cases of occasional constipation.[1]

Dosage

Dosages for oral administration (adults) for traditional uses recommended in standard herbal reference texts are given below.

Dried bark 0.5–2.5 g.[G6]

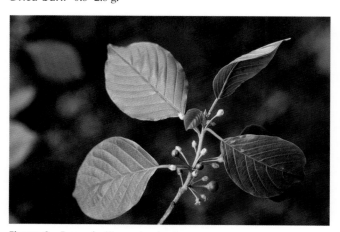

Figure 2 Frangula (*Frangula alnus*).

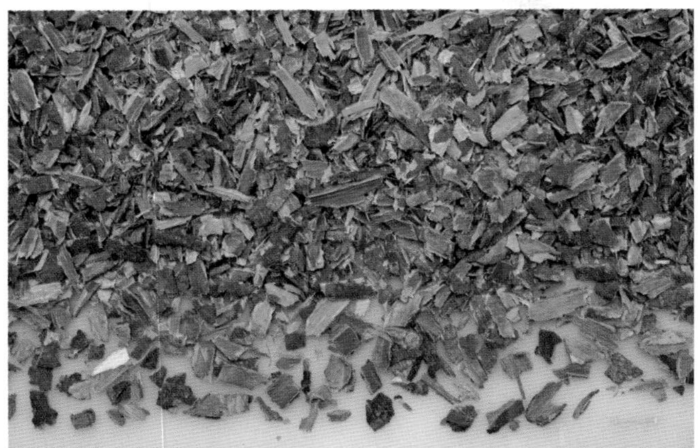

Figure 3 Frangula – dried drug substance (bark).

Liquid extract 2–5 mL (1 : 1 in 25% alcohol) three times daily.[G7]

Pharmacological Actions

The pharmacological activity of frangula can be attributed to the anthraquinone glycoside constituents. The laxative action of these compounds is well recognised (*see* Senna).

Side-effects, Toxicity

See Senna for side-effects and toxicity associated with anthraquinones.[G20]

The EMEA HMPC Community Herbal Monograph for frangula includes the following information.[1] There are no studies on single dose toxicity, on repeated dose toxicity, on reproductive toxicity or on carcinogenicity. Different frangula extracts were shown to be genotoxic in several *in vitro* systems (bacterial mutation, chromosomal aberration and DNA-repair in mammalian cells). No increases in mutations were observed in a gene mutation assay with mammalian cells. For emodin, the main laxative principle of frangula, signs of a genotoxic potential were observed in several systems (bacteria and mammalian cells *in vitro*). Other anthraquinone constituents also gave positive results in limited experiments.

Contra-indications, Warnings

See Senna for contra-indications and warnings associated with anthraquinones.

The EMEA HMPC Community Herbal Monograph for frangula states the following contra-indications and warnings.[1]

Contra-indications Not to be used in cases of intestinal obstruction and stenosis, atony, inflammatory colon diseases (e.g. Crohn's disease, ulcerative colitis), appendicitis, abdominal pain of unknown origin, severe dehydration states with water and electrolyte depletion.

Precautions As with all laxatives, frangula bark should not be given when any undiagnosed acute or persistent abdominal symptoms are present. If laxatives are needed every day, the cause of the constipation should be investigated. Long-term use of laxatives should be avoided. Use for more than two weeks requires medical supervision. Chronic use may cause pigmentation of the colon (pseudomelanosis coli) which is harmless and reversible after drug discontinuation.

Abuse, with diarrhoea and consequent fluid and electrolyte losses, may cause: dependence, with possible need for increased dosages, disturbance of the water and electrolyte (mainly hypokalaemia) balance, an atonic colon with impaired function. Intake of anthranoid containing laxatives exceeding short-term use may result in an aggravation of constipation.

Hypokalaemia can result in cardiac and neuromuscular dysfunction, especially if cardiac glycosides, diuretics or corticosteroids are taken. Chronic use may result in albuminuria and haematuria.

In chronic constipation, stimulant laxatives are not an acceptable alternative to a changed diet.

Interaction with other medicaments and other forms of interaction. Hypokalaemia (resulting from long-term laxative abuse) potentiates the action of cardiac glycosides and interacts with antiarrhythmic drugs and drugs which induce reversion to sinus rhythm (e.g. quinidine). Concomitant use with other drugs inducing hypokalaemia (e.g. thiazide diuretics, adrenocorticosteroids and liquorice root) may enhance electrolyte imbalance.

Pregnancy and lactation The use of stimulant laxatives, particularly unstandardised preparations, is not generally recommended during pregnancy (*see* Senna).

The EMEA HMPC Community Herbal Monograph for frangula includes the following information on use during pregnancy and lactation.

Pregnancy Frangula is not recommended during pregnancy.[1]

There are no reports of undesirable or damaging effects during pregnancy and on the foetus when used at the recommended dosage schedule. However, experimental data concerning a genotoxic risk of several anthranoids, e.g. emodin and physcion, and frangula extract are not counterbalanced by sufficient studies to eliminate a possible risk.[1]

Lactation Frangula is not recommended during breast feeding, as there are insufficient data on the excretion of its metabolites in breast milk. Excretion of the active principles of frangula in breast milk has not been investigated. However, small amounts of active metabolites (e.g. rhein) from other anthranoids are known to be excreted in breast milk. A laxative effect in breastfed babies has not been reported.[1]

Preparations

Proprietary single-ingredient preparations

France: Depuratif des Alpes. *Switzerland:* Elixir frangulae compositum.

Proprietary multi-ingredient preparations

Australia: Granocol; Normacol Plus. *Austria:* Artin; Gallesyn; Gallesyn; Laxalpin; Laxolind; Mag Kottas Krauterexpress Abfuhrtee; Mag Kottas May-Cur-Tee; Planta Lax; Waldheim Abfuhrdragees mild. *Belgium:* Grains de Vals; Normacol Plus. *Canada:* Constipation; Herbalax. *Czech Republic:* Abfuhr-Heilkrautertee; Cholagol; Reduktan; The Salvat. *Denmark:* Ferroplex-frangula. *France:* Dragees Fuca; Dragees Vegetales Rex; Mediflor Tisane Antirhumatismale No 2; Mediflor Tisane Circulation du Sang No 12. *Germany:* Abdomilon. *Hong Kong:* Hepatofalk; Normacol Plus. *Hungary:* Cholagol. *India:* Kanormal. *Ireland:* Normacol Plus. *Israel:* Encypalmed; Rekiv. *Italy:* Draverex; Fave di Fuca; Lactolas; Neoform.

Mexico: Normacol. *Netherlands:* Roteroblong Maagtabletten. *New Zealand:* Granocol; Normacol Plus. *Portugal:* Normacol Plus. *South Africa:* Normacol Plus. *Singapore:* Normacol Plus. *Spain:* Normacol Forte. *Switzerland:* Colosan plus; Lapidar 10; Linoforce; LinoMed; Padma-Lax; Padmed Laxan; Phyto-Laxia; Phytolaxin. *UK:* Herbulax; Lustys Herbalene; Natravene; Normacol Plus.

Reference

1 European Medicines Agency. Committee on Herbal Medicinal Products. Community Herbal Monograph on *Rhamnus frangula* L., Cortex. London, 26 October 2006. Doc Ref. EMEA/HMPC/76307/2006

F

Fucus

Summary and Pharmaceutical Comment

Kelp is a generic term that strictly speaking refers to *Laminaria* and *Macrocystis* species of brown seaweeds, although in practice it may be used in reference to other species of brown algae including *Nereocystis* and *Fucus*. The species *Fucus vesiculosus* is reported to be commonly used in the preparation of kelp products.(G60) The principal constituents of seaweeds are polysaccharides. For brown seaweeds the major polysaccharide is alginic acid (algin). Fucoidan, present in all brown algae, is thought to refer to a number of related polysaccharide esters whose main sugar component is fucose. The traditional uses of kelp in obesity and goitre are presumably attributable to the iodine content, although the self-diagnosis and treatment of these conditions with a herbal remedy is not suitable. There have been no documented studies supporting the traditional use of kelp in rheumatic conditions. In view of the iodine content and potential accumulation of toxic elements, excessive ingestion of kelp is inadvisable. Doubt over the quality of commercial seaweed preparations has been reported.

Species (Family)

Fucus vesiculosus L. and other *Fucus* species (Fucaceae)

Synonym(s)

Black Tang, Bladderwrack, Kelp, Kelpware, Rockweed, Seawrack

Brown seaweeds refer to species of *Fucus*, *Ascophyllum*, *Laminaria* and *Macrocystis*. 'Kelps' refer to species of *Laminaria* and *Macrocystis*, although kelp is often used in reference to species of *Fucus*.

Part(s) Used

Thallus (whole plant)

Pharmacopoeial and Other Monographs

BHC 1992(G6)
BHP 1996(G9)
BP 2007 (kelp)(G84)
Martindale 35th edition(G85)
Ph Eur 2007 (kelp)(G81)

Legal Category (Licensed Products)

GSL(G37)

Constituents

The following is compiled from several sources, including General References G2 and G6.

Carbohydrates Polysaccharides: alginic acid (algin) as the major component; fucoidan and laminarin (sulfated polysaccharide esters).(1)

Iodine Content of various *Laminaria* species has been reported as 0.07–0.76% of dry weight.(2)

Other constituents Various vitamins and minerals, particularly ascorbic acid (vitamin C) (0.013–0.077% of fresh material).(2)

Food Use

Seaweeds are commonly included in the diet of certain populations. The gelling properties of alginic acid, the major polysaccharide in brown seaweeds, including fucus, are extensively utilised in the dairy and baking industries to improve texture, body and smoothness of products.(1) Fucus is listed by the Council of Europe as a natural source of food flavouring (category N2). This category indicates that fucus can be added to foodstuffs in small quantities, with a possible limitation of an active principle (as yet unspecified) in the final product.(G16)

Herbal Use

Fucus is stated to possess antihypothyroid, anti-obesity and antirheumatic properties. Traditionally, it has been used for lymphadenoid goitre, myxoedema, obesity, arthritis and rheumatism.(G2, G6, G7, G8, G64)

Polysaccharides

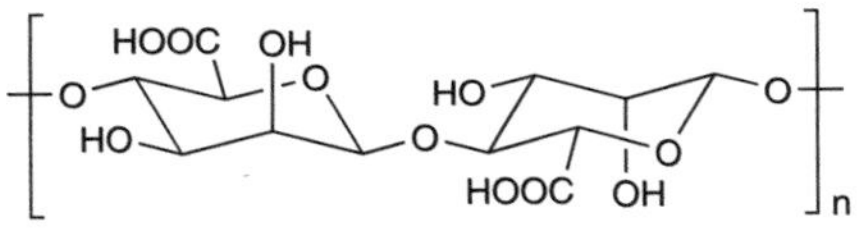

alginic acid (240 kD)
β 1→ 4 linked mannuronic acid polymer

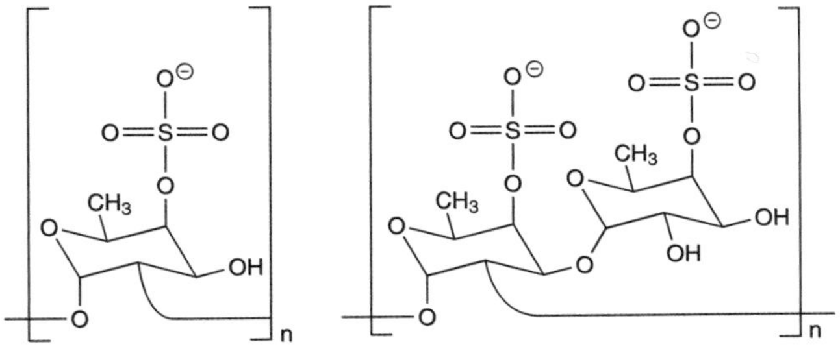

fucoidin (133 kD)
sulphated L-fucose

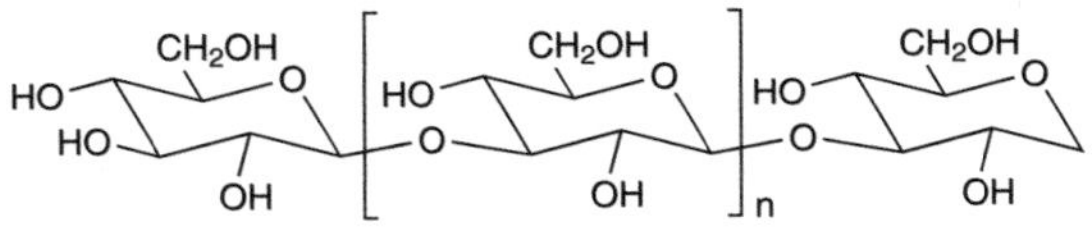

laminarin
β 1→ 3 linked glucose polymer with branching

Figure 1 Selected constituents of fucus.

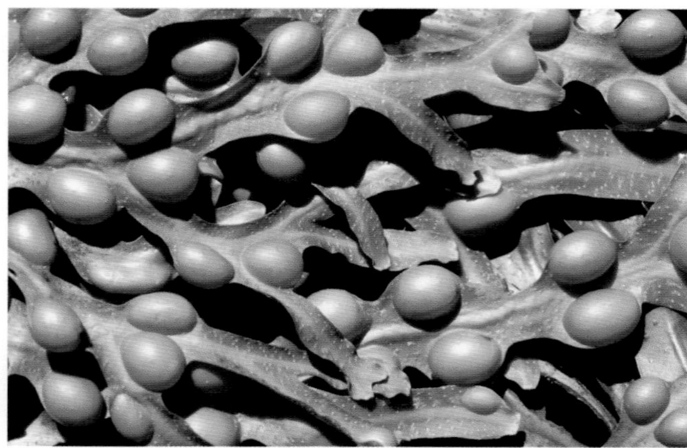

Figure 2 Fucus (*Fucus vesiculosus*).

Dosage

Dosages for oral administration (adults) for traditional uses recommended in standard herbal reference texts are given below.

Dried thallus 5–10 g as an infusion three times daily.[G6, G7]

Liquid extract 4–8 mL (1 : 1 in 25% alcohol) three times daily.[G6, G7]

Pharmacological Actions

There is a paucity of information documented specifically for *Fucus vesiculosus*, although pharmacological activities are recognised for individual constituents and other brown seaweed species.

Alginic acid is a hydrophilic colloidal substance that swells to approximately 25–35 times its original bulk in an alkaline environment and as such exerts a bulk laxative action.[3] It is stated to compare favourably with the carboxylic type of cation exchange resins. The colloidal properties of alginates have been utilised in wound dressings and skin grafts.[3]

Anticoagulant properties have been documented for brown seaweeds.[3] The glucose polymer laminarin has been identified as the anticoagulant principle in a *Laminaria* species.[4] A fucoidan fraction has been isolated from *Fucus vesiculosus* with 40–50% blood anticoagulant activity of heparin.[5]

The iodine content of seaweeds is well recognised. The low incidence of goitre amongst maritime people has been attributed to the inclusion of seaweeds in their diet.[3, 4] Similarly, the traditional use of *Fucus vesiculosus* in 'slimming teas' is thought to be attributable to the effect of iodine on hypothyroidism.[4]

Extracts of various brown seaweeds including *Ascophyllum nodosum* and *Fucus vesiculosus* have been reported to exhibit a high *in vitro* inhibitory activity towards mammalian digestive enzymes (α-amylase, trypsin and lipase) isolated from the porcine pancreas.[6] Activity was attributed to high molecular weight (30 000–100 000) polyphenols.[6]

Inhibitory effects of laminarin sulfate on lipidaemia and atherosclerosis (*in vivo*, rabbit) have been partially attributed to the *in vitro* inhibition of lipid synthesis observed in cultured chick aortic cells.[7]

Hypotensive activity observed in rats intravenously administered extracts of commercial seaweed (*Laminaria* species) preparations has been attributed to their histamine content.[8] However, histamine concentrations varied considerably between preparations, and authentic specimens of the *Laminaria* species were devoid of histamine.

Kelp extracts have antiviral activity[9] and laminarin is reported to have exhibited some tumour-inhibiting actions.[1]

Clinical studies

There is a lack of clinical research assessing the effects of fucus and rigorous randomised controlled clinical trials are required.

Side-effects, Toxicity

There is a lack of clinical safety and toxicity data for fucus preparations and further investigation of these aspects is required.

Hyperthyroidism has been associated with the ingestion of kelp and is attributable to the iodine content in the plant.[10, 11] Typical symptoms of hyperthyroidism (weight loss, sweating, fatigue, frequent soft stools) were exhibited by a 72-year-old woman following ingestion of a commercial kelp product for six months.[10] Laboratory tests confirmed the hyperthyroidism although no pre-existing evidence of thyroid disease was found and the condition resolved in six months following discontinuation of the tablets. Analysis of the kelp tablets reported an iodine content of 0.7 mg/tablet representing a daily intake of 2.8–4.2 mg iodine.[10] Clinically evident hyperthyroidism developed in an otherwise healthy woman following the daily ingestion of six 200-mg kelp tablets.[11] Symptoms gradually resolved on cessation of therapy.

The association between halogen salts and acneiform eruptions is well established.[12] Ingestion of kelp products has been associated with the worsening of pre-existing acne and the development of acneiform eruptions, which improved following withdrawal of the tablets.[12]

The ability of marine plants to accumulate heavy metals and other toxic elements is recognised, and the uptake of various radioactive compounds by seaweeds has been reported.[3, 13, 14] Fifteen samples of kelp-containing dietary supplements have been analysed for their iodine and arsenic contents.[15] The levels of arsenic were low in all but one product. The iodine levels varied widely, even between different samples of the same product, and in some products the iodine levels were high in relation to safe daily intake.

Brown algae (*Ascophyllum nodosum* and *Fucus vesiculosus*) have been found to be capable of synthesising volatile halogenated organic compounds (VHOCs).[16] VHOCs are considered to be troublesome pollutants because land plants and animals have difficulty in degrading the compounds which consequently persist in terrestrial ecosystems.[16] VHOCs released into the seawater predominantly contain bromine with iodine-containing compounds showing a slower rate of turnover.[16] Concentration of iron by brown seaweeds has been attributed to fucoidan, and alginic acid exhibits a high specificity for the binding of strontium.[13] Elevated urinary arsenic concentrations (138 and 293 μg/24 hour) in two female patients have been associated with the ingestion of kelp tablets. Subsequent analysis of the arsenic content of various kelp preparations revealed concentrations ranging from 16 to 58 μg/g product.[17, 18] The botanical source of the kelp in the products was not stated.[18]

Ascophyllum nodosum is commonly added to animal foodstuffs as a source of vitamin and minerals, with beneficial results reported for dairy cattle, sheep, pigs and poultry.[13] Feeding studies using *A. nodosum* have highlighted an atypical toxic response for rabbits compared with that of rats and pigs.[13, 19] Addition of *A. nodosum* to the diet of rabbits (at 5–10%) caused a severe drop in haemoglobin content, serum iron concentrations and packed cell volume, leading to weight loss and death in two-thirds of the animals.[13] No differences in renal and liver function, and in lipid metabolism were found between test and control animals.[13] Similar, but much milder, toxicity has also been observed in rabbits fed *Fucus serratus*.[19] Subsequent studies incorporating *A. nodosum* into the feed of rats and pigs failed to demonstrate the toxic effects observed in rabbits.[19] The toxic components in *A. nodosum* have been reported to be non-extractable with chloroform, ethanol, water and 20% sodium carbonate solution, remaining in the insoluble residue.[19]

Contra-indications, Warnings

The iodine content in kelp may cause hyper- or hypothyroidism. In view of this, ingestion of kelp preparations by children is inadvisable. The iodine content in kelp has also been associated with acneiform eruptions and aggravation of pre-existing acne. In general, brown seaweeds are known to concentrate various heavy metals and other toxic elements. Elevated urinary arsenic concentrations have been traced to the ingestion of kelp tablets. Prolonged ingestion of kelp may reduce gastrointestinal iron absorption (binding properties of fucoidan), resulting in a slow reduction in haemoglobin, packed cell volume and serum iron concentrations. Prolonged ingestion may also affect absorption of sodium and potassium ions (alginic acid) and cause diarrhoea.

Drug interactions None documented. However, the potential for preparations of fucus to interact with other medicines administered concurrently, particularly those with similar or opposing effects, should be considered. Because of its iodine content, fucus should be used with caution in individuals receiving treatment for existing abnormal thyroid function.

Pregnancy and lactation The safe use of kelp products during pregnancy and lactation has not been established. In view of the potential actions on the thyroid gland and possible contamination with toxic elements, the use of kelp should be avoided.

Preparations

Proprietary multi-ingredient preparations

UK: Fenneherb Slim Aid; Napiers Slimming Tablets; Reducing (Slimming) Tablets.

References

1 Wood CG. Seaweed extracts. A unique ocean resource. *J Chem Ed* 1974; 51: 449–452.

2 Algae as food for man. In: Chapman VJ, ed. *Seaweeds and their Uses*. London: Methuen, 1970: 115.

3 Whistler RL, ed. *Industrial Gums*, 2nd edn. New York: Academic Press, 1973: 13.

4 Burkholder PR. Drugs from the sea. *Armed Forces Chem J* 1963; 17: 6, 8, 10, 12–16.

5 Doner LW. Fucoidan. In: Whistler RL, ed. *Industrial Gums*, 2nd edn. New York: Academic Press, 1973: 115–121.

6 Barwell CJ *et al*. Inhibitors of mammalian digestive enzymes in some species of marine brown algae. *Br Phycol J* 1983; 18: 200.

7 Murata K. Suppression of lipid synthesis in cultured aortic cells by laminaran sulfate. *J Atheroscl Res* 1969; 10: 371–378.

8 Funayama S, Hikino H. Hypotensive principle of Laminaria and allied seaweeds. *Planta Med* 1981; 41: 29–33.

9 Kathan RH. Kelp extracts as antiviral substances. *Ann N Y Acad Sci* 1965; 130: 390–397.

10 Shilo S, Hirsch HJ. Iodine-induced hyperthyroidism in a patient with a normal thyroid gland. *Postgrad Med J* 1986; 62: 661–662.

11 Smet PAGM de *et al*. Kelp in herbal medicines: hyperthyroidism. *Ned Tijdschr Geneeskd* 1990; 134: 1058–1059.

12 Harrell BL, Rudolph AH. Kelp diet: A cause of acneiform eruption. *Arch Dermatol* 1976; 112: 560.

13 Blunden G, Jones RT. Toxic effects of *Ascophyllum nodosum* as a rabbit food additive. In: Food – Drugs from the Sea Proceedings 1972. Washington: Marine Technology Society, 1972: 267–293.

14 Hodge VF *et al*. Rapid accumulation of plutonium and polonium on giant brown algae. *Health Phys* 1974; 27: 29–35.

15 Norman JA *et al*. Human intake of arsenic and iodine from seaweed-based food supplements and health foods available in the UK. *Food Additives Contaminants* 1987; 5: 103–109.

16 Halocarbons. Natural pollution by algal seaweeds. *Chem Br* 1985: 513–514.

17 Walkiw O, Douglas DE. Health food supplements prepared from kelp – a source of elevated urinary arsenic. *Can Med Assoc J* 1974; 111: 1301–1302.

18 Walkiw O, Douglas DE. Health food supplements prepared form kelp – a source of elevated urinary arsenic. *Clin Toxicol* 1975; 8: 325–331.

19 Jones RT *et al*. Effects of dietary *Ascophyllum nodosum* on blood parameters of rats and pigs. *Botanica Marina* 1979; 22: 393–394.

Fumitory

Summary and Pharmaceutical Comment

Fumitory is characterised by isoquinoline alkaloids which represent the principal active ingredients. Animal studies support some of the traditional uses, but there is a lack of rigorous clinical research assessing the effects of preparations of fumitory. Fumitory should not be used in home-made ophthalmic preparations. In view of the active constituents and the lack of safety data, excessive ingestion of fumitory should be avoided.

Species (Family)

Fumaria officinalis L. (Fumariaceae)

Synonym(s)

Common Fumitory, Fumitory

Part(s) Used

Herb

Pharmacopoeial and Other Monographs

BHC 1992[G6]
BHP 1996[G9]
BP 2007[G84]
Complete German Commission E[G3]
Martindale 35th edition[G85]
Ph Eur 2007[G81]

Legal Category (Licensed Products)

GSL[G37]

Constituents

The following is compiled from several sources, including General References G2 and G6.

Alkaloids Isoquinoline-type. Protopines including protopine (fumarine) as the major alkaloid and cryptopine,[1,2] protoberberines including aurotensine, stylopine, sinactine and *N*-methylsinactine,[3] spirobenzylisoquinolines including fumaritine, fumaricine and fumariline,[4,5] benzophenanthridines including sanguinarine,[6] and indenobenzazepines including fumaritridine and fumaritrine.[6,7]

Flavonoids Glycosides of quercetin including isoquercitrin, rutin and quercetrin-3,7-diglucoside-3-arabinoglucoside.[8,9]

Acids Chlorogenic, caffeic and fumaric acids.[8]

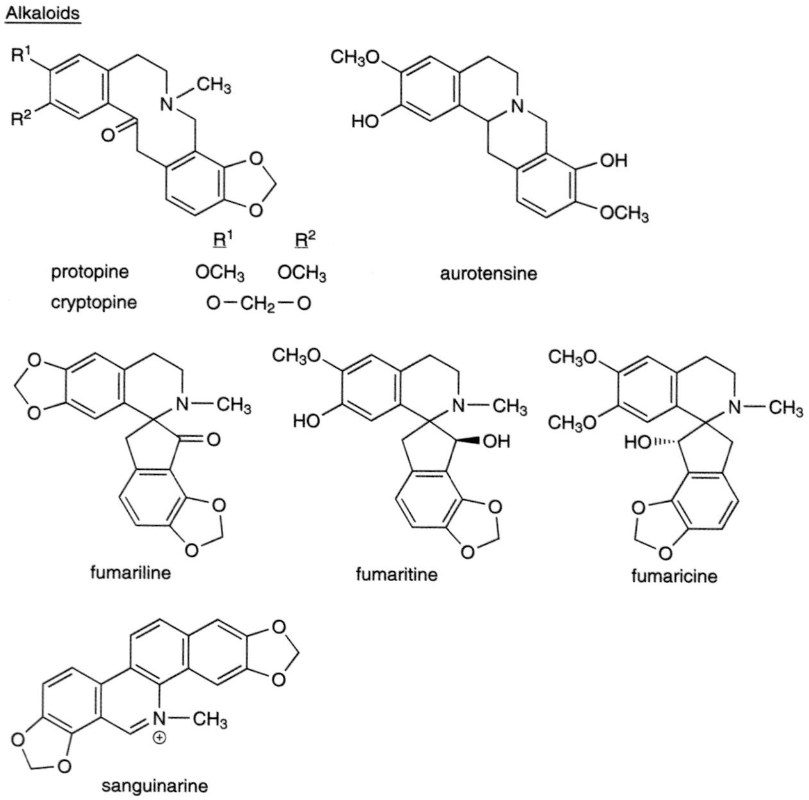

Alkaloids

	R^1	R^2
protopine	OCH_3	OCH_3
cryptopine	$O-CH_2-O$	

aurotensine

fumariline

fumaritine

fumaricine

sanguinarine

Figure 1 Selected constituents of fumitory.

Other constituents Bitter principles, mucilage and resin.

Food Use

Fumitory is listed by the Council of Europe as a natural source of food flavouring (category N3). This category indicates that fumitory can be added to foodstuffs in the traditionally accepted manner, although there is insufficient information available for an adequate assessment of potential toxicity.[G16]

Herbal Use

Fumitory is stated to possess weak diuretic and laxative properties and to act as a cholagogue. Traditionally, it has been used to treat cutaneous eruptions, conjunctivitis (as an eye lotion) and, specifically, chronic eczema.[G2, G6, G7, G8, G64]

Dosage

Dosages for oral administration (adults) for traditional uses recommended in standard herbal reference texts are given below.

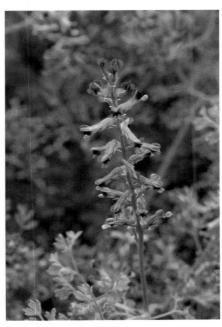

Figure 2 Fumitory (*Fumaria officinalis*).

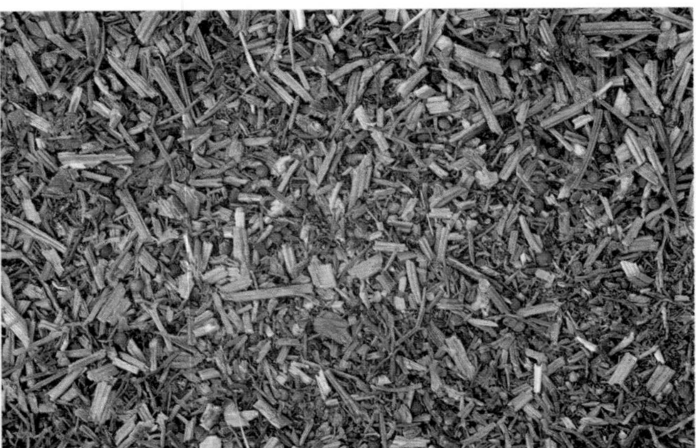

Figure 3 Fumitory – dried drug substance (herb).

Herb 2–4 g as an infusion three times daily.[G6, G7]

Liquid extract 2–4 mL (1 : 1 in 25% alcohol) three times daily.[G6, G7]

Tincture 1–4 mL (1 : 5 in 45% alcohol) three times daily.[G6, G7]

Pharmacological Actions

In vitro and animal studies

In *in vivo* (rats) studies, preparations of the herb had no effect on normal choloresis but modified bile flow that had been artificially increased or decreased.[10] Antispasmodic activity on smooth muscle has been reported.[11] Extracts inhibited formation of gall-bladder calculi in animals.[12] The major alkaloid protopine has antihistaminic,[13] hypotensive, bradycardic and sedative activities in small doses,[14] whereas larger doses cause excitation and convulsions.[14] Bactericidal activity against the Gram-positive organisms *Bacillus anthracis* and *Staphylococcus* have been reported.[14]

Clinical studies

There is a lack of clinical research assessing the effects of fumitory and rigorous randomised controlled clinical trials are required.

Clinical studies involving 105 patients with biliary disorders claimed favourable results.[15] However, the methodological limitations of these studies do not allow the reported effects to be attributed to administration of fumitory.

Side-effects, Toxicity

None documented. However, there is a lack of clinical safety and toxicity data for fumitory and further investigation of these aspects is required.

Contra-indications, Warnings

None documented.

Drug interactions None documented. However, the potential for preparations of fumitory to interact with other medicines administered concurrently, particularly those with similar or opposing effects, should be considered.

Pregnancy and lactation The safety of fumitory during pregnancy and lactation has not been established. In view of lack of pharmacological and toxicity data, the use of fumitory during pregnancy and lactation should be avoided.

Preparations

Proprietary single-ingredient preparations

Austria: Bilobene; Oddibil. *Brazil:* Oddibil. *France:* Oddibil. *Germany:* Bilobene. *Hungary:* Bilobene.

Proprietary multi-ingredient preparations

Austria: Hepabene; Oddispasmol. *Czech Republic:* Hepabene. *France:* Actibil; Bolcitol; Depuratif Parnel; Depuratum; Schoum. *Hungary:* Hepabene. *Italy:* Soluzione Schoum. *Russia:* Hepabene (Гепабене). *Spain:* Natusor Hepavesical; Odisor; Solucion Schoum. *UK:* Echinacea; Skin Cleansing.

References

1 Sener B. Turkish species of *Fumaria* L. and their alkaloids. VII Alkaloids from *Fumaria officinalis* L. and *F. cilicica* Hansskn. *Gazi Univ Eczacilik Fak Derg* 1985; 2: 45–49.
2 Hermansson J, Sandberg F. Alkaloids of *Fumaria officinalis*. *Acta Pharm Suec* 1973; 10: 520–522.
3 Mardirossian ZH *et al*. Alkaloids of *Fumaria officinalis*. *Phytochemistry* 1983; 22: 759–761.
4 MacLean DB *et al*. Structure of three minor alkaloids of *Fumaria officinalis*. *Can J Chem* 1969; 47: 3593–3599.
5 Murav'eva DA *et al*. Isolation of fumaritine from *Fumaria officinalis*. *Khim Farm Zh* 1974; 8: 32–34.
6 Forgacs P *et al*. Alcaloides des Papavéracées II: Composition chimique de dix-sept espèces de *Fumaria*. *Plantes Med Phytother* 1986; 20: 64–81.
7 Forgacs P *et al*. Composition chimique des Fumariacées. Alcaloides de quatorze espèces de *Fumaria*. *Plantes Med Phytother* 1982; 16: 99–115.
8 Massa V *et al*. Sur les pigments phenoliques du *Fumaria officinalis* L. *Trav Soc Pharm Montpellier* 1971; 31: 233–236.
9 Torck M *et al*. Flavonoids of *Fumaria officinalis* L. *Ann Pharm Fr* 1971; 29: 591–596.
10 Boucard M, Laubenheimer B. Action du nébulisat de fumeterre sur le débit bilaire du rat. *Therapie* 1966; 21: 903–911.
11 Reynier M *et al*. Action du nébulisat de fumeterre officinal sur la musculature lisse. Contribution à l'étude du mécanisme de son activité thérapeutique. *Trav Soc Pharm Montpellier* 1977; 37: 85–102.
12 Lagrange E, Aurousseau M. Effect of spray-dried product of *Fumaria officinalis* on experimental gall bladder lithiasis in mice. *Ann Pharm Fr* 1973; 31: 357–362.
13 Abdul Habib Dil. Activité anti-histaminique de la fumarine. *Therapie* 1973; 28: 767–774.
14 Preininger V. The pharmacology and toxicology of the papaveraceae alkaloids. In: RHF Manske, ed. *The Alkaloids XV.* London: Academic Press, 1975: 207–261.
15 Fiegel G. Die amphocholoretische Wirkung der *Fumaria officinalis*. *Z Allgemeinmed Landarzt* 1971; 34: 1819–1820.

Garlic

Summary and Pharmaceutical Comment

There is a vast scientific literature on the chemistry, pharmacology and clinical properties of garlic. Experimental studies have focused mainly on the cardiovascular and anticancer effects of garlic and its constituents, as well as its antimicrobial properties. Clinical studies have investigated mainly the anti-atherosclerotic and cholesterol- and lipid-lowering effects of garlic preparations. Generally, these studies report beneficial results for garlic, although the evidence at present is insufficient to recommend garlic as routine treatment for hypercholesterolaemia. *In vitro* and animal studies provide supporting evidence for some of the clinical properties of garlic and its constituents.

Garlic is characterised by its sulfur-containing constituents. Pharmacological activities documented for garlic are also associated with these compounds. It is recognised that allicin, the unstable compound formed by enzymatic action of allinase on alliin when the garlic clove is crushed, is required for the antimicrobial activity that has been demonstrated by garlic. However, serum concentrations of allicin achieved in humans following oral ingestion of garlic are unclear. The hypolipidaemic and antithrombotic actions documented for garlic have been attributed to many of the degradation products of alliin.

One of the difficulties in comparing studies that have investigated the efficacy of garlic, is establishing the concentration of active principles present in the garlic preparations used. It has been reported that the percentage of active constituents in fresh garlic may vary by a factor of 10. Many commercial garlic preparations are standardised on content of sulfur-containing constituents, particularly to alliin, or on allicin yield. Dried garlic powder contains both alliin and allinase and therefore has an allicin-releasing potential. Garlic preparations produced by heat or solvent extraction processes are stated to contain alliin but to be devoid of allinase and therefore have no allicin releasing potential. Garlic oil macerates and steam distillation products are rich in secondary alliin metabolites, such as ajoene. However, it is unclear to what extent these secondary compounds are formed in the body following the ingestion of garlic and whether, therefore, these products exhibit the pharmacological actions of fresh garlic.

Fermented garlic preparations are considered to be practically devoid of the active sulfur-containing compounds. Many 'odourless' garlic preparations are available: obviously one should establish if these products are odourless due to the formulation of the product or because they are devoid of the odoriferous, active principles. Further randomised controlled clinical trials with standardised preparations are required to establish the true usefulness of garlic in reducing serum lipids, blood pressure, platelet aggregation and exerting an antimicrobial effect. Therapeutic doses of garlic should not be given to those whose blood clots slowly and caution is recommended for patients on anticoagulant therapy.

Species (Family)

Allium sativum L. (Alliaceae/Liliaceae)

Synonym(s)

Ajo, Allium

Part(s) Used

Bulb (clove)

Pharmacopoeial and Other Monographs

BHP 1996[G9]
BP 2007[G84]
BPC 1949[G11]
Complete German Commission E[G3]
ESCOP 2003[G76]
Martindale 35th edition[G85]
Ph Eur 2007[G81]
USP29/NF24[G86]
WHO year volume 1[G63]

Legal Category (Licensed Products)

GSL[G37]

Constituents

This material is compiled from several sources including References 1–3 and General References G6 and G52.

Enzymes Allinase, peroxidases, myrosinase and others (e.g. catalases, superoxide dismutases, arginases, lipases).[2,3]

Volatile oils 0.1–0.36%. Sulfur-containing compounds including alliin, compounds produced enzymatically from alliin including allicin (diallyl thiosulfinate), allylpropyl disulfide, diallyl disulfide, diallyl trisulfide; ajoene and vinyldithiines (secondary products of alliin produced non-enzymatically from allicin); *S*-allylmercaptocysteine (ASSC) and *S*-methylmercaptocysteine (MSSC); terpenes include citral, geraniol, linalool, α- and β-phellandrene.

Other constituents Proteins (e.g. glutamyl peptides), amino acids (e.g. arginine, glutamic acid, asparagic acid, methionine, threonine), minerals, vitamins, trace elements, lipids, prostaglandins (A_2, D_2, E_2, $F_{1\alpha}$, F_2).[2,4]

Allicin and other sulfur-containing compounds are formed from alliin by the enzyme alliinase when garlic is crushed or chopped. (Alliin and alliinase are separated while the cells of a garlic bulb are intact, but crushing and chopping damage the cells of the bulb, allowing alliin and alliinase to come into contact with each other.)[G56] It is considered that 1 mg alliin is equivalent to 0.45 mg allicin.[G52] Commercial garlic preparations are often standardised on content of sulfur-containing constituents, particularly to alliin, or on allicin yield.

Garlic powder contains not less than 0.45% allicin calculated with reference to the dried drug.[G28]

G

Food Use

Garlic is used extensively as a food and as an ingredient in foods. It is listed by the Council of Europe as a natural source of food flavouring (category N1). This category indicates that there are no restrictions on the use of garlic in foods.(G16) Previously, garlic has been listed as GRAS (Generally Recognised As Safe).(G41)

Herbal Use

Garlic is stated to possess diaphoretic, expectorant, antispasmodic, antiseptic, bacteriostatic, antiviral, hypotensive and anthelmintic properties, and to be a promoter of leukocytosis. Traditionally, it has been used to treat chronic bronchitis, respiratory catarrh, recurrent colds, whooping cough, bronchitic asthma, influenza and chronic bronchitis.(G2, G6, G32, G34, G49, G64) Modern use of garlic and garlic preparations is focused on their reputed antihypertensive, anti-atherogenic, antithrombotic, antimicrobial, fibrinolytic, cancer preventive and lipid-lowering effects.

Dosage

Dosages for oral administration (adults) for traditional uses recommended in standard herbal and older pharmaceutical reference texts are given below.

Dried bulb 2–4 g three times daily;(G6) fresh garlic 4 g daily.(G3)

Tincture 2–4 mL (1 : 5 in 45% alcohol) three times daily.(G6)

Oil 0.03–0.12 mL three times daily.(G6)

Juice of Garlic (BPC 1949) 2–4 mL.(G11)

Syrup of Garlic (BPC 1949) 2–8 mL.(G11)

Clinical trials assessing the effects of garlic powder tablets on various parameters, including total serum cholesterol concentrations, triglyceride concentrations, blood pressure, platelet aggregation, vascular resistance, fibrinolysis and measures of peripheral arterial occlusive disease, have generally involved the administration of doses of 600–900 mg daily for 4–24 weeks.(G56) For prophylaxis of atherosclerosis, ESCOP (European Scientific Cooperative on Phytotherapy) states a dosage 0.5–1.0 g dried garlic powder daily (approximately equivalent to alliin 6–10 mg and allicin 3–5 mg).(G52)

Sulfur compounds

alliin (*S*-allyl-L-cysteine sulfoxide)

allinase

allylsulfenic acid

allicin

(*E*)-ajoene

(*Z*)-ajoene

thioacrolein

diallyldisulfide

2-vinyl-4H-1,3-dithiin

3-vinyl-4H-1,2-dithiin

diallyltrisulfide

Figure 1 Selected constituents of garlic.

Pharmacological Actions

In vitro and animal studies

Many pharmacological properties have been documented for garlic and its constituents *in vitro* and *in vivo* (animals), including antihypertensive, lipid-lowering, anti-atherogenic, antithrombotic, fibrinolytic, antioxidant, anticarcinogenic, antitumorigenic, immunomodulatory and antimicrobial activities. The pharmacological properties of garlic are attributed mainly to its sulfur-containing compounds. An extensive review of the pharmacological properties of garlic and its constituents is beyond the scope of this monograph, although many studies are summarised below.

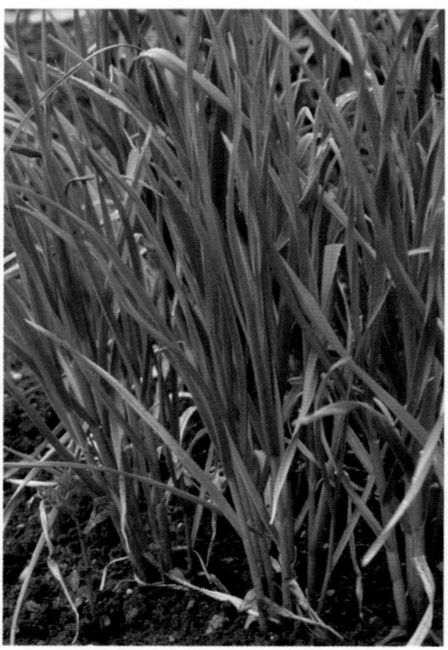

Figure 2 Garlic (*Allium sativum*).

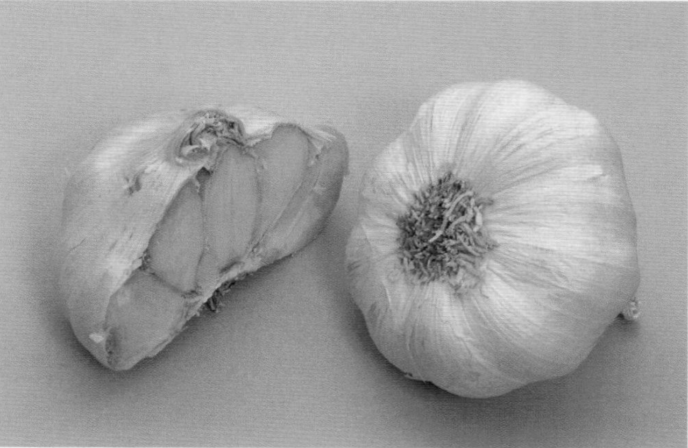

Figure 3 Garlic – dried drug substance (bulb).

The pharmacological activities of garlic and its constituents have been summarised in many reviews.[3, 5–21, G5, G56]

Pharmacokinetics The available literature on the metabolism and pharmacokinetics of the constituents of garlic in animals has been reviewed.[3, G18]

In an *ex vivo* study, allicin showed a marked first-pass clearance effect in isolated perfused rat liver.[3] In rats, alliin and allicin were administered orally at doses of 8 mg/kg.[22] Absorption of alliin and allicin was complete after 10 minutes and 30–60 minutes, respectively. The mean total urinary and faecal excretion of allicin after 72 hours was 85.5% of the dose. No unchanged alliin or allicin was detected in urine, suggesting rapid and extensive metabolism of these constituents.[3] Pharmacokinetic studies of the garlic constituent *S*-allyl-L-cysteine administered orally to rats at doses of 12.5, 25 and 50 mg/kg have reported bioavailability of 64%, 77% and 98%, respectively.[23] Peak plasma concentrations of *S*-allyl-L-cysteine occurred at one hour, and the half-life of *S*-allyl-L-cysteine was 2.33 hours following oral administration of 50 mg/kg to rats.

Anti-atherosclerotic and cholesterol- and lipid-lowering effects The effects of garlic and its constituents on cholesterol biosynthesis *in vitro* and in animal models of hypercholesterolaemia are well documented.[3]

Several *in vitro* studies have shown that garlic and its sulfur-containing constituents inhibit cholesterol biosynthesis in cultured hepatocytes.[24–28] In other *in vitro* studies, garlic extracts were shown to inhibit fatty acid and triglyceride synthesis.[29, 30]

The step(s) in the cholesterol biosynthetic pathway inhibited by garlic, and the constituents of garlic causing inhibition have not been definitively established. Several mechanisms of action for the effects of garlic constituents on cholesterol and lipid synthesis have been proposed, including inhibition of hydroxymethylglutaryl-CoA (HMG-CoA) reductase activity and other enzymes, such as lanosterol-14-demethylase, involved in cholesterol biosynthesis.[3] Other proposed mechanisms include reduction in triacylglycerol biosynthesis via a reduction in tissue concentrations of NADPH, increase in hydrolysis of triacylglycerols via increased lipase activity and inactivation of enzymes involved in lipid synthesis via an interaction with enzyme thiol groups.[6, 8, 31] More recently, fresh garlic extract and the constituents *S*-allylcysteine, diallyl trisulfide and diallyl disulfide were shown to inhibit human squalene monooxygenase, an enzyme catalysing a step in cholesterol biosynthesis.[32] Another *in vitro* study reported that *S*-allylcysteine, *S*-propylcysteine and *S*-ethylcysteine inhibit triglyceride biosynthesis in part by decreasing *de novo* fatty acid synthesis via inhibition of fatty acid synthase.[30]

The anti-atherogenic, anti-atherosclerotic and cholesterol- and lipid-lowering effects of garlic and its constituents have been documented in several animal models (e.g. rabbits, rats, chickens, pigs) of atherosclerosis, hypercholesterolaemia and hyperlipidaemia.[3] For example, a reduction in both blood and tissue lipid concentrations in hypercholesterolaemic animals fed a diet supplemented with dried garlic powder, garlic oil, or allicin has been documented.[6, 33] Garlic has also been reported to reduce hepatic triglyceride and cholesterol concentrations in rats, and to reduce aortic lipid deposition and atheromatous lesions in rabbits fed a high-fat diet.[6] Several studies have reported hypolipidaemic effects for garlic oil following administration to rats and rabbits fed a fat-rich diet to induce hyperlipidaemia.[3] Administration of aged garlic extract to rabbits fed a 1% cholesterol-enriched diet for six weeks reduced the surface area of the thoracic aorta covered by fatty streaks (atherosclerosis) and significantly reduced aortic arch cholesterol, although plasma cholesterol concentrations were not reduced.[34] Allicin administration has been reported to reduce significantly the formation of fatty streaks in mice fed a cholesterol-rich diet, compared with control mice (no allicin treatment).[35]

The cholesterol-lowering effect of garlic is thought to be dose-related; proposed mechanisms of action include inhibition of lipid synthesis and increased excretion of neutral and acidic sterols.[6, 8] An *in vitro* study reported that aged garlic extract may exert its anti-atherogenic effects via inhibition of smooth muscle proliferation and phenotypic change, and by an effect on lipid accumulation in the artery wall.[34]

Antithrombotic and fibrinolytic activities Antithrombotic activity is well documented for garlic in both *in vitro* and *in vivo* (animal) studies.[3] Antithrombotic effects have been documented for fresh garlic, garlic powder and garlic oils.[3]

G

Increased serum fibrinogen concentrations together with a decrease in blood coagulation time and fibrinolytic activity are associated with a high-fat diet and enhance thrombosis.[6] Garlic has been shown to have a beneficial effect on all of these parameters. Garlic has been shown to inhibit platelet aggregation[36, 37] caused by several inducers such as ADP, collagen, arachidonic acid, adrenaline (epinephrine) and calcium ionophore A23187.[38] Antiplatelet activity has been documented for garlic in *in vitro* studies using human platelets.[5, 39]

Several mechanisms have been proposed by which garlic is thought to exert an anti-aggregatory action. These include inhibition of thromboxane synthesis via cyclooxygenase and lipoxygenase inhibition,[8] inhibition of membrane phospholipase activity and incorporation of arachidonic acid into platelet membrane phospholipids,[40] intraplatelet mobilisation of calcium uptake and inhibition of calcium uptake into platelets.[38] Garlic oil has been reported to reduce artificial surface adhesion of platelets *in vitro*.[41] Certain garlic constituents also affect processes preceding platelet aggregation, such as activation of platelets.[3]

Garlic is thought to contain more than one inhibitor of platelet aggregation and release; allicin is considered to be the major inhibitor.[3, 42] Other studies have investigated the role of ajoene (a secondary degradation product of alliin) as an inhibitor of platelet aggregation and release.[3, 43] Ajoene inhibits platelet aggregation caused by various inducers.[44, 45] Its action is noted to be dose-dependent and reversible both *in vitro* and *in vivo*.[43] It has been suggested that this latter feature may be of clinical significance in instances where a rapid inhibition of platelet aggregation is required with subsequent reversal, such as chronic haemodialysis and coronary bypass surgery.[43] It has been proposed that ajoene exerts its anti-aggregatory effect by altering the platelet membrane via an interaction with sulfhydryl groups.[46] The inhibitory action of ajoene on granule release from platelets is thought to involve alteration of the microviscosity in the inner part of the plasma membrane.[47] Ajoene is reported to synergistically potentiate the anti-aggregatory action of prostacyclin, forskolin, indometacin and dipyridamole,[48] and to potentiate the inhibitory action of prostaglandin I_2 (PGI_2) on platelet aggregation.[21] Approximately 96% inhibition of prostaglandin synthetase and 100% inhibition of lipoxygenase has been described for ajoene *in vitro*.[40] Structure–activity investigations suggested that an allylic structure in the open disulfide ring is required for activity.[40]

Antioxidant effects Antioxidant properties have been documented for garlic *in vitro* and *in vivo* (animals).[3] Garlic constituents inhibit the formation of free radicals, support endogenous radical-scavenging mechanisms, enhance cellular antioxidant enzymes (e.g. superoxide dismutase, catalase, glutathione peroxidase), protect low-density lipoprotein from oxidation by free radicals, and inhibit the activation of the oxidant-induced transcription factor nuclear factor kappa B (NF-κB).[3, 18]

Garlic powder was reported to inhibit the production of superoxide by phorbol ester-activated human granulocytes *in vitro* (IC_{50} 390 μg/mL),[49] whereas alliin did not inhibit superoxide production in this model. It was suggested that allicin may be the constituent of garlic responsible for the observed oxygen-radical scavenging properties. *In vitro*, aged garlic extract and *S*-allylcysteine inhibited low-density lipoprotein oxidation and protected pulmonary artery endothelial cells against injury induced by oxidised low-density lipoprotein.[50] In subsequent studies using bovine pulmonary artery endothelial cells and murine macrophages, it was shown that aged garlic extract inhibited oxidised low-density lipoprotein-induced release of peroxides.[51] *In vivo* studies have reported reductions in liver lipid peroxidation and inhibition of ethanol-induced mitochondrial lipid peroxidation in rats fed garlic oil.[3]

The antioxidant properties are of interest in relation to the antiarteriosclerotic, antihepatotoxic and anticancer effects of garlic and its constituents. For example, oxidation of low-density lipoprotein plays an important role in the initiation and progression of atherosclerosis.[50]

Antihypertensive effects Several studies involving animal models (e.g. dogs, rats) of hypertension have reported hypotensive effects of garlic preparations.[3] A hypotensive effect in dogs administered garlic extract has been documented; prior administration of antagonists to known endogenous hypotensive substances such as histamine, acetylcholine, serotonin and kinins did not affect the hypotensive effect.[52] Spontaneously hypertensive rats fed standardised dry garlic powder 1 mg/kg for nine months exhibited lower blood pressure than control rats (150 versus 205 mmHg, respectively).[53] By contrast, an ethanolic extract of garlic (1–2 g and 4–8 g daily) fed to spontaneously hypertensive rats did not lead to a reduction in blood pressure.[54]

Anticarcinogenic and antitumorigenic activities Many *in vitro* and animal studies have documented anticancer activities of garlic and its constituents.[3, 14, 15] These studies indicate that allicin, allicin-derived compounds and other compounds unrelated to allicin contribute to the anticancer effects of garlic.

In several animal models, garlic has been shown to inhibit carcinogenesis and to protect against the development of experimentally induced tumours.[3, 14, 15] For example, aged garlic extract significantly inhibited the growth of Sarcoma-180 and LL/2 lung carcinoma cells transplanted into mice.[55] Garlic powder and its constituents *S*-allylcysteine and diallyl disulfide inhibited *N*-methyl-*N*-nitrosourea-induced mammary carcinogenesis in rats,[56] and fresh garlic (250 mg/kg orally, three times weekly) suppressed 4-nitroquinoline-1-oxide–induced carcinogenesis in rat tongue.[57] Inhibition of benzo[*a*]pyrene-induced neoplasia of the fore stomach and lung in female mice has been documented for four allyl group-containing derivatives in garlic.[58] Structure–activity requirements underlined the importance of the unsaturated allyl groups for activity. Saturated analogues containing propyl instead of allyl groups were devoid of activity.

In vitro studies using human tumour cell lines have reported that garlic powder and garlic extract inhibited the growth of a human lymphatic leukaemia cell line (CCRF CEM) in a concentration-dependent manner at concentrations down to 30 μg/mL.[59] Also, a combination of garlic extract and garlic powder inhibited the growth of human hepatoma (HepG02) cells and human colorectal carcinoma (Caco2) cells in a concentration-dependent manner, although no activity was observed on these tumour cell lines with garlic extract or powder alone.[59] Synthetic diallyl disulfide inhibited tumour cell growth in four human breast cancer cell lines.[60] Growth inhibition occurred regardless of oestrogen receptor status.

Evidence indicates that there are several mechanisms by which garlic and its constituents may exert anticancer effects, such as inhibition of carcinogen formation, modulation of carcinogen metabolism, inhibition of mutagenesis and genotoxicity, increased apoptosis and inhibition of angiogenesis.[20]

Garlic has been shown to inhibit the synthesis of *N*-nitroso compounds (there is a view that *N*-nitroso compounds are possible carcinogens for humans).[14] Also, in rats pretreated with dimethylbenz[*a*]anthracene (DMBA) and fed a diet supplemented with garlic powder, the occurrence of DNA adducts in mammary tissue was significantly inhibited, compared with control.[61] (DMBA initiates and promotes cancer, and alkylation of DNA is thought to be an important step in carcinogenesis.) Dietary garlic has also been shown to suppress the occurrence of DNA adducts caused by *N*-nitroso compounds.[62]

Another possible explanation is that garlic constituents may modify drug-metabolising enzymes, which would have the effect of altering the bioactivation of carcinogens.[14] Glutathione-*S*-transferase activity has been shown to increase in rat and mouse tissues after administration of garlic powder or its sulfur-containing constituents.[3, 14, 15] Certain garlic constituents, e.g. diallyl sulfide, may depress the activity of some hepatic cytochrome P450 (CYP) enzymes, such as CYP2E1 and CYP2A6,[3, 14, 15, 63] although other studies have shown that garlic constituents induce the activity of other CYP enzymes.[3, 17] In rats, the antimutagenic properties of sulfur-containing compounds from garlic, e.g. diallyl disulfide and diallyl sulfide, against the carcinogens styrene oxide and 4-nitroquinoline-1-oxide and a benzo[*a*]pyrene compound have been shown to be associated with induction of phase II enzymes.[64]

A study in mice with transitional cell carcinoma (TCC) of the bladder reported that injection of liquid extract of garlic at the site of tumour transplantation led to a significant reduction in the incidence of TCC in this model.[65] Furthermore, garlic extract together with suicide-gene therapy significantly inhibited tumour growth (as determined by evidence of apoptosis following histomorphological and immunohistochemical studies) compared with control (no gene therapy).

Effects of garlic constituents on the immune system have been documented *in vitro* and *in vivo*; these effects may contribute, at least in part, to the anticancer effects of garlic (*see* Pharmacological Actions, Immunomodulatory activity).

Immunomodulatory activity Immunostimulant activity has been described for a high molecular weight protein fraction obtained from an aged garlic extract.[66] The fraction was found to strongly stimulate mice peritoneal macrophages *in vitro*, and to stimulate carbon clearance in mice *in vivo*. It has been suggested that garlic may suppress tumour cell growth by the stimulation of immunoresponder cells.[55, 66, 67]

In vitro and/or *in vivo* (animal) studies have found that garlic has several immune-enhancing effects, such as stimulation of lymphocyte proliferation and macrophage phagocytosis, induction of macrophage- and lymphocyte-infiltration into transplanted tumours, and stimulation of interferon-γ release.[67] Other effects on the immune system documented for garlic and/

or its constituents include increased natural killer cell activity and increased interleukin-2 production by garlic fractions *in vitro*,[68] and increased numbers of antibody-forming cells in mice spleens following administration of standardised garlic powder.[3] Other studies demonstrated that, *in vitro*, aged garlic extract, compared with control, enhanced the proliferation of spleen cells in a concentration-dependent manner, increased production of cytokines (including interleukin-2 and tumour necrosis factor α) and enhanced natural killer cell activity of a T cell fraction of mouse splenic cells against YAC-1 after incubation for 24 hours.[55] Also, compared with control, aged garlic extract significantly inhibited the growth of sarcoma-180 and LL/2 lung carcinoma cells transplanted into mice, and significant increases in natural killer cell activity of spleen were observed in splenic cells from sarcoma-bearing mice treated with aged garlic extract, compared with those from control mice.[55,69]

Antimicrobial activity Antimicrobial activity (including antibacterial, antiviral, antifungal, antiprotozoal and antiparasitic activites) is well documented for garlic.[3,7] The *in vitro* antimicrobial activity of garlic is considered to be mainly due to allicin.[3]

In vitro studies have demonstrated that bacteria sensitive to garlic include species from *Staphylococcus*, *Escherichia*, *Proteus*, *Salmonella*, *Providencia*, *Citrobacter*, *Klebsiella*, *Hafnia*, *Aeromonas*, *Vibrio* and *Bacillus* genera.[7,70] In these studies, *Pseudomonas aeruginosa* was found not to be sensitive to garlic.[7,70] *In vitro* studies have also shown that allicin has significant antibacterial activity against several species, including *Bacillus subtilis*, *Staphylococcus aureus*, *Staphylococcus faecalis*, *Escherichia coli*, *Proteus mirabilis*, *Salmonella typhi* and *Vibrio cholerae*.[70]

In other *in vitro* studies, garlic oil and four diallyl sulfide constituents, including diallyl disulfide, showed activity against antibiotic-resistant *Pseudomonas aeruginosa* and *Klebsiella pneumoniae*,[71] and against *S. aureus*, methicillin-resistant *S. aureus*, *Candida* spp. and *Aspergillus* spp.[72]

Garlic has also been documented to inhibit growth in 30 strains (consisting of 17 species) of mycobacteria, including *Mycobacterium tuberculosis*.[73] *In vitro*, both aqueous garlic extract and ethanolic garlic extract inhibited the growth of *M. avium* complex (MAC) strains isolated from patients with or without acquired immune deficiency syndrome (AIDS).[74] Aqueous garlic extract at concentrations of 2–5 mg/mL inhibited the growth of clinical isolates of *Helicobacter pylori* from patients with chronic gastritis or duodenal ulcer.[75] The minimum inhibitory concentration to inhibit 90% of growth (MIC_{90}) was 5 mg/mL. Sulfur-containing compounds from garlic (diallyl sulfide and diallyl disulfide, produced from alliin) were shown to decrease growth of *H. pylori* isolates from patients with peptic ulcer.[76] It has been proposed that garlic inhibits bacterial cell growth by primarily inhibiting RNA synthesis.[77]

Broad-spectrum activity against fungi has been documented for garlic including the genera *Microsporum*, *Epidermophyton*, *Trichophyton*, *Rhodo torula*, *Torulopsis*, *Trichosporon*, *Cryptococcus neoformans* and *Candida*, including *Candida albicans*.[7]

Garlic extract has been reported to be more effective than nystatin against pathogenic yeasts, especially *Candida albicans*.[7] Inhibition of lipid synthesis is thought to be an important factor in the anticandidal activity of garlic, with a disulfide-containing component such as allicin thought to be the main active component.[78] Garlic has been found to inhibit the growth and toxin production of *Aspergillus parasiticus*.[79]

Allicin produced from synthetic alliin with alliinase isolated from garlic cloves inhibited the destruction of baby hamster kidney cells by trophozoites of the protozoan parasite *Entamoeba histolytica in vitro*.[80] Allicin also inhibited the cysteine proteinase activities of intact *E. histolytica* trophozoites. *In vitro* activity against *Giardia intestinalis* has also been documented for whole garlic extract (IC_{50} 0.3 mg/mL) and for several of its constituents, particularly allyl alcohol and allyl mercaptan (IC_{50} 7 μg/mL and 37 μg/mL, respectively).[81]

In vitro antiviral activity against parainfluenza type 3, herpes simplex type 1 and influenza B has been documented.[82,83] Activity was attributed to allicin or an allicin derivative. Garlic was reported to be ineffective towards coxsackie B1 virus.[84]

Antihepatotoxic effects Antihepatotoxic activity *in vitro* and *in vivo* has been reported for garlic and its constituents.[3] Garlic oil[85] and some of its constituents, namely alliin, *S*-allylmercaptocysteine (ASSC) and *S*-methylmercaptocysteine (MSSC) reduced carbon tetrachloride (CCl_4)- and galactosamine-induced hepatotoxicity *in vitro*.[85] Other *in vitro* studies have shown that *S*-allylcysteine, *S*-propylcysteine and *S*-allylmercaptocysteine neutralised CCl_4-induced hepatotoxicity, and that *S*-allylcysteine and *S*-allylmercaptocysteine prevent liver damage induced by hepatotoxins in acute hepatitis in mice.[3,86]

An *in vitro* study in rat hepatocytes found that diallyl sulfide (0.5 and 2 mmol/L) and diallyl disulfide (0.5 and 1 mmol/L) protected against DNA damage induced by aflatoxin B_1, compared with control.[87] In this model, diallyl sulfide and diallyl disulfide appeared to exert a hepatoprotective effect via increased activity of glutathione-*S*-transferase and glutathione peroxidase activity.

Other activities Garlic oil and juice have been reported to protect against isoprenaline-induced myocardial necrosis in rats.[88] Oral administration of garlic extract 100, 200 or 400 mg/kg to rats given oral lead acetate 5 mg/kg daily for six weeks was found to reduce tissue lead concentrations, compared with those in control rats.[89] A diet containing 2% aged garlic extract was reported to protect against intestinal damage induced by oral methotrexate and 5-fluorouracil administered to rats for 4–5 days, compared with a control diet.[90]

A study in senescence-accelerated mice found that *S*-allylcysteine, present in aged garlic extract, administered in the diet for eight months (40 mg/kg/diet daily) significantly attenuated the decrease in the conditioned avoidance response, compared with a diet lacking *S*-allylcysteine.[91] It was suggested that the findings indicate that dietary supplementation with *S*-allylcysteine may reduce age-related learning disabilities and cognitive disorders in senescence-accelerated mice.

Hypoglycaemic activity has been documented for an alcoholic garlic extract following oral administration to rabbits (dose equivalent to 50 g dry garlic powder). Fifty-nine per cent activity compared to that of 500 mg tolbutamide was observed.[92]

Garlic has been documented to cause both smooth muscle relaxation and contraction.[37,52,84] Garlic oil has been reported to depress gastrointestinal movements induced by charcoal meal and castor oil.[84] In mice, garlic has also inhibited acetylcholine- and PGE_2-induced contraction of the rat gastric fundus, with the most active components exhibiting the weakest antiplatelet aggregatory activity.[37] Garlic has also elicited contractions on the rat uterus and the guinea-pig ileum *in vitro*.[52] Both actions were blocked by flufenamic acid, but not by atropine or cyproheptadine, indicating a prostaglandin-like mode of action.

In vitro, ajoene was found to inhibit the release of lipopolysaccharide-induced prostaglandin E_2 in macrophages in a concentration-dependent manner.[93] This effect was reported to be due to inhibition of cyclooxygenase 2 (COX-2) activity by ajoene.

Clinical studies

Pharmacokinetics The available literature on the metabolism and pharmacokinetics of the constituents of garlic in humans has been reviewed.[3, 94, G18]

Addition of allicin to fresh whole blood results in conversion of allicin to allyl mercaptan and other compounds produced from allicin, such as diallyl trisulfide and ajoene, have also been shown to form allyl mercaptan in blood.[3] Sulfur-containing compounds, such as diallyl disulfide, diallyl sulfide, dimethyl sulfide and mercapturic acids, have been isolated and identified in human urine following the ingestion of garlic.[3, 95] A subsequent study detected *N*-acetyl-*S*-allyl-L-cysteine (allylmercapturic acid) in the urine of volunteers (n = 6) who had ingested two garlic tablets containing 100 mg garlic extract (Kwai).[96] The mean (standard deviation) elimination half-life of allylmercapturic acid was estimated to be 6 (1.3) hours.

It has been reported that the flavour of human breast milk is altered when lactating women consume foods containing sulfur-containing compounds, such as garlic (*see* Contra-indications, Warnings; Pregnancy and lactation).[97] Also, garlic ingestion by pregnant women significantly alters the odour of their amniotic fluid (*see* Contra-indications, Warnings; Pregnancy and lactation),[98] suggesting that the odorous components of garlic are present. Evidence for this comes from a placebo-controlled study involving 10 healthy pregnant women undergoing routine amniocentesis. The odour of samples of amniotic fluid from women who ingested capsules containing garlic extract was judged to be 'stronger' or more 'garlic-like' than that of samples from women who had ingested placebo capsules.

Pharmacodynamics Several of the pharmacological activities documented for garlic and its constituents *in vitro* and *in vivo* (animals) have also been reported in clinical studies (*see* Pharmacological Actions, Therapeutic effects).

Numerous studies have assessed the effects of the administration of garlic preparations in hypercholesterolaemia.[3] Many, but not all, of these studies have documented the effects of garlic administration in lowering serum cholesterol and triglyceride concentrations. Clinical studies have also documented fibrinolytic activity associated with garlic administration and effects on platelet function.[99, 100]

Therapeutic effects

Anti-atherosclerotic and cholesterol- and lipid- lowering effects Numerous studies have investigated the effects of garlic preparations in lowering raised serum cholesterol concentrations, and the findings of these studies have been reviewed in several meta-analyses.[101–104]

A meta-analysis of five randomised, placebo-controlled trials involving mostly patients with serum cholesterol concentrations greater than 5.17 mmol/L who received preparations of garlic extract at doses of 600–1000 mg daily for 8–24 weeks reported that garlic significantly reduced total serum cholesterol concentrations by about 9% (net reduction over placebo), compared with placebo ($p < 0.001$).[101] Another meta-analysis included 16 trials involving patients with a range of disorders (such as hyperlipidaemia, coronary heart disease and hypertension) as well as healthy volunteers, and compared garlic preparations (e.g. fresh garlic, garlic oil, garlic extract, dried garlic powder) with garlic-free diet, placebo or other agents (two studies used bezafibrate or a reserpine/diuretic combination as the comparator treatment).[102] This analysis reported a mean difference of −0.77 mmol/L (95% confidence interval (CI) −0.65, −0.89) in reduction of total serum cholesterol concentrations between garlic recipients and those receiving placebo or a garlic-free diet (net reduction over placebo: 12%). Analysis of data from the eight trials that assessed garlic powder preparations indicated that garlic powder administration significantly reduced serum triglyceride concentrations, compared with placebo (net reduction: 13%). It was stated, however, that several trials had methodological flaws, and that there was not enough evidence to recommend garlic as an effective lipid-lowering agent for routine use. The results of a subsequent randomised placebo-controlled trial involving 115 patients with moderate hyperlipidaemia (which showed no difference between garlic and placebo)[103] were included in a re-analysis[103] of the meta-analysis described above.[102] This analysis showed that the effect of garlic in reducing serum cholesterol concentrations remained statistically significant, compared with placebo, but that the size of the effect was reduced.

Several randomised, double-blind, placebo-controlled trials[105–108] have been published since the meta-analyses described above. One of these studies[105] has been criticised for its choice of garlic preparation.[109]

Several of these trials[105–107] were included in the most recent meta-analysis of randomised clinical trials of garlic preparations involving patients with hypercholesterolaemia.[104] This meta-analysis included 13 randomised, double-blind, placebo-controlled trials of garlic monopreparations involving 796 patients with coronary heart disease (n = 1 trial), hyperlipoproteinaemia (2), hypercholesterolaemia (7), hypertension (1), familial hyperlipidaemia in children (1) and healthy volunteers (1). Ten of the trials assessed the effects of a standardised garlic powder preparation (Kwai) at doses of 600–900 mg daily for 8–24 weeks; the other three trials tested garlic oil or spray dried powder. Ten trials reported differences favouring garlic over placebo in the reduction of total serum cholesterol concentrations, although these differences were statistically significant in only three studies. Overall, meta-analysis indicated a significant difference in the reduction of total cholesterol concentrations favouring garlic over placebo (−0.41 mmol/L; 95% CI −0.66 mmol/L, −0.15 mmol/L; $p < 0.01$), equivalent to a net reduction in total cholesterol concentrations of 5.8%. It was stated that although these findings indicated that garlic is more beneficial than placebo in reducing serum cholesterol concentrations, the size of the effect is small. Furthermore, several studies had methodological limitations.[104]

Another randomised, double-blind, placebo-controlled trial has been published since the meta-analysis described above. This study assessed the effects of garlic powder (tablets) 500 mg and 1000 mg daily, or placebo, for 12 weeks in 53 patients with moderate hypercholesterolaemia (baseline low-density lipoprotein cholesterol (LDL-C) 130–190 mg/dL).[108] At the end of the study there were no significant differences in the absolute mean change in LDL-C between the three groups (mean (SD) values were: 0.0 (4.3) mg/dL, 1.4 (4.8) mg/dL and −10.1 (6.8) mg/dL for the placebo, garlic powder 500 mg and garlic powder 1000 mg groups, respectively).

Another meta-analysis, which aimed to summarise the evidence for the effects of garlic on several cardiovascular-related factors, considered 45 randomised controlled trials of at least four weeks' duration.[110] It was reported that after one and three months, garlic treatment may lead to small reductions in total cholesterol concentrations (0.03–0.45 mmol/L and 0.32–0.66 mmol/L, respectively). However, no effect was noted for pooled six-month data. Changes in cholesterol concentrations were paralleled by changes in low-density lipoprotein and triglyceride concentrations.

A randomised, double-blind, placebo-controlled trial explored the anti-atherosclerotic effect of garlic powder 900 mg daily for 48 months in 280 patients with advanced atherosclerotic plaques and an established risk factor for arteriosclerosis (e.g. high systolic blood pressure, hypercholesterolaemia, diabetes mellitus, smoking).[111] It was reported that continuous garlic intake significantly reduced the increase in arteriosclerotic plaque volume, compared with placebo. However, the robustness of the findings of this study is difficult to assess independently as no exact p-value is given.

A Cochrane systematic review of garlic for the treatment of peripheral arterial occlusive disease identified only one eligible randomised, placebo-controlled trial.[112] The trial involved 78 participants with peripheral arterial occlusive disease (lower limb atherosclerosis) who received garlic, or placebo, for 12 weeks. At the end of the study, the difference in the increase in pain-free walking distance between the two groups was found to be statistically non-significant.

An open study involved 101 healthy adults aged 50–80 years who had taken a standardised garlic powder preparation at a dose of at least 300 mg daily for at least two years and 101 age- and sex-matched subjects.[113] Measures of the elastic properties of the aorta were compared for the two groups. Pulse-wave velocity and elastic vascular resistance were reported to be reduced significantly in the garlic group, compared with the control group. These findings suggest that long-term use of garlic powder to attenuate age-related increases in aortic stiffness is worth further study.

Antithrombotic and fibrinolytic effects Several placebo-controlled studies have documented fibrinolytic effects for garlic preparations in clinical studies involving patients with coronary heart disease, hyperlipidaemia and hypercholesterolaemia, and healthy volunteers.[3] Several studies involved the administration of ether-extracted garlic oil 20 mg daily for up to 90 days, whereas several others involved the administration of garlic powder 600–1500 mg daily for up to 28 days. Most, but not all, of these studies reported significant increases in fibrinolytic activity in garlic recipients, compared with placebo recipients.

An open, uncontrolled study explored the effects of garlic consumption (one fresh chopped clove daily for 16 weeks) in eight healthy male volunteers.[114] After 16 weeks, garlic consumption was reported to reduce significantly serum thromboxane B_2 and cholesterol concentrations, compared with baseline values.

Antioxidant effects Blood samples from 31 individuals who participated in a randomised, placebo-controlled trial involving 115 patients with moderate hyperlipidaemia who received a standardised garlic powder preparation 900 mg daily for six months (which showed no difference between garlic and placebo)[103] were analysed to explore the effects of garlic treatment on the resistance of low-density lipoprotein to oxidation.[115] There were no significant differences between garlic and placebo recipients in low-density lipoprotein composition. Thus, garlic administration did not reduce the susceptibility of low-density lipoprotein to oxidation. This finding contrasts with some of the results of a double-blind, placebo-controlled study involving 23 patients with coronary artery disease who received a standardised garlic powder preparation (Kwai tablets) 300 mg three times daily, or placebo, for four weeks.[116] The study reported that garlic powder administration reduced the atherogenicity of low-density lipoprotein. At the end of the study, the ability of low-density lipoprotein to induce intracellular cholesterol accumulation was decreased by 38%, compared with baseline values. Decreases in the susceptibility of low-density lipoprotein to oxidation and in low-density lipoprotein-stimulated cell proliferation (an indicator of low-density lipoprotein atherogenicity) were also documented.

The effects of standardised garlic powder tablets (Sapec; alliin 1.3%, allicin 0.6%) 900 mg daily for two months on oxidative stress status were explored in an open, uncontrolled study involving 25 healthy volunteers.[117] At the end of the study, a reduction in serum malondialdehyde concentrations was observed, compared with baseline values. It was stated that this finding indicates that standardised garlic powder may have antioxidant activity in humans.

G

Antihypertensive effects A meta-analysis of randomised controlled trials of garlic preparations assessed the evidence for the effects of garlic on blood pressure.[118] Eight trials involving 415 participants were included in the review, all of which had tested the effects of an allicin-standardised garlic powder preparation (Kwai tablets) at doses of 600–900 mg daily for 4–52 weeks. Overall, the absolute change in mean systolic blood pressure was 7.7 mmHg greater for the garlic group, compared with the placebo group (95% CI 4.3–11.0). However, only three trials specifically involved subjects with hypertension and, as reported by other meta-analyses of trials of garlic preparations, several trials had methodological limitations. Thus, it was stated that there was insufficient evidence to recommend garlic treatment for routine management of hypertension.

Another overview of trials reported that the effects of garlic treatment on blood pressure are 'insignificant'.[110]

A Cochrane systematic review that aimed to assess the efficacy of garlic preparations in preventing pre-eclampsia and its complications found only one placebo-controlled trial.[119] The study investigated the effects of a dry garlic powder preparation 800 mg daily (equivalent to 2000 μg allicin daily) taken orally for eight weeks by 100 primigravid women at 28 to 32 weeks' gestation and who were deemed to be at moderate risk for pre-eclampsia. There was no statistically significant difference between the garlic and placebo groups in gestational hypertension or pre-eclampsia. Further, the trial was deemed to be of uncertain quality as the method of random allocation to treatment group was not described.[119]

Anticancer effects The protective effects of garlic consumption against various cancers (including colon, stomach, larynx, breast and endometrial) have been explored in several epidemiological studies, and their findings have been summarised.[3, 120] Most, but not all, of these studies suggest that garlic consumption may have a protective effect, particularly against cancers of the gastro-intestinal tract.[3, 120] However, the findings should be interpreted cautiously, as bias and/or confounding cannot be excluded, and there are other methodological issues, for example, most studies did not distinguish between consumption of raw or cooked garlic.

Antimicrobial effects An epidemiological study comprising a dietary interview and measurement of serum *H. pylori* antibodies was conducted among 214 adults in a low-risk area of Shandong

Province in China.[121] The findings suggested a protective effect of garlic consumption against *H. pylori* infection.

An open, uncontrolled study involving 34 patients with tinea pedis explored the effectiveness of ajoene cream (0.4% w/w).[122] After seven days' treatment, complete cure of the infection was recorded for 27 (79%) participants. The remaining seven patients experienced complete cure after a further seven days' treatment. All patients were evaluated for recurrence of infection 90 days after the end of treatment; all found to be infection free as determined by negative cultures for the fungus.

Other effects A reduction in blood sugar concentrations and an increase in insulin have been observed following allylpropyl disulfide administration to normal volunteers, whereas another study reported that garlic exhibits hypoglycaemic actions in diabetic patients but not in controls.[5] It has also been reported that garlic can prevent tolbutamide- and adrenaline-induced hyperglycaemia.[5]

A randomised, placebo-controlled, crossover trial involving 100 Swedish participants working in a tick-endemic area found that administration of garlic powder 1200 mg daily for eight weeks resulted in fewer tick bites than did placebo administration.[123]

An open, uncontrolled study involving 15 patients with hepatopulmonary syndrome explored the effects of treatment with capsules containing a standardised garlic powder preparation for at least six months.[124] Improvements in arterial oxygenation and symptoms were documented for several participants. The effects of garlic powder treatment in patients with hepatopulmonary syndrome require further study.

Side-effects, Toxicity

Clinical data

Garlic is generally considered to be non-toxic.[8, 125] Adverse effects that have been documented in humans include a burning sensation in the mouth and gastrointestinal tract, nausea, diarrhoea and vomiting.[8]

A meta-analysis of 13 randomised, double-blind, placebo-controlled trials of garlic monopreparations, 10 of which assessed the effects of a standardised garlic powder preparation (Kwai) at doses of 600–900 mg daily for 8–24 weeks (*see* Pharmacological Actions; Therapeutic effects) reported that few adverse events were documented in the included trials.[104] The frequency and nature of adverse events reported for garlic were similar to those for placebo. The most common adverse events reported were 'garlic breath', body odour and gastrointestinal symptoms.

The allergenic potential of garlic is well recognised, and allergens have been identified as diallyl disulfide, allylpropyl sulfide and allicin (the latter may be an irritant).[126] A garlic antigen in the serum of affected patients has also been identified.[43] Cases of contact dermatitis resulting from occupational exposure to garlic have been reported.[43, 127, G51] A case of garlic allergy associated with ingestion of raw or cooked garlic has been documented.[128] There is an isolated report of multifaceted dermatitis artefacta associated with local application of garlic by a 19-year-old individual.[129] Garlic burns following local application of garlic have also been documented (*see* Contra-indications, Warnings).[130, 131]

Garlic may enhance existing anticoagulant therapy; a potential interaction between garlic and warfarin has been documented (*see* Contra-indications, Warnings; Drug interactions).[132, 133] Case reports have suggested that garlic supplementation may increase the risk of bleeding in patients undergoing surgery.[G21]

Preclinical data

Erratic pulse rates, abnormal ECGs, weight loss, lethargy and weakness, soft faeces, dehydration and tender skin on fore- and hindlimbs have been observed in spontaneously hypertensive rats administered garlic extract at 0.25 and 0.5 mL/kg every 6 hours for 28 days.[134] The effects were most pronounced in animals receiving doses two or three times a day. Conversely, acute toxicity studies for garlic extract in mice and rats have reported LD_{50} values for various routes of administration (by mouth, intraperitoneal injection, intravenous injection) as all greater than 30 mL/kg.[125] Early studies, in 1944, reported LD_{50} values for allicin in mice as 120 mg/kg (subcutaneous injection) and 60 mg/kg (intravenous injection).[43] Results of chronic toxicity studies are stated to be conflicting.[43] High doses are reported to cause anaemia due to both decreased haemoglobin synthesis and haemolysis.[43] A chronic toxicity study in rats given a garlic extract (2 g/kg) five times a week for six months, reported no toxic symptoms.[135] High doses were found to decrease food consumption slightly, but did not inhibit weight gain. There were no significant differences in urinary, haematological or serological examinations, and no toxic symptoms in histopathological examinations. Genotoxicity studies using the micronucleus test have reported both positive[136] and negative[137] findings. No evidence of mutagenicity has been reported when assessed using the Ames and Ree assay.[136]

Slight cytotoxic signs have been observed at high doses in Hep2 and Chinese hamster embryo primary cultured cells.[136]

Contra-indications, Warnings

In view of the pharmacological actions documented for garlic, there may be an increased risk of bleeding with use of garlic supplements in patients undergoing surgery.[G21] Gastrointestinal irritation may occur particularly if the clove is eaten raw by individuals not accustomed to ingesting garlic.

Drug interactions In view of the documented pharmacological actions of garlic, the potential for preparations of garlic to interfere with other medicines administered concurrently, particularly those with similar (such as antiplatelet and anticoagulant agents) or opposing effects, should be considered.

Other interactions A study involving healthy volunteers detected *N*-acetyl-*S*-allyl-L-cysteine (allylmercapturic acid) in their urine following ingestion of garlic tablets (*see* Clinical studies, Pharmacokinetics).[96] As allylmercapturic acid is used as a biomarker for monitoring human exposure to allylhalides and other chemicals leading to allylmercapturic acid excretion, it was suggested that garlic consumption may interfere with and confound this monitoring process.

Pregnancy and lactation Garlic is reputed to act as an abortifacient and to affect the menstrual cycle, and is also reported to be utero-active.[G30] *In vitro* uterine contraction has been documented.[84] (*see* Contra-indications, Warnings; Pregnancy and lactation)

Studies have shown that consumption of garlic by lactating women alters the odour of their breast milk and the suckling behaviour of their infants.[97] Further evidence for this comes from a blinded, placebo-controlled study involving 30 nursing women.[138] The results indicated that infants who had no prior exposure to garlic odour in their mothers' milk spent more time breast feeding after their mothers ingested garlic capsules than did infants whose mothers had repeatedly consumed garlic. Findings from a placebo-controlled study involving 10 healthy pregnant women undergoing routine amniocentesis indicate that the odorous components of garlic can be found in amniotic fluid following garlic consumption.[98] The odour of samples of amniotic fluid from women who ingested capsules containing garlic extract was judged to be 'stronger' or more 'garlic-like' than that of samples from women who had ingested placebo capsules. The effects of *in utero* exposure to garlic odour and on the neonate's behaviour towards exposure to garlic-flavoured human breast milk are not known.

There are no experimental or clinical reports on adverse effects during pregnancy or lactation.[G19] In view of this, doses of garlic greatly exceeding amounts used in foods should not be taken during pregnancy and lactation.

Preparations

Proprietary single-ingredient preparations

Argentina: Ajomast; Alliocaps. *Australia:* Garlix; Macro Garlic. *Austria:* Kwai. *Canada:* Kwai; Kyolic. *Germany:* benicur; Ilja Rogoff Forte; Kwai; Sapec; Strongus. *Italy:* Kwai. *Malaysia:* Kyolic. *Portugal:* Alho Rogoff. *UK:* Garlimega; Kwai; Kyolic. *USA:* GarliPure. *Venezuela:* Kwai.

Proprietary multi-ingredient preparations

Argentina: Ajo 1000 + C; Ajolip; Exail; Varisedan. *Australia:* Garlic Allium Complex; Garlic and Horseradish + C Complex; Gartech; Herbal Cold & Flu Relief; Lifesystem Herbal Formula 7 Liver Tonic; Liver Tonic Herbal Formula 6; Odourless Garlic; Odourless Garlic; Procold; Proesten; Protol; Proyeast; Silybum Complex. *Austria:* Rutiviscal. *Canada:* Kyolic 101; Kyolic 102; Kyolic 103; Kyolic 104; Kyolic 106. *France:* Arterase. *Germany:* Ilja Rogoff; Lipidavit. *Malaysia:* Echinacea Plus; Horseradish Plus; Total Man. *Mexico:* Supravital. *Switzerland:* Allium Plus; Keli-med; Triallin. *UK:* AllerClear; Antifect; Cardioace; Clogar; Fishogar; Hay Fever & Sinus Relief; Hayfever & Sinus Relief; Höfels One-A-Day Cardiomax; Höfels One-A-Day Garlic; Höfels One-A-Day Garlic with Parsley; Höfels One-A-Day Ginger, Ginkgo and Garlic; Lane's Sage and Garlic Catarrh Remedy; Napiers Cold Tablets; Sinus and Hay Fever Tablets. *USA:* GarLife; Heart Health.

References

1 Block E. The chemistry of garlic and onions. *Sci Am* 1985; 252: 114–119.
2 Sendl A. *Allium sativum* and *Allium ursinum*: Part 1. Chemistry, analysis, history, botany. *Phytomedicine* 1995; 4: 323–339.
3 Koch HP, Lawson LD, eds. *Garlic. The Science and Therapeutic Application of* Allium sativum *L. and Related Species*, 2nd edn. Baltimore, Maryland: Williams and Wilkins, 1996.
4 Al-Nagdy SA *et al.* Evidence for some prostaglandins in *Allium sativum* extracts. *Phytother Res* 1988: 2: 196–197.
5 Ernst E. Cardiovascular effects of garlic (*Allium sativum*): a review. *Pharmatherapeutica* 1987; 5: 83–89.
6 Lau BHS *et al. Allium sativum* (garlic) and atherosclerosis: a review. *Nutr Res* 1983; 3: 119–128.
7 Adetumbi M, Lau BHS. *Allium sativum* (garlic) – a natural antibiotic. *Med Hypoth* 1983; 12: 227–237.
8 Fulder S. Garlic and the prevention of cardiovascular disease. *Cardiol Pract* 1989; 7: 30–35.
9 Pizzorno JE, Murray MT. *A Textbook of Natural Medicine*. Seattle, WA: John Bastyr College Publications, 1985 (looseleaf).
10 Hamon NW. Garlic and the genus *Allium. Can Pharm J* 1987; 120: 493–498.
11 Fenwick GR, Hanley AB. The genus *Allium. CRC Crit Rev Food Sci Nutr* 1985; 22: 199–376 and 23: 1–73.
12 McElnay JC, Li Wan Po A. Garlic. *Pharm J* 1991; 246: 324–326.
13 Reuter HD. *Allium sativum* and *Allium ursinum*: Part 2. Pharmacology and medicinal application. *Phytomedicine* 1995; 2: 73–91.
14 Milner JA, Garlic: its anticarcinogenic and antitumorigenic properties. *Nutr Rev* 1996; 54: S82–S86.
15 Lea MA. Organosulfur compounds and cancer. In: *American Institute for Cancer Research. Dietary Phytochemicals in Cancer Prevention and Treatment*. New York: Plenum Press, 1996.
16 Ali M *et al.* Garlic and onions: their effect on eicosanoid metabolism and its clinical relevance. *Prostaglandins Leukot Essent Fatty Acids* 2000; 62: 55–73.
17 Yang CS *et al.* Mechanisms of inhibition of chemical toxicity and carcinogenesis by diallyl sulfide (DAS) and related compounds from garlic. *J Nutr* 2001; 131 (Suppl. Suppl.3): S1041–S1045.
18 Borek C. Antioxidant health effects of aged garlic extract. *J Nutr* 2001; 131 (Suppl. Suppl.3): S1010–S1015.
19 Yeh Y-Y, Liu L. Cholesterol-lowering effect of garlic extracts and organosulfur compounds: human and animal studies. *J Nutr* 2001; 131 (Suppl. Suppl.3): S989–S993.
20 Le Bon A-M, Siess M-H. Organosulfur compounds from *Allium* and the chemoprevention of cancer. *Drug Metab Drug Interact* 2001; 17: 51–79.
21 Afzal M *et al.* Garlic and its medicinal potential. *Inflammopharmacology* 2000; 8: 123–148.
22 Lachmann G *et al.* Untersuchungen zur Pharmakokinetik der mit 35S markierten Knoblauchinhaltsstoffe Alliin, Allicin und Vinyldithiine. *Arzneimittelforschung* 1994; 44: 734–743.
23 Nagae S *et al.* Pharmacokinetics of the garlic compound *S*-allylcysteine. *Planta Med* 1994; 60: 214–217.
24 Qureshi AA *et al.* Inhibition of cholesterol and fatty acid biosynthesis in liver enzymes and chicken hepatocytes by polar fractions of garlic. *Lipids* 1983; 18: 343–348.
25 Gebhardt R. Multiple inhibitory effects of garlic extracts on cholesterol biosynthesis in hepatocytes. *Lipds* 1993; 28: 613–619.
26 Gebhardt R *et al.* Inhibition of cholesterol biosyntheis by allicin and ajoene in rat hepatocytes and Hep G2 cells. *Biochim Biophys Acta* 1994; 1213: 57–62.
27 Gebhardt R. Amplification of palmitate-induced inhibition of cholesterol biosynthesis in cultured rat hepatocytes by garlic-derived organosulfur compounds. *Phytomedicine* 1995; 2: 29–34.
28 Gebhardt R, Beck H. Differential inhibitory effects of garlic-derived organosulfur compounds on cholesterol biosynthesis in primary rat hepatocytes. *Lipids* 1996; 31: 1269–1276.
29 Yeh Y-Y, Yeh S-M. Garlic reduces plasma lipids by inhibiting hepatic cholesterol and triacylglycerol synthesis. *Lipids* 1994; 29: 189–193.
30 Liu L, Yeh Y-Y. Water-soluble organosulfur compounds of garlic inhibit fatty acid and triglyceride synthesis in cultured rat hepatocytes. *Lipids* 2001; 36: 395–400.
31 Adoga GI. The mechanism of the hypolipidemic effect of garlic oil extract in rats fed on high sucrose and alcohol diets. *Biochem Biophys Res Commun* 1987; 142: 1046–1052.
32 Gupta N, Porter TD. Garlic and garlic-derived compounds inhibit human squalene monooxygenase. *J Nutr* 2001; 131: 1662–1667.
33 Kamanna VS, Chandrasekhara N. Effect of garlic (*Allium sativum* Linn.) on serum lipoproteins and lipoprotein cholesterol levels in Albino rats rendered hypercholesterolemic by feeding cholesterol. *Lipids* 1982; 17: 483–488.
34 Campbell JH *et al.* Molecular basis by which garlic suppresses atherosclerosis. *J Nutr* 2001; 131 (Suppl. Suppl.3): S1006–S1009.
35 Abramowitz D. Allicin-induced decrease in formation of fatty streaks (atherosclerosis) in mice fed a cholesterol-rich diet. *Coronary Artery Dis* 1999; 10: 515–519.
36 Boullin DJ. Garlic as a platelet inhibitor. *Lancet* 1981; i: 776–777.
37 Gaffen JD *et al.* The effect of garlic extracts on contractions of rat gastric fundus and human platelet aggregation. *J Pharm Pharmacol* 1984; 36: 272–274.

38 Srivastava KC, Winslows JB. Evidence for the mechanism by which garlic inhibits platelet aggregation. *Prostaglandins Leukot Med* 1986; 22: 313–321.
39 Apitz-Castro A *et al.* Effects of garlic extract and of three pure components isolated from it on human platelet aggregation, arachidonate metabolism, release reaction and platelet ultrastructure. *Thromb Res* 1983; 32: 155–169.
40 Wagner H *et al.* Effects of garlic constituents on arachidonate metabolism. *Planta Med* 1987; 53: 305–306.
41 Sharma CP, Nirmala NV. Effects of garlic extract and of three pure components isolated from it on human platelet aggregation, arachidonate metabolism, release reaction and platelet ultrastructure – comments. *Thromb Res* 1985; 37: 489–490.
42 Mohammad SF, Woodward SC. Characterization of a potent inhibitor of platelet aggregation and release reaction isolated from *Allium sativum* (garlic). *Thromb Res* 1986; 44: 793–806.
43 Symposium on the chemistry, pharmacology and medicinal applications of garlic. *Cardiol Pract* 1989; 7: 1–15.
44 Srivastava KC, Tyagi OD. Effects of a garlic-derived principle (ajoene) on aggregation and arachidonic acid metabolism in human blood platelets. *Prostaglandins Leukot Essent Fatty Acids* 1993; 49: 587–595.
45 Jamaluddin MP *et al.* Ajoene inhibition of platelet aggregation: possible mediation by a hemoprotein. *Biochem Biophys Res Commun* 1988; 153: 479–486.
46 Block E *et al.* Antithrombotic organosulfur compounds from garlic: structural, mechanistic, and synthetic studies. *J Am Chem Soc* 1986; 108: 7045–7055.
47 Rendu F *et al.* Ajoene, the antiplatelet compound derived from garlic, specifically inhibits platelet release reaction by affecting the plasma membrane internal microviscosity. *Biochem Pharmacol* 1989; 38: 1321–1328.
48 Apitz-Castro R *et al.* Ajoene. The antiplatelet principle of garlic, synergistically potentiates the antiaggregatory action of prostacyclin, forskolin, indomethacin and dypiridamole on human platelets. *Thromb Res* 1986; 42: 303–311.
49 Siegers C-P *et al.* Effects of garlic preparations on superoxide production by phorbol ester activated granulocytes. *Phytomedicine* 1999; 6: 13–16.
50 Ide N, Lau BHS. Garlic compounds protect vascular endothelial cells from oxidised low density lipoprotein-induced injury. *J Pharm Pharmacol* 1997; 49: 908–911.
51 Ide N, Lau BHS. Aged garlic extract attentuates intracellular oxidative stress. *Phytomedicine* 1999; 6: 125–131.
52 Rashid A, Khan HH. The mechanism of hypotensive effect of garlic extract. *J Pak Med Ass* 1974; 35: 357–362.
53 Jacob J *et al.* Antihypertensive und Kardioprotektive Effekte von Knoblaucherpulver (*Allium sativum*). *Med Welt* 1991; 42: 39–41.
54 Kiviranta J *et al.* Effects of onion and garlic extracts on spontaneously hypertensive rats. *Phytother Res* 1989; 3: 132–135.
55 Kyo E *et al.* Immunomodulation and antitumour activities of aged garlic extract. *Phytomedicine* 1998; 5: 259–267.
56 Schaffer EM *et al.* Garlic and associated allyl sulfur components inhibit *N*-methyl-*N*-nitrosourea induced rat mammary carcinogenesis. *Cancer Lett* 1996; 102: 199–204.
57 Balasenthil S *et al.* Prevention of 4-nitroquinoline-1-oxide-induced rat tongue carcinogenesis by garlic. *Fitoterapia* 2001; 72: 524–531.
58 Sparnins VL *et al.* Effects of organosulfur compounds from garlic and onions on benzo[*a*]pyrene-induced neoplasia and glutathione S-transferase activity in the mouse. *Carcinogenesis* 1988; 9: 131–134.
59 Siegers C-P *et al.* The effects of garlic preparations against human tumor cell proliferation. *Phyto medicine* 1999; 6: 7–11.
60 Nakagawa H *et al.* Growth inhibitory effects of diallyl disulphide on human breast cancer cell lines. *Carcinogenesis* 2001; 22: 891–897.
61 Liu JZ *et al.* Inhibition of 7,12-dimethylbenz(a)anthracene induced mammary tumours and DNA adducts by garlic powder. *Carcinogenesis* 1992; 13: 1847–1851.
62 Lin X-Y *et al.* Dietary garlic suppresses DNA adducts caused by *N*-nitroso compounds. *Carcinogenesis* 1994; 15: 349–352.
63 Fujita K-I, Kamataki T. Screening of organosulfur compounds as inhibitors of human CYP2A6. *Drug Metab Disposition* 2001; 29: 983–989.
64 Guyonnet D *et al.* Antimutagenic activity of organosulfur compounds from Allium is associated with phase II enzyme induction. *Mutat Res Genet Toxicol Environ Mutagen* 2001; 495: 135–145.
65 Moon D-G *et al.* *Allium sativum* potentiates suicide gene therapy for murine transitional cell carcinoma. *Nutr Cancer* 2000; 38: 98–105.
66 Hirao Y *et al.* Activation of immunoresponder cells by the protein fraction from aged garlic extract. *Phytother Res* 1987; 1: 161–164.
67 Lamm DL, Riggs DR. Enhanced immunocompetence by garlic: role in bladder cancer and other malignancies. *J Nutr* 2001; 131 (Suppl. Suppl.3): S1067–S1070.
68 Burger RA *et al.* Enhancement of *in vitro* human immune function by *Allium sativum* L. (garlic) fractions. *Int J Pharmacog* 1993; 31: 169–174.
69 Kyo E *et al.* Immunomodulatory effects of aged garlic extract. *J Nutr* 2001; 131 (Suppl. Suppl.3): S1075–S1079.
70 Ahsan M, Islam SN. Garlic: a broad spectrum antibacterial agent effective against common pathogenic bacteria. *Fitoterapia* 1996; 67: 374–376.
71 Tsao S-M, Yin M-C. *In vitro* activity of garlic oil and four diallyl sulphides against antibiotic-resistant *Pseudomonas aeruginosa* and *Klebsiella pneumoniae*. *J Antimicrob Chemother* 2001; 47: 665–670.
72 Tsao S-M, Yin M-C. *In vitro* antimicrobial activity of four diallyl sulphides occurring naturally in garlic and Chinese leek oils. *J Med Microbiol* 2001; 50: 646–649.
73 Delaha ED, Garagusi VF. Inhibition of mycobacteria by garlic extract (*Allium sativum*). *Antimicrob Agents Chemother* 1985; 27: 485–486.
74 Deshpande RG *et al.* Inhibition of *Mycobacterium avium* complex isolates from AIDS patients by garlic (*Allium sativum*). *J Antimicrob Chemother* 1993; 32: 623–626.
75 Cellini L *et al.* Inhibition of *Helicobacter pylori* by garlic extract (*Allium sativum*). *FEMS Immunol Med Microbiol* 1996; 13: 273–277.
76 Chung JG *et al.* Effects of garlic compounds diallyl sulfide and diallyl disulfide on arylamine N-acetyltransferase activity in strains of *Helicobacter pylori* from peptic ulcer patients. *Am J Chin Med* 1998; 26: 353–364.
77 Feldberg RS *et al.* In vitro mechanism of inhibition of bacterial cell growth by allicin. *Antimicrob Agents Chemother* 1988; 32: 1763–1768.
78 Adetumbi M *et al.* *Allium sativum* (garlic) inhibits lipid synthesis by *Candida albicans*. *Antimicrob Agents Chemother* 1986; 30: 499–501.
79 Graham HD, Graham EJF. Inhibition of *Aspergillus parasiticus* growth and toxin production by garlic. *J Food Safety* 1987; 8: 101–108.
80 Ankri S *et al.* Allicin from garlic strongly inhibits cysteine proteinases and cytopathic effects of *Entamoeba histolytica*. *Antimicrob Agents Chemother* 1997; 41: 2286–2288.
81 Harris JC *et al.* The microaerophilic flagellate *Giardia intestinalis*: *Allium sativum* (garlic) is an effective antigiardial. *Microbiology* 2000; 146: 3119–3127.
82 Hughes BG *et al.* Antiviral constituents from *Allium sativum*. *Planta Med* 1989; 55: 114.
83 Tsai Y *et al.* Antiviral properties of garlic: *In vitro* effects on influenza B, Herpes simplex and Coxsackie viruses. *Planta Med* 1985; 51: 460–461.
84 Joshi DJ *et al.* Gastrointestinal actions of garlic oil. *Phytother Res* 1987; 1: 140–141.
85 Hikino H *et al.* Antihepatotoxic actions of *Allium sativum* bulbs. *Planta Med* 1986; 52: 163–168.
86 Nakagawa S *et al.* Prevention of liver damage by aged garlic extract and its components in mice. *Phytother Res* 1989; 3: 50–53.
87 Sheen L-Y *et al.* Effect of diallyl sulfide and diallyl disulfide, the active principles of garlic, on the aflatoxin B_1-induced DNA damage in primary rat hepatocytes. *Toxicol Lett* 2001; 122: 45–52.
88 Saxena KK *et al.* Effect of garlic pretreatment on isoprenaline-induced myocardial necrosis in albino rats. *Indian J Physiol Pharmacol* 1980; 24: 233–236.
89 Senapati SK *et al.* Effect of garlic (*Allium sativum* L.) extract on tissue lead level in rats. *J Ethnopharmacol* 2001; 76: 229–232.
90 Horie T *et al.* Alleviation by garlic of antitumor drug-induced damage to the intestine. *J Nutr* 2001; 131 (Suppl. Suppl.3): S1071–S1074.
91 Nishiyama N *et al.* Ameliorative effect of S-allylcysteine, a major thioallyl constituent in aged garlic extract, on learning deficits in senescence-accelerated mice. *J Nutr* 2001; 131 (Suppl. Suppl.3): S1093–S1095.

92 Brahmachari HD, Augusti KT. Orally effective hypoglycaemic agents from plants. *J Pharm Pharmacol* 1962; 14: 254–255.
93 Dirsch VM, Vollmar AM. Ajoene, a natural product with non-steroidal anti-inflammatory drug (NSAID)-like properties? *Biochem Pharmacol* 2001; 61: 587–593.
94 Koch HP. Metabolismus und pharmakokinetik der Inhaltsstoffe des Knoblauchs: was Wissen wir darüber? *Z Phytother* 1992; 13: 83–90.
95 Jandke J, Spiteller G. Unusual conjugates in biological profiles originating from consumption of onions and garlic. *J Chromatog* 1987; 421: 1–8.
96 De Rooij BM *et al.* Urinary excretion of *N*-acetyl-*S*-allyl-L-cysteine upon garlic consumption by human volunteers. *Arch Toxicol* 1996; 70: 635–639.
97 Mennella JA, Beauchamp GK. Maternal diet alters the sensory qualities of human milk and the nursling's behavior. *Pediatrics* 1991; 88: 737–744.
98 Mennella JA *et al* Garlic ingestion by pregnant women alters the odor of amniotic fluid. *Chem Senses* 1995; 20: 207–209.
99 Bordia A *et al.* Effect of garlic (*Allium sativum*) on blood lipids, blood sugar, fibrinogen and fibrinolytic activity in patients with coronary artery disease. *Prostaglandins Leukot Essent Fatty Acids* 1998; 58: 257–263.
100 Steiner M, Lin RS. Changes in platelet function and susceptibility of lipoproteins to oxidation associated with administration of aged garlic extract. *J Cardiovasc Pharmacol* 1998; 31: 904–908.
101 Warshafsky S *et al.* Effect of garlic on total serum cholesterol. A meta-analysis. *Ann Intern Med* 1993; 119: 599–605.
102 Silagy C, Neil A. Garlic as a lipid lowering agent – a meta-analysis. *J R Coll Phys Lond* 1994; 28: 2–8.
103 Neil HAW *et al.* Garlic powder in the treatment of moderate hyperlipidaemia: a controlled trial and meta-analysis. *J R Coll Phys Lond* 1996; 30: 329–334.
104 Stevinson C *et al.* Garlic for treating hypercholesterolaemia. A meta-analysis of randomized clinical trials. *Ann Intern Med* 2000; 133: 420–429.
105 Berthold HK *et al.* Effect of a garlic oil preparation on serum lipoproteins and cholesterol metabolism. A randomized controlled trial. *JAMA* 1998; 279: 1900–1902.
106 Issacsohn JL *et al.* Garlic powder and plasma lipids and lipoproteins. A multicenter, randomized, placebo-controlled trial. *Arch Intern Med* 1998; 158: 1189–1194.
107 Adler AJ, Holub BJ. Effect of garlic and fish-oil supplementation on serum lipid and lipoprotein concentrations in hypercholesterolaemic men. *Am J Clin Nutr* 1997; 65: 445–450.
108 Gardner CD *et al.* The effect of a garlic preparation on plasma lipid levels in moderately hypercholesterolaemic adults. *Atherosclerosis* 2001; 154: 213–220.
109 Lawson LD. Effect of garlic on serum lipids. *JAMA* 1998; 280: 1568.
110 Ackermann RT *et al.* Garlic shows promise for improving some cardiovascular risk factors. *Arch Intern Med* 2001; 161: 813–824.
111 Koscielny J *et al.* The anti-atherosclerotic effect of *Allium sativum. Atherosclerosis* 1999; 144: 237–249.
112 Jepson RG *et al.* Garlic for peripheral arterial occlusive disease (Cochrane review). In: The Cochrane Library, Issue 3, 2001. Oxford: Update Software.
113 Breithaupt-Grögler K *et al.* Protective effect of chronic garlic intake on elastic properties of aorta in the elderly. *Circulation* 1997; 96: 2649–2655.
114 Ali M, Thomson M. Consumption of a garlic clove a day could be beneficial in preventing thrombosis. *Prostaglandins Leukot Essent Fatty Acids* 1995; 53: 211–212.
115 Byrne DJ *et al.* A pilot study of garlic consumption shows no significant effect on markers of oxidation or sub-fraction composition of low-density lipoprotein including lipoprotein(a) after allowance for non-compliance and the placebo effect. *Clin Chim Acta* 1999; 285: 21–33.
116 Orekhov AN *et al.* Garlic powder tablets reduce atherogenicity of low density lipoprotein. A placebo-controlled double-blind study. *Nutr Metab Cardiovasc Dis* 1996; 6: 21–31.
117 Grune T *et al.* Influence of *Allium sativum* on oxidative stress status – a clinical investigation. *Phytomedicine* 1996; 2: 205–207.
118 Silagy CA, Neil HAW. A meta-analysis of the effect of garlic on blood pressure. *J Hypertens* 1994; 12: 463–468.
119 Meher S, Duley L. *Garlic for preventing pre-eclampsia and its complications (Review).* Cochrane Database of Systematic Reviews 2006, Issue 3. Art. No. CD006065.
120 Ernst E. Can *Allium* vegetables prevent cancer? *Phytomedicine* 1997; 4: 79–83.
121 You W-C *et al. Helicobacter pylori* infection, garlic intake and precancerous lesions in a Chinese population at low risk of gastric cancer. *Int J Epidemiol* 1998; 27: 941–944.
122 Ledezma E *et al.* Efficacy of ajoene, an organosulphur compound from garlic, in the short-term therapy of tinea pedis. *Mycoses* 1996; 39: 393–395.
123 Stjernberg L, Berglund J. Garlic as an insect repellant. *JAMA* 2000; 284: 831.
124 Abrams GA, Fallon MB. Treatment of hepatopulmonary syndrome with *Allium sativum* L. (Garlic): a pilot trial. *J Clin Gastroenterol* 1998; 27: 232–235.
125 Nakagawa S *et al.* Acute toxicity test of garlic extract. *J Toxicol Sci* 1984; 9: 57–60.
126 Papageorgiou C *et al.* Allergic contact dermatitis to garlic (*Allium sativum* L.) Identification of the allergens: The role of mono-, di-, and trisulfides present in garlic. *Arch Dermatol Res* 1983; 275: 229–234.
127 Lautier R, Wendt V. Contact allergy to Alliaceae/case-report and literature survey. *Dermatosen* 1985; 33: 213–215.
128 Asero R *et al.* A case of garlic allergy. *J Allergy Clin Immunol* 1998; 101: 427–428.
129 Hallel-Halevy D *et al.* Multifaceted dermatitis caused by garlic. *J Eur Acad Dermatol Venereol* 1997; 9: 185–187.
130 Farrell AM, Staughton RCD. Garlic burns mimicking herpes zoster. *Lancet* 1996; 347: 1195.
131 Rafaat M, Leung AKC. Garlic burns. *Pediatr Dermatol* 2000; 17: 475–476.
132 Sunter W. Warfarin and garlic. *Pharm J* 1991; 246: 722.
133 Baxter K, ed. *Drug Interactions*, 7th edn. London: Pharmaceutical Press, 2006.
134 Ruffin J, Hunter SA. An evaluation of the side-effects of garlic as an antihypertensive agent. *Cytobios* 1983; 37: 85–89.
135 Sumiyoshi H *et al.* Chronic toxicity test of garlic extract in rats. *J Toxicol Sci* 1984; 9: 61–75.
136 Yoshida S *et al.* Mutagenicity and cytotoxicity tests of garlic. *J Toxicol Sci* 1984; 9: 77–86.
137 Abraham SK, Kesavan PC. Genotoxicity of garlic, turmeric and asafoetida in mice. *Mutat Res* 1984; 136: 85–88.
138 Mennella JA, Beauchamp GK. The effects of repeated exposure to garlic-flavoured milk on the nursling's behavior. *Pediatr Res* 1993; 34: 805–808.

Gentian

Summary and Pharmaceutical Comment

The major constituents of pharmacological importance in gentian are the bitter principles; limited information is available on the other compounds present. The herbal uses of gentian are supported by the known properties of the bitter principles present in the root. Excessive doses should be avoided in view of the lack of toxicity data.

Species (Family)

Gentiana lutea L. (Gentianaceae)

Synonym(s)

Bitterwort, Bitter Root, Gentiana, Yellow Gentian

Part(s) Used

Rhizome, root

Pharmacopoeial and Other Monographs

BHC 1992[(G6)]
BHP 1996[(G9)]
BP 2007[(G84)]
Complete German Commission E[(G3)]
ESCOP 2003[(G76)]
Martindale 35th edition[(G85)]
Ph Eur 2007[(G81)]

Legal Category (Licensed Products)

GSL[(G37)]

Constituents

The following is compiled from several sources, including General References G2, G6 and G62.

Alkaloids Pyridine-type. Gentianine 0.6–0.8%, gentialutine.

Bitters Major component is secoiridoid glycoside gentiopicroside (also known as gentiamarin and gentiopicrin) 2%, with lesser amounts of amarogentin (0.01–0.04%) and swertiamarine.[(1)] Gentianose (a trisaccharide bitter principle). The glycosides

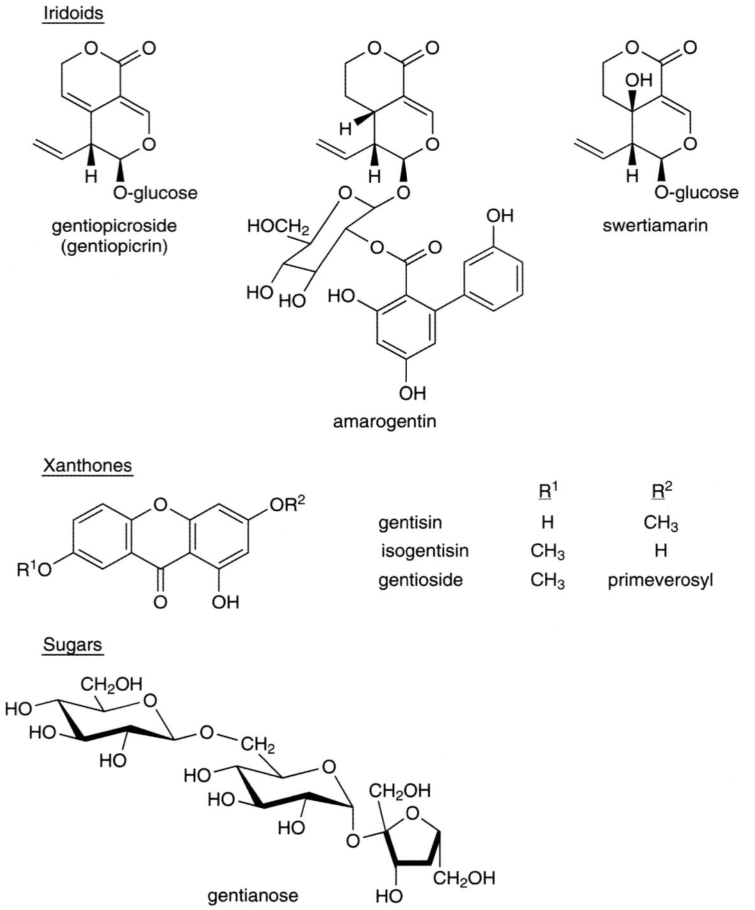

Iridoids

gentiopicroside (gentiopicrin)

amarogentin

swertiamarin

Xanthones

	R^1	R^2
gentisin	H	CH_3
isogentisin	CH_3	H
gentioside	CH_3	primeverosyl

Sugars

gentianose

Figure 1 Selected constituents of gentian.

amaropanin and amaroswerin are reported to be present in the related species *Gentiana pannonica*, *Gentiana punctata* and *Gentiana purpurea*, but are absent from *Gentiana lutea*.

Xanthones Gentisein, gentisin (gentianin), isogentisin and 1,3,7-trimethoxyxanthone.

Other constituents Carbohydrates (e.g. gentiobiose, sucrose and other common sugars), pectin, tannin (unspecified), triterpenes (e.g. β-amyrin, lupeol) and volatile oil (trace).

Food Use

Gentian (root, herbs and preparations) is listed by the Council of Europe as a natural source of food flavouring (category N4, with limits on xanthones) (*see* Appendix 3, Table 1).[G17] Previously, in the USA, gentian has been approved for food use.[G41]

Herbal Use

Gentian is stated to possess bitter, gastric stimulant, sialogogue and cholagogue properties. Traditionally, it has been used for anorexia, atonic dyspepsia, gastrointestinal atony, and specifically for dyspepsia with anorexia. The German Commission E approved use for digestive disorders such as loss of appetite, fullness and flatulence.[G3] Gentian is used in combination with angelica root and caraway fruit or with ginger and wormwood for loss of appetite and peptic discomfort.[G3]

Dosage

Dosages for oral administration (adults) for traditional uses recommended in standard herbal reference texts are given below.

Dried rhizome/root 0.6–2 g as an infusion or decoction three times daily.[G6]

Tincture 1–4 mL (1 : 5 in 45% alcohol) three times daily.[G6]

Pharmacological Actions

In vitro and animal studies

The pharmacological activites of gentian root have been reviewed.[G52] A summary of this information is provided below.

Root extracts have antifungal activity, and are reported to stimulate phagocytic activity of human lymphocytes, indicating immunostimulant activity.[G52] Choleretic properties have been documented for gentian,[G41] and gentianine has been reported to possess anti-inflammatory activity.[G22] The bitter principles stimulate secretion of gastric juices and bile, thus aiding appetite and digestion. Elevation of gastric secretion by up to 30% has been reported following the administration of gentian tincture to dogs. An infusion given orally to sheep as a single daily dose (5 g) stimulated enzyme secretion in the small intestine. A root extract (12 mg/kg/day) applied by gavage to rats for three days elevated bronchosecretion. A standardised extract perfused into the stomachs of anaesthetised rats increased gastric secretion in a dose-dependent manner. Lower doses caused no changes in gastric pH, whereas higher doses increased pH from 4.25 to 4.85. A dose of 0.5 mL/kg did not affect the incidence of gastric ulceration in rats.

Clinical studies

There is a lack of clinical research assessing the effects of gentian and rigorous randomised controlled clinical trials are required.

In an open, uncontrolled study, a single dose of an alcoholic extract of gentian (equivalent to 0.2 g), given to 10 healthy volunteers, was reported to result in a stimulation of gastric juice secretion.[2] Gall-bladder emptying was increased and prolonged whilst protein and fat digestion was enhanced. Nineteen patients with inflammatory conditions of the gastrointestinal tract (colitis, Crohn's disease, non-specific inflammation) and elevated secretory immunoglobulin A (IgA) concentrations and eight healthy individuals were treated with gentian tincture (3 × 20 drops/day) for eight days.[G52] IgA concentrations decreased in both groups.[G52] However, the methodological limitations of these studies do not allow the observed effects to be attributed to administration of gentian.

Side-effects, Toxicity

Extracts of gentian are considered to be non-toxic, and are generally well-tolerated,[G52] although clinical safety and toxicity data for gentian are limited and further investigation of these aspects is required.

Preclinical data

An acute oral LD_{50} value in mice was reported to be 25 mL/kg of extract (37% ethanol, bitterness value: 200 Swiss Pharmacopoeia units/g), and was the same as that of 37% ethanol. Rabbits treated with gentian extract (12.6 mg/day for three days) showed no toxic or abnormal concentration of serum parameters, with the exception of slightly higher erythrocyte concentrations in treated animals. Gentian may occasionally cause headache in some individuals.[G3] Mutagenic activity in the Ames test (*Salmonella typhimurium* TA100 with S9 mix) has been documented for gentian, with gentisin and isogentisin identified as mutagenic components.[3] Gentian root 100 g was reported to yield approximately 100 mg total mutagenic compounds, of which gentisin and isogentisin comprised approximately 76 mg.[3]

Contra-indications, Warnings

Gentian is stated to be contra-indicated in individuals with high blood pressure,[G60] although no rationale is given for this statement, and in individuals with hyperacidity, gastric or duodenal ulcers.[G52, G3]

Drug interactions None documented. However, the potential for preparations of gentian to interact with other medicines administered concurrently, particularly those with similar or opposing effects, should be considered.

Pregnancy and lactation Gentian is reputed to affect the menstrual cycle,[G22, G60] and it has been stated that gentian should not be used in pregnancy.[G60] In view of this and the documented mutagenic activity, gentian is best avoided in pregnancy and lactation.

Preparations

Proprietary single-ingredient preparations

Germany: Enziagil Magenplus.

Proprietary multi-ingredient preparations

Australia: Calmo; Digest; Digestaid; Digestive Aid; Extralife Sleep-Care; Pacifenity; Relaxaplex. *Austria:* Abdomilon N; Brady's-Magentropfen; China-Eisenwein; Mariazeller; Montana; Montana N; Original Schwedenbitter; Sigman-Haustropfen; Sinupret. *Brazil:* Digestar; Estomafitino; Gotas Digestivas; Xarope Iodo-Suma. *Canada:* Herbal Laxative; Herbal Nerve. *Czech Republic:* Biotussil; Dr Theiss Schweden Krauter; Dr Theiss Schwedenbitter; Naturland Grosser Swedenbitter; Sinupret. *France:* Elixir Grez; Quintonine. *Germany:* Abdomilon; Abdomilon N; Amara-Pascoe; Amara-Tropfen; Gallexier; Gastrosecur; Klosterfrau Melisana; Schwedentrunk Elixier; Sedovent; Sinupret; Solvopret; ventri-loges N. *Hong Kong:* Sinupret. *Hungary:* Sinupret. *Italy:* Amaro Medicinale; Caramelle alle Erbe Digestive. *Russia:* Herbion Drops for the Stomach (Гербион Желудочные Капли); Original Grosser Bittner Balsam (Оригинальный Большой Бальзам Биттнера); Sinupret (Синупрет). *South Africa:* Amara; Enzian Anaemodoron Drops; Helmontskruie; Lewensessens; Versterkdruppels; Wonderkroonessens. *Singapore:* Sinupret. *Spain:* Depurativo Richelet. *Switzerland:* Demonatur Gouttes pour le foie et la bile; Gastrosan; Padma-Lax; Padmed Laxan; Sinupret; Strath Gouttes pour l'estomac. *Thailand:* Pepsitase; Sinupret. *UK:* Acidosis; Appetiser Mixture; DigestAid; Indigestion Mixture; Kalms; Quiet Tyme; Scullcap & Gentian Tablets; Stomach Mixture.

References

1 Verotta L. Isolation and HPLC determination of the active principles of *Rosmarinus officinalis* and *Gentiana lutea*. *Fitoterapia* 1985; 56: 25–29.

2 Glatzel vonH, Hackenberg K. Röntgenologische untersuchungen der wirkungen von bittermitteln auf die verdauunogsorgane. *Planta Med* 1967; 15: 223–232.

3 Morimoto I *et al*. Mutagenic activities of gentisin and isogentisin from Gentianae radix (Gentianaceae). *Mutat Res* 1983; 116: 103–117.

Ginger

Summary and Pharmaceutical Comment

The chemistry of ginger is well documented with respect to the oleo-resin and volatile oil. Oleo-resin components are considered to be the main active principles in ginger and documented pharmacological actions generally support the traditional uses. In addition, a number of other pharmacological activities have been documented, including hypoglycaemic, antihypercholesterolaemic, anti-ulcer and inhibition of prostaglandin synthesis, all of which require further investigation. The use of ginger as a prophylactic remedy against motion sickness is contentious. It seems likely that ginger may act by a local action on the gastrointestinal tract, rather than by a centrally mediated mechanism.

Species (Family)

Zingiber officinale Roscoe (Zingiberaceae)

Synonym(s)

Gan Jiang, Zingiber

Part(s) Used

Rhizome

Pharmacopoeial and Other Monographs

BHC 1992[(G6)]
BHP 1996[(G9)]
BP 2007[(G84)]
BPC 1973[(G12)]
ESCOP 2003[(G76)]
Martindale 35th edition[(G85)]
Ph Eur 2007[(G81)]
USP29/NF24[(G86)]
WHO 1999 volume 1[(G63)]

Legal Category (Licensed Products)

GSL[(G37)]

Constituents

The following is compiled from several sources, including Reference 1 and General References G2 and G6.

Carbohydrates Starch (major constituent, up to 50%).

Lipids 6–8%. Free fatty acids (e.g. palmitic acid, oleic acid, linoleic acid, caprylic acid, capric acid, lauric acid, myristic acid, pentadecanoic acid, heptadecanoic acid, stearic acid, linolenic acid, arachidic acid);[(2)] triglycerides, phosphatidic acid, lecithins; gingerglycolipids A, B and C.[(3)]

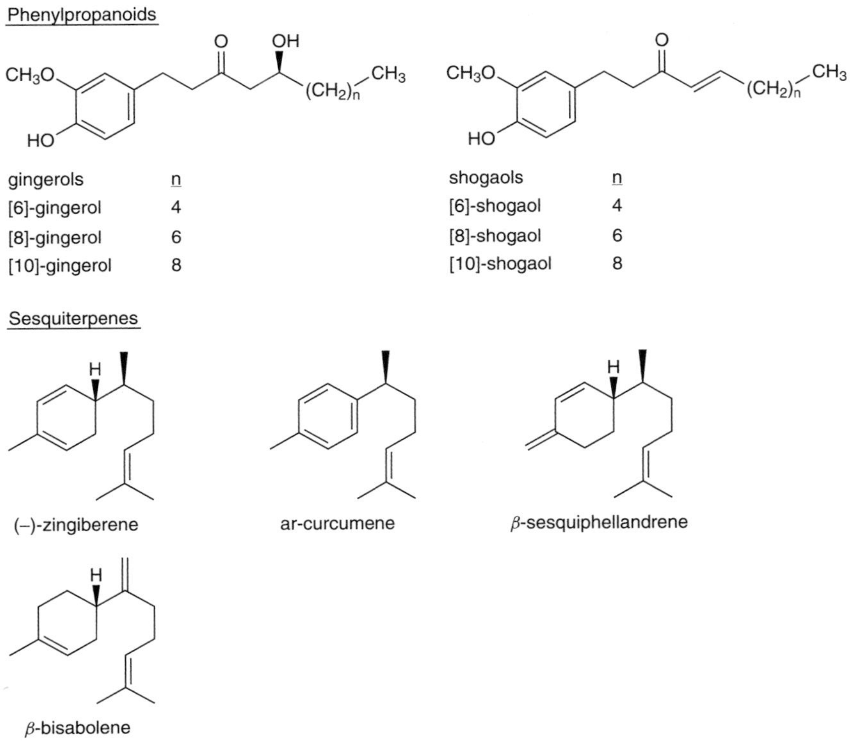

Phenylpropanoids

gingerols	n
[6]-gingerol	4
[8]-gingerol	6
[10]-gingerol	8

shogaols	n
[6]-shogaol	4
[8]-shogaol	6
[10]-shogaol	8

Sesquiterpenes

(–)-zingiberene

ar-curcumene

β-sesquiphellandrene

β-bisabolene

Figure 1 Selected constituents of ginger.

G

Oleo-resin Gingerol homologues (major, about 33%) including derivatives with a methyl side-chain,[4] shogaol homologues (dehydration products of gingerols), zingerone (degradation product of gingerols), 1-dehydrogingerdione,[5] 6-gingesulfonic acid[3] and volatile oils.

Volatile oils 1–3%. Complex, predominately hydrocarbons. β-Bisabolene and zingiberene (major); other sesquiterpenes include zingiberol, zingiberenol, *ar*-curcumene, β-sesquiphellandrene, β-sesquiphellandrol (*cis* and *trans*); numerous monoterpene hydrocarbons, alcohols and aldehydes (e.g. phellandrene, camphene, geraniol, neral, linalool, *d*-nerol).

Other constituents Amino acids (e.g. arginine, aspartic acid, cysteine, glycine, isoleucine, leucine, serine, threonine and valine), protein (about 9%), resins, diterpenes (galanolactone),[6] vitamins (especially nicotinic acid (niacin) and vitamin A), minerals.[2]

The material contains not less than 4.5% of alcohol (90%)-soluble extractive and not less than 10% of water-soluble extractive.[G15]

G

Food Use

Ginger is listed by the Council of Europe as a natural source of food flavouring (category N2). This category indicates that ginger can be added to foodstuffs in small quantities, with a possible limitation of an active principle (as yet unspecified) in the final product.[G16] It is used widely in foods as a spice. Previously, ginger has been listed as GRAS (Generally Recognised As Safe).[G41]

Herbal Use

Ginger is stated to possess carminative, diaphoretic and antispasmodic properties. Traditionally, it has been used for colic, flatulent dyspepsia, and specifically for flatulent intestinal colic.[7, G2, G6, G32, G64] Modern interest in ginger is focused on its use in the prevention of nausea and vomiting, particularly motion (travel) sickness, as a digestive aid, and as an adjunctive treatment for inflammatory conditions, such as osteoarthritis and rheumatoid arthritis.

Dosage

Dosages for oral administration (adults) for traditional uses recommended in standard herbal reference texts are given below.

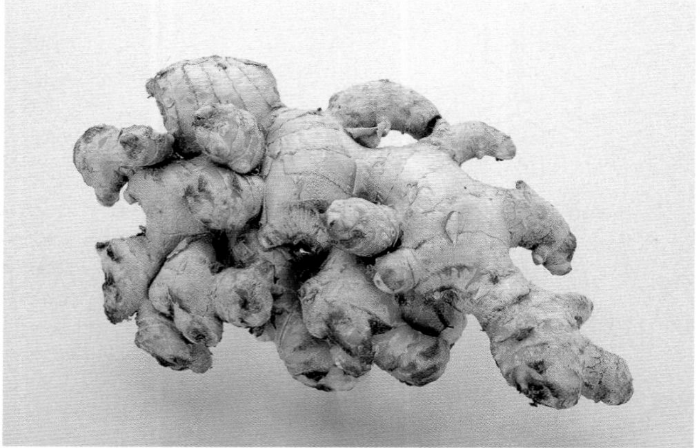

Figure 2 Ginger – dried drug substance (rhizome).

Anti-emetic

Powdered rhizome Single dose of 1–2 g,[G6] 30 minutes before travel for prevention of motion sickness,[G52] or 0.5 g, two to four times daily.[G63]

Other uses

Powdered rhizome 0.25–1 g, three times daily.[G6]

Tincture 1.5–3 mL (1 : 5) three times daily,[G6] 1.7–5 mL daily.[G50]

Pharmacological Actions

Several pharmacological activities, including anti-emetic, antithrombotic, antimicrobial, anticancer, antioxidant and anti-inflammatory properties, have been documented for preparations of ginger in *in vitro* and/or animal studies. Also, ginger has been reported to have hypoglycaemic, hypo- and hypertensive, cardiac, prostaglandin and platelet aggregation inhibition, antihypercholesterolaemic, cholagogic and stomachic properties.

Clinical studies have focused mainly on the effects of ginger in the prevention of nausea and vomiting.

In vitro and animal studies

In vitro studies have demonstrated that constituents of ginger, such as 6-, 8- and 10-gingerols and galanolactone, have antiserotonergic activity.[6, 8]

Anti-emetic activity and effects on gastrointestinal motility The older literature contains examples of studies documenting the antiemetic effects of ginger extract *in vivo* (e.g. dogs).[9] Oral administration of constituents of ginger (certain shogaols and gingerols at doses of 100 mg/kg body weight) inhibited emesis induced by oral administration of copper sulfate in leopard and ranid frogs.[10] Emetic latency was reported to be prolonged by over 150% by a trichloromethane extract of ginger at a dose of 1 g/kg body weight.

The anti-emetic activity of ginger extracts has also been assessed in dogs.[11] Acetone and ethanolic extracts of ginger, administered intragastrically at doses of 25, 50, 100 and 200 mg/kg, protected against cisplatin-induced emesis (3 mg/kg administered intravenously 30 minutes before ginger extract), compared with control. However, ginger extracts were less effective in preventing emesis than the 5-HT_3 receptor antagonist granisetron, and were ineffective against apomorphine-induced emesis.

Compared with control, an acetone extract of ginger at doses of 200 and 500 mg/kg administered orally reversed the delay in gastric emptying induced by intraperitoneal cisplatin 10 mg/kg in rats.[12] Ginger juice (2 and 4 mL/kg) had a similar effect. A 50% ethanolic extract of ginger also reversed the cisplatin-induced delay in gastric emptying, although only at a dose of 500 mg/kg. In mice, oral administration of an acetone extract of ginger (75 mg/kg), 6-shogaol (2.5 mg/kg) and 6-, 8- and 10-gingerol (5 mg/kg) enhanced the transportation of a charcoal meal, indicating enhancement of gastrointestinal motility.[13]

Anti-ulcer activity The effect of ginger (acetone extract) and zingiberene on hydrochloric acid/ethanol-induced gastric lesions in rats has been examined.[14] 6-Gingerol and zingiberene, both 100 mg/kg body weight by mouth, significantly inhibited gastric lesions by 54.5% and 53.6%, respectively. The total extract inhibited lesions by 97.5% at 1 g/kg. Oral administration of both aqueous and methanol ginger extracts to rabbits has been reported to reduce gastric secretions (gastric juice volume, acid and pepsin output).[15] Both extracts were found to be comparable with cimetidine (50 mg/kg) with respect to gastric juice volume; the aqueous extract was comparable with cimetidine and superior to the methanol extract for pepsin output, and the methanol extract superior to both the aqueous extract and comparable to cimetidine for acid output. In rats, 6-gingerol, 6-shogaol and 6-gingesulfonic acid at doses of 150 mg/kg protected against hydrochloric acid/ethanol-induced gastric lesions, compared with control.[3] 6-Gingesulfonic acid 300 mg/kg provided almost 100% protection against gastric lesions in this model. Other studies in rats found that oral administration of an ethanolic extract of ginger (500 mg/kg) inhibited gastric lesions induced by ethanol (80%), hydrochloric acid (0.6 mol/L), sodium hydroxide (0.2 mol/L), and 25% sodium chloride, compared with control.[16] The same dose of extract protected against gastric mucosal damage induced by the non-steroidal anti-inflammatory drugs (NSAIDs) indometacin and aspirin in rats. In pylorus-ligated rats, oral administration of acetone and ethanol extracts of ginger inhibited gastric secretion.[17] These extracts, at doses of 62 mg/kg, also protected against the development of stress-induced lesions, although to a lesser extent than cimetidine.

Antiplatelet activity 6-Gingerol, 6- and 10-dehydrogingerdione, 6- and 10-gingerdione have been reported to be potent inhibitors of prostaglandin biosynthesis (PG synthetase) *in vitro*, with the latter four compounds stated to be more potent than indometacin.[18] Concentration-dependent inhibition of platelet aggregation, *in vitro*, induced by ADP, adrenaline, collagen and arachidonic acid has been described for an aqueous ginger extract.[19] Ginger was also found to reduce platelet synthesis of prostaglandin-endoperoxides, thromboxane and prostaglandins. A good correlation was reported between concentrations of the extract required to inhibit platelet aggregation and concentrations necessary to inhibit platelet thromboxane synthesis.[19]

Anti-atherosclerotic and antioxidant activity Ginger oleoresin, by intragastric administration, has been reported to inhibit elevation in serum and hepatic cholesterol concentrations in rats by impairing cholesterol absorption.[20] Antihypercholesterolaemic activity has also been documented for dried ginger rhizome when given to both rats fed a cholesterol-rich diet and those with existing hypercholesterolaemia.[21] Fresh ginger juice was not found to have an effect on serum cholesterol concentrations within four hours of administration. In addition, serum cholesterol concentrations were not greatly increased within four hours of cholesterol administration.

An ethanol (50%) extract of ginger administered orally at a dose of 500 mg/kg to hyperlipidaemic rabbits led to a significant reduction in blood serum cholesterol concentrations, compared with those in control rabbits.[22] In a study in rabbits fed cholesterol for 10 weeks, administration of an ethanolic extract of ginger (200 mg/kg orally) decreased raised serum and tissue concentrations of cholesterol, serum triglycerides and serum lipoproteins.[23]

An ethanolic ginger extract, standardised to contain 40 mg/g gingerols, shogaols and zingerone, and 90 mg/g total polyphenols, was reported to inhibit low-density lipoprotein oxidation and to reduce the development of atherosclerosis in atherosclerotic mice, when compared with control.[24] In rats fed a high-fat diet for 10 weeks, an aqueous preparation of ginger powder administered orally at doses of 35 and 70 mg/kg demonstrated antioxidant activity, as measured by raised tissue concentrations of thiobarbituric acid reactive substances and hydroperoxides, and reduced activities of superoxide dismutase and catalase.[25]

The antioxidant activity of ginger constituents has been documented *in vitro*.[26]

Anti-inflammatory activity Constituents of ginger have been shown to have anti-inflammatory activity *in vitro*. In a study in intact human airway epithelial cells (A549 cells), 8-paradol and 8-shogaol inhibited cyclooxygenase 2 (COX-2) enzyme activity in a concentration-dependent manner (IC_{50} values ranged from 1 to 25 µmol/L).[27] In other studies, an acetone extract of ginger inhibited inflammation of the chorioallantoic membrane of fertilised hen's eggs in a concentration-dependent manner.[28] In another assay, the extract exhibited anti-inflammatory properties by inhibiting the release of nitric oxide in a concentration-dependent manner.[28] Ginger oil has demonstrated anti-inflammatory activity in a study in rats with severe chronic adjuvant arthritis induced by injection of 0.05 mL of a suspension of dead *Mycobacterium tuberculosis* bacilli.[29] Ginger oil 33 mg/kg administered orally for 26 days caused a significant suppression of paw and joint swelling, compared with control (no ginger oil).

Several other studies describe anti-inflammatory activity for ginger constituents.[26]

Antimicrobial activity *In vitro* activity against rhinovirus IB has been reported for sesquiterpenes isolated from ginger rhizomes.[1] The most active compound was β-sesquiphellandrene (IC_{50} 0.44 µmol/L). *In vitro* anthelmintic activity against *Ascaridia galli* Schrank has been documented for the volatile oil of *Zingiber purpureum* Roxb.[30] Activity exceeding that of piperazine citrate was exhibited by the oxygenated compounds fractionated from the volatile oil.

Anticancer activity Extracts of ginger or constituents of ginger have been shown to have cancer chemopreventive and cytotoxic or cytostatic activity *in vitro* and *in vivo* (animals). Application of an ethanolic extract of fresh ginger in a mouse skin tumorigenesis model (SENCAR mice) resulted in significant inhibition of 12-O-tetradecanoylphorbol-13-acetate (TPA)-induced induction of epidermal ornithine decarboxylase, cyclooxygenase and lipoxygenase activities in a concentration-dependent manner.[31] Preapplication of ginger extract also inhibited TPA-induced epidermal oedema and hyperplasia. Application of ginger extract 30 minutes before application of two tumour inducers to the skin of SENCAR mice protected against skin tumour incidence, compared with control. In another mouse model, topical application of 6-gingerol or 6-paradol before application of tumour inducers attenuated skin papillomagenesis.[32] Other studies also describe the cancer chemopreventive potential of ginger and its constituents.[26]

In vitro, incubation of 6-gingerol with human promyelocytic leukaemia (HL-60) cells resulted in inhibitory effects on cell viability and DNA synthesis.[33] Microscopic examination of the incubated cells provided evidence of the induction of apoptosis by 6-gingerol.

Other activities In rats, the anxiolytic effects of pretreatment with a combination preparation of standardised extracts of ginger and *Ginkgo biloba* administered intragastrically at doses between 0.5 and 100 mg/kg were assessed in the elevated plus-maze test.[34] The combination was found to have an anxiolytic effect at lower doses, but appeared to have an anxiogenic effect at higher doses.

A hypoglycaemic effect in both non-diabetic and alloxan-induced diabetic rabbits and rats has been documented for fresh ginger juice administered orally. The effect was stated to be significant in the diabetic animals.[35]

The pharmacological actions of 6-shogaol and capsaicin have been compared.[36] Both compounds caused rapid hypotension followed by a marked pressor response, bradycardia, and apnoea in rats after intravenous administration. The pressor response was thought to be a centrally acting mechanism. Contractile responses in isolated guinea-pig trachea with both compounds, and positive inotropic and chronotropic responses in isolated rat atria with 6-shogaol were thought to involve the release of an unknown active substance from nerve endings.[36] A potent, positive inotropic action on isolated guinea-pig atria has been documented and gingerols were identified as the cardiotonic principles.[37]

A cholagogic action in rats has been described for an acetone extract of ginger administered intraduodenally.[38] 6-Gingerol and 10-gingerol were reported to be the active components, the former more potent with a significant increase in bile secretion still apparent four hours after administration.

Utero-activity has been described for a phenolic compound isolated from *Zingiber cassumunar* Roxb.[39] The compound was found to exhibit a dose-related relaxant effect on the non-pregnant rat uterus *in situ*; the uterine response from pregnant rats was stated to vary with the stage of pregnancy, the post-implantation period being the most sensitive. The compound was thought to act by a similar mechanism to that of papaverine.[39]

Clinical studies

Clinical trials of ginger have focused mainly on its effects on the prevention and treatment of nausea and vomiting of various causes. Other clinical studies have assessed the effects of ginger preparations on gastrointestinal motility and on platelet function, and in vertigo and inflammatory conditions, such as osteoarthritis. Several of these studies are described below.

Nausea and vomiting and effects on gastrointestinal motility Ginger has been reported to be effective as a prophylactic against seasickness.[40,41] Ingestion of powdered ginger root 1 g was found to significantly reduce the tendency to vomit and experience cold sweating in 40 naval cadets, compared with 39 cadets who received placebo.[40] Powdered ginger root 1.88 g has been reported to be superior to dimenhydrinate 100 mg in preventing the gastrointestinal symptoms of motion sickness induced by a rotating chair.[41] However, a second study reported ginger (500 mg powdered, 1 g powdered/fresh) to be ineffective in the prevention of motion sickness induced by a rotating chair.[42] The study concluded hyoscine 600 μg and dexamfetamine 10 mg to be the most effective combination, with dimenhydrinate 50 mg as the over-the-counter motion sickness medication of choice.[42]

A systematic review of six randomised controlled trials of ginger preparations included three trials involving patients with post-operative nausea and vomiting, and three further trials in patients with seasickness (motion sickness), morning sickness (emesis of pregnancy) and cancer chemotherapy-induced nausea (one trial in each condition).[43] Two of the three studies assessing the effects of ginger in post-operative nausea and vomiting found that ginger was more effective than placebo and as effective as metoclopramide in reducing nausea. However, when the data from the three studies were pooled, the difference between the ginger and placebo groups was statistically non-significant.[43]

A randomised, double-blind, crossover trial involving women with nausea of pregnancy assessed the effects of capsules of powdered ginger root 250 mg, or placebo, administered orally four times daily for four days.[44] It was reported that symptom relief was significantly greater during treatment with ginger than with placebo, and that significantly more women stated a preference for ginger treatment than for placebo (as later disclosed). A more recent randomised, double-blind trial involving 70 women with nausea and vomiting of pregnancy assessed the effectiveness of capsules of powdered fresh ginger root 250 mg four times daily, or placebo, for four days.[45] At the end of the study, ginger recipients had significantly lower scores for nausea and fewer vomiting episodes than did the placebo group.

Studies involving healthy volunteers have investigated the effects of ginger on gastric emptying as a possible mechanism for the anti-emetic effects of ginger. A randomised, double-blind, placebo-controlled, crossover trial involving 16 volunteers assessed the effects of capsules containing powdered ginger 1 g for one week, followed by a one-week wash-out period before crossing over to the opposite arm of the study.[46] Gastric emptying was measured using a paracetamol absorption technique by comparing the effects of ginger administration on mean and peak plasma paracetamol concentrations. The results indicated that the rate of absorption of oral paracetamol was not affected by simultaneous ingestion of ginger. Another randomised, double-blind, placebo-controlled trial involving 12 healthy volunteers assessed the effects of ginger rhizome extract on fasting and postprandial gastroduodenal motility.[47] The results of this study indicated that oral administration of ginger improved gastroduodenal motility in both the fasting state and after a test meal.

A randomised, double-blind, placebo-controlled, crossover trial involving eight healthy volunteers tested the effects of powdered ginger root 1 g on experimentally induced vertigo.[48] One hour after ginger or placebo administration, participants' vestibular system was stimulated by water irrigation of the left ear. It was reported that ginger significantly reduced vertigo, when compared with placebo.

Other effects In a randomised, double-blind, placebo-controlled, crossover trial involving 75 patients with osteoarthritis of the knee or hip, the effects of capsules of ginger extract 170 mg three times daily were compared with those of ibuprofen 400 mg three times daily, or placebo, for three weeks with a one-week wash-out period between each treatment period.[49] At the end of the study, data for the 56 evaluable participants indicated that there was no strong evidence of an effect for ginger extract over that of placebo on parameters of pain.

A reduction in joint pain and improvement in joint movement in seven rheumatoid arthritis sufferers has been documented for ginger, with a dual inhibition of cyclooxygenase and lipoxygenase pathways reported as a suggested mechanism of action.[50,51] Patients took either fresh ginger in amounts ranging from 5–50 g or powdered ginger 0.1–1.0 g daily.

A placebo-controlled study assessed the effects of two doses of ginger powder (4 g daily for three months, and 10 g as a single dose) on platelet aggregation and fibrinolytic activity in patients with coronary artery disease (CAD).[52] The results indicated that long-term administration of ginger powder did not affect ADP- and epinephrine (adrenaline)-induced platelet aggregation and had no effects on fibrinolytic activity or fibrinogen concentrations, compared with placebo administration. By contrast, administration of a single dose of ginger powder to 10 patients with CAD produced a significant reduction in platelet aggregation, compared with placebo administration (n = 10 patients with CAD).

In a study involving seven women, oral raw ginger 5 g reduced thromboxane B_2 concentrations in serum collected after clotting,[50] thus indicating a reduction in eicosanoid synthesis (associated with platelet aggregation).

Side-effects, Toxicity

Clinical data

None documented. However, there is a lack of clinical safety and toxicity data for ginger and further investigation of these aspects is required. Ginger oil is stated to be non-irritating and non-sensitising although dermatitis may be precipitated in hypersensitive individuals. Phototoxicity is not considered to be of significance.[53]

Preclinical data

Ginger oil is stated to be of low toxicity[G58] with acute LD_{50} values (rat, by mouth; rabbit, dermal) reported to exceed 5 g/kg.[53]

Mutagenic activity has been documented for an ethanolic ginger extract, gingerol and shogaol in *Salmonella typhimurium* strains TA100 and TA1535 in the presence of metabolic activation (S9 mix) but not in TA98 or TA1538 with or without S9 mix.[54] Zingerone was found to be non-mutagenic in all four strains with or without S9 mix, and was reported to suppress mutagenic activity of gingerol and shogaol. Ginger juice has been reported to exhibit antimutagenic activity, whereas mutagenic activity has been described for 6-gingerol in the presence of known chemical mutagens.[55] It was suggested that certain mutagens may activate the mutagenic activity of 6-gingerol so that it is not suppressed by antimutagenic components present in the juice.[55]

Contra-indications, Warnings

Drug interactions In view of the documented pharmacological actions of ginger, the potential for preparations of ginger to interfere with other medicines administered concurrently, particularly those with similar or opposing effects, should be considered.

Ginger has been reported to possess both cardiotonic and antiplatelet activity *in vitro* and hypoglycaemic activity in *in vivo* studies. An oleo-resin component, 6-shogaol has been reported to affect blood pressure (initially decrease then increase) *in vivo*. The clinical significance of these findings, if any, is unclear.

Pregnancy and lactation Ginger is reputed to be an abortifacient[G30] and utero-activity has been documented for a related species. Doses of ginger that greatly exceed the amounts used in foods should not be taken during pregnancy or lactation.

Preparations

Proprietary single-ingredient preparations

Australia: Travacalm Natural. *Canada:* Gravol Natural Source. *Germany:* Zintona. *Switzerland:* Zintona. *UK:* Travel Sickness; Zinaxin.

Proprietary multi-ingredient preparations

Australia: Bioglan Ginger-Vite Forte; Bioglan Psylli-Mucil Plus; Boswellia Complex; Boswellia Compound; Broncafect; Cal Alkyline; Digestive Aid; Dyzco; Extralife Arthri-Care; Feminine Herbal Complex; Ginkgo Plus Herbal Plus Formula 10; Herbal Cleanse; Herbal Digestive Formula; Lifesystem Herbal Plus Formula 11 Ginkgo; PC Regulax; Peritone; PMS Support; PMT Complex; Travelaide. *Austria:* Mariazeller. *Brazil:* Broncol. *Canada:* Cayenne Plus; Chase Kolik Gripe Water. *Czech Republic:* Naturland Grosser Swedenbitter. *France:* Evacrine. *Germany:* Fovysat; Gallexier; Gastrosecur; Klosterfrau Melisana. *India:* Carmicide; Happy'tizer; Tummy Ease; Well-Beeing. *Italy:* Donalg; Pik Gel. *Malaysia:* Dandelion Complex; Total Man; Zinaxin Plus. *Russia:* Doktor Mom (Доктор Мом); Doktor Mom Herbal Cough Lozenges (Доктор Мом Растительные Пастилки От Кашля); Maraslavin (Мараславин); Original Grosser Bittner Balsam (Оригинальный Большой Бальзам Биттнера). *South Africa:* Helmontskruie; Lewensessens; Wonderkroonessens. *Singapore:* Artrex. *Switzerland:* Padma-Lax; Padmed Laxan; Tisane pour les problemes de prostate. *Thailand:* Flatulence Gastulence; Zinaxin Plus. *UK:* Arheumacare; Digestive; Dr Scurr's Zinopin; Golden Seal Indigestion Tablets; Höfels One-A-Day Ginge; Höfels One-A-Day Ginger, Ginkgo and Garlic; HRI Golden Seal Digestive; Indian Brandee; Indigestion Relief; Napiers Digestion Tablets; Napiers Monthly Calm Tea; Neo Baby Gripe Mixture; Neo Gripe Mixture; Nervous Dyspepsia Tablets; Traveleeze; Wind & Dyspepsia Relief; Zinopin. *USA:* Herbal Energy; Heart Health; My Favorite Multiple; Liver Formula. *Venezuela:* Jengimiel; Jengimiel.

References

1 Denyer CV *et al*. Isolation of antirhinoviral sesquiterpenes from ginger (*Zingiber officinale*). *J Nat Prod* 1994; 57: 658–662.
2 Lawrence BM, Reynolds RJ. Major tropical spices – ginger (*Zingiber officinale* Rosc.). *Perf Flav* 1984; 9: 1–40.
3 Yoshikawa M *et al*. 6-Gingesulfonic acid, a new anti-ulcer principle, and gingerglycolipids A, B and C, three new monoacyldigalactosylglycerols from Zingiberis rhizoma originating in Taiwan. *Chem Pharm Bull* 1992; 40: 2239–2241.
4 Chen C-C *et al*. Chromatographic analyses of gingerol compounds in ginger (*Zingiber officinale* Roscoe) extracted by liquid carbon dioxide. *J Chromatogr* 1986; 360: 163–174.
5 Charles R *et al*. New gingerdione from the rhizomes of *Zingiber officinale*. *Fitoterapia* 2000; 71: 716–718.
6 Huang Q *et al*. Anti-5-hydroxytryptamine3 effect of galanolactone, diterpenoid isolated from ginger. *Chem Pharm Bull* 1991; 39: 397–399.
7 Langner E *et al*. Ginger: history and use. *Adv Ther* 1998; 15: 25–44.
8 Yamahara J *et al*. Active components of ginger exhibiting anti-serotonergic action. *Phytother Res* 1989; 3: 70–71.
9 Chang H-M, But PP-H, eds. *Pharmacology and Applications of Chinese Materia Medica*, vol 1. Singapore: World Scientific Publishing, 1986: 366–369.
10 Kawai T *et al*. Anti-emetic principles of *Magnolia obovata* bark and *Zingiber officinale* rhizome. *Planta Med* 1994; 60: 17–20.
11 Sharma SS *et al*. Antiemetic activity of ginger (*Zingiber officinale*) against cisplatin-induced emesis in dogs. *J Ethnopharmacol* 1997; 57: 93–96.
12 Sharma SS, Gupta YK. Reversal of cisplatin-induced delay in gastric emptying in rats by ginger (*Zingiber officinale*). *J Ethnopharmacol* 1998; 62: 49–55.
13 Yamahara J *et al*. Gastrointestinal motility enhancing effect of ginger and its active constituents. *Chem Pharm Bull* 1990; 38: 430–431.
14 Yamahara J *et al*. The anti-ulcer effect in rats of ginger constituents. *J Ethnopharmacol* 1988; 23: 299–304.
15 Sakai K *et al*. Effect of extracts of Zingiberaceae herbs on gastric secretion in rabbits. *Chem Pharm Bull* 1989; 37: 215–217.
16 Al-Yahya MA *et al*. Gastroprotective activity of ginger *Zingiber officinale* Rosc., in albino rats. *Am J Chin Med* 1998; 17: 51–56.
17 Sertie JAA *et al*. Preventive anti-ulcer activity of the rhizome extract of *Zingiber officinale*. *Fitoterapia* 1992; 63: 55–59.
18 Kiuchi F *et al*. Inhibitors of prostaglandin biosynthesis from ginger. *Chem Pharm Bull* 1982; 30: 754–757.
19 Srivastava KC. Effects of aqueous extracts of onion, garlic and ginger on platelet aggregation and metabolism of arachidonic acid in the blood vascular system: in vitro study. *Prostaglandins Leukot Med* 1984; 13: 227–235.

G

20 Gujral S *et al*. Effect of ginger (*Zingiber officinale* Roscoe) oleorosin on serum and hepatic cholesterol levels in cholesterol fed rats. *Nutr Rep Int* 1974; 17: 183–189.
21 Giri J *et al*. Effect of ginger on serum cholesterol levels. *Indian J Nutr Diet* 1984; 21: 433–436.
22 Sharma I *et al*. Hypolipidaemic and antiatherosclerotic effects of *Zingiber officinale* in cholesterol fed rabbits. *Phytother Res* 1996; 10: 517–518.
23 Bhandari U *et al*. The protective action of ethanolic ginger (*Zingiber officinale*) extract in cholesterol fed rabbits. *J Ethnopharmacol* 1998; 61: 167–171.
24 Fuhrman B *et al*. Ginger extract consumption reduces plasma cholesterol, inhibits LDL oxidation and attenuates development of atherosclerosis in atherosclerotic, apolipoprotein E-deficient mice. *J Nutr* 2000; 130: 1124–1131.
25 Jeyakumar SM *et al*. Antioxidant activity of ginger (*Zingiber officinale* Rosc) in rats fed a high fat diet. *Med Sci Res* 1999; 27: 341–344.
26 Surh Y-J *et al*. Chemoprotective properties of some pungent ingredients present in red pepper and ginger. *Mutat Res* 1998; 402: 259–267.
27 Tjendraputra E *et al*. Effect of ginger constituents and synthetic analogues on cyclooxygenase-2 enzyme in intact cells. *Bioorg Chem* 2001; 29: 156–163.
28 Schuhbaum H *et al*. Anti-inflammatory activity of *Zingiber officinale* extracts. *Pharm Pharmacol Lett* 2000; 2: 82–85.
29 Sharma JN *et al*. Suppressive effects of eugenol and ginger oil on arthritic rats. *Pharmacology* 1994; 49: 314–318.
30 Taroeno *et al*. Anthelmintic activities of some hydrocarbons and oxygenated compounds in the essential oil of *Zingiber purpureum*. *Planta Med* 1989; 55: 105.
31 Katiyar SK *et al*. Inhibition of tumor promotion in SENCAR mouse skin by ethanol extract of *Zingiber officinale* rhizome. *Cancer Res* 1996; 56: 1023–1030.
32 Surh Y-J *et al*. Anti-tumor-promoting activities of selected pungent phenolic substances in ginger. *J Environ Pathol Toxicol Oncol* 1999; 18: 131–139.
33 Lee E, Surh Y-J. Induction of apoptosis in HL-60 cells by pungent vanilloids, [6]-gingerol and [6]-paradol. *Cancer Lett* 1998; 134: 163–168.
34 Hasenohrl RU *et al*. Anxiolytic-like effect of combined extracts of *Zingiber officinale* and *Ginkgo biloba* in the elevated plus-maze. *Pharmacol Biochem Behav* 1996; 53: 271–275.
35 Sharma M, Shukla S. Hypoglycaemic effect of ginger. *J Res Ind Med Yoga Homoeopath* 1977; 12: 127–130.
36 Suekawa M *et al*. Pharmacological studies on ginger. V. Pharmacological comparison between (6)-shogaol and capsaicin. *Folia Pharmac Jpn* 1986; 88: 339–347.
37 Shoji N *et al*. Cardiotonic principles of ginger (*Zingiber officinale* Roscoe). *J Pharm Sci* 1982; 71: 1174–1175.
38 Yamahara J *et al*. Cholagogic effect of ginger and its active constituents. *J Ethnopharmacol* 1985; 13: 217–225.
39 Kanjanapothi D *et al*. A uterine relaxant compound from *Zingiber cassumunar*. *Planta Med* 1987; 53: 329–332.
40 Grontved A *et al*. Ginger root against seasickness. A controlled trial on the open sea. *Acta Otolaryngol* 1988; 105: 45–49.
41 Mowrey DB, Clayson DE. Motion sickness, ginger, and psychophysics. *Lancet* 1982; i: 655–657.
42 Wood CD *et al*. Comparison of efficacy of ginger with various antimotion sickness drugs. *Clin Res Pract Drug Reg Affairs* 1988; 6: 129–136.
43 Ernst E, Pittler MH. Efficacy of ginger for nausea and vomiting. A systematic review of randomised clinical trials. *Br J Anaesthesia* 2000; 84: 367–371.
44 Fischer-Rasmussen W *et al*. Ginger treatment of hyperemesis gravidarum. *Eur J Obs Gyn Reprod Biol* 1990; 38: 19–24.
45 Vutyavanich T *et al*. Ginger for nausea and vomiting in pregnancy: randomised, double-masked, placebo-controlled trial. *Obstet Gynecol* 2001; 97: 577–582.
46 Phillips S *et al*. *Zingiber officinale* does not affect gastric emptying rate. A randomised, placebo-controlled, crossover trial. *Anaesthesia* 1993; 48: 393–395.
47 Micklefield GH *et al*. Effects of ginger on gastroduodenal motility. *Int J Clin Pharmacol Ther* 1999; 37: 341–346.
48 Grontved A, Hentzer E. Vertigo-reducing effect of ginger root. A controlled clinical study. *ORL J Otorhinolaryngol* 1986; 48: 282–286.
49 Bliddal H *et al*. A randomized, placebo-controlled, cross-over study of ginger extracts and ibuprofen in osteoarthritis. *Osteoarthritis Cartilage* 2000; 8: 9–12.
50 Srivastava KC. Effect of onion and ginger consumption on platelet thromboxane production in humans. *Prostaglandins Leukot Essent Fatty Acids* 1989; 35: 183–185.
51 Srivastava K *et al*. Ginger and rheumatic disorders. *Med Hypoth* 1989; 29: 25–28.
52 Bordia A *et al*. Effect of ginger (*Zingiber officinale* Rosc.) and fenugreek (*Trigonella foenumgraecum* L.) on blood lipids, blood sugar and platelet aggregation in patients with coronary artery disease. *Prostaglandins Leukot Essent Fatty Acids* 1997; 56: 379–384.
53 Opdyke DLJ. Ginger oil. *Food Cosmet Toxicol* 1974; 12: 901–902.
54 Nagabhushan M *et al*. Mutagenicity of ginergol and shogaol and antimutagenicity of zingerone in salmonella/microsome assay. *Cancer Lett* 1987; 36: 221–233.
55 Nakamura H, Yamamoto T. Mutagen and anti-mutagen in ginger, *Zingiber officinale*. *Mutat Res* 1982; 103: 119–126.

Ginkgo

Summary and Pharmaceutical Comment

There is a vast scientific literature describing the pharmacological effects of ginkgo leaf extracts and their constituents. These data provide some supporting evidence for the modern clinical uses of standardised ginkgo leaf extracts.

Also, standardised ginkgo leaf extracts are among the herbal preparations that have undergone most extensive clinical investigation. The effects of ginkgo extracts in dementia have been tested clinically mostly in trials involving patients with cognitive deficiency, Alzheimer's disease and/or multi-infarct dementia. Some high-quality studies involving patients with dementia have reported significant beneficial effects for standardised ginkgo leaf extracts. However, systematic reviews/meta-analysis of all relevant randomised, double-blind, placebo-controlled trials have reported modest effects for ginkgo extract, compared with placebo, and have concluded that further high-quality studies are required to establish the benefits of ginkgo in dementia. Small randomised, double-blind, placebo-controlled trials investigating the cognitive enhancing effects of ginkgo extracts in healthy volunteers have reported conflicting results. Further study is required to determine whether ginkgo extracts are of value in cognitively intact individuals. The available evidence does not demonstrate that ginkgo extracts are effective in patients with tinnitus. A meta-analysis of trials of standardised ginkgo leaf extract in peripheral arterial occlusive disease found that ginkgo significantly improved pain-free walking distance, although the clinical relevance of the extent of improvement is questionable.

Data from clinical trials and post-marketing surveillance studies indicate that standardised extracts of ginkgo leaf are well tolerated when used at recommended doses and according to other guidance. However, there are reports of bleeding associated with the use of ginkgo leaf preparations and until further information is available, ginkgo should not be used in patients with previous or existing bleeding disorders unless the potential benefits outweigh the potential harms. In view of the lack of conclusive evidence for the efficacy of ginkgo leaf in the various conditions for which it is used, and the serious nature of the potential harm, it is extremely unlikely that the benefit–harm balance would be in favour of such patients using ginkgo leaf preparations.

In view of the documented pharmacological actions of ginkgo, the potential for preparations of ginkgo leaf to interfere with other medicines administered concurrently, particularly those with similar (such as anticoagulant and antiplatelet agents) or opposing effects, should be considered.

Ginkgo should not be used during pregnancy and breastfeeding. In view of the intended uses of ginkgo and the documented pharmacological actions of ginkgo, it is not suitable for self-treatment.

Species (Family)

Ginkgo biloba L. (Ginkgoaceae)

Synonym(s)

Fossil Tree, Kew Tree, Maidenhair Tree, Yin Xing (whole plant), Yin Xing Ye (leaves), Bai Guo (seeds), *Salisburia adiantifolia* Sm., *S. biloba* (L.) Hoffmans

Part(s) Used

Leaf

Pharmacopoeial and Other Monographs

AHP[G1]
BHP 1996[G9]
BP 2007[G84]
Complete German Commission E[G3]
Martindale 35th edition[G85]
Ph Eur 2007[G81]
USP29/NF24[G86]
WHO volume 1 1999[G63]

Legal Category (Licensed Products)

Ginkgo is not included in the GSL.[G37]

Constituents

The following is compiled from several sources, including References 1 and 2.

Leaf

Amino acids 6-Hydroxykynurenic acid (2-carboxy-4-one-6-hydroxyquinoline), a metabolite of tryptophan.[3–5]

Flavonoids Dimeric flavones (e.g. amentoflavone, bilobetin, ginkgetin, isoginkgetin, sciadopitysin);[6] flavonols (e.g. quercetin, kaempferol) and their glycosides[3,7] and coumaroyl esters.

Proanthocyanidins Terpenoids Sesquiterpenes (e.g. bilobalide), diterpenes (e.g. ginkgolides A, B, C, J, M, which are unique cage molecules,[8,9,G48] and triterpenes (e.g. sterols).

Other constituents Benzoic acid, ginkgolic acids, 2-hexenal, polyprenols (e.g. di-*trans*-poly-*cis*-octadecaprenol), sugars, waxes,[1] a peptide.[10]

Seeds

Alkaloids Ginkgotoxin (4-*O*-methylpyridoxine).[11]

Amino acids Cyanogenetic glycosides Ginkgolic acids. Ginkbilobin.[12]

Quality of plant material and commercial products

According to the British and European Pharmacopoeias, ginkgo consists of the dried leaves of *Ginkgo biloba* L. It contains not less than 0.5% of flavonoids expressed as flavone glycosides (M_r 757) and calculated with reference to the dried drug.

Standardised extracts of *G. biloba* leaves are standardised on the content of ginkgo flavonoid glycosides (22–27%; determined as quercetin, kaempferol and isorhamnetin), and terpene lactones (5–7%; comprising around 2.8–3.4% ginkgolides A, B and C, and 2.6–3.2% bilobalide, and less than 5 ppm ginkgolic acids).[G3, G56]

As with other herbal medicinal products, there is variation in the qualitative and quantitative composition of ginkgo leaf crude plant material and commercial ginkgo leaf preparations.

An analytical study of 27 products containing ginkgo leaf available in the USA including 24 products that were stated to be 'standardised'.[13] For 17 of these, the content of ginkgo flavonoid glycosides and/or terpene lactones was greater than the stated amount. Also, only seven products contained ginkgolic acids at a concentration of < 500 parts per million (ppm); the concentration of ginkgolic acids in nine products was $> 25\,000$ ppm. Differences in pharmaceutical quality between different ginkgo leaf products lead to varying *in vitro* dissolution and *in vivo* bioavailability (*see* Pharmacological Actions, Pharmacokinetics).[14]

Food Use

Ginkgo biloba is not used in foods.

Herbal Use

Ginkgo has a long history of medicinal use, dating back to 2800 BC. Traditional Chinese medicine used the seeds (kernel/nuts) for therapeutic purposes. The seed is used in China as an antitussive, expectorant and anti-asthmatic, and in bladder inflammation.[1, 11, G50] In China, the leaves of *Ginkgo biloba* were also used in asthma and in cardiovascular disorders,[1] although the leaves have little history of traditional use in the West. Today, standardised concentrated extracts of *G. biloba* leaves are marketed in several European countries, and are used in cognitive deficiency, intermittent claudication (generally resulting from peripheral arterial occlusive disease), and vertigo and tinnitus of vascular origin (*see* Pharmacological Actions, Clinical studies).[G3, G32, G56, G63]

Dosage

Dosages for oral administration (adults) for traditional uses recommended in older and contemporary standard herbal reference texts are given below.

Cognitive deficiency

Leaf extract 120–240 mg dry extract orally in two or three divided doses.[G3]

Peripheral arterial occlusive disease and vertigo/tinnitus

Leaf extract 120–160 mg dry extract orally in two or three divided doses.[G3]

Diterpenes

	R1	R2	R3
ginkgolide A	OH	H	H
ginkgolide B	OH	OH	H
ginkgolide C	OH	OH	OH
ginkgolide J	OH	H	OH
ginkgolide M	H	OH	OH

bilobalide

Flavonoids

	R
kaempferol	H
quercetin	OH

amentoflavone

Amino acids

6-hydroxykynurenic acid

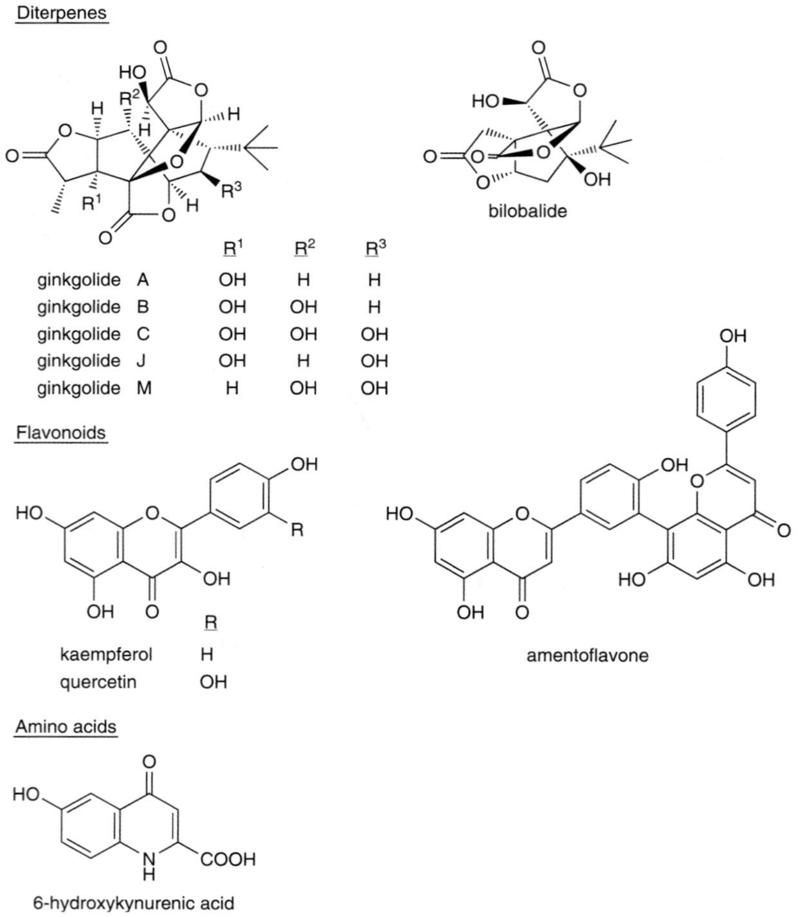

Figure 1 Selected constituents of ginkgo.

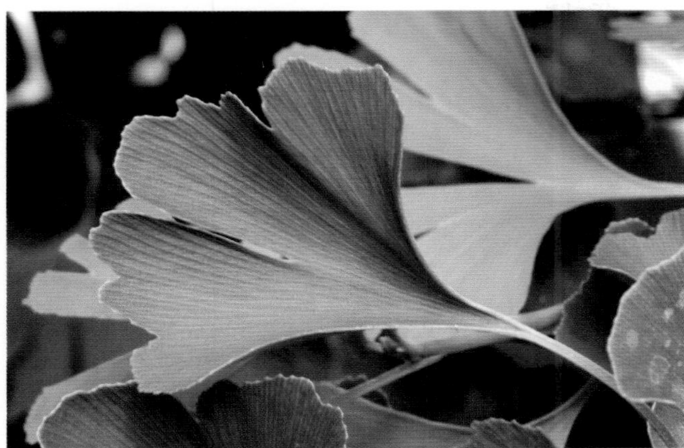

Figure 2 Ginkgo (*Ginkgo biloba*).

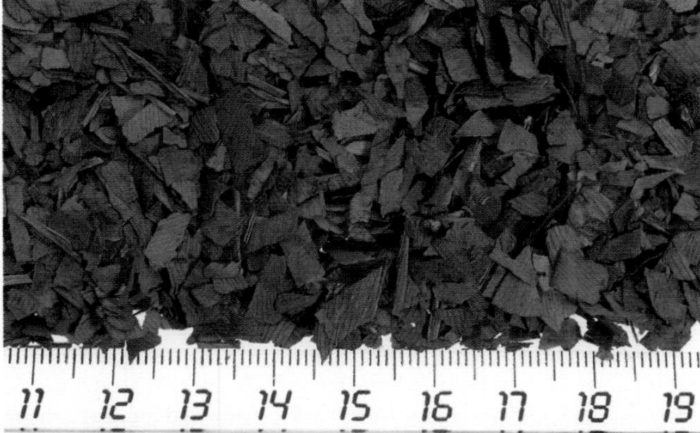

Figure 3 Ginkgo – dried drug substance (leaf).

Clinical trials of standardised extracts of *G. biloba* leaves (EGb-761, Willmar Schwabe GmbH and LI-1370, Lichtwer Pharma GmbH) in patients with cognitive deficiency have generally used oral doses ranging from 120–240 mg daily, usually for 8–12 weeks, although some studies have continued treatment for up to 24 or 52 weeks.[G56] Clinical trials in peripheral arterial occlusive disease used oral doses of 120–160 mg extract daily for 3–6 months.[G56]

Pharmacological Actions

In vitro and animal studies

There is a vast literature describing basic scientific research relating to the effects of ginkgo. Several pharmacological activities have been documented for ginkgo leaf extracts and/or their constituents. These include effects on behaviour, learning and memory, cardiovascular activities, effects on blood flow and antioxidant activity. The most important active principles of ginkgo extract include the ginkgo flavonoid glycosides and the terpene lactones.[1] Ginkgo has been described as having polyvalent action, i.e. the combined activity of several of its constituents is likely to be responsible for its effects.[15]

The pharmacological activities of ginkgo have been reviewed,[1,8,9,15–17] and other texts bring together several studies in specific areas, e.g. neuroprotective effects.[18] A summary of some of the literature on the *in vitro* and *in vivo* (animals) effects of ginkgo leaf is given below.

Effects on behaviour, learning and memory The effects of a standardised extract of ginkgo leaf (EGb-761) on learning and memory, and on behaviour in relation to ageing and in recovery from brain injury, have been well studied.[15] Animal models (rats and mice) designed to test aspects of learning and memory (e.g. acquisition and retention) have documented improvements in animals treated with oral, intraperitoneal or subcutaneous EGb-761, compared with controls.[15] Studies involving rats reported improvements in acquisition and retention in older (24-month-old), but not younger (eight-month-old) rats. Other experiments involving rats of different ages have found that older rats (12- and 18-months old) showed improved performance in an eight-arm radial maze test following oral administration of EGb-761 30 or 60 mg/kg/day, whereas performance was stable among young rats (eight weeks old) following EGb-761 administration.[15] EGb-761 200 mg/kg administered orally to rats aged more than 26 months old led to significant improvements in aspects of cognitive behaviour.[19] *In-vivo* studies have also shown that oral administration of EGb-761 (50 or 100 mg/kg/day for three weeks) to rats prevented the short-term memory-impairing effects of scopolamine administered intraperitoneally (0.125 mg/kg).[15]

The anxiolytic effects of a range of doses (0.01–10 mg/kg) of combination preparations containing different mixture ratios of standardised extracts of ginkgo leaf and ginger root have been tested in rats using the elevated plus-maze test.[20] Compared with controls, rats treated with the combination preparation (mixture ratio of ginger extract to ginkgo extract, 2.5 : 1; 1 mg/kg, intragastrically) spent increased amounts of time in the open arms of the maze, whereas the behaviour of rats treated with preparations of a mixture ratio of 1 : 1 and 1 : 2.5 did not change.

Several studies have reported that treatment with EGb-761, compared with control, aids recovery of function following brain injury, as demonstrated by behavioural tests in rats who had undergone bilateral frontal lobotomy or septohippocampal deafferentation, and in rat models of cortical hemiplegia.[15]

It has been suggested that the effects of EGb-761 in the experimental animal models described above may involve aspects of neuronal plasticity, e.g. neuronal regeneration.[15] Studies in rats have investigated, for example, the effects of EGb-761 administration on expression of neurotrophins and apolipoprotein E, and on behavioural recovery, following entorhinal cortex lesions, and on regeneration of primary olfactory neurons following olfactory bulbectomy. Research investigating the effects of EGb-761 on neuronal plasticity has been summarised.[1,15,21]

Cardiovascular and haemorheological activities Studies investigating the molecular mechanisms that may contribute to the vasoregulatory (vasodilatation and vasoconstriction) effects of standardised ginkgo leaf extract (EGb-761) have been described.[15,22] *In vitro* experiments using isolated rabbit aorta suggested that possible mechanisms include effects on cyclic-GMP phosphodiesterase, prostaglandin I_2 and nitric oxide (NO). *Ex vivo* studies using isolated guinea-pig heart showed that EGb-761 led to a concentration-dependent increase in coronary blood flow. In studies involving isolated rat heart and in anaesthetised rabbits, EGb-761 administration has been reported to protect against myocardial ischaemia–reperfusion injury; the antioxidant and free-radical scavenging effects of EGb-761 (*see* Pharmacological Actions, Antioxidant activity) may be important in this regard.[15] One study using isolated rat hearts suggested that the cardioprotective effects were due to the terpenoid constituents of EGb-761, and that the mechanism was independent of direct free radical-scavenging activity.[23] An *in vitro* study with endothelial cells suggested that the anti-ischaemic activity of EGb-761 may be due partly to the effects of the constituent bilobalide in protecting mitochondrial activity.[24]

The effects of ginkgo leaf extract have been studied in normal rats and those with ischaemic brain damage with middle cerebral artery occlusion.[25] Oral administration of ginkgo extract 100 mg/kg was reported to increase cerebral blood flow in normal rats, but the increase was less marked in rats with cerebral artery occlusion.

In-vitro studies using human blood cells have documented effects of EGb-761 on several haemorheological parameters.[15] For example, *in vitro*, EGb-761 normalised changes in erythrocyte viscosity and in the viscoelastic properties of the erythrocyte membrane induced by standard metabolic challenge (pH 6.8; 380 mosmol/L) in six human blood donors. In other *in vitro* experiments, EGb-761 protected against hydrogen peroxide-induced damage in human erythrocytes. In studies using blood from patients with circulatory disorders, incubation with EGb-761 was reported to decrease erythrocyte aggregation. *In vitro* experiments using human neutrophils have found that EGb-761 at a concentration of 10 μmol/L inhibits release of hydrogen peroxide from these cells. The effects of EGb-761 on inhibition of human platelet aggregation elicited by substances such as thrombin and collagen have been documented.[15] A study using blood donated by healthy volunteers (n = 35) reported that a standardised extract of ginkgo leaf inhibited ADP- and collagen-induced platelet aggregation in platelet-rich plasma, gel-filtered platelets and in whole blood in a concentration-dependent manner.[26]

Platelet-activating factor antagonism Ginkgolides have been reported to competitively inhibit the binding of platelet-activating factor (PAF) to its membrane receptor.[8, 9, 27]

Ginkgolide B antagonises thrombus formation induced by PAF and, in guinea-pigs, it also induces a rapid curative thrombolysis. A protective effect is exerted by ginkgolides on PAF-induced bronchoconstriction and airway hyperactivity in immunoanaphylaxis and in antigen-induced bronchial provocation tests. Oral or intravenous injection of ginkgolide B antagonises cardiovascular impairments and bronchoconstriction induced by PAF. Ginkgolide B does not appear to interfere with cyclooxygenase, but at an earlier step involving PAF receptors and phospholipase activation. Eosinophil infiltration occurs in asthma and in allergic reactions, the number of eosinophils increasing during late phase. Since PAF is a potent activator of eosinophil function, it has been argued that ginkgolide B may interfere with the late-phase response.[27]

Pre-administration of ginkgolide B (1–5 mg/kg, intravenous) to rats has been reported to reduce PAF-induced decreases in diastolic and systolic arterial blood pressure in anaesthetised normotensive rats; this effect has also been reported in this animal model when ginkgolide B is administered shortly after PAF administration.[15]

Ginkgolide B has also been documented to have some beneficial effects in endotoxic shock; PAF is believed by some to be implicated in shock states. In anaesthetised guinea-pigs, intravenous administration of ginkgolide B (1 or 6 mg/kg) prior to injection of *Salmonella typhimurium* endotoxin reduced the initial rapid decrease in blood pressure, and intravenous administration of ginkgolide B during the prolonged phase of shock (1 hour after endotoxin administration) immediately and dose dependently reversed the decrease in blood pressure.[15] Other studies have found that ginkgolide B reduced arterial blood pressure in the secondary, but not the early, phase following administration of *Escherichia coli* endotoxin.[15]

Antioxidant activity The free radical-scavenging effects and antioxidant activity of EGb-761 *in vitro* are well documented.[15] EGb-761 scavenges several reactive oxygen species, including hydroxyl, superoxide and peroxyl radicals.[15, 28, 29] In rat cerebellar neurons and cerebellar granule cells, ginkgo extract was reported to protect against oxidative stress induced by hydrogen peroxide, another reactive oxygen species.[30, 31] In cultures of rat hippocampal cells, incubation with EGb-761 protected against cell death induced by β-amyloid, protected against toxicity induced by hydrogen peroxide, and blocked β-amyloid-induced events, such as accumulation of reactive oxygen species.[32] Bilobalide has also been documented to protect neurons against oxidative stress induced by reactive oxygen species *in vitro*.[33] Experiments in gerbils have suggested that the neuroprotective effects of gingko extract may be due to inhibition of nitric oxide formation.[34]

Other studies which have described neuroprotective effects of EGb-761 have suggested that antioxidant activity may be involved.[16] *In vitro*, a standardised ginkgo leaf extract was found to inhibit photo-induced formation of cholesterol oxides in a concentration-dependent manner.[35]

Antioxidant activity has been documented for EGb-761 *in vivo*. In rats, treatment with EGb-761 increased the concentrations of circulating and cellular polyunsaturated fatty acids, and reduced erythrocyte cell lysis induced by hydrogen peroxide.[36] Also in rats, oral administration of EGb-761 was reported to increase activity of the enzymes catalase and superoxide dismutase in the hippocampus, striatum and substantia nigrum.[37] Other data collected in this study suggested a decrease in lipid peroxidation in rat hippocampus in EGb-761-treated rats. In another study in rats, EGb-761 (200 mg/kg/day for four weeks) protected against carbon tetrachloride-induced (1.5 mL/kg) liver damage, as determined by malondialdehyde concentrations (a breakdown product of lipid peroxidation).[38]

Other activities *In-vivo* studies have suggested that EGb-761 may protect against chemically induced carcinogenesis. In mice, oral administration of EGb-761 (150 mg/kg daily for two weeks), compared with control, was reported to reduce tumour multiplicity; however, the inhibitory effect was not statistically significant.[39] It was also reported that EGb-761-treatment reduced the cardiotoxicity of doxorubicin.

EGb-761 and ginkgolide B have been shown to inhibit peripheral-type benzodiazepine receptor (PBR) expression and cell proliferation in the human breast cancer cell line MDA-231, which is known to be rich in PBR.[40] By contrast, the proliferation of MCF-7 breast cancer cells, which are low in PBR, was not affected.

In rats, oral administration of standardised ginkgo leaf extract 300 mg/kg was shown to ameliorate nephrotoxicity induced by administration of gentamicin 80 mg/kg.[41]

In-vitro studies have shown that ginkgolic acids have cytotoxic activity.[42] Incubation of a human keratinocyte cell line with a preparation of ginkgolic acids (containing 99% ginkgolic acids) at concentrations of $\geqslant$ 30 mg/L for 18 hours increased the proportion of apoptotic cells from around 6% to around 80%.[43]

Mean (95% confidence interval) IC_{50} values for ginkgolic acids and a standardised ginkgolic-acid-free (< 5ppm) extract of ginkgo leaf (EGb-761) for human keratinocyte cells and rhesus monkey kidney tubular epithelial cells, respectively, were: ginkgolic acids, 21.8 mg/L (20.6–23.0) and 4.6 mg/L (3.7–5.6), respectively; ginkgo extract, 889 mg/L (859–938) and 1481 mg/L (1439–1523), respectively.[43] The ginkgolic acid mixture (containing five alkylphenols at concentrations of 47%, 43% and 3% for three compounds) was obtained from the heptane-soluble fraction of a 60% w/w acetone extract of *G. biloba* leaf.

Oestrogenic activity *in vitro* has been documented for a *G. biloba* leaf extract (Meditec Korea Pharm. Co Ltd, Korea; not further specified) and several of its flavonoid constituents. In competitive radiolabelled ligand binding assays, ginkgo leaf extract and the flavonoid constituents quercetin, kaempferol and isorhamnetin bound to both oestrogen receptor (ER) ER-alpha and ER-beta receptors, although they showed a greater affinity for ER-beta receptors. At certain concentrations, ginkgo extract and the flavonoid constituents induced the proliferation of ER-positive MCF-7 human breast cancer cells; this effect was blocked by incubation with tamoxifen.[44] The clinical relevance of these findings has not been established.

Aqueous extracts of dried ginkgo leaves have been reported to inhibit monoamine oxidases (MAO) A and B.[45] A study investigating the effects of bilobalide on gamma-aminobutyric acid (GABA) concentrations and on glutamic acid decarboxylase activity in mouse brain found that GABA concentrations and glutamic acid decarboxylase activity were significantly higher in animals treated orally with bilobalide 30 mg/kg daily for four days.[46] However, there were no differences between treated and control mice with regard to glutamate concentrations.

Several *in-vivo* studies have documented adaptive effects for EGb-761.[22]

A peptide isolated from the leaves of *Ginkgo biloba* has been reported to have antifungal activity against several fungi, including *Pellicularia sasakii* and *Alternaria alternata*.[10]

Three long-chain phenols, anacardic acid, bilobol and cardanol, isolated from seeds of *G. biloba* are active against Sarcoma 180 ascites in mice.[47]

Clinical studies

Pharmacokinetics The pharmacokinetics of constituents of standardised extracts of ginkgo leaf are reasonably well documented.[1, 17, 48, G21] Mean bioavailabilities of ginkgolide A, ginkgolide B and bilobalide following oral administration of ginkgo extract 120 mg to fasting healthy volunteers were 80%, 88% and 79%, respectively. Food intake increased the time taken to reach peak concentration (suggesting slower absorption), but did not affect bioavailability.[1, G18] Peak concentrations of ginkgolides A and B and bilobalide observed in fasting volunteers ranged from 16.5 to 33.3 ng/mL, and from 11.5 to 21.1 ng/mL in volunteers who had consumed food.[1]

Maximum plasma concentrations of total ginkgolides A and B and bilobalide following oral administration of a ginkgo leaf extract (Ginkgoselect) and a phospholipid complex of ginkgo leaf (Ginkgoselect Phytosome), both providing 9.6 mg total terpene lactones, were 85.0 and 181.8 μg/mL, for ginkgo extract and the phospholipid complex, respectively.[49] Times to maximum concentration were 120 minutes and 180–240 minutes for ginkgo extract and the phospholipid complex, respectively, whereas the mean elimination half-life of each of the terpene lactones investigated was within the range 120-180 minutes.

In a randomised, crossover study, 12 healthy individuals received ginkgo leaf extract 40 mg twice daily and 80 mg once daily for 7 days, with a wash-out period of 21 days between the different dosage regimens.[50] It was reported that the twice-daily dosage regimen, compared with the once-daily regimen, resulted in a significantly longer half-life and mean residence time for ginkgolide B, although the maximum plasma concentration was higher with the once-daily dosage regimen. Time to maximum plasma concentration for ginkgolide B was 2.3 hours for administration of ginkgo leaf extract according to either dosage regimen. In another study involving healthy individuals given a single oral dose of ginkgo leaf extract, mean values for the absorption rate constant, elimination rate constant, absorption half-life, elimination half-life and time to maximum plasma concentration for the flavonoid constituents quercetin and kaempferol were 0.61 and 0.55 per hour, 0.37 and 0.30 per hour, 1.51 and 1.56 hours, 2.17 and 2.76 hours, and 2.30 and 2.68 hours, respectively.[51]

Urinary excretion of ginkgolides A and B, and bilobalide, is around 70%, 50% and 30%, respectively, of the dose administered orally.[G18]

Different ginkgo leaf extracts have different *in-vitro* dissolution rates resulting in differences in bioavailability in humans.[14]

G

Therapeutic effects Most clinical trials of ginkgo have explored its effects in the treatment of cognitive deficiency or cerebral insufficiency,[52, G56] a term used to describe a collection of symptoms thought to arise from an age-related reduction in cerebral blood flow. These symptoms include forgetfulness, poor concentration, poor perception, debilitation, dizziness, fatigue, sleep disturbances, listlessness, depressed mood, headache, mood swings, restlessness, tinnitus, anxiety, hearing loss and disorientation.[52, G56] Several studies have tested the effects of standardised ginkgo leaf extracts on cognitive function in patients with Alzheimer's disease[53] and/or multi-infarct dementia.[54] Both are conditions which share several symptoms (e.g. memory impairment) with cerebral insufficiency. Several other trials have explored the effects of ginkgo extracts on cognitive ability in individuals with no history of significant cognitive impairment. A few studies have explored the effects of ginkgo on tinnitus alone.[55]

Clinical research with ginkgo extracts has also focused on effects in improving pain-free walking distance in patients with intermittent claudication/peripheral arterial occlusive disease.[56, G56] Other studies have explored the effects of ginkgo in patients with chronic venous insufficiency, antidepressant-related sexual dysfunction, seasonal affective disorder (SAD), and symptoms of depression.

Almost all clinical trials of ginkgo have investigated the effects of the standardised ginkgo leaf extracts EGb-761 and LI-1370.

Cognitive deficiency, dementia in Alzheimer's disease, multi-infarct dementia A Cochrane systematic review of studies assessing *G. biloba* leaf preparations in cognitive impairment and dementia included 33 randomised, double-blind, controlled trials.[57] All but one of the included studies investigated the effects of standardised ginkgo leaf extracts EGb-761 and LI-1370 at oral doses ranging from 80–600 mg daily and typically 200 mg daily. The study that did not use either of these preparations assessed an ethanolic extract of ginkgo leaves (drug-to-extract ratio 4 : 1, standardised for total flavone glycosides 0.20 mg/mL and total ginkgolides 0.34 mg/mL) at doses lower than those used in the other 32 studies.

Meta-analyses showed that ginkgo at doses less than 200 mg daily for less than 12 weeks, compared with placebo, was associated with benefits in clinical global improvement as assessed by physicians: odds ratio (OR; 95% confidence interval (CI)) 15.32 (5.90–39.80; $p < 0.0001$); a similar result was found for ginkgo > 200 mg daily for 24 weeks (OR 2.16, 95% CI 1.11–4.20; $p = 0.02$). Significant improvements in cognition, assessed using various scales, were also found for ginkgo (any dose) at 12, 24 and 52 weeks, when compared with placebo (p = 0.0008, 0.03 and < 0.01 for 12, 24 and 52 weeks, respectively),[57] and significant improvements in ability to perform activities of daily living were seen with ginkgo (doses < 200 mg daily), compared with placebo, at 12, 24 and 52 weeks ($p \leqslant 0.01$, $p = 0.05$ and $p \leqslant 0.01$, respectively). The conclusions of the review were that there is some evidence of improvements in cognition and function associated with treatment with a standardised extract of ginkgo leaf. However, many of the early trials included in the review had methodological limitations, and the three most recent trials showed inconsistent results. There is a need for a large rigorous randomised, placebo-controlled trial to establish the benefits of ginkgo in cognitive impairment.[57]

G

A review of controlled clinical trials of ginkgo in patients with cerebral insufficiency identified 40 studies.[52] Generally, trials tested oral doses of standardised extracts of ginkgo leaf of 120 mg daily administered for at least four to six weeks. Most trials reported significant results or positive (but not statistically significant) trends in favour of ginkgo, compared with control. However, it was reported that most trials were of poor methodological quality; only eight studies were considered to be well-conducted. All of these eight studies reported statistically significant results for ginkgo, compared with placebo. Nevertheless, further randomised, double-blind, controlled trials involving larger numbers of patients were deemed necessary.[52]

Many controlled studies of the ginkgo extracts EGb-761 and LI-1370 were conducted before new guidelines for testing the efficacy of nootropic drugs were developed.[G56] Details of two studies that did meet the methodological criteria described in the guidelines (both of which were included in the Cochrane systematic review described above) are given below.

In a randomised, double-blind, placebo-controlled trial, after a four-week placebo run-in period, 216 patients with mild-to-moderate primary degenerative dementia of the Alzheimer type, or multi-infarct dementia, received standardised ginkgo leaf extract (EGb-761) 120 mg orally twice daily, or placebo, for 24 weeks.[58] At the end of the study, data for 156 patients were eligible for analysis. There were significantly more responders to treatment (defined as a response to at least two of the three primary outcome measures – a psychopathological assessment, an assessment of cognitive performance and a behavioural assessment of activities of daily life) in the ginkgo group, compared with the placebo group (28% versus 10% of ginkgo and placebo recipients, respectively; $p = 0.005$). The difference was also statistically significant in an intention-to-treat analysis (23% versus 10% of ginkgo and placebo recipients, respectively; $p = 0.005$).

A randomised, double-blind, placebo-controlled study involved 327 patients with mild-to-severe dementia related to Alzheimer's disease or multi-infarct dementia.[59] Participants received standardised ginkgo leaf extract (EGb-761) 40 mg orally three times daily ($n = 166$), or placebo ($n = 161$), for 52 weeks, and underwent a battery of assessments at 12, 26 and 52 weeks. The primary outcome measures were the Alzheimer's Disease Assessment Scale Cognitive Subscale (Adas-Cog), the Geriatric Evaluation by Relative's Rating Instrument (GERRI) and the Clinical Global Impression of Change (CGIC). In an intention-to-treat analysis ($n = 309$), ginkgo recipients scored significantly better than did placebo recipients on the Adas-Cog and the GERRI ($p = 0.04$ and $p = 0.004$, respectively). A slight worsening on the CGIC was observed for both groups. The average end-points for the intention-to-treat analysis were 38.6 and 34.6 weeks for the ginkgo and placebo groups, respectively.

Another systematic review of randomised, double-blind, placebo-controlled trials assessing the effects of standardised ginkgo leaf extracts on cognitive function in patients with Alzheimer's disease, characterised according to recognised criteria, included four studies.[53] These involved oral administration of ginkgo extract 120 or 240 mg daily for 12–26 weeks, and involved a total of 212 patients each in the ginkgo and placebo groups. A meta-analysis of the results of the four studies indicated a modest effect for ginkgo, compared with placebo (difference of 3% on the Adas-Cog).

Another systematic review included nine randomised, double-blind, placebo-controlled trials of standardised ginkgo leaf extracts in patients with dementia of the Alzheimer type and/or multi-infarct dementia.[54] The review included two studies described above.[58,59] Studies generally involved the administration of oral doses of ginkgo extract 120 or 240 mg daily for 6–12 weeks, although two studies involved a 24-week[48] or 52-week[49] administration period. One study involved the administration of intravenous infusions of ginkgo extract 200 mg four times per week for four weeks. It was reported that, overall, the studies provided evidence to support the efficacy of standardised ginkgo leaf extracts in the symptomatic treatment of dementia. However, methodological limitations of several of the included studies (e.g. poorly defined inclusion and exclusion criteria and method of randomisation, treatment period less than six months, small sample sizes) were also emphasised. It was concluded that further studies are required to establish the benefits of ginkgo in dementia.[54]

The study included in the Cochrane review described above that did not assess the effects of EGb-761 or LI-1370 assessed the effects of an alcohol/water extract of fresh leaves of ginkgo (drug extract ratio 1 : 4; total flavonoid glycosides 0.20 mg/mL, total ginkgolides 0.34 mg/mL) in a randomised, double-blind, placebo-controlled trial involving patients with age-related impairment of memory and/or concentration.[60] Participants received undiluted ginkgo extract ($n = 77$), diluted ginkgo extract (1 : 1 with placebo) ($n = 82$), or placebo ($n = 82$), 40 drops (1.9 mL) three times daily for 24 weeks. At the end of the treatment period, a check for blinding indicated that participants were unable to identify the treatment they received. There were no statistically significant differences between the three groups in subjective perceptions of memory and concentration, and in the following objective measures: the Expended Mental Control Test (a measure of attention and concentration), and Rey test parts 1 and 2 (which measure short-term memory and learning curve, and long-term memory and recognition, respectively). However, a significant difference between groups was observed in the Benton test of visual retention-revised (a measure of short-term visual memory) – increases in baseline scores of 18%, 26% and 11% were recorded for the high-dose ginkgo, low-dose ginkgo and placebo groups, respectively ($p = 0.0076$).[60]

Cognitive enhancement in healthy volunteers Ginkgo has been tested for its cognitive enhancing effects in healthy (i.e. cognitively intact) individuals in addition to investigations into its effects in patients with cognitive deficiency.

A systematic review of double-blind, placebo-controlled trials assessing the effects of preparations of *G. biloba* leaf on cognitive function in healthy individuals included nine such trials.[61] The trials were considered to be of good methodological quality. The review found no evidence of substantial or consistent effects for ginkgo, compared with placebo, on objective measures of cognitive function. Several of the studies included in the review, as well as new trials published since, and those assessing combination preparations containing *G. biloba* leaf extract, are summarised below.

In a double-blind, placebo-controlled, cross-over study, 20 healthy volunteers aged 19–24 years received a standardised extract of ginkgo leaf (GK501) at doses of 120 mg, 240 mg and 360 mg.[62] A battery of tests used to assess cognitive performance was carried out immediately before and at 1, 2.5, 4 and 6 hours after ginkgo administration. It was reported that with doses of ginkgo extract of 240 and 360 mg, there was a statistically significant improvement in 'speed of attention' (a measure of reaction time) from 2.5 hours up to 6 hours (the last measurement point) after ginkgo administration.

In a randomised, double-blind, placebo-controlled, crossover study, eight healthy female volunteers (mean age 32 years) were given a standardised extract of *G. biloba* leaf at doses of 120, 240 and 600 mg.[63] One hour after treatment, volunteers undertook a series of psychological tests. Memory was found to be significantly improved with *G. biloba* leaf 600 mg, compared with placebo.

A randomised, double-blind, placebo-controlled, crossover trial involving 31 volunteers aged 30–59 years tested the effects of a standardised extract of ginkgo leaf (LI-1370) 50 mg three times daily, 100 mg three times daily, 120 mg each morning, 240 mg each morning, and placebo, each taken for two days followed by a wash-out period of at least five days.[64] A battery of tests to assess memory and cognitive and psychomotor performance was carried out 30 minutes before ginkgo administration and then hourly for 12 hours. It was reported that there was a 'marginally significant' effect of treatment, compared with placebo, in a test assessing short-term memory, although the p-value given for this was greater than 0.05 ($p = 0.053$). Post-hoc analyses suggested that ginkgo extract 120 mg each morning was associated with better performance in this test than other doses of ginkgo extract (including ginkgo extract 50 mg three times daily) and placebo. There were no statistically significant effects of treatment on immediate and delayed word recall and choice reaction time.

In two separate randomised, double-blind, placebo-controlled studies, healthy individuals received a single 120 mg dose of ginkgo leaf extract (LI-1370), or placebo ($n = 52$) or ginkgo leaf extract 120 mg daily, or placebo, for six weeks ($n = 40$) before undergoing tests to assess cognitive function.[65] Single-dose ginkgo extract significantly improved performance in tests of attention ($p < 0.05$), when compared with placebo, but no significant improvements were observed following longer-term administration. Similarly, in a randomised, double-blind, placebo-controlled study involving healthy individuals who received ginkgo leaf extract (mean dose 185 mg/day, determined subsequently when the preparation was found to contain only 65% of the content stated) for 13 weeks, no improvements were observed in alleviation of post-prandial state decrement ('post-lunch dip') and chemosensory function with ginkgo, compared with placebo.[66] In a double-blind, placebo-controlled, crossover study involving 15 healthy individuals, *G. biloba* leaf extract 360 mg as a single oral dose had significant effects on certain aspects of electroencephalogram recordings, such as reductions in frontal theta and beta activity, when compared with placebo.[67] These findings suggest that *G. biloba* leaf extract can directly modulate cerebroelectrical activity.[67]

Other studies have assessed the effects of a combination preparation of *G. biloba* leaf and *Panax ginseng* on cognitive function in healthy younger individuals. In a double-blind, placebo-controlled, crossover study, 20 healthy individuals received single doses of *G. biloba* leaf extract (GK501) 120, 240 and 360 mg, or placebo, and a combination of *G. biloba* leaf extract and *P. ginseng* root extract at doses of 120 and 200, 240 and 400, and 360 and 600 mg, respectively, or placebo.[68] Statistically significant improvements in one cognitive performance test (serial threes) were observed with all three ginkgo doses, compared with placebo ($p < 0.05$ for each), but there were no statistically significant improvements in other tests. Following administration of the combination preparation, there were statistically significant improvements in certain tests at certain timepoints, but these results were not consistent for all doses tested and across all timepoints measured in the study.

Other studies have assessed the cognitive-enhancing effects of ginkgo extracts in older volunteers. In a randomised, double-blind, placebo-controlled trial, 48 cognitively intact individuals aged over 55 years received a standardised ginkgo leaf extract (EGb-761) 60 mg three times daily, or placebo, for six weeks.[69] A battery of neuropsychological tests was carried out before treatment and at the end of the study. Ginkgo extract recipients experienced a significant improvement in tests assessing speed of processing abilities, compared with placebo recipients ($p < 0.03$). However, no statistically significant differences between the ginkgo extract and placebo groups were evident for tests assessing memory.

In a questionnaire survey, the effects of administration of a standardised ginkgo leaf extract (LI-1370) 120 mg daily for four months on the activities of daily living were assessed in volunteers aged 32–97 years (mean (SD) 68.9 (8.4) years).[70] Volunteers were recruited via a magazine editorial. Of 8557 initial respondents, 5028 were eligible for the survey. In total, 1000 volunteers (who were not currently using any ginkgo products) were said to be randomly allocated to receive ginkgo extract; all other respondents were allocated to the no-treatment control group, unless they had stated that they only wished to receive ginkgo. It was reported that ginkgo extract recipients achieved significantly better scores than the control group on a scale assessing ability to perform activities of daily living, self-assessment of ability to cope, and visual analogue scales for mood and sleep. However, for several reasons, the results of this study should be interpreted cautiously. For example, the study was carried out by post, therefore investigators did not meet participants at any time, the study was not truly randomised, the study was open, the control group did not receive placebo tablets, and there was no check on compliance.

At the end of the study, 1570 individuals continued in a follow-up study in which they selected whether or not to receive ginkgo treatment.[71] After six months, data collected using a postal questionnaire indicated that there were statistically significant differences between groups (individuals received ginkgo or no treatment during the initial four-month study, and ginkgo or no treatment during the six-month follow-up study, creating four groups) in scores for activities of daily living and mood; benefits were associated with longer use of ginkgo. The design of this study, however, does not allow definitive conclusions to be drawn.

In a randomised, double-blind, placebo-controlled, parallel group trial in which 64 healthy volunteers with neurasthenic complaints received a combination preparation containing *G. biloba* leaf extract and *P. ginseng* root extract at doses of 30 and 50 mg, respectively, 60 and 100 mg, respectively, and 120 and 200 mg, respectively, or placebo, twice daily, for 12 weeks, participants in the higher-dose ginkgo–ginseng group, compared with the placebo group, achieved significantly higher scores in tests designed to assess cognitive function ($p = 0.008$).[72]

In contrast, several other studies assessing the effects of combination preparations containing *G. biloba* leaf extract and other herbal ingredients on cognitive function have reported no statistically significant effects.

The effects of a combination preparation of *G. biloba* and *P. ginseng* on memory were assessed in a randomised, double-blind, placebo-controlled, multicentre, parallel group trial involving 256 healthy volunteers aged 38 to 67 years (mean (SD), 56 (7) years).[73] Participants received a preparation containing *G. biloba* leaf extract 60 mg and *P. ginseng* root extract 100 mg, twice daily, 120 and 200 mg, respectively, once daily, or placebo, for 12 weeks. Assessments were undertaken at weeks 4, 8, 12 and 14 of the study. At the end of the study, the primary outcome variable the Quality of Memory Index was significantly improved in the treatment group, compared with the placebo group ($p = 0.026$). No statistically significant effects were seen with respect to the secondary outcome variables power and continuity of attention, and speed of memory processes.[73]

A lack of effect for a combination preparation containing *G. biloba* leaf extract and *P. ginseng* (Gincosan), administered at doses of 120 and 200 mg daily, respectively, for 12 weeks, was also reported following a randomised, double-blind, placebo-controlled trial involving 57 post-menopausal women.[74] A randomised, double-blind, placebo-controlled trial involving 85 healthy individuals aged 19 to 68 years (mean age 41.8 years) found no statistically significant effects on cognitive function for a combination preparation containing *G. biloba* leaf extract and *Bacopa monniera*, when compared with placebo.[75]

Tinnitus and hearing loss Tinnitus and hearing loss are two of the symptoms of dementia.[G56] Several studies have assessed the effects of ginkgo on these conditions alone.

A meta-analysis of randomised, double-blind, placebo-controlled trials of *G. biloba* leaf preparations for tinnitus included six such trials involving a total of 1318 participants.[76] Four studies involved oral administration of tablets of ginkgo leaf extract at doses of 30 to 150 mg daily typically for 12 weeks, one study used a liquid preparation of ginkgo leaf and one study involved administration of a ginkgo leaf preparation 200 mg by intravenous infusion followed by oral administration of 80 mg twice daily for 12 weeks. The review did not find any statistically significant difference between ginkgo and placebo with respect to the proportion of participants experiencing benefit.[76] A Cochrane systematic review of *G. biloba* for tinnitus used stricter inclusion criteria and hence included only two trials.[77] The conclusions of the review were that the limited evidence available did not demonstrate that *G. biloba* leaf was effective for the treatment of tinnitus.

A new randomised, double-blind, placebo-controlled trial assessing *G. biloba* in tinnitus has been published since the Cochrane review. This trial was included in the broader review described above.[76] In the study, 66 adults with tinnitus as their only or main presenting complaint to a general otolaryngology outpatient clinic received a sustained-release *G. biloba* leaf preparation 120 mg daily, or placebo, for 12 weeks. Among the 60 individuals who completed the study, there were no statistically significant improvements in the primary outcome measures (Tinnitus Handicap Inventory, Glasgow Health Status Inventory, average hearing threshold) for the ginkgo group, compared with the placebo group ($p > 0.1$ for each).[76]

A previous systematic review of randomised, controlled trials of ginkgo extracts in tinnitus included five studies – four studies compared ginkgo extracts with placebo, and one study compared ginkgo extract with conventional drugs. Three trials tested the standardised ginkgo leaf extract EGb-761; full details of other extracts tested in the other studies are not given in the review. The review concluded that, overall, the studies identified provided evidence to support ginkgo extracts as a treatment for tinnitus, but that further investigation was required to fully establish the benefits. Typically, at least two of the studies had methodological flaws.[55]

Two of the reviews described above included a double-blind, controlled trial that tested the effects of a standardised ginkgo leaf extract (LI-1370) 50 mg, or placebo, three times daily for 12 weeks in 1121 individuals, aged 18–70 years, with tinnitus who were otherwise healthy.[78] Participants were recruited via advertisements placed in the UK national press and in a British Tinnitus Association's publication. The main outcome measure was participants' self-assessment of tinnitus (loudness and 'how troublesome') before, during and after treatment, carried out via postal questionnaires and telephone calls. Participants were paired where possible (489 pairs, i.e. 978 of 1121 participants were matched) and then randomly allocated to active or placebo. At the end of the study, the results indicated that ginkgo extract (LI-1370) 50 mg three times daily was 'no more effective than placebo in treating tinnitus'.[78] The design of this study has been criticised. For example, participants did not have face-to-face contact with an investigator at any time during the study.[79]

In a randomised, controlled trial, 28 patients with untreated sudden loss of hearing received intravenous infusions of 6% hydroxyethyl starch (HES), or intravenous and oral ginkgo extract, for 10 days.[80] There were no statistically significant differences between the two groups in improvements in hearing. Further studies involving larger numbers of participants are required.[80]

Peripheral arterial occlusive disease/intermittent claudication The effects of standardised extracts of ginkgo have been investigated in patients with Fontaine stage II peripheral arterial occlusive disease. This condition is characterised by the onset of pain, as a result of oxygen deficit in the leg muscles, on walking distances greater than around 30–300 metres.[G56] The rationale for using ginkgo in this condition is for its effects in improving blood flow.

A meta-analysis of randomised, double-blind, placebo-controlled trials of ginkgo extract for the treatment of intermittent claudication included eight studies that assessed effects on walking distance.[56] The trials involved a total of 415 patients who received a standardised extract of ginkgo leaf at doses of 120 or 160 mg daily, or placebo, for 6, 12 (one trial each) or 24 weeks. The pooled results from all trials indicated a statistically significant increase in pain-free walking distance for ginkgo-treated patients, compared with placebo recipients (weighted mean difference (WMD): 34 metres; 95% confidence intervals (CI): 26–43 metres). A similar result was obtained when results for the six studies of good methodological quality were pooled (WMD: 37 metres; 95% CI: 26–47 metres). It is questionable whether the extent of these increases in pain-free walking distance is clinically relevant.[56]

Chronic venous insufficiency and venous ulcers A randomised, double-blind, placebo-controlled trial assessed the protective effects of a combination preparation (Ginkgor Forte) containing a standardised extract of ginkgo (2.3%), troxerutine (48.85%) and heptaminol (48.85%) against venous wall injury in 48 female patients with chronic venous insufficiency.[81] Ginkgor Forte

625 mg daily, or placebo, was given for four weeks. In total, 42 patients completed the study, but only 28 were included in the final analysis because of protocol violations. Circulating endothelial cell (CEC) count was used as a measure of injury to the vascular endothelium (CEC counts are raised in patients with chronic venous insufficiency).[81] After four weeks' treatment, CEC counts decreased significantly in both the treatment and placebo groups (by 14.5% and 8.4%, respectively), compared with baseline values (p = 0.0021 and p = 0.0146, respectively). The mean change in CEC count after four weeks' treatment was reported to be significantly greater for the treatment group, compared with the placebo group (p = 0.039).

In another double-blind trial, 213 patients with chronic venous or mixed ulcers located at the malleolus (rounded protuberance on ankle joint) received ginkgo extract 160 mg daily, or placebo, together with standard care (elastic stockings, local dressings and cleansing of ulcers) for 12 weeks.[1] At the end of the study, ginkgo extract recipients, compared with placebo recipients, showed a significant reduction in ulcer area.

Asthma, PAF antagonism Intradermal injections of PAF induce a biphasic inflammatory response similar to that observed in sensitised individuals subjected to moderate doses of allergen. A single dose of a mixture of ginkgolides has been reported to antagonise this response.[82] Oral administration of ginkgolides resulted in a reduction of eosinophil infiltration in atopic patients given intracutaneous injections of PAF.[82]

In a randomised, double-blind, crossover study, 80 and 120 mg capsules containing a standardised mixture of ginkgolides A, B and C (ratio of 40 : 40 : 20) were given as a single oral dose two hours before challenge by intradermal PAF/histamine. Both dose ranges inhibited flare which was maximal after five minutes. Within 15–30 minutes wheal volume was reduced, with the greatest effect being observed for the higher dose treatments. The protection was still present eight hours after oral dosing.[8] Similar inhibition of PAF was observed for platelet aggregation with single oral doses of 80 and 120 mg extract which were given two hours before blood withdrawal. The ginkgolide mixture given orally also blocked PAF-induced airway hyper-responsiveness.

Antagonism of the effects of PAF by a standardised mixture of ginkgolides was assessed in a double-blind, placebo-controlled crossover study in six healthy subjects aged 25–35 years.[83] Wheal and flare responses to PAF examined two hours after ingestion of 80 mg and 120 mg of ginkgolide mixture were inhibited in a dose-related manner. Both doses significantly inhibited PAF-induced platelet aggregation in platelet-rich plasma.[83]

A randomised, double-blind, crossover study involved patients with atopic asthma who were challenged with their specific dust or pollen antigen.[8] After 6.5 hours, participants were subjected to a provocation test with acetylcholine so that the treatment of later stages of an asthma attack could be assessed. Mixed ginkgolide standardised extract, 40 mg three times daily, or placebo, were given during the three days before the test and a final single dose of 120 mg of extract was given two hours before the challenge. The results suggested that ginkgolides were effective in both the early phase and the late phase of airway hyperactivity.[8]

A study involving six patients with a history of exercise-induced asthma assessed the effects of a specific PAF antagonist (BN 52063, a standardised mixture of ginkgolides A, B and C, ratio of 40 : 40 : 20) on the response to isocapnic hyperventilation with dry cold air.[84] Participants were randomised to receive BN 52063 240 mg orally two hours before cold air challenge, 2.4 mg by metered dose inhaler 30 minutes before cold air challenge, or placebo. It was reported that oral BN 52063 did not reduce bronchoconstriction during challenge. A significant increase in airways resistance was observed after inhalation of BN 52063. In another study, six patients with a history of exercise-induced asthma received BN 52063 120 mg orally twice daily, 1 mg by spinhaler three times daily, or placebo, for three days, then, on the test day, 240 mg orally three hours before exercise challenge, 5 mg by spinhaler one hour before challenge, or placebo, respectively. With oral treatment, the prolonged reduction in peak expiratory flow was significantly attenuated ($p < 0.05$).[84]

Antidepressant-related sexual dysfunction Two randomised, double-blind, placebo-controlled trials have assessed the effects of ginkgo leaf preparations on sexual function in individuals with antidepressant-related sexual dysfunction. One study involved administration of ginkgo leaf extract (120 mg daily for weeks one to two, 160 mg daily for weeks three to four and 240 mg daily for weeks five to eight; n = 37 participants),[85] and another study involved 240 mg daily for 12 weeks (n = 24).[86] Neither of the studies found statistically significant differences in sexual function between participants in the ginkgo and placebo groups.

Two open, uncontrolled studies have explored the effects of ginkgo extract in sexual dysfunction associated with treatment with antidepressant drugs.[87, 88]

Acute ischaemic stroke A Cochrane systematic review of randomised or quasi-randomised controlled trials assessing the effects of *G. biloba* leaf preparations in acute ischaemic stroke identified 14 such studies of which ten, involving a total of 792 participants, provided outcome data.[89] Meta-analysis of the nine trials that used a dichotomous outcome variable (improvement or no improvement in neurological deficit) showed a higher proportion of ginkgo recipients experienced neurological improvement than did placebo recipients (odds ratio, 95% CI: 2.66, 1.79–3.94; $p < 0.00001$). However, all of these trials were deemed to be of poor methodological quality. The one trial that was of good methodological quality used a continous scale for outcome; this showed no statistically significant improvement in neurological deficit for ginkgo recipients compared with placebo recipients (weighted mean difference (fixed effects model), 95% CI: 0.81, −8.9–10.52). The conclusions of the review were that there is no evidence from high-quality clinical trials to support the use of *G. biloba* extract in the treatment of patients with acute ischaemic stroke.[89]

Visual disorders A Cochrane review of the effects of ginkgo extract in age-related macular degeneration identified one randomised, controlled trial involving 20 patients.[90] The study design did not include blinding of the assessment of outcome. The review concluded that the effects of ginkgo extract in preventing progression of age-related macular degeneration had not yet been adequately assessed.

A randomised, double-blind, placebo-controlled, crossover trial involving 27 participants with bilateral visual field damage resulting from normal tension glaucoma assessed the effects of oral administration of a standardised ginkgo leaf extract (flavonoid glycosides 24%, terpene lactones 6%) 40 mg three times daily for four weeks.[91] The trial reported statistically significant improvements in visual field indices with ginkgo treatment, compared with baseline values, but did not report statistical analyses comparing ginkgo with placebo.

Other conditions Several randomised, double-blind, placebo-controlled trials have assessed the effects of ginkgo leaf preparations in preventing acute mountain sickness, and have reported conflicting results. In a four-arm study in which 614 participants received a standardised ginkgo leaf extract (flavonoid glycosides 24%, terpene lactones 6%) 120 mg twice daily, acetazolamide 250 mg, both agents, or placebo, for three to four doses before ascent, ginkgo was no better than placebo in preventing acute mountain sickness among the 487 participant who completed the trial (incidence for ginkgo, acetozolamide, ginkgo plus acetazolamide, and placebo: 35, 12, 14 and 34%, respectively).[92] A similar study also found no statistically significant differences in outcomes between ginkgo (120 mg twice daily for five days before mountain ascent) and placebo recipients.[93] In contrast, in a randomised, double-blind, placebo-controlled trial involving 26 individuals who received ginkgo leaf extract 60 mg, or placebo, three times daily starting 24 hours before rapid mountain ascent a significantly lower proportion of ginkgo recipients compared with placebo recipients developed severe acute mountain sickness (17% versus 64%, respectively; $p = 0.021$), although there was no statistically significant difference between the ginkgo and placebo groups in overall incidence of acute mountain sickness (58.3% versus 92.9% for ginkgo and placebo, respectively; $p = 0.07$).[94] The study, however, involved only small numbers of participants and it is possible that it did not have sufficient statistical power to detect a difference between the two groups if one existed.

In a randomised, double-blind, controlled trial, 27 patients with seasonal affective disorder (SAD) received standardised extract of ginkgo leaf (Bio-Biloba, containing flavone glycosides 24 mg and terpene lactones 6 mg) one tablet twice daily ($n = 15$), or placebo ($n = 12$), for 10 weeks or until development of depression requiring treatment.[95] All participants began the trial during October to December; assessments were carried out at baseline and on termination of study medication. Six of the 15 ginkgo recipients and two of the 12 placebo recipients terminated the study treatment because of emerging symptoms of SAD ('winter depression'). It was reported that this difference between groups was not statistically significant, according to Fisher's exact test. Also, there were no statistically significant differences between groups on the Montgomery–Asberg Depression Rating Scale, the ATYP scale (for symptoms of hypersomnia, hyperphagia and carbohydrate craving) and on self-assessed symptoms (energy, tiredness, appetite, carbohydrate craving, depressed mood). The results of this study cannot be considered definitive because of the small sample size of the study and other limitations.[95]

A placebo-controlled trial involving 165 women with premenstrual syndrome explored the effects of standardised ginkgo leaf extract (EGb-761) 160 mg daily, or placebo, taken from day 16 of the menstrual cycle to day 5 of the following cycle, for two cycles.[96] Both groups experienced improvements in symptoms, compared with baseline values, although ginkgo recipients, compared with placebo recipients, were reported to experience significantly greater improvements in breast tenderness (as evaluated by the physician).

The effects of ginkgo extract have been explored in patients with schizophrenia. The rationale for this is based on the theory that excess free radical formation may occur in patients with schizophrenia, since superoxide dismutase (SOD) concentrations have been reported to be higher in certain tissues in such patients. (SOD is an enzyme that detoxifies superoxide radicals.) In a double-blind, placebo-controlled trial, 82 inpatients with chronic schizophrenia (illness for at least five years) were 'divided randomly' to receive haloperidol 0.25 mg/kg daily, with or without ginkgo extract 360 mg daily, for 12 weeks.[97] At the end of the study, mean SOD concentrations (expressed as ng/mL haemoglobin) were reported to be significantly lower, compared with baseline values, for ginkgo recipients (mean (SD): 815.8 (697.8) and 596.7 (148.3), respectively; $p = 0.021$). In participants who received haloperidol only, mean (SD) SOD concentrations fell from 780.4 (605.4) at baseline to 617.6 (189.7) at the end of the study, although this decrease was reported to be statistically non-significant. A between-group comparison was not reported. Mean (SD) SOD concentrations in a group of 30 age- and sex-matched healthy volunteers were 515.8 (70.4).[97]

The effects of a preparation comprising *Ginkgo biloba* dimeric flavonoids in a 1 : 2 complex with phosphatidylcholine (GBDF-Phytosome) on the microcirculation of the skin have been investigated using various techniques including, infrared photo-pulse plethysmography, laser doppler flowmetry, high-performance contact thermography and computerised videothermography.[98] In a controlled study, small numbers of healthy individuals and volunteers with acrocyanosis or cellulitis were treated with 0.5 mL of a cream (oil-in-water emulsion) containing 3% GBDF-Phytosome or an oil-in-water emulsion of 2% phosphatidylcholine (control). Participants who received the GBDF-Phytosome preparation were reported to experience significant increases in capillary blood flow and skin temperature, compared with baseline values, whereas no significant changes were observed for the control group. No between-group comparisons were reported.[98] These preliminary findings suggest that the effects of this preparation on skin microcirculation may deserve further investigation.

The effects of ginkgo have been assessed in Raynaud's disease. In a randomised, double-blind, placebo-controlled trial undertaken in wintertime, 22 participants (mostly women) aged 18 to 52 years and with primary Raynaud's disease (i.e. without associated connective tissue disease) received a standardised (not further specified) *G. biloba* leaf extract (Seredrin, Health Perception Ltd, UK) 120 mg, or placebo, three times daily for ten weeks. Data from three participants were excluded from the analysis for legitimate reasons. Analysis of data from the remaining 19 participants showed that ginkgo treatment, compared with placebo, was associated with a greater reduction in the mean number of attacks of Raynaud's disease per week (mean (standard deviation) number of attacks before and after treatment, respectively: ginkgo, 13.2 (16.5) and 5.8 (8.3); placebo, 14.6 (10.7) and 10.7 (12.3); $p = 0.000005$).[99] No statistically significant differences between the two groups were observed for haemorheological parameters, including mean fibrinogen plasma concentrations and platelet aggregation.

Ginkgo has been investigated for its effects in treating vitiligo; the rationale for this is centred around the antioxidant (oxidative stress is now thought to be involved in pathogenesis of vitiligo) and anti-inflammatory properties of ginkgo.[100] In a randomised, double-blind, placebo-controlled trial, 52 patients with slow-spreading vitiligo received *G. biloba* leaf extract 40 mg (standardised for flavonoid glycosides 9.6 mg; Ginkocer, Ranbaxy, India) three times daily. Treatment was continued where response was considered adequate (arrest of disease progression in participants with unstable disease, and some repigmentation in existing lesions) for up to six months. Data from 47 participants were included in the analysis; a report of the study does not describe adequately why or when five participants withdrew from the study. Cessation of active progression of depigmentation occurred in a greater proportion of ginkgo recipients than placebo recipients ($p = 0.006$).[100]

A preliminary study explored the effects of ginkgo in the treatment of cocaine dependence, the rationale for this being that chronic cocaine use is associated with cognitive deficits and that the use of nootropic agents, such as ginkgo, may improve cognitive function and reduce the frequency of relapse.[101] In a randomised, double-blind, placebo-controlled trial, 44 cocaine-dependent individuals aged 18 to 60 years received a standardised ginkgo leaf extract (EGb-761) 120 mg, or placebo, twice daily for eight weeks; a third arm of the study received piracetam 2.4 g twice daily. At the end of the study, there were no statistically significant differences between the ginkgo and placebo groups with respect to any of the outcome measures assessed, including physician-assessed clinical global impression scores, Addiction Severity Index scores, urine toxicology screens and treatment retention.[101] As the study involved only small numbers of participants and as a sample size calculation was not performed, it is possible that the study did not have sufficient statistical power to be able to detect a difference between the groups if one existed.

In a study involving patients with end-stage renal disease who had been undergoing peritoneal dialysis for at least six months, participants were randomised to receive ginkgo leaf extract (Ginexin, SK Pharmaceuticals, Korea; not further specified) 160 mg daily for eight weeks, or no treatment.[102] At the end of the study, ginkgo treatment was associated with a statistically significant reduction in plasma D-dimer concentrations (a marker of intravascular coagulation), compared with baseline values,[102] although no statistical comparison with the no-treatment control group was reported. No statistically significant changes in other haemostatic factors, including plasma fibrinogen concentrations, international normalised ratio (INR), von Willebrand's factor and albumin were observed following ginkgo treatment, compared with baseline values, although again, no statistical comparisons with the no-treatment control group were reported. The hypothesis that ginkgo treatment improves the coagulation profile without changing other haemostatic factors in patients with end-stage renal disease who undergo peritoneal dialysis requires testing in rigorous randomised controlled clinical trials.

A phase II (open, uncontrolled) study explored the effects of standardised ginkgo leaf extract (EGb-761) given in combination with 5-fluorouracil (5-FU) in 44 patients with advanced progressive colorectal cancer who had previously received 5-FU.[103] The rationale for including ginkgo extract in the regimen was based on its reputed ability to increase local blood flow. Thus, it was hypothesised that ginkgo extract might 'enhance local tumour blood flow and thus improve the distribution of 5-FU'. In the study, participants received ginkgo extract 350 mg in 250 mL saline intravenously over 30 minutes on days 1–6, and 5-FU 500 mg/m^2 in 250 mL saline intravenously over 30 minutes on days 2–6. The regimen was repeated every three weeks until recurrence of tumour progression. Data from 32 patients who had received at least two courses of treatment were eligible for analysis. Of these patients, 69% experienced progression of disease, 25% experienced no change, and 6.3% (n = 2) were in partial remission.[103]

Side-effects, Toxicity

Clinical data

Clinical data on safety aspects of *G. biloba* leaf preparations are available from several sources, including clinical trials, postmarketing surveillance-type studies and spontaneous reports of suspected adverse drug reactions. Available data indicate that standardised extracts of ginkgo leaf are well tolerated when used at recommended doses and according to other guidance.[52, G21] However, there are reports of bleeding associated with the use of ginkgo leaf preparations (*see* Side-effects, Toxicity; Haemorrhage).

A Cochrane systematic review of studies assessing *G. biloba* leaf preparations in cognitive impairment and dementia included 33 randomised, double-blind, controlled trials.[57] All but one of the included studies investigated the effects of standardised ginkgo leaf extracts EGb-761 and LI-1370 at oral doses ranging from 80–600 mg daily and typically 200 mg daily. The study that did not use either of these preparations assessed an ethanolic extract of ginkgo leaves (drug-to-extract ratio 4 : 1, standardised for total flavone glycosides 0.20 mg/mL and total ginkgolides 0.34 mg/mL) at doses lower than those used in the other 32 studies. Meta-analyses showed that there were no statistically significant differences between ginkgo (any dose) treatment and placebo in the proportion of trial participants experiencing adverse events, and the numbers of participants withdrawing from the studies.[57]

G

A systematic review of nine randomised, double-blind, placebo-controlled trials of standardised ginkgo leaf extracts in patients with dementia of the Alzheimer type and/or multi-infarct dementia concluded that, overall, the frequency of adverse effects reported for ginkgo was not markedly different than that for placebo.[54] The largest trial included in this review involved 327 patients with mild-to-severe dementia related to Alzheimer's disease or multi-infarct dementia who received standardised ginkgo leaf extract (EGb-761) 40 mg orally three times daily (n = 166), or placebo (n = 161), for 52 weeks.[59] It was reported that there was no statistically significant differences between ginkgo and placebo in the number of participants reporting adverse events, or in the frequency and severity of adverse events. Of 188 adverse events reported during the study, 97 were reported by ginkgo recipients and 91 by placebo recipients. However, clinical trials generally only have the statistical power to detect common, acute adverse effects.

Similar findings were reported in another systematic review/meta-analysis which included eight randomised, double-blind, placebo-controlled trials of ginkgo extract for the treatment of intermittent claudication, involving a total of 415 patients who received standardised extract of ginkgo leaf at doses of 120 or 160 mg daily, or placebo, for up to 24 weeks.[56] Five of the eight studies included reported (rarely) mild, transient adverse events occurring in ginkgo recipients; the remaining three studies, comprising almost 50% of the total number of patients, did not report any adverse events.

A postmarketing surveillance study involving 10 815 patients who received a standardised extract (LI-1370) of ginkgo leaf reported that the frequency of adverse effects was 1.7%.[G56] Adverse effects reported with standardised extracts of ginkgo leaf are generally mild, and include nausea, headache, gastrointestinal upset and diarrhoea; allergic skin reactions occur rarely.[104, G21, G56]

The World Health Organization's Uppsala Monitoring Centre (WHO-UMC; Collaborating Centre for International Drug Monitoring) receives summary reports of suspected adverse drug reactions from national pharmacovigilance centres of over 70 countries worldwide. To the end of the year 2005, the WHO-UMC's Vigisearch database contained a total of 594 reports, describing a total of 1178 adverse reactions, for products reported to contain *G. biloba* only as the active ingredient (*see* Table 1).[105] This number may include case reports described below. Reports originated from 23 different countries. The total number of reactions (i.e. not individual cases; one case may describe several

G

Table 1 Summary of spontaneous reports (*n* = 594) of suspected adverse drug reactions associated with single-ingredient *Ginkgo biloba* preparations held in the Vigisearch database of the World Health Organization's Uppsala Monitoring Centre for the period up to end of 2005.[a, b, 105]

System organ class. **Adverse drug reaction name (number)**	**Total**
Application site disorders.	2
Body as a whole – general disorders. Including allergic reaction (4); asthenia (6); back pain (5); fatigue (8); fever (22); hyperpyrexia (4); malaise (13); pain (3); pallor (3); rigors (28); syncope (4); therapeutic response decreased (3)	130
Cardiovascular disorders, general. Including hypertension (15); hypotension (8); hypotension, postural (4); circulatory failure (13)	48
Central and peripheral nervous system disorders. Including ataxia (5); coma (5); convulsions (11); convulsions, grand mal (3); dizziness (21); headache (35); neuropathy (3); paraesthesia (9); paralysis (3); tremor (3); vertigo (10)	137
Collagen disorders.	3
Endocrine disorders.	1
Foetal disorders.	1
Gastrointestinal system disorders. Including abdominal pain (19); diarrhoea (33); dyspepsia (9); flatulence (3); gastrointestinal haemorrhage (4); gastric ulcer, haemorrhagic (3); haematemesis (4); melaena (4); nausea (37); vomiting (30)	166
Hearing and vestibular disorders. Including tinnitus (4)	9
Heart rate and rhythm disorders. Including arrhythmia (5); bradycardia (5); palpitation (4); tachycardia (15)	43
Liver and biliary system disorders. Including gamma-GT increased (6); hepatic function abnormal (4); hepatic cirrhosis (4); hepatitis (11); hepatocellular damage (4); bilirubinaemia (3); jaundice (6); hepatic enzymes increased (10); SGOT increased (7); SGPT increased (14)	73
Metabolic and nutritional disorders. Including acidosis (3); hyponatraemia (7)	23
Musculo-skeletal system disorders. Including arthralgia (11); myalgia (4); skeletal pain (3)	28
Myo-endo pericardial and valve disorders.	4
Neonatal and infancy disorders.	1
Neoplasm.	2
Platelet, bleeding and clotting disorders. Including haematoma (6); haemorrhage NOS (4); prothrombin decreased (8); prothrombin increased (4); purpura (19); purpura thrombocytopenic (3); thrombocytopenia (10)	58
Psychiatric disorders. Including aggressive reaction (5); agitation (5); amnesia (3); anxiety (3); anorexia (5); confusion (17); depression (8); hallucination (10); insomnia (8); somnolence (3)	
Red blood cell disorders. Including anaemia (10); pancytopenia (3)	18
Reproductive disorders, female and male.	8
Resistance mechanism disorders.	4
Respiratory system disorders. Including dyspnoea (8); epistaxis (9)	32
Skin and appendages disorders. Including angioedema (8); bullous eruption (3); eczema (7); epidermal necrolysis (3); erythema multiforme (4); Stevens-Johnson syndrome (6); photosensitivity reaction (5); pruritus (28); rash (13); rash, erythematous (34); rash, maculopapular (5); rash, psoriaform (3); sweating increased (8); urticaria (15)	165
Special senses other, disorders.	1
Urinary system disorders. Including face oedema (4)	16
Vascular (extracardiac) disorders. Including cerebral haemorrhage (7); cerebrovascular disorder (3); haemorrhage, intracranial (5); flushing (6)	36
Vision disorders. Including conjunctivitis (5); vision abnormal (10)	26
White cell and res disorders. Including agranulocytosis (5); leucopenia (6); leukocytosis (11)	25
Other reactions described using terms not included in database	30
Total number of suspected adverse drug reactions	1178

[a]Specific reactions described where *n* = 3 or more
[b]Caveat statement. These data were obtained from the Vigisearch database held by the WHO Collaborating Centre for International Drug Monitoring, Uppsala, Sweden. The information is not homogeneous at least with respect to origin or likelihood that the pharmaceutical product caused the adverse reaction. Any information included in this report does not represent the opinion of the World Health Organization

reactions) included 58 reactions associated with platelet, bleeding and clotting disorders (*see* Table 1); other reactions include gastrointestinal haemorrhage, haematemesis and melaena (*n* = 4 each), bloody diarrhoea (1), haemorrhagic gastric ulcer (3), epistaxis (9), haemoptysis (2), post-operative haemorrhage (3), cerebral, subarachnoid or intracranial haemorrhage (13), cerebral infarction or cerebrovascular disorder (5) and ocular or retinal haemorrhage (3). (These data were obtained from the Vigisearch database held by the WHO Collaborating Centre for International Drug Monitoring, Uppsala, Sweden. The information is not homogeneous at least with respect to origin or likelihood that the pharmaceutical product caused the adverse reaction. Any information included in this report does not represent the opinion of the World Health Organization.)

Haemorrhage Reports of bleeding and associated disorders included in the WHO-UMC's Vigisearch database are discussed above. There are several case reports in the literature of bleeding associated with ingestion of *Ginkgo biloba* extracts. A systematic review of published case reports describing bleeding associated with ginkgo use identified 15 published case reports (including a new report published in the same paper by the authors of the systematic review). Most of the cases involved serious adverse effects, including intracranial bleeding (*n* = 8 episodes, two required surgical evacuation, two patients experienced permanent neurologic defects, and one patient died), and ocular bleeding (*n* = 4, all returned to baseline vision although one patient required surgery).[106] Where stated, the duration ginkgo exposure before onset of the adverse event varied from less than two weeks' exposure for the two cases of spontaneous hyphema, less than two months' exposure for two cases of intracranial bleeding, and more than six months' exposure for eight other cases. In most cases, there were other risk factors for bleeding, including clinical risk factors and use of other medicines known to increase the risk of bleeding.[106] In addition, most of the case reports do not adequately describe the ginkgo preparation implicated and, typically, in the rare cases that a sample of the product is available, no chemical analysis of the product is undertaken. Since most of the reports originate from countries where ginkgo products are sold as unlicensed dietary supplements, the possibility that poor or variable pharmaceutical quality of products plays a role in these cases cannot be ruled out.

Reports identified by the review include those describing a 70-year-old man who experienced spontaneous bleeding from the iris into the anterior chamber of the eye one week after he began taking standardised ginkgo extract 80 mg daily;[107] a 61-year-old man who had taken ginkgo extract 120 mg or 160 mg daily for six months who experienced a subarachnoid haemorrhage;[108] a 33-year-old woman who began experiencing increasingly severe headaches, as well as double vision and nausea and vomiting, over several months, and who had been consuming standardised ginkgo extract 120 mg daily for two years;[109] a 59-year-old man who experienced vitreous haemorrhage after undergoing a liver transplant and who had been consuming a ginkgo product before and during his operation and subsequent recovery period;[110] a 34-year-old man who experienced post-operative bleeding following a laparoscopic cholecystectomy and who had been taking two ginkgo tablets daily (not further specified);[111] a 56-year-old man who experienced a cerebral haemorrhage and who had been taking ginkgo leaf extract 40 mg three times daily for 18 months;[112] a 65-year-old woman who experienced retrobulbar haemorrhage and who had been taking ginkgo leaf extract 40 mg three times daily for two years.[113] A causal relationship between ginkgo ingestion and bleeding in these cases has not been definitively established.

A new report published since the systematic review describes a 77-year-old woman who experienced persistent post-operative bleeding from the wound after undergoing a total hip arthroplasty.[114] Four weeks post-operatively it was found that the woman had been taking ginkgo leaf extract (not further specified) 120 mg daily. Ginkgo use was stopped and the patient's wound healed within ten weeks.

Other effects There is a report of acute myoglobinuria in a 29-year-old man who was a regular weight-trainer and who had been taking a combination preparation containing extracts of ginkgo (200 mg), guarana (*Paullinia cupana*, 500 mg) and kava (*Piper methysticum*, 100 mg).[115] The man was admitted to an intensive care unit with severe muscle pain and blood creatine kinase and myoglobin concentrations of 100 500 IU/L (normal values: 0–195) and 10 000 ng/mL (normal values: 0–90), respectively. Signs and symptoms subsided within six weeks. The relevance, if any, of ginkgo ingestion to the man's condition, is unclear.

Contact or ingestion of the fruit pulp has produced severe allergic reactions including erythema, oedema, blisters and itching.[82] The seed contains the toxin 4-O-methylpyridoxine which is reported to be responsible for 'gin-nan' food poisoning in Japan and China.[11] The main symptoms are convulsion and loss of consciousness and lethality is estimated in about 27% of cases in Japan, infants being particularly vulnerable.

Contra-indications, Warnings

In view of the intended uses of ginkgo and the documented pharmacological actions of ginkgo, it is not suitable for self-treatment.

There are reports of haemorrhagic reactions associated with the use of ginkgo leaf preparations. Until further information is available, it is reasonable to advise that ginkgo should not be used in patients with previous or existing bleeding disorders unless the potential benefits outweigh the potential harms. In view of the lack of conclusive evidence for the efficacy of ginkgo leaf in the various conditions for which it is used, and the serious nature of the potential harm, it is extremely unlikely that the benefit–harm balance would be in favour of such patients using ginkgo leaf preparations. Oestrogenic activity *in vitro* has been documented for a *G. biloba* leaf extract.[44] The clinical relevance of this finding has not been established.

The fruit pulp has produced severe allergic reactions and should not be handled or ingested. The seed causes severe adverse effects when ingested.

Drug interactions In view of the documented pharmacological actions of ginkgo the potential for preparations of ginkgo leaf to interfere with other medicines administered concurrently, particularly those with similar or opposing effects, should be considered. In particular, ginkgo extract should only be used with caution in patients taking anticoagulant and/or antiplatelet agents.

Inhibition of the activity of certain human cytochrome P450 (CYP) drug metabolising enzymes, particularly CYP2C9 and, to a lesser extent CYP1A2, CYP2E1 and CYP3A4, has been described for a standardised extract of ginkgo leaf (EGb-761) in *in-vitro* studies,[116] and other *in vitro* experiments have reported moderate inhibition of CYP3A4 and CYP2C9 activity by *G. biloba* and/or its isolated constituents.[117, 118] A flavonoid fraction and most of its subfractions showed strong inhibition of the CYP enzymes CYP2C9, CYP1A2, CYP2E1 and CYP3A4 ($IC_{50} < 40\ \mu g/mL$), whereas a terpenoid fraction inhibited activity of CYP2C9 only.[116] The flavonol aglycones kaempferol, quercetin, apigenin and others, but not the terpene lactone and flavonoid glycoside constituents of ginkgo leaf, were found to be potent inhibitors of CYP1A2 and CYP3A.[119]

An *in vivo* (rats) study found that a standardised extract of ginkgo leaf (EGb-761) 100 mg/kg body weight administered orally for four days was associated with increased CYP P450 enzymes in the liver and increased the metabolism of endogenous steroids.[120] The latter finding, however, has not been confirmed in drug interactions studies involving healthy volunteers. A standardised extract of ginkgo leaf (EGb-761) administered orally at a dose of 240 mg daily for 28 days,[120] and a ginkgo leaf extract 240 mg daily for 14 days,[121] had no statistically significant effects, compared with baseline values, on the profile of endogenous steroids in healthy individuals.[120, 121]

Other drug interaction studies involving healthy individuals report conflicting results with respect to the inhibition or induction of CYP enzymes by ingestion of ginkgo leaf preparations. Studies have found that ginkgo leaf extract was associated with certain changes in the pharmacokinetics of nifedipine,[122] and omeprazole,[123] but not digoxin,[124] donepezil,[125] and warfarin.[126]

In a drug-interaction study involving 12 healthy individuals, administration of a standardised extract of ginkgo leaf (EGb-761) administered orally at a dose of 120 mg twice daily for 14 days was not associated with any statistically significant changes, compared with baseline values, in the pharmacokinetics of the probe CYP 2D6 substrate dextromethorphan; ginkgo administration was associated with a statistically significant change, compared with baseline values, in the area under the plasma concentration time curve for the CYP3A4 substrate alprazolam, but as there was no statistically significant change in the elimination half-life of alprazolam, it is unlikely that ginkgo had an inductive effect on CYP3A4.[127]

Pregnancy and lactation No studies appear to have been reported on the effects of *G. biloba* leaf extracts or ginkgolides in pregnant or lactating women. In view of the many pharmacological actions documented and the lack of toxicity data, use of ginkgo during pregnancy and breastfeeding should be avoided.

Preparations

Proprietary single-ingredient preparations

Argentina: Clarvix; Kalter; Tanakan. *Australia:* Proginkgo. *Austria:* Cerebokan; Ceremin; Gingohexal; Gingol; Tebofortan; Tebonin. *Belgium:* Memfit; Tanakan; Tavonin. *Brazil:* Binko; Clibium; Dinaton; Equitam; Gibilon; Ginbiloba; Gincolin; Ginkoba; Ginkobil; Ginkofarma; Ginkogreen; Ginkolab; Ginkoplus; Gyncobem; Kiadon; Kirsan; Mensana; Tanakan; Tebonin. *Chile:* Kiadon; Memokit; Nokatar; Rokan. *Czech Republic:* Tebokan. *France:* Ginkogink; Tanakan; Tramisal. *Germany:* Alz; Duogink; Gincuran; Gingiloba; Gingium; Gingobeta; Gingopret; Ginkobil; Ginkodilat; Ginkokan; Ginkopur; Isoginkgo; Kaveri; Rokan; Tebonin. *Greece:* Tanacain; Tebokan. *Hong Kong:* Ebamin; Ginkolin; Tanakan. *Hungary:* Gingium; Ginkgold; Tanakan; Tebofortan; Tebonin. *Italy:* Ginkoba. *Malaysia:* Gincare; Tanakan. *Mexico:* Bilogink; Kolob; Tanakan; Tebonin; Vasodil. *Netherlands:* Tavonin. *Portugal:* Abolibe; Biloban; Gincoben; Ginkoftal; Vasactife. *Russia:* Bilobil (Билобил); Tanakan (Танакан). *Singapore:* Ginkapran; Ginkosen; Tanakan. *Spain:* Fitokey Ginkgo; Tanakene. *Switzerland:* Demonatur Ginkgo; Geriaforce; Gingosol; Symfona; Tanakene; Tebokan. *Thailand:* Tanakan. *UK:* Ginkovital. *USA:* BioGinkgo. *Venezuela:* Kiadon; Tanakan.

Proprietary multi-ingredient preparations

Argentina: Centellase de Centella Queen; Flebitol; GB 100; Herbaccion Celfin; Herbaccion Memory; SCV 300; Venoful; VNS 45. *Australia:* Bilberry Plus Eye Health; Bioglan Vision-Eze; Bioglan Zellulean with Escin; Extralife Extra-Brite; Extralife Eye-Care; Extralife Leg-Care; Eye Health Herbal Plus Formula 4; For Peripheral Circulation Herbal Plus Formula 5; Gingo A; Ginkgo Biloba Plus; Ginkgo Complex; Ginkgo Plus Herbal Plus Formula 10; Herbal Arthritis Formula; Herbal Capillary Care; Lifechange Circulation Aid; Lifechange Multi Plus Antioxidant; Lifesystem Herbal Formula 6 For Peripheral Circulation; Lifesystem Herbal Plus Formula 11 Ginkgo; Lifesystem Herbal Plus Formula 5 Eye Relief; Prophthal; Vig; Vig. *Brazil:* Composto Anticelulitico; Derm'attive Solaire; Traumed. *Canada:* Ginkoba. *Chile:* Celltech Gold; Gincosan; Mentania; Sebium AKN. *Czech Republic:* Gincosan; Ginkor Fort. *France:* Ginkor Fort; Ginkor; Parogencyl prevention gencives; Photoderm Flush. *Germany:* Perivar. *Hong Kong:* Flavo-C; Ginkor Fort. *Hungary:* Ginkor Fort. *Italy:* Angioton; Forticrin; Ginkoba Active; Ginkoftal; Ginkoret; Memoactive; Memorandum; Pik Gel; Pulsalux; Varicofit; Vasobrain Plus; Vasobrain; Vasopt; Vertiginkgo. *Malaysia:* Ginkor Fort; Total Man. *Russia:* Ginkor Fort (Гинкор Форт); Ginkor Gel (Гинкор Гель). *Singapore:* Ginkgo-PS. *Switzerland:* Allium Plus; Arterosan Plus; Capsules-vital; Gincosan; Triallin. *Thailand:* Ginkor Fort. *UK:* Actimind; Boots Alternatives Sharp Mind; I-Sight; Nature's Garden; ProBrain; Rutin Compound Tablets. *USA:* Dorofen; Gentaplex; Healthy Eyes; Mental Clarity.

References

1 Van Beek TA *et al*. *Ginkgo biloba* L. *Fitoterapia* 1998; 69: 195–244.
2 Van Beek TA, ed. *Ginkgo. The Genus Ginkgoaceae*. Amsterdam: Harwood Academic Publishers, 1998.
3 Victoire C *et al*. Isolation of flavonoid glycosides from *Ginkgo biloba* leaves. *Planta Med* 1988; 54: 245–247.
4 Schenne A, Holzl J. 6-Hydroxykynurensaure, die erste N- haltige Verbindung aus den Blattern von *Ginkgo biloba*. *Planta Med* 1986; 52: 235–236.
5 Nasr C, *et al*. *2-Quinoline carboxylic acid-4,6-dihydroxy from* Ginkgo biloba. Paper presented at the Phytochemical Society of Europe Symposium: Biologically Active Natural Products, Lausanne, 1986, p. 9.
6 Briancon-Scheid F *et al*. HPLC separation and quantitative determination of biflavones in leaves from *Ginkgo biloba*. *Planta Med* 1983; 49: 204–220.
7 Vanhaelen M, Vanhaelen-Fastre R. Kaempferol-3-O-β-glucoside (astragalin) from *Ginkgo biloba*. *Fitoterapia* 1988; 59: 511.
8 Braquet P. The ginkgolides: potent platelet-activating factor antagonists isolated from *Ginkgo biloba* L.: Chemistry, pharmacology and clinical applications. *Drugs of the Future* 1987; 12: 643–699.
9 Anonymous. Extract of *Ginkgo biloba* (EGb-761). *Presse Med* 1986; 15: 1438–1598.
10 Huang X *et al*. Characteristics and antifungal activity of a chitin binding protein from *Ginkgo biloba*. *FEBS* 2000; 478: 123–126.
11 Wada K *et al*. Studies on the constitution of edible medicinal plants. 1. Isolation and identification of 4-O-methylpyridoxine, toxic principle from the seed of *Ginkgo biloba* L. *Chem Pharm Bull* 1988; 36: 1779–1782.
12 Wang H, Ng TB. Ginkbilobin, a novel antifungal protein from *Ginkgo biloba* seeds with sequence similarity to embryo-abundant protein. *Biochem Biophys Res Commun* 2000; 279: 407–411.
13 Kressmann S. Pharmaceutical quality of different *Ginkgo biloba* brands. *J Pharm Pharmacol* 2002; 54: 661–669.
14 Kressmann S *et al*. Influence of pharmaceutical quality on the bioavailability of active components from *Ginkgo biloba* preparations. *J Pharm Pharmacol* 2002; 45(11): 1507–1514.
15 DeFeudis FV. *Ginkgo biloba. From Chemistry to Clinic*. Wiesbaden, Germany: Ullstein Medical, 1998.
16 Clostre F, De Feudis FV, eds. *Cardiovascular Effects of Ginkgo biloba Extract (EGb761). Advances in Ginkgo biloba Extract Research*, vol 3. Paris: Elsevier, 1994: 1–162.
17 Reuter HD. *Ginkgo biloba* – botany, constituents, pharmacology and clinical trials. *Br J Phytother* 1995/6; 4: 3–20.
18 Christen Y, ed. *Ginkgo biloba Extract (EGb-761) as a Neuroprotective Agent: From Basic Studies to Clinical Trials. Advances in Ginkgo biloba Extract Research*, vol 8. Paris: Elsevier, 2001.
19 Winter JC. The effects of an extract of Ginkgo biloba, EGb-761, on cognitive behaviour and longevity in the rat. *Physiol Behav* 1998; 63: 425–433.
20 Hasenöhrl RU *et al*. Dissociation between anxiolytic and hypomnestic effects for combined extracts of *Zingiber officinale* and *Ginkgo biloba*, as opposed to diazepam. *Pharmacol Biochem Behav* 1998; 59: 527–535.
21 Christen Y *et al*., eds. *Effects of Ginkgo biloba Extract (EGb-761) on Neuronal Plasticity. Advances in Ginkgo biloba Extract Research*, vol 5. Paris: Elsevier, 1996.
22 Papadopoulos V *et al*. *Adaptive Effects of Ginkgo biloba Extract (EGb-761). Advances in Ginkgo biloba Extract Research*, vol 6. Paris: Elsevier, 1997.
23 Liebgott T *et al*. Complementary cardioprotective effects of flavonoid metabolites and terpenoid constituents of *Ginkgo biloba* extract (EGb-761) during ischemia and reperfusion. *Basic Res Cardiol* 2000; 95: 368–377.
24 Janssens D *et al*. Protection by bilobalide of the ischaemia-induced alterations of the mitochondrial respiratory activity. *Fund Clin Pharmacol* 2000; 14: 193–201.
25 Zhang WR *et al*. Protective effect of Ginkgo extract on rat brain with transient middle cerebral artery occlusion. *Neurol Res* 2000; 22: 517–521.
26 Dutta-Roy AK *et al*. Inhibitory effect of *Ginkgo biloba* extract on human platelet aggregation. *Platelets* 1999; 10: 298–305.

27 Hosford D, *et al*. Natural antagonists of platelet-activating factor. *Phytother Res* 1988; 2: 1–17.
28 Maitra I *et al*. Peroxyl radical scavenging activity of *Ginkgo biloba* extract EGb-761. *Biochem Pharmacol* 1995; 49: 1649–1655.
29 Lee S-L *et al*. Superoxide scavenging effect of *Ginkgo biloba* extract on serotonin-induced mitogenesis. *Biochem Pharmacol* 1998; 56: 527–533.
30 Oyama Y *et al*. *Ginkgo biloba* extract protects brain neurons against oxidative stress induced by hydrogen peroxide. *Brain Res* 1996; 712: 349–352.
31 Wei T *et al*. Hydrogen peroxide-induced oxidative damage and apoptosis in cerebellar granule cells: protection by *Ginkgo biloba* extract. *Pharmacol Res* 2000; 41: 427–433.
32 Bastianetto S *et al*. The ginkgo biloba extract (EGb-761) protects hippocampal neurons against cell death induced by β-amyloid. *Eur J Neurosci* 2000; 12: 1882–1890.
33 Zhou L-J, Zhu X-Z. Reactive oxygen species-induced apoptosis in PC12 cells and protective effect of bilobalide. *J Pharmacol Exp Ther* 2000; 293: 982–988.
34 Calapai G *et al*. Neuroprotective effects of *Ginkgo biloba* extract in brain ischaemia are mediated by inhibition of nitric oxide synthesis. *Life Sci* 2000; 67: 2673–2683.
35 Rasetti MF *et al*. Extracts of *Ginkgo biloba* L. leaves and *Vaccinium myrtillus* L. fruits prevent photo-induced oxidation of low density lipoprotein cholesterol. *Phytomedicine* 1996/97; 3: 335–338.
36 Drieu K *et al*. Effect of the extract of *Ginkgo biloba* (EGb-761) on the circulating and cellular profiles of polyunsaturated fatty acids: correlation with the anti-oxidant properties of the extract. *Prostaglandins Leukot Essent Fatty Acids* 2000; 63: 293–300.
37 Bridi R *et al*. The antioxidant activity of standardized extract of *Ginkgo biloba* (EGb-761) in rats. *Phytother Res* 2001; 15: 449–451.
38 Bahcecioglu IH *et al*. Protective effect of *Ginkgo biloba* extract on CCl_4-induced liver damage. *Hepatol Res* 1999; 15: 215–224.
39 Agha AM *et al*. Chemopreventive effect of *Ginkgo biloba* extract against benzo(a)pyrene-induced fore stomach carcinogenesis in mice: amelioration of doxorubicin cardiotoxicity. *J Exp Clin Cancer Res* 2001; 20: 39–50.
40 Papadopoulos V *et al*. Drug-induced inhibition of the peripheral-type benzodiazepine receptor expression and cell proliferation in human breast cancer cells. *Anticancer Res* 2000; 20: 2835–2848.
41 Naidu MUR *et al*. *Ginkgo biloba* extract ameliorates gentamicin-induced nephrotoxicity in rats. *Phytomedicine* 2000; 7: 191–197.
42 Siegers CP. Cytotoxicity of alkylphenols from *Ginkgo biloba*. *Phytomedicine* 1999; 6: 281–283.
43 Hecker H *et al*. *In vitro* evaluation of the cytotoxic potential of alkylphenols from *Ginkgo biloba* L. *Toxicology* 2002; 177: 167–177.
44 Oh SM, Chung KH. Estrogenic activities of *Ginkgo biloba* extracts. *Life Sci* 2004; 74: 1325–1335.
45 White HL *et al*. Extracts of *Ginkgo biloba* leaves inhibit monoamine oxidase. *Life Sci* 1996; 58: 1315–1321.
46 Sasaki K *et al*. Effects of bilobalide on gamma-aminobutyric acid levels and glutamic acid decarboxylase in mouse brain. *Eur J Pharmacol* 1999; 367: 165–173.
47 Itokawa H *et al*. Antitumour principles from *Ginkgo biloba* L. *Chem Pharm Bull* 1987; 35: 3016–3020.
48 Biber A. Pharmacokinetics of *Ginkgo biloba* extracts. *Pharmacopsychiatry* 2003; 36 (Suppl. Suppl.1):S32–37.
49 Mauri P *et al*. Liquid chromatographic/atmospheric pressure chemical ionization mass spectrometry of terpene lactones in plasma of volunteers dosed with *Ginkgo biloba* L. extracts. *Rapid Comm Mass Spec* 2001; 15(12): 929–934.
50 Drago F *et al*. Pharmacokinetics and bioavailability of a *Ginkgo biloba* extract. *J Ocular Pharmacol Ther* 2002; 18(2): 197–202.
51 Wang FM *et al*. Disposition of quercetin and kaempferol in human following an oral administration of *Ginkgo biloba* extract tablets. *Eur J Drug Metab Pharmacokinetics* 2003; 28(3): 173–177.
52 Kleijnen J, Knipschild P. *Ginkgo biloba* for cerebral insufficiency. *Br J Clin Pharmacol* 1992; 34: 352–358.
53 Oken BS *et al*. The efficacy of *Ginkgo biloba* on cognitive function in Alzheimer disease. *Arch Neurol* 1998; 55: 1409–1415.
54 Ernst E, Pittler MH. *Ginkgo biloba* for dementia. A systematic review of double-blind, placebo-controlled trials. *Clin Drug Invest* 1999; 17: 301–308.
55 Ernst E, Stevinson C. *Ginkgo biloba* for tinnitus: a review. *Clin Otolaryngol* 1999; 24: 164–167.
56 Pittler MH, Ernst E. *Ginkgo biloba* extract for the treatment of intermittent claudication: a meta-analysis of randomized trials. *Am J Med* 2000; 108: 276–281.
57 Birks J, Grimley Evans J. *Ginkgo biloba* for cognitive impairment and dementia. The Cochrane Database of Systematic Reviews 2002, Issue 4. Art. No. CD003120.
58 Kanowski S *et al*. Proof of efficacy of the *Ginkgo biloba* special extract EGb-761 in outpatients suffering from mild to moderate primary degenerative dementia of the Alzheimer type or multi-infarct dementia. *Pharmacopsychiatry* 1996; 29: 47–56.
59 Le Bars P *et al*. A placebo-controlled, double-blind, randomized trial of an extract of *Ginkgo biloba* for dementia. *JAMA* 1997; 278: 1327–1332.
60 Brautigam MRH *et al*. Treatment of age-related memory complaints with *Ginkgo biloba* extract: a randomized double blind placebo-controlled study. *Phytomedicine* 1998; 5: 425–434.
61 Canter PH, Ernst E. *Ginkgo biloba*: a smart drug? A systematic review of controlled trials of the cognitive effects of ginkgo biloba extracts in healthy people. *Psychopharmacology Bull* 2002; 36(3): 108–123.
62 Kennedy DO *et al*. The dose-dependent cognitive effects of acute administration of *Ginkgo biloba* to healthy young volunteers. *Psychopharmacology* 2000; 151: 416–423.
63 Subhan Z, Hindmarsh I. The psychopharmacological effects of *Ginkgo biloba* extract in normal healthy volunteers. *Int J Clin Pharmacol Res* 1984; 4: 89–93.
64 Rigney U *et al*. The effects of acute doses of standardized *Ginkgo biloba* extract on memory and psychomotor performance in volunteers. *Phytother Res* 1999; 13: 408–415.
65 Elsabagh S *et al*. Differential cognitive effects of *Ginkgo biloba* after acute and chronic treatment in healthy young volunteers. *Psychopharmacology* 2005; 179: 437–446.
66 Mattes R, Pawlik MK. Effects of *Ginkgo biloba* on alertness and chemosensory function in healthy adults. *Human Psychopharmacol* 2004; 19: 81–90.
67 Kennedy DO *et al*. Electroencephalograph effects of single doses of *Ginkgo biloba* and *Panax ginseng* in healthy young volunteers. *Pharmacol Biochem Behav* 2003; 75: 701–709.
68 Scholey AB, Kennedy DO. Acute, dose-dependent cognitive effects of *Ginkgo biloba*, *Panax ginseng* and their combination in healthy young volunteers: differential interactions with cognitive demand. *Hum Psychopharmacol Clin Exp* 2002; 17: 3544.
69 Mix JA, Crews WD. An examination of the efficacy of *Ginkgo biloba* extract EGb-761 on the neuropsychological functioning of cognitively intact older adults. *J Altern Complement Med* 2000; 6: 219–229.
70 Cockle SM *et al*. The effects of *Ginkgo biloba* extract (LI-1370) supplementation on activities of daily living in free living older volunteers: a questionnaire survey. *Hum Psychopharmacol* 2000; 15: 227–235.
71 Trick L *et al*. The effects of *Ginkgo biloba* extract (LI-1370) supplementation and discontinuation on activities of daily living and mood in free living older volunteers. *Phytotherapy Res* 2004; 18: 531–537.
72 Wesnes KA *et al*. The cognitive, subjective, and physical effects of a *Ginkgo biloba/Panax ginseng* combination in healthy volunteers with neurasthenic complaints. *Psychopharmacol Bull* 1997; 33(4): 677–683.
73 Wesnes KA *et al*. The memory enhancing effects of a *Ginkgo biloba/Panax ginseng* combination in healthy middle-aged volunteers. *Psychopharmacology* 2000; 152: 353–361.
74 Hartley DE *et al*. Gincosan (a combination of *Ginkgo biloba* and *Panax ginseng*): the effects on mood and cognition of 6 and 12 weeks' treatment in post-menopausal women. *Nutritional Neurosci* 2004; 7: 325–333.
75 Nathan PJ *et al*. Effects of a combined extract of *Ginkgo biloba* and *Bacopa monniera* on cognitive function in healthy humans. *Human Psychopharmacol* 2004; 19: 91–96.
76 Rejali D *et al*. *Ginkgo biloba* does not benefit patients with tinnitus: a randomized placebo-controlled double-blind trial and meta-analysis of randomized trials. *Clin Otolaryngol* 2004; 29: 226–231.

G

77 Hilton M, Stuart E. Ginkgo biloba *for tinnitus*. The Cochrane Database of Systematic Reviews 2004, Issue 2. Art. No.: CD003852. pub2.
78 Drew S, Davies E. Effectiveness of *Ginkgo biloba* in treating tinnitus: double blind, placebo controlled trial. *BMJ* 2001; 322: 73–75.
79 Ernst E. Marketing studies and scientific research must be distinct. *BMJ* 2001; 322: 1249.
80 Bukovics K *et al*. Vergleich von Ginkgo biloba und 6% HES 200/0,5 in der Behandlung des akuten Hörsturzes. *J Pharmakol Ther* 1999; 2: 48–56.
81 Janssens D *et al*. Increase in circulating endothelial cells in patients with primary chronic venous insufficiency: protective effect of Ginkor Fort in a randomized double-blind, placebo-controlled clinical trial. *J Cardiovasc Pharmacol* 1999; 33: 7–11.
82 Pizzorno JE, Murray MT. *A Textbook of Natural Medicine*. Seattle, WA: John Bastyr College Publications, 1985 (looseleaf).
83 Chung KF. Effect of a ginkgolide mixture (BN 52063) in antagonising skin and platelet responses to platelet activating factor in man. *Lancet* 1987; i: 248–251.
84 Wilkens JH *et al*. Effects of a PAF-antagonist (BN 52063) on bronchoconstriction and platelet activation during exercise-induced asthma. *Br J Clin Pharmacol* 1990; 29: 85–91.
85 Kang BJ *et al*. A placebo-controlled, double-blind trial of *Ginkgo biloba* for antidepressant-induced sexual dysfunction. *Human Psychopharmacol* 2002; 17: 279–284.
86 Wheatley D. Triple-blind, placebo-controlled trial of *Ginkgo biloba* in sexual dysfunction due to antidepressant drugs. *Human Psychopharmacol* 2004; 19: 545–548.
87 Cohen AJ, Bartlik B. *Ginkgo biloba* for antidepressant-induced sexual dysfunction. *J Sex Marital Ther* 1998; 24: 139–143.
88 Wheatley D. *Ginkgo biloba* in the treatment of sexual dysfunction due to antidepressant drugs. *Hum Psychopharmacol* 1999; 14: 511–513.
89 Zeng X *et al*. Ginkgo biloba for acute ischaemic stroke. The Cochrane Database of Systematic Reviews 2005, Issue 4. Art. No. CD003691. pub2.
90 Evans JR. *Ginkgo biloba* extract for age-related macular degeneration (Cochrane review). In: *The Cochrane Library*, Issue 3, 2001. Oxford: Update Software, 2001.
91 Quaranta L *et al*. Effect of *Ginkgo biloba* extract on preexisting visual field damage in normal tension glaucoma. *Ophthalmology* 2003; 110: 359–364.
92 Gertsch JH *et al*. on behalf of the Prevention of High Altitude Illness Trial Research Group. Randomised, double-blind, placebo controlled comparison of ginkgo biloba and acetazolamide for prevention of acute mountain sickness among Himalayan trekkers: the prevention of high altitude illness trial (PHAIT). *BMJ* 2004; 328: 797.
93 Chow T *et al*. *Ginkgo biloba* and acetazolamide prophylaxis for acute mountain sickness. *Arch Intern Med* 2005; 165: 296–301.
94 Gertsch JH *et al*. *Ginkgo biloba* for the prevention of severe acute mountain sickness (AMS) starting one day before rapid ascent. *High Alt Med Biol* 2002; 3(1): 29–37.
95 Lingjaerde O *et al*. Can winter depression be prevented by *Ginkgo biloba* extract? A placebo-controlled trial. *Acta Psychiatr Scand* 1999; 100: 62–66.
96 Tamborini A, Taurelle R. *Rev Fr Gynecol Obstet* 1993; 88: 147. Cited by Bone K. Treatment of congestive symptoms of premenstrual syndrome with ginkgo. *Br J Phytother* 1995/96; 4: 46.
97 Zhang XY *et al*. The effect of extract of *Ginkgo biloba* added to haloperidol on superoxide dismutase in inpatients with chronic schizophrenia. *J Clin Psychopharmacol* 2001; 21: 85–88.
98 Bombardelli E *et al*. Activity of phospholipid-complex of *Ginkgo biloba* dimeric flavonoids on the skin microcirculation. *Fitoterapia* 1996; 67: 265–273.
99 Muir AH. *et al*. The use of *Ginkgo biloba* in Raynaud's disease: a double-blind placebo-controlled trial. *Vascular Med* 2002; 7: 265–267.
100 Parsad D *et al*. Effectiveness of oral *Ginkgo biloba* in treating limited, slowly spreading vitiligo. *Clin Exp Dermatol* 2003; 28: 285–287.
101 Kampman K *et al*. A pilot trial of piracetam and *Ginkgo biloba* for the treatment of cocaine dependence. *Addictive Behav* 2003; 28: 437–448.
102 Kim SH *et al*. Effects of *Ginkgo biloba* on haemostatic factors and inflammation in chronic peritoneal dialysis patients. *Phytotherapy Res* 2005; 19: 546–548.
103 Hauns B *et al*. Phase II study of combined 5-fluorouracil/*Ginkgo biloba* extract (GBE 761 ONC) therapy in 5-fluorouracil pretreated patients with advanced colorectal cancer. *Phytother Res* 2001; 15: 34–38.
104 DeFeudis FV. Safety of EGb-761-containing products. In: DeFeudis FV, ed. *Ginkgo biloba Extract (EGb-761). Pharmacological Activities and Clinical Applications*. Amsterdam: Elsevier, 1991.
105 Vigibase, WHO Adverse Reactions database, Uppsala Monitoring Centre [accessed January 20, 2006].
106 Bent S *et al*. Spontaneous bleeding associated with *Ginkgo biloba*. A case report and systematic review of the literature. *J Gen Intern Med* 2005; 20: 657–661.
107 Rosenblatt M, Mindel J. Spontaneous hyphema associated with ingestion of *Ginkgo biloba* extract. *N Engl J Med* 1997; 336: 1108.
108 Vale S. Subarachnoid haemorrhage associated with *Ginkgo biloba*. *Lancet* 1998; 352: 36.
109 Rowin J, Lewis SL. Spontaneous bilateral subdural hematomas associated with chronic *Ginkgo biloba* ingestion. *Neurology* 1996; 46: 1775–1776.
110 Hauser D *et al*. Bleeding complications precipitated by unrecognized *Ginkgo biloba* use after liver transplantation. *Transpl Int* 2002; 15: 377–379.
111 Fessenden JM *et al*. *Ginkgo biloba*: a case report of herbal medicine and bleeding postoperatively from a laparoscopic cholecystectomy. *American Surg* 2001; 67: 33–35.
112 Benjamin J *et al*. A case of cerebral haemorrhage – can *Ginkgo biloba* be implicated? *Postgrad Med J* 2001; 77: 112–113.
113 Fong KCS, Kinnear PE. Retrobulbar haemorrhage associated with chronic *Ginkgo biloba* ingestion. *Postgrad Med J* 2003; 79: 531–532.
114 Bebbington A *et al*. Persistent bleeding after total hip arthroplasy caused by herbal self-medication. *J Arthroplasty* 2005; 20(1): 125–126.
115 Donadio V *et al*. Myoglobinuria after ingestion of extracts of guarana, *Ginkgo biloba* and kava. *Neurol Sci* 2000; 21: 124.
116 Gaudineau C *et al*. Inhibition of human P450 enzymes by multiple constituents of the *Ginkgo biloba* extract. *Biochem Biophys Res Comm* 2004; 318: 1072–1078.
117 Yale SH, Glurich I. Analysis of the inhibitory potential of *Ginkgo biloba*, *Echinacea purpurea*, and *Serenoa* repens on the metabolic activity of cytochrome P450 3A4, 2D6, and 2C9. *J Alt Comp Med* 2005; 11(3): 433–439.
118 He N, Edeki T. The inhibitory effects of herbal components on CYP2C9 and CYP3A4 catalytic activites in human liver microsomes. *Am J Therapeut* 2004; 11(3): 206–212.
119 Von Moltke LL *et al*. Inhibition of human cytochromes P450 by components of *Ginkgo biloba*. *J Pharm Pharmacol* 2004; 56(8): 1039–1044.
120 Chatterjee SS *et al*. Influence of the Ginkgo extract EGb-761 on rat liver cytochrome P450 and steroid metabolism and excretion in rats and man. *J Pharm Pharmacol* 2005; 57(5): 641–650.
121 Markowitz JS *et al*. Effect of *Ginkgo biloba* extract on plasma steroid concentrations in healthy volunteers: a pilot study. *Pharmacotherapy* 2005; 25(10): 1337–1340.
122 Yoshioka M *et al*. Studies on interactions between functional foods or dietary supplements and medicines. IV. Effects of *Ginkgo biloba* leaf extract on the pharmacokinetics and pharmacodynamics of nifedipine in healthy volunteers. *Biol Pharm Bull* 2004; 27(12): 2006–2009.
123 Yin OQ *et al*. Pharmacogenetics and herb-drug interactions: experience with *Ginkgo biloba* and omeprazole. *Pharmacogenetics* 2004; 14(12): 841–850.
124 Mauro VF *et al*. Impact of *Ginkgo biloba* on the pharmacokinetics of digoxin. *Am J Therapeut* 2003; 10: 247–251.
125 Yasui-Furokori N *et al*. The effects of *Ginkgo biloba* extracts on the pharmacokinetics and pharmacodynamics of donepezil. *J Clin Pharmacol* 2004; 44(5): 538–542.
126 Jiang X *et al*. Effect of ginkgo and ginger on the pharmacokinetics and pharmacodynamics of warfarin in healthy subjects. *Br J Clin Pharmacol* 2005; 59: 425–432.
127 Markowitz JS *et al*. Multiple-dose administration of *Ginkgo biloba* did not affect cytochrome P-450 2D6 or 3A4 activity in normal volunteers. *J Clin Psychopharmacol* 2003; 23(6): 576–581.

Ginseng, Eleutherococcus

Summary and Pharmaceutical Comment

Phytochemical studies have revealed that there is no one constituent type that is characteristic of Eleutherococcus ginseng. Studies have shown that components thought to represent the main active constituents ('eleutherosides') consist of a heterogeneous mixture of common plant constituents, including carbohydrates, coumarins, lignans, phenylpropanoids and triterpenoids.

Since the 1950s, many studies (animal and human) have been carried out in Russia, and more recently in Western countries, to investigate the reputed adaptogen properties of Eleutherococcus ginseng. (An adaptogen is a substance that is defined as having three characteristics, namely lack of toxicity, non-specific action, and a normalising action.)

Preclinical studies have indicated that preparations of *E. senticosus* and/or its isolated constituents has a range of pharmacological properties; results of these studies provide some supporting evidence for adaptogenic properties for certain *E. senticosus* preparations, although pharmacological explanations for the observed actions are less well understood.

Clinical trials of *E. senticosus* preparations have focused on assessing effects related to the reputed adaptogenic properties of this herbal medicinal product, although rigorous clinical investigations are limited. Studies have tested different *E. senticosus* preparations, which vary qualitatively and quantitatively in their phytochemical composition, administered according to different dosage regimens, and to different study populations (e.g. healthy volunteers, older patients with hypertension), making interpretation of the results difficult. At present there is insufficient evidence to support definitely the efficacy of specific *E. senticosus* preparations in the various indications for which it is used and/or has been tested.

Similarly, there are only limited clinical data on safety aspects of *E. senticosus* preparations. The clinical trials of *E. senticosus* root preparations available have typically involved only very small numbers of patients and been of short duration, so have the statistical power only to detect very common, acute adverse effects. Rigorous investigation of safety aspects of well-characterised *E. senticosus* root preparations administered orally at different dosages, including the effects of long-term treatment, is required.

In view of the many pharmacological actions documented for ginseng, and the lack of safety and toxicity data, the use of *E. senticosus* during both pregnancy and breastfeeding should be avoided.

Species (Family)

Eleutherococcus senticosus (Rupr. & Maxim.) Maxim. (Araliaceae)

Synonym(s)

Acanthopanax senticosus (Rupr. & Maxim.) Maxim., Devil's Shrub, Eleuthero, *Hedera senticosa* Rupr. & Maxim., Siberian Ginseng, Touch-Me-Not, Wild Pepper

Part(s) Used

Root

Pharmacopoeial and Other Monographs

BHC 1992[G6]
BHMA 2003[G66]
BHP 1996[G9]
BP 2007[G84]
Complete German Commission E[G3]
ESCOP 2003[G76]
Martindale 35th edition[G85]
Ph Eur 2007[G81]
WHO volume 2[G70]

Legal Category (Licensed Products)

Eleutherococcus ginseng is not included in the GSL.[G37]

Constituents

Carbohydrates Polysaccharides (glycans); some have been referred to as eleutherans.[1] Galactose, methyl-α-D-galactose (eleutheroside C), glucose, maltose, sucrose.

Coumarins Isofraxidin-7-glucoside (eleutheroside B_1), 7-ethylumbelliferone.[2]

Lignans (−)-Syringaresinol-4′,4″-di-*O*-β-D-glucopyranoside (eleutheroside E), episyringaresinol-4″-*O*-β-D-glucopyranoside (eleutheroside E_2),[3] 7*SR*,8*RS*-dihydrodehydroconiferyl alcohol, dehydrodiconiferyl alcohol, 7,8-*trans*-diconiferylalcohol-4-*O*-β-D-glucopyranoside, *meso*-secoisolariciresinol, (−)-syringaresinol-4-*O*-β-D-glucopyranoside,[2] sesamin.

Phenylpropanoids Syringin (eleutheroside B), coniferyl alcohol, coniferyl aldehyde, 5′-*O*-caffeoylquinic acid (chlorogenic acid), 1′,5′-*O*-dicaffeoylquinic acid, 4′,5′-*O*-dicaffeoylquinic acid.[4]

Triterpenoids Daucosterol (eleutheroside A), β-hederin (eleutheroside K),[5, 6, G6] 3β-{*O*-β-D-glucopyranosyl-(1→3)-*O*-β-D-galactopyranosyl-(1→4)-[*O*-α-L-rhamnopyranosyl-(1→2)]-*O*-β-D-glucuronopyranosyl}-16α-hydroxy-13β,28-epoxyoleanane,[1] 3β-{*O*-α-L-rhamnopyranosyl-(1→4)-*O*-α-L-rhamnopyranosyl-(1→4)-[*O*-α-L-rhamnopyranosyl-(1→2)]-*O*-β-D-glucopyranosyl-(1→x)-*O*-β-D-glucuronopyranosyl}-16α-hydroxy-13β,28-epoxyoleanane.[6, 7]

Essential oil 0.8%. Individual components not documented.

Other parts of the plant

Stem (−)-Sesamin, isofraxidin, syringaresinol, eleutheroside B, eleutheroside E, 5-hydroxymethylfurfural, isovanillin.[8]

Leaves Flavonoids, including hyperin (quercetin-3-*O*-β-galactoside), quercetin, quercitrin, rutin,[9] and four 3,4-seco-lupan-type triterpenoids.[10]

Quality of plant material and commercial products

According to the British and European Pharmacopoeias, Eleutherococcus ginseng consists of the whole or cut, dried, underground organs of *E. senticosus* (Rupr. Et Maxim.) Maxim.[G81, G84] Eleutherosides A to G are present in roots at concentrations of 0.6–0.9% and in stems at concentrations of 0.6–1.5%.[5] An HPLC method for determining the eleutheroside content of *E. senticosus* roots, which involves the use of ferulic acid rather than eleutherosides B and E (which are very expensive) as an external standard, has been developed and validated.[11] Methods previously reported for the isolation and quantitative analysis of *E. senticosus* root material include centrifugal partition chromatography with HPLC,[12] and reversed-phase HPLC.[13]

As with other herbal medicinal products, there is variation in the qualitative and quantitative composition of commercial eleutherococcus preparations. Analysis of 25 'ginseng' products available for purchase from a health-food store in the USA included 11 products labelled as containing *E. senticosus*. All 11 products contained the correct species, as determined by LC-MS/MS (liquid chromatography/mass spectrometry) analysis identifying the presence of eleutherosides B and E and absence of ginsenosides (apart from the two products which were labelled as also containing *Panax ginseng*). However, there was wide variation between products in the content of these eleutherosides, as determined by HPLC (high-performance liquid chromatography).[14] In products containing powdered *E. senticosus*, eleutheroside B and E content per 100 g of product ranged from 0.009–0.155% and from 0.032–1.122%, respectively, thus total eleutheroside content (B plus E) varied 43-fold between products. With liquid preparations, there was a 200-fold variation in total (B plus E) eleutheroside content between products (0.003–0.551% per 100 g product). For the six products which provided

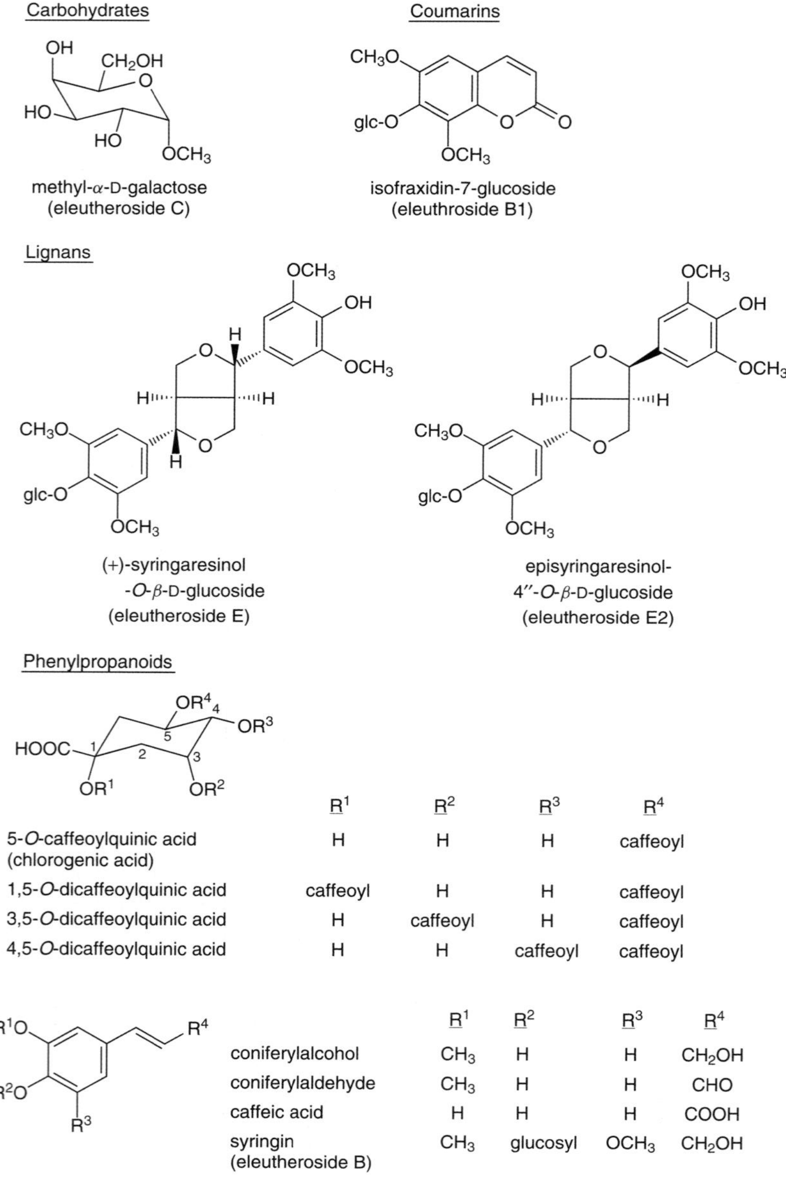

Figure 1 Selected constituents of Eleutherococcus ginseng.

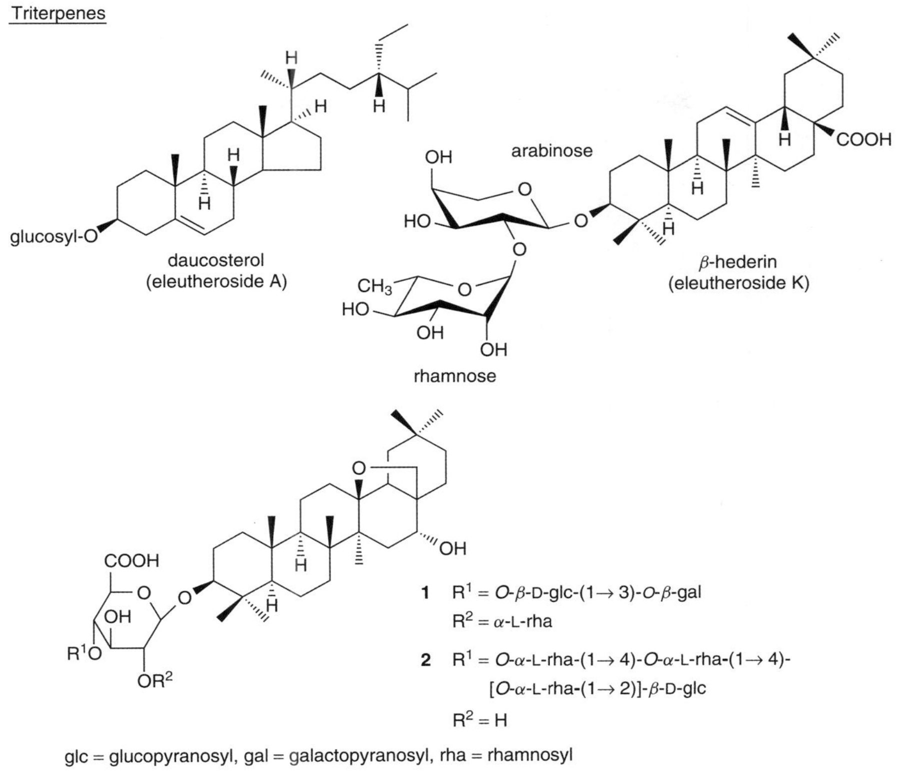

Triterpenes

daucosterol (eleutheroside A)

β-hederin (eleutheroside K)

arabinose

rhamnose

1 R^1 = O-β-D-glc-(1→ 3)-O-β-gal
R^2 = α-L-rha

2 R^1 = O-α-L-rha-(1→ 4)-O-α-L-rha-(1→ 4)-[O-α-L-rha-(1→ 2)]-β-D-glc
R^2 = H

glc = glucopyranosyl, gal = galactopyranosyl, rha = rhamnosyl

Figure 2 Selected constituents of Eleutherococcus ginseng.

quantitative information on the product label, the actual eleutheroside content varied from 12–328% of that stated on the label. Earlier work involving analysis of commercial products purchased in the USA and Canada found that the eleutheroside B concentrations in *E. senticosus* capsules, powder and liquid preparations varied from 0.01–0.03% w/w, 0.01–1.00% w/w, and 0.03–0.13 mg/mL, respectively, and that eleutheroside E concentrations varied from 0.04–0.16% w/w, 0.06–0.66% w/w, and 0.01–1.62 mg/mL, respectively.(13)

Food Use

Eleutherococcus ginseng is not used in foods.

Herbal Use

Eleutherococcus ginseng does not have a traditional herbal use in the UK, although it has been used for many years in the former Soviet Union. Like *Panax ginseng*, Eleutherococcus ginseng is claimed to be an adaptogen in that it increases the body's resistance to stress and builds up general vitality.(G6, G8, G49)

Dosage

Dosages for oral administration (adults) recommended in older standard herbal reference texts are the same for several traditional uses. Dry root 0.6–3 g daily for up to one month has been recommended.(G6, G49) Russian studies in healthy human subjects have involved the administration of an ethanolic extract in doses ranging from 2–16 mL one to three times daily, for up to 60 consecutive days.

Clinical trials of *E. senticosus* have assessed the effects of different preparations administered orally according to different dosage regimens. A rigorous trial involving individuals with chronic fatigue investigated the effects of a standardised extract of *E. senticosus* root providing 2.24 mg eleutherosides (B and E) daily for two months.(15) Studies conducted in Russia and involving healthy human subjects have involved the administration of an ethanolic extract (not further specified) at doses ranging from 2–16 mL one to three times daily, orally, for up to 60 consecutive days.(5) Doses administered to non-healthy individuals ranged from 0.5–6.0 mL given one to three times daily for up to 35 days. In both groups, multiple dosing regimens were separated by an extract-free period of two to three weeks.(5)

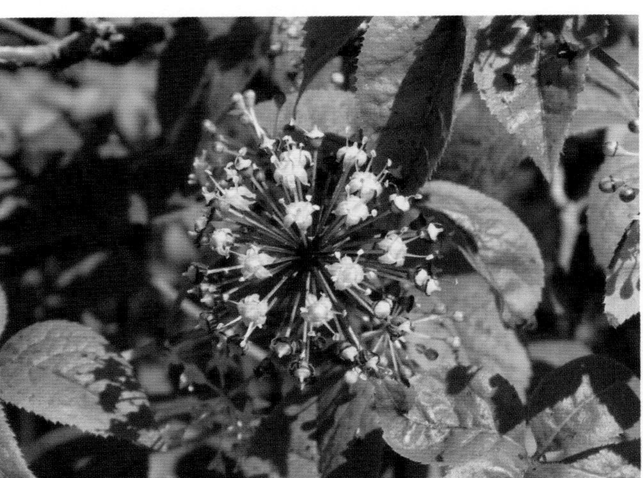

Figure 3 Eleutherococcus ginseng (*Eleutherococcus senticosus*).

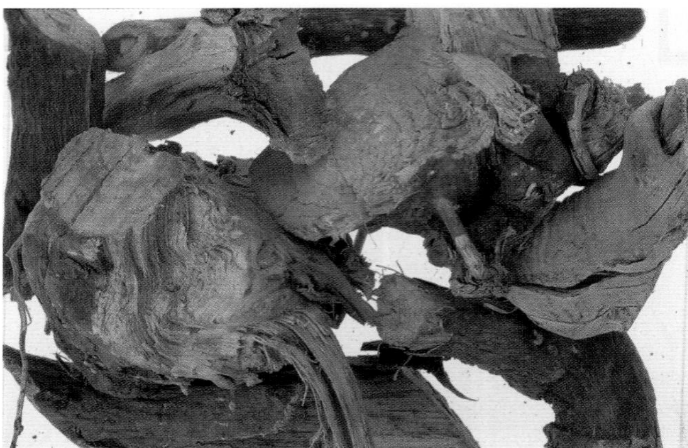

Figure 4 Eleutherococcus ginseng – dried drug substance (root).

G

Pharmacological Actions

The so-called adaptogenic properties of eleutherococcus were first extensively investigated in the countries of the former USSR. Pharmacological studies on extracts of eleutherococcus started in the 1950s. The majority of the early literature on eleutherococcus has been published in Russian and therefore difficulty is encountered in obtaining translations. A review of the literature up to the early 1980s[5] describes the chemistry and toxicity of eleutherococcus and documents results of *in vitro*, *in vivo* and human studies involving the oral administration of an ethanolic extract. More recently, the concept of adaptogens as it relates to eleutherococcus and its chemical constituents has been reviewed.[16] Preparations of eleutherococcus root and/or their isolated constituents have been reported to have several properties *in vitro* and/or *in vivo*, including anticancer, antiviral, hypoglycaemic and immunomodulant activities, although robust evidence of these effects from clinical studies is generally lacking.

In vitro and animal studies

The following represents a summary of the results of preclinical studies investigating the effects of eleutherococcus. It draws on data included in a review[5] as well as on more recent papers published in English. Used here, 'ginseng' refers to eleutherococcus unless indicated otherwise.

Antiviral and antibacterial activities *In vitro* antiviral activity against RNA-type viruses (human rhinovirus, respiratory syncytial virus and influenza A virus) has been demonstrated with an ethanolic extract of ginseng root. No effect was noted in cells infected with DNA-type viruses (adenovirus 5 and herpes simplex type 1 virus).[17]

Hypoglycaemic activity Hypoglycaemic activity has been documented both in normal animals and in those with induced hyperglycaemia (rabbit, mouse), but with little effect on alloxan-induced hyperglycaemia (rat).[5, 18] Hypoglycaemic activity (mice, intraperitoneal injection) of an aqueous ginseng extract has been attributed to polysaccharide components termed eleutherans A–G.[19]

Central nervous system effects Sedative actions (rat, mouse), CNS-stimulant effects (intravenous/subcutaneous injection, rabbit), and a decrease/increase in barbiturate sleeping time has been reported using an aqueous extract of ginseng root.[5, 20]

Immunostimulant, antitoxic actions Numerous *in vitro* and *in vivo* studies have examined the immunomodulatory effects of ginseng. Oral administration of eleutherococcus root prepared as a decoction inhibited mast-cell dependent anaphylaxis in mice.[21] Similar results were obtained using the same animal model for a water extract of ginseng obtained from cell culture.[22] An ethanol extract of *E. senticosus* root inhibited the release of interleukin (IL)-4, IL-5, and IL-12 from human peripheral blood lymphocytes in *in vitro* experiments using human whole blood.[23] The release of IL-6 was stimulated by higher concentrations of the ginseng preparation and inhibited with lower concentrations, suggesting that ginseng root has immunomodulatory rather than immunosuppressive or immunostimulant activity.[23] In other *in-vitro* experiments using human peripheral blood, lower concentrations of an ethanol extract of ginseng root enhanced the proliferation of human lymphocytes, whereas higher concentrations had an antiproliferative effect.[24]

In contrast to the findings described above, *in-vitro* studies using mouse macrophages found that an aqueous extract of ginseng root did not stimulate the expression of a range of cytokines investigated.[25] Increased resistance to induced listeriosis infection (mouse, rabbit) with prophylactic ginseng administration and reduced resistance with simultaneous administration, stimulation of specific antiviral immunity (guinea-pig, mouse), regulation of complement titre and lysozyme activity post immunisation have been documented.[5] *In vitro*, a combination preparation containing *E. senticosus* extract (11.6 mg, standardised for eleutheroside E 1 mg) and *Andrographis paniculata* extract (plant parts not specified) enhanced phytohaemagglutin-induced proliferation of human peripheral blood lymphocytes, whereas the preparation inhibited the spontaneous proliferation of human peripheral blood lymphocytes.[26]

Immunomodulatory effects have been reported for polysaccharide components isolated from *E. senticosus* (plant part not stated),[27] and from cell culture of *E. senticosus*.[28] Polysaccharide administration (100 mg/kg for six days) stimulated phagocytic activity in mice and (following repeated administration of 40 mg/kg) suppressed propogation of human tubercular bacillus in two animal models.[27] Polysaccharide isolated from cell culture increased the proliferation and differentiation of B-cells and increased the cytokine production of macrophages *in vitro*.[28] Immunostimulant activity *in vitro* (using granulocyte, carbon clearance and lymphocyte-transformation tests) has been documented for other high molecular weight polysaccharide components.[29, 30]

Effects on overall performance A beneficial action on parameters indicative of stress or on overall work capacity in mice has been reported for eleutherococcus root bark,[31] although a lack of adaptogenic response has also been shown in mice receiving ginseng infusions.[32, 33] In one study, mice receiving a commercial concentrated extract of ginseng exhibited significantly more aggressive behaviour.[32] Ginseng is claimed to result in a more economical utilisation of glycogen and high-energy phosphorus compounds, and in a more intense metabolism of lactic and pyruvic acids during stress.[5] The adaptogenic effect of ginseng may involve regulation of energy, nucleic acid, and protein metabolism in tissues.[5] It may also be that ginseng limits the binding of stress hormones to their receptors by inhibiting catechol-O-methyltransferase.[34] These hypotheses requires testing in order to elucidate possible mechanisms of action for constituents of ginseng root.

Cardiovascular activity 3,4-Dihydroxybenzoic acid (DBA) has been identified as an anti-aggregatory component in Eleutherococcus ginseng.[1] Compared with aspirin, activity of DBA was comparable to collagen- and ADP-induced platelet aggregation, but less potent versus arachidonic acid-induced platelet aggregation.[1] Ginseng root also showed an endothelium-dependent vasorelaxant effect *in vitro*. Depending on the vessel size, this was mediated either by nitrous oxide or endothelium-derived hyperpolarising factor.[35]

Effect on reproductive capacity Ginseng has been reported to improve the reproductive capacity of bulls and cows, and to have no adverse effects on the various blood parameters (haemoglobin, total plasma protein, albumin and globulin, protein coefficient) measured.[5] A preparation of ginseng root increased the motility of human sperm *in vitro*.[36]

Anticancer and cytotoxic effects An aqueous extract of ginseng root showed additive antiproliferative effects with cytarabine *in vitro* against leukaemia cells.[37] In *in-vitro* experiments using human peripheral blood, an ethanol extract of ginseng root displayed cytotoxic activity against human lymphocytes when applied to the system at a high concentration.[24]

Steroidal activity Gonadotrophic activity in immature male mice (intraperitoneal injection), oestrogenic activity in immature female mice, and an anabolic effect in immature rats (intraperitoneal injection) has been reported.[5]

Other activities An aqueous extract of ginseng root administered orally to rats for 30 days (100 or 200 mg/kg body weight daily) before intravenous administration of lipopolysaccharide (LPS) led to reductions in LPS-induced increases in nitric oxide concentrations and lipid peroxidation, and reduced concentrations of indicators of renal dysfunction.[38] An aqueous extract of ginseng cell culture was found to reduce weight gain, serum LDL cholesterol concentrations and triglyceride accumulation in obese mice.[39] Ginseng root stimulated erythropoiesis during paradoxical sleep deprivation in mice by modulation of brain neurotransmitters.[40]

Other actions documented for ginseng include an increase in catecholamine concentrations in the brain, adrenal gland and urine,[5] and a variable effect on induced hypothermia (rabbit, rat, mouse).[5]

Other parts of the plant

Several of the activities described above for eleutherococcus root have also been described for other parts of the plant, such as leaves and stem bark.

The antibacterial activity of three compounds isolated by methanolic extraction from the dried leaves of ginseng was tested against various Gram-positive and Gram-negative bacteria. Chiisanogenin, but not hyperin or chiisanoside, demonstrated moderate antibacterial activity against *Bacillus subtilis*, *Staphylococcus epidermidis*, *S. aureus*, *Proteus vulgaris* and *Salmonella typhimurium*, with minimum inhibitory concentrations ranging from 50–100 μg/ml.[41]

Oral administration of eleutherococcus stem prepared as a decoction inhibited mast-cell dependent anaphylaxis in mice.[42] A beneficial action on parameters indicative of stress or on overall work capacity in rats has been reported for phenolic compounds isolated from eleutherococcus stem bark.[43]

Preparations of other parts of the plant and/or their isolated constituents have also been reported to have certain cardiovascular efffects. The triterpenoid chiisanogenin from the leaves of *E. senticosus* has been shown to be 50 times as potent as aspirin in inhibiting U46619-induced platelet aggregation and 10–20 times as potent in inhibiting adrenaline- and arachidonic acid–induced aggregation.[44] An aqueous extract of ginseng stem bark protected against the effects of transient focal cerebral ischaemia in rats, an effect apparently mediated by microglial activation and inhibition of cyclooxygenase-2.[45] An increase in lipoprotein lipase activity was observed in adipocytes cultured with an aqueous extract of dried ginseng leaves.[46]

Aqueous or alcoholic extracts of the stem of ginseng have shown hepatoprotective[47, 48] and antioxidant properties[47] *in vivo*. Anti-inflammatory and antinociceptive effects were noted with an ethyl acetate extract of ginseng stem bark in rats: these were attributed to the *in vivo* conversion of liriodendrin to syringaresinol.[49] Preparations of other parts of the plant and/or their isolated constituents have been reported to have certain anticancer effects. Fractionated glycoproteins from an aqueous extract of ginseng stem bark inhibited lung metastasis in mice both prophylactically and therapeutically. This effect was mediated by activation of macrophages and natural killer (NK) cells.[50, 51] In studies using a stem bark extract, sesamin was identified as the component with antitumour activity *in vitro* in human stomach cancer cells.[52]

Ethanol-induced apoptosis in a human neuroblastoma cell line (SK-N-MC) was inhibited by an aqueous extract of ginseng (plant part not stated) *in vitro*.[53] In rats, an ethanolic extract of ginseng stem bark and one of its components, sesamin, showed cytoprotective properties against Parkinson's disease induced by 1-methyl-4-phenyl-1,2,3,6-tetrahydropyridine (MPTP) or rotenone.[54, 55]

Clinical studies

Clinical trials of *E. senticosus* preparations have focused on assessing effects related to the reputed adaptogenic properties of this herbal medicinal product, although rigorous clinical investigations are limited. Studies have tested different *E. senticosus* preparations, including combination herbal preparations containing *E. senticosus*, which vary qualitatively and quantitatively in their phytochemical composition. Furthermore, different preparations have been administered according to different dosage regimens, and to different study populations (e.g. healthy volunteers, older patients with hypertension), making interpretation of the results difficult.

A large body of clinical research has been published in the Russian literature, making access difficult,[5] although consideration of a review of some of this work indicates that these clinical trials are unlikely to meet contemporary standards in terms of their design, analysis and reporting. Therefore, at present there is insufficient evidence to support definitively the efficacy of specific *E. senticosus* preparations in the various indications for which it is used and/or has been tested. Details of clinical trials of *E. senticosus* preparations published in the English literature are summarised below.

In a randomised, double-blind, placebo-controlled, trial, 96 individuals with chronic fatigue (unexplained fatigue of at least six months' duration and a Rand Vitality Index score of 12 or less) recruited using newspaper adverstisements and via chronic fatigue syndrome (CFS) support groups, received capsules containing a standardised extract of *E. senticosus* root providing 2.24 mg eleutherosides (B and E) daily, or placebo, for two months.[15] At the end of the study, Rand Vitality Index scores had improved in

G

both groups and there were no statistically significant differences between groups ($p > 0.05$). Sub-group analyses suggested that there was a treatment effect depending on duration and severity of fatigue at baseline, but this requires testing in larger randomised controlled trials. In a two-month, open-label extension to the initial study, all remaining participants received *E. senticosus*, although they were still unaware of their initial treatment allocation and the likely time to onset of action of *E. senticosus*. During this phase, participants who received placebo during months one and two showed a statistically significant improvement in mean Rand Vitality Index score when assessed at month four, compared with month two ($p = 0.02$), whereas participants who had received *E. senticosus* during months one and two, did not show any statistically significant improvements in Rand Vitality Index scores during the open-label phase of the study.[15]

Another randomised, double-blind, controlled trial assessed the effects of an *E. senticosus* dry extract (Centofiori, Italy; not further specified) 300 mg daily ($n = 10$), or placebo, for eight weeks on quality of life in 20 participants aged 65 years or more with hypertension and who were undergoing treatment with digitalis (not further specified).[56] After four weeks' treatment, improvements in the social functioning and mental compartment summary scores ($p < 0.05$ for both) of the SF-36 general health status questionnaire were observed, but at the eight-week endpoint, there were no statistically significant differences between groups. The study, however, has several methodological limitations, including the small sample size and lack of *a priori* hypotheses for sub-group analyses. Participants in the *E. senticosus* group were more likely than those in the placebo group to state that they had received verum (70% versus 20%); $p < 0.05$), so it is possible that unblinding occurred during the study, and this may have biased the results towards a more positive effect for *E. senticosus*. Also, total SF-36 scores were not reported, and it is possible that there was no statistically significant difference between these at the four-week assessment, thus a placebo response in both groups cannot be ruled out. A report of the study states that no statistically significant differences in blood pressure control and serum digoxin concentrations were observed, although supporting data were not provided.

Several clinical trials have explored the reputed adaptogenic effects of *E. senticosus* preparations in athletes. A placebo-controlled trial involved ten groups each comprising three male endurance athletes matched for training duration and frequency. Participants ($n = 30$) were assessed for steroidal hormone indices of stress and lymphocyte subset counts before and after six weeks' treatment with a 35% ethanolic extract of *E. senticosus* root 8 mL daily (equivalent to 4 g dried root), a 60% ethanolic extract of *Panax ginseng* root 4 mL daily (equivalent to 2 g dried root), or placebo.[57] Participants were randomly assigned to treatment within groups of three. Six groups of three completed the study, although data from laboratory tests of blood samples were available for only five groups of three athletes. At the end of the study, *E. senticosus* recipients had a significantly greater decrease in the testosterone to cortisol ratio, than did placebo recipients ($p < 0.05$); this appeared to be due to increased cortisol concentrations (which would suggest increased, rather than decreased, stress), rather than decreased testosterone concentrations. There were no significant differences between the three groups in any of the lymphocyte parameters measured, such as lymphocyte count, CD3+ cell, natural killer cell and B-cell CD20+ counts ($p > 0.05$ for all).[57] It is not clear whether the observed change in testosterone to cortisol ratio in *E. senticosus* recipients represents a genuine effect, or whether it is a spurious finding, and the effects of *E. senticosus* on steroid hormone concentrations require further investigation.

In another double-blind, controlled trial, 20 highly trained distance runners received a 30–40% ethanol extract of *E. senticosus* (not further specified) 60 drops daily, or placebo, for six weeks. Participants were matched by sex, body weight and ten-kilometre race pace and then randomly assigned as matched pairs to one of the treatment groups.[58] During the study, participants undertook five 15-minute trials of a submaximal treadmill run (at their ten-kilometre race pace) and one maximal treadmill run (i.e. to exhaustion; T_{max}). Data available for eight matched pairs did not show any statistically significant differences between groups in heart rate, oxygen consumption (VO_2), expired minute volume (VE), VE/VO_2, respiratory exchange rate, T_{max}, serum lactate concentrations and participants' rating of perceived exertion. However, because of the small sample size, the study lacked the statistical power to detect any differences between the two groups.[58]

Significant improvements in maximal oxygen uptake and oxygen pulse ($p < 0.05$ for both, compared with a no-treatment control group), and in total work capacity and maximum exhaustion time ($p < 0.05$, compared with placebo and a no-treatment control group) were observed with an ethanolic extract of *E. senticosus* 2 mL twice daily (1 mL contained 0.53 mg syringin (eleutheroside B) and 0.12 mg syringaresinol diglucoside (eleutheroside E)) in a single-blind, placebo-controlled, cross-over study involving six healthy male athletes who underwent a series of physical exercises.[59] However, the methodological limitations of the study (small sample size, no apparent random allocation to treatment, single-blind nature of assessments) preclude definitive conclusions.

A small number of other studies has assessed the effects of *E. senticosus* in healthy, young, non-athlete volunteers. In a randomised, double-blind, controlled trial, 45 volunteers received *E. senticosus* (Fon Wan Blu Giuliani, Milan, Italy; not further specified) two 'vials' daily for 30 days, and undertook the Stroop Colour-Word test as a challenge stressor before and after treatment.[60] A report of the study describes statistically significant reductions in test-induced increases in systolic blood pressure and heart rate after *E. senticosus* treatment, compared with baseline values. However, the study is flawed as no statistical comparisons were reported for the *E. senticosus* group compared with the placebo group.

A further study in 50 healthy volunteers compared the effects of a 35% ethanol extract of *E. senticosus* roots (Taigutan; 1 g extract equivalent to 1 g root, not further specified) 25 drops three times daily for 30 days ($n = 35$) with those of Echinacin (containing 80 g *Echinacea purpurea* herb fresh juice in 100 g final product) 40 drops three times daily for 30 days ($n = 15$).[61] Blood samples taken from participants before and after treatment were subjected to biochemical tests. Statistically significant reductions in concentrations of triglycerides, total cholesterol, LDL cholesterol and free fatty acids, an increase in polymorphonuclear leukocyte phagocytic activity, and increases in other components related to cellular defence were described following *E. senticosus* treatment, compared with baseline values ($p < 0.05$ for each), but not following treatment with the echinacea preparation. In a second phase of the study, 20 of the participants were randomly selected to also undertake assessment of physical fitness before and after treatment. Statistically significant increases in oxygen consumption during maximal effort and in exhaled volume were described following *E. senticosus* treatment, compared with baseline values ($p < 0.01$ for each), but not in other parameters of physical fitness nor for any of these parameters following treatment with the echinacea preparation. However, this study is also flawed as no statistical comparisons were reported for the *E. senticosus* group compared with the echinacea group, the study did not include a placebo arm, and no corrections were made for multiple statistical tests.

In a randomised, double-blind, placebo-controlled trial involving 93 individuals with herpes, a greater proportion of recipients of a standardised extract of *E. senticosus* root (400 mg daily for six months) experienced improvements in the frequency, severity and duration of episodes of herpes, than did placebo recipients (75% versus 34%; $p = 0.0002$ for each).[62]

Immunomodulatory activity has been documented for an ethanolic extract of *E. senticocus* 30–40 mL extract (eleutheroside B 0.2% w/v) daily in a double-blind, placebo-controlled trial involving healthy volunteers.[63] A significant increase in the total lymphocyte count, particularly in the T lymphocyte cell count, was observed for ginseng recipients, compared with placebo recipients. Specificity of action on the lymphocytes was confirmed by the fact that neither granulocyte nor monocyte counts were significantly altered.[63]

Several other double-blind, placebo-controlled trials, some of which involved random allocation to treatment, have investigated the effects of combination herbal preparations containing *E. senticosus* as well as *Andrographis paniculata* with or without other herbal ingredients (*Schizandra chinensis* and *Glycyrrhiza glabra*) in the treatment of upper respiratory tract infections[64, 65] and in patients with Familial Mediterranean fever.[66] Another study assessed the effects of a combination preparation containing *E. senticosus* root extract, *Adhatoda vasica* leaf extract and *Echinacea purpurea* extract (plant part not specified).[67] Reports of these studies have claimed beneficial effects for the combination preparations, compared with placebo, on the various outcome measures assessed. However, the lack of randomisation in several of these studies, and the lack of critical analysis of the results by the authors, indicate that further research is required to confirm or refute these findings. A meta-analysis of the trials of a preparation containing standardised extracts of *E. senticosus* root and *A. paniculata* herb concluded that there was evidence that the combination was effective in relieving symptoms of acute upper respiratory tract infections, but that further research was required before firm recommendations could be made.[68]

In a randomised, double-blind, placebo-controlled, cross-over trial involving 24 healthy volunteers who received a preparation of *E. senticosus* root 625 mg twice daily, a standardised *Ginkgo biloba* preparation equivalent to 28.2 mg flavonoid glycosides and 7.2 mg terpene lactones daily, a vitamin preparation, or placebo, for three months, selective memory was significantly improved in *E. senticosus* recipients compared with placebo recipients at the end of the study ($p < 0.02$).[69]

Several other studies involving small numbers of participants have assessed the effects of a preparation of the leaves of *E. senticosus* (Endurox™) which contain ciwujianosides, a series of triterpenoid glycosides chemically distinct from the eleutherosides. One uncontrolled, open-label study[70] reported beneficial effects on parameters of physical endurance, compared with baseline values, in eight men who had taken a preparation containing 800 mg *E. senticosus* leaf extract for two weeks, but three other studies with more rigorous designs (randomised, double-blind, placebo-controlled, crossover trials) found no effects for *E. senticosus* leaf extract at doses of 800 or 1200 mg taken orally for seven to ten days.[71–73] The latter three studies included only ten or fewer participants, so it is possible that they lacked the statistical power to detect any differences between the treatment and placebo groups. The available evidence indicates that *E. senticosus* leaf extract administered according to the dosage regimens tested has no beneficial effects on perfomance during exercise lasting up to two hours.[74]

Side-effects, Toxicity

Clinical data

There are only limited clinical data on safety aspects of *E. senticosus* preparations. No post-marketing surveillance-type studies were identified, and there are only a small number of clinical trials of *E. senticosus*, the majority of which are of poor methodological quality. Trials have assessed the effects of different *E. senticosus* preparations, including combination herbal preparations containing *E. senticosus*, which vary qualitatively and quantitatively in their phytochemical composition. Furthermore, different preparations have been administered according to different dosage regimens, and to different study populations (e.g. healthy volunteers, older patients with hypertension), making interpretation of the results difficult. The clinical trials of *E. senticosus* root preparations available have typically involved only very small numbers of patients and been of short duration, so have the statistical power only to detect very common, acute adverse effects. Rigorous investigation of safety aspects of well-characterised *E. senticosus* root preparations administered orally at different dosages, including the effects of long-term treatment, is required.

In a randomised, double-blind, controlled trial in which 96 individuals with chronic fatigue received capsules containing a standardised extract of *E. senticosus* root providing 2.24 mg eleutherosides (B and E) daily, or placebo, the proportions of participants experiencing adverse effects were 24% and 28% for the *E. senticosus* and placebo groups, respectively.[15] After one month's treatment, adverse effects reported by the greatest proportions of *E. senticosus* and placebo recipients were headache (10% and 8%, respectively), breast tenderness (7% and 3%, respectively) and nervousness (7% and 3%, respectively). There were no statistically significant differences in changes in mean systolic and diastolic blood pressure measurements. The frequency of adverse effects was reported to be lower for both groups during the second month of treatment.

Other studies, which involved only small numbers of participants and which had other methodological flaws, have provided conflicting data on the effects of *E. senticosus* root preparations on blood pressure measurements. One randomised, double-blind, placebo-controlled trial of an *E. senticosus* dry extract 300 mg daily for eight weeks study involved 20 participants aged 65 years or more with hypertension and who were undergoing treatment with digitalis (not further specified);[56] it was stated that no statistically significant differences in blood pressure control and serum digoxin concentrations were observed, although supporting data were not provided. Further study of the effects of well-characterised preparations of *E. senticosus* root extracts on blood pressure in different patient groups is required.

Several other clinical trial reports either did not provide any data on frequency and type of adverse effects, or stated that no adverse effects occurred during the study.

Preclinical data

Results of various animal toxicity studies have indicated ginseng to be non-toxic.[5] Many species have been exposed to extracts including mice, rats, rabbits, dogs, minks, deer, lambs, and piglets.[5] Documented acute oral LD_{50} values for various preparations include: 23 mL/kg and 14.5 g/kg (mice), and greater than 20 mL/kg (dogs) for a 33% ethanolic extract;[5,18] 31 g/kg (mice) for the powdered root; greater than 3 g/kg (mice) for an aqueous extract (equivalent to 25 g dried roots/kg).[18] No deaths occurred in mice administered single 3 g/kg doses of a freeze-dried aqueous extract.[59] Symptoms observed in dogs receiving 7.1 mL/kg doses of an ethanolic extract (sedation, ataxia, loss of righting reflex, hypopnoea, tremors, increased salivation and vomiting) were attributed to the ethanol content of the extract.[5] A chronic toxicity study reported no toxic manifestations or deaths in rats fed 5 mL/kg of an ethanolic extract for 320 days.[5]

Teratogenicity studies in male and female rats, pregnant minks, rabbits and lambs have reported no abnormalities in the offspring and no adverse effects in the animals administered the extracts. Premature death in parent female rabbits fed 13.5 mL/kg ethanolic extract daily was attributed to ethanol intoxication.[5]

Mutagenicity studies using *Salmonella typhimurium* TA100 and TA98, and the micronucleus test in mice have reported no activity for ginseng.[75] Differences in various serum biochemical parameters have been reported between test (ginseng) and control groups.[75] Parameters affected included alkaline phosphatase and gamma-glutamyl transferase enzymes (increased), serum triglycerides (decreased), and creatinine and blood urea nitrogen (increased).[75] No pathological changes were found in rats receiving a ginseng extract.[75]

Contra-indications, Warnings

The Russian literature on *E. senticosus* includes several contra-indications and warnings with respect to its use, although the scientific basis and evidence for many of these statements is not clear, and some contradict recent research. These Russian recommendations include the advice that ginseng should be avoided by premenopausal women, healthy individuals aged less than 40 years, and individuals who are highly energetic, nervous, tense, hysteric, manic or schizophrenic,[76] which at least appear to conflict with clinical research on the effects of *E. senticosus* preparations when taken by athletes (i.e. highly energetic individuals). It is also advised that *E. senticosus* should not be taken with stimulants, including coffee, antipsychotic drugs or during treatment with hormones, and that individuals considered suitable to use ginseng should abstain from alcoholic beverages, sexual activity, bitter substances and spicy foods during ginseng use.[76] It is also stated that *E. senticosus* is unsuitable for individuals with high blood pressure (180/90 mmHg or greater).[5] In general, and in view of the lack of safety data, it is appropriate to advise against the long-term or otherwise excessive use of ginseng. Some clinical studies involving long-term administration of ginseng have involved ginseng-free periods of 2–3 weeks every 30–60 days.

Drug interactions In view of the constituents of *E. senticosus*, and the pharmacological actions of *E. senticosus* preparations and their isolated constituents described following preclinical and, to a lesser extent, clinical studies, the potential for preparations of *E. senticosus* to interfere with other medicines administered concurrently, particularly those with anticoagulant, hypoglycaemic and/or hypo/hypertensive activity, should be considered.

A study involving healthy volunteers (n = 12) who received a preparation containing a standardised extract of *E. senticosus* root in addition to ground root material (one 485 mg capsule, containing approximately 2 mg eleutheroside B and 4 mg eleutheroside E, twice daily for 14 days) found that, at the end of the study, there were no statistically significant differences in the pharmacokinetic parameters of the cytochrome P4503A4 probe substrate dextromethorphan and of the CYP2D6 probe substrate alprazolam, when compared with baseline values. These findings suggest that this *E. senticosus* preparation administered according to this dosage regimen does not affect CYP3A4 and CYP2D6 activity.[77]

There is an isolated report of raised serum digoxin concentrations in a 74-year-old man who had been taking digoxin for over ten years to control atrial fibrillation. His serum digoxin concentration had been stable during this time in the range 0.9 to 2.2 nmol/L, but at a routine check-up (day 0) was found to be 5.2 nmol/L and remained high for a further two weeks despite reductions in digoxin dose and, on day 10, cessation of digoxin treatment.[78] On day 26, the patient revealed he had been taking 'Siberian ginseng' capsules since the previous summer (duration of use not specified but was at least two months) and stopped taking the product that day. His serum digoxin concentration returned to within the normal therapeutic range by day 33 (seven days after stopping the ginseng product), and digoxin treatment was restarted. A positive rechallenge was reported during which the patient's serum digoxin concentration rose to 3.2 nmol/L 52 days after re-starting the ginseng product. Positive dechallenge occurred again with the serum digoxin concentration falling to 1.2 nmol/L six days after stopping ginseng treatment. It is not stated in the report whether the patient took the same or a different ginseng product during the second episode of use, and no analysis of the product(s) concerned was carried out. For this reason, the validity of the report has been questioned.[79]

Some interference with a serum digoxin immunoassay (the fluorescence polarisation immunoassay) has been reported *in vitro* and *in vivo* (mice), leading to artificially raised measurements.[80]

Pregnancy and lactation Teratogenicity studies in various animal species have not reported any teratogenic effects for ginseng. However, in view of the many pharmacological actions documented for ginseng, the use of ginseng during both pregnancy and lactation should be avoided. It is unknown whether the pharmacologically active constituents in ginseng are secreted in the breast milk.

Preparations

Proprietary single-ingredient preparations

Canada: Benylin Energy Boosting. *Czech Republic:* Eleutherosan. *Germany:* Eleu-Kokk; Eleu; Eleutheroforce; Eleutherokokk; Konstitutin. *UK:* Elagen.

Proprietary multi-ingredient preparations

Argentina: Sigmafem. *Australia:* Astragalus Complex; Bacopa Complex; Bioglan Ginsynergy; Gingo A; Ginkgo Biloba Plus; Medinat Esten; Tyroseng. *Spain:* Energysor; Natusor Low Blood Pressure; Tonimax. *USA:* Energy Support; Menopause Support.

References

1 Yun-Choi HS *et al*. Potential inhibitors of platelet aggregation from plant sources, III. *J Nat Prod* 1987; 50: 1059–1064.

2 Makarieva TN *et al*. Lignans from *Eleutherococcus senticosus* (Siberian ginseng). *Pharm Sci* 1997; 3: 525–527.
3 Li XC *et al*. A new lignan glycoside from *Eleutherococcus senticosus*. *Planta Med* 2001; 67: 776–778.
4 Tolonen A *et al*. Identification of isomeric dicaffeoylquinic acids from *Eleutherococcus senticosus* using HPLC-ESI/TOF/MS and ^{1}H-NMR methods. *Phytochem Anal* 2002; 13: 316–328.
5 Farnsworth NR *et al*. Siberian ginseng (*Eleutherococcus senticosus*): Current status as an adaptogen. In: Wagner H *et al*., eds. *Economics and Medicinal Plant Research*, vol 1, London: Academic Press, 1985: 155–209.
6 Phillipson JD, Anderson LA. Ginseng – quality, safety and efficacy? *Pharm J* 1984; 232: 161–165.
7 Segiet-Kujawa E, Kaloga M. Triterpenoid saponins of *Eleutherococcus senticosus* roots. *J Nat Prod* 1991; 54: 1044–1048.
8 Ryu J *et al*. A benzenoid from the stem of *Acanthopanax senticosus*. *Arch Pharm Res* 2004; 27: 912–914 .
9 Chen M *et al*. Analysis of flavonoid constituents from leaves of *Acanthopanax senticosus* Harms by electrospray tandem mass spectrometry. *Rapid Comm Mass Spectrom* 2002; 16: 264–271.
10 Park SY *et al*. New 3,4-seco-lupane-type triterpene glycosides from *Acanthopanax senticosus* forma *inermis*. *J Nat Prod* 2000; 63: 1630–1633.
11 Apers S *et al*. Quality control of roots of *Eleutherococcus senticosus* by HPLC. *Phytochem Anal* 2005; 16: 55–60.
12 Slacanin I *et al*. The isolation of *Eleutherococcus senticosus* constituents by centrifugal partition chromatography and their quantitative determination by high-performance liquid chromatography. *Phytochem Anal* 1991; 2: 137–142.
13 Yat PN *et al*. An improved extraction procedure for the rapid, quantitative high-performance liquid chromatographic estimation of the main eleutherosides (B and E) in *Eleutherococcus senticosus* (Eleuthero). *Phytochem Anal* 1998; 9: 291–295.
14 Harkey MR *et al*. Variability in commercial ginseng products: an analysis of 25 preparations. *Am J Clin Nut* 2001; 73: 1101–1106.
15 Hartz AJ *et al*. Randomized controlled trial of Siberian ginseng for chronic fatigue. *Psychological Med* 2004; 34: 51–61.
16 Davydov M, Krikorian AD. *Eleutherococcus senticosus* (Rupr. & Maxim.) Maxim. (Araliaceae) as an adaptogen: a close look. *J Ethnopharmacol* 2000; 72: 345–393.
17 Glatthaar-Saalmüller B *et al*. Antiviral activity of an extract derived from roots of *Eleutherococcus senticosus*. *Antiviral Res* 2001; 50: 223–228.
18 Medon PJ *et al*. Hypoglycaemic effect and toxicity of *Eleutherococcus senticosus* following acute and chronic administration in mice. *Acta Pharmacol Sin* 1981; 2: 281–285.
19 Hikino H *et al*. Isolation and hypoglycaemic activity of eleutherans A, B, C, D, E, F, and G: Glycans of *Eleutherococcus senticosus* roots. *J Nat Prod* 1986; 49: 293–297.
20 Medon PJ *et al*. Effects of *Eleutherococcus senticosus* extracts on hexobarbital metabolism *in vivo* and *in vitro*. *J Ethnopharmacol* 1984; 10: 235–241.
21 Yi JM *et al*. *Acanthopanax senticosus* root inhibits mast cell-dependent anaphylaxis. *Clinica Chimica Acta* 2001; 312: 163–168.
22 Jeong HJ *et al*. Inhibitory effects of mast cell-mediated allergic reactions by cell cultured Siberian ginseng. *Immunopharmacol Immunotoxicol* 2001; 23: 107–117.
23 Schmolz MW *et al*. The synthesis of Rantes, G-CSF, IL-4, IL-5, IL-6, IL-12 and IL-13 in human whole-blood cultures is modulated by an extract from *Eleutherococcus senticosus* L. roots. *Phytother Res* 2001; 15: 268–270.
24 Borchers AT*et al*. Comparative effects of three species of ginseng on human peripheral blood lymphocyte proliferative responses. *Int J Immunother* 1998; XIV: 143–152.
25 Wang H *et al*. Asian and Siberian ginseng as a potential modulator of immune function: an in vitro cytokine study using mouse macrophages. *Clinica Chimica Acta* 2003; 327: 123128.
26 Panossian A *et al*. Effect of andrographolide and Kan Jang – fixed combination of extract SHW-10 and extract SHE-3 – on proliferation of human lymphocytes, production of cytokines and immune activation markers in the whole blood cells culture. *Phytomedicine* 2002; 9: 598–605.
27 Shen ML *et al*.. Immunopharmacological effects of polysaccharides from *Acanthopanax senticosus* on experimental animals. *Int J Immunopharmacol* 1991; 13: 549–554.
28 Han SB *et al*. Toll-like receptor-mediated activation of B cells and macrophages by polysaccharide isolated from cell culture of *Acanthopanax senticosus*. *Int Immunopharmacol* 2003; 3: 1301–1312.
29 Wagner H *et al*. Immunstimulierend wirkende Polysaccharide (heteroglykane) aus höheren Pflanzen. *Arzneimittelforschung* 1985; 35: 1069.
30 Wagner H. Immunostimulants from medicinal plants. In: Chang HM *et al*., eds. *Advances in Chinese Medicinal Materials Research*. Singapore: World Scientific, 1985: 159.
31 Kimura Y, Sumiyoshi M. Effects of various *Eleutherococcus senticosus* cortex on swimming time, natural killer activity and corticosterone level in forced swimming stressed mice. *J Ethnopharmacol* 2004; 95: 447–453.
32 Lewis WH *et al*. No adaptogen response of mice to ginseng and *Eleutherococcus* infusions. *J Ethnopharmacol* 1983; 8: 209–214.
33 Martinez B, Staba EJ. The physiological effects of *Aralia*, *Panax* and *Eleutherococcus* on exercised rats. *Jpn J Pharmacol* 1984; 35: 79–85.
34 Gaffney BT *et al*. *Panax ginseng* and *Eleutherococcus senticosus* may exaggerate an already existing biphasic response to stress via inhibition of enzymes which limit the binding of stress hormones to their receptors. *Medical Hypotheses* 2001; 56: 567–572.
35 Kwan CY *et al*. Vascular effects of Siberian ginseng (*Eleutherococcus senticosus*): endothelium-dependent NO- and EDHF-mediated relaxation depending on vessel size. *Naumyn Schmiedebergs Arch Pharmacol* 2004; 369: 473–480.
36 Liu J *et al*. Effects of several Chinese herbal aqueous extracts on human sperm motility *in vitro*. *Andrologia* 2004; 36: 78–83.
37 Hacker B, Medon PJ. Cytotoxic effects of *Eleutherococcus senticosus* aqueous extracts in combination with N^6-(Δ^2-isopentenyl)-adenosine and 1-β-D-arabinofuranosylcytosine against L1210 leukemia cells. *J Pharm Sci* 1984; 73: 270–272.
38 Yokozawa T *et al*. Protective effects of Acanthopanax Radix extract against endotoxemia induced by lipopolysaccharide. *Phytotherapy Res* 2003; 17: 353–357.
39 Cha YS *et al*. *Acanthopanax senticosus* extract prepared from cultured cells decreases adiposity and obesity indices in C57BL/6J mice fed a high fat diet. *J Med Food* 2004; 7: 422–429.
40 Provalova NV *et al*. Mechanisms underling the effects of adaptogens on erythropoiesis during paradoxical sleep deprivation. *Bull Exp Biol Med* 2002; 133: 428–432.
41 Lee S *et al*.. Antibacterial compounds from the leaves of *Acanthopanax senticosus*. *Arch Pharm Res* 2003; 26: 40–42.
42 Yi JM *et al*. Effect of *Acanthopanax senticosus* stem on mast cell-dependent anaphylaxis. *J Ethnopharmacol* 2002; 79: 347–352.
43 Nishibe S *et al*. Phenolic compounds from stem bark of *Acanthopanax senticosus* and their pharmacological effect in chronic swimming stressed rats. *Chem Pharm Bull* 1990; 38: 1763–1765.
44 Jin JL *et al*. Platelet anti-aggregating triterpenoids from the leaves of *Acanthopanax senticosus* and the fruits of *A. sessiliflorus*. *Planta Med* 2004; 70: 564–566.
45 Bu Y *et al*. Siberian ginseng reduces infarct volume in transient focal cerebral ischaemia in Sprague-Dawley rats. *Phytother Res* 2005; 19: 1167–1169.
46 Yang JY *et al*. Effect of *Acanthopanax senticosus* on lipoprotein lipase in 3T3-L1 adipocytes. *Phytother Res* 2004; 18: 160–163.
47 Lee S *et al*. Anti-oxidant activities of *Acanthopanax senticosus* stems and their lignan components. *Arch Pharm Res* 2004; 27: 106–110.
48 Park EJ, *et al*. Water-soluble polysaccharide from *Eleutherococcus senticosus* stems attenuates fulminant hepatic failure induced by D-galactosamine and lipopolysaccharide in mice. *Basic Clin Pharmacol Toxicol* 2004; 94: 298–304.
49 Jung HJ *et al*. *In vivo* anti-inflammatory and antinociceptive effects of liriodendrin isolated from the stem bark of *Acanthopanax senticocus*. *Planta Med* 2003; 69: 610–616.
50 Yoon TJ *et al*. Anti-metastatic activity of *Acanthopanax senticosus* extract and its possible immunological mechanism of action. *J Ethnopharmacol* 2004; 93: 247–253.
51 Ha ES *et al*. Anti-metastatic activity of glycoprotein fractionated from *Acanthopanax senticosus*, involvement of NK-cell and macrophage activation. *Arch Pharm Res* 2004; 27: 217–224.

52 Hibasami H *et al*. Induction of apoptosis by *Acanthopanax senticosus* HARMS and its component, sesamin in human stomach cancer KATO III cells. *Oncol Rep* 2000; 7: 1213–1216.
53 Jang MH *et al*. Protective effect of *Acanthopanax senticosus* against ethanol-induced apoptosis of human neuroblastoma cell line SK-N-MC. *Am J Chinese Med* 2003; 31: 379–388.
54 Fujikawa T *et al*. *Acanthopanax senticosus* Harms as a prophylactic for MTMP-induced Parkinson's disease in rats. *J Ethnopharmacol* 2005; 97: 375–381.
55 Fujikawa T *et al*.. Effect of sesamin in *Acanthopanax senticosus* HARMS on behavioral dysfunction in rotenone-induced parkinsonian rats. *Biol Pharm Bull* 2005; 28: 169–172.
56 Cicero AFG *et al*.. Effects of Siberian ginseng (*Eleutherococcus senticosus* Maxim.) on elderly quality of life: a randomized clinical trial. *Arch Gerontol Geriatr* 2004; 9 (Suppl. Suppl.): 69–73.
57 Gaffney BT *et al*. The effects of *Eleutherococcus senticosus* and *Panax ginseng* on steroidal hormone indices of stress and lymphocyte subset numbers in endurance athletes. *Life Sciences* 2001; 70: 431–442.
58 Dowling EA *et al*. Effect of *Eleutherococcus senticosus* on submaximal and maximal exercise performance. *Med Sci Sports Exercise* 1996; 28: 482–489.
59 Asano K *et al*. Effect of *Eleutherococcus senticosus* extract on human physical working capacity. *Planta Med* 1986; 52: 175.
60 Facchinetti F *et al*.. *Eleutherococcus senticosus* reduces cardiovascular stress response in healthy subjects: a randomized, placebo-controlled trial. *Stress Health* 2002; 18: 11–17.
61 Szołomicki S *et al*. The influence of active components of *Eleutherococcus senticosus* on cellular defence and physical fitness in man. *Phytotherapy Res* 2000; 14: 30–35.
62 Williams M. Immunoprotection against herpes simplex type II infection by eleutherococcus root extract. *Int J Alt Comp Med* 1995; 13: 9–12.
63 Bohn B *et al*. Flow-cytometric studies with *Eleutherococcus senticosus* extract as an immunomodulatory agent. *Arzneimittelforschung* 1987; 37: 1193–1196.
64 Melchior J *et al*. Double-blind, placebo-controlled pilot and phase III study of activity of standardized *Andrographis paniculata* herba Nees extract fixed combination (Kan Jang) in the treatment of uncomplicated upper-respiratory tract infection. *Phytomedicine* 2000; 7: 341–350.
65 Gabrielan ES *et al*. A double-blind, placebo-controlled study of *Andrographis paniculata* fixed combination Kan Jang in the treatment of acute upper respiratory tract infections including sinusitis. *Phytomedicine* 2002; 9: 589–597.
66 Amaryan G *et al*. Double-blind, placebo-controlled, randomized, pilot clinical trial of ImmunoGuard® – a standardized fixed combination of *Andrographis paniculata* Nees, with *Eleutherococcus senticosus* Maxim, *Schizandra chinensis* Bail. and *Glycyrrhiza glabra* L. extracts in patients with familial Mediterranean fever. *Phytomedicine* 2003; 10: 271–285.
67 Narimanian M *et al*. Randomized trial of a fixed combination of herbal extracts containing *Adhatoda vasica*, *Echinacea purpurea* and *Eleutherococcus senticosus* in patients with upper respiratory tract infections. *Phytomedicine* 2005; 12: 539–547.
68 Poolsup N *et al*. *Andrographis paniculata* in the symptomatic treatment of uncomplicated upper respiratory tract infection: a systematic review of randomized controlled trials. *C Clin Pharm Ther* 2004; 29: 37–45.
69 Winther K *et al*. Russian root (Siberian ginseng) improves cognitive functions in middle-aged people, whereas Ginkgo biloba seems effective only in the elderly. *J Neurol Sci* 1997; 150: S90.
70 Wu YN *et al*. Effect of ciwujia (Radix acanthopanacis senticosus) preparation on human stamina. *J Hyg Res* 1996; 25: 57–61.
71 Cheuvront SN *et al*. Effect of Endurox™ on metabolic responses to submaximal exercise. *Int J Sport Nut* 1999; 9: 434–442.
72 Plowman SA *et al*. The effects of Endurox on the physiological responses to stair-stepping exercise. *Res Q Exercise Sport* 1999; 70: 385–388.
73 Eschbach LC The effect of Siberian ginseng (*Eleutherococcus senticosus*) on substrate utilization and performance during prolonged cycling. *Int J Sport Nut Exercise Metab* 2000; 10: 444–451.
74 Goulet EDB, Dionne IJ. Assessement of the effects of *Eleutherococcus senticosus* on endurance performance. *Int J Sport Nut Exercise Metab* 2000; 14: 75–83.
75 Hirosue T *et al*. Mutagenicity and subacute toxicity of *Acanthopanax senticosus* extracts in rats. *J Food Hyg Soc Jpn* 1986; 27: 380–386.
76 Baldwin CA *et al*. What pharmacists should know about ginseng. *Pharm J* 1986; 237: 583.
77 Donovan JL *et al*. Siberian ginseng (*Eleutherococcus senticosus*) effects on CYP2D6 and CYP3A4 activity in normal volunteers. *Drug Metabolism Disposition* 2003; 31: 519–522.
78 McRae S. Elevated serum digoxin levels in a patient taking digoxin and Siberian ginseng. *Can Med Ass J* 1996; 155: 293–295.
79 Awang DVC. Siberian ginseng toxicity may be case of mistaken identity. *Can Med Ass J* 1996; 155: 1237.
80 Dasgupta A. Effect of Asian and Siberian ginseng on serum digoxin measurement by five digoxin immunoasays. *Am J Clin Pathol* 2003; 119: 298–303.

G

Ginseng, Panax

Summary and Pharmaceutical Comment

The chemistry of *Panax ginseng* root is well documented. Research has focused mainly on the saponin components (ginsenosides), which are generally considered to be the main active constituents, although pharmacological actions have been documented for certain non-saponin components, principally polysaccharides. Many of the pharmacological actions documented for ginseng, at least in preclinical studies, directly oppose one another and this has been attributed to the actions of the individual ginsenosides. For example, ginsenoside R_{b-1} exhibits CNS-depressant, hypotensive and tranquillising actions whilst ginsenoside R_{g-1} exhibits CNS-stimulant, hypertensive and anti-fatigue actions. These opposing actions are thought to explain the 'adaptogenic' reputation of ginseng, that is the ability to increase the overall resistance of the body to stress and to balance bodily functions. Preclinical studies have indicated that preparations of *Panax* species and/or their isolated constituents have a range of pharmacological properties; results of these studies provide some supporting evidence for the traditional uses and adaptogenic properties for certain *Panax* species preparations, although pharmacological explanations for the observed actions are less well understood.

Clinical trials of *Panax* species preparations have focused on assessing effects related to the reputed adaptogenic properties of this herbal medicinal product, although rigorous clinical investigations are limited. Studies have tested different preparations of different *Panax* species and different commercial products (which vary qualitatively and quantitatively in their phytochemical composition) administered according to different dosage regimens, and to different study populations making interpretation of the results difficult. At present there is insufficient evidence to support definitely the efficacy of specific *Panax* species preparations in the various indications for which they are used and/or have been tested.

Similarly, there are only limited clinical data on safety aspects of *Panax* species preparations. Clinical trials of *Panax* species root preparations typically have involved small numbers of patients and been of short duration, so have the statistical power only to detect very common, acute adverse effects. The available evidence suggests that preparations of *Panax* species root are well-tolerated when used for limited periods of time at recommended doses. Rigorous investigation of safety aspects of well-characterised *Panax* species root preparations administered orally at different dosages, including the effects of long-term treatment, is required. In view of the many pharmacological actions documented, the potential for preparations of *Panax* species to interfere with other medicines administered concurrently, particularly those with similar or opposing effects, should be considered. In general, and in view of the lack of safety data, it is appropriate to advise against the long-term or otherwise excessive use of *Panax* species.

The use of *Panax* species during both pregnancy and breastfeeding should be avoided.

Species (Family)

Various *Panax* species (Araliaceae) including:
**Panax ginseng* Meyer
†*Panax quinquefolius* L.
‡*Panax notoginseng* (Burk.) Chen ex C.Y. Wu

This monograph focuses on *P. ginseng*, although some information on other *Panax* species is also included.

Synonym(s)

**P. quinquefolius* var. *coreensis* Sieb., *P. schin-seng* T. Nees, *P. schin-seng* var. *coraiensis* T. Nees, *P. versus* Oken, Ren Shen, Asian Ginseng, Chinese Ginseng, Korean Ginseng, Oriental Ginseng
†*P. quinquefolius* var. *americanus* Raf., *P. quinquefolius* var. *obovatus* Raf., *P. cuneataus* Raf., *P. americanus* var. *elatus* Raf., American Ginseng
‡*Aralia quinquifolia* var. *notoginseng* (Burk.), *P. pseudoginseng* var. *notoginseng* (Burk.) Hoo & Tseng, San Qi, Sanchi Ginseng, Tienchi Ginseng

Part(s) Used

Root. White ginseng represents the peeled and sun-dried root whilst red ginseng is unpeeled, steamed and dried.

Pharmacopoeial and Other Monographs

BHC 1992[(G6)]
BHP 1996[(G9)]
BP 2007[(G84)]
Complete German Commission E[(G3)]
Martindale 35th edition[(G85)]
Ph Eur 2007[(G81)]
USP29/NF24[(G86)]

Legal Category (Licensed Products)

GSL[(G37)]

Constituents

The following is compiled from several sources, including General References G2 and G6.

Terpenoids Complex mixture of compounds (ginsenosides or panaxosides) involves three aglycone structural types – two tetracyclic dammarane-type sapogenins (protopanaxadiol and protopanaxatriol) and a pentacyclic triterpene oleanolic acid-type. Different naming conventions have been used for these compounds. In Japan, they are known as ginsenosides and are represented by R_x where 'x' indicates a particular saponin. For example, R_a, R_{b-1}, R_c, R_d, R_{g-1}. In Russia, the saponins are referred to as panaxosides and are represented as panaxoside X where 'X' can be A–F. The suffixes in the two systems are not equivalent and thus panaxoside A does not equal R_a but R_{g-1}.[(1)]

The saponin content varies between different *Panax* species. For example, in *P. ginseng* the major ginsenosides are R_{b-1}, R_c and R_{g-1} whereas in *P. quinquefolis* R_{b-1} is the only major ginsenoside.[(1)]

Other constituents Volatile oil (trace) mainly consisting of sesquiterpenes including panacene, limonene, terpineol, eucalyptol, α-phellandrene and citral,[2] sesquiterpene alcohols including the panasinsanols A and B, and ginsenol,[3,4] polyacetylenes,[5,6] sterols, polysaccharides (mainly pectins and glucans),[7] starch (8–32%), β-amylase,[8] free sugars, vitamins (B_1, B_2, B_{12}, panthotenic acid, biotin), choline (0.1–0.2%), fats, minerals.

The sesquiterpene alcohols are stated to be characteristic components of *Panax ginseng* in that they are absent from the volatile oils of other *Panax* species.[4]

Quality of plant material and commercial products

According to the British and European Pharmacopoeias, *Panax ginseng* consists of the whole or cut dried root, designated as white ginseng, treated with steam and then dried, designated red ginseng, of *Panax ginseng* C.A.Meyer.[G81,G84] As with other herbal medicinal products, there is variation in the qualitative and quantitative composition of crude plant material obtained from *Panax* species and commercial *Panax ginseng* preparations and those derived from other *Panax* species.

Thirty seven commercial samples of root from *P. ginseng* (n = 22), *P. quinquefolius* (n = 10) and *P. notoginseng* (n = 5) obtained from herbal outlets in Taiwan were analysed to determine their respective chemical profiles.[9] The saponin content of *P. notoginseng* and *P. quinquefolius* was higher than that of *P. ginseng*, although statistical analyses to support this were not performed. Mean total saponin (R_{b-1}, R_{b-2}, R_c, R_d, R_e, R_f, R_{g-1}) contents for *P. notoginseng*, *P. quinquefolius* wild, *P. quinquefolius* cultivated, *P. ginseng* white, and *P. ginseng* red were 118.7, 58.0, 43.1, 5.2 and 5.9 mg/g, respectively. Variations in total saponin content within species and types of ginseng were also found: *P. notoginseng* 23.8–30.7, *P. quinquefolius* wild 8.7–24.0, *P. quinquefolius* cultivated 8.4–19.5, *P. ginseng* white 3.5–9.0, and *P. ginseng* red 3.9–7.2 mg/g.[9] In another analytical study, the saponin content of 47 samples of ginseng obtained from 12 *Panax taxa* was examined using reverse-phase high-performance liquid chromatography. Material from *P. ginseng* was found to have the lowest total saponin content (5.8–15.6 mg/g).[10]

Analysis using gas chromatography (GC) and GC-mass spectrometry of best-selling commercial preparations of *Panax* species purchased from pharmacies and health-food stores in European countries, Argentina, Canada, China and the USA found variations in their saponin content: *P. ginseng*, pure root preparations, 1.9–8.1% (n = 14); *P. ginseng*, extract preparations, 4.9–13.3% (n = 20); *P. quinquefolius*, 5.2% (n = 1); *P. notoginseng*, 7.5% (n = 1).[11]

Analysis of 25 'ginseng' products available for purchase from a health-food store in the USA included eight products labelled as containing *Panax ginseng*, four labelled as containing *P. quinquefolius*, one labelled as containing *P. notoginseng*, and three labelled as containing mixtures of different species.[12] All of the products labelled as containing *Panax* species contained ginsenosides, although total ginsenoside content varied: monopreparations of

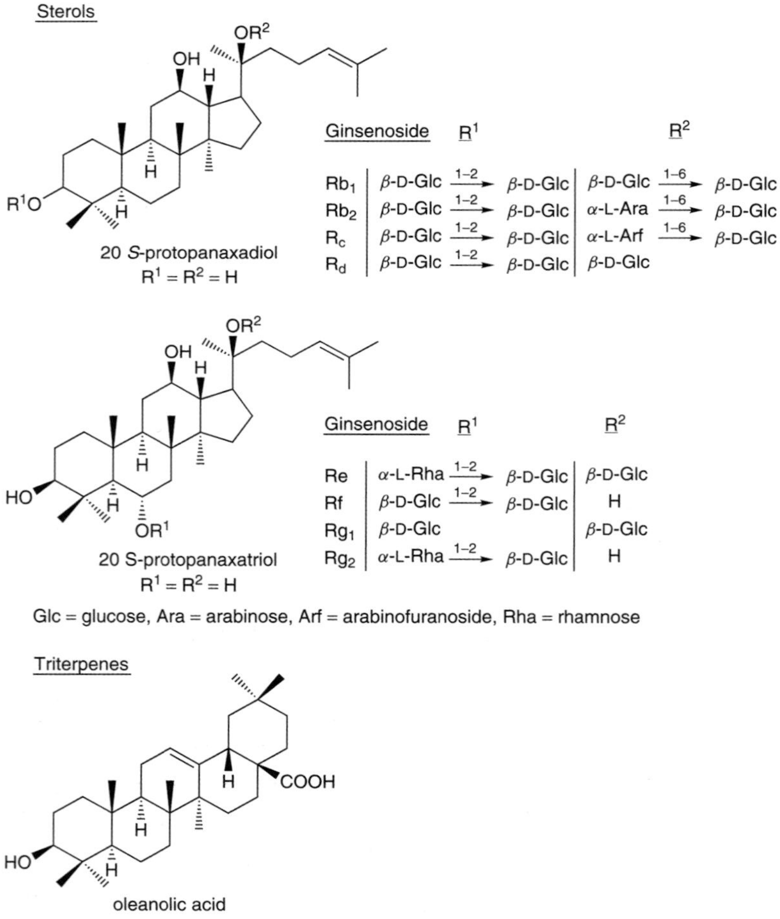

Sterols

20 *S*-protopanaxadiol
$R^1 = R^2 = H$

Ginsenoside	R^1	R^2
Rb_1	β-D-Glc $\xrightarrow{1-2}$ β-D-Glc	β-D-Glc $\xrightarrow{1-6}$ β-D-Glc
Rb_2	β-D-Glc $\xrightarrow{1-2}$ β-D-Glc	α-L-Ara $\xrightarrow{1-6}$ β-D-Glc
R_c	β-D-Glc $\xrightarrow{1-2}$ β-D-Glc	α-L-Arf $\xrightarrow{1-6}$ β-D-Glc
R_d	β-D-Glc $\xrightarrow{1-2}$ β-D-Glc	β-D-Glc

20 S-protopanaxatriol
$R^1 = R^2 = H$

Ginsenoside	R^1	R^2
Re	α-L-Rha $\xrightarrow{1-2}$ β-D-Glc	β-D-Glc
Rf	β-D-Glc $\xrightarrow{1-2}$ β-D-Glc	H
Rg_1	β-D-Glc	β-D-Glc
Rg_2	α-L-Rha $\xrightarrow{1-2}$ β-D-Glc	H

Glc = glucose, Ara = arabinose, Arf = arabinofuranoside, Rha = rhamnose

Triterpenes

oleanolic acid

Figure 1 Selected constituents of *Panax ginseng*.

powdered *P. ginseng*, 0.29–3.36 mg/100 g product (n = 6); monopreparations of powdered *P. quinquefolius*, 1.24–2.91 mg/100 g product (n = 2); monopreparation of powdered *P. notoginseng*, 4.27 mg/100 g product (n = 1); liquid monopreparations of *P. ginseng*, 0.44–0.69 mg/100 mL product (n = 2); liquid monopreparations of *P. quinquefolius*, 0.78–1.30 mg/100 mL product (n = 2). Of the 16 products containing *Panax* species, seven were labelled as containing a specific concentration of ginsenosides, yet the actual content deviated from the labelled amount, containing 18.0–136.8% of the amount stated on the label.(12) All but one of these products contained a lower concentration of ginsenosides than the labelled amount.

In 2005, the USA Department of the Interior Fish and Wildlife Service determined that wild *P. quinquefolius* root must be at least ten years old and have four 'prongs' or leaves before it can be legally exported from the USA.(13) This decision extended the previous five-year minimum age limit determined by the Convention on International Trade in Endangered Species (CITES).(14)

Food Use

Ginseng (*P. ginseng*) is listed by the Council of Europe as a natural source of food flavouring (category N2). This category indicates that ginseng can be added to foodstuffs in small quantities, with a possible limitation of an active principle (as yet unspecified) in the final product.(G16)

Herbal Use

Ginseng (*P. ginseng*) is stated to possess thymoleptic, sedative, demulcent and stomachic properties, and is reputed to be an aphrodisiac. Traditionally, it has been used for neurasthenia, neuralgia, insomnia, hypotonia, and specifically for depressive states associated with sexual inadequacy.(G2, G6, G8, G64)

P. ginseng and other *Panax* species have been used traditionally in Chinese medicine for many thousands of years. Uses include as a stimulant, tonic, diuretic and stomachic,(15) but typically the different species have different clinical uses. Traditionally, use has been divided into two categories: short-term – to improve stamina, concentration, healing process, stress resistance, vigilance and work efficiency in healthy individuals, and long-term – to improve well-being in debilitated and degenerative conditions especially those associated with old age.

Dosage

Traditionally, dosage recommendations differ for short-term use by healthy individuals and long-term use by elderly or debilitated persons.

Short-term (for younger and healthy individuals) 0.5–1.0 g root daily, as two divided doses, for a course generally lasting 15–20 days and with a treatment-free period of approximately two weeks between consecutive courses. Doses are recommended to be taken in the morning, two hours before a meal, and in the evening, not less than two hours after a meal.(15)

Long-term (for older individuals and those with poor health) 0.4–0.8 g root daily. Doses may be taken continuously.(1)

In China, doses used traditionally and currently are typically 3–9 g root powder daily taken as a decoction.(16)

Dosages used in clinical trials vary depending on the *Panax* species, type of preparation and indication under investigation. Several studies have assessed the effects of a standardised extract of *P. ginseng* root (G115) at doses of 100–400 mg daily for 4–12 weeks.

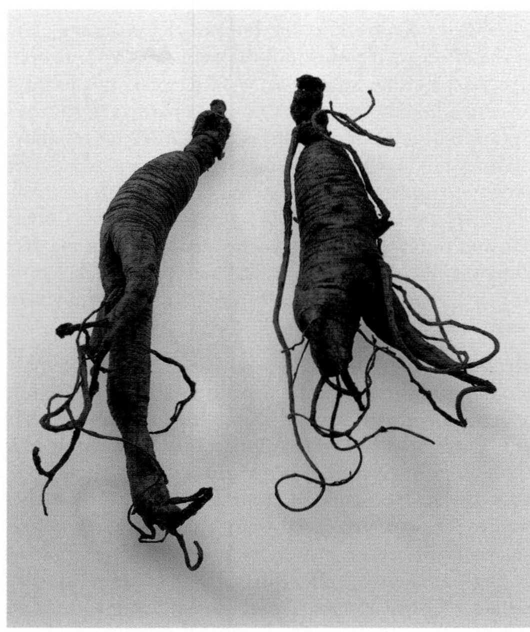

Figure 2 *Panax ginseng* – dried drug substance (root).

Pharmacological Actions

In the 1950s, early studies on ginseng reported its ability to improve both physical endurance and mental ability in animals and humans.(17) In addition, the 'tonic' properties of ginseng were confirmed by the observation that doses taken for a prolonged period of time increased the overall well-being of an individual, measured by various parameters such as appetite, sleep and absence of moodiness, resulting in an increased work efficiency.(10) Since then, numerous studies have investigated the complex pharmacology of ginseng in both animals and humans. The saponin glycosides (ginsenosides/panaxosides) are generally recognised as the main active constituents in ginseng, although pharmacological activities have also been associated with non-saponin components.

The following sections on preclinical and clinical studies are intended to give an indication of the type of research that has been published for ginseng rather than to provide a comprehensive bibliography of ginseng research papers.

In vitro and animal studies

Pharmacokinetics There are only limited data on the pharmacokinetics of the constituents of *P. ginseng*. Ginsenosides R_{g-1}, R_{b-1} and R_{b-2} have been detected in the gastrointestinal tract of rats following oral administration of *P. ginseng* root, although absorption rates are low.(18–21)

Corticosteroid-like activity Many of the activities exhibited by *Panax ginseng* have been compared with corticosteroid-like actions and results of endocrinological studies have suggested that the ginsenosides may primarily augment adrenal steroidogenesis via an indirect action on the pituitary gland.(22) Ginsenosides have increased adrenal cAMP in intact but not in hypophysectomised rats and dexamethasone, a synthetic glucocorticoid that provides positive feedback at the level of the pituitary gland, has blocked the effect of ginsenosides on pituitary corticotrophin and adrenal corticosterone secretion.[22] Hormones produced by the pituitary and adrenal glands are known to play a significant role in the adaptation capabilities of the body.[23] Working capacity is one of the indices used to measure adaptation ability and ginseng has been shown to increase the working capacity of rats following single (132%) and seven-day (179%) administration (intraperitoneal). Furthermore, seven-day administration of ginseng decreased the reduction seen in working capacity when the pituitary–adrenocortical system is blocked by prior administration of hydrocortisone.[23]

Hypoglycaemic activity Hypoglycaemic activity has been documented for ginseng and attributed to both saponin and polysaccharide constituents. *In vitro* studies using isolated rat pancreatic islets have shown that ginsenosides promote an insulin release which is independent of extracellular calcium and which utilises a different mechanism to that of glucose.[24] In addition, *in vivo* studies in rats have reported that a *P. ginseng* extract increases the number of insulin receptors in bone marrow and reduces the number of glucocorticoid receptors in rat brain homogenate.[25] Both of these actions are thought to contribute to the antidiabetic action of *P. ginseng*, in view of the known diabetogenic action of adrenal corticoids and the knowledge that the number of insulin receptors generally decreases with ageing.[25]

Hypoglycaemic activity observed in both normal and alloxan-induced hyperglycaemic mice administered *P. ginseng* or *P. quinquefolium* (intraperitoneal) has also been attributed to non-saponin but uncharacterised principles[26–29] or to glycan (polysaccharide) components.[30–34] Glycans isolated from Korean or Chinese *P. ginseng* (A–E) were found to possess stronger hypoglycaemic activity than those isolated from Japanese *P. ginseng* (Q–U).[34] Proposed mechanisms of action have included elevated plasma insulin concentration due to an increase of insulin secretion from pancreatic islets, and enhancement of insulin sensitivity.[32] However, these mechanisms do not explain the total hypoglycaemic activity that has been exhibited by the polysaccharides and further mechanisms are under investigation.[32]

The effect of panaxans A and B from *P. ginseng* roots on the activities of key enzymes participating in carbohydrate metabolism has been studied.[29] DPG-3-2, a non-saponin component, has been shown to stimulate insulin biosynthesis in pancreatic preparations from various hyperglycaemic (but not normoglycaemic) animals; ginsenosides R_{b-1} and R_{g-1} were found to decrease islet insulin concentrations to an undetectable level.[27]

Cardiovascular activity Individual saponins from *P. notoginseng* have been reported to have different actions on cardiac haemodynamics.[35] For instance R_g, $R_{g\text{-}1}$ and total flower saponins have increased cardiac performance whilst R_b and total leaf saponins have decreased it; calcium antagonist activity has been reported for R_b but not for R_g; R_b but not R_g has produced a protective effect on experimental myocardial infarction in rabbits.[35] Negative chronotropic and inotropic effects *in vitro* have been observed for ginseng saponins and a mechanism of action similar to that of verapamil has been suggested.[36] *In vitro* studies on the isolated rabbit heart have reported an increase in coronary blood flow together with a positive inotropic effect.[37] Anti-arrhythmic action on aconitine and barium chloride (rat) and adrenaline (rabbit)-induced arrhythmias, and prolongation of RR, PR and QT_c intervals (rat), have been documented for saponins $R_{c\text{-}1}$ and $R_{d\text{-}1}$ from *P. notoginseng*. The mode of action was thought to be similar to that of amiodarone.[38] Ginsenosides (i.p.) have been reported to protect mice against metabolic disturbances and myocardial damage associated with conditions of severe anoxia.[39]

P. notoginseng has produced a marked hypotensive response together with bradycardia following intravenous administration to rats. The dose-related effect was blocked by many antagonists suggesting multi-site activity.[37] Higher doses were found to cause vasoconstriction rather than vasodilation in renal, mesenteric and femoral arteries.[37]

The total ginseng saponin fraction (*Panax* species not specified) has been reported to be devoid of haemolytic activity. However, individual ginsenosides have been found to exhibit either haemolytic or protective activities. Protective ginsenosides include R_c, $R_{b\text{-}2}$ and R_e, whereas haemolytic saponins have included R_g, R_h and R_f.[40] The number and position of sugars attached to the sapogenin moiety was thought to determine activity.[40] Haemostatic activity has also been documented.[41]

Oral administration of *P. ginseng* to rats fed a high cholesterol diet reduced serum cholesterol and triglycerides, increased high-density lipoprotein (HDL) cholesterol, decreased platelet adhesiveness, and decreased fatty changes to the liver.[42] *P. ginseng* has also been reported to reduce blood coagulation and enhance fibrinolysis.[43] Panaxynol and the ginsenosides R_o, $R_{g\text{-}1}$ and $R_{g\text{-}2}$ have been documented as the main antiplatelet components in *P. ginseng* inhibiting aggregation, release reaction and thromboxane formation *in vitro*.[43] Anti-inflammatory activity and inhibition of thromboxane B_2 have previously been described for panaxynol.[43] Anticomplementary activity *in vitro* (human serum) has been documented for *P. ginseng* polysaccharides with highest activity observed in strongly acidic polysaccharide fractions.[7]

Effects on neurotransmitters Studies in rats have shown that a standardised *P. ginseng* extract (G115) inhibits the development of morphine tolerance and physical dependence, of a decrease in hepatic glutathione concentrations, and of dopamine receptor sensitivity without antagonising morphine analgesia, as previously documented for the individual saponins.[44] The inhibition of tolerance was thought to be associated with a reduction in morphinone production, a toxic metabolite which irreversibly blocks the opiate receptor sites, and with the activation of morphinone–glutathione conjugation, a detoxication process. The mechanism of inhibition of physical dependence was unclear but thought to be associated with changed ratios of adrenaline, noradrenaline, dopamine and serotonin in the brain.[44]

A total ginsenoside fraction has been reported to inhibit the uptake of various neurotransmitters into rat brain synaptosomes in descending order of gamma-aminobutyrate and noradrenaline, dopamine, glutamate and serotonin.[45–47] The fraction containing ginsenoside R_d was most effective. Uptake of metabolic substrates 2-deoxy-D-glucose and leucine was only slightly affected and therefore it was proposed that the *P. ginseng* extracts were acting centrally rather than locally as surface active agents.

Studies in rats have indicated that the increase in dopaminergic receptors in the brain observed under conditions of stress is prevented by pretreatment with *P. ginseng*.[48]

Hepatoprotective activity Antoxidant and detoxifying activities have been documented.[49] Protection against carbon tetrachloride- and galactosamine-induced hepatotoxicity has been observed in cultured rat hepatocytes for specific ginsenosides (oleanolic acid and dammarane series).[49,50] However, at higher doses certain ginsenosides from both series were found to exhibit simultaneous cytotoxic activity.

Cytotoxic and antitumour activity Cytotoxic activity (ED_{50} 0.5 μg/mL) versus L1210 has been documented for polyacetylenes isolated from *P. ginseng* root.[5,6,51] The antitumour effect of ginseng polysaccharides in tumour-bearing mice has been associated with an immunological mechanism of action.[52] Ginseng polysaccharides have been reported to increase the lifespan of tumour-bearing mice and to inhibit the growth of tumour cells *in vivo*, although cytocidal action was not seen *in vitro*.[52] Antitumour activity *in vitro* versus several tumour cell lines has been documented for a polyacetylene, panaxytriol, from *P. ginseng*.[53]

Antiviral activity Antiviral activity (versus Semliki forest virus; 34–40% protection) has been documented for *P. ginseng* extract (G115, Pharmaton) administered orally to rats.[54] The extract also enhanced the level of protection afforded by 6-MFA, an interferon-inducing agent of fungal origin.[54] *P. ginseng* has been found to induce *in vitro* and *in vivo* production of interferon and to augment the natural killer and antibody dependent cytotoxic activities in human peripheral lymphocytes.[54,55] In addition, *P. ginseng* enhances the antibody-forming cell response to sheep red blood cells in mice and stimulates cell mediated immunity both *in vitro* and *in vivo*.[54,55] In view of these observations, it has been proposed that the antiviral activity of *P. ginseng* may be immunologically mediated.[54,55]

Clinical studies

Clinical trials of preparations of *P. ginseng* and other *Panax* species have focused on assessing effects related to the reputed adaptogenic properties of this herbal medicinal product, although rigorous clinical investigations are limited. Studies have tested different *Panax* species preparations, including combination herbal preparations containing *P. ginseng*, which vary qualitatively and quantitatively in their phytochemical composition. Furthermore, different preparations have been administered according to different dosage regimens, and to different study populations making interpretation of the results difficult. A large body of clinical research has been published in the Chinese and other Asian literature, making access difficult, although many of these studies are unlikely to meet contemporary Western standards in terms of their design, analysis and reporting.[16] Therefore, at present there is insufficient evidence to support definitively the efficacy of specific *Panax* species preparations in the various indications for which they are used and/or have been tested. Details of several clinical trials of ginseng (*Panax* spp.) preparations published in the English literature are summarised below.

Effects on physical performance Several studies have found that preparations of *P. ginseng* do not improve physical performance in healthy adults. In a randomised, double-blind, placebo-controlled trial, 38 healthy adults received an aqueous extract of *P. ginseng* (G115, Pharmaton SA, Lugano, Switzerland) 200 mg twice daily for eight weeks.[56] Participants underwent exhaustive exercise testing before and after the intervention; recovery from exercise was also monitored. At the end of the study, data from 27 participants were available for analysis. No statistically significant differences in physical performance and heart rate recovery were detected between the ginseng and placebo groups.[56] Similar randomised, double-blind, placebo-controlled studies have found that treatment with *P. ginseng* root extract (G115) 200 mg daily for eight weeks had no statistically significant effects on maximal work performance, oxygen uptake during resting, exercise and recovery, respiratory exchange ratio, minute ventilation, heart rate and blood lactic acid concentrations in 19 healthy adult females ($p > 0.05$ for each),[57] and no effect on oxygen consumption, respiratory exchange ratio, minute ventilation, heart rate, blood lactic acid concentrations and perceived exertion in 36 healthy adult males who received *P. ginseng* root extract (G115) 200 or 400 mg daily for eight weeks.[58] In a further randomised, double-blind, placebo-controlled trial involving 28 healthy adults, administration of *P. ginseng* root extract (not further specified) 200 mg daily for three weeks had no statistically significant effects on maximal exercise capacity, total exercise time, work load, plasma lactate concentrations, haematocrit, heart rate and perceived exertion.[59] As all of these studies involved only small numbers of participants it is possible that they did not have sufficient statistical power to detect a difference between the treatment and placebo groups if one exists.

Effects on cognitive performance Several studies have examined the effects of preparations of *P. ginseng* root, typically the commercial product G115, alone, or in combination with other herbal ingredients, on cognitive performance. Generally, these studies have involved healthy volunteers, and trials evaluating the effects of *P. ginseng* root preparations on patients with impaired cognitive function are lacking. Further research examining the effects of acute and longer-term administration of preparations of *P. ginseng* and other *Panax* species in both healthy individuals and patients with impaired cognitive function are required.[60] In a double-blind, placebo-controlled, crossover study involving 15 healthy individuals, *P. ginseng* root extract (G115) 200 mg as a single oral dose had significant effects on certain aspects of electroencephalogram recordings, such as reductions in frontal theta and beta activity, when compared with placebo.[61] These findings suggest that *P. ginseng* root extract can directly modulate cerebroelectrical activity.[61]

In a double-blind, placebo-controlled, crossover study, 30 healthy individuals received capsules containing *P. ginseng* extract (G115) 200 or 400 mg as a single dose before undergoing a battery of tests designed to assess cognitive performance.[62] A statistically significant improvement in one test of cognitive performance (serial sevens) was observed with the lower ginseng dose, compared with placebo, but no statistically significant difference was observed with the higher dose, and there were no statistically significant differences in other tests of cognitive performance for either dose.[62] There was a statistically significant improvement in scores for mental fatigue for both doses when measured after the third battery of tests, but this finding was not consistent when measured at other timepoints.

In another double-blind, placebo-controlled, crossover study, 28 healthy individuals received single doses of *P. ginseng* root extract (G115) 200 mg, an ethanolic extract of guarana (*Paullinia cupana*) 75 mg, both herbal preparations, or placebo, with a one-week wash-out period between each; participants undertook a battery of cognitive performance tests before and after treatments.[63] Administration of *P. ginseng* root extract, compared with placebo, led to statistically significant improvements in some (e.g. speed of attention, speed of memory, secondary memory) but not all (e.g. accuracy of attention, working memory, Bond-Lader mood scales) tests of cognitive performance, although improvements were not observed at every timepoint measured after administration. In some tests, administration of both ginseng and guarana led to greater improvements than did ginseng alone.[63] In similar experiments, 20 healthy individuals received single doses of *P. ginseng* root extract (G115) 200, 400, 600 mg, or placebo, and a combination of *P. ginseng* root extract and *Ginkgo biloba* leaf extract at doses of 200 and 120, 400 and 240, 600 and 360 mg, respectively, or placebo.[64] Statistically significant improvements in one cognitive performance test (serial sevens) were observed with administration of *P. ginseng* root extract 400 mg, compared with placebo, but reduced performance in this test was seen following administration of the 200 mg dose. Following administration of the combination preparation, statistically significant improvements in certain tests at certain timepoints, but these results were not consistent for all doses tested and across all timepoints measured in the study.

The effects of the same combination preparation of *P. ginseng* and *G. biloba* on memory were assessed in a randomised, double-blind, placebo-controlled, multicentre, parallel group trial involving 256 healthy volunteers aged 38–67 years (mean (SD), 56 (7) years).[65] Participants received a preparation containing *P. ginseng* root extract and *G. biloba* leaf extract 100 and 60 mg, respectively, twice daily, 200 and 120 mg, respectively, once daily, or placebo, for 12 weeks. Assessments were undertaken at weeks 4, 8, 12 and 14 of the study. At the end of the study, the primary outcome variable the Quality of Memory Index was significantly improved in the treatment group, compared with the placebo group (p = 0.026). No statistically significant effects were seen with respect to the secondary outcome variables power and continuity of attention, and speed of memory processes.[65]

In a randomised, double-blind, placebo-controlled, parallel group trial, 64 healthy volunteers with neurasthenic complaints received a combination preparation containing *P. ginseng* root extract and *G. biloba* leaf extract at doses of 50 and 30 mg, respectively, 100 and 60 mg, respectively, 200 and 120 mg, respectively, or placebo, twice daily, for 12 weeks.[66] At the end of the study, participants in the higher-dose ginseng–ginkgo group, compared with the placebo group, achieved significantly higher scores in tests designed to assess cognitive function ($p = 0.008$).

Hypoglycaemic activity Most studies investigating hypoglycaemic activity of ginseng preparations have assessed effects in healthy (non-diabetic) individuals. In a randomised, single-blind (the study may have been conducted double-blind but this was not specifically stated), placebo-controlled, crossover trial, nine individuals with type-2 diabetes mellitus (mean (standard deviation, SD) glycosylated haemoglobin HbA_{1c} 0.08 (0.005); reference range for well-controlled type-2 diabetes mellitus, 0.065–0.075) received a capsule containing 'American' ginseng (*P. quinquefolius*, containing protopanaxadiols R_{b-1} 1.53%, R_{b-2} 0.06%, R_c 0.24%, R_d 0.44%, and protopanaxatriols R_{g-1} 0.1%, R_e 0.83%;[67] Chai-Na-Ta Corp, British Columbia, Canada) as a single dose both 40 minutes before a 25 g oral glucose challenge and, on a separate occasion, at the same time as the oral glucose challenge.[68] Incremental glycaemia at 45 minutes was significantly lower following ginseng treatment with either regimen (i.e. given with or before glucose challenge) than it was following placebo administration ($p < 0.05$ for both). In similar experiments involving non-diabetic individuals, a statistically significant reduction in incremental glycaemia was only observed when ginseng was administered 40 minutes before glucose challenge.[68] Further experiments in non-diabetic individuals indicated that the effect on postprandial glycaemia was not dose-dependent as glucose tolerance was similar following administration of doses of ginseng ranging from 1–9 g.[69,70] However, the effect of *P. quinquefolius* was time-dependent as reductions in postprandial glycaemia were observed only with administration of *P. quinquefolius* 40, 80 and 120 minutes,[69,70] but not 0, 10 and 20 minutes, before glucose challenge.[70] In another similar randomised, blinded, placebo-controlled, crossover trial involving non-diabetic individuals, no effect on post-prandial glycaemia was observed following oral administration 40 minutes before glucose challenge of 6 g of the same commercial *P. quinquefolius* preparation, but obtained from a different batch.[67] This conflicting result may be due to the lower ginsenoside content of the latter product (containing protopanaxadiols R_{b-1} 0.65%, R_{b-2} 0.02%, R_c 0.11%, R_d 0.12%, and protopanaxatriols R_{g-1} 0.08%, R_e 0.67%).[67]

Other similar studies involving non-diabetic individuals have reported different and less consistent results for preparations of *P. ginseng*. In two randomised, single-blind, placebo-controlled, crossover studies, 11 individuals received capsules containing 500 mg three-year-old powdered whole root of *P. ginseng* (containing protopanaxadiols R_{b-1} 0.18%, R_{b-2} 0.09%, R_c 0.07%, R_d 0.02%, and protopanaxatriols R_{g-1} 0.16%, R_e 0.17% and R_f 0.12%) at a single dose of 1, 2, 3, 6 and 9 g 40 minutes before glucose challenge.[71] No statistically significant differences were observed for the treatment versus placebo groups. Furthermore, when results for all *P. ginseng* groups were pooled, the 2-hour plasma glucose concentration was higher in the *P. ginseng* group than in the placebo group. These findings are in contrast to effects observed for *P. quinquefolius*, and could be explained by differences in the ginsenoside content of preparations derived from the two species.[71]

In a double-blind, placebo-controlled, crossover study in which 30 non-diabetic individuals received capsules containing *P. ginseng* extract (G115) 200 or 400 mg as a single dose before undergoing a battery of tests designed to assess cognitive performance,[62] statistically significant reductions in blood glucose concentrations occurred for both doses of ginseng at all measured post-treatment timepoints ($p < 0.01$ for all).

Immunomodulatory activity In a randomised, double-blind, placebo-controlled trial, 38 healthy adults received an aqueous extract of *P. ginseng* (G115, Pharmaton SA, Lugano, Switzerland) 200 mg twice daily for eight weeks.[56] Participants underwent exhaustive exercise testing before and after the intervention in order to effect immunosuppression. At the end of the study, data from 27 participants were available for analysis. No statistically significant differences in secretory immunoglobulin A (IgA; the primary immunoglobulin contained in secretions of the mucosal immune system) parameters were detected between the *P. ginseng* and placebo groups, indicating that the *P. ginseng* preparation had no effect on mucosal immunity.[56]

A randomised, double-blind, placebo-controlled trial involving 60 healthy individuals assessed the effects of two different extracts of *P. ginseng* on immune parameters.[72] Participants received an aqueous extract of *P. ginseng* (not further specified) 100 mg, a standardised extract of *P. ginseng* (G115) 100 mg, or placebo, twice daily for eight weeks. Analysis of participants' blood samples taken before and after four and eight weeks of treatment indicated that both extracts had statistically significant effects on various immune parameters, compared with baseline values,[72] although from a report of the study, it is not clear whether or not these changes were statistically significant when compared with values for the placebo group.

Cancer prevention A small number of epidemiological studies have explored the effects of ginseng use on prevention of cancer. A case–control study involving all cases of newly diagnosed cancer during a one-year time period at a major hospital cancer centre in Korea included 905 cases and 905 age, sex and date of admission matched controls.[73] Of the 905 cases, 62% had a history of 'ginseng' (not further specified) use (determined by face-to-face interviews using a structured questionnaire), compared with 75% in the control group ($p < 0.01$). The odds ratio (95% confidence interval) (OR; 95% CI) for cancer in relation to ginseng intake was 0.56 (0.45 to 0.69). This study was subsequently extended to include a total of 1987 case–control pairs.[74] Ginseng users had a lower risk of cancer, compared with non-users (OR 0.50; 95% CI 0.44 to 0.58); ORs (95% CI) for being diagnosed with cancer differed for use of different types of ginseng; the lowest being for fresh ginseng extract 0.37 (0.29 to 0.46), white ginseng powder 0.30 (0.22 to 0.41) and red ginseng extract 0.20 (0.08 to 0.50). No decrease in risk was seen with use of fresh ginseng slices, fresh ginseng juice and white ginseng tea: OR (95% CI), 0.79 (0.63–1.01), 0.71 (0.49–1.03), 0.69 (0.45–1.07), respectively.(74) ORs were lowest for ovarian (0.15), larynx (0.18), oesophageal (0.20) and panceatic (0.22) cancers.

The questionnaire used in the case–control studies described above was used to determine ginseng use in a cohort study involving 4634 people aged over 40 years.[75] In this study, 54.7% of cancer cases had a history of ginseng use, compared with 71.2% of individuals without cancer. The relative risk (RR; 95% CI) for cancer was reduced with ginseng intake (0.40, 0.28–0.56; $p < 0.05$). When evaluted by intake of type of ginseng, the RR was significantly reduced with ginseng extract (0.31, 0.13–0.74) and multiple combinations of ginseng preparations (0.34, 0.20–0.53), but not for other types of ginseng.[75] The available evidence for the cancer preventive effect of ginseng preparations in humans is inconclusive, and further methodologically rigorous research is required.[76,77]

Quality of life The effects of different preparations of *P. ginseng* root on quality-of-life measures have been asssessed in several randomised, controlled trials involving different participant groups, including healthy individuals, post-menopausal women and patients with diabetes. A systematic review of trials published by the end of the year 2002 included nine studies, of which eight involved a placebo control group, four involved the administration of monopreparations of *P. ginseng* root, and five involved combination preparations of *P. ginseng* and vitamins/minerals.[78] The review did not provide details of the specific *P. ginseng* preparations tested in the trials, only that doses ranged from 80–400 mg daily and that studies lasted from two to nine months. These variations in products tested, together with differences in study design, outcome measures evaluated, and participant groups involved, make overall interpretation of the results difficult and, to some extent, invalid. All but one of the included studies reported improvement in at least one quality-of-life measure, or a subscale, but there were conflicting findings. In essence, at present, evidence of a beneficial effect for *P. ginseng* on quality-of-life measures is inconclusive. Further research is needed to establish the effects, if any, of preparations of *P. ginseng* root and other *Panax* species on quality of life. Furthermore, results of trials should be considered in the context of the chemical profile of individual preparations, since this is likely to differ qualitatively and quantitatively between products. One of the studies included in the review described above found that *P. ginseng* root extract (G115) 200 or 400 mg daily for eight weeks had no statistically significant effects on psychological well-being, as assessed using the Positive Affect Negative Affect Scale, in a randomised, double-blind, placebo-controlled trial involving 83 healthy younger adults (mean age 26 years).[79]

Other effects The effects of an aqueous extract of *P. ginseng* roots on blood alcohol clearance were assessed in an open study involving 14 healthy men aged 25–35 years; each participant served as his own control.[80] Participants consumed a single dose of alcohol (25% ethanol 72 g per 65 kg body weight) over 45 minutes with and without *P. ginseng* root extract 3 g/kg body weight. Blood samples taken 40 minutes after the end of the period of alcohol ingestion showed blood alcohol concentrations of 0.18% and 0.11% for the control and treatment periods, respectively ($p < 0.001$). The design of this study does not allow the observed effects to be attributed to ginseng administration, and the hypothesis that *P. ginseng* increases blood alcohol clearance requires testing in methodologically rigorous randomised, controlled trials.

Side-effects, Toxicity

G

Clinical data

There are only limited clinical data on safety aspects of preparations of *P. ginseng* and other *Panax* species. There is a lack of formal post-marketing surveillance-type studies, and existing pharmacoepidemiological studies typically have assessed potential benefits and not risks of harm(s). There is a substantial number of placebo-controlled clinical trials of preparations of *P. ginseng* and other *Panax* species, although many of these have methodological limitations, including lack of randomisation and/or double-blinding. Trials have assessed the effects of different preparations, including combination herbal preparations containing different *Panax* species, which vary qualitatively and quantitatively in their phytochemical composition. Furthermore, different preparations have been administered according to different dosage regimens, and to different study populations (e.g. healthy volunteers, patients with hypertension), making interpretation of the results difficult. The clinical trials of *Panax* species root preparations available typically have involved small numbers of patients and been of short duration (typically four to 12 weeks), so have the statistical power only to detect very common, acute adverse effects. Rigorous investigation of safety aspects of correctly identified, well-characterised *Panax* species root preparations administered orally at different dosages, including the effects of long-term treatment, is required.

A systematic review of data available up to May 2001 relating to adverse events of monopreparations of *P. ginseng* preparations identified 48 placebo-controlled trials, 14 trials with an active control group, and 20 uncontrolled studies.[81] Of these, 42 trials involved healthy individuals and athletes, and the remainder involved older individuals, postmenopausal women or patients with hypertension, respiratory diseases, hepatitis, erectile dysfunction. Thirteen placebo-controlled studies provided sufficiently detailed information on reported adverse events. Six of these studies, mostly involving healthy individuals, had assessed the effects of a *P. ginseng* root extract (G115) typically at a dose of 200 mg daily for three to 16 weeks, although one study lasted for two years. Five other placebo-controlled studies assessed the effects of red *P. ginseng* root taken for around two to 12 weeks (one study involved administration for one year), and in two other studies, the species and type of ginseng were not clearly specified. Adverse events reported generally were similar in type and frequency to those reported for the placebo groups.[81] Nine placebo-controlled trials, four of which assessed a *P. ginseng* root extract (G115), stated that no adverse events occurred during the study period.

Placebo-controlled trials of *P. ginseng* published since the systematic review was conducted, and placebo-controlled trials assessing the effects of preparations of *P. quinquefolius*, typically have not provided detailed information on the occurrence of adverse events. One study stated that there was no difference in symptoms, mostly gastrointestinal adverse events, between the *P. quinquefolius* and placebo groups reported during the study,[67] whereas another study assessing *P. quinquefolius* stated that no adverse effects occurred during the study.[70]

The systematic review also identified publications describing 27 case reports associated with the use of 'ginseng', although for 22 reports no information was provided on the type (i.e. red or white *P. ginseng*), preparation and dosage of *P. ginseng* ingested, and it is unlikely that any chemical analysis of the products ingested was undertaken. Four cases of agranulocytosis initially attributed to use of *P. ginseng*-containing products, were later attributed to undeclared ingredients (aminopyrine and phenylbutazone) detected in the products.[81] For many of the cases, there were other factors, including concurrent medications and cessation of treatment effects, that could explain the observed effects. The cases included six reports of mastalgia, two of post-menopausal vaginal bleeding and one of metrorrhagia (uterine bleeding at irregular intervals, usually for prolonged period of time) in women who had ingested or applied (one case of vaginal bleeding was associated with use of a 'ginseng' face cream[82]) 'ginseng' products. Several of the reports describe positive dechallenge and/or rechallenge. Most of these reports, however, are from the older literature and involved the use of unlicensed, poorly described products; a causal association with *Panax* species has not been established, and the relevance of these reports to products marketed currently is not clear. Two cases of mania have also been described. One involved a 35-year-old woman with depressive illness who was stabilised on treatment with lithium and amitriptyline and who stopped lithium treatment and began taking ginseng (not further specified).[83] The second report described a 26-year-old-man with no history of psychiatric illness who experienced a manic episode two months after starting treatment with red *P. ginseng* root 500 to 750 mg daily on five days per week.[84] Analysis of the product found no evidence of notable contaminants.

The World Health Organization's Uppsala Monitoring Centre (WHO-UMC; Collaborating Centre for International Drug Monitoring) receives summary reports of suspected adverse drug reactions from national pharmacovigilance centres of over 70 countries worldwide. A systematic review of information available up to May 2001 relating to adverse effects associated with *P. ginseng* summarised reports from the WHO-UMC database describing a total of 168 adverse reactions associated with monopreparations of ginseng.[81] However, this number of reports relates to unspecified 'ginseng' preparations, not necessarily preparations of *P. ginseng*. To the end of the year 2005, the WHO-UMC's database contained only nine reports, describing a total of 20 adverse reactions, for monopreparations specified as *P. ginseng*.[85]

In a phase 1 study involving healthy males aged 18–35 years who received an extract of *P. ginseng* root (21.4 mg/mL; standardised for ginsenosides 10.5%) 20 mL twice daily for ten days, no adverse effects on fertility parameters, including volume of ejaculate, number of spermatozoids per millilitre, and proportions of active, inactive, normokinetic, dyskinetic and akinetic spermatozoids, were observed, compared with baseline values.[86]

In 1979, two studies referred to a 'ginseng abuse syndrome' (GAS) which emphasised that most side-effects documented for 'ginseng' were associated with the ingestion of large doses together with other psychomotor stimulants, including tea and coffee. GAS was defined as diarrhoea, hypertension, nervousness, skin eruptions and sleeplessness; other symptoms occasionally observed included amenorrhoea, decreased appetite, depression, euphoria, hypotension and oedema.[87,88] However, these two studies have been widely criticised over the variety of ginseng and other preparations used, and over the lack of authentication of the ginseng species ingested.[1,G19]

A review of the Russian literature describes symptoms of overdose as those exhibited by individuals allergic to ginseng, namely palpitations, insomnia and pruritus, together with heart pain, decrease in sexual potency, vomiting, haemorrhagic diathesis, headache and epistaxis, and that ingestion of very large doses has been reported to be fatal.[15] The primary publications upon which these statements are based have not been used here, so the quality of the reports, including their descriptions of the ginseng preparations implicated, has not been assessed here.

Preclinical data

Results documented for toxicity studies carried out in a number of animal species using standardised extracts (SE) indicate *P. ginseng* to be of low toxicity.[89–93]

Single doses of up to 2 g SE have been administered to mice and rats with no toxic effects observed.[92] LD_{50} values (p.o.) in mice and rats have been estimated at 2 g/kg and greater than 5 g/kg.[89] In addition, LD_{50} values (i.p., mice) have been estimated for individual ginsenosides as 305 mg/kg (R_{b-2}), 324 mg/kg (R_d), 405 mg/kg (R_e), 410 mg/kg (R_c), 1110 mg/kg (R_{b-1}), 1250 mg/kg (R_{g-1}), and 1340 mg/kg (R_f); an LD_{50} (i.v., mice) of 3806 mg/kg has been estimated for the saponins R_{c-1} and R_{d-1}.[89]

Doses of approximately 720 mg of a *P. ginseng* extract (G115) have been administered orally to rats for 20 days with no toxicological effects documented.[93]

Daily doses of up to 15 mg G115/kg body weight have been administered orally to dogs for 90 days with no toxic effects documented. An initial increase in excitability which disappeared after two to three weeks was the only observation reported in rats fed 200 mg G115/kg body weight for 25 weeks.[92]

P. quinquefolius has been reported to be devoid of mutagenic potential when investigated versus *Salmonella typhimurium* strain TM677.[94]

Contra-indications, Warnings

The older literature includes statements that the use of *P. ginseng* is contra-indicated during acute illness, haemorrhage and during the acute period of coronary thrombosis,[1] and it has been recommended that *P. ginseng* should be avoided by individuals who are highly energetic, nervous, tense, hysteric, manic or schizophrenic, and that *P. ginseng* should not be taken with stimulants, including coffee, antipsychotic drugs or during treatment with hormones.[1,G49] The scientific basis and evidence for many of these statements is not clear. However, in view of their documented pharmacological activities, *Panax* species preparations should be used with caution in patients with diabetes and cardiovascular disorders. In general, and in view of the lack of safety data, it is appropriate to advise against the long-term or otherwise excessive use of *Panax* species.

Drug interactions In view of the pharmacological actions of *Panax* species preparations and their isolated constituents described following preclinical and, to a lesser extent, clinical studies, the potential for preparations of *Panax* species to interfere with other medicines administered concurrently, particularly those with anticoagulant, hypoglycaemic and/or cardiovascular activity, should be considered.

Two cases of a suspected interaction between 'ginseng' and phenelzine have been documented. One report described insomnia, headache and tremulousness in a 64-year-old woman who began taking a 'ginseng' tea in addition to her existing phenelzine treatment; the woman previously had used 'ginseng' tea alone without experiencing any adverse effects,[95] and three years after the first epidsode of concurrent use of phenelzine and 'ginseng' tea, the woman ingested 'ginseng' capsules and experienced similar symptoms.[96] A second report described a 42-year-old woman for whom treatment with phenelzine was initiated because of major depressive illness. The woman was also receiving triazolam and lorazepam and began self-treatment with unspecified preparations of ginseng and bee pollen.[97] She experienced headaches, irritability and visual hallucinations. A causal relationship with use of *Panax* species in these cases cannot be established.

There is an isolated case report of a suspected interaction between *P. ginseng* and warfarin involving a 47-year-old-man with an aortic heart valve who was receiving warfarin for thromboprophylaxis. Two weeks after the man began treatment with a *P. ginseng* root extract (Ginsana), his international normalised ratio (INR) fell to 1.5, having previously been stable for nine months.[98] On stopping use of the *P. ginseng* preparation, his INR returned to within the target range.

In a randomised, open-label, crossover study, 12 healthy male individuals received a single dose of warfarin 25 mg alone or after seven days' treatment with capsules containing *P. ginseng* root (containing extract equivalent to 500 mg root; standardised for ginsenosides 8.93 mg, as ginsenoside R_{g-1}) two or three times daily.[99] There were no statistically significant differences in area under the plasma-concentration time curve (AUC), elimination half-life ($t_{1/2}$), total clearance, volume of distribution, maximal plasma concentration (C_{max}) and time to maximal concentration for either *R*-warfarin or *S*-warfarin when warfarin was taken following *P. ginseng* treatment, compared with values for ingestion of warfarin alone. There were also no statistically significant differences in protein binding of *R*- and *S*-warfarin, or in warfarin pharmacodynamics as assessed using INR values, following *P. ginseng* administration. By contrast, another drug interaction study involving healthy volunteers found that a preparation of *P. quinquefolius* root reduced the anticoagulant effect of warfarin. In a randomised, double-blind, placebo-controlled trial, 20 healthy individuals received powdered root of *P. quinquefolius* (containing R_{b-1} 1.93%, R_{b-2} 0.20%, R_c 0.61%, R_d 0.42%, R_e 1.68% and R_{g-1} 0.35%) 1 g twice daily, or placebo, for three weeks; treatment was taken for a total of three weeks, beginning four days after oral administration of warfarin 5 mg daily for three days, concurrently with a second three-day period of warfarin administration, and for four days after the second period of warfarin exposure.[100] There was a significantly greater reduction in the magnitude of the INR, the primary outcome measure, in the *P. quinquefolius* group, compared with that in the placebo group ($p = 0.0012$).

The contrasting findings for *P. ginseng* root and *P. quinquefolius* root preparations could be explained by differences in their chemical composition, particularly ginsenoside content. The effects of different *Panax* species preparations on warfarin pharmacokinetics in patients receiving warfarin treatment or prophylaxis require investigation.

In another drug interaction study involving healthy individuals ($n = 20$), participants received a *P. ginseng* root extract preparation (Ginsana, Pharmaton, Connecticut, USA; standardised for ginsenosides 4%) 100 mg twice daily for 14 days.[101] Data collected over a one-week period before *P. ginseng* administration provided a within-subject control group. At the end of the study, there were no statistically significant changes in the 6-β-hydroxycortisol : cortisol ratio following *P. ginseng* administration, compared with baseline values, suggesting that *P. ginseng* did not induce CYP3A enzyme activity.[101] By contrast, in *in vitro* experiments, a *P. ginseng* root extract (G115; standardised for 4% ginsenosides) and a *P. quinquefolius* root extract (standardised for 10% total ginsenosides) both inhibited CYP1A1, CYP1A2 and CYP1B1 activities in a concentration-dependent manner.[102] *P. quinquefolius* root extract was 45-fold more potent than *P. ginseng* root extract in inhibiting CYP1A2. The ginsenosides R_{b-1}, R_{b-2}, R_c, R_d, R_e, R_f and R_{g-1}, added to the system either individually or as a mixture, at concentrations reflecting those at which the ginseng extracts caused inhibition, did not affect CYP1A and B enzyme activities. These findings led to the suggestion that other ginsenosides could be responsible for the inhibitory effects on the CYP enzymes investigated, or that the effects could be due to other compounds, such as tannins, as these were not removed from the extracts.[102]

G

Pregnancy and lactation No fetal abnormalities have been observed in rats and rabbits administered a standardised *P. ginseng* extract (40 mg/kg, p.o.) from day 1 to day 15 of pregnancy.[92] *P. ginseng* has also been fed to two successive generations of rats in doses of up to 15 mg G115/kg body weight/day (equivalent to approximately 2700 mg *P. ginseng* extract) with no teratogenic effects observed.[89] However, the safety of *P. ginseng* during pregnancy has not been established in humans and therefore its use should be avoided. Similarly, there are no published data concerning the secretion of pharmacologically active constituents from *P. ginseng* into the breast milk and use of *P. ginseng* during lactation is therefore best avoided. However, a more recent study which investigated the effect of ginsenoside R_{b-1} on the development of rat embryos during organogenesis *in vitro* found that median total morphological scores were significantly lower for embryos exposed to ginsenoside R_{b-1} at concentrations of 30 μg/mL, compared with those for control embryos ($p < 0.05$).[103] The clinical relevance of these findings is not known. The effects of ginsenoside R_{b-1} and other ginsenosides, including the possibility of additive effects, on embryogensis requires further investigation.

The safety of *P. ginseng* during pregnancy has not been established in humans. Similarly, there are no published data concerning the secretion of pharmacologically active constituents from *P. ginseng* into the breast milk. In view of the lack of safety data and the findings described above, and until further information is available, the use of *P. ginseng* preparations during pregnancy and breastfeeding should be avoided.

Preparations

Proprietary single-ingredient preparations

Argentina: Ginsana; Herbaccion Bioenergizante. *Australia:* Herbal Stress Relief. *Austria:* Ginsana. *Belgium:* Ginsana. *Brazil:* Ginsana; Ginsex. *Canada:* Ginsana. *Czech Republic:* Ginsana. *France:* Gerimax Tonique. *Germany:* Ardey-aktiv; Coriosta Vitaltonikum N; Ginsana; Hevert-Aktivon Mono; IL HWA; Orgaplasma. *Italy:* Ginsana. *Malaysia:* Ginsana. *Mexico:* Raigin; Rutying; Sanjin Royal Jelly. *Portugal:* Ginsana. *Russia:* Gerimax Ginseng (Геримакс Женьшень); Ginsana (Гинсана). *Singapore:* Ginsana. *Spain:* Bio Star. *Switzerland:*

Ginsana; KintaVital. *Thailand:* Ginsana; Ginsroy. *UK:* Korseng; Red Kooga.

Proprietary multi-ingredient preparations

Argentina: Dynamisan; Herbaccion Ginseng Y Magnesio; Optimina Plus; Total Magnesiano con Ginseng; Total Magnesiano con Vitaminas y Minerales; Vifortol. *Australia:* Bioglan Ginsynergy; Extralife Extra-Brite; Ginkgo Biloba Plus; Ginkgo Complex; Glycyrrhiza Complex; Infant Tonic; Irontona; Nervatona Plus; Panax Complex; Vig; Vig; Vitatona. *Austria:* Gerimax Plus; ProAktiv. *Brazil:* Gerin; Poliseng. *Canada:* Damiana-Sarsaparilla Formula; Energy Plus; Ginkoba. *Chile:* Gincosan; Mentania. *Czech Republic:* Gincosan. *France:* Nostress; Thalgo Tonic; Tonactil. *Germany:* Ginseng-Complex "Schuh"; Peking Ginseng Royal Jelly N. *Hong Kong:* Cervusen. *Italy:* Alvear con Ginseng; Apergan; Bioton; Fon Wan Ginsenergy; Forticrin; Fosfarsile Forte; Fosfarsile Forte; Four-Ton; Ginsana Ton; Neoplus; Ottovis. *Malaysia:* 30 Plus; Adult Citrex Multivitamin + Ginseng + Omega 3; Total Man. *Russia:* Doppelherz Ginseng Aktiv (Доппельгерц Женьшень Актив); Doppelherz Vitalotonik (Доппельгерц Виталотоник). *South Africa:* Activex 40 Plus. *Singapore:* Gin-Vita. *Spain:* Energysor; Redseng Polivit; Ton Was; Vigortonic. *Switzerland:* Biovital Ginseng; Burgerstein TopVital; Geri; Gincosan; Imuvit; Supradyn Vital 50+; Triallin. *Thailand:* Imugins; Imuvit; Multilim RG; Revitan. *UK:* Actimind; Red Kooga Co-Q-10 and Ginseng; Regina Royal Concorde; Seven Seas Ginseng; Vitegin Capsules; Wellman. *USA:* Energy Support; Mental Clarity.

G

References

1 Baldwin CA *et al.* What pharmacists should know about ginseng. *Pharm J* 1986; 237: 583–586.
2 Chung BS. Studies on the components of Korean ginseng (II) On the composition of ginseng essential oils. *Kor J Pharmacog* 1976; 7: 41–44.
3 Iwabuchi H *et al.* Studies on the sesquiterpenoids of *Panax ginseng* C. A. Meyer III. *Chem Pharm Bull* 1989; 37: 509–510.
4 Iwabuchi H *et al.* Studies on the sesquiterpenoids of *Panax ginseng* C. A. Meyer II. Isolation and structure determination of ginsenol, a novel sesquiterpene alcohol. *Chem Pharm Bull* 1988; 36: 2447–2451.
5 Ahn B-Z *et al.* Acetylpanaxydol and panaxydolchlorohydrin, two new poly-ynes from Korean ginseng with cytotoxic activity against L1210 cells. *Arch Pharm (Weinheim)* 1989; 322: 223–226.
6 Fujimoto Y, Satoh M. A new cytotoxic chlorine-containing polyacetylene from the callus of *Panax ginseng. Chem Pharm Bull* 1988; 36: 4206–4208.
7 Gao Q-P *et al.* Chemical properties and anti-complementary activities of polysaccharide fractions from roots and leaves of *Panax ginseng. Planta Med* 1989; 55: 9–12.
8 Yamasaki K *et al.* Purification and characterization of β-amylase from ginseng. *Chem Pharm Bull* 1989; 37: 973–978.
9 Chuang WC *et al.* A comparative study on commercial samples of ginseng radix. *Planta Med* 1995; 61: 459–465.
10 Zhu S *et al.* Comparative study on triterpene saponins of Ginseng drugs. *Planta Med* 2004; 70(7): 666–677.
11 Cui JF. Identification and quantification of ginsenosides in various commercial ginseng preparations. *Eur J Pharm Sci* 1995; 3: 77–85.
12 Harkey MR *et al.* Variability in commercial ginseng products: an analysis of 25 preparations. *Am J Clin Nutr* 2001; 73: 1101–1106.
13 United States Department of the Interior Fish and Wildlife Service. *Convention permit applications for wild American ginseng harvested in 2005.* August 3, 2005.
14 Convention on International Trade in Endangered Species of Wild Fauna and Flora. *Notification to the Parties. No. 2000/018.* Geneva, 29 February 2000.
15 Baranov AI. Medicinal uses of ginseng and related plants in the Soviet Union: recent trends in the Soviet literature. *J Ethnopharmacol* 1982; 6: 339–353.
16 Dharmananada S. The nature of ginseng. Traditional use, modern research and the question of dosage. *HerbalGram* 2002; 54: 34–51.
17 Brekhman II. *Panax* ginseng-1. *Med Sci Service* 1967; 4: 17–26.
18 Takino Y *et al.* Studies on the absorption, distribution, excretion and metabolism of ginseng saponins. I. Quantitative analysis of ginsenoside Rg1 in rats. *Chem Pharm Bull* 1982; 30(6): 2196–2201.
19 Odani T *et al.* Studies on the absorption, distribution, excretion and metabolism of ginseng saponins. III. The absorption, distribution and excretion of ginsenoside Rb1 in rats. *Chem Pharm Bull* 1983; 31(3): 1059–1066.
20 Odani T *et al.* Studies on the absorption, distribution, excretion and metabolism of ginseng saponins. IV. Decompostion of ginsenoside Rg1 and -Rb1 in the digestive tract of rats. *Chem Pharm Bull* 1983; 31 (10): 3691–3697.
21 Karikura M *et al.* Studies on the absorption, distribution, excretion and metabolism of ginseng saponins. V. The decomposition products of ginsenoside Rb2 in the large intestine of rats. *Chem Pharm Bull* 1990; 38(10): 2859–2861.
22 Li TB *et al.* Effects of ginsenosides, lectins and *Momordica charantia* insulin-like peptide on corticosterone production by isolated rat adrenal cells. *J Ethnopharmacol* 1987; 21: 21–29.
23 Filaretov AA *et al.* Role of pituitary-adrenocortical system in body adaptation abilities. *Exp Clin Endocrinol* 1988; 92: 129–136.
24 Guodong L, Zhongqi L. Effects of ginseng saponins on insulin release from isolated pancreatic islets of rats. *Chin J Integr Trad Western Med* 1987; 7: 326.
25 Yushu H, Yuzhen C. The effect of *Panax ginseng* extract (GS) on insulin and corticosteroid receptors. *J Trad Chin Med* 1988; 8: 293–295.
26 Kimura M *et al.* Pharmacological sequential trials for the fractionation of components with hypoglycemic activity in alloxan diabetic mice from *Ginseng radix. J Pharm Dyn* 1981; 4: 402–409.
27 Waki I *et al.* Effects of a hypoglycemic component of *Ginseng radix* on insulin biosynthesis in normal and diabetic animals. *J Pharm Dyn* 1982; 5: 547–554.
28 Avakian EV *et al.* Effect of *Panax ginseng* extract on energy metabolism during exercise in rats. *Planta Med* 1984; 50: 151–154.
29 Suzuki Y, Hikino H. Mechanisms of hypoglycemic activity of panaxans A and B, glycans of *Panax ginseng* roots: effects on the key enzymes of glucose metabolism in the liver of mice. *Phytother Res* 1989; 3: 15–19.
30 Oshima Y *et al.* Isolation and hypoglycemic activity of quinquefolans A, B, and C, glycans of *Panax quinquefolium* roots. *J Nat Prod* 1987; 50: 188–190.
31 Konno C, Hikino H. Isolation and hypoglycemic activity of panaxans M, N, O and P, glycans of *Panax ginseng* roots. *Int J Crude Drug Res* 1987; 25: 53–56.
32 Suzuki Y, Hikino H. Mechanisms of hypoglycemic activity of panaxans A and B, glycans of *Panax ginseng* roots: effects of plasma level, secretion, sensitivity and binding of insulin in mice. *Phytother Res* 1989; 3: 20–24.
33 Konno C *et al.* Isolation and hypoglycaemic activity of panaxans A, B, C, D and E, glycans of *Panax ginseng* roots. *Planta Med* 1984; 50: 434–436.
34 Konno C *et al.* Isolation and hypoglycaemic activity of panaxans Q, R, S, T and U, glycans of *Panax ginseng* roots. *J Ethnopharmacol* 1985; 14: 69–74.
35 Manren R *et al.* Calcium antagonistic action of saponins from *Panax notoginseng* (sanqi-ginseng). *J Trad Chin Med* 1987; 7: 127–130.
36 Wu J-X, Chen J-X. Negative chronotropic and inotropic effects of *Panax saponins. Acta Pharmacol Sin* 1988; 9: 409–412.
37 Lei X-L *et al.* Cardiovascular pharmacology of *Panax notoginseng* (Burk) F.H. Chen and *Salvia militiorrhiza. Am J Chin Med* 1986; 14: 145–152.
38 Li XJ, Zhang BH. Studies on the antiarrhythmic effects of panaxatriol saponins (PTS) isolated from *Panax notoginseng. Acta Pharm Sin* 1988; 23: 168–173.
39 Yunxiang F, Xiu C. Effects of ginsenosides on myocardial lactic acid, cyclic nucleotides and ultrastructural myocardial changes of anoxia on mice. *Chin J Integr Trad Western Med* 1987; 7: 326.

40 Namba T *et al*. Fundamental studies on the evaluation of the crude drugs. (I). Hemolytic and its protective activity of ginseng saponins. *Planta Med* 1974; 28: 28–38.
41 Kosuge T *et al*. Studies on antihemorrhagic principles in the crude drugs for hemostatics. I. On hemostatic activities of the crude drugs for hemostatics. *Yakugaku Zasshi [J Pharm Soc Jpn]* 1981; 101: 501–503.
42 Yamamoto M, Kumagai M. Anti-atherogenic action of *Panax ginseng* in rats and in patients with hyperlipidemia. *Planta Med* 1982; 45: 149–166.
43 Kuo S-C *et al*. Antiplatelet components in *Panax ginseng*. *Planta Med* 1990; 56: 164–167.
44 Kim H-S *et al*. Antinarcotic effects of the standardized ginseng extract G115 on morphine. *Planta Med* 1990; 56: 158–163.
45 Tsang D *et al*. Ginseng saponins: Influence on neurotransmitter uptake in rat brain synaptosomes. *Planta Med* 1985; 51: 221–224.
46 Kobayashi S *et al*. Inhibitory actions of phospholipase A_2 and saponins including ginsenoside Rb_1 and glycyrrhizin on the formation of nicotinic acetylcholine receptor clusters on cultured mouse myotubes. *Phytother Res* 1990; 4: 106–111.
47 Tsang D *et al*. Ginenoside modulates K^+ stimulated noradrenaline release from rat cerebral cortex slices. *Planta Med* 1986; 52: 266–268.
48 Saksena AK *et al*. Effect of *Withania somnifera* and *Panax ginseng* on dopaminergic receptors in rat brain during stress. *Planta Med* 1989; 55: 95.
49 Nakagawa S *et al*. Cytoprotective activity of components of garlic, ginseng and ciuwjia on hepatocyte injury induced by carbon tetrachloride *in vitro*. *Hiroshima J Med Sci* 1985; 34: 303–309.
50 Hikino H *et al*. Antihepatotoxic actions of ginsenosides from *Panax ginseng* roots. *Planta Med* 1985; 51: 62–64.
51 Ahn B-Z, Kim SI. Heptadeca-1,8*t*-dien-4,6-diin-3,10-diol, ein weiteres, gegen L1210 – Zellen cytotoxisches Wirkprinzip aus der Koreanischen Ginsengwurzel. *Planta Med* 1988; 54: 183.
52 Qian B-C *et al*. Effects of ginseng polysaccharides on tumor and immunological function in tumor-bearing mice. *Acta Pharmacol Sin* 1987; 8: 277–288.
53 Matsunaga H *et al*. Studies on the panaxytriol of *Panax ginseng* C.A. Meyer. Isolation, determination and antitumor activity. *Chem Pharm Bull* 1989; 37: 1279–1281.
54 Singh VK *et al*. Combined treatment of mice with *Panax ginseng* extract and interferon inducer. *Planta Med* 1983; 47: 235–236.
55 Singh VK *et al*. Immunomodulatory activity of *Panax ginseng* extract. *Planta Med* 1984; 50: 462–465.
56 Engels HJ *et al*. Effects of ginseng on secretory IgA, performance, and recovery from interval exercise. *Med Sci Sports Exercise* 2003; 35(4): 690–696.
57 Engels HJ *et al*. Failure of chronic ginseng supplementation to affect work performance and energy metabolism in healthy adult females. *Nutrition Res* 1996; 16(8): 1295–1305.
58 Engels HJ, Wirth JC. No ergogenic effects of ginseng (*Panax ginseng* C.A.Meyer) during graded maximal aerobic exercise. *J Am Diet Assoc* 1997; 97: 1110–1115.
59 Allen JD *et al*. Ginseng supplementation does not enhance healthy young adults' peak aerobic exercise performance. *J Am Coll Nut* 1998; 17(5): 462–466.
60 Kennedy DO, Scholey AB. Ginseng: potential for the enhancement of cognitive performance and mood. *Pharmacol Biochem Behav* 2003; 75: 687–700.
61 Kennedy DO *et al*. Electroencephalograph effects of single doses of *Ginkgo biloba* and *Panax ginseng* in healthy young volunteers. *Pharmacol Biochem Behav* 2003; 75: 701–709.
62 Reay JL *et al*. Single doses of Panax ginseng (G115) reduce blood glucose levels and improve cognitive performance during sustained mental activity. *J Psychopharmacol* 2005; 19(4): 357–365.
63 Kennedy DO *et al*. Improved cognitive performance in human volunteers following administration of guarana (*Paullinia cupana*) extract: comparison and interaction with *Panax ginseng*. *Pharmacol Biochem Behav* 2004; 79: 401–411.
64 Scholey AB, Kennedy DO. Acute, dose-dependent cognitive effects of *Ginkgo biloba*, *Panax ginseng* and their combination in healthy young volunteers: differential interactions with cognitive demand. *Hum Psychopharmacol Clin Exp* 2002; 17: 35–44.
65 Wesnes KA *et al*. The memory enhancing effects of a *Ginkgo biloba/Panax ginseng* combination in healthy middle-aged volunteers. *Psychopharmacology* 2000; 152: 353–361.
66 Wesnes KA *et al*. The cognitive, subjective, and physical effects of a *Ginkgo biloba/Panax ginseng* combination in healthy volunteers with neurasthenic complaints. *Psychopharmacol Bull* 1997; 33(4): 677–683.
67 Sievenpiper JL *et al*. Variable effects of American ginseng: a batch of American ginseng (*Panax quinquefolius* L.) with a depressed ginsenoside profile does not affect postprandial glycemia. *Eur J Clin Nut* 2003; 57: 243–248.
68 Vuksan V *et al*. American ginseng (*Panax quinquefolius* L.) reduces postprandial glycemia in nondiabetic subjects and subjects with type 2 diabetes mellitus. *Arch Intern Med* 2000; 160: 1009–1013.
69 Vuksan V *et al*. American ginseng improves glycemia in individuals with normal glucose tolerance: effect of dose and time escalation. *J Am Coll Nut* 2000; 19(6): 738–744.
70 Vuksan V *et al*. American ginseng (*Panax quinquefolius* L.) attenuates postprandial glycemia in a time-dependent but not dose-dependent manner in healthy individuals. *Am J Clin Nutr* 2001; 73: 753–758.
71 Sievenpiper JL *et al*. Null and opposing effects of Asian ginseng (*Panax ginseng* C.A.Meyer) on acute glycemia: results of two acute dose escalation studies. *J Am Coll Nutr* 2003; 22(6): 524–532.
72 Scaglione F *et al*. Immunomodulatory effects of two extracts of *Panax ginseng* C.A.Meyer. *Drugs Exptl Clin Res* 1990; 16(10): 537–542.
73 Yun TK, Choi SY. A case-control study of ginseng intake and cancer. *Int J Epidemiol* 1990; 19(4): 871–876.
74 Yun TK, Choi SY. Preventive effect of ginseng intake against various human cancers: a case-control study on 1987 pairs. *Cancer Epidemiol Biomarkers Prev* 1995; 4(4): 401–408.
75 Yun TK, Choi SY. Non-organ specific cancer prevention of ginseng: a prospective study in Korea. *Int J Epidemiol* 1998; 27: 359–364.
76 Yun TK *Panax ginseng* – a non-organ-specific cancer preventive. *Lancet Oncol* 2001; 2: 49–55.
77 Shin HR *et al*. The cancer-preventive potential of *Panax ginseng*: a review of human and experimental evidence. *Cancer Causes Control* 2000; 11: 565–576.
78 Coleman CI *et al*. The effects of *Panax ginseng* on quality of life. *J Clin Pharm Ther* 2003; 28: 5–15.
79 Cardinal BJ, Engels H-J. Ginseng does not enhance psychological well-being in healthy young adults: results of a double-blind, placebo-controlled, randomized clinical trial. *J Am Diet Assoc* 2001; 101: 655–660.
80 Lee FC *et al*. Effects of *Panax ginseng* on blood alcohol clearance in man. *Clin Exp Pharmac Physiol* 1987; 14: 543–546.
81 Coon JT, Ernst E. *Panax ginseng*. A systematic review of adverse effects and drug interactions. *Drug Safety* 2002; 25(5): 323–344.
82 Hopkins MP *et al*. Ginseng face cream and unexplained vaginal bleeding. *Am J Obstet Gynecol* 1988; 159: 1121–1122.
83 Gonzalez-Seijo JC *et al*. Manic episode and ginseng: report of a possible case. *J Clin Psychopharmacol* 1995; 15: 447–448.
84 Engelberg D *et al*. A case of ginseng-induced mania. *J Clin Psychopharmacol* 2001; 21(5): 535–537.
85 Vigibase, WHO Adverse Reactions database, Uppsala Monitoring Centre [accessed January 24, 2006].
86 Mkrtchyan A *et al*. A phase I clinical study of *Andrographis paniculata* fixed combination Kan Jang™ versus ginseng and valerian on the semen quality of healthy male subjects. *Phytomedicine* 2005; 12: 403–409.
87 Siegel RK. Ginseng abuse syndrome – problems with the panacea. *JAMA* 1979; 241: 1614–1615.
88 Siegel RK. Ginseng and high blood pressure. *JAMA* 1980; 243: 3.
89 Berté F. *Toxicological investigation of the standardized ginseng extract G115 after unique administration [LD_{50}]*. Manufacturer's data, on file. 1982, pp. 1–12.
90 Hess FG *et al*. Reproduction study in rats of ginseng extract G115. *Food Chem Toxicol* 1982; 20: 189–192.
91 Hess FG *et al*. Effects of subchronic feeding of ginseng extract G115 in beagle dogs. *Food Chem Toxicol* 1983; 21: 95–97.
92 Trabucchi E. *Toxicological and pharmacological investigation of Geriatric Pharmaton. Manufacturer's data on file*. 1971, pp. 1–22.
93 Savel J. *Toxicological report on Geriatric Pharmaton. Manufacturer's data on file*. 1971, pp. 1–31.

G

94 Chang YS *et al*. Evaluation of the mutagenic potential of American ginseng (*Panax quinquefolius*). *Planta Med* 1986; 52: 338.
95 Shader RI, Greenblatt DJ. Phenelzine and the dream machine: ramblings and reflections [abstract]. *J Clin Psychopharmacol* 1985; 5: 65.
96 Shader RI *et al*. Bees, ginseng and MAOIs revisited. *J Clin Psychopharmacol* 1988; 8: 235.
97 Jones BD *et al*. Interaction of ginseng with phenelzine. *J Clin Psychopharmacol* 1987; 7: 201–202.
98 Janetzky K, Morreale AP. Probable interaction between warfarin and ginseng. *Am J Health Syst Pharm* 1997; 54: 692–693.
99 Jiang X *et al*. Effect of St John's wort and ginseng on the pharmacokinetics and pharmacodynamics of warfarin in healthy subjects. *Br J Clin Pharmacol* 2004; 57(5): 592–599.
100 Yuan CS *et al*. American ginseng reduces warfarin's effect in healthy patients. A randomized, controlled trial. *Ann Intern Med* 2004; 141: 23–27.
101 Anderson GD *et al*. Drug interaction potential of soy extract and *Panax ginseng*. *J Clin Pharmacol* 2003; 43: 643–648.
102 Chang TKH *et al*. *In vitro* effect of standardized ginseng extracts and individual ginsenosides on the catalytic activity of human CYP1A1, CYP1A2, and CYP1B1. *Drug Metab Disp* 2002; 30: 378–384.
103 Chan LY *et al*. An in-vitro study of ginsenoside Rb1-induced teratogenicity using a whole rat embryo model. *Human Reproduction* 2003; 18(10): 2166–2168.

Golden Seal

Summary and Pharmaceutical Comment

Golden seal is characterised by the isoquinoline alkaloid constituents. These compounds, primarily hydrastine and berberine, represent the main active components of golden seal. Several activities have been documented for the alkaloid constituents and many of these support the traditional herbal uses of the root. However, rigorous clinical investigations of efficacy and safety are limited. In view of the pharmacological properties of the alkaloid constituents, excessive use of golden seal should be avoided.

Species (Family)

Hydrastis canadensis L. (Ranunculaceae)

Synonym(s)

Xanthorhiza simplicissima Marsh., Yellow Root

Part(s) Used

Rhizome, root

Pharmacopoeial and Other Monographs

AHP(G1)
BHC 1992(G6)
BHP 1996(G9)
BP 2007(G84)
Martindale 35th edition(G85)
Ph Eur 2007(G81)
USP29/NF24(G86)

Legal Category (Licensed Products)

GSL(G37)

Alkaloids

hydrastine

berberine

canadine

Figure 1 Selected constituents of golden seal.

Constituents

The following is compiled from several sources, including General References G6, G40 and G62.

Alkaloids Isoquinoline-type. 2.5–6.0%. Hydrastine (major, 1.5–4.0%), berberine (0.5–6.0%), berberastine (2–3%), and canadine (1%), with lesser amounts of related alkaloids including candaline and canadaline.(1–3)

Other constituents Chlorogenic acid, carbohydrates, fatty acids (75% saturated, 25% unsaturated), volatile oil (trace), resin, meconin (meconinic acid lactone).

Food Use

Golden seal is not used in foods, although it is reported to be used in herbal teas.(G41) The concentration of berberine permitted in foods is limited to 0.1 mg/kg, and 10 mg/kg in alcoholic beverages.(G16)

Herbal Use

Golden seal is stated to be a stimulant to involuntary muscle, and to possess stomachic, oxytocic, antihaemorrhagic and laxative properties. Traditionally it has been used for digestive disorders, gastritis, peptic ulceration, colitis, anorexia, upper respiratory catarrh, menorrhagia, post-partum haemorrhage, dysmenorrhoea, topically for eczema, pruritus, otorrhoea, catarrhal deafness and tinnitus, conjunctivitis, and specifically for atonic dyspepsia with hepatic symptoms.(G6, G7, G8)

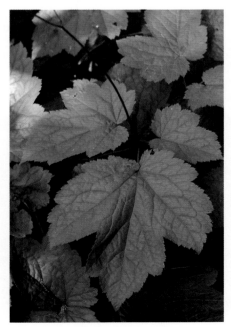

Figure 2 Golden seal (*Hydrastis canadensis*).

Dosage

Dosages for oral administration (adults) for traditional uses recommended in older and contemporary standard herbal and/or pharmaceutical reference texts are given below.

Dried rhizome 0.5–1.0 g as a decoction three times daily.[G6, G7]

Liquid extract of Hydrastis (BPC 1949) 0.3–1.0 mL.

Tincture of Hydrastis (BPC 1949) 2–4 mL.

Pharmacological Actions

The pharmacological activity of golden seal is attributed to the isoquinoline alkaloid constituents, primarily hydrastine and berberine,[3, 4] which are reported to have similar properties.[G41] Antibiotic, immunostimulant, anticonvulsant, sedative, hypotensive, uterotonic, choleretic and carminative activities have been described for berberine.[3]

G

In vitro and animal studies

Limited work has been documented for golden seal, although the pharmacology of berberine and hydrastine is well studied.

The total alkaloid fraction of golden seal has been reported to exhibit anticonvulsant activity in smooth muscle preparations (e.g. mouse intestine, uterus).[5] However, *in vitro*, canadine is reported to exhibit uterine stimulation in guinea-pig and rabbit tissues.[4] Berberine, canadine and hydrastine are all stated to exhibit utero-activity.[G30]

Berberine and hydrastine have produced a hypotensive effect in laboratory animals following intravenous administration.[6, 7, G41] High doses of hydrastine are documented to produce an increase in blood pressure.[7] *In vitro*, berberine has been reported to decrease the anticoagulant action of heparin in canine and human blood.[7]

Berberine is reported to exert a stimulant action on the heart and to increase coronary blood flow, although higher doses are stated to inhibit cardiac activity.[7]

Antimuscarinic and antihistamine actions have been documented for berberine.[7]

In rats, berberine has exhibited antipyretic activity three times as effective as aspirin.[3]

Berberine potentiated barbiturate sleeping time, but did not exhibit any analgesic or tranquillising effects.[7]

A broad spectrum of antimicrobial activity against bacteria, fungi, and protozoa has been reported for berberine. Sensitive organisms include *Staphylococcus* spp., *Streptococcus* spp., *Chlamydia aureus*, *Corynebacterium diphtheriae*, *Salmonella typhi*, *Diplococcus pneumoniae*, *Pseudomonas aeruginosa*, *Shigella dysenteriae*, *Trichomonas vaginalis*, *Neisseria gonorrhoeae*, *Neisseria meningitidis*, *Treponema pallidum*, *Giardia lamblia* and *Leishmania donovani*.[3] Berberine is reported to be effective against diarrhoeas caused by enterotoxins such as *Vibrio cholerae* and *Escherichia coli*.[7] *In vivo* and *in vitro* studies in hamsters and rats have reported significant activity for berberine against *Entamoeba histolytica*.[3]

Anticancer activity has been reported for berberine in B1, KB and PS tumour systems.[G22] In addition, berberine sulfate was found to inhibit the action of teleocidin, a known tumour promoter, on the formation of mouse skin tumours initiated with 7,12-dimethylbenz[*a*]anthracene.[5]

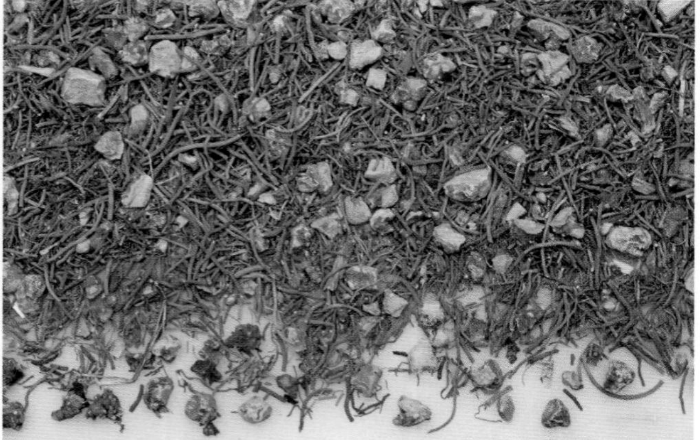

Figure 3 Golden seal – dried drug substance (rhizome, root).

Clinical studies

There is a lack of clinical research assessing the effects of golden seal and rigorous randomised controlled clinical trials are required. Berberine is stated to be effective in the treatment of acute diarrhoea on the basis of data from several clinical studies.[3] It has been found effective against diarrhoeas caused by *Escherichia coli*, *Shigella dysenteriae*, *Salmonella paratyphi* B, *Klebsiella*, *Giardia lamblia* and *Vibrio cholerae*.[3] Berberine has been used to treat trachoma, an infectious ocular disease caused by *Chlamydia trachomatis*, which is a major cause of blindness and impaired vision in developing countries.[3]

Clinical studies have shown berberine to stimulate bile and bilirubin secretion and to improve symptoms of chronic cholecystitis, and to correct raised concentrations of tyramine in patients with liver cirrhosis.[3]

Further investigation is required to determine whether or not the effects described for berberine also occur with golden seal.

Side-effects, Toxicity

There is a lack of clinical safety and toxicity data for golden seal and further investigation of these aspects is required. The alkaloid constituents are potentially toxic and symptoms of golden seal poisoning include stomach upset, nervous symptoms and depression; large quantities may even be fatal.[8] High doses of hydrastine are reported to cause exaggerated reflexes, convulsions, paralysis and death from respiratory failure.[4] The root may cause contact ulceration of mucosal surfaces.

Contra-indications, Warnings

Golden seal is contra-indicated in individuals with raised blood pressure.[G7, G22, G49] The alkaloid constituents of golden seal are potentially toxic and excessive use should be avoided.

Drug interactions None documented. However, in view of the documented pharmacological actions of golden seal and the alkaloid constituents, the potential for preparations of golden seal to interact with other medicines administered concurrently, particularly those with similar or opposing effects, should be considered.

Pregnancy and lactation Golden seal is contra-indicated for use during pregnancy.[3, G7, G49] Berberine, canadine, hydrastine and hydrastinine have all been reported to produce uterine stimulant activity.[G30] It is not known whether the alkaloids are excreted in breast milk. The use of golden seal during lactation should be avoided.

Preparations

Proprietary single-ingredient preparations

Germany: Gingivitol N.

Proprietary multi-ingredient preparations

Australia: Euphrasia Complex; Herbal Cleanse; Hydrastis Complex; Sambucus Complex; Urapro; Urinase. *Brazil:* Bromidrastina. *Canada:* Echinacea Goldenseal Formula. *France:* Climaxol. *Spain:* Proctosor; Solucion Schoum. *UK:* Digestive; Golden Seal Indigestion Tablets; HRI Golden Seal Digestive; Wind & Dyspepsia Relief. *USA:* Immune Support.

References

1 Gleye J *et al*. La canadaline: nouvel alcaloide d'*Hydrastis canadensis*. *Phytochemistry* 1974; 13: 675–676.

2 El-Masry S *et al*. Colorimetric and spectrophotometric determination of *Hydrastis* alkaloids in pharmaceutical preparations. *J Pharm Sci* 1980; 69: 597–598.

3 Pizzorno JE, Murray MT. *Hydrastis canadensis*, *Berberis vulgaris*, *Berberis aquitolium* and other berberine containing plants. In: *Textbook of Natural Medicine*. Seattle: John Bastyr College Publications, 1985 (looseleaf).

4 Genest K, Hughes DW. Natural products in Canadian pharmaceuticals iv. *Hydrastis canadensis*. *Can J Pharm Sci* 1969; 4: 41–45.

5 Nishino H *et al*. Berberine sulphate inhibits tumour-promoting activity of teleocidin in two-stage carcinogenesis on mouse skin. *Oncology* 1986; 43: 131–134.

6 Wisniewski W, Gorta T. Effect of temperature on the oxidation of hydrastine to hydrastinine in liquid extracts and rhizomes of *Hydrastis canadensis* in the presence of air and steam. *Acta Pol Pharm* 1969; 26: 313–317.

7 Preininger V. The pharmacology and toxicology of the Papaveraceae alkaloids. In: Manske RHF, Holmes HL, eds. *The Alkaloids*, vol 15. New York: Academic Press, 1975: 239.

8 Hardin JW, Arena JM. *Human Poisoning from Native and Cultivated Plants*, 2nd edn. Durham, North Carolina: Duke University Press, 1974.

Gravel Root

Summary and Pharmaceutical Comment

The chemistry of gravel root is poorly studied and no scientific evidence was located to justify the herbal uses. In view of the very limited information on the chemistry and pharmacological and toxicological effects of gravel root, excessive use and use during pregnancy and lactation should be avoided.

G

Species (Family)

Eupatorium purpureum L. (Asteraceae/Compositae)

Synonym(s)

E. trifoliatum L., Joe-Pye Weed, Kydney Root, Purple Boneset

Part(s) Used

Rhizome, root

Pharmacopoeial and Other Monographs

BHP 1983[G7]
Martindale 35th edition[G85]

Legal Category (Licensed Products)

GSL[G37]

Constituents

The following is compiled from several sources, including General References G20 and G40.

Little information is available on the chemistry of gravel root. It is stated to contain euparin (a benzofuran compound), eupatorin (a flavonoid), resin and volatile oil.

Other plant parts The herb is reported to contain echinatine, an unsaturated pyrrolizidine alkaloid.[1]

Food Use

Gravel root is not used in foods.

Herbal Use

Gravel root is stated to possess antilithic, diuretic and antirheumatic properties. Traditionally, it has been used for urinary calculus, cystitis, dysuria, urethritis, prostatitis, rheumatism, gout, and specifically for renal or vesicular calculi.[G7,G64]

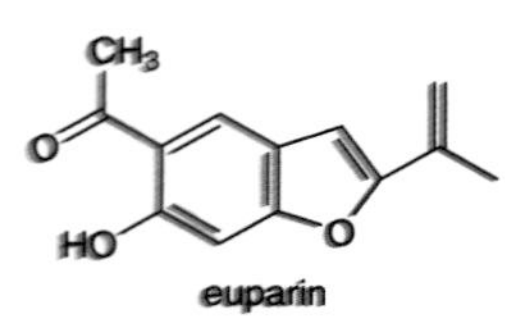

Benzofurans

CH_3

HO

euparin

Figure 1 Selected constituents of gravel root.

Dosage

Dosages for oral administration (adults) for traditional uses recommended in standard herbal reference texts are given below.

Dried rhizome/root 2–4 g as a decoction three times daily.[G7]

Liquid extract 2–4 mL (1 : 1 in 25% alcohol) three times daily.[G7]

Tincture 1–2 mL (1 : 5 in 40% alcohol) three times daily.[G7]

Pharmacological Actions

None documented.

Clinical studies

There is a lack of clinical research assessing the effects of gravel root and rigorous randomised controlled clinical trials are required.

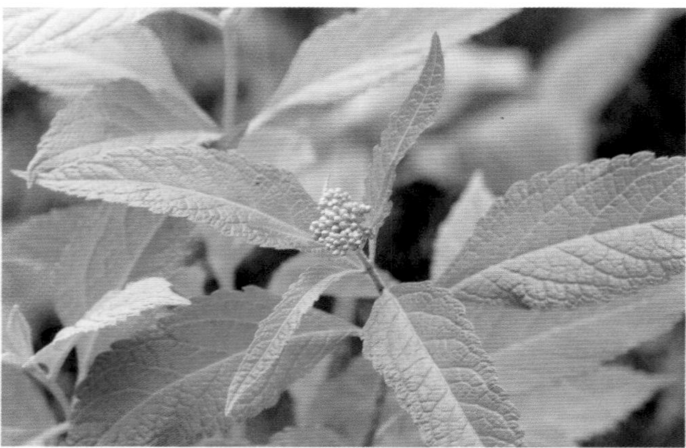

Figure 2 Gravel root (*Eupatorium purpureum*).

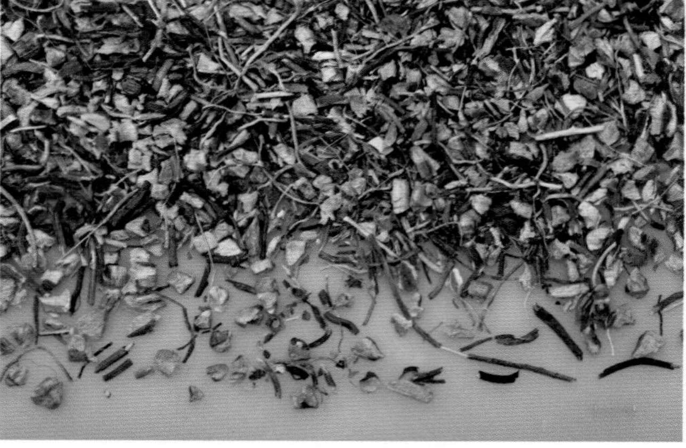

Figure 3 Gravel root – dried drug substance (root).

Side-effects, Toxicity

None documented although there is a lack of clinical safety and toxicity data for gravel root and further investigation of these aspects is required. Pyrrolizidine alkaloids are constituents of many species of *Eupatorium*.[1, G20] Pyrrolizidine alkaloids with an unsaturated pyrrolizidine nucleus are reported to be hepatotoxic in both animals and humans (*see* Comfrey). An unsaturated pyrrolizidine alkaloid, echinatine, has been reported for the aerial parts of gravel root.

Contra-indications, Warnings

None documented. However, there is very limited chemical and pharmacological information available for gravel root and this should be considered when assessing whether or not use of gravel root is appropriate.

Drug interactions None documented. However, there is very limited chemical and pharmacological information available for gravel root and the potential for preparations of gravel root to interact with other medicines administered concurrently should be considered.

Pregnancy and lactation The safety of gravel root has not been established. In view of the lack of phytochemical, pharmacological and toxicological information the use of gravel root during pregnancy and lactation should be avoided.

Preparations

Proprietary multi-ingredient preparations

UK: Backache.

G

Reference

1 *Pyrrolizidine Alkaloids. Environmental Health Criteria 80*. Geneva: WHO, 1988.

Ground Ivy

Summary and Pharmaceutical Comment

The chemistry of ground ivy is well studied. Documented pharmacological activities for constituents of ground ivy support some of the herbal uses, although there is a lack of clinical research assessing the effects of ground ivy and rigorous randomised controlled clinical trials are required. In view of the lack of safety and toxicity data, and the reported cytotoxic activity of ursolic acid, excessive use of ground ivy and use during pregnancy and lactation should be avoided.

Species (Family)

Glechoma hederacea L. (Labiatae)

Synonym(s)

Nepeta hederacea (L.) Trevis, *N. glechoma* Benth.

Part(s) Used

Herb

Pharmacopoeial and Other Monographs

BHC 1992[G6]
BHP 1996[G9]
Martindale 35th edition[G85]

Legal Category (Licensed Products)

GSL[G37]

Constituents

The following is compiled from several sources, including General Reference G6.

Amino acids Asparagic acid, glutamic acid, proline, tyrosine and valine.

Flavonoids Flavonol glycosides (e.g. hyperoside, isoquercitrin, rutin) and flavone glycosides (e.g. luteolin diglucoside, cosmosyin, cynaroside and cosmoriin).[1]

Steroids β-Sitosterol.

Terpenoids Oleanolic acid, α-ursolic acid, β-ursolic acid.[2]

Volatile oils 0.03–0.06%. Various terpenoid components including *p*-cymene, linalool, limonene, menthone, α-pinene, β-pinene, pinocamphone, pulegone and terpineol; glechomafuran (a sesquiterpene).[3]

Other constituents Palmitic acid and other fatty acids, rosmarinic acid, succinic acid, bitter principle (glechomin), choline, gum, diterpene lactone (marrubiin), saponin, tannin and wax.

Food Use

Ground ivy is listed by the Council of Europe as a natural source of food flavouring (category N3). This category indicates that ground ivy can be added to foodstuffs in the traditionally accepted manner, although there is insufficient information available for an adequate assessment of potential toxicity.[G16]

Herbal Use

Ground ivy is stated to possess mild expectorant, anticatarrhal, astringent, vulnerary, diuretic and stomachic properties. Traditionally, it has been used for bronchitis, tinnitus, diarrhoea, haemorrhoids, cystitis, gastritis, and specifically for chronic bronchial catarrh.[G6, G7, G8, G49, G64]

Dosage

Dosages for oral administration (adults) for traditional uses recommended in standard herbal reference texts are given below.

Dried herb 2–4 g as an infusion three times daily.[G6, G7]

Liquid extract 2–4 mL (1 : 1 in 25% alcohol) three times daily.[G6, G7]

Pharmacological Actions

In vitro and animal studies

In vivo anti-inflammatory activity has been reported for an ethanolic extract of ground ivy, which was stated to exhibit a moderate inhibition (27%) of carrageenan-induced rat paw oedema.[4]

Ursolic acid analogues, 2α- and 2β-hydroxyursolic acid, have been documented to provide significant ulcer-protective activity in mice.[5]

The astringent activity documented for ground ivy has been attributed to rosmarinic acid, a polyphenolic acid.[6]

Glechomin and marrubiin are stated to be bitter principles, and α-terpineol is known to be an antiseptic component of volatile oils.[G48, G49]

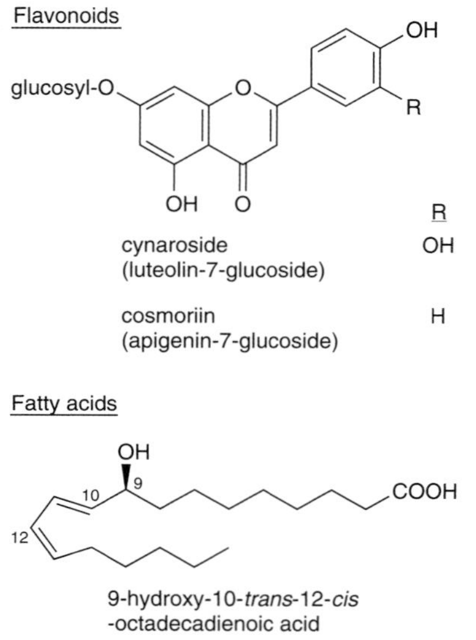

Flavonoids

	R
cynaroside (luteolin-7-glucoside)	OH
cosmoriin (apigenin-7-glucoside)	H

Fatty acids

9-hydroxy-10-*trans*-12-*cis*-octadecadienoic acid

Figure 1 Selected constituents of ground ivy.

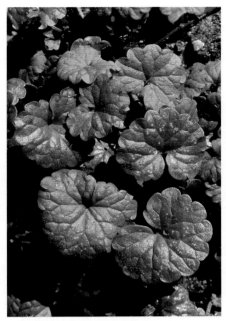

Figure 2 Ground ivy (*Glechoma hederacea*).

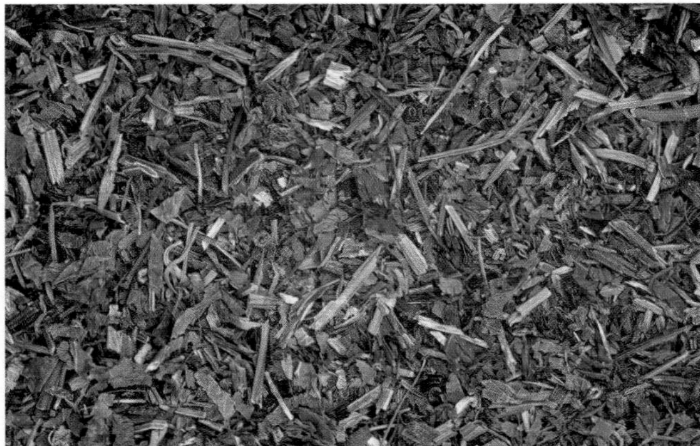

Figure 3 Ground ivy – dried drug substance (herb).

Anti-inflammatory and astringent properties are generally associated with flavonoids and tannins, respectively. Anti-inflammatory properties have been documented for rosmarinic acid (*see* Rosemary).

In vitro antiviral activity against the Epstein–Barr virus has been documented for ursolic acid.[7] Both oleanolic and ursolic acids were found to inhibit tumour production by TPA in mouse skin, with activity comparable to that of retinoic acid, a known tumour-promoter inhibitor.[7]

Significant cytotoxic activity has also been reported for ursolic acid in lymphocytic leukaemia (P-388, L-1210) and human lung carcinoma (A-549), and marginal activity in KB cells, human colon (HCT-8), and mammary (MCF-7) tumour cells.[8]

Clinical studies

There is a lack of clinical research assessing the effects of ground ivy and rigorous randomised controlled clinical trials are required.

Side-effects, Toxicity

There is a lack of clinical safety and toxicity data for ground ivy and further investigation of these aspects is required.

Poisoning in cattle and horses has been documented in Eastern Europe.[9] Symptoms include accelerated weak pulse, difficulty in breathing, conjunctival haemorrhage, elevated temperature, dizziness, spleen enlargement, dilation of the caecum, and gastroenteritis revealed at post-mortem. Antitumour and cytotoxic activities have been reported for oleanolic and ursolic acids (*see* Pharmacological Actions, *In vitro* and animal studies).

Ground ivy volatile oil contains many terpenoids and terpene-rich volatile oils are irritant to the gastrointestinal tract and kidneys. Pulegone is an irritant, hepatotoxic, and abortifacient principle of the volatile oil of pennyroyal. However, in comparison with pennyroyal the overall yield of volatile oil is much less (0.03–0.06% in ground ivy and 1–2% in pennyroyal).

Contra-indications, Warnings

Ground ivy is contra-indicated in epilepsy[G7] although no rationale for this statement has been found. Excessive doses may be irritant to the gastrointestinal mucosa and should be avoided by individuals with existing renal disease.

Drug interactions None documented. However, the potential for preparations of ground ivy to interact with other medicines administered concurrently, particularly those with similar or opposing effects, should be considered.

Pregnancy and lactation The safety of ground ivy has not been established. In view of the lack of toxicity data and the possible irritant and abortifacient action of the volatile oil, the use of ground ivy during pregnancy and lactation should be avoided.

Preparations

Proprietary multi-ingredient preparations

UK: Gerard House Water Relief Tablets; Water Naturtabs.

References

1 Zieba J. Isolation and identification of flavonoids from *Glechoma hederacea*. *Pol J Pharmacol Pharm* 1973; 25: 593–597.

2 Zieba J. Isolation and identification of nonheteroside triterpenoids from *Glechoma hederacea*. *Pol J Pharmacol Pharm* 1973; 25: 587–592.

3 Stahl E, Datta SN. New sesquiterpenoids of the ground ivy (*Glechoma hederacea*). *Justus Liebigs Ann Chem* 1972; 757: 23–32.

4 Mascolo N *et al*. Biological screening of Italian medicinal plants for anti-inflammatory activity. *Phytother Res* 1987; 1: 28–31.

5 Okuyama E *et al*. Isolation and identification of ursolic acid-related compounds as the principles of *Glechoma hederacea* having an antiulcerogenic activity. *Shoyakugaku Zasshi* 1983; 37: 52–55.

6 Okuda T *et al*. The components of tannic activities in Labiatae plants. I. Rosmarinic acid from Labiatae plants in Japan. *Yakugaku Zasshi* 1986; 106: 1108–1111.

7 Tokuda H *et al*. Inhibitory effects of ursolic and oleanolic acid on skin tumor promotion by 12-O-tetradecanoylphorbol-13-acetate. *Cancer Lett* 1986; 33: 279–285.

8 Lee K-H *et al*. The cytotoxic principles of *Prunella vulgaris*, *Psychotria serpens*, and *Hyptis capitata*: Ursolic acid and related derivatives. *Planta Med* 1988; 54: 308.

9 MAFF. *Poisonous Plants in Britain*. London: HMSO, 1984: 139.

Guaiacum

Summary and Pharmaceutical Comment

Guaiacum is characterised by the resin fraction of the heartwood and much has been documented on the constituents (principally lignans) of the resin, although little is known regarding other constituents. No scientific information was found to justify the herbal use of guaiacum as an antirheumatic or anti-inflammatory agent. In view of the lack of toxicity data, excessive use of guaiacum and use during pregnancy and lactation should be avoided.

Species (Family)

Guaiacum officinale L. (Zygophyllaceae)
Guaiacum sanctum L.

Synonym(s)

Guaiac, Guajacum, Guayacar, Lignum Vitae, Palo Santo

Part(s) Used

Resin obtained from the heartwood

Pharmacopoeial and Other Monographs

BHC 1992[G6]
BHP 1996[G9]
Complete German Commission E[G3]
Martindale 35th edition[G85]

Legal Category (Licensed Products)

GSL[G37]

Constituents

The following is compiled from several sources, including General Reference G6.

Resins 15–20%. Guaiaretic acid, dehydroguaiaretic acid, guaiacin, isoguaiacin, α-guaiaconic acid (lignans), furoguaiacin and its monomethyl ether, furoguaiacidin, tetrahydrofuroguaiacin-A and tetrahydrofuroguaiacin-B (furano-lignans), furoguaia oxidin (enedione lignan).[1–4]

Steroids β-Sitosterol.

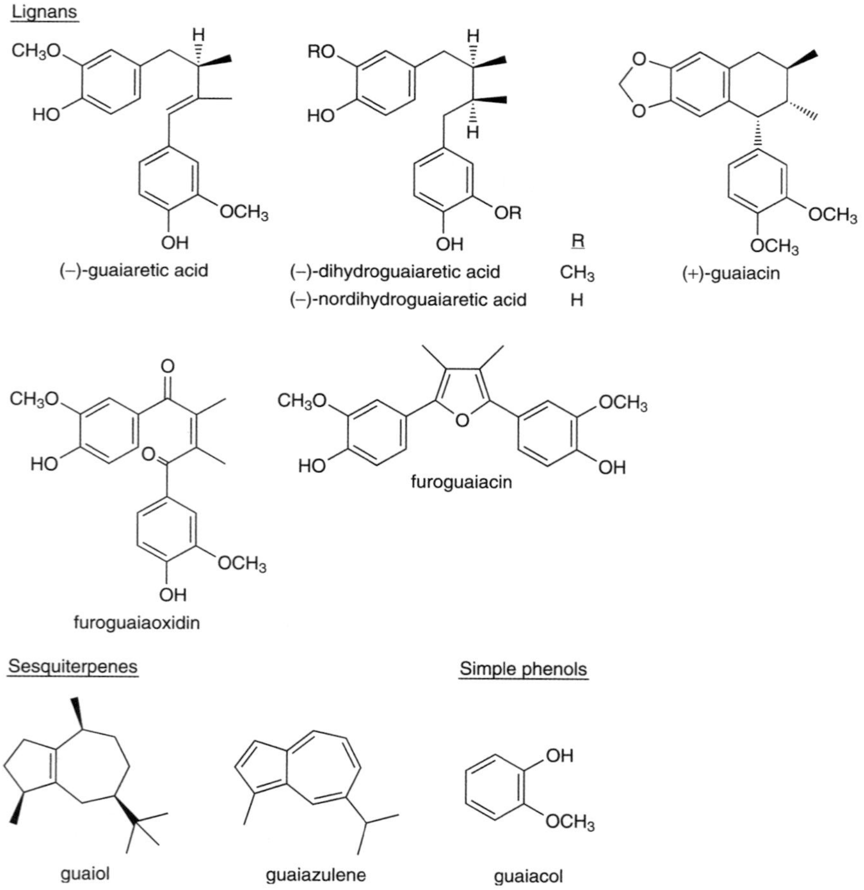

Lignans

(−)-guaiaretic acid

(−)-dihydroguaiaretic acid — R = CH_3
(−)-nordihydroguaiaretic acid — R = H

(+)-guaiacin

furoguaiaoxidin

furoguaiacin

Sesquiterpenes

guaiol

guaiazulene

Simple phenols

guaiacol

Figure 1 Selected constituents of guaiacum.

Terpenoids Saponins, oleanolic acid.[5,6] Sesquiterpenes, including guaiol and guaiazulene.

Food Use

Guaiacum is listed by the Council of Europe as a natural source of food flavouring (category N2). This category indicates that guaiacum can be added to foodstuffs in small quantities, with a possible limitation of an active principle (as yet unspecified) in the final product.[G16]

Herbal Use

Guaiacum is stated to possess antirheumatic, anti-inflammatory, diuretic, mild laxative and diaphoretic properties. Traditionally, it has been used for subacute rheumatism, prophylaxis against gout, and specifically for chronic rheumatism and rheumatoid arthritis.[G6, G7, G8, G64]

Dosage

Dosages for oral administration (adults) for traditional uses recommended in older standard herbal and/or pharmaceutical reference texts are given below.

Dried wood 1–2 g as a decoction three times daily.[G6, G7]

Liquid extract 1–2 mL (1 : 1 in 80% alcohol) three times daily.[G6, G7]

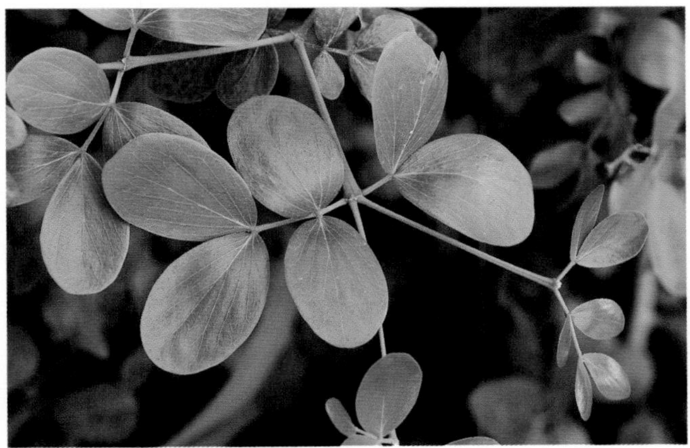

Figure 2 Guaiacum (*Guaiacum officinale*).

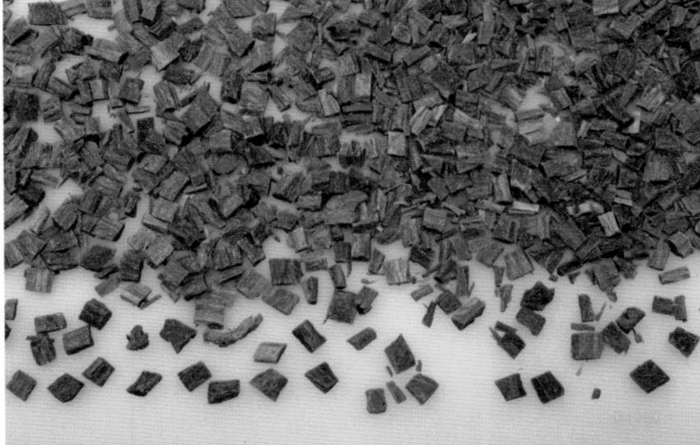

Figure 3 Guaiacum – dried drug substance (wood).

Tincture of Guaiacum (BPC 1934) 2–4 mL.

Pharmacological Actions

In vitro and animal studies

None documented. Antimicrobial properties are associated with lignans and much has been documented for nordihydroguaiaretic acid, the principal lignan constituent in chaparral (*see* Chaparral).

Clinical studies

There is a lack of clinical research assessing the effects of guaiacum and rigorous randomised controlled clinical trials are required.

Side-effects, Toxicity

There is a lack of clinical safety and toxicity data for guaiacum and further investigation of these aspects is required.

Guaiacum resin has been reported to cause contact dermatitis.[G51] The resin is documented to be of low toxicity; the oral LD_{50} in rats is greater than 5 g/kg body weight.[G48]

Contra-indications, Warnings

It is recommended that guaiacum is avoided by individuals with hypersensitive, allergic or acute inflammatory conditions.[G49]

Drug interactions None documented. However, there is limited pharmacological information for guaiacum, and the potential for preparations of guaiacum to interact with other medicines administered concurrently should be considered.

Pregnancy and lactation The safety of guaiacum during pregnancy has not been established. In view of this, and the overall lack of pharmacological and toxicological data, the use of guaiacum during pregnancy and lactation should be avoided.

Preparations

Proprietary multi-ingredient preparations

Australia: Boswellia Compound; Guaiacum Complex. *Switzerland:* Pommade au Baume. *UK:* Gerard House Reumalex; Rheumatic Pain Relief; Rheumatic Pain Remedy; Rheumatic Pain.

References

1 King FE, Wilson JG. The chemistry of extractives from hardwoods. Part XXXVI. The lignans of *Guaiacum officinale* L. *J Chem Soc* 1964; 4011–4024.

2 Kratochvil JF *et al.* Isolation and characterization of α-guaiaconic acid and the nature of guaiacum blue. *Phytochemistry* 1971; 10: 2529–3251.

3 Majumder PL, Bhattacharyya M. Structure of furoguaiacidin: a new furanoid lignan of the heartwood of *Guaiacum officinale* L. *Chem Ind* 1974; 77–78.

4 Majumder P, Bhattacharyya M. Furoguaiaoxidin – a new enedione lignan of *Guaiacum officinale*: a novel method of sequential introduction of alkoxy functions in the 3- and 4-methyl groups of 2,5-diaryl-3,4-dimethylfurans. *JCS Chem Commun* 1975; 702–703.

5 Ahmad VU *et al.* Officigenin, a new sapogenin of *Guaiacum officinale*. *J Nat Prod* 1984; 47: 977–982.

6 Ahmad VU *et al.* Guaianin, a new saponin from *Guaiacum officinale*. *J Nat Prod* 1986; 49: 784–786.

Hawthorn

Summary and Pharmaceutical Comment

Hawthorn is characterised by its phenolic constituents, in particular the flavonoid components to which many of the pharmacological properties associated with hawthorn have been attributed. The phytochemistry of hawthorn fruit and hawthorn leaf with flower are, in general, qualitatively similar, although separate monographs for the fruit (berries) and leaf with flowers appear in the British Pharmacopoeia and European Pharmacopoeia.(G81, G84) Pharmacological actions documented following preclinical and clinical studies support some of the traditional uses of hawthorn, although clinical evidence is limited to preparations containing hawthorn leaf with flower.

A systematic review and meta-analysis of 13 randomised, double-blind, placebo-controlled trials of standardised extracts of hawthorn leaf and flower in patients with chronic heart failure found that the products assessed were beneficial as adjunctive treatments in patients with chronic heart failure, but there is insufficient evidence to support the use of hawthorn extract alone in the treatment of chronic heart failure. Further well-designed randomised controlled trials are necessary to confirm the findings.

Data from randomised controlled trials and post-marketing surveillance studies suggest that the hawthorn preparations assessed are well-tolerated when taken at recommended dosages. However, results cannot necessarily be extrapolated to other hawthorn products, which may differ qualitatively and quantitatively in their chemical content. Further well-designed post-marketing surveillance studies are required to assess the safety of hawthorn extracts, including with long-term use. In view of the documented pharmacological actions of hawthorn the potential for preparations of hawthorn to interfere with other medicines administered concurrently, particularly those with similar or opposing effects, including antihypertensive, antihypotensive, and inotropic agents, should be considered. Hawthorn fruit or hawthorn leaf and flower are contraindicated during pregnancy and breastfeeding.

Species (Family)

**Crataegus laevigata* (Poir.) DC. (Rosaceae)
†*Crataegus monogyna* Jacq.

Synonym(s)

**C. oxyacanthoides* Thuill., *C. oxyacantha* auct.
†*Crataegus oxyacantha* L., nom. ambig.

Part(s) Used

Fruit, leaf, flower

Pharmacopoeial and Other Monographs

American Herbal Pharmacopoeia(G1)
BHP 1996(G9)
BP 2007(G84)
BHMA 2003(G66)
Complete German Commission E(G3)
ESCOP 2003(G76)
Martindale 35th edition(G85)
Ph Eur 2007(G81)
WHO volume 2(G70)

Legal Category (Licensed Products)

Hawthorn is not included in the GSL.(G37)

Constituents

The following is compiled from several sources, including General References G1 and G2.

Amines Phenylethylamine, *O*-methoxyphenethylamine and tyramine.(1)

Flavonoids Up to 1%.(G81) Flavonol (e.g. kaempferol, quercetin) and flavone (e.g. apigenin, luteolin) derivatives, rutin, hyperoside, vitexin glycosides, orientin glycosides.(2–5) The fruits contain relatively more hyperoside and the leaves relatively more vitexin glycosides.(G75)

Tannins Proanthocyanins (catechin-type oligomers).(6, 7)

Other constituents Cyanogenetic glycosides and saponins.

Quality of plant material and commercial products

As with other herbal medicinal products, there can be variation in the qualitative and quantitative composition of hawthorn crude plant material and commercial preparations of hawthorn fruit and/or leaf with flower. According to the British and European Pharmacopoeias, hawthorn leaf with flower consists of the whole or cut, dried flower-bearing tops of *C. laevigata* or *C. monogyna* (or rarely certain other *Crataegus* species), and contains not less than 1.5% of flavonoids, expressed as hyperoside and calculated with reference to the dried drug.(G81, G84) Detailed descriptions of hawthorn berry and leaf with flower for use in botanical, microscopic and macroscopic identification have been published, along with qualitative and quantitative methods for the assessment of hawthorn berry and leaf with flower raw material.(G1)

Aqueous-alcoholic (40–70% ethanol or methanol) extracts of hawthorn leaf with flower obtained from several different manufacturers were reported to have a similar profile of constituents (procyanidins, flavonoids, total vitexin and total phenols) both qualitatively and quantitatively, whereas an aqueous extract was stated to have a lower concentration of procyanidins, flavonoids and total phenols, and a similar total vitexin content.(8) However, no statistical analyses were described to support these findings and there were in fact also substantial quantitative variations between aqueous-alcoholic extracts in content of procyanidins (8.7–13.5%), flavonoids calculated as hyperoside (1.1–3.4%), vitexin-2"-*O*-rhamnoside and hyperoside (5.7–7.9%), total vitexins (4.1–4.9%) and total phenols (19.5–25.6%); values for these constituents for the aqueous extract were 8.0%, 0.7%, 5.6%, 4.1% and 14.0%, respectively. Further work showed that all the extracts had a relaxant effect on norepinephrine (noradrenaline)-induced contractions of guineapig aortic rings *in vitro*, achieving relaxations of 29–44% of baseline values. EC_{50} (effective concentration) values were between 4.2–9.8 mg/mL for the aqueous-alcoholic extracts and 22.4 mg/mL for the aqueous extract, although maximum effects were similar for all extracts.[8] The positive control milrinone had a significantly greater effect than any of the extracts (EC_{50} 1.3 mg/mL). Basic statistical analyses indicated that there were no statistically significant differences between the aqueous-alcoholic extracts in terms of their relaxant effects, indicating pharmacological equivalence. However, more sophisticated analysis allowing for multiple analyses indicated that the effects of the 40% ethanol and 55% methanol extracts differed significantly from those of the other aqueous-alcoholic extracts. These findings provide some support for the equivalence of 40–70% ethanol or methanol extracts of hawthorn leaf with flower,[8] although this would be strengthened by more consistent results in further studies. The equivalence of preparations of hawthorn fruit also requires investigation.

Food Use

Hawthorn is not commonly used in foods. It is listed by the Council of Europe as a natural source of food flavouring (category N2). This category indicates that hawthorn can be added to foodstuffs in small quantities, with a possible limitation of an active principle (as yet unspecified) in the final product.[G16]

Herbal Use

Hawthorn fruit is stated to possess cardiotonic, coronary vasodilator and hypotensive properties. Traditionally, it has been used for cardiac failure, myocardial weakness, paroxysmal tachycardia, hypertension, arteriosclerosis and Buerger's disease.[G3, G7] The German Commission E did not approve therapeutic use of the fruit.[G3] Modern interest in hawthorn is focused on the use of hawthorn leaf with flower in reduced cardiac performance.[G3]

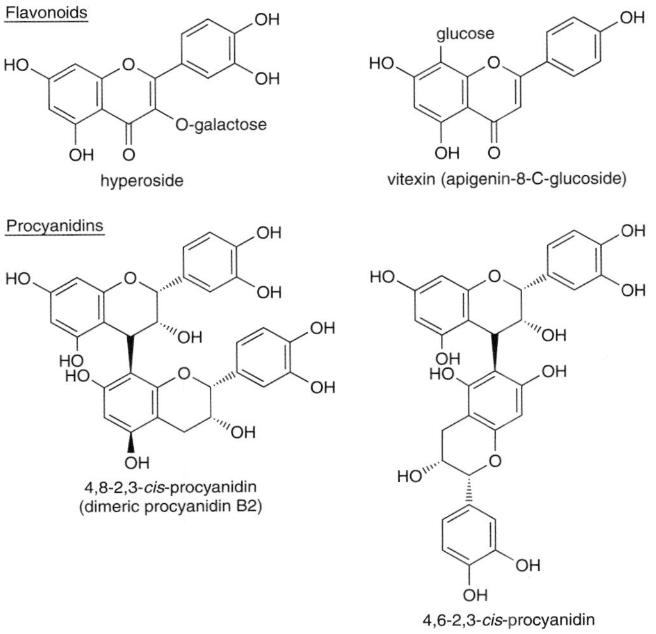

Flavonoids

hyperoside

vitexin (apigenin-8-C-glucoside)

Procyanidins

4,8-2,3-*cis*-procyanidin (dimeric procyanidin B2)

4,6-2,3-*cis*-procyanidin

Figure 1 Selected constituents of hawthorn.

Dosage

Dosages for oral administration (adults) for traditional uses recommended in older standard herbal reference texts are given below.

Fruit

Dried fruit 0.3–1.0 g as an infusion three times daily.[G7]

Liquid extract 0.5–1.0 mL (1 : 1 in 25% alcohol) three times daily.[G7]

Tincture 1–2 mL (1 : 5 in 45% alcohol) three times daily.[G7]

Leaf with flower For the treatment of decreasing cardiac efficiency corresponding to functional stage II of the New York Heart Association 160–900 mg aqueous-alcoholic extract (ethanol 45% v/v or methanol 70% v/v; drug to extract ratio 4–7 : 1, with defined flavonoid and/or procyanidin content corresponding to 3.5–19.8 mg flavonoids, calculated as hyperoside, and 30–168.7 mg

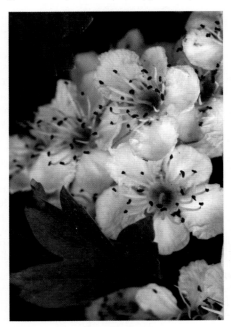

Figure 2 Hawthorn (*Crataegus laevigata*).

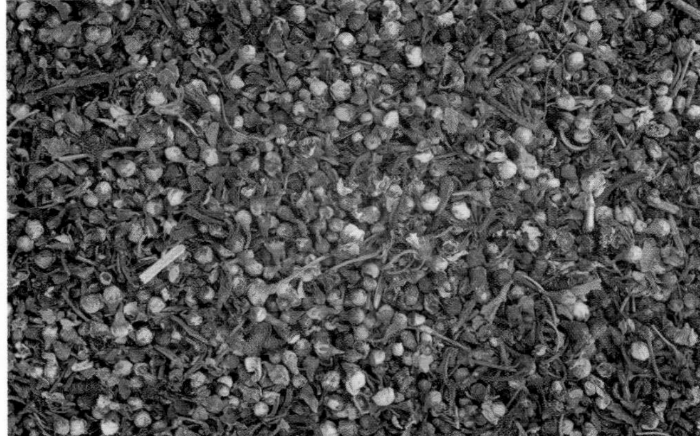

Figure 3 Hawthorn – dried drug substance (fruit and leaf).

procyanidins, calculated as epicatechin) daily, in two to three divided doses.[G3]

Clinical trials of hawthorn leaf with flower in patients with different stages of heart failure (according to the NYHA classification) mainly have assessed the effects of a standardised extract (WS-1442, containing 18.8% oligomeric procyanidins) administered orally at doses ranging from 160–1800 mg daily for up to 16 weeks.

Pharmacological Actions

In vitro and animal studies

Pharmacokinetics There are only limited data available on the pharmacokinetics of constituents of hawthorn preparations. In male rats given an 80% ethanol extract of the fruits of *C. pinnatifida* Bge. var major N.E.Br. containing (−)-epicatechin15.8%, chlorogenic acid 3.4%, hyperoside 2.7% and isoquercitrin 2.0% at a dose of 220 mg/kg by intravenous injection, pharmacokinetic parameters for these compounds were (expressed as mean (standard deviation)): plasma drug concentration, 142.8 (16.2), 33.1 (6.1), 38.8 (6.0) and 26.7 (4.9), respectively; elimination half-life ($t_{1/2}$), 74.2 (10.0), 18.9 (1.8), 18.1 (1.1) and 11.1 (2.2) minutes, respectively; area under the plasma-concentration time curve (AUC), 2204.5 (261.0), 526.1 (37.4), 358.8 (18.0) and 216.0 (11.5) μg/min/mL, respectively; clearance, 16.0 (2.0), 14.3 (1.0), 16.7 (0.8) and 20.9 (1.1) mL/min/kg, respectively.[9] The plasma drug concentration, $t_{1/2}$, AUC and urinary excretion were significantly higher, and the volume of distribution and total body clearance were significantly lower, following intravenous injection of the extract than following intravenous injection of the individual four compounds at doses matching those in the extract ($p < 0.05$ for all). Following oral administration of a similar dose of the extract and the individual compounds, only epicatechin was absorbed, and there were no statistically significant differences in its pharmacokinetic parameters after administration as part of an extract or as the pure compound. A possible explanation for these findings is that other constituents of hawthorn extract may influence the pharmacokinetics of the constituents studied.[9]

Cardiovascular activity Cardiovascular activity has been documented for hawthorn and attributed to the flavonoid components, in particular the procyanidins.

A dry ethanol (45%) extract of hawthorn leaf with flower (drug-to-extract ratio 4–6.6 : 1, standardised for oligomeric procyanidins 18.75%; WS-1442) at a dose 100 mg/kg orally by gavage daily for seven days significantly improved cardiac function and reduced infarct size in a rat model of prolonged ischaemia and reperfusion, compared with control ($p < 0.05$).[10] In other experiments, hawthorn extracts and/or isolated constituents increased coronary blood flow both *in vitro* (in the guinea-pig heart) and *in vivo* (in the cat, dog and rabbit), reduced blood pressure *in vivo* (in cat, dog, rabbit and rat models), increased (head, skeletal muscle and kidney) and reduced (skin, gastrointestinal tract) peripheral blood flow *in vivo* (in the dog) and reduce peripheral resistance *in vivo* (in the dog).[6, 11–16] The hypotensive activity of hawthorn has been attributed to a vasodilation action rather than via adrenergic, muscarinic or histaminergic receptors.[15] Beta-adrenoceptor blocking activity (versus adrenaline-induced tachycardia) has been exhibited *in vivo* in the dog and *in vitro* in the frog heart using flower, leaf and fruit extracts standardised for their procyanidin content.[6] A direct relationship was found between the concentration of procyanidin and observed actions.

Negative chronotropic and positive inotropic actions have been observed *in vitro* using the guinea-pig heart and attributed to flavonoid and proanthocyanidin fractions.[17] A positive inotropic effect has also been exhibited by amine constituents *in vitro* using guinea-pig papillary muscle.[1]

Hawthorn extracts have also been reported to lack any effect on the heart rate and muscle contractility in studies that have observed an effect on blood pressure in the dog and rat.[14, 15] Hawthorn extracts have exhibited some prophylactic anti-arrhythmic activity in rabbits administered intravenous aconitine.[18] Extracts infused after aconitine did not affect the induced arrhythmias. *In vitro*, vitexin rhamnoside has been reported to have no effect on the action of ouabain and aconitine.[18] A crude extract of *Crataegus pinnatifidia* Bge. var *major* N.E.Br. and the flavonoid vitexin rhamnoside have been reported to exert a protective action on experimental ischaemic myocardium in anaesthetised dogs.[19] The extracts were observed to decrease left ventricular work, decrease the consumption of oxygen index, and increase coronary sinus blood oxygen concentrations, resulting in a decrease in oxygen consumption and balance of oxygen metabolism. In contrast to other studies, an increase in coronary blood flow was not observed. The authors attributed these opposing results to the variation in concentrations of active constituents between the different plant parts. *In vitro*, vitexin rhamnoside has been reported to exert a protective action towards cardiac cells deprived of oxygen and glucose.[20]

Other activities A mild CNS-depressant effect has been documented in mice that received oral administration of hawthorn flower extracts.[21] An increase in barbiturate sleeping time and a decrease in spontaneous basal motility were the most noticeable effects.

Free radicals have been linked with the ageing process. When fed to mice, a hawthorn fruit (*C. pinnatifidia*) extract has been reported to enhance the action of superoxide dismutase (SOD), which promotes the scavenging of free radicals.[22] An inhibition of lipid peroxidation, which can be caused by highly reactive free radicals, was also documented.[22] The pharmacological actions of leaf with flowers include increase in cardiac contractility, increase in coronary blood flow and myocardial circulation, protection from ischaemic damage and decrease of peripheral vascular resistance.[G52]

Clinical studies

Heart failure and other cardiovascular disorders Clinical trials of preparations of hawthorn mainly have assessed the effects of standardised extracts of the leaf and flower in patients with different stages of heart failure, according to the NYHA classification. There have been at least 13 randomised, double-blind, placebo-controlled trials of hawthorn extracts involving patients with NYHA heart failure classes I to III. The results of at least ten other studies have been published, but these have assessed the effects of combination preparations of hawthorn or were not conducted according to a randomised, placebo-controlled design. Most randomised, double-blind, placebo-controlled trials have assessed the effects of a dry 45% ethanol extract of hawthorn leaves with flowers (WS-1442; drug-to-extract ratio 4–6 : 1, containing 18.8% oligomeric procyanidins). Several other trials have compared the effects of another extract of hawthorn leaf with flower (LI-132; standardised for 2.2% flavonoids) with those of placebo, or the angiotensin converting enzyme (ACE) inhibitor captopril.

A systematic review and meta-analysis included 13 randomised, double-blind, placebo-controlled trials of standardised extracts of hawthorn leaf and flower in patients with chronic heart failure. Ten trials tested the extract WS-1442 administered orally at doses ranging from 160 to 1800 mg daily for three to 16 weeks, whereas the other three trials assessed the extract LI-132 at doses of 300, 600 or 900 mg daily for four or eight weeks; in several trials, participants were also receiving concurrent standard treatments, such as diuretics, although a number of trials excluded patients who were already receiving diuretics, glycosides, calcium antagonists and ACE inhibitors, and in some studies it was not clear whether or not participants received concomitant medications.[23] Eight trials, involving a total of 632 participants, provided data that were suitable for meta-analysis. Data from four trials (n = 310 participants), which assessed maximal workload, showed that hawthorn extracts were superior to placebo (weighted mean difference (WMD), 95% confidence interval (CI): 7 Watt, 3 to 11 Watt; $p < 0.01$), and data from six trials which assessed the systolic blood pressure–heart rate product (systolic blood pressure in mmHg multiplied by heart rate per minute divided by 100) showed that this outcome was reduced to a greater extent in hawthorn recipients than placebo recipients (WMD, 95% CI: -20, -32 to -8). Of the five trials that were not included in the meta-analysis, three reported statistically significant effects for hawthorn extracts, compared with placebo, with respect to primary outcome measures, and two reported no statistically differences for hawthorn extracts, compared with placebo.[23]

The review concluded that hawthorn extracts are beneficial as adjunctive treatments in patients with chronic heart failure, but there is insufficient evidence to support the use of hawthorn extract alone in the treatment of chronic heart failure. Furthermore, as some of the trials did not score highly in an assessment of their methodological quality and as, overall, the studies involved relatively small numbers of patients, further well-designed randomised controlled trials are necessary to confirm the findings. Also, the observed effects cannot necessarily be extrapolated to hawthorn preparations other than those tested in the trials described above.

The largest trial included in the meta-analysis was a randomised, double-blind, placebo-controlled trial initially involving 209 patients with chronic stable NYHA class III heart failure who received hawthorn extract WS-1442 900 or 1800 mg daily, or placebo, for 16 weeks. At the end of the study, for the 139 patients who were eligible for analysis, the maximum tolerated workload during bicycle exercise was significantly greater for the higher dose hawthorn group, compared with the placebo group ($p < 0.05$).[24]

In another randomised, double-blind, controlled trial, 40 patients with chronic heart failure (NYHA class II) received a combination preparation containing extracts of hawthorn and passionflower (standardised on flavone and proanthocyanidin content) 2 mL three times daily, or placebo, for 42 days.[25] Significant improvements were noted for the treatment group, compared with placebo, in exercise capacity, heart rate at rest, diastolic blood pressure during exercise, and concentrations of total plasma cholesterol and low-density lipids ($p < 0.05$ for each). There were no statistically significant differences between groups in maximum exercise capacity, breathlessness, and physical performance.

In a non-randomised, double-blind, controlled trial, the effects of a standardised extract of hawthorn leaf and flower (LI-132) 900 mg daily were compared with those of the ACE inhibitor captopril 37.5 mg daily for eight weeks in 132 patients with chronic stable NYHA class II heart failure. During the study, exercise tolerance increased significantly in both groups, compared with baseline values ($p < 0.001$), and the blood pressure–heart rate product and incidence and severity of symptoms decreased in both groups; there were no statistically significant differences between the groups.[26]

The effectiveness (i.e. effects when used in general practice) of a hawthorn extract (WS-1442) were assessed in a prospective, non-interventional, cohort study involving 952 patients with heart failure (NYHA class II). Of these, 588 patients received the hawthorn extract either alone or in addition to standard treatment, and 364 patients received standard treatment alone. Interim results for 533 patients from whom 130 pairs of patients matched for certain cardiac and demographic characteristics at baseline suggested that fatigue ($p = 0.036$), stress dyspnoea ($p = 0.020$) and, marginally, palpitations ($p = 0.048$) were significantly less marked in the hawthorn extract cohort than in the comparative cohort.[27] However, final results of the study are required before conclusions can be drawn.

A preliminary randomised, double-blind, placebo-controlled trial assessed the effects of a hawthorn extract 500 mg daily, alone and in combination with a magnesium supplement 600 mg daily, for ten weeks in 36 patients with mild hypertension. Reductions in systolic and diastolic blood pressure were observed in all groups, and there were no statistically significant differences between groups.[28] However, it is possible that as the study involved only small numbers of participants that it did not have adequate statistical power to detect any differences between groups.

Data pooled from two randomised, controlled, crossover studies each involving 24 participants with orthostatic dysregulation who received one of three doses of an oral combination preparation containing an ethanol extract of hawthorn berries, D-camphor and menthol on four separate days indicated a statistically significant effect for higher dose of the combination preparation, compared with placebo, with respect to mean arterial pressure, and systolic and diastolic blood pressure.[29]

Other conditions The effects of a combination preparation containing *C. oxyacantha*, *Eschscholtzia californica* and magnesium were assessed in a randomised, double-blind, placebo-controlled trial involving 264 participants with mild-to-moderate anxiety disorders with associated functional disturbances. Participants received the combination preparation (n = 130), or placebo (n = 134), two tablets twice daily for three months. At the end of the study, reductions in Hamilton anxiety scale scores were significantly greater for the treatment group than for the placebo group.[30]

Side-effects, Toxicity

Clinical data

Data from randomised controlled trials and post-marketing surveillance studies suggest that hawthorn preparations are well-tolerated when taken at recommended dosages. While these studies provide some useful data for the hawthorn products assessed, their results cannot necessarily be extrapolated to other manufacturers' hawthorn products, which may differ qualitatively and quantitatively in their chemical content. In addition, clinical trials are designed primarily to assess efficacy, not safety, and have the statistical power only to detect common, acute adverse effects. Further well-designed post-marketing surveillance studies are required to assess the safety of hawthorn extracts, including with long-term use.

A systematic review and meta-analysis included 13 randomised, double-blind, placebo-controlled trials of standardised extracts of hawthorn leaf and flower in patients with chronic heart failure (*see* Pharmacological Actions, Clinical studies), of which 12 trials reported data on adverse events. Of these, nine trials tested the extract WS-1442 administered orally at doses ranging from 160–1800 mg daily for three to 16 weeks, whereas the other three trials assessed the extract LI-132 at doses of 300, 600 or 900 mg daily for four or eight weeks.[23] The systematic review reported that in five trials no adverse events occurred in the hawthorn groups and that in the seven other trials, 39 adverse events, most commonly, dizziness/vertigo (n = 8 cases), occurred among around 300 hawthorn recipients. However, the review did not state whether or not the number and type of adverse events occurring in the hawthorn groups were different to those for the placebo groups. In the largest trial included in the systematic review, the frequency of dizziness was lower in the higher dose hawthorn group than in the lower dose hawthorn and placebo groups.[24]

H

In two post-marketing surveillance studies involving over 4500 patients with NYHA class I or II heart failure who received hawthorn extract (WS-1442[31]) 900 mg daily for eight or 24 weeks, adverse events were reported by 1.3%[32] and 1.4%[31] of participants. Adverse events reported included hot flushes, stomach complaints, palpitations, dizziness, dyspnoea, headache and epistaxis.[32]

Preclinical data

General symptoms of acute toxicity observed in a number of animal models (e.g. guinea-pig, frog, tortoise, cat, rabbit, rat) have been documented as bradycardia and respiratory depression leading to cardiac arrest and respiratory paralysis.[11–13] Acute toxicity (LD_{50}) of isolated constituents (mainly flavonoids) has been documented as 50–2600 mg/kg (by intravenous injection) and 6 g/kg (by mouth) in various animal preparations.[11–13] The documented acute toxicity of commercial hawthorn preparations has also been reviewed.[11–13]

Contra-indications, Warnings

In view of the nature of the actions documented for hawthorn, there is a view that preparations of hawthorn berries and leaves with flowers are not suitable for self-medication.

Drug interactions In view of the documented pharmacological actions of hawthorn, the potential for preparations of hawthorn to interfere with other medicines administered concurrently, particularly those with similar or opposing effects, including antihypertensive, antihypotensive, and inotropic agents, should be considered.

In an open-label, randomised, crossover study involving healthy volunteers who received digoxin 0.25 mg for ten days and digoxin 0.25 mg in addition to an extract of hawthorn leaves and flowers (WS-1442) 450 mg twice daily (equivalent to 168.6 mg oligomeric procyanidins) for three weeks with a three-week wash-out period, there were no statistically significant differences between digoxin alone and digoxin plus hawthorn extract in any of the measured pharmacokinetic parameters.[33] Digoxin concentrations were lower in the digoxin plus hawthorn group and, although this did not reach statistical significance ($p = 0.054$), it is possible that the study did not have sufficient statistical power to detect a difference. Furthermore, the study involved healthy volunteers, and the effects of co-administration of digoxin and hawthorn extract in patients with heart failure requires investigation.

Pregnancy and lactation Certain hawthorn extracts exhibit activity on uterine tissue (reductions in tone and motility) *in vitro* and *in vivo* (animals).[11–13] The clinical relevance of these findings is not known. In view of the these and other pharmacological activities described for hawthorn, together with the lack of information on the use of hawthorn during pregnancy and breastfeeding, preparations containing hawthorn fruit or hawthorn leaf and flower are contra-indicated during these periods.

Preparations

Proprietary single-ingredient preparations

Austria: Bericard; Crataegan; Crataegutt. *Brazil:* Dekatin. *Chile:* Cratenox. *Czech Republic:* Caj z Hlohu; Cardiplant; Hloh-List S. *France:* Aubeline; Cardiocalm; Spasmosedine. *Germany:* Ardeycordal mono; Basticrat; Born; Chronocard N; Cordapur Novo; Corocrat; Craegium; Cratae-Loges; Crataegutt; Crataegysat F; Crataepas; Esbericard novo; Faros; Kneipp Pflanzen-Dragees Weissdorn; Koro-Nyhadin; Kytta-Cor; Lomacard; Natucor; Orthangin novo; Oxacant-mono; Regulacor-POS; Senicor; Steicorton; Stenocrat mono. *Hungary:* Crataegutt. *Russia:* Novo-Passit (Ново-Пассит). *Switzerland:* Cardiplant; Crataegisan; Crataegitan; Faros; Vitacor.

Proprietary multi-ingredient preparations

Argentina: Hepatodirectol; Passacanthine; Sequals G. *Australia:* Asa Tones; Bioglan Bioage Peripheral; Coleus Complex; Dan Shen Compound; For Peripheral Circulation Herbal Plus Formula 5; Gingo A; Ginkgo Biloba Plus; Ginkgo Complex; Lifechange Circulation Aid; Lifesystem Herbal Formula 6 For Peripheral Circulation; Multi-Vitamin Day & Night. *Austria:* Omega; Rutiviscal; Virgilocard; Wechseltee St Severin. *Belgium:* Natudor; Sedinal; Seneuval. *Brazil:* Calman; Calmazin; Calmiplan; Floriny; Pasalix; Passi Catha; Passiflora Composta; Passiflorine; Sedalin; Serenus; Sominex. *Chile:* Armonyl. *Czech Republic:* Alvisan Neo; Fytokliman Planta; Hertz- und Kreislauftee; Hypotonicka; Novo-Passit; Valofyt Neo. *France:* Biocarde; Euphytose; Mediflor Tisane Calmante Troubles du Sommeil No 14; Mediflor Tisane Circulation du Sang No 12; Natudor; Neuroflorine; Nicoprive; Nocvalene; Passiflorine; Passinevryl; Quinisedine; Sedatif Tiber; Sedopal; Spasmine; Sympaneurol; Sympathyl; Sympavagol; Tranquital; Vagostabyl. *Germany:* Antihypertonicum S; Biovital Aktiv; Biovital Aktiv; Biovital Classic; Bomacorin; Cardio-Longoral; Chlorophyl liquid "Schuh"; Convallocor-SL; Convastabil; Fovysat; Ginseng-Complex "Schuh"; Ilja Rogoff; Korodin; Oxacant-sedativ; Passin; Protecor; Salus Herz-Schutz-Kapseln; Septacord; Tornix. *Hungary:* Biovital; Biovital. *Israel:* Nerven-Dragees; Passiflora. *Italy:* Anevrasi; Lenicalm; Noctis; Parvisedil; Passiflorine; Sedatol; Sedatol; Sedofit; Sedopuer F. *Mexico:* Ifupasil. *Monaco:* Neuropax. *Portugal:* Neurocardol. *Russia:* Doppelherz Vitalotonik (Доппельгерц Виталотоник); Herbion Drops for the Heart (Гербион Сердечные Капли). *Spain:* Natusor High Blood Pressure; Natusor Somnisedan; Passiflorine; Sedasor; Sedonat; Tensiben. *Switzerland:* Arterosan Plus; Cardiaforce; Circulan; Dragees pour le coeur et les nerfs; Dragees sedatives Dr Welti; Ipasin; Phytomed Cardio; Strath Gouttes pour le coeur; Tisane pour le coeur et la circulation; Triallin; Valverde Coeur. *UK:* Tranquil. *Venezuela:* Cratex; Equaliv; Eufytose; Pasidor; Pasifluidina; Passiflorum. *USA:* Heart Health; My Favorite Multiple.

References

1 Wagner H, Grevel J. Cardioactive drugs IV. Cardiotonic amines from *Crataegus oxyacantha*. *Plant Med* 1982; 45: 99–101.
2 Nikolov N *et al*. New flavonoid glycosides from *Crataegus monogyna* and *Crataegus pentagyna*. *Planta Med* 1982; 44: 50–53.
3 Ficarra P *et al*. High-performance liquid chromatography of flavonoids in *Crataegus oxyacantha* L. *Il Farmaco Ed Pr* 1984; 39: 148–157.
4 Ficcara P *et al*. Analysis of 2-phenyl-chromon derivatives and chlorogenic acid. II – High-performance thin layer chromatography and high-performance liquid chromatography in flowers, leaves and buds extractives of *Crataegus oxyacantha* L. *Il Farmaco Ed Pr* 1984; 39: 342–354.
5 Pietta P *et al*. Isocratic liquid chormatographic method for the simultaneous determination of *Passiflora incarnata* L. and *Crataegus monogyna* flavonoids in drugs. *J Chromatogr* 1986; 357: 233–238.
6 Rácz-Kotilla E *et al*. Hypotensive and beta-blocking effect of procyanidins of *Crataegus monogyna*. *Planta Med* 1980; 39: 239.
7 Vanhaelen M, Vanhaelen-Fastre R. TLC-densitometric determination of 2,3-*cis*-procyanidin monomer and oligomers from hawthorn (*Crataegus laevigata* and *C. monogyna*). *J Pharm Biomed Anal* 1989; 7: 1871–1875.
8 Vierling W *et al*. Investigation of the pharmaceutical and pharmacological equivalence of different hawthorn extracts. *Phytomedicine* 2003; 10: 8–16.
9 Chang Q *et al*. Comparison of the pharmacokinetics of hawthorn phenolics in extract versus individual pure compound. *J Clin Pharmacol* 2005; 45: 106–112.
10 Veveris M *et al*. Crataegus special extract WS® 1442 improves cardiac function and reduces infarct size in a rat model of prolonged coronary ischemia and reperfusion. *Life Sci* 2004; 74: 1945–1955.
11 Ammon HPT, Händel M. Crataegus, toxicology and pharmacology. Part I: Toxicity. *Planta Med* 1981; 43: 105–120.
12 Ammon HPT, Händel M. Crataegus, toxicology and pharmacology. Part II: Pharmacodynamics. *Planta Med* 1981; 43: 209–239.
13 Ammon HPT, Händel M. Crataegus, toxicology and pharmacology. Part III: Pharmacodynamics and pharmacokinetics. *Planta Med* 1981; 43: 313–322.
14 Lièvre M *et al*. Assessment in the anesthetized dog of the cardiovascular effects of a pure extract (hyperoside) from hawthorn. *Ann Pharm Fr* 1985; 43: 471–477.
15 Abdul-Ghani A-S *et al*. Hypotensive effect of *Crateagus oxyacantha*. *Int J Crude Drug Res* 1987; 25: 216–220.
16 Petkov V. Plants with hypotensive, antiatheromatous and coronarodilatating action. *Am J Chin Med* 1979; 7: 197–236.
17 Leukel A *et al*. Studies on the activity of *Crataegus* compounds upon the isolated guinea pig heart. *Planta Med* 1986; 52: 65.
18 Thompson EB *et al*. Preliminary study of potential antiarrhythmic effects of *Crataegus monogyna*. *J Pharm Sci* 1974; 63: 1936–1937.
19 Lianda L *et al*. Studies on hawthorn and its active principle. I. Effect on myocardial ischemia and hemodynamics in dogs. *J Trad Chin Med* 1984; 4: 283–288.
20 Lianda L *et al*. Studies on hawthorn and its active principle. II. Effects on cultured rat heart cells deprived of oxygen and glucose. *J Trad Chin Med* 1984; 4: 289–292.
21 Della Loggia R *et al*. Depressive effect of *Crataegus oxyacantha* L. on central nervous system in mice. *Sci Pharm* 1983; 51: 319–324.
22 Dai Y-R *et al*. Effect of extracts of some medicinal plants on superoxide dismutase activity in mice. *Planta Med* 1987; 53: 309–310.
23 Pittler MH, *et al*. Hawthorn extract for treating chronic heart failure: meta-analysis of randomized trials. *Am J Med* 2003; 114: 665–674.
24 Tauchert M. Efficacy and safety of crataegus extract WS® 1442 in comparison with placebo in patients with chronic stable New York Heart Association class-III heart failure. *Am Heart J* 2002; 143: 910–915.
25 von Eiff M *et al*. Hawthorn/Passionflower extract and improvement in physical exercise capacity of patients with dyspnoea Class II of the NYHM functional classification. *Acta Ther* 1994; 20: 47–66.
26 Tauchert M *et al*. [Effectiveness of the hawthorn extract LI 132 compared with the ACE inhibitor captopril. Multicentre, double-blind study in 132 patients with NYHA stage II cardiac insufficiency]. *Münch Med Wochenschr* 1994; 136 (Suppl. Suppl.1):S27–S33 [German].
27 Habs M. Prospective, comparative cohort studies and their contribution to the benefit assessments of therapeutic options: heart failure treatment with and without hawthorn special extract WS® 1442. *Forsch Komplementärmed Klass Naturheilkd* 2004; 11 (Suppl. Suppl.1): 36–39.
28 Walker AF Promising hypotensive effect of hawthorn extract: a randomized, double-blind, pilot study of mild essential hypertension. *Phytotherapy Res* 2002; 16: 48–54.
29 Belz GG *et al*. Camphor-Crataegus berry extract combination dose-dependently reduces tilt induced fall in blood pressure in orthostatic hypotension. *Phytomedicine* 2002; 9: 581–588.
30 Hanus M, *et al*. Double-blind, randomised, placebo-controlled study to evaluate the efficacy and safety of a fixed combination containing two plant extracts (*Crataegus oxyacantha* and *Eschscholtzia californica*) and magnesium in mild-to-moderate anxiety disorders. *Curr Med Res Opinion* 2004; 20(1): 63–71.
31 Tauchert M *et al*.. High-dose crataegus (hawthorn) extract WS® 1442 in the treatment of NYHA stage II heart failure. *Herz* 1999; 24: 465–474.
32 Schmidt U, *et al*. High dosed therapy with crataegus extract in patients suffering from heart failure NYHA stage I and II. *Z Phytother* 1998; 19: 22–30.
33 Tankanow R, *et al*. Interaction study between digoxin and a preparation of hawthorn (*Crataegus oxyacantha*). *J Clin Pharmacol* 2003; 43: 637–642.

Holy Thistle

Summary and Pharmaceutical Comment

The chemistry of holy thistle is well documented and the available pharmacological data support most of the stated uses. However, there is a lack of clinical research assessing efficacy and safety of preparations of holy thistle. In view of the lack of toxicity data, excessive use of holy thistle and use during pregnancy and lactation should be avoided.

Species (Family)

Cnicus benedictus L. (Asteraceae/Compositae)

Synonym(s)

Blessed Thistle, Carbenia Benedicta, *Carbenia benedicta* (L.) Arcang., Carduus Benedictus, Cnicus

Part(s) Used

Herb

Pharmacopoeial and Other Monographs

BHC 1992[G6]
BHP 1996[G9]
Complete German Commission E[G3]
Martindale 35th edition[G85]

Legal Category (Licensed Products)

GSL[G37]

Constituents

The following is compiled from several sources, including General References G2, G6, G30, G40 and G62.

Lignans Arctigenin, nortracheloside, 2-acetyl nortracheloside and trachelogenin.[1]

Polyenes Several polyacetylenes.[2]

Steroids Phytosterols (e.g. *n*-nonacosan, sitosterol, sitosteryl glycoside, stigmasterol).[3]

Tannins Type unspecified (8%).

Terpenoids Sesquiterpenes including cnicin 0.2–0.7%,[4] yielding salonitenolide as aglycone,[5] and artemisiifolin. Shoot and flowering head are reported to be devoid of cnicin.[4] Triterpenoids including α-amyrenone, α-amyrin acetate, α-amyrin, multiflorenol, multiflorenol acetate and oleanolic acid.[3]

Volatile oils Many components, mainly hydrocarbons.[6]

Other constituents Lithospermic acid, mucilage, nicotinic acid and nicotinamide complex, resin.

Food Use

Holy thistle is listed by the Council of Europe as natural source of food flavouring (category N2). This category indicates that holy thistle can be added to foodstuffs in small quantities, with a possible limitation of an active principle (as yet unspecified) in the final product.[G16] Previously in the USA, holy thistle was permitted for use in alcoholic beverages.[G65]

Herbal Use

Holy thistle is stated to possess bitter stomachic, antidiarrhoeal, antihaemorrhagic, febrifuge, expectorant, antibiotic, bacteriostatic, vulnerary and antiseptic properties. Traditionally, it has been used for anorexia, flatulent dyspepsia, bronchial catarrh, topically for gangrenous and indolent ulcers, and specifically for atonic dyspepsia, and enteropathy with flatulent colic.[G6, G64]

Dosage

Dosages for oral administration (adults) for traditional uses recommended in standard herbal reference texts are given below.

Dried flowering tops 1.5–3.0 g as an infusion three times daily.[G6, G7]

Liquid extract 1.5–3.0 mL (1 : 1 in 25% alcohol) three times daily.[G6, G7]

Pharmacological Actions

In vitro and animal studies

Antibacterial activity has been reported for an aqueous extract of the herb, for cnicin, and for the volatile oil.[6–9] Activity has been

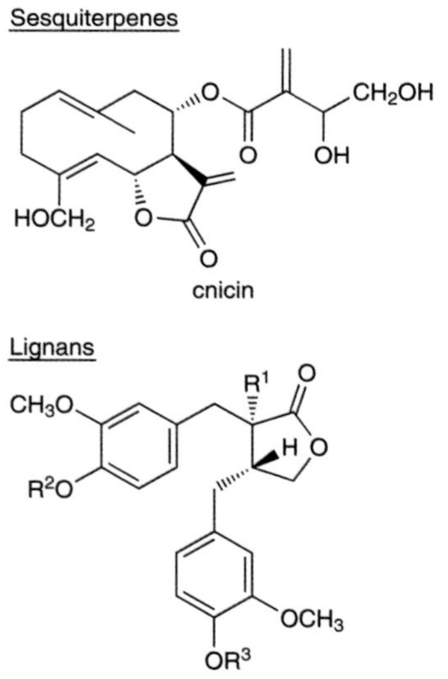

Sesquiterpenes

cnicin

Lignans

	R^1	R^2	R^3
(–)-arctigenin	H	H	CH_3
trachelogenin	OH	H	CH_3
nortracheloside	OH	Glucose	H
2-acetylnor-tracheloside	O-Acetyl	Glucose	H

Figure 1 Selected constituents of holy thistle.

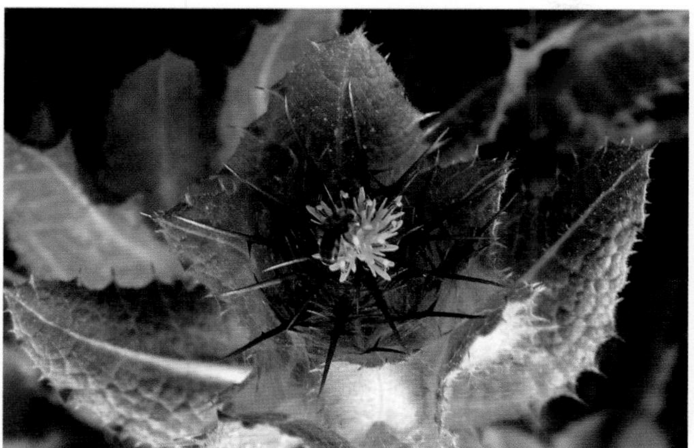

Figure 2 Holy thistle (*Cnicus benedictus*).

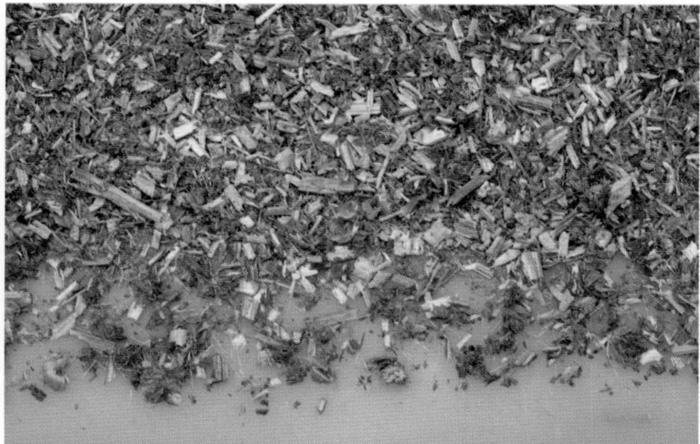

Figure 3 Holy thistle – dried drug substance (herb).

documented against *Bacillus subtilis*, *Brucella abortus*, *Brucella bronchoseptica*, *Escherichia coli*, *Proteus* species, *Pseudomonas aeruginosa*, *Staphylococcus aureus* and *Streptococcus faecalis*. The antimicrobial activity of holy thistle has been attributed to cnicin and to the polyacetylene constituents.[9]

Cnicin has exhibited *in vivo* anti-inflammatory activity (carrageenan-induced rat-paw oedema test) virtually equipotent to indometacin.[4] Antitumour activity has been documented in mice against sarcoma 180 for the whole herb,[8] and against lymphoid leukaemia for cnicin;[8] cnicin has also been reported to exhibit *in vitro* activity against KB cells.[8] An α-methylene-γ-lactone moiety is thought to be necessary for the antibacterial and antitumour activities of cnicin.[8]

Lithospermic acid is thought to be responsible for the antigonadotrophic activity documented for holy thistle.[G30] The sesquiterpene lactone constituents are stated to be bitter principles.[G62]

Tannins are generally known to possess astringent properties.

Clinical studies

There is a lack of clinical research assessing the effects of holy thistle and rigorous randomised controlled clinical trials are required.

Side-effects, Toxicity

None documented. However, there is a lack of clinical safety and toxicity data for holy thistle and further investigation of these aspects is required.

The toxicity of cnicin has been studied in mice: the acute oral LD_{50} was stated to be 1.6–3.2 mmol/kg body weight and intraperitoneal administration was reported to cause irritation of tissue. In the writhing test, cnicin was found to cause abdominal pain with an ED_{50} estimated as 6.2 mmol/kg.[4]

Antitumour activity has been documented for the whole herb and for cnicin (*see* Pharmacological Actions; *In vitro* and animal studies).

Contra-indications, Warnings

None documented for holy thistle. Plants containing sesquiterpene lactones with an α-methylene-γ-lactone moiety are generally considered to be allergenic, although no documented hypersensitivity reactions to holy thistle were located. Holy thistle may cause an allergic reaction in individuals with a known hypersensitivity to other members of the Compositae (e.g. chamomile, ragwort, tansy).

Drug interactions None documented. However, the potential for preparations of holy thistle to interact with other medicines administered concurrently, particularly those with similar or opposing effects, should be considered.

Pregnancy and lactation The safety of holy thistle has not been established. In view of the lack of toxicity data, excessive use of holy thistle during pregnancy and lactation should be avoided.

Preparations

Proprietary multi-ingredient preparations

Austria: Mariazeller. *Brazil:* Digestron. *Czech Republic:* Ungolen. *Germany:* Gallexier; Gastritol. *Russia:* Original Grosser Bittner Balsam (Оригинальный Большой Бальзам Биттнера). *South Africa:* Essens Amara of Groen Amara. *Switzerland:* Gastrosan. *UK:* Bio-Strath Artichoke Formula; Sure-Lax (Herbal).

References

1 Vanhaelen M, Vanhaelen-Fastré R. Lactonic lignans from *Cnicus benedictus*. *Phytochemistry* 1975; 14: 2709.
2 Vanhaelen-Fastré R. Constituents polyacetyleniques de *Cnicus benedictus* L. *Planta Med* 1974; 25: 47–59.
3 Ulubelen A, Berkan T. Triterpenic and steroidal compounds of *Cnicus benedictus*. *Planta Med* 1977; 31: 375–377.
4 Schneider G, Lachner I. A contribution to analytics and pharmacology of Cnicin. *Planta Med* 1987; 53: 247–251.
5 Vanhaelen-Fastré R, Vanhaelen M. Presence of salonitenolide in *Cnicus benedictus*. *Planta Med* 1974; 26: 375–379.
6 Vanhaelen-Fastré R. Constitution and antibiotical properties of the essential oil of *Cnicus benedictus*. *Planta Med* 1973; 24: 165–175.
7 Cobb E. Antineoplastic agent from *Cnicus benedictus*. British Patent 1,335,181 (Cl.A61k) 24 Oct 1973, Appl.54,800/69 (via *Chemical Abstracts* 1975; 83: 48189j).
8 Vanhaelen-Fastré R. Antibiotic and cytotoxic activities of cnicin isolated from *Cnicus benedictus*. *J Pharm Belg* 1972; 27: 683–688.
9 Vanhaelen-Fastré R. *Cnicus benedictus*: Separation of antimicrobial constituents. *Plant Med Phytother* 1968; 2: 294–299.

Hops

Summary and Pharmaceutical Comment

The chemistry of hops is well documented and is characterised by the bitter acid components of the oleo-resin. Documented pharmacological activities support the herbal uses, although evidence from robust clinical studies is limited. Excessive use of hops and use during pregnancy and lactation should be avoided in view of the limited toxicity data.

Species (Family)

Humulus lupulus L. (Cannabaceae/Moraceae)

Synonym(s)

Humulus, Lupulus

Part(s) Used

Strobile

Pharmacopoeial and Other Monographs

BHC 1992[(G6)]
BHP 1996[(G9)]
BP 2007[(G84)]
Complete German Commission E[(G3)]
ESCOP 2003[(G76)]
Martindale 35th edition[(G85)]
Ph Eur 2007[(G81)]

Legal Category (Licensed Products)

GSL[(G37)]

Constituents

The following is compiled from several sources, including General References G2, G6 and G52.

Flavonoids Astragalin, kaempferol, quercetin, quercitrin and rutin.

Chalcones Isoxanthohumol, xanthohumol, 6-isopentenylnaringenin, 3′-(isoprenyl)-2′, 4-dihydroxy-4′, 6′-dimethoxychalcone, 2′,6′-dimethoxy-4, 4′-dihydroxychalcone.[(1)]

Oleo-resin 15-30%. Bitter principles (acylphloroglucides) in a soft and hard resin. The lipophilic soft resin consists mainly of α-acids (e.g. humulone, cohumulone, adhumulone, prehumulone, posthumulone), β-acids (e.g. lupulone, colupulone, adlupulone), and their oxidative degradation products including 2-methyl-3-buten-2-ol[(2, 3, G52)] The hard resin contains a hydrophilic δ-resin and χ-resin.

Tannins 2–4%. Condensed; gallocatechin identified.[(4)]

Volatile oils 0.3–1.0%. More than 100 terpenoid components identified; primarily (at least 90%) β-caryophyllene, farnescene and humulene (sesquiterpenes), and myrcene (monoterpene).

Other constituents Amino acids, phenolic acids, gamma-linoleic acids, lipids and oestrogenic substances (disputed).[(5)]

It has been stated that only low amounts of 2-methyl-3-buten-2-ol, the sedative principle identified in hops, are present in sedative tablets containing hops.[(2)] However, it is thought that 2-methyl-3-buten-2-ol is formed *in vivo* by metabolism of the α-bitter acids and, therefore, the low amount of 2-methyl-3-buten-2-ol in a preparation may not indicate low sedative activity.[(6)] Interestingly, relatively high concentrations of 2-methyl-3-buten-2-ol were found in bath preparations, suggesting that high concentrations of 2-methyl-3-buten-2-ol may be achieved in both tea and bath products containing hops.[(2)]

Food Use

Hops are listed by the Council of Europe as a natural source of food flavouring (category N2). This category indicates that hops can be added to foodstuffs in small quantities, with a possible limitation of an active principle (as yet unspecified) in the final product.[(G16)] Previously, hops has been listed as GRAS (Generally Recognised As Safe).[(G65)]

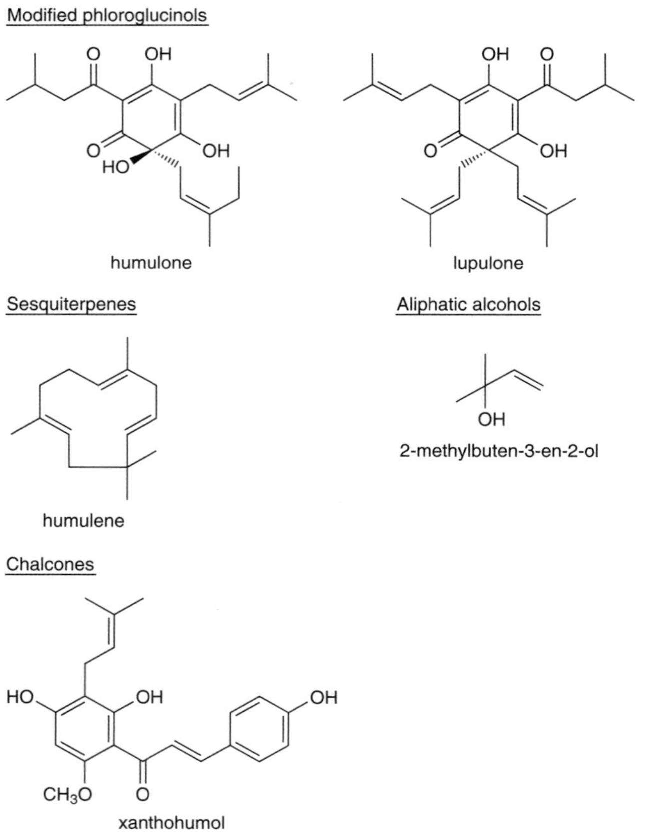

Figure 1 Selected constituents of hops.

Herbal Use

Hops are stated to possess sedative, hypnotic and topical bactericidal properties. Traditionally, they have been used for neuralgia, insomnia, excitability, priapism, mucous colitis, topically for crural ulcers, and specifically for restlessness associated with nervous tension headache and/or indigestion. The German Commission E approved use for mood disturbances such as restlessness and anxiety as well as sleep disturbances.[G3] Hops are used in combination with valerian root for nervous sleeping disorders and conditions of unrest.[G3]

Dosage

Dosages for oral administration (adults) for traditional uses recommended in contemporary standard herbal reference texts are given below.

Dried strobile 0.5 g as an infusion two to four times daily.[G76]

Liquid extract 0.5–2.0 mL (1 : 1 in 45% alcohol) up to three times daily.[G76]

Tincture 1–2 mL (1 : 5 in 60% alcohol) up to three times daily.[G76]

Pharmacological Actions

In vitro and animal studies

Antibacterial activity, mainly against Gram-positive bacteria, has been documented for hops, and attributed to the humulone and lupulone constituents.[7] The activity of the bitter acids against Gram-positive bacteria is thought to involve primary membrane leakage. Resistance of Gram-negative bacteria to the resin acids is attributed to the presence of a phospholipid-containing outer membrane, as lupulone and humulone are inactivated by serum phospholipids.[7] Structure–activity studies have indicated the requirement of a hydrophobic molecule and a six-membered central ring for such activity.[8]

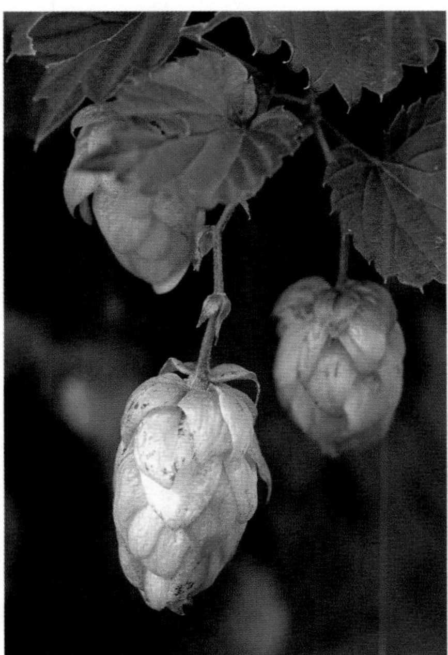

Figure 2 Hops (*Humulus lupulus*).

The humulones and lupulones are thought to possess little activity towards fungi or yeasts. However, antifungal activity has been documented for the bitter acids towards *Trichophyton*, *Candida*, *Fusarium* and *Mucor* species.[9] Flavonone constituents have also been documented to possess antifungal activity towards *Trichophyton* and *Mucor* species, and antibacterial activity towards *Staphylococcus aureus*.[10]

Antispasmodic activity has been documented for an alcoholic hops extract on various isolated smooth muscle preparations.[11] Hops have been reported to exhibit hypnotic and sedative properties.[G41] 2-Methyl-3-buten-2-ol, a bitter acid degradation product, has been identified as a sedative principle in hops.[2,3] 2-Methyl-3-buten-2-ol has been shown to possess narcotic properties in mice and motility depressant activity in rats, with the latter not attributable to a muscle-relaxant effect.[12] It has also been suggested that isovaleric acid residues present in hops may contribute towards the sedative action. In mice, hops extract administered intraperitoneally (100, 250, 500 mg/kg) 30 minutes prior to a series of behavioural tests, resulted in a dose-dependent suppression of spontaneous locomotor at doses of 250 mg/kg for up to one hour.[13] The time for mice to be able to remain on a rota rod was decreased by 59% and 65% at doses of 250 mg/kg and 500 mg/kg, respectively. The time of onset of convulsions and survival time after administration of pentylenetetrazole (100 mg/kg) was significantly lengthened. Hops extract (35 mg/kg, intraperitoneal administration) produced a dose-dependent increase in sleeping time in mice treated with pentobarbitol. An antinociceptive effect was noted by increased latency of licking forepaws in hotplate tests and hypothermic activity observed from a time-dependent fall of rectal temperature at a dose of 500 mg/kg.[13]

Hops have previously been reported to possess oestrogenic constituents.[5] However, when a number of purified components, including the volatile oil and the bitter acids, were examined using the uterine weight assay in immature female mice, no oestrogenic activity was found.[5]

Clinical studies

Clinical research assessing the effects of hops is limited and rigorous randomised controlled clinical trials are required.

Clinical studies have generally assessed hops given in combination with one or more additional herbs. For example, hops has been reported to improve sleep disturbances when given in combination with valerian (*see* Valerian, Clinical studies).[14]

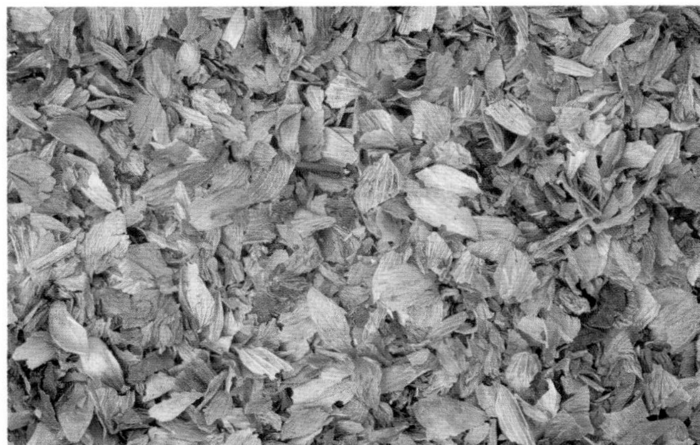

Figure 3 Hops – dried drug substance (strobile).

Hops, in combination with chicory and peppermint, has been documented to relieve pain in patients with chronic cholecystitis (calculous and non-calculous).[15] A herbal product containing a mixture of plant extracts, including hops and uva-ursi, and alpha-tocopherol acetate was reported to improve irritable bladder and urinary incontinence.[16] However, these observations require confirmation in robust clinical studies.

Side-effects, Toxicity

There is a lack of clinical safety and toxicity data for hops and further investigation of these aspects is required.

Respiratory allergy caused by the handling of hop cones has been documented;[17] a subsequent patch test using dried, crushed flowerheads proved negative. Positive patch test reactions have been documented for fresh hop oil, humulone, and lupulone. Myrcene, present in the fresh oil but readily oxidised, was concluded to be the sensitising agent in the hop oil.[G51] Contact dermatitis to hops has long been recognised[G51] and is attributed to the pollen.[G41]

Small doses of hops are stated to be non-toxic.[G42] Large doses administered to animals by injection have resulted in a soporific effect followed by death, with chronic administration resulting in weight loss before death.[G39]

Contra-indications, Warnings

Allergic reactions have been reported for hops, although only following external contact with the herb and oil.

Drug interactions None documented. However, the potential for preparations of hops to interact with other medicines administered concurrently, particularly those with similar or opposing effects, should be considered. There are some conflicting data on the oestrogenic activity of hops,[5] although 8-prenylnaringenin, documented as a constituent of hops, has been shown to have oestrogenic activity in preclinical studies.[G76] Concern has been expressed that herbs with oestrogenic effects may stimulate breast cancer growth and oppose action of competitive oestrogen receptor antagonists such as tamoxifen.[18] However, this requires confirmation.

Pregnancy and lactation *In vitro* antispasmodic activity on the uterus has been documented. In view of this and the lack of toxicity data, the use of hops during pregnancy and lactation should be avoided.

Preparations

Proprietary single-ingredient preparations

Russia: Novo-Passit (Ново-Пассит). *Switzerland:* Klosterfrau Nervenruh Dragees.

Proprietary multi-ingredient preparations

Australia: Extralife Sleep-Care; Humulus Compound; Natural Deep Sleep; Pacifenity; Passiflora Complex; Passionflower Plus; Prosed-X; Relaxaplex. *Austria:* Baldracin; Baldrian AMA; Hova; Montana; Nervenruh; Nerventee St Severin; Sedadom; Wechseltee St Severin. *Canada:* Herbal Sleep Aid; Herbal Sleep Well. *Chile:* Valupass. *Czech Republic:* Baldracin; Detsky Caj s Hermankem; Fytokliman Planta; Novo-Passit; Sanason; Schlaf-Nerventee N; Species Nervinae Planta; Valofyt Neo; Visinal. *France:* Nostress. *Germany:* Ardeysedon; Avedorm duo; Baldrian-Dispert Nacht; Baldriparan N Stark; Biosedon; Boxocalm; Cefasedativ; Dormeasan; Dormoverlan; Gutnacht; Ilja Rogoff; Klosterfrau Beruhigungs Forte; Kytta-Sedativum; Leukona-Beruhigungsbad; Luvased; Moradorm S; Nervendragees; Nervenkapseln; Nervinfant N; Nervoregin forte; Pascosedon; Schlaf- und Nerventee; Sedacur; Sedaselect D; Selon; Sensinerv forte; Valdispert comp; Valeriana mild; Valverde Baldrian Hopfen bei Einschlafstorungen und zur Beruhigung; Vivinox Day. *Hungary:* Hova. *Israel:* Nerven-Dragees. *Italy:* Emmenoiasi. *Mexico:* Nervinetas. *Russia:* Doppelherz Vitalotonik (Доппельгерц Виталотоник); Sanason (Санасон). *South Africa:* Avena Sativa Comp. *Switzerland:* Baldriparan; Dormeasan; Dragees pour le coeur et les nerfs; Dragees pour le sommeil; Dragees sedatives Dr Welti; Hova; Hyperiforce comp; Nervinetten; ReDormin; Relaxo; Soporin; Tisane calmante pour les enfants; Tisane pour le sommeil et les nerfs; Valverde Coeur; Valverde Sommeil; Zeller Sommeil. *UK:* Anased; Avena Sativa Comp; Boots Alternatives Sleep Well; Boots Sleepeaze Herbal Tablets; Calmanite Tablets; Fenneherb Newrelax; Gerard House Serenity; Gerard House Somnus; HRI Calm Life; HRI Night; Kalms Sleep; Kalms; Napiers Sleep Tablets; Napiers Tension Tablets; Natrasleep; Newrelax; Nodoff; Nytol Herbal; Quiet Days; Quiet Life; Quiet Nite; Quiet Tyme; Relax B+; Sleepezy; Slumber; Sominex Herbal; Stressless; Unwind Herbal Nytol; Valerina Night-Time; Ymea. *Venezuela:* Lupassin; Nervinetas.

References

1 Song-San S *et al.* Chalcones from *Humulus lupulus*. *Phytochemistry* 1989; 28: 1776–1777.

2 Hänsel R *et al.* The sedative-hypnotic principle of hops. 3. Communication: Contents of 2-methyl-3-butene-2-ol in hops and hop preparations. *Planta Med* 1982; 45: 224–228.

3 Wohlfart R *et al.* Detection of sedative–hypnotic hop constituents, V: Degradation of humulones and lupulones to 2-methyl-3-buten-2-ol, a hop constituent possessing sedative-hypnotic activity. *Arch Pharm (Weinheim)* 1982; 315: 132–137.

4 Gorissen H *et al.* Separation and identification of (+)-gallocatechin in hops. *Arch Int Physiol Biochem* 1968; 76: 932–934.

5 Fenselau C, Talalay P. Is oestrogenic activity present in hops? *Food Cosmet Toxicol* 1973; 11: 597–603.

6 Hänsel R, Wohlfart R. Narcotic action of 2-methyl-3-butene-2-ol contained in the exhalation of hops. *Z Naturforsch* 1980; 35: 1096–1097.

7 Teuber M, Schmalreck AF. Membrane leakage in *Bacillus subtilis* 168 induced by the hop constituents lupulone, humulone, isohumulone and humulinic acid. *Arch Mikrobiol* 1973; 94: 159–171.

8 Schmalreck AF *et al.* Structural features determining the antibiotic potencies of natural and synthetic hop bitter resins, their precursors and derivatives. *Can J Microbiol* 1975; 21: 205–212.

9 Mizobuchi S, Sato Y. Antifungal activities of hop bitter resins and related compounds. *Agric Biol Chem* 1985; 49: 399–405.

10 Mizobuchi S, Sato Y. A new flavanone with antifungal activity isolated from hops. *Agric Biol Chem* 1984; 48: 2771–2775.

11 Caujolle F *et al.* Spasmolytic action of hop (*Humulus lupulus*). *Agressologie* 1969; 10: 405–10.

12 Wohlfart R *et al.* The sedative-hypnotic principle of hops. 4. Communication: Pharmacology of 2-methyl-3-buten-2-ol. *Planta Med* 1983; 48: 120–123.

13 Lee KM *et al.* Effects of *Humulus lupulus* extract on the central nervous system in mice. *Planta Med* 1993; 59: A691.

14 Müller-Limmroth W, Ehrenstein W. Untersuchungen über die Wirkung von Seda-Kneipp auf den Schlaf schlafgestörter Menschen. *Med Klin* 1977; 72: 1119–1125.

15 Chakarski I *et al.* Clinical study of a herb combination consisting of *Humulus lupulus*, *Cichorium intybus*, *Mentha piperita* in patients

with chronic calculous and non-calculous cholecystitis. *Probl Vatr Med* 1982; 10: 65–69.
16 Lenau H *et al.* Wirksamkeit und Verträglichkeit von Cysto Fink bei Patienten mit Reizblase und/oder Harninkontinenz. *Therapiewoche* 1984; 34: 6054.
17 Newmark FM. Hops allergy and terpene sensitivity: An occupational disease. *Ann Allergy* 1978; 41: 311–312.
18 Baxter KB, ed. *Stockley's Drug Interactions*, 7th edn. London: Pharmaceutical Press, 2006.

Horehound, Black

Summary and Pharmaceutical Comment

Limited information is available on the chemistry of black horehound. A small number of studies have investigated pharmacological properties of isolated constituents and this information goes some way towards supporting some of the traditional uses, although there is a lack of basic experimental and clinical research into the effects of preparations of black horehound. In view of the lack of data on pharmacological effects, efficacy and safety, the appropriateness of medicinal use of black horehound should be considered. Excessive use, at least, should be avoided. The use of black horehound during pregnancy and breastfeeding should be avoided. The potential for black horehound to interact with other medicines should be considered.

Species (Family)

Ballota nigra L. (Labiatae)

Synonym(s)

Ballota, *Ballota foetida* Lam.

Part(s) Used

Herb

Pharmacopoeial and Other Monographs

BHP 1996[G9]
BP 2007[G84]

Legal Category (Licensed Products)

Black horehound is not included in the GSL.[G37]

Constituents

Diterpenes Ballotinone (7-oxomarrubiin),[1] ballotenol,[2] preleosibirin,[3] 13-hydroxyballonigrinolide, ballonigrin,[4,5] and 7-α-acetoxymarrubiin.[6]

Flavonoids Lactoylated flavonoids 7-O-(2S-β-D-glucopyranosyloxypropanoyl)-luteolin and 7-*O*-(2S-hydroxypropanoyl)-luteolin (luteolin-7-lactate),[7] apigenin-7-glucoside, vicenin-2.[8]

Phenylpropanoids Verbascoside (acteoside), forsythoside B, arenarioside, ballotetroside, alyssonoside, lavandulifoliside, angoroside, caffeoylmalic acid.[5,7,9–12]

Essential oil *B. nigra* ssp. foetida 0.02%, major components β-caryophyllene and germacrene D.[13]

Related species Diterpenes from *B. africana*, *B. andreuzziana*, *B. aucheri*, *B. hispanica*, *B. inaequidens*, *B. pseudodictamnus*, *B. lanata*, *B. rupestris* and *B. saxatilis*, and flavonoids from *B. acetabulosa*, *B. glandulissima*, *B. hirsuta*, *B. inequidens*, *B. pseudodictamnus* and *B. saxatilis*.[14]

Food Use

Black horehound is listed by the Council of Europe as a natural source of food flavouring (category N3). This category indicates that black horehound can be added to foodstuffs in the traditionally accepted manner, although insufficient information is available for an adequate assessment of potential toxicity.[G16]

Herbal Use

Black horehound is stated to possess anti-emetic, sedative and mild astringent properties. Traditionally, it has been used for nausea, vomiting, nervous dyspepsia, and specifically for vomiting of central origin.[G7, G64]

Dosage

Dosages for oral administration (adults) for traditional uses recommended in standard herbal reference texts are given below.

Dried herb 2–4 g as an infusion three times daily.[G7]

Liquid extract 1–3 mL (1 : 1 in 25% alcohol) three times daily.[G7]

Tincture 1–2 mL (1 : 10 in 45% alcohol) three times daily.[G7]

Pharmacological Actions

There is a lack of basic experimental and clinical research into the effects of preparations of black horehound, although a small

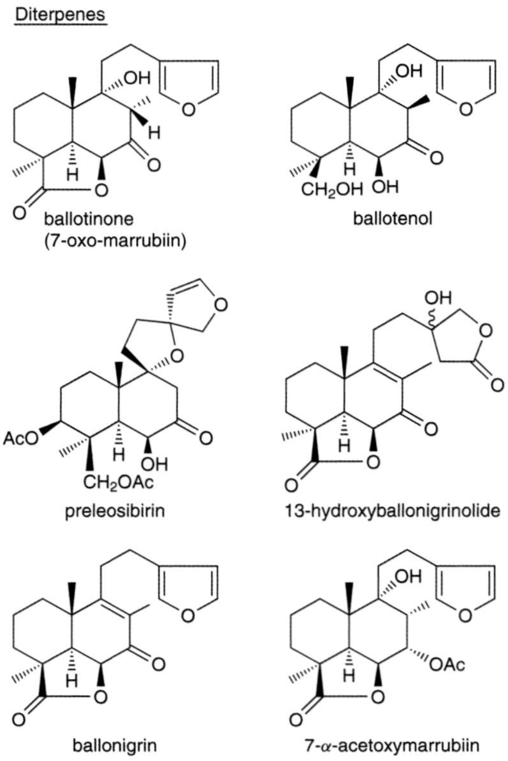

Diterpenes

ballotinone (7-oxo-marrubiin)

ballotenol

preleosibirin

13-hydroxyballonigrinolide

ballonigrin

7-α-acetoxymarrubiin

Figure 1 Selected constituents of black horehound.

number of studies has investigated pharmacological properties of isolated constituents.

In-vitro and animal studies

Certain phenylpropanoid derivatives isolated from the aerial parts of black horehound show pharmacological properties *in vitro*, including antibacterial, antioxidant and neurosedative activities. The phenylpropanoid glycosides arenarioside, forsythoside B and verbascoside, and the non-glycosidic phenylpropanoid caffeoylmalic acid bind to benzodiazepine, dopaminergic and morphinic receptors *in vitro*.[8] In radiolabelled ligand receptor binding assays using rat brain preparations, IC_{50} (concentrations required for 50% inhibition of radioligand binding) values for these compounds for each of the three receptor types were all < 5.0 mg/mL. By contrast, ballotetroside did not show any affinity for binding to the receptors studied.

Arenarioside, forsythoside B and verbascoside inhibited the growth of one strain of the Gram-negative bacterium *Proteus mirabilis* and two strains of the Gram-positive bacterium *Staphylococcus aureus*, including a methicillin-resistant strain of *S. aureus* (minimum inhibitory concentration to prevent visible growth = 128 μg/mL).[12] Arenarioside also inhibited the growth of one strain of *P. mirabilis* when incubated at a concentration of 64 μg/mL. The compounds tested did not show any activity against *Enterococcus faecalis*, and the Gram-negative bacteria *Pseudomonas aeruginosa*, *Escherichia coli*, *Enterobacter aerogenes*, *Klebsiella pneumoniae* and *K. oxytoca*.[12]

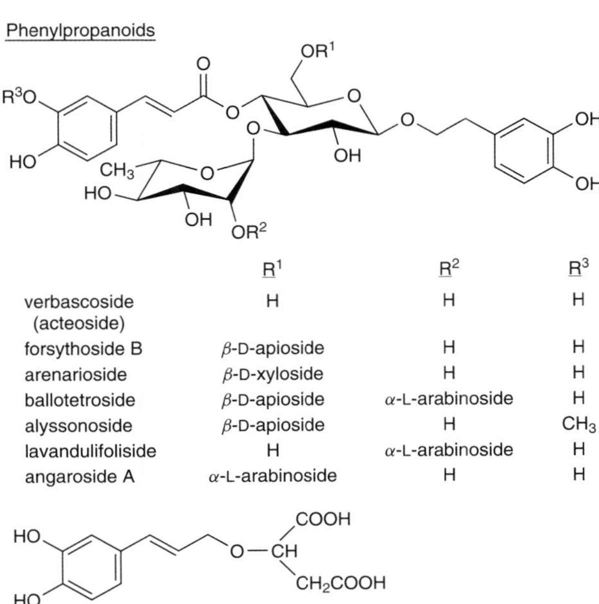

Figure 2 Selected constituents of black horehound.

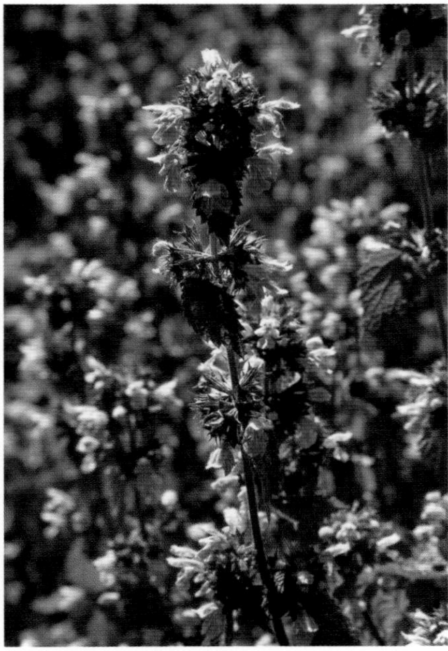

Figure 3 Black horehound (*Ballota nigra*).

Arenarioside, forsythoside B and verbascoside, as well as ballotetroside, another phenylpropanoid glycoside isolated from the aerial parts of black horehound, have antioxidant properties *in vitro*.[11] These compounds inhibited copper ion-induced oxidation of low-density lipoproteins (LDL) with ED_{50} (efficacious concentration) values of 1.8, 1.0, 1.0 and 7.5 μmol/L, respectively. (LDL oxidation may be involved in the pathogenesis of atherosclerosis.) By comparison, quercetin, a known inhibitor of copper ion-induced LDL oxidation had an ED_{50} value of 2.3 μmol/L. Further experiments showed that whereas quercetin chelated copper ions, the phenylpropanoid glycosides tested did not, indicating that their inhibition of copper ion-induced LDL oxidation is independent of any capacity for copper ion chelation[11]

In further experiments involving cell-free systems, arenarioside, ballotetroside, forsythoside B and verbascoside, as well as the non-glycosidic phenylpropanoid caffeoylmalic acid, demonstrated a concentration-dependent scavenging capacity towards several reactive oxygen species (ROS).[8] For each of the compounds, the

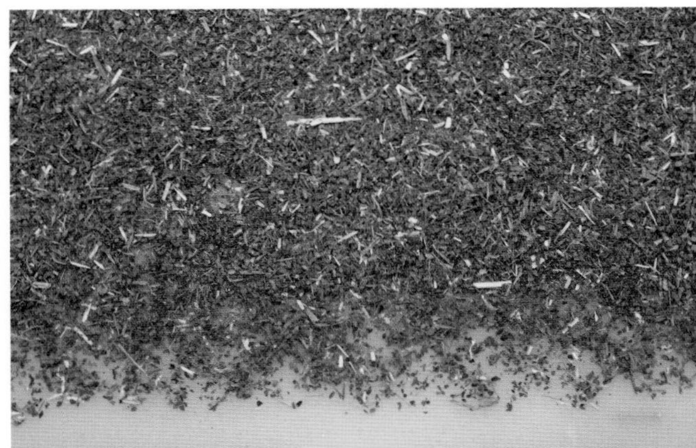

Figure 4 Black horehound – dried drug substance (herb).

greatest ROS scavenging activity was seen for hydrogen peroxide and hypochlorous acid (concentrations required for 50% inhibition were $\leqslant$ 5.0 mg/L for all compounds, except ballotetroside, $<$ 12 mg/L). Concentration-dependent inhibitions of ROS production by phorbol ester-stimulated PMNs were also seen in cellular systems following incubation with forsythoside B, verbascoside and caffeoylmalic acid, whereas arenarioside and ballotetroside showed little or no activity.[8]

Clinical studies

There is a lack of clinical research assessing the effects of black horehound and rigorous randomised controlled clinical trials are required.

Side-effects, Toxicity

None documented. However, there is a lack of clinical safety and toxicity data for black horehound and further investigation of these aspects is required.

In *in vitro* experiments, the release of lactate dehydrogenase from polymorphonuclear neutrophils (PMN), an indicator of toxicity, was maintained below 20% following incubation with arenarioside, ballotetroside, forsythoside B, verbascoside and caffeoylmalic acid at concentrations ranging from 0.1 to 200 mg/L.[8] A report of the study states that this effect was not significant ($p < 0.01$), although it is not clear what was the control.

Contra-indications, Warnings

None documented.

Drug interactions None documented. However, the potential for preparations of black horehound to interact with other medicines administered concurrently, particularly those with similar or opposing effects, should be considered.

Pregnancy and lactation Black horehound is reputed to affect the menstrual cycle although the scientific basis for this statement is not clear.[G30] In view of the lack of phytochemical, pharmacological and toxicity data, the use of black horehound during pregnancy and breastfeeding should be avoided.

References

1 Savona G *et al*. Structure of ballotinone, a diterpenoid from *Ballota nigra*. *J Chem Soc Perkin Trans 1* 1976; 1607–1609.
2 Savona G *et al*. The structure of ballotenol, a new diterpenoid from *Ballota nigra*. *J Chem Soc Perkin Trans 1* 1977; 497–499.
3 Bruno M *et al*. Preleosibirin, a prefuranic labdane diterpene from *Ballota nigra* subsp. *foetida*. *Phytochemistry* 1986; 25: 538–539.
4 Seidel V *et al*. Isolation from *Ballota nigra* L. of 13-hydroxyballonigrinolide, a diterpene useful for the standardization of the drug. *J Pharm Belg* 1996; 51: 72–73.
5 Seidel V *et al*. Diterpène esters hétérosidiques phénylpropanoïques de *Ballota nigra* L. *Ann Pharm Franc* 1998; 56: 31–35.
6 Savona G *et al*. Structures of three new diterpenoids from Ballota species. *J Chem Soc Perkin Trans 1* 1997; 5: 322–324.
7 Bertrand MO *et al*. Two major flavonoids from *Ballota nigra*. *Biochem Syst Ecol* 2000; 28: 1031–1033.
8 Daels-Rakotoarison DA *et al*. Neurosedative and antioxidant activitites of phenylpropanoids from *Ballota nigra*. *Arzneim Forsch* 2000; 50: 16–23.
9 Seidel V *et al*. Phenylpropanoid glycosides from *Ballota nigra*. *Planta Med* 1996; 62: 186–187.
10 Seidel V *et al*. A phenylpropanoid glycoside from *Ballota nigra*. *Phytochemistry* 1997; 44(4): 691–693.
11 Seidel V, *et al*. Phenylpropanoids from *Ballota nigra* L. inhibit *in vitro* LDL peroxidation. *Phytotherapy Res* 2000; 14: 93–98.
12 Didry N *et al*. Isolation and antibacterial activity of phenylpropanoid derivatives from *Ballota nigra*. *J Ethnopharmacol* 1999; 67: 197–202.
13 Bader A *et al*. Composition of the essential oil of *Ballota undulata*, *B. nigra* ssp. *foetida* and *B. saxatilis*. *Flavour Frag Journal* 2003; 18: 502–504.
14 Sever Yilmiz B, Saltan Çitoğlu G.[Chemical constituents of *Ballota L.* species]. *Ankara Ecz Fak Derg* 2003; 32: 37–53 [Turkish].

Horehound, White

Summary and Pharmaceutical Comment

The chemistry of white horehound is well documented. Limited pharmacological information is available, although expectorant properties have been reported which support some of the herbal uses. There is a lack of robust clinical research assessing the efficacy and safety of white horehound. In view of the lack of toxicity data and suggested cardioactive properties, excessive use of white horehound and use during pregnancy and lactation should be avoided.

Species (Family)

Marrubium vulgare L. (Labiatae)

Synonym(s)

Common Hoarhound, Hoarhound, Horehound, Marrubium

Part(s) Used

Flower, leaf

Pharmacopoeial and Other Monographs

BHC 1992[(G6)]
BHP 1996[(G9)]
BP 2007[(G84)]
Complete German Commission E[(G3)]
Martindale 35th edition[(G85)]

Legal Category (Licensed Products)

GSL [(G37)]

Constituents

The following is compiled from several sources, including General References G2, G6 and G62.

Diterpenes

premarrubiin
marrubiin
marrubenol
vulgarol

Figure 1 Selected constituents of white horehound.

Alkaloids Pyrrolidine-type. Betonicine 0.3%, the *cis*-isomer turicine.

Flavonoids Apigenin, luteolin, quercetin, and their glycosides.[(1)]

Terpenoids Diterpenes including marrubiin 0.3–1.0%, a lactone, as the main component with lesser amounts of various alcohols (e.g. marrubenol, marrubiol, peregrinol and vulgarol). Marrubiin has also been stated to be an artefact formed from a precursor, premarrubiin, during extraction.[(2)]

Volatile oils Trace. Bisabolol, camphene, *p*-cymene, limonene, β-pinene, sabinene and others,[(2)] a sesquiterpene (unspecified).

Other constituents Choline, saponin (unspecified), β-sitosterol (a phytosterol), waxes (C_{26}-C_{34} alkanes).

Food Use

White horehound is listed by the Council of Europe as a natural source of food flavouring (category N2). This category indicates that white horehound can be added to foodstuffs in small quantities, with a possible limitation of an active principle (as yet unspecified) in the final product.[(G16)] Previously, white horehound has been listed as GRAS (Generally Recognised As Safe).[(G65)]

Herbal Use

White horehound is stated to possess expectorant and antispasmodic properties. Traditionally, it has been used for acute or chronic bronchitis, whooping cough, and specifically for bronchitis with non-productive cough.[(G2, G6, G7, G8, G64)]

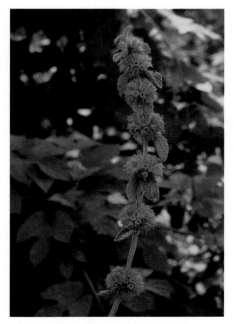

Figure 2 White horehound (*Marrubium vulgare*).

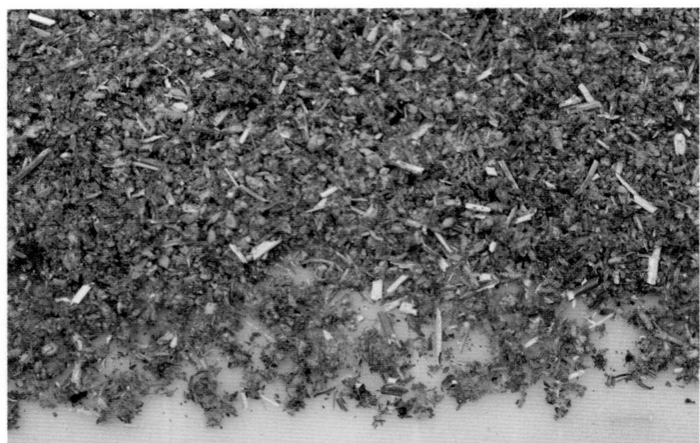

Figure 3 White horehound – dried drug substance (leaf).

H

Dosage

Dosages for oral administration (adults) for traditional uses recommended in standard herbal reference texts are given below.

Dried herb 1–2 g as an infusion three times daily.[G6, G7]

Liquid extract 2–4 mL (1 : 1 in 20% alcohol) three times daily.[G6, G7]

Pharmacological Actions

In vitro and animal studies

Aqueous extracts have been reported to exhibit an antagonistic effect towards 5-hydroxytryptamine *in vivo* in mice, and *in vitro* in guinea-pig ileum and rat uterus tissue.[3] Expectorant and vasodilative properties have been documented for the volatile oil.[4] However, the main active expectorant principle in white horehound is reported to be marrubiin, which is stated to stimulate secretions of the bronchial mucosa.[G60] Marrubiin has also been stated to be cardioactive, possessing anti-arrhythmic properties, although higher doses are reported to cause arrhythmias.[G60] Marrubin acid (obtained from the saponification of marrubiin) has been documented to stimulate bile secretion in rats, whereas marrubiin was found to be inactive.[5] White horehound is stated to possess bitter properties (BI 65 000 compared to gentian BI 10 000–30 000) with marrubiin as the main active component.[G62]

Large doses of white horehound are purgative.[G10, G60] The volatile oil has antischistosomal activity.[6]

Clinical studies

There is a lack of clinical research assessing the effects of white horehound and rigorous randomised controlled clinical trials are required.

Side-effects, Toxicity

There is a lack of clinical safety and toxicity data for white horehound and further investigation of these aspects is required.

The plant juice of white horehound is stated to contain an irritant principle, which can cause contact dermatitis.[G51]

No documented toxicity studies were located for the whole plant, although an LD_{50} (rat, by mouth) value for marrubin acid is reported as 370 mg/kg body weight.[5]

Contra-indications, Warnings

None documented. Cardioactive properties and an antagonism of 5-hydroxytryptamine have been documented in animals. However, the clinical relevance, if any, of these findings is unclear.

Drug interactions None documented. However, the potential for preparations of white horehound to interact with other medicines administered concurrently, particularly those with similar or opposing effects, should be considered.

Pregnancy and lactation White horehound is reputed to be an abortifacient and to affect the menstrual cycle.[G30] Uterine stimulant activity in animals has been documented.[G30] In view of this and the lack of safety data, the use of white horehound during pregnancy and lactation should be avoided.

Preparations

Proprietary multi-ingredient preparations

UK: Rob-Bron Tablets.

References

1 Kowalewski Z, Matlawska I. Flavonoid compounds in the herb of *Marrubium vulgare* L. *Herba Pol* 1978; 24: 183–186.

2 Henderson MS, McCrindle R. Premarrubiin. A diterpenoid from *Marrubium vulgare* L. *J Chem Soc* 1969; (C): 2014.

3 Cahen R. Pharmacologic spectrum of *Marrubium vulgare*. *C R Soc Biol* 1970; 164: 1467–1472.

4 Karryev MO *et al*. Some therapeutic properties and phytochemistry of common horehound. *Izv Akad Nauk Turkm SSR Ser Biol Nauk* 1976; 3: 86–88.

5 Krejcí I, Zadina R. Die Gallentreibende Wirkung von Marrubiin und Marrabinsäure. *Planta Med*; 1959; 7: 1–7.

6 Saleh MM, Glombitza KW. Volatile oil of *Marrubium vulgare* and its anti-schistosomal activity. *Planta Med* 1989; 55: 105.

Horse-chestnut

Summary and Pharmaceutical Comment

Horse-chestnut is traditionally characterised by its saponin components, in particular aescin, which represents a mixture of compounds. However, horse-chestnut also contains other pharmacologically active constituents, including coumarins and flavonoids. Many of the documented activities can be attributed to the saponin and flavonoid constituents in horse-chestnut. The traditional use of horse-chestnut in peripheral vascular disorders is supported by data from preclinical studies in which anti-inflammatory and capillary stabilising effects have been observed. There is evidence from randomised, double-blind, controlled clinical trials to support the use of horse-chestnut seed extract in the treatment of symptoms of chronic venous insufficiency but confirmation from more robust studies is required. In view of the limited information on safety and toxicity, excessive use of horse-chestnut and use during pregnancy and lactation should be avoided.

Species (Family)

Aesculus hippocastanum L. (Hippocastanaceae)

Synonym(s)

Aesculus

Part(s) Used

Seed

Pharmacopoeial and Other Monographs

BHP 1996[(G9)]
ESCOP 2003[(G76)]
Martindale 35th edition[(G85)]
USP29/NF24[(G86)]

Legal Category (Licensed Products)

GSL (for external use only)[(G37)]

Constituents

The following is compiled from several sources, including General References G52, G59 and G62.

Coumarins Aesculetin, fraxin (fraxetin glucoside), scopolin (scopoletin glucoside).

Flavonoids Flavonol (kaempferol, quercetin) glycosides including astragalin, isoquercetrin, rutin; leucocyanidin (quercetin derivative).

Saponins French pharmacopoeial standard, not less than 3% aescin. A mixture of saponins collectively referred to as 'aescin' (3–10%); α- and β-aescin as major glycosides.

Tannins Type unspecified but likely to be condensed in view of the epicatechin content (formed during hydrolysis of condensed tannins).

Other constituents Allantoin, amino acids (adenine, adenosine, guanine), choline, citric acid, phytosterol.

Food Use

Horse-chestnut is not used in foods.

Herbal Use

Traditionally, horse-chestnut has been used for the treatment of varicose veins, haemorrhoids, phlebitis, diarrhoea, fever and enlargement of the prostate gland. The German Commission E approved use for treatment of chronic venous insufficiency in the legs.[(G3)]

Dosage

Dosages for oral administration (adults) for traditional uses recommended in older and contemporary standard herbal and/or pharmaceutical reference texts are given below.

Fruit 0.2–1.0 g three times daily.[(G49)]

Preparations Extracts equivalent to 50–150 mg triterpenes calculated as aescin, in divided doses.[(G52)]

Pharmacological Actions

Documented studies have concentrated on the actions of the saponins, in particular, aescin.

In vitro and animal studies

Anti-inflammatory and anti-oedema effects Anti-inflammatory activity in rats has been documented for both a fruit extract and the saponin fraction.[(1–4)] Anti-inflammatory activity in the rat has been reported to be greater for a total horse-chestnut extract compared to aescin. In addition, an extract excluding aescin also exhibited activity, suggesting that horse-chestnut contains anti-inflammatory agents other than aescin.[(5)] No difference in activity was noted when the horse-chestnut extracts were administered prior to and after dextran (inflammatory agent). It has been proposed that aescin affects the initial phase of inflammation by exerting a 'sealing' effect on capillaries and by reducing the number and/or diameter of capillary pores.[(3)]

Effects on venous tone Horse-chestnut extract (16% aescin, 0.2 mg/mL) and also aescin (0.1 mg/mL) induced contractions in isolated bovine and human veins.[(G52)] Concentration-dependent contractions of isolated canine veins were observed with a horse-chestnut extract (16% aescin, 5×10^{-4} mg/mL).[(G52)] A standardised extract (16% aescin, 50 mg, given intravenously) increased femoral venous pressure in anaesthetised dogs, and decreased cutaneous capillary hyperpermeability in rats (200 mg/kg, given orally).[(G52)]

H

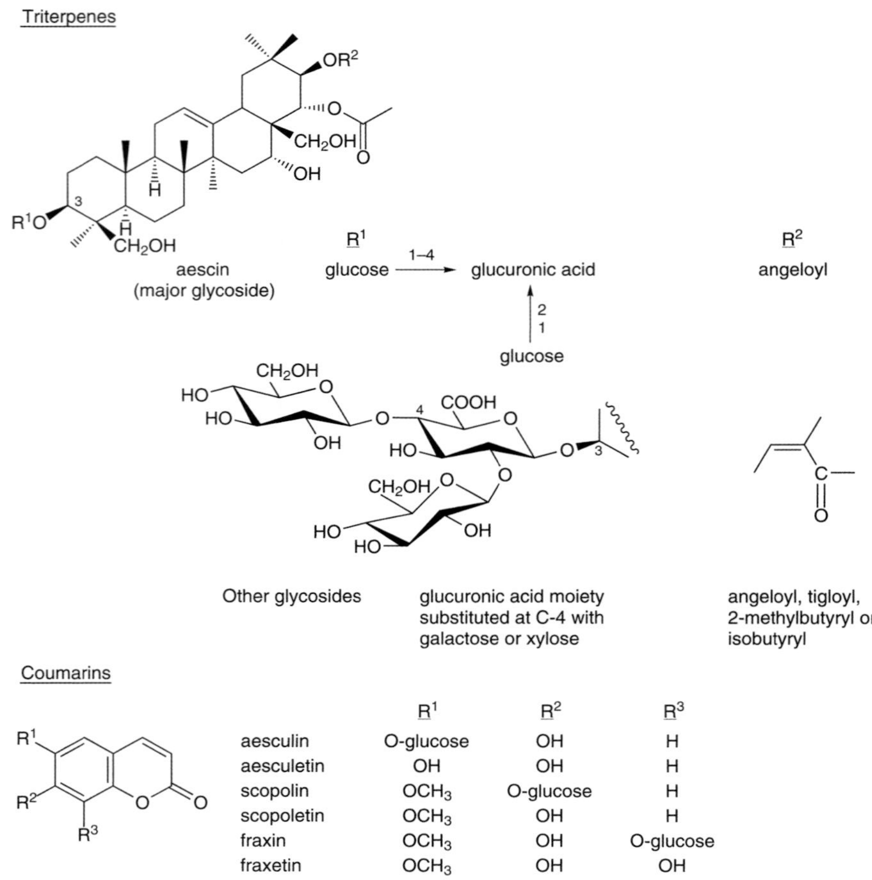

Figure 1 Selected constituents of horse-chestnut.

In addition, the saponin fraction has been reported to exhibit analgesic and antigranulation activities in rats,(3) to reduce capillary permeability,(6) and to produce an initial hypotension followed by a longer lasting hypertension in anaesthetised animals.(4) Prostaglandin production by venous tissue is thought to be involved in the regulation of vascular reactivity.(7) Prostaglandins of the E series are known to cause relaxation of venous tissues whereas those of the F_{α} series produce contraction. Increased venous tone induced by aescin *in vitro* was found to be associated with an increased $PGF_{2\alpha}$ synthesis in the venous tissue.

Other activities *In vitro*, aescin has been documented to inhibit hyaluronidase activity (IC_{50} 150 μmol/L).(G52)

A saponin fraction of horse-chestnut has been reported to contract isolated rabbit ileum.(3)

Antiviral activity *in vitro* against influenza virus (A_2/Japan 305) has been described for aescin.(8)

Metabolism studies of aescin in the rat have concluded that aescin toxicity is reduced by hepatic metabolism.(9)

Flavonoids and tannins are generally recognised as having anti-inflammatory and astringent properties, respectively.

Clinical studies

Chronic venous insufficiency Several studies have assessed the effects of horse-chestnut seed extract in patients with chronic venous insufficiency, a common condition which causes oedema of the lower leg.

A Cochrane systematic review of randomised, double-blind, controlled trials of horse-chestnut seed extract in chronic venous insufficiency included 17 studies: ten placebo-controlled trials and seven studies comparing horse-chestnut seed extract with reference medication (O-β-hydroxyethylrutosides, pycnogenol) or compression therapy.(10) Trials involved the administration of horse-chestnut seed extract equivalent to 50–150 mg aescin daily for two to 16 weeks. Collectively, results of placebo-controlled studies indicated that horse-chestnut seed extract was superior to placebo with respect to leg pain (weighted mean difference (95% confidence interval (CI)) in 100 mm visual analogue scale scores: 42.40 mm (34.90–49.90; six trials), oedema and pruritus resulting from chronic venous insufficiency.(10) Trials comparing horse chestnut seed extract with other treatment approaches indicated that the herbal preparation was as effective in relieving symptoms of chronic venous insufficiency. The review concluded that horse-chestnut seed extract is an effective short-term treatment for symptoms of chronic venous insufficiency, but that because of methodological limitations of existing studies, further well-designed clinical trials are required for confirmation of the observed effects.(10)

Other effects Glycosaminoglycan hydrolyses are enzymes involved in the breakdown of substances (proteoglycans) that determine capillary rigidity and pore size (thus influencing the passage of macromolecules into the surrounding tissue). Proteoglycans also interact with collagen, stabilising the fibres and regulating their correct biosynthesis.(11) The activity of these enzymes was found to be raised in patients with varicosis, compared with healthy patients. In a study involving 15 patients with varicosis treated with horse-chestnut extract (900 mg daily) for 12 days, the activity of these enzymes was significantly reduced.[11] However, this observation requires confirmation in larger, robust clinical studies.

In a randomised, double-blind, placebo-controlled study involving 70 healthy individuals with haematomas, a topical gel (2% aescin) reduced sensitivity to pressure on affected areas.[G52]

The cosmetic applications of horse-chestnut have been reviewed;[12] these effects are attributed to properties associated with the saponin constituents.

Side-effects, Toxicity

Clinical data

There is a lack of clinical safety and toxicity data for horse-chestnut and further investigation of these aspects is required.

Two incidences of toxic nephropathy have been reported and were stated as probably secondary to the ingestion of high doses of aescin.[13] In Japan, where horse-chestnut has been used as an anti-inflammatory drug after surgery or trauma, hepatic injury has been described in a male patient who received an intramuscular injection of a proprietary product containing horse-chestnut.[14] Liver function tests showed a mild abnormality and a diagnosis of giant cell tumour of bone (grade 2) by bone biopsy was made. Other side-effects stated to have been reported for the product include shock, spasm, mild nausea, vomiting and urticaria.[14] However, a causal association with horse-chestnut use in this case has not been established.

Preclinical data

A proprietary product containing horse-chestnut (together with phenopyrazone and cardiac glycoside-containing plant extracts) has been associated with the development of a drug-induced autoimmune disease called 'pseudolupus syndrome' in Germany and Switzerland.[15,16] The individual component in the product responsible for the syndrome was not established.

The effect of aescin, both free and albumin-bound, on renal tubular transport processes has been studied in the isolated, artificially perfused frog kidney.[17] Aescin was found to primarily affect tubular, rather than glomerular, epithelium and it was noted that binding to plasma protein (approximately 50%) protects against this nephrotoxicity. Aescin was thought to be neither secreted nor reabsorbed in the tubules, and the concentration of unbound aescin filtered through the kidney (13%) was considered to be too low to have toxic effects. The authors commented that the symptoms of acute renal failure in humans are caused primarily by interference with glomeruli and in view of this, the nephrotoxic potential of aescin is probably only relevant when the kidneys are already damaged and also if the aescin is displaced from its binding to plasma protein.[17]

It has been noted that death occurs rapidly in animals given large doses of aescin, due to massive haemolysis. Death is more prolonged in animals given smaller doses of aescin.[4]

LD_{50} values for aescin have been estimated in mice, rats and guinea-pigs and range from 134 to 720 mg/kg (by mouth) and from 1.4 to 15.2 mg/kg (intravenous injection).[G49] The total saponin fraction has been reported to be less toxic in mice (intraperitoneal injection) compared to the isolated aescin mixture (LD_{50} 46.5 mg/kg and 9.5 mg/kg, respectively).[3] The haemolytic index of horse-chestnut is documented as being 6000, compared with 9500 to 12 500 for aescin.[G62] Daily doses in rats (100 mg/kg, orally) of a standardised extract of horse-chestnut (16% aescin) did not produce teratogenic effects, and the extract was negative in the Ames test with *Salmonella typhimurium* TA98 without actuation.[G52]

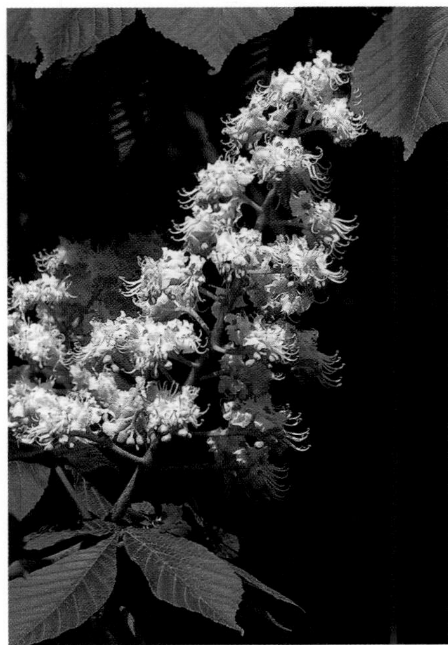

Figure 2 Horse-chestnut (*Aesculus hippocastanum*).

Contra-indications, Warnings

Horse-chestnut may be irritant to the gastrointestinal tract due to the saponin constituents. Saponins are generally recognised to possess haemolytic properties, but are not usually absorbed from the gastrointestinal tract following oral administration. As a precaution, horse-chestnut should be avoided by patients with existing renal or hepatic impairment.

Drug interactions None documented. However, the potential for preparations of horse-chestnut to interact with other medicines administered concurrently, particularly those with similar or opposing effects, should be considered. Horse-chestnut has coumarin constituents, although those detected so far do not

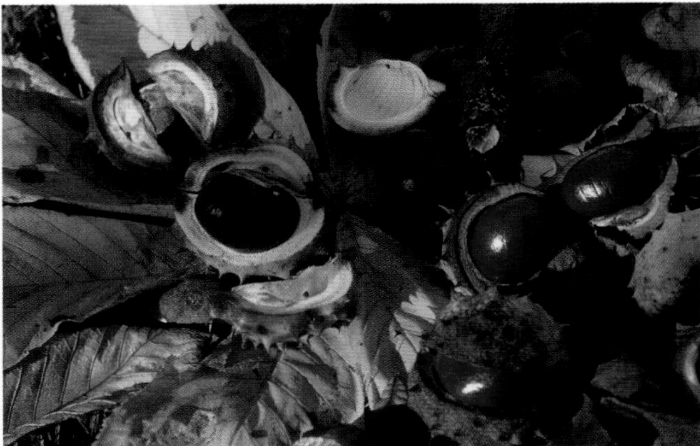

Figure 3 Horse-chestnut – dried drug substance (seed).

possess the minimum structural requirements for anti-coagulant activity. There is evidence from preclinical studies that aescin, the main saponin component in horse-chestnut, binds to plasma protein. However, it is not clear if this has clinical relevance in terms of affecting binding of other drugs.

Pregnancy and lactation The safety of horse-chestnut during pregnancy and lactation has not been established. In view of the pharmacologically active constituents present in horse-chestnut, use during pregnancy and lactation should be avoided.

Preparations

Proprietary single-ingredient preparations

Argentina: Grafic Retard; Herbaccion Venotonico; Nadem; Venastat; Venostasin. *Austria:* Aesculaforce; Provenen; Venosin; Venostasin. *Belgium:* Venoplant. *Brazil:* Varilise; Venafort; Venostasin. *Chile:* Venastat. *Czech Republic:* Venitan. *Germany:* Aescorin Forte; Aescusan; Aescuven; Concentrin; Essaven; Heweven Phyto; Hoevenol; Noricaven; Plissamur; Sklerovenol N; Venalot novo; Venen-Dragees; Venen-Fluid; Venen-Tabletten; Venen-Tropfen N; Venentabs; Veno-biomo; Venodura; Venoplant; Venopyronum; Venostasin. *Hungary:* Venastat. *Italy:* Flebostasin. *Mexico:* Venastat. *Spain:* Plantivenol; Varicid. *Switzerland:* Aesculaforce; AesculaMed; Phlebostasin; Venavit N; Venostasin.

Proprietary multi-ingredient preparations

Argentina: Nadem Forte; Venoful; VNS 45. *Australia:* Bioglan Cirflo; Bioglan Zellulean with Escin; Extralife Leg-Care; Herbal Capillary Care; Proflo. *Austria:* Dilaescol; Heparin Comp. *Belgium:* Rectovasol. *Brazil:* Castanha de India Composta; Digestron; Hemorroidex; Mirorroidin; Novarrutina; Proctosan; Supositorio Hamamelis Composto; Traumed; Varizol; Venocur Triplex. *Chile:* Proctoplex. *Czech Republic:* Heparin-Gel. *France:* Arterase; Climaxol; Creme Rap; Evarose; Fluon; Hemorrogel; Histo-Fluine P; Intrait de Marron d'Inde P; Mediflor Tisane Circulation du Sang No 12; Opo-Veinogene; Phlebosedol; Phytomelis; Veinophytum; Veinostase; Veinotonyl. *Germany:* Aescusan; Amphodyn; Cefasabal; Cycloven Forte N; Diu Venostasin; Fagorutin Rosskastanien-Balsam N; Heparin Comp; Intradermi; PC 30 V; Sportupac M; Traumacyl; Varicylum-S; Venen Krauter NT; Venen-Salbe N; Venengel; Weleda Hamorrhoidalzapfchen. *Italy:* Capill Venogel; Capill; Centella Complex; Centella Complex; Centeril H; Centeril H; Flavion; Inflamase; Pik Gel; Proctopure; Varicogel; Venactive; Venoplus. *Mexico:* Almodin. *South Africa:* Stibium Comp. *Spain:* Contusin; Roidhemo; Ruscimel. *Switzerland:* Demoven N; Ipasin; Strath Gouttes pour les veines.

References

1 Farnsworth NR, Cordell GA. A review of some biologically active compounds isolated from plants as reported in the 1974–75 literature. *Lloydia* 1976; 39: 420–455.
2 Benoit PS *et al*. Biological and phytochemical evaluation of plants. XIV. Antiinflammatory evaluation of 163 species of plants. *Lloydia* 1976; 39: 160–171.
3 Cebo B *et al*. Pharmacological properties of saponin fractions from Polish crude drugs: *Saponaria officinalis*, *Primula officinalis*, and *Aesculus hippocastanum*. *Herba Pol* 1976; 22: 154–162.
4 Vogel G *et al*. Untersuchungen zum Mechanismus der therapeutischen und toxischen Wirkung des Rosskastanien-saponins aescin. *Arzneimittelforschung* 1970; 20: 699–705.
5 Tsutsumi S, Ishizuka S. Anti-inflammatory effects of the extract *Aesculus hippocastanum* and seed. *Shikwa-Gakutto* 1967; 67: 1324–1328.
6 De Pascale V *et al*. Effect of an escin-cyclonamine mixture on capillary permeability. *Boll Chim Farm* 1974; 113: 600–614.
7 Longiave D *et al*. The mode of action of aescin on isolated veins: Relationship with $PGF_2\alpha$. *Pharmacol Res Commun* 1978; 10: 145–153.
8 Rao SG, Cochran KW. Antiviral activity of triterpenoid saponins containing acylated β-amyrin aglycones. *J Pharm Sci* 1974; 63: 471.
9 Rothkopf M. Effects of age, sex and phenobarbital pretreatment on the acute toxicity of the horse chestnut saponin aescin in rats. *Naunyn-Schmied archpharm* 1977; 297 (Suppl. Suppl.): R18.
10 Pittler MH, Ernst E. Horse-chestnut seed extract for chronic venous insufficiency (Review). 2006, Issue 1. Art. No.: CD003230.10.1002/14651858.CD003230.pub2
11 Kreysel HW *et al*. A possible role of lysosomal enzymes in the pathogenesis of varicosis and the reduction in their serum activity by Venostasin[R]. *Vasa* 1983; 12: 377– 382.
12 Proserpio G *et al*. Cosmetic uses of horse-chestnut (*Aesculum hippocastanum*) extracts, of escin and of the cholesterol/escin complex. *Fitoterapia* 1980; 51: 113–128.
13 Grasso A, Corvaglia E. Two cases of suspected toxic tubulonephrosis due to escine. *Gazz Med Ital* 1976; 135: 581–584.
14 Takegoshi K *et al*. A case of Venoplant[R]-induced hepatic injury. *Gastroenterol Japonica* 1986; 21: 62–65.
15 Grob P *et al*. Drug-induced pseudolupus. *Lancet* 1975; ii: 144–148.
16 Russell AS. Drug-induced autoimmune disease. *Clin Immunol Allergy* 1981; 1: 57–76.
17 Rothkopf M *et al*. Animal experiments on the question of the renal toleration of the horse chestnut saponin aescin. *Arzneimittelforschung* 1977; 27: 598–605.

Horseradish

Summary and Pharmaceutical Comment

The chemistry of horseradish is well established and it is recognised as one of the richest plant sources of peroxidase enzymes.[(G48)] Little pharmacological information was located, although the isothiocyanates and peroxidases probably account for the reputed circulatory stimulant and wound-healing actions, respectively. The oil is one of the most hazardous of all essential oils and it is not recommended for either external or internal use.[(G58)] Horseradish should not be ingested in amounts exceeding those used in foods.

Species (Family)

Armoracia rusticana P. Gaertin., B. Mey. & Scherb.

Synonym(s)

Armoracia lapathifolia, *Cochlearia armoracia* L., *Nasturtium armoracia* (L.) Fr.

Part(s) Used

Root

Pharmacopoeial and Other Monographs

Complete German Commission E[(G3)]
Martindale 35th edition[(G85)]

Legal Category (Licensed Products)

GSL[(G37)]

Constituents

The following is compiled from several sources, including General References G40, G58 and G62.

Coumarins Aesculetin, scopoletin.[(1)]

Phenols Caffeic acid derivatives and lesser amounts of hydroxycinnamic acid derivatives. Concentrations of acids are reported to be much lower in the root than in the leaf.[(1)]

Volatile oils Glucosinolates (mustard oil glycosides) gluconasturtiin and sinigrin (*S*-glucosides), yielding phenylethylisothiocyanate and allylisothiocyanate after hydrolysis. Isothiocyanate content estimated as 12.2–20.4 mg/g freeze dried root.[(2, 3)] Other isothiocyanate types include isopropyl, 3-butenyl, 4-pentenyl, phenyl, 3-methylthiopropyl and benzyl derivatives.[(4)]

Other constituents Ascorbic acid, asparagin, peroxidase enzymes, resin, starch and sugar.

Other plant parts Kaempferol and quercetin have been documented for the leaf.

Food Use

Horseradish is listed by the Council of Europe as a natural source of food flavouring (category N2). This category indicates that horseradish can be added to foodstuffs in small quantities, with a possible limitation of an active principle (as yet unspecified) in the final product.[(G16)] Previously horseradish has been listed as GRAS (Generally Recognised As Safe).[(G57)] Horseradish is commonly used as a food flavouring.

Herbal Use

Horseradish is stated to possess antiseptic, circulatory and digestive stimulant, diuretic and vulnerary properties.[(G42, G49, G64)] Traditionally, it has been used for pulmonary and urinary infection, urinary stones, oedematous conditions, and externally for application to inflamed joints or tissues.[(G49)]

Dosage

Dosages for oral administration (adults) for traditional uses recommended in older herbal reference texts are given below.

Root (fresh) 2–4 g before meals.[(G49)]

Pharmacological Actions

In vitro and animal studies

A marked hypotensive effect in cats has been documented for horseradish peroxidase, following intravenous administration.[(5)] The effect was completely blocked by aspirin and indometacin, but was not affected by antihistamines. It was concluded that horseradish peroxidase acts by stimulating the synthesis of arachidonic acid metabolites.

Glucosinolates

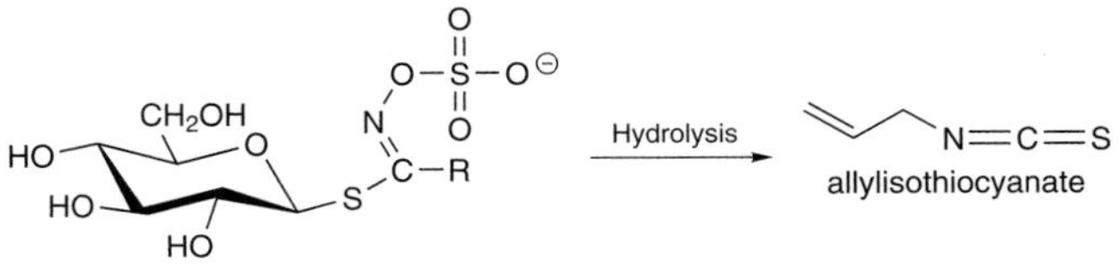

Hydrolysis → allylisothiocyanate

	R
sinigrin (prop-2-enylglucosinolate)	$-CH_2CH{=}CH_2$
gluconasturtin (2-phenylethylglucosinolate)	$-CH_2CH_2C_6H_5$

Coumarins

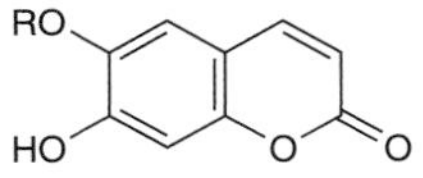

	R
aesculin	glucose
aesculetin	H

Figure 1 Selected constituents of horseradish.

H

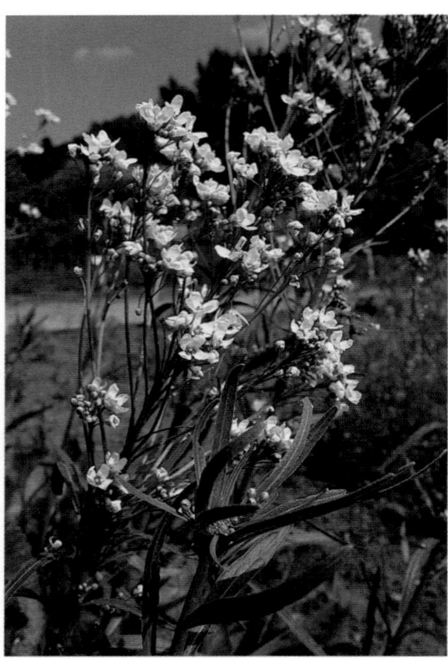

Figure 2 Horseradish (*Armoracia rusticana*).

Clinical studies

There is a lack of clinical research assessing the effects of horseradish.

Side-effects, Toxicity

There is a lack of clinical safety and toxicity data for horseradish and further investigation of these aspects is required.

Isothiocyanates are reported to have irritant effects on the skin and also to be allergenic.(G51, G58) Animal poisoning has been documented for horseradish. Symptoms described include inflammation of the stomach or rumen, and excitement followed by collapse.(G33)

Contra-indications, Warnings

It is stated that horseradish may depress thyroid function, and should be avoided by individuals with hypothyroidism or by those receiving thyroxine.(G42, G49) No rationale for this statement is included, except that this action is common to all members of the cabbage and mustard family.

Drug interactions None documented. However, the potential for preparations of horseradish to interact with other medicines

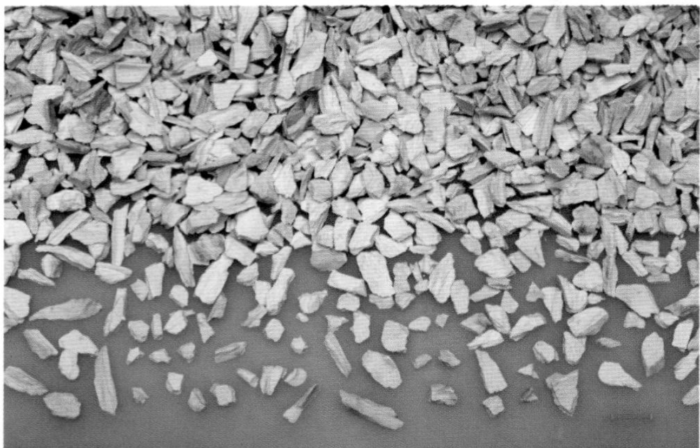

Figure 3 Horseradish – dried drug substance (root).

administered concurrently, particularly those with similar or opposing effects, should be considered.

Pregnancy and lactation Allylisothiocyanate is extremely toxic and a violent irritant to mucous membranes.(G58) In view of this, use of horseradish should be avoided during pregnancy and lactation.

Preparations

Proprietary multi-ingredient preparations

Australia: Garlic and Horseradish + C Complex; Garlic, Horseradish, A & C Capsules; Procold. *Germany:* Angocin Anti-Infekt N. *Malaysia:* Horseradish Plus. *Switzerland:* Kernosan Elixir; Sanogencive. *UK:* Mixed Vegetable Tablets.

References

1 Stoehr H, Herrman K. Phenolic acids of vegetables. III. Hydroxycinnamic acids and hydroxybenzoic acids of root vegetables. *Z Lebensm-Unters Forsch* 1975: 159: 219–224.

2 Hansen H. Content of glucosinolates in horseradish (*Armoracia rusticana*). *Tidsskr Planteavl* 1974; 73: 408–410.

3 Kojima M. Volatile components of *Wasabia japonica*. II. Volatile components other than isothiocyanates. *Hakko Kogaku Zasshi* 1971; 49: 650–653.

4 Kojima M *et al*. Studies on the volatile components of *Wasabia japonica, Brassica juncea*, and *Cocholearia armoracia* by gas chromatography-mass spectrometry. *Yakugaku Zasshi* 1973; 93: 453–459.

5 Sjaastad OV *et al*. Hypotensive effects in cats caused by horseradish peroxidase mediated by metabolites of arachidonic acid. *J Histochem Cytochem* 1984; 32: 1328–1330.

Hydrangea

Summary and Pharmaceutical Comment

Limited information is available on the chemistry of hydrangea, although related species have been investigated more thoroughly.[G41] No scientific evidence was located to justify the herbal uses. In view of the lack of toxicity data, excessive use of hydrangea and use during pregnancy and lactation should be avoided.

Species (Family)

Hydrangea arborescens L. (Saxifragaceae)

Synonym(s)

Mountain Hydrangea, Seven Barks, Smooth Hydrangea, Wild Hydrangea

Part(s) Used

Rhizome, Root

Pharmacopoeial and Other Monographs

BHP 1996[G9]
Martindale 35th edition[G85]

Legal Category (Licensed Products)

GSL[G37]

Constituents

The following is compiled from several sources, including General Reference G40.

Limited information is available on the chemistry of hydrangea. It is stated to contain carbohydrates (e.g. gum, starch, sugars), flavonoids (e.g. kaempferol, quercetin, rutin), resin, saponins, hydrangin and hydrangenol, a stilbenoid,[1] and to be free from tannins.

Food Use

Hydrangea is not used in foods. Previously in the USA, hydrangea has been listed as a 'Herb of Undefined Safety'.[G22]

Herbal Use

Hydrangea is stated to possess diuretic and antilithic properties. Traditionally, it has been used for cystitis, urethritis, urinary calculi, prostatitis, enlarged prostate gland, and specifically for urinary calculi with gravel and cystitis.[G7, G64]

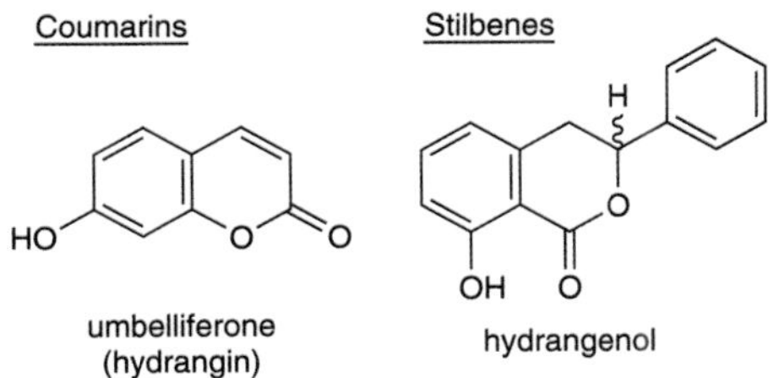

Figure 1 Selected constituents of hydrangea.

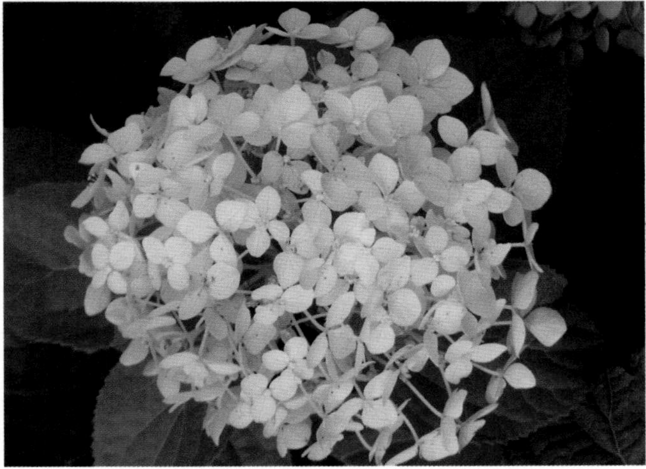

Figure 2 Hydrangea (*Hydrangea arborescens*).

Dosage

Dosages for oral administration (adults) for traditional uses recommended in standard herbal reference texts are given below.

Dried rhizome/root 2–4 g as a decoction three times daily.[G7]

Liquid extract 2–4 mL (1 : 1 in 25% alcohol) three times daily.[G7]

Tincture 2–10 mL (1 : 5 in 45% alcohol) three times daily.[G7]

Pharmacological Actions

In vitro and animal studies

None documented for hydrangea. Synthesised hydrangenol derivatives have been reported to possess anti-allergic properties,

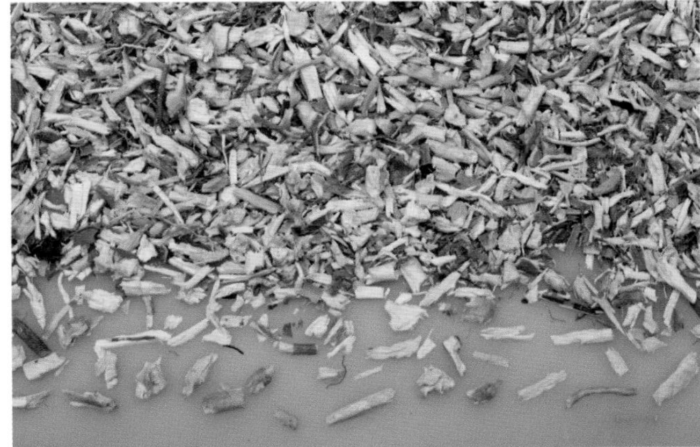

Figure 3 Hydrangea – dried drug substance (rhizome).

H

exhibiting a strong inhibitory action towards hyaluronidase activity and histamine release.[2]

Clinical studies

There is a lack of clinical research assessing the effects of hydrangea and rigorous randomised controlled clinical trials are required.

Side-effects, Toxicity

There is a lack of clinical safety and toxicity data for hydrangea and further investigation of these aspects is required.

Hydrangea has been reported to cause contact dermatitis,[G51] and it is stated that hydrangin may cause gastroenteritis.[G22] Symptoms of overdose are described as vertigo and a feeling of tightness in the chest.[G22]

H

Contra-indications, Warnings

None documented.

Drug interactions None documented. However, the potential for preparations of hydrangea to interact with other medicines administered concurrently should be considered.

Pregnancy and lactation The safety of hydrangea has not been established. In view of the lack of phytochemical, pharmacological and toxicity data, the use of hydrangea during pregnancy and lactation should be avoided.

Preparations

Proprietary multi-ingredient preparations

UK: Antiglan; Backache.

References

1 Harborne JB, Baxter H. *Phytochemical Dictionary.* London: Taylor and Francis, 1993.
2 Kakegawa H *et al.* Inhibitory effects of hydrangeol derivatives on the activation of hyaluronidase and their anti-allergic activities. *Planta Med* 1988; 54: 385–389.

Hydrocotyle

Summary and Pharmaceutical Comment

The chemistry of hydrocotyle is well studied and its pharmacological activity seems to be associated with the triterpenoid constituents. Documented preclinical studies support the herbal use of hydrocotyle as a dermatological agent although robust clinical studies are lacking. In view of the lack of toxicity data, excessive ingestion of hydrocotyle and use during pregnancy and lactation should be avoided.

Species (Family)

Centella asiatica (L.) Urban (Apiaceae Umbelliferae)

Synonym(s)

Asiatic Pennywort, Centella, Gotu Kola, *Hydrocotyle asiatica* L., *Hydrocotyle lurida* Hance, Indian Pennywort, Indian Water Navelwort, Ji Xue Cao

Part(s) Used

Herb

Pharmacopoeial and Other Monographs

BHP 1983[G7]
Martindale 35th edition[G85]
WHO volume 1 1999[G63]

Legal Category (Licensed Products)

GSL (for external use only)[G37]

Constituents

The following is compiled from several sources, including General Reference G60.

Amino acids Alanine and serine (major components), aminobutyrate, aspartate, glutamate, histidine, lysine and threonine.[1] The root contains greater quantities than the herb.[1]

Flavonoids Quercetin, kaempferol and various glycosides.[2–4]

Terpenoids Triterpenes, asiaticoside, centelloside, madecassoside, brahmoside and brahminoside (saponin glycosides). Aglycones are referred to as hydrocotylegenin A–E;[5] compounds A–D are reported to be esters of the triterpene alcohol R_1-barrigenol.[5,6] Asiaticentoic acid, centellic acid, centoic acid and madecassic acid.

Volatile oils Various terpenoids including β-caryophyllene, *trans*-β-farnesene and germacrene D (sesquiterpenes) as major components, α-pinene and β-pinene. The major terpenoid is stated to be unidentified.

Other constituents Hydrocotylin (an alkaloid), vallerine (a bitter principle), fatty acids (e.g. linoleic acid, linolenic acid, lignocene, oleic acid, palmitic acid, stearic acid), phytosterols (e.g. campesterol, sitosterol, stigmasterol),[7] resin and tannin.

The underground plant parts of hydrocotyle have been reported to contain small quantities of at least 14 different polyacetylenes.[8–10]

Food Use

Hydrocotyle is not used in foods.

Herbal Use

Hydrocotyle is stated to possess mild diuretic, antirheumatic, dermatological, peripheral vasodilator and vulnerary properties. Traditionally it has been used for rheumatic conditions, cutaneous affections, and by topical application, for indolent wounds, leprous ulcers, and cicatrisation after surgery.[G7, G64]

Dosage

Dosages for oral administration (adults) for traditional uses recommended in standard herbal reference texts are given below.

Dried leaf 0.6 g as an infusion three times daily.[G7]

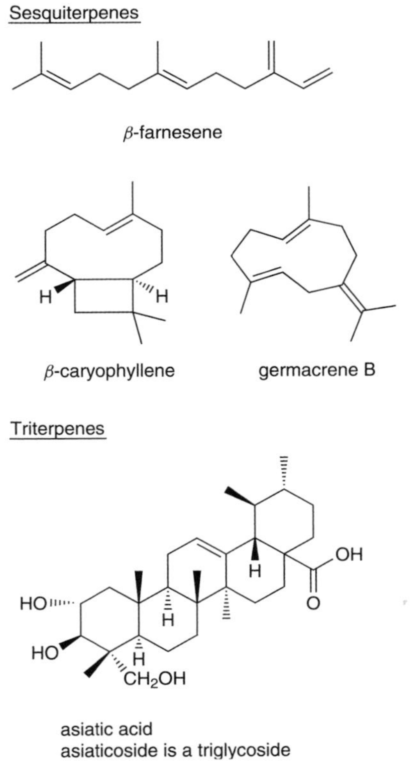

Sesquiterpenes

β-farnesene

β-caryophyllene

germacrene B

Triterpenes

HO
HO
H
H
H
CH_2OH
OH
O

asiatic acid
asiaticoside is a triglycoside

Figure 1 Selected constituents of hydrocotyle.

H

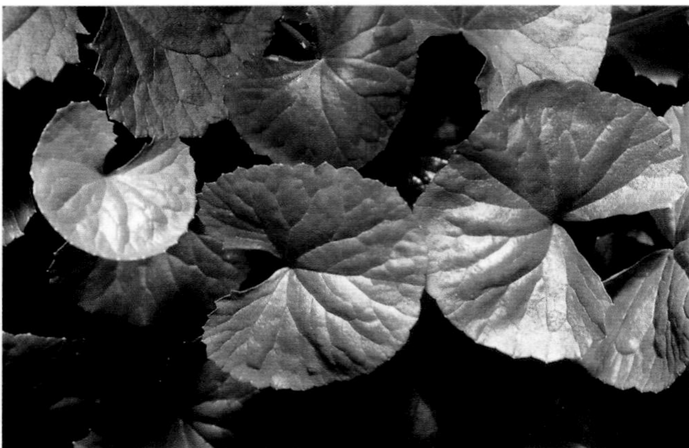

Figure 2 Hydrocotyle (*Centella asiatica*).

Pharmacological Actions

In vitro and animal studies

The triterpenoids are regarded as the active principles in hydrocotyle.[7] Asiaticoside is reported to possess wound-healing ability, by having a stimulating effect on the epidermis and promoting keratinisation.[11] Asiaticoside is thought to act by an inhibitory action on the synthesis of collagen and mucopolysaccharides in connective tissue.[11]

Both asiaticoside and madecassoside are documented to be anti-inflammatory, and the total saponin fraction is reported to be active in the carrageenan rat paw oedema test.[12]

In vivo studies in rats have shown that asiaticoside exhibits a protective action against stress-induced gastric ulcers, following subcutaneous administration,[13] and accelerates the healing of chemical-induced duodenal ulcers, after oral administration.[14] It was thought that asiaticoside acted by increasing the ability of the rats to cope with a stressful situation, rather than via a local effect on the mucosa.[13]

In vivo studies in mice and rats using brahmoside and brahminoside, by intraperitoneal injection, have shown a CNS-depressant effect.[15] The compounds were found to decrease motor activity, increase hexobarbitone sleeping time, slightly decrease body temperature, and were thought to act via a cholinergic mechanism.[15] A hypertensive effect in rats was also observed, but only following large doses.[15] *In vitro* studies with brahmoside and brahminoside indicated a relaxant effect on the rabbit duodenum and rat uterus, and an initial increase, followed by a decrease, in the amplitude and rate of contraction of the isolated rabbit heart.[15] Higher doses were found to cause cardiac arrest, although subsequent intravenous administration in dogs caused no marked change in an ECG.[15]

Fresh plant juice is reported to be devoid of antibacterial activity,[16] although asiaticoside has been reported to be active versus *Mycobacterium tuberculosis*, *Bacillus leprae* and *Entamoeba histolytica*, and oxyasiaticoside was documented to be active against tubercle bacillus.[16,17] The fresh plant juice is also stated not to exhibit antitumour or antiviral activities, but to possess a moderate cytotoxic action in human ascites tumour cells.[16]

Clinical studies

Several studies describing the use of hydrocotyle to treat wounds and various skin disorders have been documented. However, these studies have important methodological limitations and preclude definitive conclusions on the effects of hydrocotyle. Robust clinical studies are required. A cream containing a hydrocotyle extract was found to be effective in the treatment of psoriasis in seven patients to whom it was applied.[18] An aerosol preparation, containing a hydrocotyle extract, was reported to improve the healing in 19 of 25 wounds that had proved refractory to other forms of treatment.[11] A hydrocotyle extract containing asiaticoside (40%), asiatic acid (29–30%), madecassic acid (29–30%) and madasiatic acid (1%) was stated to be successful as both a preventive and curative treatment, when given to 227 patients with keloids or hypertrophic scars.[19] The effective dose in adults was reported to be between 60 and 90 mg. It was proposed that the triterpene constituents in the hydrocotyle extract act in a similar manner to cortisone, with respect to wound healing, and interfere with the metabolism of abnormal collagen.[19]

Pharmacokinetics There are only very limited data on the pharmacokinetics of constituents of hydrocotyle.

The triterpene constituents are reported to be metabolised primarily in the faeces in a period of 24–76 hours, with a small percentage metabolised via the kidneys.[19] An extract containing asiatic acid, madecassic acid, madasiatic acid and asiaticoside reached peak plasma concentrations in 2–4 hours, irrespective of whether it is administered in tablet, oily injection or ointment formulations.[19]

Side-effects, Toxicity

Clinical data

There is a lack of clinical research assessing the effects of hydrocotyle and rigorous randomised controlled clinical trials are required.

A burning sensation was reported by four of 20 patients during the period of application of an aerosol preparation containing hydrocotyle.[11] However, it is not clear whether other components in the formulation contributed to this reaction. Ingestion of hydrocotyle is stated to have produced pruritus over the whole body.[G51]

Preclinical data

In vitro antifertility activity against human and rat sperm has been described for the total saponin fraction.[17] Asiaticoside and brahminoside are thought to be the active components, although no spermicidal or spermostatic action could be demonstrated for

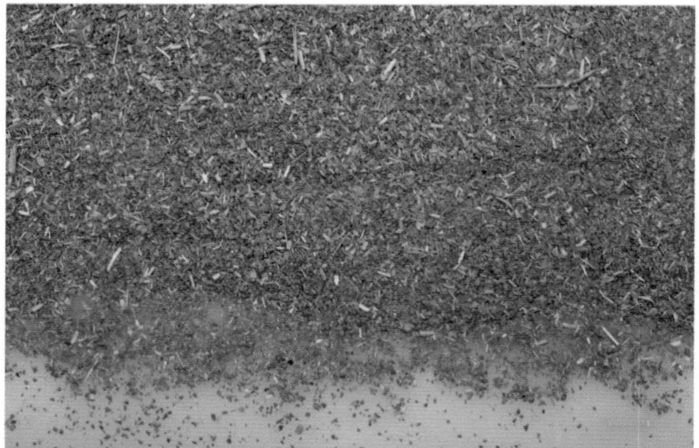

Figure 3 Hydrocotyle – dried drug substance (herb).

the pure saponins.[17] A crude hydrocotyle extract has been reported to significantly reduce the fertility of female mice when administered orally.[10] No mechanism of action was investigated.

Teratogenicity studies in the rabbit have reported negative findings for a hydrocotyle extract containing asiatic acid, madecassic acid, madasiatic acid and asiaticoside.[19]

Contra-indications, Warnings

It is stated that hydrocotyle may produce photosensitisation.[G7]

Drug interactions None documented. However, the potential for preparations of hydrocotyle to interact with other medicines administered concurrently, particularly those with similar or opposing effects, should be considered. There is limited evidence from preclinical studies that brahmoside and brahminoside, constituents of hydrocotyle, have CNS depressant activity.[15]

Pregnancy and lactation Hydrocotyle is reputed to be an abortifacient and to affect the menstrual cycle.[G30] Relaxation of the isolated rat uterus has been documented for brahmoside and brahminoside.[15] Triterpene constituents have been reported to lack any teratological effects in rabbits.[19] However, in view of the lack of toxicity data, the use of hydrocotyle during pregnancy and lactation should be avoided.

Preparations

Proprietary single-ingredient preparations

Austria: Madecassol. *Belgium:* Madecassol. *Brazil:* Centella-Vit. *Chile:* Celulase Plus; Celulase; Centabel; Escar T; Madecassol. *France:* Madecassol. *Greece:* Madecassol. *Hong Kong:* Madecassol. *Italy:* Centellase. *Mexico:* Madecassol. *Portugal:* Madecassol. *Singapore:* Centellase; Centica. *Spain:* Blastoestimulina. *Venezuela:* Litonate; Madecassol; Triffadiane.

Proprietary multi-ingredient preparations

Argentina: Celu-Atlas; Centella Queen Complex; Centella Queen Reductora; Centellase de Centella Queen; Centellase Gel; Clevosan; Clevosan; Clevosan; Estri-Atlas; Garcinol Max; Ginal Cent; Ginkan; Herbaccion Celfin; Lidersoft; Mailen; Moragen; No-Gras; Ovumix; Pentol; Redudiet; Vagicural Plus; Venoful; VNS 45. *Australia:* Extralife Leg-Care. *Brazil:* Composto Anticelulitico; Composto Emagrecedor; Derm'ative 10; Emagrevit. *Chile:* Celulase Con Neomicina; Cicapost; Dermaglos Plus; Escar T-Neomicina; Madecassol Neomicina. *France:* Calmiphase; Fadiamone; Madecassol Neomycine Hydrocortisone. *Italy:* Angioton; Angioton; Capill Venogel; Capill; Centella Complex; Centella Complex; Centeril H; Centeril H; Dermilia Flebozin; Emmenoiasi; Flebolider; Gelovis; Neomyrt Plus; Osmogel; Pik Gel; Varicofit; Venactive. *Malaysia:* Total Man. *Mexico:* Madecassol C; Madecassol N. *Monaco:* Akildia. *Portugal:* Antiestrias. *Spain:* Blastoestimulina; Blastoestimulina; Blastoestimulina; Cemalyt; Nesfare.

References

1 George VK, Gnanarethinam JL. Free amino acids in *Centella asiatica*. *Curr Sci* 1975; 44: 790.
2 Rzadkowska-Bodalska H. Flavonoid compounds in herb pennywort (*Hydrocotyle vulgaris*). *Herba Pol* 1974; 20: 243–246.
3 Voigt G *et al*. Zur Struktur der Flavonoide aus *Hydrocotyle vulgaris* L. *Pharmazie* 1981; 36: 377–379.
4 Hiller K *et al*. Isolierung von Quercetin-3-O-(6-O-α-L-arabinopyranosyl)-β-D-galaktopyranosid, einem neuen Flavonoid aus *Hydrocotyle vulgaris* L. *Pharmazie* 1979; 34: 192–193.
5 Hiller K *et al*. Saponins of *Hydrocotyle vulgaris*. *Pharmazie* 1971; 26: 780.
6 Hiller K *et al*. Zur Struktur des Hauptsaponins aus *Hydrocotyle vulgaris* L. *Pharmazie* 1981; 36: 844–846.
7 Asakawa Y *et al*. Mono- and sesquiterpenoids from *Hydrocotyle* and *Centella* species. *Phytochemistry* 1982; 21: 2590–2592.
8 Bohlmann F, Zdero C. Polyacetylenic compounds. 230. A new polyyne from Centella species. *Chem Ber* 1975; 108: 511–514.
9 Schulte KE *et al*. Constituents of medical plants. XXVII. Polyacetylenes from *Hydrocotyle asiatica*. *Arch Pharm (Weinheim)* 1973; 306: 197–209.
10 Gotu Kola. *Lawrence Review of Natural Products*, 1988.
11 Morisset T *et al*. Evaluation of the healing activity of hydrocotyle tincture in the treatment of wounds. *Phytother Res* 1987; 1: 117–121.
12 Jacker H-J *et al*. Zum antiexsudativen Verhalten einiger Triterpensaponine. *Pharmazie* 1982; 37: 380–382.
13 Ravokatra A, Ratsimamanga AR. Action of a pentacyclic triterpenoid, asiaticoside, obtained from *Hydrocotyle madagascariensis* or *Centella asiatica* against gastric ulcers of the Wistar rat exposed to cold (2°). *C R Acad Sci (Paris)* 1974; 278: 1743–1746.
14 Ravokatra A *et al*. Action of asiaticoside extracted from hydrocyte on duodenal ulcers induced with mercaptoethylamine in male Wistar rats. *C R Acad Sci (Paris)* 1974; 278: 2317–2321.
15 Ramaswamy AS *et al*. Pharmacological studies on *Centella asiatica* Linn. (*Brahma manduki*) (N.O. Umbelliferae). *J Res Indian Med* 1970; 4: 160–175.
16 Lin Y-C *et al*. Search for biologically active substances in Taiwan medicinal plants. 1. Screening for anti-tumor and anti-microbial substances. *Chin J Microbiol* 1972; 5: 76–81.
17 Oliver-Bever B. *Medicinal Plants in Tropical West Africa*. Cambridge: Cambridge University Press, 1986.
18 Natarajan S, Paily PP. Effect of topical *Hydrocotyle asiatica* in psoriasis. *Indian J Dermatol* 1973; 18: 82–85.
19 Bossé J-P *et al*. Clinical study of a new antikeloid agent. *Ann Plast Surg* 1979; 3: 13–21.

Ispaghula

Summary and Pharmaceutical Comment

The characteristic component of ispaghula is the mucilage which provides it with its bulk laxative action. Many of the herbal uses are therefore supported, although no published information was located to justify the use of ispaghula in cystitis or infective skin conditions. Adverse effects and precautions generally associated with bulk laxatives apply to ispaghula. Clinical evidence exists for hypocholesterolaemic activity.

The EMEA Committee on Herbal Medicinal Products (HMPC) draft Community Herbal Monographs for ispaghula husk[G82] and seed[G83] include the following therapeutic indications: (a) treatment of habitual constipation; (b) conditions in which easy defecation with soft stools is desirable, e.g. in cases of painful defecation after rectal or anal surgery, anal fissures and haemorrhoids;[G82, G83] and for ispaghula husk, (c) in patients for whom an increased daily fibre intake may be advisable, e.g. as an adjuvant in constipation-predominant irritable bowel syndrome, and as an adjuvant to diet in hypercholesterolaemia.[G82] Bulk laxatives lower the transit time through the gastrointestinal tract and may affect the absorption of concurrently administered drugs. Concomitant use with thyroid hormones and medicines known to inhibit peristalsis should only be under medical supervision.[G82, G83]

Ispaghula seed and husk may be used during pregnancy and lactation.

Species (Family)

Plantago ovata Forssk. (Plantaginaceae)

Synonym(s)

Blond Psyllium, Indian Plantago, Ispagol, Ispaghul, Pale Psyllium, Spogel

Part(s) Used

Seed, husk

Pharmacopoeial and Other Monographs

BHC 1992[G6]
BHP 1996[G9]
BP 2007[G84]
Complete German Commission E (Psyllium, Blonde)[G3]
EMEA HMPC Community Herbal Monographs[G82, G83]
ESCOP 2003[G76]
Martindale 35th edition[G85]
Ph Eur 2007[G81]
WHO volume 1 1999[G63]
USP29/NF24[G86]

Legal Category (Licensed Products)

GSL[G37]

Constituents

The following is compiled from several sources, including General References G2, G6, G52 and G59.

Alkaloids Monoterpene-type. (+)-Boschniakine (indicaine), (+)-boschniakinic acid (plantagonine) and indicainine.

Mucilages 10–30%. Mucopolysaccharide consisting mainly of a highly branched arabinoxylan with a xylan backbone and branches of arabinose, xylose and 2-*O*-(galacturonic)-rhamnose moieties. Present mainly in the seed husk.

Other constituents Aucubin (iridoid glucoside), sugars (fructose, glucose, sucrose), planteose (trisaccharide), protein, sterols (campesterol, β-sitosterol, stigmasterol), triterpenes (α- and β-amyrin), fatty acids (e.g. linoleic, oleic, palmitic, stearic), tannins.

Food Use

In food manufacture, ispaghula may be used as a thickener or stabiliser.[G41]

Herbal Use

Ispaghula is stated to possess demulcent and laxative properties. Traditionally, ispaghula has been used in the treatment of chronic constipation, dysentery, diarrhoea and cystitis.[G2, G4, G6–G8, G32, G43, G52, G64] Topically, a poultice has been used for furunculosis. The German Commission E approved use for chronic constipation and disorders in which bowel movements with loose stools are desirable, e.g. patients with anal fistulas, haemorrhoids, preg-

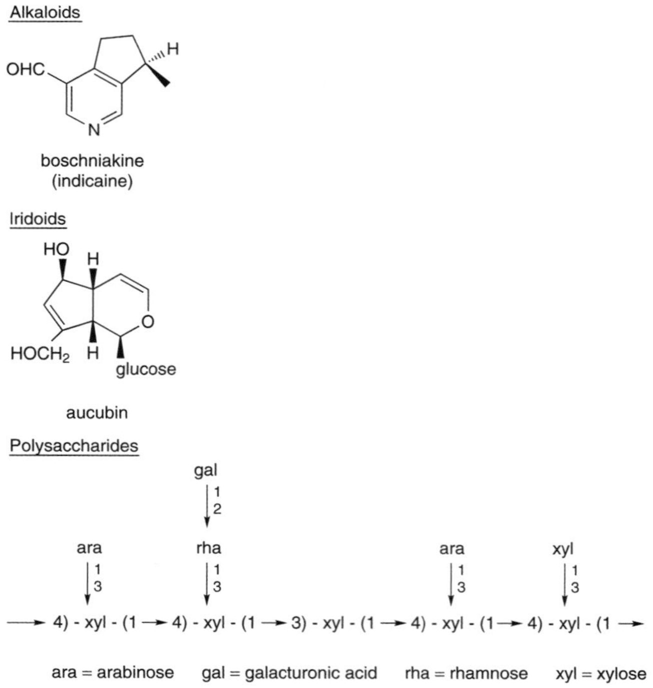

Alkaloids

boschniakine (indicaine)

Iridoids

aucubin

Polysaccharides

→ 4) - xyl - (1 → 4) - xyl - (1 → 3) - xyl - (1 → 4) - xyl - (1 → 4) - xyl - (1 →

ara = arabinose gal = galacturonic acid rha = rhamnose xyl = xylose

Figure 1 Selected constituents of ispaghula.

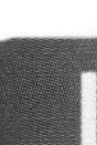

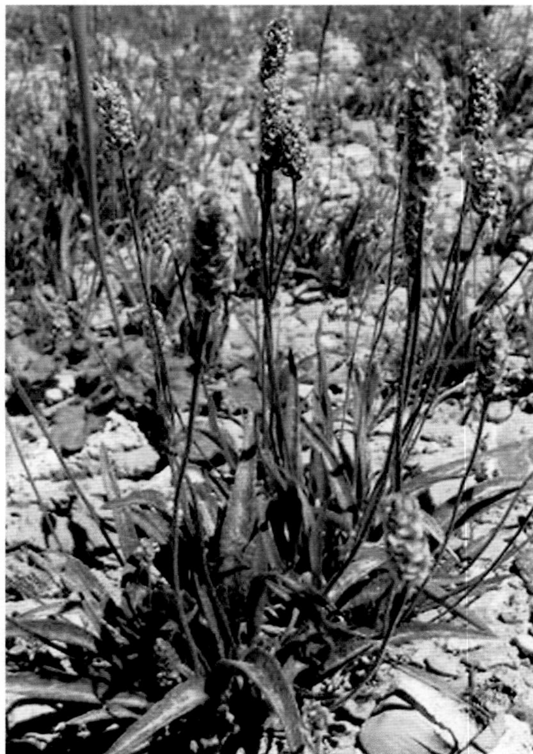

Figure 2 Ispaghula (*Plantago ovata*).

nancy, secondary medication in the treatment of various forms of diarrhoea and in the treatment of irritable bowel syndrome.(G3)

The European Medicines Agency (EMEA) Committee on Herbal Medicinal Products (HMPC) has adopted a Community Herbal Monograph for ispaghula husk(G82) and seed.(G83) The draft monographs include the following therapeutic indications under well-established use: (a) treatment of habitual constipation; (b) conditions in which easy defaecation with soft stools is desirable, e.g. in cases of painful defaecation after rectal or anal surgery, anal fissures and haemorrhoids;(G82, G83) and for ispaghula husk, (c) in patients for whom an increased daily fibre intake may be advisable, e.g. as an adjuvant in constipation-predominant irritable bowel syndrome, and as an adjuvant to diet in hypercholesterolaemia.(G82)

Dosage

Dosages for oral administration (adults) for traditional uses recommended in older and contemporary standard herbal reference texts are given below.

Seeds 5–10 g (3 g in children) three times daily;(G6, G7) 12–40 g per day, husk 4–20 g;(G3) 3–5 g.(G43) Children 6–12 years, half adult dose. Children under six years, treat only under medical supervision.(G52) Seeds should be soaked in warm water for several hours before taking.

Liquid extract 2–4 mL (1 : 1 in 25% alcohol) three times daily.(G6, G7)

Husk 3–5 g.(G46) Seeds and husk should be soaked in warm water for several hours before administration.

The EMEA HMPC Community Herbal Monographs advise the following dosages.

Ispaghula husk, indications (a) and (b) (see Herbal Use)(G82) Adults, elderly, adolescents aged over 12 years: 7–11 g daily in divided doses. Children aged 6–12 years: 3–8 g daily in divided doses.

Ispaghula husk, indication (c) (see Herbal Use)(G82) Adults, elderly, adolescents aged over 12 years: 7–20 g daily in one to three divided doses.

Ispaghula seed, indications (a) and (b) (see Herbal Use)(G83) Adults, elderly, adolescents aged over 12 years: 25–40 g daily in one to three divided doses. Children aged 6–12 years: 12–25 g daily in one to three divided doses.

Pharmacological Actions

The principal pharmacological actions of ispaghula can be attributed to the mucilage component.

In vitro and animal studies

An alcoholic extract lowered the blood pressure of anaesthetised cats and dogs, inhibited isolated rabbit and frog hearts, and stimulated rabbit, rat and guinea-pig ileum.(G41) The extract exhibited cholinergic activity.(G41) A mild laxative action has also been reported in mice administered iridoid glycosides, including aucubin.[1] Four-week supplementation of a fibre-free diet with ispaghula seeds (100 or 200 g/kg) was compared with that of the husks and wheat bran in rats.[2] The seeds increased faecal fresh weight by up to 100% and faecal dry weight by up to 50%. Total faecal bile acid secretion was stimulated, and β-glucuronidase activity reduced, by ispaghula. The study concluded that ispaghula acts as a partly fermentable, dietary fibre supplement increasing stool bulk, and that it probably has metabolic and mucosa-protective effects.

Ispaghula husk depressed the growth of chickens by 15% when added to their diet at 2%.(G41)

Ispaghula seed powder is stated to have strongly counteracted the deleterious effects of adding sodium cyclamate (2%), FD & C Red No. 2 (2%), and polyoxyethylene sorbitan monostearate (4%) to the diet of rats.(G41)

Clinical studies

Ispaghula is used as a bulk laxative.(G3, G43, G52) The swelling properties of the mucilage enable it to absorb water in the gastrointestinal tract, thereby increasing the volume of the faeces

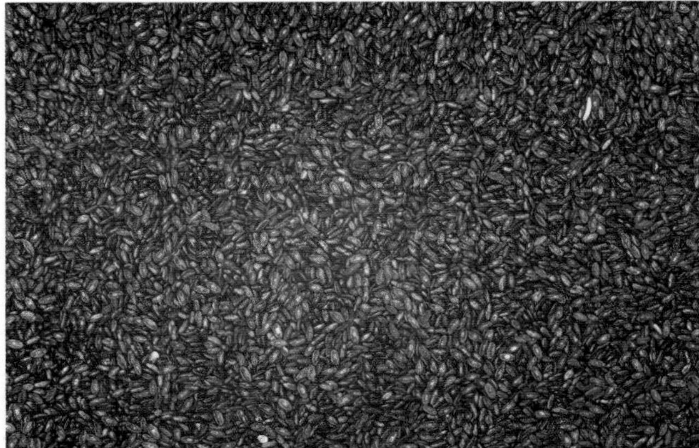

Figure 3 Ispaghula – dried drug substance (seed).

and promoting peristalsis. Bulk laxatives are often used for the treatment of chronic constipation and when excessive straining must be avoided following ano rectal surgery or in the management of haemorrhoids. Ispaghula is also used in the management of diarrhoea and for adjusting faecal consistency in patients with colostomies and in patients with diverticular disease or irritable bowel syndrome.

Laxative effect Ispaghula increases water content of stools and total stool weight in patients,[3] thus promoting peristalsis and reducing mouth-to-rectum transit time.[4] In a short-term study, 42 adults with constipation ($\leqslant$3 bowel movements per week) received either ispaghula (7.2 g/day) or ispaghula plus senna (6.5 g + 1.5 g/day).[5] Both treatments increased defecation frequency, and wet and dry stool weights, improved stool consistency, and gave subjective relief.

A randomised, double-blind, double-dummy, multicentre study involved 170 subjects with chronic idiopathic constipation.[6] The study included a two-week baseline (placebo) phase, followed by two weeks' treatment with ispaghula (Metamucil) 5.1 g, twice daily or docusate sodium 100 mg twice daily. Compared with docusate, ispaghula significantly increased stool water content (0.01% versus 2.33% for docusate and ispaghula, respectively; p = 0.007), and total stool output (271.9 g/week versus 359.9 g/week for docusate and ispaghula, respectively; p = 0.005). Furthermore, bowel movement frequency was significantly greater for ispaghula, compared with docusate. It was concluded that ispaghula has greater overall laxative efficacy than docusate in patients with chronic constipation.[6]

Antidiarrhoeal effect An open, randomised, crossover trial involving 25 patients with diarrhoea compared the effects of loperamide with those of ispaghula and calcium.[7] Nineteen patients completed both periods of treatment. The results indicated that both treatments halved stool frequency. Ispaghula and calcium were reported to be significantly better than loperamide with regard to urgency and stool consistency.[7]

Nine volunteers with phenolphthalein-induced diarrhoea were treated in random sequence with placebo, ispaghula (Konsyl), calcium polycarbophyl or wheat bran.[8] Wheat bran and calcium polycarbophyl had no effect on faecal consistency or on faecal viscosity. By contrast, ispaghula made stools firmer and increased faecal viscosity. In a dose–response study involving six subjects, 9, 18 and 30 g ispaghula per day caused a near-linear increase in faecal viscosity.[8]

The effects of ispaghula have been explored in children. In an open, uncontrolled study, 23 children with chronic non-specific diarrhoea were treated with an unrestricted diet for one week, and then treated with ispaghula (Metamucil) for two weeks (one tablespoonful twice daily). Seven patients responded to the unrestricted diet and 13 were said to respond to ispaghula treatment.[9]

Hypocholesterolaemic effects In a double-blind, placebo-controlled, parallel-group study, 26 men with mild-to-moderate hypercholesterolaemia (serum cholesterol concentration: 4.86–8.12 mmol/L) received ispaghula (Metamucil) 3.4 g, or cellulose placebo, three times daily at meal times for eight weeks.[10] At the end of the study, serum cholesterol concentrations were reduced by 14.8% in the treated group, low-density lipoprotein (LDL) cholesterol by 20.2% and ratio of LDL to high-density lipoprotein (HDL) cholesterol by 14.8%, compared with baseline values. There were no significant changes in serum lipid concentrations with placebo treatment, compared with baseline values. Differences in serum cholesterol concentrations between the two groups were statistically significant after four weeks (p-value not reported).

A double-blind, placebo-controlled, parallel trial study compared the effects of ispaghula (Metamucil 5.1 g, daily) and placebo in 118 patients (aged 21–70 years old) with primary hypercholesterolaemia (total serum cholesterol $\geqslant$5.7 mmol/L).[11] Thirty-seven participants maintained a high-fat diet and 81 a low-fat diet. Treated patients in both low- and high-fat diet groups showed small significant decreases ($p < 0.05$) in total cholesterol and LDL cholesterol levels (5.8% and 7.2%, respectively, for high-fat diets; 4.2% and 6.4%, respectively, for low-fat diets). No significant differences were seen in LDL cholesterol response for treated patients on either diet.

In a randomised, double-blind, crossover study, 20 males (mean (SD) age 44 (4) years) with moderate hypercholesterolaemia (mean (SD) total cholesterol concentration 265 (17) mg/dL, LDL 184 (15) mg/dL) were randomised to receive a 40-day course of ispaghula (Metamucil) 15 g daily, or placebo (cellulose).[12] There was a wash-out period of more than 10 days between treatments. Ispaghula lowered LDL cholesterol (168 mg/dL) more than did cellulose placebo (179 mg/dL), decreased relative cholesterol absorption, and increased the fractional turnover of both chenodeoxycholic acid and cholic acid. Bile acid synthesis increased in subjects whose LDL cholesterol was lowered by more than 10%. It was concluded that ispaghula lowers LDL cholesterol primarily by stimulation of bile acid synthesis.[12]

A meta-analysis of eight published and four unpublished studies carried out in four countries reviewed the effect of consumption of ispaghula-enriched cereal products on blood cholesterol, and LDL and HDL cholesterol concentrations.[13] Overall, the trials included 404 adults with mild-to-moderate hypercholesterolaemia (5.17–7.8 mmol/L) who consumed low-fat diets. The meta-analysis indicated that subjects who consumed ispaghula cereal had lower total cholesterol and LDL cholesterol than subjects who ate control cereal concentrations (differences of 0.31 mmol/L (5%) and 0.35 mmol/L (9%), respectively). HDL cholesterol concentrations were not affected in subjects eating ispaghula cereal.

Another meta-analysis included eight studies involving a total of 384 patients with hypercholesterolaemia who received ispaghula and 272 subjects who received cellulose placebo.[14] Compared with placebo, consumption of 10.2 g ispaghula per day for $\geqslant$8 weeks lowered serum total cholesterol concentrations by 4% ($p < 0.0001$) and LDL cholesterol by 7% ($p < 0.0001$), but did not affect serum HDL cholesterol or triacyl glycerol concentrations. The ratio of apolipoprotein (apo) B to apo A-1 was lowered by 6% ($p < 0.05$), relative to placebo, in subjects consuming a low-fat diet.[14] It was concluded that ispaghula is a useful adjunct to a low-fat diet in individuals with mild-to-moderate hypercholesterolaemia.

A randomised, placebo-controlled, multicentre study evaluated the long-term effectiveness of ispaghula husk as an adjunct to diet in treatment of primary hypercholesterolaemia.[15] Men and women with hypercholesterolaemia followed the American Heart Association Step 1 diet for eight weeks prior to treatment. Individuals with LDL cholesterol concentrations between 3.36 and 4.91 mmol/L were randomly assigned to receive either ispaghula (Metamucil 5.1 g) or cellulose placebo twice daily for 26 weeks whilst continuing diet therapy. Overall, 163 participants completed the full protocol, 133 receiving ispaghula and 30 receiving cellulose placebo. Serum total and LDL cholesterol concentrations were 4.7% and 6.7% lower, respectively, in the ispaghula group than in the placebo group after 24–26 weeks ($p < 0.001$).

A randomised, double-blind, placebo-controlled crossover trial assessed the effects of ispaghula in lowering elevated LDL cholesterol concentrations in 20 children (aged 5–17 years).[16] Children with LDL cholesterol concentrations of >2.84 mmol/L after three months on a low-fat, low-cholesterol diet received five weeks' treatment with a ready-to-eat cereal containing water-soluble ispaghula husk (6 g/day) or placebo. The results indicated that there were no significant differences in total cholesterol, LDL cholesterol or HDL cholesterol concentrations between the two groups.

In a similar 12-week study, 50 children (aged 2–11 years) with LDL cholesterol concentrations ⩾110 mg/dL received either cereal enriched with ispaghula (3.2 g soluble fibre per day) or plain cereal whilst maintaining a low-fat diet.[17] Total cholesterol decreased by 21 mg/dL for the ispaghula group in comparison with 11.5 mg/dL for the control group ($p < 0.001$). LDL cholesterol also decreased by 23 mg/dL for the treated group in comparison with 8.5 mg/dL for the placebo group ($p < 0.01$).

The effect of adding water-soluble fibre to a diet low in total fats, saturated fat and cholesterol to treat hypercholesterolaemic children and adolescents has been reviewed.[18] The review summarised that reductions in LDL cholesterol concentrations ranged from 0–23%. This wide range may be related to dietary intervention and to clinical trial conditions. It was proposed that additional trials with larger numbers of well-defined subjects are needed.

Hypoglycaemic effect Several studies have shown that ispaghula husk lowered blood glucose concentrations due to delayed intestinal absorption.[G52] In one crossover study, 18 patients with non-insulin-dependent diabetes received ispaghula (Metamucil) or placebo twice (immediately before breakfast and dinner) during each 15-hour crossover phase.[19] For meals eaten immediately after ispaghula ingestion, maximum post-prandial glucose elevation was reduced by 14% at breakfast and 20% at dinner, relative to placebo. Postprandial serum insulin concentrations measured after breakfast were reduced by 12%, relative to placebo. Second-meal effects after lunch showed a 31% reduction in postprandial glucose elevation, relative to placebo. No significant differences in effects were noted between patients whose diabetes was controlled by diet alone and those whose diabetes was controlled by oral hypoglycaemic drugs. It was concluded that the results indicate that ispaghula as a meal supplement reduces proximate and second-meal postprandial glucose and insulin in non-insulin dependent diabetics.[19]

Other effects Ispaghula husk has been used to treat small numbers of patients with left-sided diverticular disease.[4] Marked motility was observed for the right colon, but was not as pronounced for the left colon. The effects of ispaghula in this condition may be worth further investigation.

In an open, randomised, multicentre trial, 102 patients with ulcerative colitis (three months in remission, salicylate-treated, colitis over 20 cm) received ispaghula (10 g twice daily; $n = 35$), oral mesalazine (500 mg three times daily; $n = 37$) or ispaghula plus mesalazine ($n = 30$) for one year.[20] Assessment, including endoscopy, was carried out at 3, 6, 9 and 12 months. The results suggested that ispaghula may be equivalent to mesalazine in maintaining remission in ulcerative colitis. However, this requires further investigation in a randomised, double-blind study.

Side-effects, Toxicity

In common with all bulk laxatives, ispaghula seed and husk may increase or cause flatulence, although this usually disappears in the course of treatment. There is a risk of abdominal distension and intestinal or oesophageal obstruction, particularly if ispaghula seed or husk is swallowed dry or without sufficient fluid. Allergic reactions, including (rarely) anaphylactic reactions, may occur.[G3, G83, G84]

Contra-indications, Warnings

The EMEA HMPC Community Herbal Monographs include the following information. Ispaghula seed and husk should not be used by patients with: a sudden change in bowel habit that persists for more than two weeks; undiagnosed rectal bleeding; failure to defecate following the use of a laxative; abnormal constrictions in the gastrointestinal tract; diseases of the oesophagus and cardia; potential or existing intestinal blockage (ileus); paralysis of the intestine or megacolon; poorly controlled diabetes mellitus; known hypersensitivity to ispaghula seed or husk.[G82, G83]

Ispaghula seed and husk should not be used by patients with faecal impaction and undiagnosed abdominal symptoms, abdominal pain, nausea and vomiting (unless advised by a doctor).[G82] Where ispaghula seed or husk is used in constipation, the use of ispaghula husk should be discontinued and medical advice sought if the constipation does not resolve within three days of starting treatment, if abdominal pain occurs and/or if there is any irregularity in the faeces. Where ispaghula seed or husk is used as an adjuvant to diet in hypercholesterolaemia this should be under medical supervision.[G82] Ispaghula seed and ispaghula husk should always be taken with a sufficient amount of fluid: for each 1 g of the herbal substance, at least 30 mL of fluid (water, milk or fruit juice) should be used to prepare a mixture. Taking these preparations without adequate fluid may cause them to swell and block the throat or oesophagus and may cause choking. Intestinal obstructions may occur if an adequate fluid intake is not maintained. Ispaghula should not be taken by anyone who has had difficulty in swallowing or any throat problems. If chest pain, vomiting or difficulty in swallowing or breathing is experienced after taking the preparation, immediate medical attention should be sought. The treatment of the debilitated patient requires medical supervision. The treatment of elderly patients should be supervised. Preparations of ispaghula seed and ispaghula husk should be taken during the day and at least 30 minutes away from intake of other medicines.[G82, G83]

Drug and other interactions Bulk laxatives lower the transit time through the gastrointestinal tract and therefore may affect the absorption of other drugs.[G45] Absorption of concurrently administered drugs may be delayed. The EMEA HMPC Community Herbal Monographs include the following information. Enteral absorption of concomitantly administered medicines such as minerals (e.g. calcium, iron, lithium, zinc), vitamins (B_{12}), cardiac glycosides and coumarin derivatives may be delayed. For this reason the product should not be taken within 0.5–1 hour of other medicines. If the product is taken together with meals in the case of insulin-dependent diabetics, it may be necessary to reduce the insulin dose. Ispaghula seed and husk should only be used concomitantly with thyroid hormones under medical supervision as the dose of thyroid hormones may need to be adjusted. In order to reduce the risk of gastrointestinal obstruction, ispaghula seed and husk should only be used with medicines known to inhibit peristalsis (e.g. loperamide, opioids and opioid-like agents) under medical supervision.(G82, G83)

Pregnancy and lactation Ispaghula seed and husk may be used during pregnancy and lactation.

Preparations

Proprietary single-ingredient preparations

Argentina: Agiofibras; Konsyl; Lostamucil; Metamucil; Motional; Mucofalk; Plantaben. *Australia:* Agiofibe; Ford Fibre; Fybogel; Metamucil. *Austria:* Agiocur; Laxans; Metamucil. *Belgium:* Colofiber. *Brazil:* Agiofibra; Metamucil; Plantaben. *Canada:* Laxucil; Metamucil; Mucillium; Novo-Mucilax; Prodiem Plain. *Chile:* Euromucil; Fibrasol; Metamucil; Plantaben. *Denmark:* Vi-Siblin. *Finland:* Agiocur; Laxamucil; Vi-Siblin. *France:* Mucivital; Spagulax Mucilage; Spagulax; Transilane. *Germany:* Agiocur; Flosa; Flosine; Metamucil; Mucofalk; Pascomucil. *Hong Kong:* Agiocur; Metamucil; Mucofalk; Naturlax. *India:* Isogel. *Ireland:* Fybogel. *Israel:* Agiocur; Konsyl; Mucivital. *Italy:* Agiofibre; Fibrolax; Planten. *Malaysia:* Mucofalk. *Mexico:* Agiofibra; Fibromucil; Hormolax; Metamucil; Mucilag; Plantaben; Siludane. *Monaco:* Psylia. *Netherlands:* Metamucil; Mucofalk; Regucol; Volcolon. *Norway:* Lunelax; Vi-Siblin. *New Zealand:* Isogel; Metamucil; Mucilax. *Portugal:* Agiocur; Mucofalk. *South Africa:* Agiobulk; Agiogel; Fybogel. *Singapore:* Fybogel; Mucilin; Mucofalk. *Spain:* Biolid; Cenat; Laxabene; Metamucil; Plantaben. *Sweden:* Lunelax; Vi-Siblin. *Switzerland:* Agiolax mite; Laxiplant Soft; Metamucil; Mucilar. *Thailand:* Agiocur; Fybogel; Metamucil; Mucilin. *UK:* Fibrelief; Fybogel; Isogel; Ispagel; Regulan. *USA:* Fiberall; Hydrocil Instant; Konsyl-D; Konsyl; Metamucil; Reguloid; Syllact.

Proprietary multi-ingredient preparations

Argentina: Agiolax; Isalax Fibras; Kronolax; Medilaxan; Mermelax; Rapilax Fibras; Salutaris. *Australia:* Agiolax; Bioglan Psylli-Mucil Plus; Herbal Cleanse; Nucolox; PC Regulax. *Austria:* Agiolax. *Belgium:* Agiolax. *Brazil:* Agiolax; Plantax. *Canada:* Prodiem Plus. *Chile:* Bilaxil. *Finland:* Agiolax. *France:* Agiolax; Filigel; Imegul; Jouvence de l'Abbe Soury; Parapsyllium; Schoum; Spagulax au Citrate de Potassium; Spagulax au Sorbitol. *Germany:* Agiolax. *Hong Kong:* Agiolax. *Ireland:* Fybogel Mebeverine. *Israel:* Agiolax. *Italy:* Agiolax; Duolaxan; Fibrolax Complex; Sedatol; Sedatol; Soluzione Schoum. *Mexico:* Agiolax. *Netherlands:* Agiolax. *Norway:* Agiolax. *Portugal:* Agiolax; Excess. *South Africa:* Agiolax. *Spain:* Agiolax; Solucion Schoum. *Sweden:* Agiolax; Vi-Siblin S. *Switzerland:* Agiolax; Mucilar Avena. *Thailand:* Agiolax. *UK:* Anased; Fibre Dophilus; Fibre Plus; Fybogel Mebeverine; HRI Calm Life; Manevac; Nodoff; Nytol Herbal; Slumber. *USA:* Perdiem; Senna Prompt. *Venezuela:* Agiolax; Avensyl; Fiberfull; Fibralax; Senokot con Fibra.

References

1 Inouye H *et al*. Purgative activities of iridoid glycosides. *Planta Med* 1974; 25: 285–288.

2 Leng-Peschlow E. *Plantago ovata* seeds as dietary fibre supplement: physiological and metabolic effects in rats. *Br J Nutr* 1991; 66: 331–349.

3 Stevens J *et al*. Comparison of the effects of psyllium and wheat bran on gastrointestinal transit time and stool characteristics. *J Am Diet Assoc* 1988; 88: 323–326.

4 Thorburn HA *et al*. Does ispaghula husk stimulate the entire colon in diverticular disease? *Gut* 1992; 33: 352–356.

5 Marlett JA *et al*. Comparative laxation of psyllium with and without senna in an ambulatory constipated population. *Am J Gastroenterol* 1987; 82: 333–337.

6 McRorie JW *et al*. Psyllium is superior to docusate sodium for treatment of chronic constipation. *Aliment Pharmacol Ther* 1998; 12: 491–497.

7 Qvitzau S *et al*. Treatment of chronic diarrhoea: loperamide versus ispaghula husk and calcium. *Scand J Gastroenterol* 1988; 23: 1237–1240.

8 Eherer AJ *et al*. Effect of psyllium, calcium polycarbophil, and wheat bran on secretory diarrhea induced by phenolphthalein. *Gastroenterology* 1993; 104: 1007–1012.

9 Smalley JR *et al*. Use of psyllium in the management of chronic nonspecific diarrhea of childhood. *J Pediatr Gastroenterol Nutr* 1982; 1: 361–363.

10 Anderson JW *et al*. Cholesterol-lowering effects of psyllium hydrophilic mucilloid for hypercholesterolemic men. *Arch Intern Med* 1988; 148: 292–296.

11 Sprecher DL *et al*. Efficacy of psyllium in reducing serum cholesterol levels in hypercholesterolemic patients on high- or low-fat diets. *Ann Intern Med* 1993; 119: 545–554.

12 Everson GT *et al*. Effects of psyllium hydrophilic mucilloid on LDL-cholesterol and bile acid synthesis in hypercholesterolemic men. *J Lipid Res* 1992; 33: 1183–1192.

13 Olson BH *et al*. Psyllium-enriched cereals lower blood total cholesterol and LDL cholesterol, but not HDL cholesterol, in hypercholesterolemic adults: results of a meta-analysis. *J Nutr* 1997; 127: 1973–1980.

14 Anderson JW *et al*. Cholesterol-lowering effects of psyllium intake adjunctive to diet therapy in men and women with hypercholesterolemia: meta-analysis of 8 controlled trials. *Am J Clin Nutr* 2000; 71: 472–479.

15 Anderson JW *et al*. Long-term cholesterol-lowering effects of psyllium as an adjunct to diet therapy in the treatment of hypercholesterolaemia. *Am J Clin Nut* 2000; 71: 1433–1438.

16 Dennison BA, Levine DM. Randomized, double-blind, placebo-controlled, two-period crossover clinical trial of psyllium fiber in children with hypercholesterolemia. *J Pediatr* 1993; 123: 24–29.

17 Williams CL *et al*. Soluble fiber enhances the hypocholesterolemic effect of the step I diet in childhood. *J Am College Nutr* 1995; 14: 251–257.

18 Kwiterovich Jr PO. The role of fiber in the treatment of hypercholesterolemia in children and adolescents. *Pediatrics* 1995; 96: 1005–1009.

19 Pastors JG *et al*. Psyllium fiber reduces rise in postprandial glucose and insulin concentrations in patients with non-insulin-dependent diabetes. *Am J Clin Nutr* 1991; 53: 1431–1435.

20 Fernández-Bañares F *et al*. Randomised clinical trial of *Plantago ovata* efficacy as compared to mesalazine in maintaining remission in ulcerative colitis. *Gastroenterology* 1997; 112: A971.

Jamaica Dogwood

Summary and Pharmaceutical Comment

Jamaica dogwood is characterised by various isoflavone constituents, to which the antispasmodic properties described for the wood have been attributed. In addition, sedative and narcotic activities have been documented following preclinical studies, thus supporting the reputed herbal uses. However, there is a lack of clinical research assessing the efficacy and safety of Jamaica dogwood. Although Jamaica dogwood is reported to be of low toxicity in various animal species, it is also documented as toxic to humans.[G51] In view of this, excessive use of Jamaica dogwood and use during pregnancy and lactation should be avoided.

Species (Family)

Piscidia piscipula L. Sarg. (Leguminosae)

Synonym(s)

Erythina piscipula L., Fish Poison Bark, *Ichthyomethia communis* S.F. Blake, *I. piscipula* (L.) Hitchc., *I. piscipula* (L.) Hitchc., var. *typica* Stehle & L. Quentin, *P. inebrians* Medik, *P. erythina* L., *P. toxicaria* Salisb., *Robinia alata* Mill., West Indian Dogwood

Part(s) Used

Root bark

Pharmacopoeial and Other Monographs

BHC 1992[G6]
BHP 1996[G9]
Martindale 35th edition[G85]

Legal Category (Licensed Products)

GSL[G37]

Constituents

The following is compiled from several sources, including General References G6 and G40.

Acids Piscidic acid (*p*-hydroxybenzyltartaric) and its mono and diethyl esters,[1] fukiic acid and the 3′-O-methyl derivative; malic acid, succinic acid, and tartaric acid.

Isoflavonoids Ichthynone, jamaicin, piscerythrone, piscidone and others. Milletone, isomillettone, dehydromillettone, rotenone and sumatrol (rotenoids), and lisetin.[2–5]

Glycosides Piscidin, reported to be a mixture of two compounds, saponin glycoside (unidentified).[6]

Other constituents Alkaloid (unidentified, reported to be from the stem), resin, volatile oil 0.01%, β-sitosterol, tannin (unspecified).[6]

Food Use

Jamaica dogwood is stated by the Council of Europe to to be toxicologically unacceptable for use as a natural food flavouring.[G16]

Herbal Use

Jamaica dogwood is stated to possess sedative and anodyne properties. Traditionally, it has been used for neuralgia, migraine, insomnia, dysmenorrhoea, and specifically for insomnia due to neuralgia or nervous tension.[G6, G7, G8, G64]

Dosage

Dosages for oral administration (adults) for traditional uses recommended in older and contemporary standard herbal and/or pharmaceutical reference texts are given below.

Dried root bark 1–2 g as a decoction three times daily.[G6, G7]

Liquid extract 1–2 mL (1 : 1 in 30% alcohol) three times daily.[G6, G7]

Liquid Extract of Piscidia (BPC 1934) 2–8 mL.

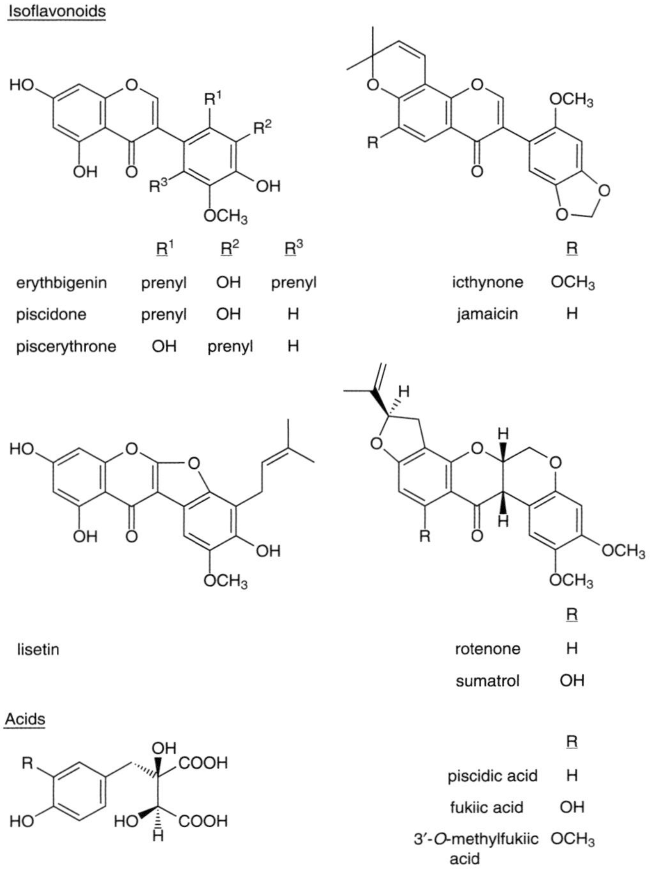

Figure 1 Selected constituents of Jamaica dogwood.

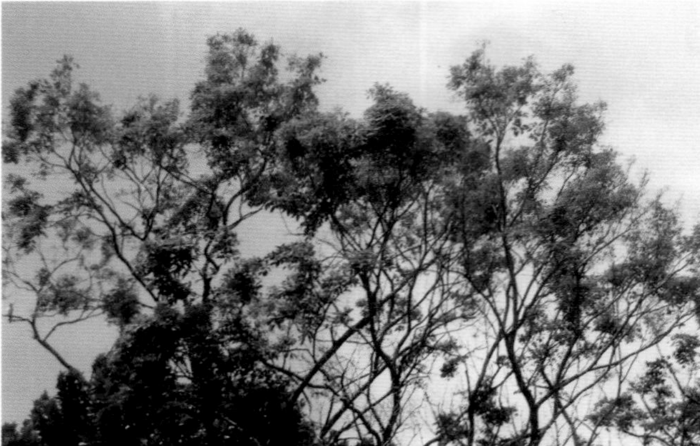

Figure 2 Jamaica dogwood (*Piscidia piscipula*).

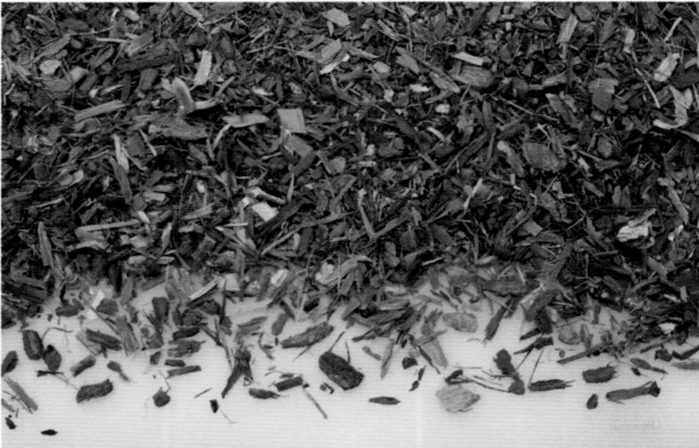

Figure 3 Jamaica dogwood – dried drug substance (root bark).

Pharmacological Actions

In vitro and animal studies

Results of early studies reported Jamaica dogwood to possess weak cannabinoid and sedative activities in the mouse, guinea-pig and cat.[6–8] In addition, *in vitro* antispasmodic activity on rabbit intestine, and guinea-pig and rat uterine muscle[6, 9, 10] were noted and *in vivo* utero-activity in the cat and monkey were documented.[6, 7, 10, 11] In some instances, *in vitro* antispasmodic activity was found to be comparable to, or greater than, that observed for papaverine.

More recent work has supported these findings and reported that the antispasmodic activity of Jamaica dogwood on uterine smooth muscle is attributable to two isoflavone constituents, one being equipotent to papaverine.[11]

Jamaica dogwood extracts have also been documented to exhibit antitussive, antipyretic, and anti-inflammatory activities in various experimental animals.[7]

Rotenone is an insecticide that has been used in agriculture for the control of lice, fleas, and as a larvicide.[G45] Jamaica dogwood has been used extensively throughout Central and South America as a fish poison;[6] the wood contains two piscicidal principles, rotenone and ichthynone.

Rotenone has reportedly exhibited anticancer activity towards lymphocytic leukaemia and human epidermoid carcinoma of the nasopharynx.[G22]

Clinical studies

There is a lack of clinical research assessing the effects of Jamaica dogwood and rigorous randomised controlled clinical trials are required.

Side-effects, Toxicity

There is a lack of clinical safety and toxicity data for Jamaica dogwood and further investigation of these aspects is required.

Symptoms of overdose are stated to include numbness, tremors, salivation and sweating.[G22]

Jamaica dogwood has been found to be toxic when administered parenterally to rats and rabbits, but non-toxic when given orally, with doses exceeding 90 g dried extract/kg tolerated.[6] An LD_{50} (mice, intravenous injection) of an unidentified saponin constituent has been reported as 75 µg/kg body weight.[9] Oral doses of up to 1.5 mg/kg were stated to have no effect.[6]

Jamaica dogwood is stated to be irritant and toxic to humans.[G51] Rotenone is documented to be carcinogenic.[G22]

Contra-indications, Warnings

None documented. However, in view of the available information, Jamaica dogwood should be used with caution.

Drug interactions None documented. However, the potential for preparations of Jamaica dogwood to interact with other medicines administered concurrently, particularly those with similar or opposing effects, should be considered. There is limited evidence from preclinical studies that Jamaica dogwood has sedative activity.

Pregnancy and lactation Jamaica dogwood has been reported to exhibit a potent depressant action on the uterus both *in vitro* and *in vivo*. In view of this and the general warnings regarding the use of Jamaica dogwood, it should not be used during pregnancy and lactation.

References

1 Bridge W *et al.* Constituents of 'Cortex Piscidiae Erythrinae'. Part I. The structure of piscidic acid. *J Chem Soc* 1948; 257.

2 Falshaw CP *et al.* The Extractives of Piscidia Erythrina L. III. The constitutions of lisetin, piscidone and piscerythrone. *Tetrahedron* 1966; Suppl 7: 333–348.

3 Redaelli C, Santaniello E. Major isoflavonoids of the Jamaican dogwood *Piscidia erythrina. Phytochemistry* 1984; 23: 2976–2977.

4 Delle Monache F *et al.* Two isoflavones from *Piscidia erythrina. Phytochemistry* 1984; 23: 2945–2947.

5 Harborne JB, Mabry TJ, eds. *The Flavonoids.* New York: Chapman and Hall, 1982: 606.

6 Costello CH, Butler CL. An investigation of *Piscidia erythrina* (Jamaica Dogwood). *J Am Pharm Assoc* 1948; 37: 89–96.

7 Aurousseau M *et al.* Certain pharmacodynamic properties of *Piscidia erythrina. Ann Pharm Fr* 1965; 23: 251–257.

8 Della-Loggia R *et al.* Evaluation of the activity on the mouse CNS of several plant extracts and a combination of them. *Riv-Neurol* 1981; 51: 297–310.

9 Pilcher JD *et al.* The action of the so-called female remedies on the excised uterus of the guinea-pig. *Arch Intern Med* 1916; 18: 557–583.

10 Pilcher JD, Mauer RT. The action of female remedies on the intact uteri of animals. *Surg Gynecol Obstet* 1918; 97–99.

11 Della Loggia R *et al.* Isoflavones as spasmolytic principles of *Piscidia erythrina. Prog Clin Biol Res* 1988; 280: 365–368.

Java Tea

Summary and Pharmaceutical Comment

The reported pharmacological activities of Java tea are mainly associated with the lipophilic flavonoids, benzochromene and, to a lesser extent, diterpene constituents.

Documented scientific evidence from *in vitro* and animal studies provides some supportive evidence for some of the traditional uses of Java tea. However, there is a lack of clinical data and well-designed, controlled clinical trials involving adequate numbers of patients are required. Furthermore, studies investigating the active principles responsible for specific pharmacological activities and their mechanisms of action are necessary.

There have been reports of adulteration/botanical substitution occurring with *Orthosiphon*.(G2)

In view of the lack of toxicity and safety data, excessive use of Java tea, and use during pregnancy and lactation, should be avoided.

Species (Family)

Orthosiphon aristatus var. *aristatus* (Blume) Miq. (Labiatae/Lamiaceae)

Synonym(s)

Kumis Kucing (Indonesian, Malay), *Orthosiphon aristatus* Miq., *Orthosiphon spicatus* (Thunb.) Bak., *O. stamineus* Benth.

Part(s) Used

Fragmented dried leaves, tops of stems

Pharmacopoeial and Other Monographs

BHP 1996(G9)
BP 2007(G84)
Complete German Commission E(G3)

Benzochromenes

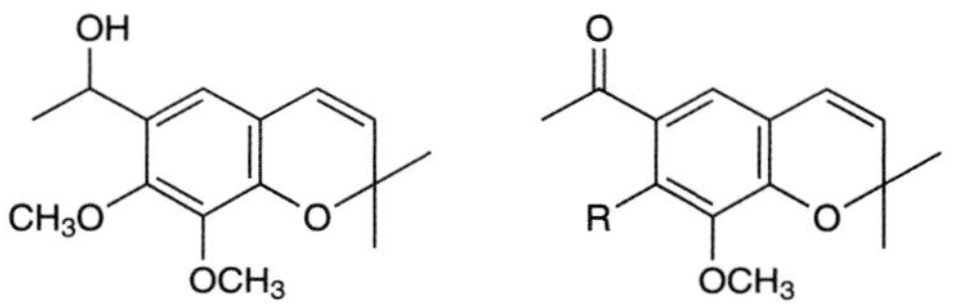

orthochromene A

	R
methylripariochromene A	OCH_3
acetovanillochromene	H

Flavonoids

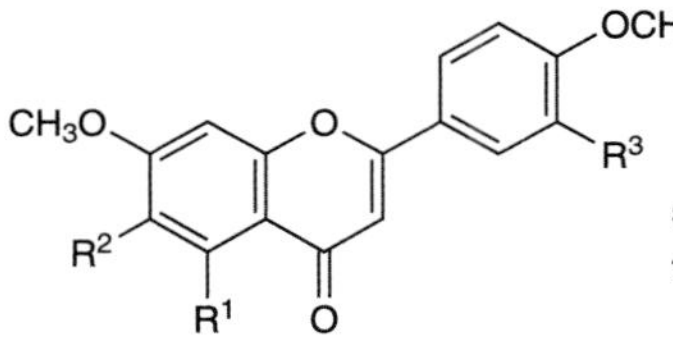

	R^1	R^2	R^3
sinensetin	OCH_3	OCH_3	OCH_3
tetramethyl-scutellarin	OCH_3	OCH_3	H
eupatorin	OH	OCH_3	OH
5-hydroxy-6,7,3′,4′-tetramethylflavone	OH	OCH_3	OCH_3
3′-hydroxy-5,6,7,4′-tetramethoxyflavone	OCH_3	OCH_3	OH
salvigenin	OH	OCH_3	H
trimethylapigenin	OCH_3	H	H
tetramethyllutein	OCH_3	H	OCH_3

Phenylpropanoids

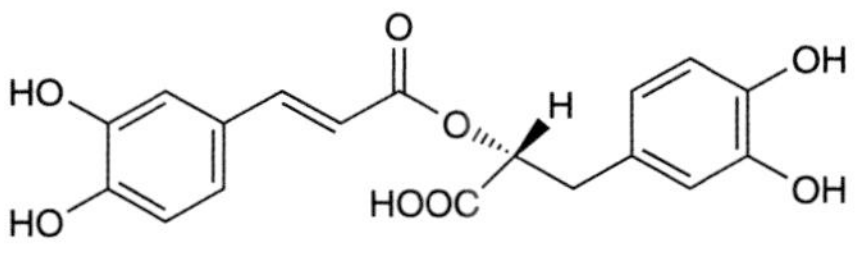

rosmarinic acid

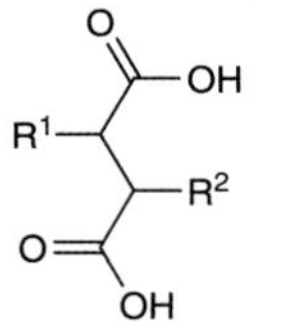

	R^1	R^2
caffeoyl tartrate	caffeoyl	H
di-caffeoyl tartrate	caffeoyl	caffeoyl

Figure 1 Selected constituents of java tea.

ESCOP 2003[G76]
Martindale 35th edition[G85]
Ph Eur 2007[G81]

Legal category (Licensed Products)

Java tea is not included in the GSL.

Constituents

The following is compiled from several sources, including General References G2 and G52.

Benzochromenes Orthochromene A,[1] methylripariochromene A[2] and acetovanillochromene.[1,3]

Diterpenes Numerous closely related pimarane-type diterpenes, including orthosiphonones A and B,[1] orthosiphols A, B, E to I, M, N, P, R, S, T,[4,5] staminol A[5] neo-orthosiphols A and B[3,6,7] neo-orthosiphone A,[8] norstaminolactone A, norstaminols B and C, norstaminone A,[7] and seco-orthosiphols A to C.[9]

Essential oil 0.02–0.7%. Various compounds including β-elemene, β-caryophyllene, α-humulene, β-caryophyllene oxide, can-2-one and palmitic acid.[10]

Flavonoids Sinensetin, tetramethylscutellarein, eupatorin, 5-hydroxy-6,7,3′,4′-tetramethoxyflavone, 3′-hydroxy-5,6,7,4′-tetramethoxyflavone, salvigenin, trimethylapigenin, tetramethoxyluteolin[11] nine flavonoids which are methylated derivatives of scutellarein (5,6,7,4′-tetramethoxyflavone) or 6-hydroxyluteolin (5,6,7, 3′,4′-pentahydroxyflavone), quercetin-3-O-glucoside, kaempferol-3-O-glucoside,[3,12–15] 4′,5,6,7-tetramethoxyflavone, 3′,4′,5,6,7-pentamethoxyflavone.[16]

Phenylpropanoids Rosmarinic acid (major), caffeoyl tartrate, dicaffeoyltartrate, four caffeic acid depsides (1–4).[13]

Other constituents Inositol, phytosterols (e.g. β-sitosterol),[11,13] esculetin (a coumarin), potassium salts.

Food Use

Java tea is not used in foods.

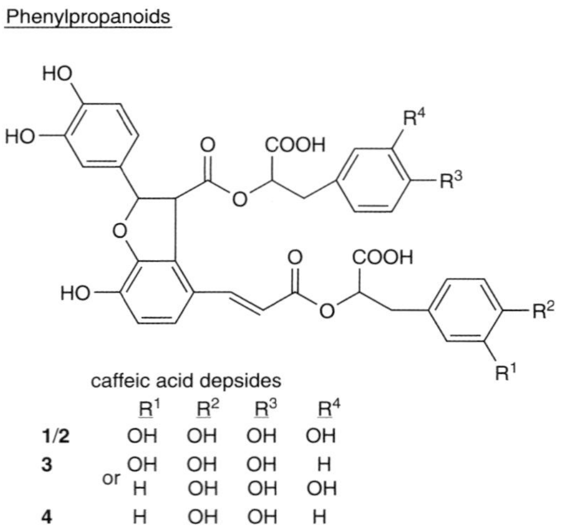

Phenylpropanoids

caffeic acid depsides

	R^1	R^2	R^3	R^4
1/2	OH	OH	OH	OH
3	OH	OH	OH	H
or	H	OH	OH	OH
4	H	OH	OH	H

Figure 2 Selected constituents of java tea.

Diterpenes

orthosiphonone A

orthosiphonone B

	R^1	R^2
orthosiphol A	Ac	H
orthosiphol B	H	Ac

	R^1	R^2	R^3
orthosiphol F	Ac	H	Bz
orthosiphol G	Ac	H	H
orthosiphol H	Ac	Ac	Bz

	R
neoorthosiphol A	H
staminol A	Ac

neoorthosiphol B

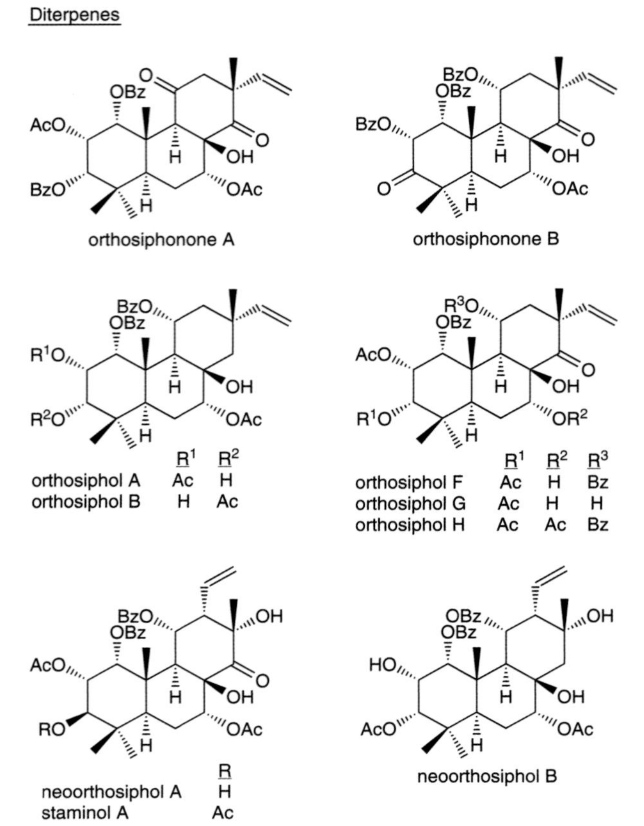

Figure 3 Selected constituents of java tea.

Herbal Use

Java tea has traditionally been used in Java for the treatment of hypertension and diabetes.[1,6,17,G35] It has also been used in folk medicine for bladder and kidney disorders, gallstones, gout and rheumatism. Java tea is stated to have diuretic properties.[18]

Dosage

Dosage for oral administration (adults) for traditional uses recommended in contemporary standard herbal reference texts are given below.

Dried material 2–3 g in 150 mL water two to three times daily as an infusion.[G52]

Pharmacological Actions

In vitro and animal studies

Diuretic effects Several studies in rats have reported diuretic activity of extracts of *O. stamineus* and *O. aristatus*[18–20] and of flavonoids (sinensetin and a tetramethoxyflavone) isolated from *O. aristatus*.[21] Intraperitoneal administration of a hydroalcoholic extract of *O. stamineus* to rats caused a significant diuresis over the following 2–24 hours compared with controls.[18] The effect was similar to that observed following intraperitoneal administration of hydrochlorothiazide (10 mg/kg).[18] Oral administration of an aqueous extract of *O. aristatus* increased ion excretion to a similar extent as did furosemide, although no diuretic action was noted.[20]

Oral administration of methylripariochromene A (100 mg/kg) has been shown to increase urinary volume in fasted rats for three hours after oral administration; the increase in urine volume was similar to that observed with oral administration of hydrochlorothiazide (25 mg/kg).[17] Sodium, potassium and chloride ion excretion was increased with methylripariochromene A (100 mg/kg), although urinary sodium ion excretion did not increase. A mechanism for the diuretic action of methylripariochromene A has not yet been elucidated, although it appears to have a different mode of action to that of hydrochlorothiazide.[17]

Hypoglycaemic effects In normoglycaemic rats, oral administration of an aqueous extract of *O. stamineus* (0.5 g/kg) had no significant effect on fasting blood glucose concentrations over a 7-hour period, although administration of 1 g/kg produced a significant decrease in blood glucose concentration compared with that in a control group.[22] A hypoglycaemic effect was also observed following administration of *O. stamineus* extract (1 g/kg) to rats loaded with glucose (1.5 g/kg) and in streptozotocin-induced diabetic rats; the effect of *O. stamineus* extract in streptozotocin-induced diabetic rats was similar to that observed with glibenclamide (10 mg/kg).[22]

Antihypertensive effects Methylripariochromene A has been reported to have several pharmacological actions related to antihypertensive activity.

In stroke-prone, spontaneously hypertensive rats, subcutaneous administration of methylripariochromene A (100 mg/kg) produced a continuous reduction in systolic blood pressure and a decrease in heart rate. Methylripariochromene A also suppressed agonist-induced contractions in the rat thoracic aorta and decreased the contractile force in isolated guinea-pig atria without significantly affecting the beating (heart) rate. The mechanism of action for these antihypertensive effects of methylripariochromene A is, however, unclear.[17]

Migrated pimarane-type diterpenes (neo-orthosiphols A and B), isopimarane-type diterpenes (orthosiphols A and B, orthosiphonones A and B), benzochromenes (methylripariochromene, acetovanillochromene, orthochromene A) and flavones (tetramethylscutellarein, sinensetin) isolated from *O. aristatus* have been reported to exhibit a suppressive effect on contractile responses in the rat thoracic aorta.[3]

Cytostatic effects Sinensetin and tetramethylscutellarein have been reported to demonstrate *in vitro* cytostatic activity towards Ehrlich ascites tumour cells.[23] Growth inhibition appears to be dose dependent, with 50% inhibition occurring at concentrations of approximately 30 and 15 µg/mL for sinensetin and tetramethylscutellarein, respectively. Orthosiphols A and B have been reported to inhibit inflammation induced by the tumour promoter 12-O-tetradecanoylphorbol-13-acetate (TPA) on mouse ears.[4]

Fractions of *O. stamineus* leaves have been reported to have activity against a melanoma cell line *in vitro*.[24]

Antimicrobial effects An aqueous extract of *O. aristatus* has demonstrated antibacterial activity against two serotypes of *Streptococcus mutans* (MIC 7.8–23.4 mg/mL).[25] Other *in vitro* studies have reported a lack of antibacterial activity for flavonoids (sinensetin, tetramethylscutellarein and a tetramethoxyflavone in concentrations of 10 and 100 µg/mL) isolated from *O. aristatus* leaves against *Escherichia coli*, *Proteus mirabilis*, *Pseudomonas aeruginosa*, *Staphylococcus aureus* and *Enterococcus*.[21]

O. stamineus extract has also been shown to inhibit spore germination in six out of nine fungal species tested: *Saccharomyces pastorianus*, *Candida albicans*, *Rhizopus nigricans*, *Penicillium digitatum*, *Fusarium oxysporum* and *Trichophyton mentagrophytes*.[26]

Other effects *In vitro*, *O. spicatus* has been shown to inhibit 15-lipoxygenase, an enzyme thought to be involved in the development of atherosclerosis.[11] Furthermore, the flavonoids sinensetin and tetramethylscutellarein demonstrate dose-dependent inhibition with IC_{50} values of 114 ± 5 and 110 ± 3 µmol/L, respectively, although other flavonoids from *O. spicatus* appear to be less efficient inhibitors of 15-lipoxygenase. The inhibitory activity of the whole extract was greater than could be expected from the activities of each of its flavonoid constituents, and it has been suggested that synergism may be occurring.[11] More recent *in vitro* studies have shown that flavonoids from *O. spicatus* prevent oxidative inactivation of 15-lipoxygenase, with trimethylapigenin,

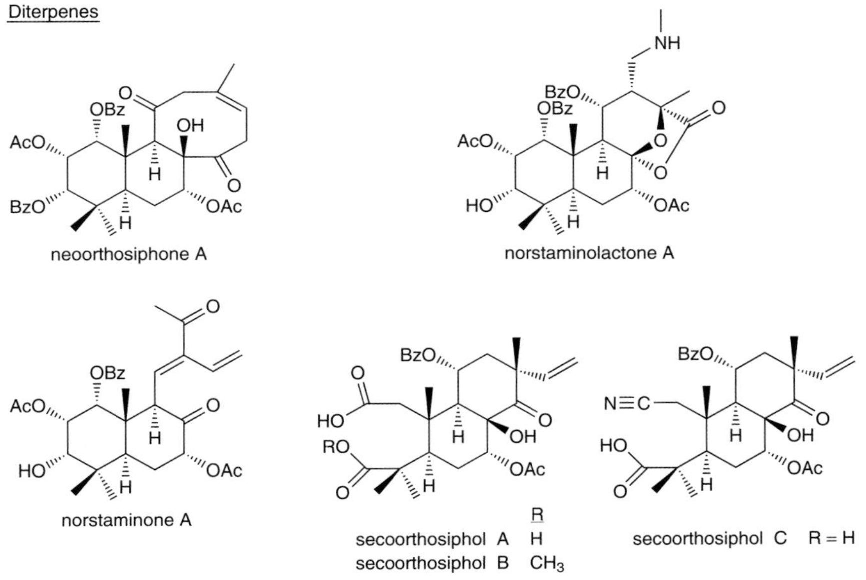

Diterpenes

neoorthosiphone A

norstaminolactone A

norstaminone A

	R
secoorthosiphol A	H
secoorthosiphol B	CH_3

secoorthosiphol C R = H

Figure 4 Selected constituents of java tea.

J

eupatorin and tetramethylluteolin showing the strongest enzyme-stabilising effects.[27] However, there was no correlation between enzyme stabilisation and enzyme inhibition.[27]

Clinical studies

Clinical investigation of preparations of Java tea is extremely limited. A randomised, double-blind, placebo-controlled, cross-over study reported no effect on 12- and 24-hour urine output or on sodium excretion in 40 healthy volunteers who received 600 mL of an infusion of *Orthosiphon* leaves daily (equivalent to 10 g dried leaves) for four days.[28] A small number of uncontrolled studies has explored the effects of preparations of Java tea and reported conflicting findings. The design of such studies does not allow the observed effects to be attributed definitively to the intervention. A study involving six healthy volunteers who drank *Orthosiphon* tea (250 mL) every six hours for one day reported an increase in urine acidity six hours after ingestion.[29]

A study involving 67 patients with uratic diathesis who received Java tea for three months reported that no effects were observed on diuresis, glomerular filtration, osmotic concentration, urinary pH, plasma content and excretion of calcium, inorganic phosphorus and uric acid.[30]

J

Side-effects, Toxicity

None documented.

Contra-indications, Warnings

None known. In view of the lack of clinical data on the use of Java tea, excessive or long-term use should be avoided. It has been recommended that adequate fluid intake (2 L or more per day) should be ensured whilst using Java tea,[G35] although the scientific basis for this statement is not clear.

Drug interactions None documented. However, in view of the documented pharmacological actions of Java tea, the potential for preparations of Java tea to interfere with other medicines administered concurrently, particularly those with similar or opposing effects, should be considered.

Pregnancy and lactation There are no data available on the use of Java tea in pregnancy and lactation. In view of the lack of toxicity data, use of Java tea during pregnancy and lactation should be avoided.

Preparations

Proprietary single-ingredient preparations

Germany: Carito mono; Diurevit Mono; Nephronorm med; Orthosiphonblatter Indischer Nierentee; Repha Orphon.

Proprietary multi-ingredient preparations

Austria: Solubitrat. *France:* Dellova; Tealine. *Germany:* Aqualibra; BioCyst; Canephron novo; Dr. Scheffler Bergischer Krautertee Blasen- und Nierentee; Harntee STADA; Harntee-Steiner; Hevert-Blasen-Nieren-Tee N; Heweberberol-Tee; Nephronorm med; Nephrubin-N; Nephrubin-N. *Spain:* Lepisor; Urisor. *Switzerland:* Bilifuge; Demonatur Dragees pour les reins et la vessie; Prosta-Caps Chassot N; Tisane pour les reins et la vessie.

References

1 Shibuya H *et al.* Indonesian medicinal plants. XXII. 1) Chemical structures of two new isopimarane-type diterpenes, orthosiphonones A and B, and a new benzochromene, orthochromene A from the leaves of *Orthosiphon aristatus* (Lamiaceae). *Chem Pharm Bull* 1999; 47: 695–698.
2 Guerin J-C, Reveillere H-P. *Orthosiphon stamineus* as a potent source of methylripariochromene A. *J Nat Prod* 1989; 52: 171–173.
3 Ohashi K *et al.* Indonesian medicinal plants. XXIII. 1) Chemical structures of two new migrated pimarane-type diterpenes, neoorthosiphols A and B, and suppressive effects on rat thoracic aorta of chemical constituents isolated from the leaves of *Orthosiphon aristatus* (Lamiaceae). *Chem Pharm Bull* 2000; 48: 433–435.
4 Masuda T *et al.* Orthosiphol A and B, novel diterpenoid inhibitors of TPA (12-O-tetradecanoylphorbol-13-acetate)-induced inflammation, from *Orthosiphon stamineus. Tetrahedron* 1992; 48: 6787–6792.
5 Stampoulis P *et al.* Staminol A, a novel diterpene from *Orthosiphon stamineus. Tetrahedron Lett* 1999; 40: 4239–4242.
6 Shibuya H *et al.* Two novel migrated pimarane-type diterpenes, neoorthosiphols A and B, from the leaves of *Orthosiphon aristatus* (Lamiaceae). *Chem Pharm Bull* 1999; 47: 911–912.
7 Awale S *et al.* Norstaminane- and isopimarane-type diterpenes of *Orthosiphon stamineus* from Okinawa. *Tetrahedron Lett* 2002; 58: 5503–5512.
8 Awale S *et al.* Neoorthosiphonone A; a nitric oxide (NO) inhibitory diterpene with new carbon skeleton from *Orthosiphon stamineus. Tetrahedron Lett* 2004; 45: 1359–1362.
9 Awale S *et al.* Secoorthosiphols A-C: three highly oxygenated secoisopimarane-type diterpenes from *Orthosiphon stamineus. Tetrahedron Lett* 2002; 43: 1473–1475.
10 Schut G, Zwaving JH. Content and composition of the essential oil of *Orthosiphon aristatus. Planta Med* 1986; 52: 240–241.
11 Lyckander IM, Malterud KE. Lipophilic flavonoids from *Orthosiphon spicatus* as inhibitors of 15-lipoxygenase. *Acta Pharm Nord* 1992; 4: 159–166.
12 Schneider G, Tan HS. Die lipophilen Flavone von *Folia Orthosiphonis. Dtsch Apoth Ztg* 1973; 113: 201.
13 Sumaryono W *et al.* Qualitative and quantitative analysis of the phenolic constituents from *Orthosiphon aristatus. Planta Med* 1991; 57: 176–180.
14 Proksch P. *Orthosiphon aristatus* (Blume) Miquel—der Katzenbart. Pflanzeninhaltsstoffe und ihre potentielle diuretische Wirkung. *Z Phytother* 1992; 13: 63–69.
15 Pietta PG *et al.* High-performance liquid chromatography with diode-array ultraviolet detection of methoxylated flavones in *Orthosiphon* leaves. *J Chromatog* 1991; 547: 439–442.
16 Bombardelli E *et al.* Flavonoid constituents of *Orthosiphon stamineus. Fitoterapia* 1972; 43: 35.
17 Matsubara T *et al.* Antihypertensive actions of methylripariochromene A from *Orthosiphon aristatus*, an Indonesian traditional medicinal plant. *Biol Pharm Bull* 1999; 22: 1083–1088.
18 Beaux D *et al.* Effect of extracts of *Orthosiphon stamineus* Benth, *Hieracium pilosella* L., *Sambucus nigra* L., and *Arctostaphylos uva-ursi* (L.) Spreng. in rats. *Phytother Res* 1998; 12: 498–501.
19 Casadebaig-Lafon J. Elaboration d'extraits végétaux adsorbés, réalisation d'extraits secs d'*Orthosiphon stamineus* Benth. *Pharm Acta Helv* 1989; 64: 220–224.
20 Englert J, Harnischfeger G. Diuretic action of aqueous *Orthosiphon* extract in rats. *Planta Med* 1992; 58: 237–238.
21 Schut GA, Zwaving JH. Pharmacological investigation of some lipophilic flavonoids from *Orthosiphon aristatus. Fitoterapia* 1993; 64: 99–102.
22 Mariam A *et al.* Hypoglycaemic activity of the aqueous extract of *Orthosiphon stamineus. Fitoterapia* 1996; 67: 465–468.
23 Malterud KE *et al.* Flavonoids from *Orthosiphon spicatus. Planta Med* 1989; 55: 569–570.
24 Estevez NA. Fractions of *Orthosiphon stamineus* Benth. leaves with antitumour activity. Preliminary results. *Rev Cuba Farm* 1980; 14: 21.
25 Chen C-P *et al.* Screening of Taiwanese drugs for antibacterial activity against *Steptococcus mutans. J Ethnopharmacol* 1989; 27: 285–295.

26 Guerin J-C, Reveillere H-P. Antifungal activity of plant extracts used in therapy. II. Study of 40 plant extracts against 9 fungi species. *Ann Pharm Franc* 1985; 43: 77–81.

27 Lyckander IM, Malterud KE. Lipophilic flavonoids from *Orthosiphon spicatus* prevent oxidative inactivation of 15-lipoxygenase. *Prostaglandins Leukot Essent Fatty Acids* 1996; 54: 239–246.

28 Du Dat D *et al*. Studies on the individual and combined diuretic effects of four Vietnamese traditional herbal remedies (*Zea mays*, *Imperata cylindrica*, *Plantago major* and *Orthosiphon stamineus*). *J Ethnopharmacol* 1992; 36: 225–231.

29 Nirdnoy M, Muangman V. Effects of *Folia orthosiphonis* on urinary stone promoters and inhibitors. *J Med Assoc Thailand* 1991; 74: 319–321.

30 Tiktinsky OL, Bablumyan YA. The therapeutic effect of Java tea and *Equisetum arvense* in patients with uratic diathesis. *Urol Nefrol* 1983; 48: 47–50.

Juniper

Summary and Pharmaceutical Comment

Some of the traditional uses documented for juniper are supported by documented pharmacological actions or known activities of documented constituents. However, there is a lack of clinical research assessing the efficacy and safety of juniper. There is evidence that the berries are abortifacient and since this is believed not to be due to the oil there must be other toxic constituents present. In view of this, use of juniper should not exceed levels specified in food legislation. Juniper is contra-indicated during pregnancy and should not be used during lactation.

Species (Family)

Juniperus communis L. (Cupressaceae)

Synonym(s)

Baccae Juniperi, Common Juniper, Genièvre, Wacholderbeeren, Zimbro

Part(s) Used

Fruit (berry)

Pharmacopoeial and Other Monographs

BHP 1996[(G9)]
BP 2007[(G84)]
Complete German Commission E[(G3)]
ESCOP 2003[(G76)]
Martindale 35th edition[(G85)]
Ph Eur 2007[(G81)]

Legal Category (Licensed Products)

GSL[(G37)]

Constituents

The following is compiled from several sources, including General References G2, G58 and G62.

Acids Diterpene acids, ascorbic acid and glucuronic acid.

Flavonoids Amentoflavone,[(1)] quercetin, isoquercitrin, apigenin and various glycosides.

Tannins Proanthocyanidins (condensed), gallocatechin and epigallocatechin.[(2)]

Volatile oils 0.2–3.42%. Primarily monoterpenes (about 58%) including α-pinene, myrcene and sabinene (major), and camphene, camphor, 1,4-cineole, *p*-cymene, α- and γ-cadinene, limonene, β-pinene, γ-terpinene, terpinen-4-ol, terpinyl acetate, α-thujene, borneol; sesquiterpenes including caryophyllene, epoxydihydrocaryophyllene and β-elemem-7α-ol.[(3, 4)]

Other constituents Geijerone (C_{12} terpenoid), junionone (monocyclic cyclobutane monoterpenoid),[(5)] desoxypodophyllotoxin (lignan),[(6)] resins and sugars.

Food Use

Juniper berries are widely used as a flavouring component in gin. Juniper is listed by the Council of Europe as a natural source of food flavouring (fruit N2, leaf and wood N3). Category N2 indicates that the berries can be added to foodstuffs in small quantities, with a possible limitation of an active principle (as yet unspecified) in the final product. Category N3 indicates that there is insufficient information available for an adequate assessment of potential toxicity to be made.[(G16)] Previously, in the USA, extracts and oils of juniper were permitted for food use.[(G65)]

Herbal Use

The German Commission E approved use for dyspepsia.[(G3)] Juniper is stated to possess diuretic, antiseptic, carminative, stomachic and antirheumatic properties. Traditionally, it has been used for cystitis, flatulence, colic, and applied topically for rheumatic pains in joints or muscles.[(G2, G7, G64)]

Monoterpenes

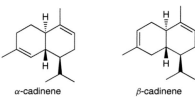

α-pinene β-pinene sabinene terpin-4-ol

Sesquiterpenes

α-cadinene β-cadinene

Flavonoids

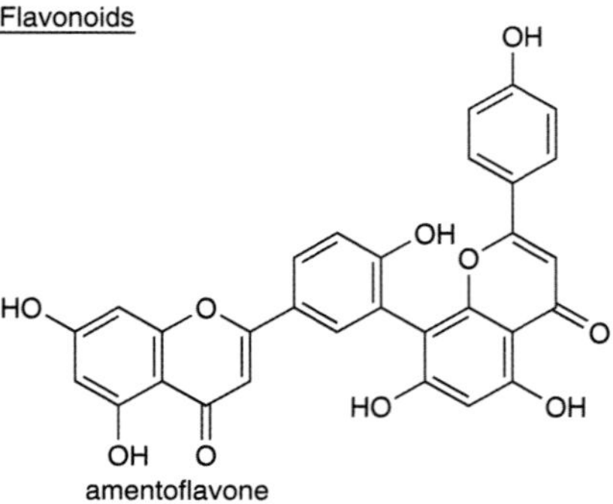

Figure 1 Selected constituents of juniper.

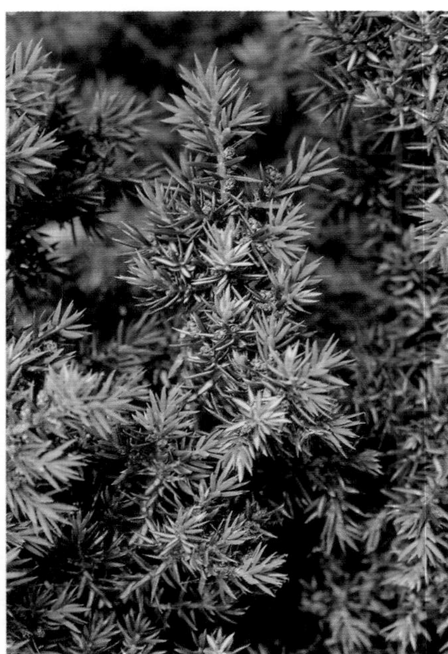

Figure 2 Juniper (*Juniperus communis*).

Dosage

Dosages for oral administration (adults) for traditional uses recommended in older and contemporary standard herbal reference texts are given below.

Dried ripe fruits 100 mL as an infusion (1 : 20 in boiling water) three times daily.[G7]

Fruit 1–2 g or equivalent three times daily; 2–10 g (equivalent to 20–100 mg of volatile oil).[G3]

Liquid extract 2–4 mL (1 : 1 in 25% alcohol) three times daily.[G7]

Tincture 1–2 mL (1 : 5 in 45% alcohol) three times daily.[G7]

Pharmacological Actions

Pharmacological actions that have been documented for juniper are primarily associated with the volatile oil components.

In vitro and animal studies

The volatile oil is stated to possess diuretic, gastrointestinal antiseptic and irritant properties.[G41]

The diuretic activity of juniper has been attributed to the volatile oil component, terpinen-4-ol, which is reported to increase the glomerular filtration rate.[G60] Terpenin-4-ol is no longer thought to be irritant to the kidneys.[G76]

An antifertility effect has been described for a juniper extract, administered to rats (300 or 500 mg, by mouth) on days 1–7 of pregnancy.[7] An abortifacient effect was also noted at both doses when the extract was administered on days 14–16 of pregnancy.[7] No evidence of teratogenicity was reported. Anti-implantation activity has been reported as 60–70%[8] and as being dose dependent.[7] Juniper is reported to have both a significant[9] and no[8] antifertility effect. A uterine stimulant activity has been documented for the volatile oil.[G30]

A potent and non-toxic inhibition of the cytopathogenic effects of herpes simplex virus type 1 in primary human amnion cell culture has been described for a juniper extract.[6, 10] The active component isolated from the active fraction was identified as a lignan, desoxypodophyllotoxin.[6] Antiviral activities documented for the volatile oil have also been partly attributed to the flavonoid amentoflavone.[1]

Anti-inflammatory activity of 60% compared to 45% for the indometacin control has been reported for juniper berry extract.[11] Both test and control were administered orally to rats (100 mg/kg and 5 mg/kg respectively) one hour before eliciting foot oedema.

A transient hypertensive effect followed by a more prolonged hypotensive effect has been reported for a juniper extract in rats (25 mg/kg, intravenous injection).[12]

A fungicidal effect against *Penicillium notatum* has been documented.[13]

Astringent activity is generally associated with tannins, which have been documented as components of juniper. An aqueous decoction of the berries has a hypoglycaemic effect in rats.[14] In rats, oral administration of an aqueous infusion (5 mL) increased chloride ion secretion by 119% and by 45% in similar experiments with rabbits.[G52]

Side-effects, Toxicity

Clinical data

There is a lack of clinical safety and toxicity data for juniper and further investigation of these aspects is required.

The volatile oil is reported to be generally non-sensitising and non-phototoxic, although slightly irritant when applied externally to human and animal skin.[G41, G58]

Dermatitic reactions have been recognised with juniper and positive patch test reactions have been documented.[15, G51] The latter are attributed to the irritant nature of the juniper extract.[15] Adverse effects following external application of the essential oil are described as burning, erythema, inflammation with blisters and oedema.[G22]

Preclinical data

The acute toxicity of juniper has been investigated in rats who were administered extracts for seven days.[11] An oral dose of 2.5 g/kg was tolerated with no mortalities or side-effects noted. A dose of 3 g/kg induced hypothermia and mild diarrhoea in 10–30% of animals.[11] An LD_{50} value (mice, intraperitoneal injection) has been stated as 3 g/kg.[4] There is evidence from

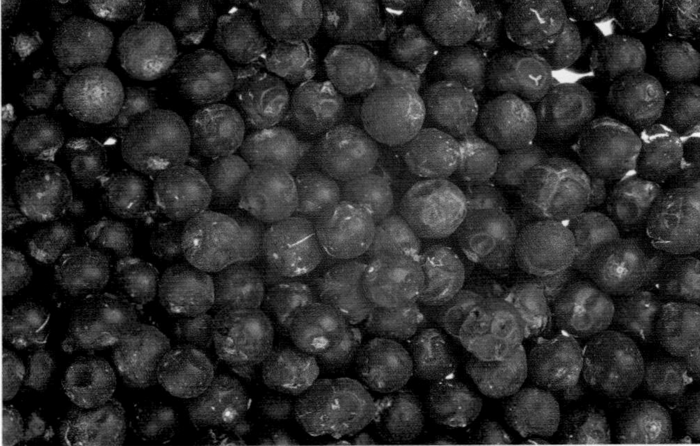

Figure 3 Juniper – dried drug substance (fruit).

preclinical studies that juniper has antifertility and abortifacient effects (*see* Pharmacological Actions, *In vitro* and animal studies).

Contra-indications, Warnings

Juniper is contra-indicated in individuals with acute or chronic inflammation of the kidney.(G76)

Drug interactions None documented. However, the potential for preparations of juniper to interact with other medicines administered concurrently, particularly those with similar or opposing effects, should be considered. There is limited evidence from preclinical studies that juniper has diuretic and hypoglycaemic effects.

Pregnancy and lactation A juniper fruit extract has exhibited abortifacient, antifertility and anti-implantation activities (*see Pharmacological Actions, In vitro* and animal studies). In view of this, juniper is contra-indicated in pregnancy.(G7, G22, G49) Juniper should not be used during lactation.

Preparations

Proprietary single-ingredient preparations

Czech Republic: Plod Jalovce.

Proprietary multi-ingredient preparations

Australia: Arthritic Pain Herbal Formula 1; Lifesystem Herbal Formula 1 Arthritic Aid; Profluid; Protemp. *Austria:* Mariazeller; St Bonifatius-Tee. *Brazil:* Pilulas De Witt's. *Canada:* Herbal Diuretic. *Czech Republic:* Abfuhr-Heilkrautertee. *France:* Depuratum; Mediflor Tisane Antirhumatismale No 2. *Germany:* Amara-Tropfen. *Italy:* Broncosedina. *South Africa:* Amara. *Switzerland:* Heparfelien; Kernosan Heidelberger Poudre; Tisane pour les reins et la vessie. *UK:* Backache; Watershed. *USA:* Natural Herbal Water Tablets; Water Pill.

J

References

1 Chandler RF. An inconspicuous but insidious drug. *Rev Pharm Can* 1986; 563–566.
2 Friedrich H, Engelshowe R. Tannin producing monomeric substances in *Juniperus communis. Planta Med* 1978; 33: 251–257.
3 Wagner H, Wolff P, eds. *New Natural Products and Plant Drugs with Pharmacological, Biological or Therapeutical Activity.* Berlin: Springer-Verlag, 1977.
4 *Fenaroli's Handbook of Flavor Ingredients*, 2nd edn. Boca Raton: CRC Press, 1975.
5 Thomas AF, Ozainne M. 'Junionone' [1-(2,2-Dimethylcyclobutyl)but-1-en-3-one], the first vegetable monocyclic cyclobutane monoterpenoid. *J C S Chem Commun* 1973; 746.
6 Markkanen T *et al.* Antiherpetic agent from juniper tree (*Juniperus communis*), its purification, identification, and testing in primary human amnion cell cultures. *Drugs Exp Clin Res* 1981; 7: 691–697.
7 Agrawal OP *et al.* Antifertility effects of fruits of *Juniperus communis. Planta Med* 1980; 40 (Suppl. Suppl.): 98–101.
8 Prakash AO *et al.* Anti-implantation activity of some indigenous plants in rats. *Acta Eur Fertil* 1985; 16: 441–448.
9 Prakash AO. Biological evaluation of some medicinal plant extracts for contraceptive efficacy. *Contracept Deliv Syst* 1984; 5: 9.
10 Marrkanen T. Antiherpetic agent(s) from juniper tree (*Juniperus communis*). Preliminary communication. *Drugs Exp Clin Res* 1981; 7: 69–73.
11 Mascolo N *et al.* Biological screening of Italian medicinal plants for anti-inflammatory activity. *Phytother Res* 1987; 1: 28–31.
12 Lasheras B *et al.* Étude pharmacologique préliminaire de *Prunus spinosa* L. Amelanchier ovalis Medikus, *Juniperus communis* L. et *Urtica dioica* L. *Plant Méd Phytothér* 1986; 20: 219–226.
13 Hejtmánková N *et al.* The antifungal effects of some Cupressaceae. *Acta Univ Palacki Olomuc Fac Med* 1973; 60: 15–20.
14 Sanchez de Medina F *et al.* Hypoglycaemic activity of Juniper berries. *Planta Med* 1994; 60: 197–200.
15 Mathias CGT *et al.* Plant dermatitis – patch test results (1975–78). Note on *Juniperus* extract. *Contact Dermatitis* 1979; 5: 336–337.

Kava

Summary and Pharmaceutical Comment

The chemistry of kava is well documented (*see* Constituents) and there is strong evidence that the kavalactone constituents are responsible for the observed pharmacological activities.

Randomised, double-blind, placebo-controlled clinical trials of certain standardised kava preparations have shown beneficial effects on measures of anxiety, although because of methodological limitations of some studies, further well-designed trials are required to confirm the anxiolytic effects. Also, most trials have been carried out with one particular standardised kava extract (containing 70% kavalactones) and it cannot be assumed that the effects shown in these studies will be produced by other kava extracts. Clinical trials involving patients with anxiety have also compared well-defined standardised kava preparations with certain standard anxiolytic agents. While these studies have suggested that the kava extracts tested may be as effective as certain standard anxiolytic agents, further investigation is necessary. Data from pharmacological studies provide supporting evidence for the anxiolytic effects of kava, although many of the other traditional uses of kava (*see* Herbal use) have not been tested scientifically. Many pharmacological studies involving individual kavalactones have investigated the effects of the synthetic kavalactone (±)-kavain, rather than the natural compound (+)-kavain. Some studies have used both the natural compound and the synthetic racemate and have reported a lack of stereospecific effect.

In placebo-controlled clinical trials, standardised kava extracts generally have been well tolerated; reported adverse events have been mild and transient and similar in nature and frequency to those reported for placebo. Clinical trials, however, can provide only limited information on the safety profile of a medicine. Spontaneous reports of hepatotoxicity associated with the use of kava preparations have arisen since the year 2000. Although the risk of serious liver toxicity is thought to be low, the reaction is idiosyncratic. Against this background, kava was prohibited in unlicensed medicines in the UK in 2003, and in the EU, all licensed kava products were removed from the market. In 2005 in the UK, evidence relating to hepatotoxicity associated with kava was reviewed and the Expert Working Group's report concluded that there was insufficient new evidence to support a change in the regulatory position, i.e. the inclusion of kava in unlicensed medicines remains prohibited. Regulatory action has also been taken in Canada and Australia (voluntary recall), and in the USA, consumers were warned of the risk of liver toxicity with use of kava-containing products.

Other adverse reactions documented for kava preparations include an ichthyosiform (scaly, non-inflammatory) skin condition, termed 'kava dermopathy', usually associated with the traditional method of preparing and ingesting kava (*see* Side-effects, Toxicity, Skin reactions).

In view of the documented pharmacological actions of kava and in view of the reported inhibitory activity against certain cytochrome P450 drug metabolising enzymes, the potential for preparations of kava root/rhizome to interfere with other medicines administered concurrently, particularly those with similar or opposing effects, should be considered.

Use of kava should be avoided during pregnancy and breastfeeding.

Although kava is prohibited in the UK and several other countries, individuals may obtain kava preparations over the Internet. Healthcare professionals should be aware that patients may be taking herbal medicinal products containing kava. Healthcare professionals should enquire about use of kava in patients presenting with symptoms of hepatotoxicity (*see* Side-effects, Toxicity, Hepatotoxicity). Adverse reactions have been reported in association with use of 'herbal ecstasy' tablets, which often contain ephedrine alkaloids, although healthcare professionals should be aware that some products have been stated to contain kava.

Species (Family)

Piper methysticum Forst. f. (Piperaceae)

Fourteen different varieties are used throughout Oceania (Polynesia, Melanesia, Micronesia).[1]

Related species

Cultivars of *P. methysticum* have been developed in some Pacific Islands from *Piper wichmannii* C. DC (syn: *Piper erectum* C. DC, *Piper arbuscula* Trelease).[2,3]

Synonym(s)

Intoxicating Pepper, Kava-kava, Kawa, Kawa-kawa, *Macropiper methysticum* (G. Forst.) Hook. & Arn., *M. latifolium* Miq., Waghi, Wati, Bari (Irian Jaya), Koniak, Keu, Oyo (Papua New Guinea)

Part(s) Used

Peeled dry rhizome (sometimes referred to incorrectly as the root)

Pharmacopoeial and Other Monographs

BHMA 2003[G66]
BHP 1996[G9]
Complete German Commission E 1998[G3]
Expanded German Commission E 2000[G4]
Martindale 35th edition[G85]
WHO volume 2 2002[G70]

Legal Category (Licensed Products)

Prohibited in unlicensed medicines in the UK.[4]

Constituents

Kavalactones Kawalactones, kavapyrones, 2-pyrones, δ-lactones with styryl or dihydrostyryl substituents.[1–3, 5–9, G56] Dried rhizomes should contain at least 3.5% kavalactones[G56] and good-quality material 5.5–8.3%.[10] Ethanol–water extracts contain 30% kavalactones, whereas acetone–water extracts contain 70%.[G56] The kavalactones occur as a complex mixture of at least 18 compounds,[5] which are of three main types: styryl enolide pyrones (e.g. kawain (= kavain), dimethoxykawain, methysticin), styryl dienolide pyrones (e.g. yangonin, desmethoxyyangonin), and dihydrostyryl enolide pyrones (e.g. dihydrokawain, dimethoxydihydrokawain, dihydromethysticin). The four major kavalactones of the rhizome are kawain (1–2%), dihydrokawain (0.6–1%), methysticin (1.2–2%) and dihydromethysticin (0.5–0.8%).[G56] Smaller quantities (<0.1%) of dimeric kavalactones (e.g. truxyangonins I, II, III) have also been isolated.[2,3]

Alkaloids/amides Cepharadione A (aporphine-type) is a minor component (4 kg yielded 1 mg).[11] Small quantities of *N*-cinnamoylpyrrolidine and its *O*-methoxy analogue are also present.[6,12,13]

Chalcones Flavokawains A, B and C.[6,9,14]

Flavonoids Pinostrobin, 5,7-dimethoxyflavanone.[14]

Steroids Sitosterol, stigmasterol, stigmastanol.[6,13]

Esters Bornyl cinnamate[13] and bornyl 3,4-methylenedioxycinnamate.[14]

Aliphatic alcohols Docosan-1-ol, dodecan-1-ol, eicosan-1-ol, hexacosan-1-ol, hexadecan-1-ol, octadecan-1-ol, *n*-tetradecanol, transphytol.[6]

Other constituents Cinnamylideneacetone,[5] long-chain fatty acids.[6]

Other parts of the plant

Stem peelings may be included as raw material in kava commerce due to the high demand for the rhizome; leaves and branches are used in folk medicine. Pipermethystine (a piperidone amide) is present in stem peelings (traces to 0.85%).[15] 3α,4α-Epoxy-5β-pipermethysticin (0.93%) was isolated from stem peelings of one cultivar, but was absent from 10 other cultivars, and the related

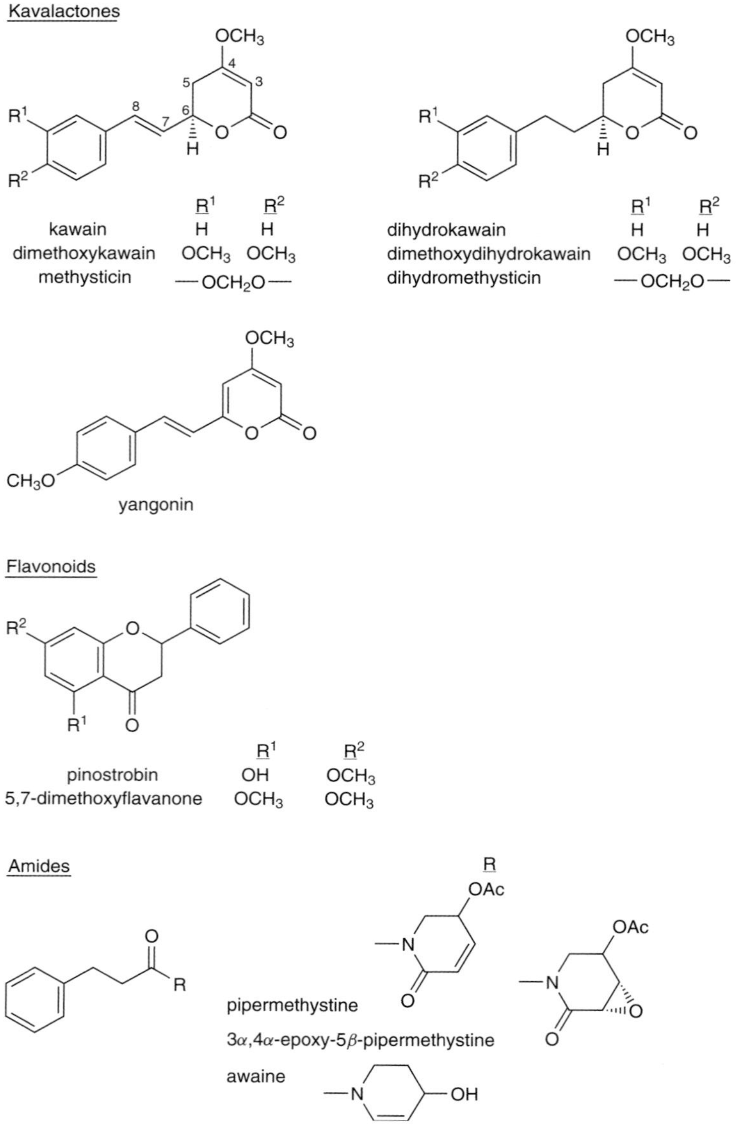

Figure 1 Selected constituents of kava.

alkaloid awaine was present in the unopened leaves of 11 cultivars (0.16–2.67%). 7,8-Dihydrokawain, 7,8-dihydromethysticin and 5,6,7,8-tetrahydroyangonin are present in stem peelings.

Other species

Kavalactones occur in *P. wichmanni* and *P. sanctum*. The latter species contains several cinnamoyl butenolides (piperolides), e.g. methylenedioxypiperolide and 7,8-epoxypiperolide.[2,3]

Food Use

Kava is used as an intoxicant drink, on either informal or ceremonial occasions, by Pacific Islanders e.g. from Fiji, Samoa and Tonga.[1,7] Some claim that it has a pleasant, cooling, aromatic taste with numbing on the tongue and is stimulating, while others refer to great bitterness with a burning sensation in the mouth. It is reputed to reduce fatigue, allay anxieties and produce a cheerful and sociable attitude. Unpleasant effects reported include dizziness, sleeping disorders, stomach pains, lethargy and skin reactions. These reported effects are taken from a wide geographical area and any differences may be due to a number of reasons including plant varieties or growing conditions.

Herbal Use

In many parts of the Pacific it is believed that kava is beneficial to health by soothing nervous conditions, inducing relaxation and sleep, counteracting fatigue, and reducing weight. Medicinal uses also include treatment of urinary tract infections, asthma, rheumatism, headache, fever, gonorrhoea and syphilis, and use as a diuretic and stomachic.[1,7,G34] The medicinal use of kava is now widespread, e.g. across Europe, North America and Australia, where it is used to treat anxiety, nervous tension, restlessness, mild depression and menopausal symptoms.[G9,G32,G50,G56,G60,G67] It has also been adopted by the Aboriginal community in parts of Australia as an intoxicating drink.[16]

The German Commission E recommended kava for the treatment of nervous anxiety, stress and restlessness.[G3] Traditional uses listed for kava rhizome in other standard herbal and pharmaceutical reference texts include cystitis, urethritis, infection or inflammation of the genitourinary tract, rheumatism and, topically, for joint pains.[G66]

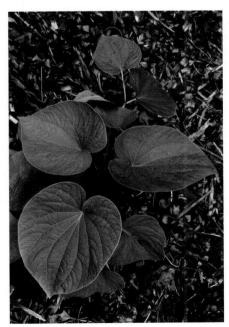

Figure 2 Kava (*Piper methysticum*).

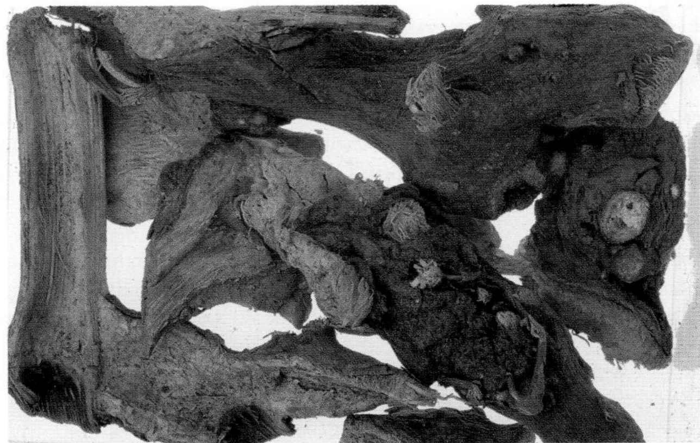

Figure 3 Kava – dried drug substance (rhizome).

Dosage

Dosages for oral administration (adults) for treatment of anxiety recommended in older and contemporary standard herbal reference texts are given below.

Dried rhizome 1.5–3 g per day.[G50] Equivalent to 60–120 mg kavalactones per day.[G3]

Liquid extract 3–6 mL per day (1 : 2 liquid extract, unspecified solvent).[G50]

Standardised preparations 100–200 mg kavalactones per day.[G50] 60 mg kavalactones 2–4 times per day in tablet form.[G50] 60–120 mg kavalactones per day.[G3]

Kava exists in numerous varieties of differing potency[7] and only preparations with standardised kavalactone content should be used for medicinal purposes. Medicinal extracts prepared with ethanol–water yield dry extracts with about 30% kavalactones content, whereas acetone–water prepared dry extracts contain about 70% kavalactones.[G56]

Dosages (adults) used in clinical trials have varied widely, but typically are those equivalent to 60–240 mg kavalactones daily by oral administration in divided doses (*see* Pharmacological Actions, Clinical studies). Duration of use of kava extracts generally should not exceed three months.[G3,G4,G56]

Pharmacological Actions

Kava has been investigated mostly for its anxiolytic effects, although other central nervous system activities, such as anticonvulsant and analgesic properties, and other effects have been documented following preclinical studies. The kavalactones are believed to be the major active constituents of kava.

In vitro and animal studies

Pharmacokinetics Uptake of the kavalactones kavain, dihydrokavain, yangonin and desmethoxyyangonin into brain tissue has been documented following intraperitoneal administration of each of these compounds at a dose of 100 mg/kg to mice.[17] Maximum concentrations of kavain and dihydrokavain were noted five minutes after administration, and these compounds were rapidly eliminated. In contrast, yangonin and desmethoxyyangonin were eliminated more slowly. All four compounds were also detected in mouse brain tissue following intraperitoneal administration of kava resin 120 mg/kg (containing kavain 36.7%, dihydrokavain 19.2%, yangonin 15% and desmethoxyyangonin 13.3%), although the concentrations of kavain and yangonin were higher than was noted following individual administration of these constituents.

Central nervous system activities Anxiolytic properties for kava extract and isolated kavalactones have been documented in an experimental model of anxiety, the chick social separation–stress procedure. In a series of experiments, kava extract (containing 30% kavalactones; 30 mg/mL per kg body weight), dihydrokavain (30 mg/mL per kg body weight) and chlordiazepoxide (5 mg/mL per kg body weight) administered intraperitoneally 30 minutes before testing significantly reduced the separation–stress effect ($p < 0.05$ for each substance).[18] However, the isolated kavalactones kavain, methysticin, dihydromethysticin, yangonin and desmethoxyyangonin administered according to the same regimen did not have a statistically significant effect. Further work using the same experimental model confirmed these findings and found that total kavalactone content was not predictive of outcome, but that a dihydrokavain content of at least 15% was necessary for anxiolytic activity.[19] In this study, the kava samples and fractions that demonstrated anxiolytic activity were reported to be without sedative effects.

K

In contrast, previous studies have reported sedative effects for kava extract. In mice, kava extract (containing 7% kavalactones) at doses of at least 50 mg/kg body weight (by intraperitoneal injection) reduced spontaneous motility to a greater extent than did control.[20] The effect was enhanced by the addition of (±)-kavain (ratio of kava extract to (±)-kavain, 1 : 0.12), although this compound had no sedative effect when administered alone. In another experimental model, kava extract 100 mg/kg body weight and (±)-kavain 12 mg/kg body weight, each administered alone, had no sedative effect, whereas a combination of the two substances significantly reduced amphetamine (5 mg/kg body weight subcutaneously)-induced hypermotility. Sedative effects have also been documented for an ethanolic extract of kava rhizome (containing 50% kavalactones) 100 mg/kg body weight administered by gastric tube and 200 mg/kg body weight intraperitoneally in the amphetamine-induced hypermotility test and barbiturate-induced sleeping time, respectively.[21]

In studies utilising the conditioned avoidance response test in rats, an experimental model used to test for antipsychotic activity, aqueous (kavalactone-free) kava extract 30–500 mg/kg body weight intraperitoneally had no statistically significant effect.[22] However, administration of kava resin at doses of 125 mg/kg intraperitoneally significantly inhibited the conditioned avoidance response, although to a lesser extent than did chlorpromazine and haloperidol.

In cats, a kava extract in arachis oil (50–100 mg kavalactones per kg body weight intraperitoneally) and the individual kavalactone (±)-kavain (10–50 mg per kg body weight intraperitoneally) were reported to be active in the amygdala complex region of the brain.[23]

Receptor binding studies with kava extracts and individual kavalactones have reported conflicting results. One series of experiments found that kava resin and individual kavalactones displayed only weak activity on $GABA_A$- and no activity on $GABA_B$-binding sites in rat brain membranes *in vitro*, and that there was no significant effect on benzodiazepine receptors following intraperitoneal administration of kava resin 150 mg/kg body weight to mice.[24] A marked effect of kavain on GABA has also been stated to be unlikely.[25] By contrast, a kavalactone-enriched ethanol/aqueous extract of kava rhizome (containing 58% kavalactones and 42% other lipid-soluble compounds) increased the density of GABA-binding sites in certain brain regions.[26] Other experiments have shown concentration- and structure-dependent effects of kavalactones on binding of bicuculline methochloride (BMC) to $GABA_A$ receptors from rat cortex preparations.[27] (+)-Kavain, (+)-methysticin and (+)-dihydromethysticin enhanced BMC binding by 18–28% at a concentration of 0.1 µmol/L, whereas (+)-dihydrokavain did so only at a concentration of 10 µmol/L, and yangonin at a concentration of 1 µmol/L; desmethoxyyangonin had no effect. Further radioreceptor assays demonstrated that these six kavalactones had no effect on the binding of flunitrazepam to benzodiazepine receptors in rat cortex preparations, indicating that the influence of kavalactones on $GABA_A$ receptors was not based upon an interaction with benzodiazepine receptors.[27]

Other *in vitro* studies have investigated the effects of kava extracts and individual kavalactones on other transmitters in the central nervous system (CNS). A kavalactone-rich kava rhizome extract (containing 68% kavalactones) was a reversible inhibitor of monoamine-oxidase B (MAO-B) in intact and disrupted platelets (inhibitory concentration IC_{50} 24 µmol/L and 1.2 µmol/L, respectively), although there were differences in MAO-B inhibition among the different synthetic kavalactones with desmethoxyyangonin and (±)-methysticin being the most potent inhibitors.[28] Differences between kavalactones in inhibition of noradrenaline (norepinephrine) uptake in synaptosomes prepared from rat cerebral cortex and hippocampus have also been documented: (±)- and (+)-kavain gave approximately equal values and both were more potent inhibitors than (+)-methysticin, although none of the compounds inhibited serotonin uptake.[29] It has been suggested, following *in vitro* studies involving ipsapirone (a serotonin-1_A receptor agonist)-induced field potential changes in guinea-pig hippocampal slices, that kavain and dihydromethysticin may modulate serotonin-1_A receptor activity, although further work is needed to identify the precise mechanism for this.[30]

In vivo studies in rats administered a single oral dose of (+)-dihydromethysticin 100 mg/kg body weight or fed (±)-kavain in the diet over a 78-day period showed that neither kavalactone regimen affected brain tissue concentrations of dopamine and serotonin, although since extracellular neurotransmitter concentrations were not measured in this study, receptor-mediated effects of kavalactones on dopaminergic and serotonergic neurons could not be excluded.[31] *In vivo* (rats), kava extract 20 and 120 mg/kg body weight intraperitoneally increased dopamine concentrations in the nucleus accumbens, although a dose of 220 mg/kg body weight led to an initial decrease followed by an increase above baseline values.[32] It was suggested that this ceiling effect may be due to yangonin which may have dopamine antagonist activity.

The development of physiological tolerance to an aqueous extract of kava administered intraperitoneally to mice has been documented, although there was no clear evidence of development of physiological or learned tolerance to kava resin.[33]

Anticonvulsant and neuroprotective activities Studies described in the older literature have documented anticonvulsant effects for kavalactones in several experimental models.[34, G50] The anticonvulsant properties of (+)-methysticin *in vitro* may arise from a direct membrane action on the excitability of neurons,[34] and *in vitro* assays have shown that (+)-methysticin,[35] (+)-kavain[36] and the synthetic kavalactone (±)-kavain[34–36] appear to interact with voltage-dependent sodium channels, and that (±)-kavain also interacts with voltage-dependent calcium channels.[37] Inhibition by (±)-kavain of veratridine-activated voltage-dependent sodium ion channels in synaptosomes from rat cerebral cortex,[38] and veratridine-induced increase in intracellular calcium ion concentrations has been described following *in vitro* studies utilising rat cerebrocortical synaptosomes.[39] Reduction in veratridine-induced glutamate release following (±)-kavain administration has been reported both *in vitro*[39] and *in vivo* in freely moving rats.[40] Substances which reduce extracellular glutamate concentrations are of interest for their potential as anticonvulsant agents.

Some of the mechanisms described above documented for certain kavalactones may also be important in neuroprotective effects reported for the synthetic kavalactone (±)-kavain. For example, the role of sodium-ion channel blockade in the neuroprotective effect of (±)-kavain against anoxia *in vitro* has been described,[41] and (±)-kavain (50, 100 or 200 mg/kg intraperitoneally) has been shown to protect nigrostriatal dopaminergic neurons against 1-methyl-4-phenyl-1,2,3,6-tetrahydropyridine (MPTP)-induced toxicity in mice, an experimental model of Parkinson's disease.[42] A neuroprotective effect against ischaemic brain damage in mice and rats has been demonstrated for kava extract (WS-1490 containing 70% kavalactones) and the individual kavalactones methysticin and dihydromethysticin, but not for kavain, dihydrokavain and yangonin. Kava extract 150 mg/kg given orally as an emulsion (polyethyleneglycol 400 and water; 20 : 80) one hour before experimentally induced ischaemia, and methysticin and dihydromethysticin (both 10 and 30 mg/kg intraperitoneally 15 minutes before induction of ischaemia), compared with control, significantly reduced the size of the infarct area in mice brains ($p < 0.05$).[43] In rats, kava extract administered according to the same regimen as used in mice significantly reduced infarct volume compared with control ($p < 0.05$).

Analgesic activity Antinociceptive activity *in vivo* (mice) in the tail immersion test has been documented for kava resin (150 mg/kg intraperitoneally) and for the individual kavalactones dihydrokawain, dihydromethysticin, kavain and methysticin at doses of 150, 275, 300 and 360 mg/kg (intraperitoneally), respectively, compared with controls.[44] Yangonin, tetrahydroyangonin, desmethoxyyangonin and dehydroyangonin had no or only a weak effect. Both kava resin (200 mg/kg, orally) and aqueous kava extract (250 mg/kg, intraperioneally) displayed antinociceptive activity in the acetic acid-induced writhing test, also in mice. In further tests using both models, naloxone failed to reverse the antinociceptive effects of kava resin or aqueous kava extract, indicating that analgesic activity of kava is achieved via non-opiate pathways.[44] Analgesic activity of dihydrokawain and dihydromethysticin has been reported previously.[45]

Other activities Kava extract has been reported to have a muscle relaxant effect in isolated frog muscles, thought to be due to a direct effect on muscle contractility.[46] Reductions in contractions of isolated guinea-pig ileum induced by carbachol and by raised extracellular potassium ion concentrations have been documented for the synthetic kavalactone (±)-kavain, although the compound had no effect on caffeine-induced contractions of ileum strips or on calcium ion-induced contractions of skinned muscles.[47] (±)-Kavain has also been reported to relax maximally contracted murine airway smooth muscle and to reduce carbachol- and potassium chloride-induced airway smooth muscle contraction.[48] Further investigation indicated that nitric oxide and cyclooxygenase-mediated events did not play a role in kavain-induced relaxation.

In contrast, a previous study found that (+)-kavain inhibited human platelet aggregation in a concentration-dependent manner *in vitro*.[49] The formation of prostaglandin E_2 and thromboxane B_2 was also inhibited in a concentration-dependent manner, suggesting that (+)-kavain is an inhibitor of cyclooxygenase.

An ethanol extract of kava and the isolated kavalactones dehydrokavain, dihydrokavain, kavain, yangonin and methysticin inhibited tumour necrosis factor alpha (TNFα) release *in vitro* from BALB/3T3 cells incubated with okadaic acid and suppressed lipopolysaccharide-induced TNFα production *in vivo* in diabetic mice following intraperitoneal administration.[50]

Antifungal activity against several microorganisms, including *Candida albicans*, has been described for a 10% aqueous kava extract.[51]

Clinical studies

Clinical trials of kava preparations have focused on investigating anxiolytic effects in various patient groups. Several trials have assessed effects in healthy volunteers, and others have explored the effects of kavain, a constituent of kava.

A Cochrane systematic review of monopreparations of kava for the treatment of anxiety included 12 randomised, double-blind, placebo-controlled trials involving a total of 700 participants.[52] All but one of these trials tested the effects of a standardised (70% kavalactones) preparation of kava rhizome (WS-1490) at various dosages but typically equivalent to 60–240 mg kavalactones daily for four weeks. Only two trials were conducted for longer than four weeks; both used a dose equivalent to 210 mg kavalactones daily given for eight weeks in one study[53] and 24 weeks in the other.[54]

Seven of the 12 trials, involving a total of 380 participants, used the total score on the Hamilton Anxiety Scale as their primary outcome measure, and provided data suitable for meta-analysis. Meta-analysis showed a reduction in anxiety scale scores in kava recipients, compared with placebo recipients (weighted mean difference: 3.9; 95% confidence interval (CI), 0.1–7.7; $p = 0.05$). All except one of these trials included participants with non-psychotic anxiety; one study involved women with anxiety associated with the climacteric (perimenopausal period). Removing this trial and the trial that did not assess the kava extract WS-1490 from the meta-analysis indicated a statistically significant reduction in anxiety scores for kava recipients compared with placebo recipients (weighted mean difference: 3.4; 95% CI, 0.5–6.4; $p = 0.02$).[52]

The five studies not included in the meta-analysis reported statistically significant improvements for kava recipients, compared with placebo recipients, on outcomes (e.g. response rates, reduction in scores on various anxiety scales).[52] These five studies were heterogeneous in that they involved different patient groups, such as women with anxiety associated with the perimenopausal period, individuals with preoperative anxiety, and outpatients with neurotic anxiety. Consequently, dosage regimens of kava varied widely (e.g. equivalent to kavalactones 60 mg in the evening and 1 hour preoperatively, to 140 mg kavalactones daily for four weeks).

The conclusions of the review were that kava extract is an effective symptomatic treatment for anxiety, but that limitations of the studies included meant that further rigorous trials were needed.[52] A similar meta-analysis, which included six rando-

K

mised, double-blind, placebo-controlled trials assessing the effects of the kava extract WS-1490 in patients with non-psychotic anxiety disorders reached a similar conclusion.[55]

Some other research has been published, but has added little to the evidence base because of methodological issues. In a randomised, double-blind, placebo-controlled, multicentre trial, 61 patients with sleep disturbances associated with anxiety, tension and restlessness states of non-psychotic origin received a kava extract (WS-1490) 200 mg daily, or placebo, for four weeks.[56] At the end of the study, statistically significant improvements in the two primary outcome measures quality of sleep and recuperative effect after sleep were observed for kava recipients, compared with the placebo group ($p = 0.007$ and 0.018, respectively; intention-to-treat analysis).

In a randomised, double-blind, placebo-controlled trial conducted entirely over the Internet, 391 adults who scored at least 40 points on the State-Trait Anxiety Inventory (STAI) State scale and who reported having sleeping problems on at least two occasions received capsules containing kava extract (each containing total kavalactones 100 mg) one three times daily, two capsules containing valerian extract (each containing valerenic acids 3.2 mg; no further details of preparation provided) one hour before bedtime, or placebo, for 28 days.[57] At the end of the study, there were no statistically significant differences between kava and placebo with respect to the primary outcome measures changes from baseline in STAI-state anxiety scores and Insomnia Severity Index scores.

K

For example, a study involving 68 perimenopausal women reported that kava extract 100 mg (containing 55% kavain) or 200 mg daily improved anxiety compared with no treatment, but participants were not masked as to their treatment allocation.[58]

Results from some clinical studies have suggested that kava extracts may be as effective as certain standard anxiolytic agents, although this requires further investigation and confirmation. In a six-week, randomised, double-blind trial involving 172 patients with non-psychotic anxiety, the standardised kava extract WS-1490 (containing 70% kavalactones) 100 mg three times daily was as effective as oxazepam 5 mg and bromazepam 3 mg, each taken three times daily.[59] Another randomised, double-blind, multicentre trial, involving 129 outpatients with generalised anxiety disorder, reported that the kava extract LI-150 400 mg (standardised to 30% kavapyrones = 120 mg) each morning for eight weeks was as effective as buspirone 5 mg twice daily and opipramol (a tricyclic antidepressant) 50 mg twice daily.[60]

A randomised, placebo-controlled study involving 40 postmenopausal women with anxiety assessed the effects of a kava extract 100 mg daily (containing 55% kavain) given in addition to hormone replacement therapy (oestrogens plus progestogens or oestrogens alone).[61] It was reported that women who received kava showed greater reductions in anxiety scores than women who received placebo. However, the study had various methodological limitations.

In a randomised, controlled study involving 54 healthy volunteers, kava extract (LI-150, equivalent to 120 mg kavalactones; $n = 18$) and valerian extract 600 mg (LI-156; $n = 18$), taken daily for one week, significantly reduced systolic blood pressure following mental stress tests, compared with baseline values, whereas no such reduction was observed in the no-treatment control group ($p < 0.001$ for both kava and valerian).[62] No effect on diastolic blood pressure was recorded for either herbal preparation, and valerian, but not kava, appeared to reduce heart rate following mental stress tests. These findings require confirmation in placebo-controlled studies, and their relevance to everyday stress needs to be investigated.[62]

Several other randomised, double-blind, controlled trials involving patients with anxiety have compared the effects of the synthetic kavalactone, (±)-kavain, administered at a dose of 200 mg three times daily for 3–4 weeks, with those of placebo,[63] or benzodiazepines, such as oxazepam.[64] One trial assessed the effects of kavain, or placebo, 200 mg three times daily for three weeks in 83 outpatients who had been treated with benzodiazepines for at least six weeks and who were undergoing benzodiazepine withdrawal.[65] Generally, these studies have reported beneficial effects for kavain, but typically have involved only small numbers of patients.

A preliminary study involving healthy individuals assessed the effects of a single 300 mg dose of a kava extract on cognitive performance and mood in a randomised, double-blind, placebo-controlled trial.[66] Some improvements in mood (in trait cheerful participants only) and cognitive performance were observed during the study, although further assessment of the effects of kava on these parameters is required.

A case series described improvements after administration of a kava extract (WS-1490) in extrapyramidal side-effects experienced by 42 patients with various psychiatric diagnoses who were receiving neuroleptic drugs.[67] The hypothesis that kava extract can reduce extrapyramidal side-effects requires testing in rigorous randomised controlled trials.

Pharmacokinetics Little is known about the clinical pharmacokinetics of kava preparations. Several metabolites of kavalactones have been detected and identified in human urine following ingestion of around 1 L of kava (prepared by the traditional method of aqueous extraction of kava rhizome) over 1 hour by healthy male volunteers before sleeping.[68] Urine samples were collected before sleeping and on rising in the morning. Kawain, dihydrokawain, desmethoxyyangonin, tetrahydroyangonin, dihydromethysticin, 11-methoxytetrahydroyangonin, yangonin, methysticin and dehydromethysticin were detected unchanged in human urine; metabolic transformations observed included reduction of the 3,4-double bond and/or demethylation of the 4-methoxyl group of the kavalactone ring. The C_{12} hydroxy analogue of yangonin (12-hydroxy-12-desmethoxyyangonin) was also detected, and it may have been formed by demethylation of yangonin and/or C_{12} hydroxylation of desmethoxyyangonin. Dihydroxylated metabolites of the kavalactones and products from ring opening of the kavalactone ring were not detected.[68]

Side-effects, Toxicity

In randomised, placebo-controlled trials involving different patient groups with anxiety, kava extracts generally have been well tolerated; adverse events reported, and their frequencies, are similar to those reported for placebo. However, clinical trials have the statistical power only to detect common, acute adverse effects.

Spontaneous reports of suspected adverse drug reactions associated with kava preparations have raised concerns over hepatotoxic reactions (*see* Hepatotoxicity).

A systematic review of eight placebo-controlled trials of kava extracts administered at doses equivalent to 55–240 mg kavalactones daily for two days to 24 weeks found that adverse events reported for both kava and placebo were most commonly gastrointestinal symptoms, tiredness, restlessness, tremor and headache.[69] Three trials included in the review, one of which tested kava extract 100 mg daily (equivalent to 55 mg kavalactones) for 24 weeks,[61] reported that adverse events were not observed in either the kava or placebo groups.

A similar finding was reported by a more recent Cochrane systematic review of monopreparations of kava for the treatment of anxiety (*see* Clinical studies).[52] This review comprised seven of the eight placebo-controlled trials from the earlier review[69] (the other trial was excluded from the Cochrane review because it tested kava extract in addition to hormone replacement therapy)[61] and five new trials.

Four of the trials, involving 30% of the total number of participants in the trials included in the review, reported that adverse events were not observed during treatment with kava extract.[52] Randomised, double-blind clinical trials comparing kava extracts with certain benzodiazepines and other anxiolytic agents have also found kava to be well tolerated. In a six-week trial involving 172 patients with non-psychotic anxiety, gastrointestinal disturbances occurred in one of 57 participants who received WS-1490 100 mg three times daily (equivalent to 210 mg kavalactones daily), whereas tiredness, vertigo and pruritus occurred in seven of the remaining 115 participants who received oxazepam 5 mg or bromazepam 3 mg, both taken three times daily.[59] In an eight-week trial involving 129 outpatients with generalised anxiety disorder, 14 of 43 (33%) participants who received the kava extract LI-150 400 mg (standardised to 30% kavalactones = 120 mg) each morning experienced adverse events, compared with 10 (24%) and 11 (26%) participants who received buspirone 5 mg twice daily and opipramol 50 mg twice daily, respectively.[60] A total of 27 adverse events was reported in the kava group, compared with 16 and 14 for buspirone and opipramol, respectively. Adverse events reported for kava included upper respiratory tract infections, gastrointestinal disorders, weight changes, skin reactions and tachycardia, all of which were also reported for buspirone and/or opipramol.

These clinical trials and systematic reviews, however, provide only limited evidence to support the safety of kava extracts since they involved only small numbers of participants, involved different patient groups, tested different doses of kava extract (typically equivalent to 60–240 mg kavalactones daily), and most were of relatively short duration, usually around four weeks. Further, most trials investigated preparations of the kava extract WS-1490, and other standardised extracts of kava and kava preparations supplied by herbal medicine practitioners have undergone considerably less assessment.

Two post-marketing surveillance studies published in the early to mid-1990s involving patients treated in one study with WS-1490 150 mg daily (equivalent to 105 mg kavalactones; n = 4049) and in the other with Antares 120 (equivalent to 120 mg kavalactones; n = 3029) reported that the frequencies of adverse events were 1.5% and 2.3%, respectively.[69] In both studies, adverse events commonly reported were mild gastrointestinal disorders and allergic reactions and, in the latter study, headaches and vertigo, which stopped when kava treatment was discontinued. A rather higher frequency of adverse events was reported during a post-marketing surveillance study carried out in Brazil.[70] Among 850 participants with anxiety who received WS-1490 100 mg three times daily (equivalent to 210 mg kavalactones daily), 16.7% reported adverse events, most commonly fatigue/tiredness, nausea, confusion and gastrointestinal upset.

The World Health Organization's Uppsala Monitoring Centre (WHO-UMC; Collaborating Centre for International Drug Monitoring) receives summary reports of suspected adverse drug reactions from national pharmacovigilance centres of over 70 countries worldwide. To the end of the year 2005, the WHO-UMC's Vigisearch database contained a total of 91 reports, describing a total of 189 adverse reactions, for products reported

Table 1 Summary of spontaneous reports (n = 91) of suspected adverse drug reactions associated with single-ingredient *Piper methysticum* preparations held in the Vigisearch database of the World Health Organization's Uppsala Monitoring Centre for the period up to end of 2005[71, a, b]

System organ class. **Adverse drug reaction name (number)**	**Total**
Body as a whole – general disorders.	16
Cardiovascular disorders, general.	1
Central and peripheral nervous system disorders. Including dizziness (4); headache (4)	15
Gastrointestinal system disorders. Including abdominal pain (4); nausea (6); vomiting (3)	18
Heart rate and rhythm disorders. Including tachycardia (3)	3
Liver and biliary system disorders. Including hepatic failure (3); hepatic function abnormal (3); hepatitis (13); hepatocellular damage (6); bilirubinaemia (4); jaundice (8); hepatic enzymes increased (6)	55
Metabolic and nutritional disorders.	3
Musculo-skeletal system disorders.	1
Platelet, bleeding and clotting disorders.	3
Psychiatric disorders. Including anxiety (5)	15
Respiratory system disorders. Including dyspnoea (3)	7
Skin and appendages disorders. Including dermatitis (3); pruritus (8); rash, erythematous (8); rash, maculopapular (4); urticaria (6)	41
Urinary system disorders. Including face oedema (4)	5
Vision disorders. Including vision abnormal (4)	6
Total number of suspected adverse drug reactions	189

[a]Specific reactions described where n = 3 or more
[b]Caveat statement. These data were obtained from the Vigisearch database held by the WHO Collaborating Centre for International Drug Monitoring, Uppsala, Sweden. The information is not homogeneous at least with respect to origin or likelihood that the pharmaceutical product caused the adverse reaction. Any information included in this report does not represent the opinion of the World Health Organization

to contain *P. methysticum* only as the active ingredient (*see* Table 1).[71] This number may include some of the case reports described in the sections below. Reports originated from nine different countries. The total number of reactions included reports describing a total of 55 reactions associated with liver and biliary system disorders (*see* Table 1), including three cases of hepatic failure and two of hepatic coma. (These data were obtained from the Vigisearch database held by the WHO Collaborating Centre for International Drug Monitoring, Uppsala, Sweden. The information is not homogeneous at least with respect to origin or likelihood that the pharmaceutical product caused the adverse reaction. Any information included in this report does not represent the opinion of the World Health Organization.)

Hepatotoxicity

Clinical data None of the clinical trials and post-marketing surveillance studies described above reported hepatotoxicity as an observed adverse event, although not all studies carried out liver function tests on participants. Seven of the 11 trials included in the Cochrane review of the kava extract WS-1490 for the treatment of anxiety (*see* Clinical studies) did involve monitoring participants' liver function (e.g. serum aspartate transaminase and alanine transaminase concentrations) and did not report any abnormalities or clinically significant changes in values obtained.[52]

Over the years 2000 and 2001, a safety concern arose regarding cases of hepatoxicity reported in association with the use of kava extracts. The signal first emerged in Switzerland, following a cluster of spontaneous reports to the medicines' regulatory authority, and was strengthened a year or so later following further spontaneous reports from Switzerland and Germany. By July 2002, a total of 68 reports of liver toxicity associated with use of kava had been received by regulatory authorities in Canada, France, the UK and USA, as well as in Switzerland and Germany,[72] and by the end of January 2005, 79 cases of liver damage associated with use of kava had been identified worldwide.[73] The severity of the liver damage described in the reports varied from abnormal liver function test results to irreversible liver failure and death; at least six patients received liver transplants, one of whom, as well as at least two other individuals, subsequently died.

Cases reported in the UK included two of raised liver function test values in men aged 40 and 48 who had taken unspecified kava preparations for three months and eight years, respectively.[74] Both stopped taking kava and their liver function test values normalised. Another UK case related to a woman (age not stated) who had taken kava 150 mg three times daily for two months, in addition to fluoxetine, and who experienced jaundice and raised liver function test values and was hospitalised for seven weeks.

K

In the UK, evidence relating to the hepatotoxicity associated with kava was reviewed in 2005 in a public consultation and later that year by the Expert Working Group set up to consider the evidence. The Expert Working Group's report was published in July 2006 and concluded that there was insufficient new evidence to support a change in the regulatory position, hence the inclusion of kava in unlicensed medicines in the UK remains prohibited.[75] The report also identified several new questions and issues that may be important with respect to hepatotoxicity of kava, including the possibility that other alkaloid and/or amide constituents may be present, and their possible contribution to hepatotoxicity, and the need for a systematic evaluation of all marketed kava products and their source material, and of the variation in the phytochemistry of kava cultivars.[75]

Earlier reviews of German data relating to hepatotoxicity associated with kava have produced conflicting opinions on causality. One review emphasised that there was no dose–response relationship for kava-associated hepatotoxicity, and that crude estimates of incidence based on primary care data suggest that any risk of hepatotoxicity is similar to that of benzodiazepines.[76] However, this conclusion is questionable since estimates of this nature can be inaccurate and misleading.

By contrast, a review of seven previously published and 29 unpublished case reports of kava-associated hepatotoxicity concluded that these data clearly showed the potential for severe, unpredictable kava-related hepatotoxicity.[77] Cases included nine individuals who developed fulminant hepatic failure, of whom six underwent successful liver transplantation (one only after retransplantation), two died after transplantation due to postoperative infectious complications, and one who was too old to undergo transplantation also died. All other cases, which comprised mostly cholestatic or necrotising hepatitis, underwent full recovery after withdrawal of kava treatment. Among these 36 reports, the relationship between kava ingestion and hepatotoxicity was considered 'certain' in three cases and 'probable' in 21.[77] Most individuals were concurrently using other medication and several were regular consumers of alcohol.

A case report from Australia describes a 56-year-old woman who developed fatigue, nausea and jaundice after taking a preparation named 'Kava 1800 Plus' one tablet three times daily for around 10 weeks.[78] Each tablet was stated to contain kavalactones 60 mg, *Passiflora incarnata* 50 mg and *Scutellaria lateriflora* 100 mg, although the latter ingredient was not identified in the product, so the precise composition of the product is unknown. She presented two weeks after first experiencing these symptoms and was hospitalised. Five days later, a biopsy revealed non-specific severe acute hepatitis with pan-acinar necrosis and collapse of hepatic lobules. She underwent liver transplantation on day 17 after admission, but the procedure was complicated and she died from progressive blood loss and circulatory failure. Subsequent examinations confirmed massive hepatic necrosis.

Until the year 2003, it was thought that kava-associated hepatoxicity occurred only with ethanolic and acetonic kava extracts. However, recent reports described hepatoxic effects associated with consumption of traditional aqueous extracts of kava root. Two cases in New Caledonia involved women aged in their fifties who started consuming kava prepared in the traditional manner as an aqueous preparation.[79] Both women developed signs and symptoms of hepatotoxicity, including icterus and raised liver function test values four or five weeks after starting kava. Neither patient consumed alcohol. Kava consumption was stopped; both patients recovered and liver function test values normalised over the following three months.[79] Subsequently, in a cross-sectional study, blood samples were collected from 27 individuals who were chronic kava drinkers, recruited from kava bars in New Caledonia. Participants had been consuming kava regularly for at least five years and had a mean intake equivalent to around 32 g kavalactones weekly or 70 mg/kg daily; 12 participants also consumed alcohol.[79] Transaminase concentrations were more than 1.5 times the upper limit of normal in three participants, and 23 participants had increases in concentration of GGT (which is not necessarily a specific marker of liver injury); alkaline phosphatase and bilirubin concentrations were within normal ranges for all subjects. Another cross-sectional study, involving indigenous people from an Arnhem Land community (Northern Territory, Australia), included 98 participants, of whom 36 had never used kava.[80] Of the 62 kava users, 14 had ingested kava within the previous 24 hours, and 10 and 15 had used kava within the previous one or two weeks, or one or two months, respectively. Investigation of liver function test values indicated that changes appeared to be reversible and started to normalise after one or two weeks of kava abstinence.[80]

Inhibition of certain cytochrome P450 (CYP) drug metabolising enzymes has been shown *in vitro* and *in vivo* for kava extracts and individual kavalactones (*see* Contra-indications, Warnings). The relevance of this for the hepatotoxic effects described for kava is not known; further work is needed to determine whether the inhibition of CYP enzymes by kava can lead to raised plasma concentrations of concurrently ingested drugs with hepatotoxic effects.

Skin reactions

An ichthyosiform (scaly, non-inflammatory), usually yellowish or whitish, skin condition termed kava dermopathy has been documented among kava users in Polynesia, Micronesia and Melanesia where powdered kava rhizome is prepared as a drink with cold water or coconut milk.[81] The condition is reversible on stopping kava. Initially, it was thought that the condition was related to niacin deficiency, but this hypothesis was rejected following a small randomised, placebo-controlled trial of nicotinamide 100 mg daily for three weeks which showed no difference between groups.[82]

Measures of health among 39 users of kava (prepared as a cold water infusion of powdered kava rhizome) were compared with those of 34 age-matched non-users of kava in an Aboriginal community in the Northern Territory in Australia.[83] Most (n = 35) were 'heavy' or 'very heavy' users of kava (310 g or more per week). It was reported that kava users were more likely to complain of poor health, and to have a scaly skin rash. However, the study had several methodological limitations (e.g. no correction for multiple statistical tests) and potential biases.

Several cases of allergic skin reactions have been reported in association with kava use. One case described a man who presented with oedema and severe non-pruritic erythema involving his upper body, head and neck, the morning after drinking several cups of 'kava tea'.[84] It was reported that the man had previously had a similar reaction to kava tea three months earlier whilst overseas and for which he was hospitalised and treated with intravenous corticosteroids. A case of systemic contact-type dermatitis following several weeks' use of kava extract (Antares), chlorprothixene (an antipsychotic agent with properties similar to those of chlorpromazine) and diazepam has been described.[85] Two further cases described a 70-year-old man and a 52-year-old woman who experienced skin eruptions (erythematous plaques and/or papules) in sebaceous gland-rich areas after using kava extract (no further details provided) for two to three weeks.[86] Both patients were reported to display reactions to kava in diagnostic allergy or skin patch tests. Generalised erythema and papules with severe itching were described in a 36-year-old woman who had taken kava extract (Antares) 120 mg daily for three weeks.[87] The rash, but not the itching, responded to short-term treatment with systemic corticosteroids, and six weeks later, patch test results for Antares were positive one day after application.

Central nervous system effects

Four cases of involuntary movements and dyskinesia associated with use of kava extracts have been reported, although causality has not been established; it has been stated that these symptoms suggest that constituents of kava may have antagonistic effects on central dopaminergic pathways.[88] In three cases, involuntary movements involving the neck, head and/or trunk, and involuntary oral and lingual dyskinesia began within a few minutes to 4 hours after ingestion of kava extracts (Laitan 100 mg or Kavasporal forte 150 mg) for anxiety. One of these cases involved a 28-year-old man who had previously experienced three episodes of acute dystonic reactions following exposure to promethazine and fluspirilene, although he denied having used these medicines in relation to the current episode. The fourth case report described a 76-year-old woman being treated with levodopa 500 mg and benserazide 125 mg for Parkinson's disease and who experienced an increase in the duration and frequency of her 'off' periods 10 days after starting Kavasporal forte 150 mg twice daily, prescribed by her physician for tension. (The 'on–off' phenomenon – sudden swings in mobility–immobility – occurs with long-term use of levodopa.) In all four cases, symptoms resolved on stopping kava or following treatment with biperiden administered intravenously.

Two other cases describe neurological symptoms following excessive use of traditional preparations of kava, i.e. as a beverage. A 27-year-old Aboriginal Australian man experienced generalised severe choreoathetosis (characterised by chorea and athetosis, a form of dyskinesia) without impairment of consciousness on three occasions after drinking large amounts of kava (precise quantity not specified).[89] Routine investigations were normal, apart from raised liver function test values (serum alkaline phosphatase 162 IU/L, normal range 35–135 IU/L; gamma-glutamyltransferase 426 IU/L, normal range <60 IU/L). His symptoms responded to treatment with diazepam administered intravenously. Disorientation was reported in a 34-year-old Tongan man, a heavy user of kava (40 bowls daily for 14 years), who had ingested further excessive amounts of kava over the previous 12 hours.[90] The man was treated in hospital with Plasmalyte intravenously and intramuscular thiamine and five hours after admission his symptoms had resolved.

In a controlled study, individuals intoxicated following kava consumption (205 g powder) experienced ataxia, tremors, sedation, blepharospasm and reduced accuracy performing a visual search task, when compared with control subjects who had not ingested kava. These results suggest that kava intoxication results in specific abnormalities of movement co-ordination and visual attention, but normal performance of complex cognitive functions.[91]

Effects on mental performance

The effects of kava extracts and the synthetic kavalactone (±)-kavain on mental performance have been explored in studies involving healthy volunteers. Preliminary studies involving small numbers of volunteers have suggested that kava extract (WS-1490 200 mg three times daily for five days) did not appear to impair memory as assessed by certain tests (e.g. word recognition) carried out under laboratory conditions.[92] In another series of tests, designed to assess mental alertness, volunteers received kava extract, Antares 120 (standardised to 120 mg kavalactones per tablet), one tablet daily, diazepam 10 mg daily, or placebo.[93] It was reported that the experiments provided evidence that kava did not cause drowsiness or lack of concentration, for example, reaction time was reduced in placebo recipients, but not kava recipients. Other research involving volunteers found that a single dose of kava extract 600 mg (LI-158; drug–extract ratio, 12.5 : 1) led to a 'moderate' increase in tiredness, compared with placebo, and as assessed using visual analogue scale scores, although statistical analysis was not reported.[94] Confirmation of these findings is required. In a battery of psychometric and other tests following administration of a range of single doses of the synthetic kavalactone (±)-kavain (200, 400 and 600 mg) and clobazam 30 mg to healthy volunteers, (±)-kavain appeared to have a sedative effect which was stated to be different to that observed with clobazam.[95] Compared with placebo, (±)-kavain, but not clobazam, improved intellectual performance, attention, concentration and reaction time.

Other reactions

There are isolated reports of myopathy and myoglobinuria associated with the use of kava preparations, although causality in these cases has not been established.

One report described dermatomyositis associated with use of kava for anxiety by a 47-year-old woman.[96] The woman, who had also been taking valproic acid for 18 months and sertraline occasionally over two years for bipolar disorder, developed a rash involving her back, neck and face, as well as muscle weakness, two weeks after taking kava (dosage not specified). She improved initially following treatment with methylprednisolone, but then developed a fever which prompted her to attend a hospital emergency department. Investigations revealed a raised serum creatine kinase concentration (8654 U/L, normal values stated as 24–170 U/L) and myopathic patterns in various muscles, and biopsy samples showed changes indicative of dermatomyositis. The woman was treated initially with parenteral prednisone, after which her creatine kinase concentration returned to normal, and also received methotrexate for five months and hydroxychloroquine. Prednisone treatment was reduced over the following year, and at one year of follow-up the woman remained symptom-free.

Another isolated report describes a 29-year-old man who experienced severe muscle pain and passed dark urine one morning a few hours after having taken a herbal product said to contain kava 100 mg, *Ginkgo biloba* extract 200 mg and guarana (which contains methylxanthines) 500 mg (daily dosage was not stated), for the first time.[97] The man was admitted to an intensive care unit and was found to have highly elevated serum creatine kinase (100 500 IU/L, normal range given as 0–195 IU/L) and myoglobin (10 000 ng/mL, normal range stated as 0–90 ng/mL) concentrations, but no renal complications. Investigations excluded metabolic myopathy as a possible cause; his signs and symptoms subsided over six weeks.

Disturbances of visual function have been reported following a study involving a 30-year-old kava-naïve male volunteer who ingested 600 mL of aqueous extract of pulverised kava 'root' (rhizome).[98] Measurements involving the man's right eye only indicated reductions in near point of accommodation and convergence, an increase in pupil diameter, and disturbance of oculomotor balance, but no effects on visual or stereoacuity or ocular refractive error. The experiment was not carried out according to a double-blind, controlled design and, therefore, the findings require further investigation.

K

A case of hypokalaemic renal tubular acidosis due to Sjögren's syndrome (a symptom complex of unknown aetiology, marked by keratoconjunctivitis sicca, xerostamia, with or without lachrymal and salivary gland enlargement, respectively, and presence of connective tissue disease, usually rheumatoid arthritis, but sometimes systemic lupus erythematosus, scleroderma or polymyositis) has been reported in a 36-year-old woman.[99] She was stated to have begun taking kava, echinacea and St John's wort two weeks before becoming ill, but the report does not provide any further details of the echinacea species contained in the product(s), nor of the types of preparations, formulations, dosages and routes of administration of any of the herbal medicines listed. The woman was hospitalised with severe generalised muscle weakness and tests revealed she had a serum potassium ion concentration of 1.3 mEq/L. She was given electrolyte replacement for four days after which the muscle weakness resolved, and was started on hydroxychloroquine 200 mg daily for 'probable' Sjögren's syndrome. The authors suggested that ingestion of echinacea may have aggravated an autoimmune disorder (*see* Echinacea, Side-effects, Toxicity) although causality has not been established.[99]

No clear evidence of an association between kava consumption and ischaemic heart disease (IHD) was found in a case–control study (using up to four randomly selected control subjects) involving 83 individuals from Aboriginal communities in Arnhem Land (Northern Territory, Australia) who were diagnosed with IHD for the first time during 1992–1997.[100] In a similar case–control study involving 115 individuals (and 415 control subjects) with pneumonia, no association between kava use and pneumonia was found.[101]

Toxicology

Incubation of the kava alkaloid pipermethystine, which occurs mostly in kava leaves and stem peelings, with human hepatoma cells resulted in a 90% loss in cell viability within 24 hours when applied at a concentration of 100 μmol/L and 65% cell death at a concentration of 50 μmol/L.[102] Further experiments indicated that pipermethystine causes cell death in part by disrupting mitochondrial function. It has been suggested that pipermethysticine could be involved in hepatoxicity associated with kava root extracts,[102] although since hepatotoxicity has been associated both with authorised commerical products (therefore made according to the principles of good manufacturing practice) and traditional aqueous extracts (which might be more easily contaminated with leaves and stem peelings) this suggestion requires further examination.

A study involving small numbers of rats administered an aqueous (water) extract of kava 'root' equivalent to kavalactones 200 or 500 mg/kg/day for 2–4 weeks found that serum concentrations of the enzymes alanine aminotransferase, aspartate aminotransferase, alkaline phosphatase and lactate dehydrogenase were not elevated following kava administration, compared with control.[103] The clinical relevance of these findings is not known.

In other toxicological studies, LD_{50} values for a standardised kava extract containing 70% kavalactones have been reported as 370 mg/kg and 16 g/kg for intraperitoneal and oral administration, respectively, in rats, and 380 mg/kg and 1.8 g/kg for intraperitoneal and oral administration, respectively, in mice.[G50]

An ethanolic extract of kava root was reported to be cytotoxic (EC_{50} approximately 50 μmol/L) in an *in vitro* system assessing viability of human hepatocytes. The kavalactones methysticin, desmethoxyyangonin and yangonin also displayed cytotoxicity in this system, with methysticin having the greatest cytotoxic activity.[104] *In vitro* cytotoxicity of kavalactones has also been described in a human lymphoblastoid cell line; the cytotoxic effect appears to be due to the parent compound and not as a result of activation of kava constituents to toxic metabolites.[105]

Contra-indications, Warnings

It has been stated that kava is contra-indicated in endogenous depression.[G3, G4] Even when administered in accordance with recommended dosage regimens, kava may adversely affect motor reflexes, and may affect ability to drive and/or operate machinery.[G3, G4]

It has been reported that there is no evidence that use of kava extracts has the potential for physical or psychological dependency to develop.[G56] However, as most clinical studies of kava extracts have been of short duration, typically around four weeks (maximum 24 weeks) and/or usually have involved only small numbers of participants, further study is required before definitive statements are made on the potential for dependency with kava.

Drug interactions There is an isolated report of a 54-year-old man who was taking alprazolam, cimetidine and terazosin and who became lethargic and disoriented three days after he began taking kava purchased from a health-food store (no further details of the kava preparation were provided).[106] The man was hospitalised and his symptoms resolved after several hours. He tested negatively for alcohol, and positively for benzodiazepines; the man stated he had not taken overdoses of either alprazolam or kava. The clinical importance and role of kava in this reaction is not known, although there is a view that concurrent use of kava and substances with central nervous system effects could lead to enhanced activity.[G3, G4]

The effects on performance of a kava extract given in combination with bromazepam have been explored in a randomised, double-blind, controlled crossover trial involving 18 healthy volunteers. Participants received a kava extract (Antares) equivalent to 120 mg kavalactones twice daily, or bromazepam 4.5 mg twice daily, or both agents, for 14 days.[107] Significant reductions in indicators of performance, such as motor coordination, were reported for recipients of both kava and bromazepam, compared with recipients of kava alone, but there was no difference between kava plus bromazepam compared with bromazepam alone.

Isolated case reports of extrapyramidal symptoms associated with use of kava extracts have led to the suggestion that constituents of kava may have dopamine antagonist effects (*see* Side-effects, Toxicity, Central nervous system effects).[88] On this basis, the potential for kava to interact with dopamine agonists or antagonists should be considered.

Inhibition of certain cytochrome P450 (CYP) drug metabolising enzymes has been shown *in vitro* and *in vivo* for kava extracts and individual kavalactones. In a randomised, open-label, crossover study, 12 healthy volunteers received kava root extract 1000 mg twice daily (subsequently found to be equivalent to total kavalactones 138 mg daily) for 28 days; probe drugs were administered before and after kava administration to assess effects on CYP enzymes.[108] Administration of the kava extract according to this dosage regimen inhibited CYP2E1, but not CYP3A4/5, CYP2D6 and CYP1A2.

In *in vitro* studies, methanolic, acetone and ethyl acetate extracts of kava rhizome significantly inhibited CYP3A4 activity, compared with control, at concentrations as low as 10 µg/mL (ethyl acetate extract).[109] In other *in vitro* experiments, several individual kavalactones were tested for their effects on the activities of CYP1A2, CYP2C9, CYP2C19 and CYP2D6, as well as CYP3A4. Desmethoxyyangonin, dihydromethysticin and methysticin produced a concentration-dependent inhibition of one or more of the CYP isoforms at concentrations of <10 µmol/L, considered as 'potent' inhibition (e.g. IC_{50} values for desmethoxyyangonin, dihydromethysticin and methysticin for CYP2C19 were 0.51, 0.43 and 0.93 µmol/L, respectively, and for dihydromethysticin and methysticin for CYP3A4 under certain assay conditions were 2.49 and 1.49 µmol/L, respectively).[110] In several cases, this degree of inhibition was greater than that shown by positive controls which are known to produce clinically significant drug interactions. Similar results have been reported for an ethanolic kava root extract and the individual kavalactones desmethoxyyangonin, dihydromethysticin and yangonin: in two *in vitro* models, both the extract and the individual kavalactones inhibited CYP1A2, CYP2C9, CYP2C19, CYP2E1 and CYP3A4 with IC_{50} values of around 10 µmol/L.[104]

Differences in CYP enzyme inhibition have been described for commercial preparations (acetone, methanol and ethanol extracts) and traditional aqueous extracts, with commercial preparations having a greater inhibitory effect than traditional preparations on CYP3A4, CYP1A2, CYP2C9 and CYP2C19.[111] Desmethoxyyangonin and dihydromethysticin induced the expression of CYP3A23 by approximately seven-fold in an *in vitro* system; other experimental results suggested that the inductive effect of these kavalactones is additively or synergistically enhanced by the presence of other kavalactones.[112] Other *in vitro* experiments have demonstrated that kava root extract and the individual kavalactones kavain, dihydrokavain, methysticin, dihydromethysticin and desmethoxyyangonin inhibit the efflux transporter P-glycoprotein.[113]

The clinical relevance of these findings is not known, although the potential for kava extracts to interact with concurrently administered drugs metabolised mainly by the CYP enzymes mentioned above should be considered.

There are conflicting results from *in vitro* studies regarding the effects of the kavalactone (+)-kavain on cyclooxygenase activity.[48, 49] One study reported that (+)-kavain inhibited human platelet aggregation *in vitro* (*see In vitro* and animal studies, Other activities], although the clinical relevance of this, if any is not known. At present, there is insufficient evidence to warn against the concurrent use of kava preparations and antiplatelet agents. The kavalactones kavain, methysticin, yangonin and desmethoxyyangonin did not inhibit alcohol dehydrogenase *in vitro* when applied to the system at concentrations of 1, 10 and 100 µmol/L.[114]

Alcohol The effects of concurrent use of kava extract and alcohol have undergone some investigation. In a randomised, double-blind, controlled trial, 20 healthy participants received kava extract (WS-1490; Laitan) 300 mg daily (equivalent to 210 mg kavalactones), or placebo, for eight days.[115] Alcohol was ingested on days one, four and eight in quantities sufficient to achieve a blood alcohol concentration of 50 mg%; participants underwent a series of tests designed to assess psychomotor performance before and after alcohol consumption. The results indicated that there was no difference in performance between the kava and placebo groups, apart from one test (concentration) in which the kava group was reported to be superior to the placebo group.[115]

A small study involving 40 healthy participants found that the concurrent ingestion of a kava beverage (350 mL of aqueous extract of Fijian kava) and alcohol 0.75 g/kg led to a greater reduction in cognitive performance, as assessed by a series of tests, compared with that observed with ingestion of alcohol alone; ingestion of kava alone did not affect cognitive performance.[116]

Studies in mice given ethanol (3.5 and 4 g/kg, intraperitoneally) and kava resin 200 or 300 mg/kg orally have demonstrated a prolongation of hypnotic effects.[117]

Pregnancy and lactation There is a lack of information on the use of kava preparations during pregnancy and breastfeeding. Given the lack of data, kava should be avoided during these periods.

Preparations

Proprietary single-ingredient preparations

Brazil: Ansiopax; Calmonex; Farmakava; Kavakan; Kavalac; Kavasedon; Laitan; Natuzilium. *Czech Republic:* Antares; Kavasedon; Leikan. *Venezuela:* Kavasedon.

Proprietary multi-ingredient preparations

USA: Calming Aid.

References

1 Singh YN, Blumenthal M. Kava an overview. *Herbalgram* 1997; 39: 33–55.

K

2 Alton J. Kava-kava (*Piper methysticum* G. Forster) in contemporary medical research [translation of reference 3]. *Eur J Herb Med* 1997; 3: 17–23.

3 Hansel R. Kava-kava (*Piper methysticum* G. Forster) in der modernen Arzneimittelforschung. *Z Phytother* 1996; 17: 180–195.

4 The Medicines for Human Use (Kava-Kava) (Prohibition) Order 2002 (SI2002/3170). London: The Stationery Office, 2003.

5 Dharmaratne HRW *et al.* Kavalactones from *Piper methysticum*, and their ^{13}C NMR spectroscopic analyses. *Phytochemistry* 2002; 59: 429–433.

6 Parmar VS *et al.* Phytochemistry of the genus *Piper*. *Phytochemistry* 1997; 46: 597–673.

7 Singh YN. Kava: an overview. *J Ethnopharmacol* 1992; 37: 13–45.

8 Shao Y *et al.* Reversed-phase high-performance liquid chromatographic method for quantitative analysis of the six major kavalactones in *Piper methysticum*. *J Chromatogr A* 1998; 825: 1–8.

9 Wu D *et al.* Cyclooxygenase enzyme inhibitory compounds with antioxidant activities from *Piper methysticum* (kava kava) roots. *Phytomed* 2002; 9: 41–47.

10 Bone K. Kava – a safe treatment for anxiety. *Br J Phytother* 1993/4; 3: 147–153.

11 Jaggy H, Achenbach H. Cepharadione A from *Piper methysticum*. *Planta Med* 1992; 58: 111.

12 Achenbach H, Karl W. Über die isolierung von zwei neuen pyrrolididen aus Rauschpfeffer (*Piper methysticum* Forst.). *Chem Ber* 1970; 103: 2535–2540.

13 Cheng D *et al.* Identification by methane chemical ionization gas chromatography/mass spectrometry of the products obtained by steam distillation and aqueous acid extraction of commercial *Piper methysticum*. *Biomed Environ Mass Spectrom* 1988; 17: 371–376.

14 Wu D *et al.* Novel compounds from *Piper methysticum* Forst (Kava Kava) roots and their effect on cyclooxygenase enzyme. *J Agric Food Chem* 2002; 50: 701–705.

15 Dragull K *et al.* Piperidine alkaloids from *Piper methysticum*. *Phytochemistry* 2003; 63: 193–198.

16 Cawte J. Psychoactive substances of the South seas: betel, kava and pituri. *Aust N Z J Psychiatry* 1985; 19: 83–87.

17 Keledjian J *et al.* Uptake into mouse brain of four compounds present in the psychoactive beverage kava. *J Pharm Sci* 1988; 77: 1003–1006.

18 Smith KK *et al.* Anxiolytic effects of kava extract and kavalactones in the chick social separation-stress paradigm. *Psychopharmacology* 2001; 155: 86–90.

19 Feltenstein MW *et al.* Anxiolytic properties of *Piper methysticum* extract samples and fractions in the chick social-separation-stress procedure. *Phytother Res* 2003; 17: 210–216.

20 Capasso A, Calignano A. Synergism between the sedative action of kava extract and D,L-kawain. *Acta Ther* 1988; 14: 249–256.

21 Capasso A, Pinto A. Experimental investigations of the synergistic-sedative effect of passiflora and kava. *Acta Ther* 1995; 21: 127–139.

22 Duffield PH *et al.* Effect of aqueous and lipid-soluble extracts of kava on the conditioned avoidance response in rats. *Arch Int Pharmacodyn* 1989; 301: 81–90.

23 Holm E *et al.* Untersuchungen zum Wirkungsprofil von D,L-kavain. Zerebrale Angriffsorte und Schlaf-Wach-Rhythmus im Tierexperiment. *Arzneim Forsch* 1991; 41: 673–683.

24 Davies LP *et al.* Kava pyrones and resin: studies on $GABA_A$, $GABA_B$ and benzodiazepine binding sites in rodent brain. *Pharmacol Toxicol* 1992; 71: 120–126.

25 Grunze H, Walden J. Kawain limits excitation in CA 1 pyramidal neurons of rats by modulating ionic currents and attenuating excitatory synaptic transmission [letter]. *Hum Psychopharm Clin Exp* 1999; 14: 63–66.

26 Jussofie A *et al.* Kavapyrone enriched extract from *Piper methysticum* as modulator of the GABA binding site in different regions of rat brain. *Psychopharmacology* 1994; 116: 469–474.

27 Boonen G, Häberlein H. Influence of genuine kavapyrone enantiomers on the $GABA_A$ binding site. *Planta Med* 1998; 64: 504–506.

28 Uebelhack R *et al.* Inhibition of platelet MAO-B by kava pyrone-enriched extract from *Piper methysticum* Forster (kava-kava). *Pharmacopsychiatry* 1998; 31: 187–192.

29 Seitz U *et al.* [3H]-Monoamine uptake inhibition properties of kava pyrones [letter]. *Planta Med* 1997; 63: 548–549.

30 Walden J *et al.* Actions of kavain and dihydromethysticin on ipsapirone-induced field potential changes in the hippocampus. *Hum Psychopharmacol* 1997; 12: 265–270.

31 Boonen G *et al.* *In vivo* effects of the kavapyrones (+)-dihydromethysticin and (+/–)-kavain on dopamine, 3,4-dihyroxyphenylacetic acid, serotonin and 5-hydrozyindoleacetic acid levels in striatal and cortical brain regions. *Planta Med* 1998; 64: 507–510.

32 Baum SS *et al.* Effect of kava extract and individual kavapyrones on neurotransmitter levels in the nucleus accumbens of rats. *Prog Neuro-Psychopharmacol Biol Psychiat* 1998; 22: 1105–1120.

33 Duffield PH, Jamieson D. Development of tolerance to kava in mice. *Clin Exp Pharmacol Physiol* 1991; 18: 571–578.

34 Gleitz J *et al.* Anticonvulsive action of (+/–)-kavain estimated from its properties on stimulated synaptosomes and Na^+ channel receptor sites. *Eur J Pharmacol* 1996; 315: 89–97.

35 Magura EI *et al.* Kava extract ingredients, (+)-methysticin and (+/–)-kavain inhibit voltage-operated Na^+-channels in rat CA1 hippocampal neurons. *Neuroscience* 1997; 81: 345–351.

36 Gleitz J *et al.* Kavain inhibits non-stereospecifically veratridine-activated Na^+ channels [letter]. *Planta Med* 1996; 62: 580–581.

37 Schirrmacher K *et al.* Effects of (+/–)-kavain on voltage-activated inward currents of dorsal root ganglion cells from neonatal rats. *Eur Neuropsychopharmacol* 1999; 9: 171–176.

38 Gleitz J *et al.* (+/–)-Kavain inhibits veratridine-activated voltage-dependent Na^+-channels in synaptosomes prepared from rat cerebral cortex. *Neuropharmacology* 1995; 34: 1133–1138.

39 Gleitz J *et al.* (+/–)-Kavain inhibits the veratridine- and KCl-induced increase in intracellular Ca^{2+} and glutamate-release of rat cerebrocortical synaptosomes. *Neuropharmacology* 1996; 35: 179–186.

40 Ferger B *et al.* *In vivo* microdialysis study of (+/–)-kavain on veratridine-induced glutamate release. *Eur J Pharmacol* 1998; 347: 211–214.

41 Gleitz J *et al.* The protective action of tetrodotoxin and (+/–)-kavain on anaerobic glycolysis, ATP content and intracellular Na^+ and Ca^{2+} of anoxic brain vesicles. *Neuropharmacology* 1996; 35: 1743–1752.

42 Schmidt N, Ferger B. Neuroprotective effects of (+/–)-kavain in the MPTP mouse model of Parkinson's disease. *Synapse* 2001; 40: 47–54.

43 Backhauss C, Krieglstein J. Extract of kava (*Piper methysticum*) and its methysticin constituents protect brain tissue against ischemic damage in rodents. *Eur J Pharmacol* 1992; 215: 265–269.

44 Jamieson DD, Duffield PH. The antinociceptive actions of kava components in mice. *Clin Exp Pharmacol Physiol* 1990; 17: 495–508.

45 Brüggemann F, Meyer HJ. Die analgetische Wirkung der Kawa-Inhaltsstoffe Dihydrokawain und Dihydromethysticin. *Arzneimittel-Forschung* 1963; 13: 407–409.

46 Singh YN. Effects of kava on neuromuscular transmission and muscle contractility. *J Ethnopharmacol* 1983; 7: 267–276.

47 Seitz U *et al.* Relaxation of evoked contractile activity of isolated guinea-pig ileum by (+/–)-kavain. *Planta Med* 1997; 63: 303–306.

48 Martin HB *et al.* Kavain inhibits murine airway smooth muscle contraction. *Planta Med* 2000; 66: 601–606.

49 Gleitz J *et al.* Antithrombotic action of the kava pyrone (+)-kavain prepared from *Piper methysticum* on human platelets. *Planta Med* 1997; 63: 27–30.

50 Hashimoto T *et al.* Isolation and synthesis of TNF-α release inhibitors from Fijian kawa (*Piper methysticum*). *Phytomedicine* 2003; 10: 309–317.

51 Blaszcyk T *et al.* Kawa-kawa als antimykotikum. *Pharmazie* 1997; 21: 32–34.

52 Pittler MH, Ernst E. Kava extract versus placebo for treating anxiety (Cochrane review). The Cochrane Database of Systematic Reviews, 2003, Issue 1. Art. No. :CD003383.

53 Warnecke G. [Psychosomatische Dysfunktionen im weiblichen Klimakterium]. *Fortschr Med* 191 109: 119–122.

54 Volz H-P, Kieser M. Kava-kava extract WS 1490 versus placebo in anxiety disorders – a randomized, placebo-controlled 25-week outpatient trial. *Pharmacopsychiatry* 1997; 30: 1–5.

55 Witte S *et al.* Meta-analysis of the efficacy of the acetonic kava-kava extract WS® 1490 in patients with non-psychotic anxiety disorders. *Phytotherapy Res* 2005; 19: 183–188.

56 Lehrl S. Clinical efficacy of kava extract WS 1490 in sleep disturbances associated with anxiety disorders. Results of a multicenter, randomized, placebo-controlled, double-blind clinical trial. *J Affect Disord* 2004; 78(2): 101–110.
57 Jacobs BP *et al.* An internet-based randomized, placebo-controlled trial of kava and valerian for anxiety and insomnia. *Medicine* 2005; 84 (4): 197–207.
58 Cagnacci A *et al.* Kava-kava administration reduces anxiety in perimenopausal women. *Maturitas* 2003; 44: 103–109.
59 Woelk H *et al.* Behandlung von Angst-Patienten. Doppelblindstudie: Kava-Spezialextrakt WS 1490 versus Benzodiazepine. *Z Allg Med* 1993; 69: 271–277.
60 Boerner RJ *et al.* Kava-kava extract LI 150 is as effective as opipramol and buspirone in generalised anxiety disorder – an 8-week randomized, double-blind, multi-centre clinical trial in 129 out-patients. *Phytomedicine* 2003; 10(Suppl IV): 38–49.
61 De Leo V *et al.* Valutazione dell'associazione di estratto di kava-kava e terapia ormonale sostitutiva nel trattamento d'ansia in postmenopausa. *Minerva Ginecol* 2000; 52: 263–267.
62 Cropley M *et al.* Effect of kava and valerian on human physiological and psychological responses to mental stress assessed under laboratory conditions. *Phytother Res* 2002; 16: 23–27.
63 Möller HJ, Heuberger L. Anxiolytische Potenz von D,L-kavain. Ergebnisse einer plazebokontrollierten Doppelblindstudie. *Münch Med Wschr* 1989; 131: 656–659.
64 Lindenberg D, Pitule-Schödel H. D,L-kavain im Vergleich zu Oxazepam bei Angstzuständen. Doppelblindstudie zur klinischen Wirksamkeit. *Fortschr Med* 1990; 108: 31–34.
65 Möller H-J *et al.* Kavain als Hilfe beim Benzodiazepin-Entzug. *Münch Med Wschr* 1992; 134: 587–590.
66 Thompson R *et al.* Enhanced cognitive performance and cheerful mood by standardized extracts of *Piper methysticum* (kava-kava). *Human Psychopharmacol* 2004; 19(4): 243–250.
67 Boerner RJ, Klement S. Attenuation of neuroleptic-induced extrapyramidal side-effects by kava special extract WS 1490. *Wiener Med Wochenschrift* 2004; 154: 21–22.
68 Duffield AM *et al.* Identification of some human urinary metabolites of the intoxicating beverage kava. *J Chromatogr* 1989; 475: 273–281.
69 Stevinson C *et al.* A systematic review of the safety of kava extract in the treatment of anxiety. *Drug Safety* 2002; 25: 251–261.
70 Neto JT. Eficácia e tolerabilidade do extrato de kava-kava WS 1490 em estados de ansiedade. Estudo multicêntrico brasileiro. *Rev Bras Med* 1999; 56: 280–284.
71 Uppsala Monitoring Centre. Vigibase, WHO Adverse Reactions database (accessed 20 January, 2006).
72 Medicines Control Agency. Consultation MLX 286: Proposals to prohibit the herbal ingredient kava-kava (*Piper methysticum*) in unlicensed medicines. Medicines Control Agency, 19 July 2002.
73 Anon. Kava-kava. The Medicines for Human Use (Kava-kava) (Prohibition) Order 2002. Herbal Safety News, Medicines and Healthcare products Regulatory Agency (http://www.mhra.gov.uk, accessed 26 January, 2006).
74 Adverse Drug Reactions On-line Information Tracking (ADROIT) system. Medicines and Healthcare products Regulatory Agency, London, UK.
75 Committee on Safety of Medicines' Expert Working Group (Kava). Report of the CSM's expert working group on the safety of kava. Medicines and Healthcare products Regulatory Agency, 2006. Available at http://www.mhra.gov.uk (accessed 25 September, 2006).
76 Schulze J *et al.* Toxicity of kava pyrones, drug safety and precautions – a case study. *Phytomedicine* 2003; 10: 68–73.
77 Stickel F *et al.* Hepatitis induced by kava (*Piper methysticum rhizoma*). *J Hepatol* 2003; 39: 62–67.
78 Gow PJ *et al.* Fatal fulminant hepatic failure induced by a natural therapy containing kava. *Med J Aust* 2003; 178: 442–443.
79 Russmann S *et al.* Hepatic injury due to traditional aqueous extracts of kava root in New Caledonia. *Eur J Gastroenterol Hepatol* 2003; 15: 1033–1036.
80 Clough AR *et al.* Liver function test abnormalities in users of aqueous kava extracts. *J Toxicol Clin Toxicol* 2003; 41(6): 821–829.
81 Norton SA, Ruze P. Kava dermopathy. *J Am Acad Dermatol* 1994; 31: 89–97.
82 Ruze P. Kava-induced dermopathy: a niacin deficiency? *Lancet* 1990; 335: 1442–1445.
83 Mathews JD *et al.* Effects of the heavy usage of kava on physical health: summary of a pilot survey in an Aboriginal community. *Med J Aust* 1988; 148: 548–555.
84 Levine R, Taylor WB. Take tea and see [letter]. *Arch Dermatol* 1988; 122: 856.
85 Süss R, Lehmann P. Hämatogenes Kontaktekzem durch pflanzliche Medikamente am Beispiel des Kavawurzelextraktes. *Hautarzt* 1996; 47: 459–461.
86 Jappe U *et al.* Sebotropic drug reaction resulting from kava-kava extract therapy: a new entity? *J Am Acad Dermatol* 1998; 38: 104–106.
87 Schmidt P, Boehncke W-H. Delayed-type hypersensitivity reaction to kava-kava extract. *Contact Dermatitis* 2000; 42: 363.
88 Schelosky L *et al.* Kava and dopamine antagonism. *J Neurol Neurosurg Psychiatry* 1995; 58: 639–640.
89 Spillane PK *et al.* Neurological manifestations of kava intoxication. *Med J Aust* 1997; 167: 172–173.
90 Chanwai LG. Kava toxicity. *Emerg Med* 2000; 12: 142–145.
91 Cairney S *et al.* Saccade and cognitive impairment associated with kava intoxication. *Human Psychopharmacol* 2003; 18(7): 525–533.
92 Münte TF *et al.* Effects of oxazepam and an extract of kava roots (*Piper methysticum*) on event-related potentials in a word recognition task. *Neuropsychobiology* 1993; 27: 46–53.
93 Gessner B, Cnota P. Untersuchung der Vigilanz nach Applikation von Kava-kava-extrakt, diazepam oder Plazebo. *Z Phytother* 1994; 15: 30–37.
94 Schulz H *et al.* The quantitative EEG as a screening instrument to identify sedative effects of single doses of plant extracts in comparison with diazepam. *Phytomedicine* 1998; 5: 449–458.
95 Saletu B *et al.* EEG-Brain mapping, psychometric and psychophysiological studies on central effects of kavain – a kava plant derivative. *Hum Psychopharmacol* 1989; 4: 169–190.
96 Guro-Razuman S *et al.* Dermatomyositis-like illness following kava-kava ingestion. *J Clin Rheumatol* 1999; 6: 342–345.
97 Donadio V *et al.* Myoglobinuria after ingestion of extracts of guarana, *Ginkgo biloba* and kava. *Neurol Sci* 2000; 21: 124.
98 Garner LF, Klinger JD. Some visual effects caused by the beverage kava. *J Ethnopharmacol* 1985; 13: 307–311.
99 Logan JL, Ahmed J. Critical hypokalemic renal tubular acidosis due to Sjögren's syndrome: association with the purported immune stimulant echinacea. *Clin Rheumatol* 2003; 22: 158–159.
100 Clough AR *et al.* Case-control study of the association between kava use and ischaemic heart disease in eastern Arnhem Land (Northern Territory) Australia. *J Epidemiol Community Health* 2004; 58: 140–141.
101 Clough AR *et al.* Case-control study of the association between kava use and pneumonia in eastern Arnhem and Aboriginal communities (Northern Territory, Australia). *Epidemiol Infect* 2003; 131(1): 627–635.
102 Nerurkar PV *et al.* *In vitro* toxicity of kava alkaloid, pipermethystine, in HepG2 cells compared to kavalactones. *Toxicolog Sci* 2004; 79: 106–111.
103 Singh YN, Devkota AK. Aqueous kava extracts do not affect liver function tests in rats. *Planta Med* 2003; 69: 496–499.
104 Zou L *et al.* Effects of kava (kava-kava, 'Awa, Yaqona, *Piper methysticum*) on c-DNA-expressed cytochrome P450 enzymes and cryopreserved hepatocytes. *Phytomedicine* 2004; 11(4): 285–294.
105 Zou L *et al.* Kava does not display metabolic toxicity in a homogeneous cellular assay. *Planta Med* 2004; 70(4): 289–292.
106 Almeida JC, Grimsley EW. Coma from the health food store: interaction between kava and alprazolam. [letter]. *Ann Intern Med* 1996; 125: 940–941.
107 Herberg K-W. Alltagssicherheit unter Kava-Kava Extrakt, Bromazepam und deren Kombination. *Z Allg Med* 1996; 72: 973–977.
108 Gurley BJ *et al.* *In vivo* effects of goldenseal, kava kava, black cohosh, and valerian on human cytochrome P450 1A2, 2D6, 2E1, and 3A4/5 phenotypes. *Clin Pharmacol Ther* 2005; 77: 415–426.
109 Unger M *et al.* Inhibition of cytochrome P450 3A4 by extracts and kavalactones of *Piper methysticum* (kava-kava). *Planta Med* 2002; 68: 1055–1058.

110 Zou L *et al*. Effects of herbal components on cDNA-expressed cytochrome P450 enzyme catalytic activity. *Life Sci* 2002; 71: 1579–1589.
111 Cote CS *et al*. Composition and biological activity of traditional and commercial kava extracts. *Biochem Biophys Res Comm* 2004; 322(1): 147–152.
112 Ma Y *et al*. Desmethoxyyangonin and dihydromethysticin are two major pharmacological kavalactones with marked activity on the induction of CYP3A23. *Drug Metab Disp* 2004; 32(11): 1317–1324.
113 Weiss J *et al*. Extracts and kavalactones of *Piper methysticum* G. Forst. (kava-kava) inhibit P-glycoprotein *in vitro*. *Drug Metab Disp* 2005; 33(11): 1580–1583.
114 Anke J *et al*. Kavalactones fail to inhibit alcohol dehydrogenase *in vitro*. *Phytomedicine* 2006; 13(3): 192–195.
115 Herberg KW. Zum Einfluss von Kava-Spezialextrakt WS 1490 in Kombination mit Ethylalkohol auf sicherheitsrelevante Leisungsparameter. *Blutalkohol* 1993; 30: 96–105.
116 Foo H, Lemon J. Acute effects of kava, alone or in combination with alcohol, on subjective measures of impairment and intoxication and on cognitive performance. *Drug Alcohol Rev* 1997; 16: 147–155.
117 Jamieson DD, Duffield PH. Positive interaction of ethanol and kava resin in mice. *Clin Exp Pharmacol Physiol* 1990; 17: 509–514.

Lady's Slipper

Summary and Pharmaceutical Comment

Virtually no phytochemical or pharmacological data are available for lady's slipper to justify its use as a herbal remedy. In view of the lack of toxicity data, excessive use and use during pregnancy and lactation should be avoided.

Species (Family)

Cypripedium parviflorum var. *pubescens* (Willd.) O.W. Knight (Orchidaceae)

Synonym(s)

American Valerian, Cypripedium, *Cypripedium calceolus* var. *pubescens* (Willd.) Correll, *Cypripedium pubescens* Willd., Nerve Root

Part(s) Used

Rhizome, root

Pharmacopoeial and Other Monographs

BHP 1983[G7]

Legal Category (Licensed Products)

GSL (Cypripedium)[G37]

Constituents

Little chemical information has been documented. Lady's slipper is stated to contain glycosides, resin, tannic and gallic acids (usually associated with hydrolysable tannins), tannins and a volatile oil.

Several quinones have been reported including cypripedin, stated to belong to a group of rare non-terpenoid phenanthraquinones and not previously isolated from natural sources.[1]

Food Use

Lady's slipper is not used in foods.

Herbal Use

Lady's slipper is stated to possess sedative, mild hypnotic, antispasmodic and thymoleptic properties. Traditionally, it has been used for insomnia, hysteria, emotional tension, anxiety states, and specifically for anxiety states with insomnia.[G7, G64]

Benzonaphthoquinone

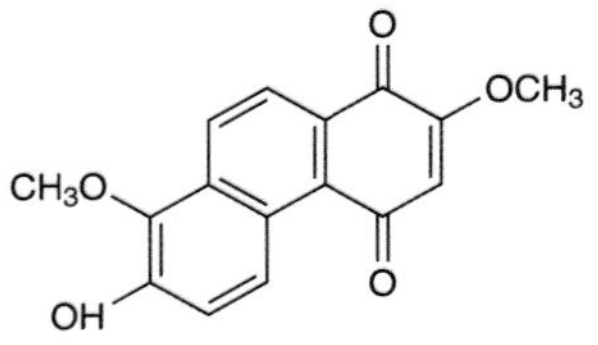

CH_3O — OH — OCH_3

cypripedin

Figure 1 Selected constituents of lady's slipper.

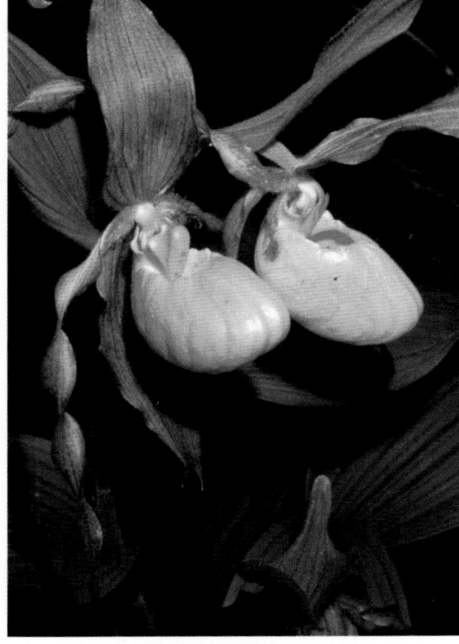

Figure 2 Lady's slipper (*Cypripedium parviflorum* var. *pubescens*).

Dosage

Dosages for oral administration (adults) for traditional uses recommended in standard herbal reference texts are given below.

Dried rhizome/root 2–4 g as an infusion three times daily.[G7]

Liquid extract 2–4 mL (1 : 1 in 45% alcohol) three times daily.[G7]

Pharmacological Actions

None documented.

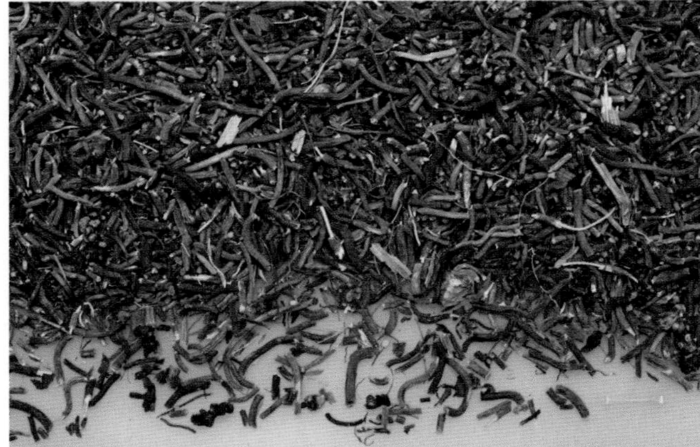

Figure 3 Lady's slipper – dried drug substance (root).

Clinical studies

There is a lack of clinical research assessing the effects of lady's slipper and rigorous randomised controlled clinical trials are required.

Side-effects, Toxicity

There is a lack of clinical safety and toxicity data for lady's slipper and further investigation of these aspects is required.

It has been stated that the roots may cause psychedelic reactions and large doses may result in giddiness, restlessness, headache, mental excitement and visual hallucinations.[G22] Lady's slipper is stated to be allergenic and contact dermatitis has been documented.[G51] The sensitising property of lady's slipper has been attributed to the quinone constituents.[1]

Contra-indications, Warnings

Lady's slipper may cause an allergic reaction in sensitive individuals.

Drug interactions None documented. However, the potential for preparations of lady's slipper to interact with other medicines administered concurrently should be considered.

Pregnancy and lactation The safety of lady's slipper has not been established. In view of the lack of phytochemical, pharmacological and toxicological information the use of lady's slipper during pregnancy and lactation should be avoided.

Reference

1 Schmalle H, Hausen BM. A new sensitizing quinone from lady slipper (*Cypripedium calceolus*). *Naturwissenschaften* 1979; 66: 527–528.

Lemon Verbena

Summary and Pharmaceutical Comment

Limited information is available on lemon verbena. Some of the traditional uses may be attributable to the volatile oil, for which many components have been identified, and to the flavone constituents. In the UK, lemon verbena is mainly used as an ingredient of herbal teas.

Species (Family)

Aloysia triphylla (L'Her.) Britton (Verbenaceae)

Synonym(s)

Aloysia citriodora (Cav.) Ort., *Lippia citriodora* (Ort.) HBK, *Verbena citriodora* Cav., *Verbena triphylla* L'Her.

Part(s) Used

Flowering top, leaf

Pharmacopoeial and Other Monographs

Martindale 35th edition[(G85)]

Legal Category (Licensed Products)

Lemon verbena is not included in the GSL.[(G37)]

Constituents

Flavonoids Flavones including apigenin, chrysoeriol, cirsimaritin, diosmetin, eupafolin, eupatorin, hispidulin, luteolin and derivatives, pectolinarigenin and salvigenin.[(1)]

Volatile oils Terpene components include borneol, cineol, citral, citronellal, cymol, eugenol, geraniol, limonene, linalool, β-pinene, nerol, and terpineol (monoterpenes), and α-caryophyllene, β-caryophyllene, myrcenene, pyrollic acid and isovalerianic acid (sesquiterpenes).[(2)]

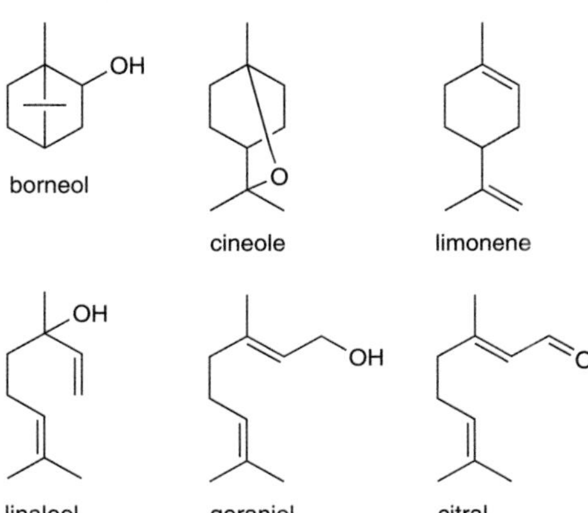

Figure 1 Selected constituents of lemon verbena.

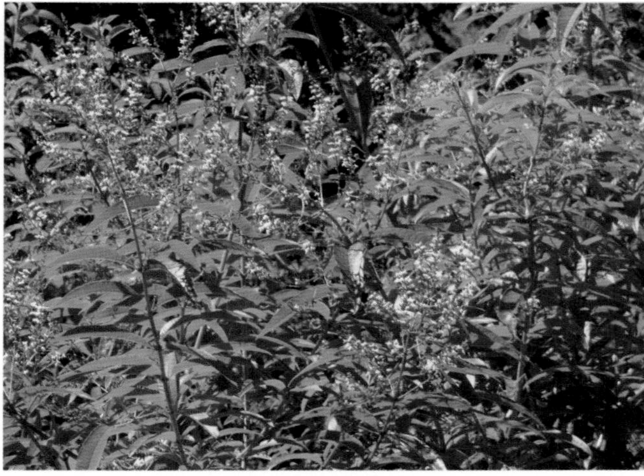

Figure 2 Lemon verbena (*Aloysia triphylla*).

Food Use

Previously, lemon verbena has been listed as GRAS (Generally Recognised As Safe) for human consumption in alcoholic beverages. Lemon verbena is also used in herbal teas.[(G57)]

Herbal Use

Lemon verbena is reputed to possess antispasmodic, antipyretic, sedative and stomachic properties. It has been used for the treatment of asthma, cold, fever, flatulence, colic, diarrhoea and indigestion.[(G38, G57, G64)]

Dosage

Dosages for oral administration (adults) for traditional uses recommended in older pharmaceutical reference texts are given below.

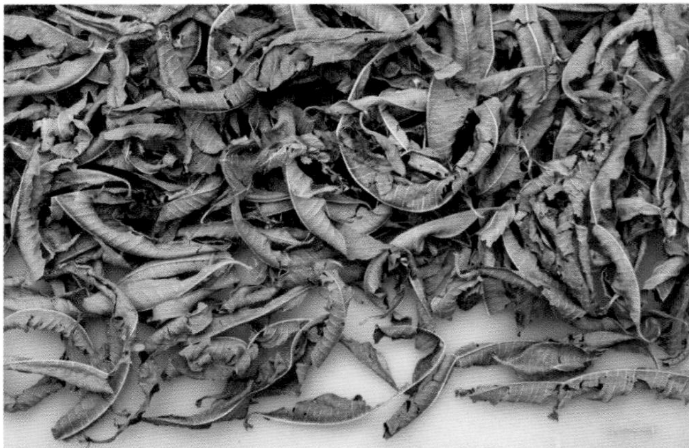

Figure 3 Lemon verbena – dried drug substance (leaf).

Decoction 45 mL taken several times daily.[G34]

Pharmacological Actions

None documented.

Clinical studies

There is a lack of clinical research assessing the effects of lemon verbena and rigorous randomised controlled clinical trials are required.

Side-effects, Toxicity

None documented. However, there is a lack of clinical safety and toxicity data for lemon verbena and further investigation of these aspects is required. Terpene-rich volatile oils are generally regarded as irritant and may cause kidney irritation during excretion.

Contra-indications, Warnings

Individuals with existing renal disease should avoid excessive doses of lemon verbena in view of the possible irritant nature of the volatile oil.

Drug interactions None documented. However, the potential for preparations of lemon verbena to interact with other medicines administered concurrently should be considered.

Pregnancy and lactation In view of the lack of pharmacological and toxicity data, and the potential irritant nature of the volatile oil, excessive doses of lemon verbena are best avoided during pregnancy and lactation.

Preparations

Proprietary multi-ingredient preparations

Spain: Agua del Carmen.

References

1 Skaltsa H, Shammas G. Flavonoids from *Lippia citriodora*. *Planta Med* 1988; 54: 465.
2 Montes M *et al*. Sur la composition de l'essence d'*Aloysia triphylla* (Cedron). *Planta Med* 1973; 23: 119–124.

Liferoot

Summary and Pharmaceutical Comment

Little information is documented for liferoot. No pharmacological studies were found to substantiate the traditional uses. The *Senecio* genus is characterised by unsaturated pyrrolizidine alkaloid constituents and the hepatotoxicity of this class of compounds is well recognised (*see* Comfrey). In view of this, liferoot is not suitable for use as a herbal medicine.

Species (Family)

Senecio aureus L. (Asteraceae/Compositae)

Synonym(s)

Golden Ragwort, Golden Senecio, Heart-leaved Groundsel, Squaw Weed

Part(s) Used

Herb

Pharmacopoeial and Other Monographs

BHP 1983[G7]
Martindale 35th edition[G85]

Legal Category (Licensed Products)

Liferoot is not included in the GSL.[G37]

Constituents

The following is compiled from several sources, including General Reference G19.

Limited information is documented regarding the constituents of liferoot, although it is well recognised that *Senecio* species contain pyrrolizidine alkaloids.

Pyrrolizidine alkaloids Floridanine, florosenine, otosenine, senecionine.[1,2]

The volatile oil composition of various *Senecio* species (but not *Senecio aureus*) has been investigated.[3]

Food Use

Liferoot is not used as a food.

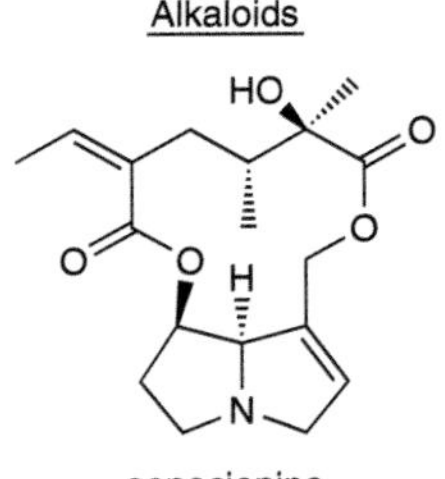

Figure 1 Selected constituents of liferoot.

Herbal Use

Liferoot is stated to possess uterine tonic, diuretic and mild expectorant properties. Traditionally, it has been used in the treatment of functional amenorrhoea, menopausal neurosis and leucorrhoea (as a douche).[G7, G64]

Dosage

Dosages for oral administration (adults) for traditional uses recommended in standard herbal reference texts are given below. However, current advice is that liferoot is not suitable for use as a herbal medicine and should not be ingested.

Herb 1–4 g as an infusion three times daily.[G7]

Liquid extract 14 mL (1 : 1 in 25% alcohol) three times daily.[G7]

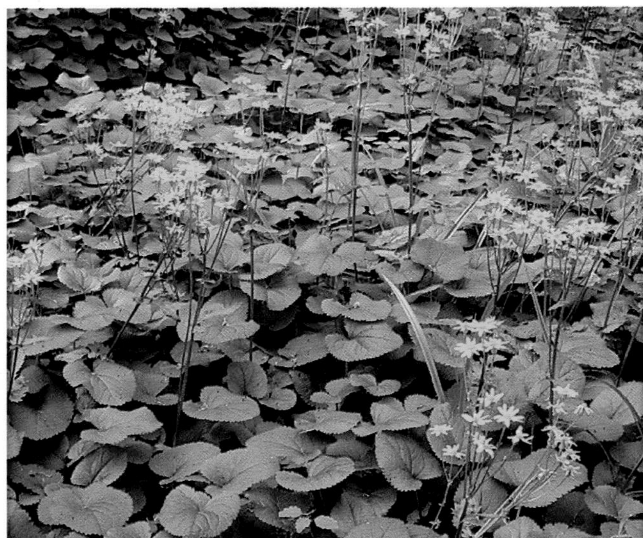

Figure 2 Liferoot (*Senecio aureus*).

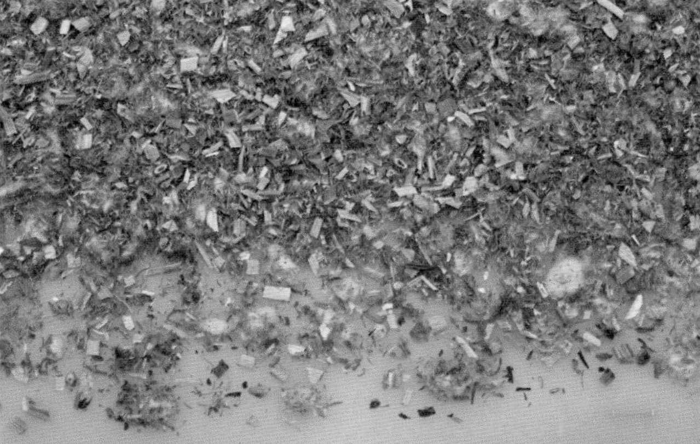

Figure 3 Liferoot – dried drug substance (herb).

Pharmacological Actions

No documented studies were located.

Side-effects, Toxicity

Liferoot contains pyrrolizidine alkaloids. The toxicity, primarily hepatic, of this class of compounds is well recognised in both animals and humans[G19] (*see* Comfrey).

Contra-indications, Warnings

In view of the hepatotoxic pyrrolizidine alkaloid constituents, liferoot should not be ingested.[G19]

Pregnancy and lactation In view of the toxic constituents, liferoot is contraindicated during pregnancy and lactation.[G49] Furthermore, liferoot is traditionally reputed to be an abortifacient, emmenagogue, and uterine tonic.[G7, G22] In animals, placental transfer and secretion into breast milk[4] has been documented for unsaturated pyrrolizidine alkaloids.

References

1 *Pyrrolizidine Alkaloids. Environmental Health Criteria 80.* Geneva: WHO, 1988.
2 Roder E *et al.* Pyrrolizidinalkaloide aus *Senecio aureus. Planta Med* 1983; 49: 57–59.
3 Dooren B *et al.* Composition of essential oils of some *Senecio* species. *Planta Med* 1981; 42: 385–389.
4 Mattocks AR. *Chemistry and Toxicology of Pyrrolizidine Alkaloids.* London: Academic Press, 1986: 1–393.

L

Lime Flower

Summary and Pharmaceutical Comment

The chemistry of lime flower is well documented. Little scientific information was located to justify the reputed herbal uses of lime flower, although some correlation can be made with the known pharmacological activities of the reported constituents. In view of the lack of toxicological data excessive use of lime flower and use during pregnancy and lactation should be avoided.

Species (Family)

**Tilia cordata* Mill. (Tiliaceae)
†*Tilia platyphyllos* Scop.
‡*Tilia* × *vulgaris* Hayne, a hybrid of the above (Tiliaceae)

Synonym(s)

Lime Tree, Linden Tree
**T. officinarum* Crantz, *T. officinarum* Crantz subsp. *officinarum* pro parte, *T. ulmifolia* Scop., *T. parvifolia* Ehrh. ex Hoffm., Small-leaved Lime
†*T. officinarum* Crantz, *T. officinarum* Crantz subsp. *officinarum* pro parte, Large-leaved Lime
‡*T.* × *europaea* auct. non L., Lime

Part(s) Used

Flowerheads

Pharmacopoeial and Other Monographs

BHC 1992[G6]
BHP 1996[G9]
BP 2007[G84]
Complete German Commission E (Linden)[G3]
Martindale 35th edition[G85]
Ph Eur 2007[G81]

Legal Category (Licensed Products)

GSL[G37]

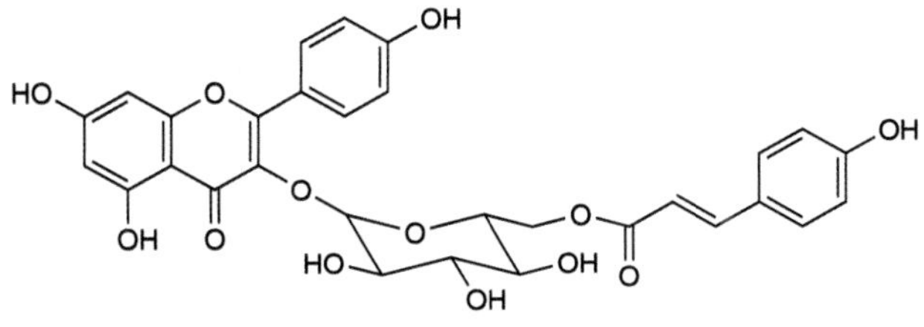

Flavonoids

tiliroside

Figure 1 Selected constituents of lime flower.

Constituents

The following is compiled from several sources, including General References G2, G6 and G62.

Acids Caffeic acid, chlorogenic acid and *p*-coumaric acid.

Amino acids Alanine, cysteine, cystine, isoleucine, leucine, phenylalanine and serine.

Carbohydrates Mucilage polysaccharides (3%). Five fractions identified yielding arabinose, galactose, rhamnose, with lesser amounts of glucose, mannose, and xylose; galacturonic and glucuronic acids;[1] gum.

Flavonoids Kaempferol, quercetin, myricetin and their glycosides.

Volatile oil Many components including alkanes, phenolic alcohols and esters, and terpenes including citral, citronellal, citronellol, eugenol, limonene, nerol, α-pinene and terpineol (monoterpenes), and farnesol (sesquiterpene).

Other constituents Saponin (unspecified), tannin (condensed) and tocopherol (phytosterol).

Food Use

Lime flower is listed by the Council of Europe as a natural source of food flavouring (category N2). This category indicates that lime flower can be added to foodstuffs in small quantities, with a possible limitation of an active principle (as yet unspecified) in the final product.[G16] Previously, lime flower has been listed as GRAS (Generally Recognised As Safe).[G65]

Herbal Use

Lime flower is stated to possess sedative, antispasmodic, diaphoretic, diuretic and mild astringent properties. Traditionally it has been used for migraine, hysteria, arteriosclerotic hypertension, feverish colds, and specifically for raised arterial pressure associated with arteriosclerosis and nervous tension.[G2, G6, G7, G8, G64]

Dosage

Dosages for oral administration (adults) for traditional uses recommended in standard herbal and/or pharmaceutical reference texts are given below.

Flowerhead 2–4 g by infusion.

Liquid extract 2–4 mL (1 : 1 in 25% alcohol).

Tincture 1–2 mL (1 : 5 in 45% alcohol).

Pharmacological Actions

In vitro and animal studies

In vitro, lime flower has been reported to exhibit antispasmodic activity followed by a spasmogenic effect on rat duodenum.[2] The actions were inhibited by atropine and papaverine, and reinforced by acetylcholine. The diaphoretic and antispasmodic properties claimed for lime flower have been attributed to *p*-coumaric acid and the flavonoids.[G39, G60] In addition, a number of actions have been associated with volatile oils including diuretic, sedative and antispasmodic effects, which may also account for some of the reputed uses of lime flower.[3–5] Volatile oils are not thought to possess any true diuretic activity, but to act as a result of certain terpenoid components having an irritant action on the kidneys during renal excretion.

Lime flower has been documented to possess a restricted range of antifungal activity.[6]

Clinical studies

There is a lack of clinical research assessing the effects of lime flower and rigorous randomised controlled clinical trials are required.

Side-effects, Toxicity

There is a lack of clinical and preclinical safety and toxicity data for lime flower and further investigation of these aspects is required.

Contra-indications, Warnings

Previously it has been advised that lime flower should be avoided by individuals with an existing cardiac disorder;[G22, G39, G60] however, the scientific basis for this statement, if any, is not known.

Drug interactions None documented. However, the potential for preparations of lime flower to interact with other medicines administered concurrently, particularly those with similar or opposing effects, should be considered.

Pregnancy and lactation The safety of lime flower has not been established. In view of the lack of toxicological data, use of lime flower during pregnancy and lactation should be avoided.

Preparations

Proprietary single-ingredient preparations

Belgium: Vibtil. *Czech Republic:* Kvet Lipy; Lipovy. *Monaco:* Vibtil.

Proprietary multi-ingredient preparations

Argentina: Armonil; Nervocalm; Sedante Dia; Serenil. *Austria:* Grippetee St Severin; St Bonifatius-Tee. *Belgium:* Natudor. *Canada:* Herbal Sleep Well. *Chile:* Calmatol; Nature Complex Reduct-Te; Recalm; Reduc-Te. *Czech Republic:* Cajova Smes pri Nachlazeni; Nontusyl; Pruduskova. *France:* Apaisance; Calmophytum; Mediflor Tisane Antirhumatismale No 2; Mediflor Tisane Calmante Troubles du Sommeil No 14; Vigilia. *Israel:* Jungborn. *Italy:* Alkagin; Lenicalm; Sedofit; Tussol. *Portugal:* Alkagin; Alkagin; Alkagin. *Spain:* Agua del Carmen; Jaquesor; Mesatil; Natusor Gripotul; Natusor Jaquesan; Natusor Sinulan; Natusor Somnisedan. *Switzerland:* Tisane contre les refroidissements; Tisane pour nourissons et enfants. *UK:* Menopause Relief; Tranquil; Wellwoman.

References

1 Kram G, Franz G. Structural investigations on the water soluble polysaccharides of lime tree flowers (*Tilia cordata* L.). *Pharmazie* 1985; 40: 501.
2 Lanza JP, Steinmetz M. Actions comparees des exraits aqueux de graines de *Tilia platyphylla* et de *Tilia vulgaris* sur l'intestin isolé de rat. *Fitoterapia* 1986; 57: 185.
3 Taddei I *et al*. Spasmolytic activity of peppermint, sage and rosemary essences and their major constituents. *Fitoterapia* 1988; 59: 463–468.
4 Svendsen AB, Scheffer JJC. *Essential Oils and Aromatic Plants. Proceedings of the 15th International Symposium on Essential Oils.* Dordrecht: Martinus Nijhoff, 1984; 225–226.
5 Sticher O. Plant mono-, di- and sesquiterpenoids with pharmacological and therapeutical activity. In: Wagner H, Wolff P, eds. *New Natural Products with Pharmacological, Biological or Therapeutical Activity.* Berlin: Springer-Verlag, 1977: 137–176.
6 Guerin J-C, Reveillere H-P. Antifungal activity of plant extracts used in therapy. I Study of 41 plant extracts against 9 fungi species. *Ann Pharm Fr* 1984; B: 553–559

Liquorice

Summary and Pharmaceutical Comment

The phytochemistry is well documented for liquorice and it is particularly characterised by triterpenoid components. Many of the traditional uses of liquorice are supported by documented pharmacological data although limited evidence of antispasmodic activity was found. Carbenoxolone, an ester derivative of a triterpenoid constituent in liquorice, is well known for its use in ulcer therapy. Much has been written concerning the steroid-type adverse effects associated with liquorice ingestion. Liquorice ingestion should therefore be avoided by individuals with an existing cardiovascular disorder and moderate consumption should be observed by other individuals.

Species (Family)

Glycyrrhiza glabra L. (Leguminosae)

Synonym(s)

Gan Cao (root/rhizome), *Glycyrrhiza glabra* L. var. *glabra*, *G. glabra* L. subsp. *glandulifera* (Waldst. & Kit.) Ponert, Licorice

Part(s) Used

Root, stolon

Pharmacopoeial and Other Monographs

BHC 1992[G6]
BHP 1996[G9]
BP 2007[G84]
Complete German Commission E[G3]
Martindale 35th edition[G85]
Ph Eur 2007[G81]
USP29/NF24[G86]
WHO volume 1 1999[G63]

Legal Category (Licensed Products)

GSL[G37]

Constituents

The following is compiled from several sources, including General References G2 and G6.

Coumarins Glycyrin, heniarin, liqcoumarin, umbelliferone, GU-7 (3-arylcoumarin derivative).[1]

Flavonoids Flavonols and isoflavones including formononetin, glabrin, glabrol, glabrone, glyzarin, glycyrol, glabridin and derivatives, kumatakenin, licoflavonol, licoisoflavones A and B, licoisoflavanone, licoricone, liquiritin and derivatives, phaseollinisoflavan;[2] chalcones including isoliquiritigenin, licuraside, echinatin, licochalcones A and B, neo-licuroside.[3]

Terpenoids Glycyrrhizin glycoside (1–24%) also known as glycyrrhizic or glycyrrhizinic acid yielding glycyrrhetinic (or glycyrrhetic) acid and glucuronic acid following hydrolysis;[4] glycyrrhetol, glabrolide, licoric acid, liquiritic acid and β-amyrin.

Volatile oils 0.047%.[5] More than 80 components identified including anethole, benzaldehyde, butyrolactone, cumic alcohol, eugenol, fenchone, furfuryl alcohol, hexanol, indole, linalool, γ-nonalactone, oestragole, propionic acid, α-terpineol and thujone[5]

Other constituents Amino acids, amines, gums, lignin, starch, sterols (β-sitosterol, stigmasterol), sugars and wax.

Other plant parts Components documented for the leaves of *G. glabra* include flavonoids (kaempferol and derivatives, isoquercetin, quercetin and derivatives, phytoalexins), coumarins (bergapten, xanthotoxin), phytoestrogen, β-sitosterol and saponaretin.[6]

Food Use

Liquorice is widely used in foods as a flavouring agent. Liquorice root is listed by the Council of Europe as a natural source of food flavouring (category N2). This category indicates that liquorice can be added to foodstuffs in small quantities, with a possible limitation of an active principle (as yet unspecified) in the final product.[G16] Previously, liquorice has been listed as GRAS (Generally Recognised As Safe).[G41]

Herbal Use

Liquorice is stated to possess expectorant, demulcent, antispasmodic, anti-inflammatory and laxative properties. Traditionally, it is also reported to affect the adrenal glands. It has been used for bronchial catarrh, bronchitis, chronic gastritis, peptic ulcer, colic and primary adrenocortical insufficiency.[G2, G6–G8, G10, G64]

Dosage

Dosages for oral administration (adults) for traditional uses recommended in older and contemporary standard herbal and/or pharmaceutical reference texts are given below.

Powdered root 1–4 g as a decoction three times daily.[G6, G7]

Liquorice Extract (BPC 1973) 0.6–2.0 g.

Pharmacological Actions

The pharmacological actions of liquorice have been reviewed.[7, 8]

In vitro and animal studies

Much has been documented regarding the steroid-type actions of liquorice (*see* Side-effects, Toxicity). Both glycyrrhizin and glycyrrhetinic acid (GA) have been reported to bind to glucocorticoid and mineralocorticoid receptors with moderate affinity, and to oestrogen receptors, sex hormone-binding globulin and corticosteroid-binding globulin with very weak affinity.[9–11] It has been suggested that glycyrrhizin and glycyrrhetinic acid may influence endogenous steroid activity via a receptor mechanism, with displacement of corticosteroids or other endogenous steroids.[9]

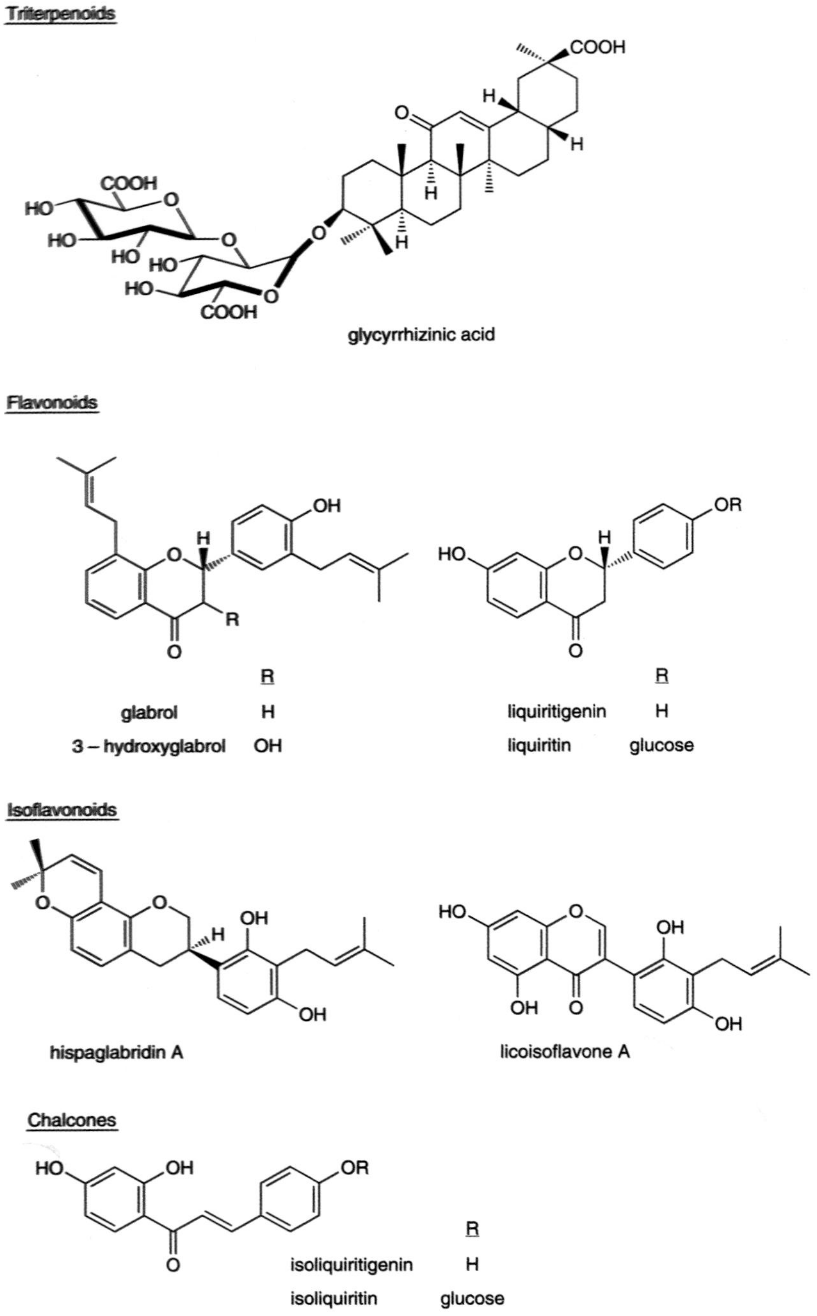

Triterpenoids

glycyrrhizinic acid

Flavonoids

	R
glabrol	H
3 – hydroxyglabrol	OH

	R
liquiritigenin	H
liquiritin	glucose

Isoflavonoids

hispaglabridin A

licoisoflavone A

Chalcones

	R
isoliquiritigenin	H
isoliquiritin	glucose

Figure 1 Selected constituents of liquorice.

The anti-oestrogenic action documented for glycyrrhizin at relatively high concentrations has been associated with a blocking effect that would be caused by glycyrrhizin binding at oestrogen receptors.[9] However, oestrogenic activity has also been documented for liquorice and attributed to the isoflavone constituents.[8] Liquorice exhibits an alternative action on oestrogen metabolism, causing inhibition if oestrogen concentrations are high and potentiation when concentrations are low.[8]

The relatively low affinity of glycyrrhizin and glycyrrhetinic acid for binding to mineralocorticoid receptors, together with the fact that liquorice does not exert its mineralocorticoid activity in adrenalectomised animals, indicates that a direct action at mineralocorticoid receptors is not the predominant mode of action.[12] It has been suggested that glycyrrhizin and glycyrrhetinic acid may exert their mineralocorticoid effect via an inhibition of 11β-hydroxysteroid dehydrogenase (11β-OHSD).[12] 11β-OHSD is a microsomal enzyme complex found predominantly in the liver and kidneys which catalyses the conversion of cortisol (potent mineralocortoid activity) to the inactive cortisone. Deficiency of 11β-OHSD results in increased concentrations of urinary free cortisol and cortisol metabolites. Glycyrrhetinic acid has been shown to inhibit renal 11β-OHSD in rats.[12] It has also been proposed that glycyrrhizin and glycyrrhetinic acid may displace cortisol from binding to transcortin.[13]

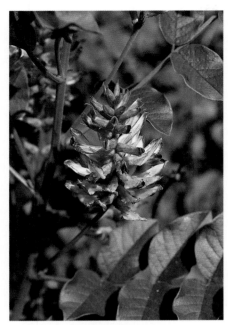

Figure 2 Liquorice (*Glycyrrhiza glabra*).

Antiplatelet activity *in vitro* has been documented for a 3-arylcoumarin derivative, GU-7, isolated from liquorice.[1] GU-7 was thought to inhibit platelet aggregation by increasing intraplatelet cyclic AMP concentration.

Isoliquiritigenin has been reported to inhibit aldose reductase, the first enzyme in the polyol pathway which reduces glucose to sorbitol.[14] Isoliquiritigenin was subsequently found to inhibit sorbitol accumulation in human red blood cells *in vitro*, and in red blood cells, the sciatic nerve and the lens of diabetic rats administered isoliquirigenin intragastrically.[14, 15] Many diabetic complications, such as cataracts, peripheral neuropathy, retinopathy and nephropathy have been associated with the polyol pathway and have shown improvement with inhibitors of aldose reductase.[14, 15]

Significant anti-inflammatory action is exhibited by glycyrrhetinic acid against UV erythema.[16] 18α-Glycyrrhetinic acid has exhibited stronger anti-inflammatory action compared to its stereoisomer 18β-glycyrrhetinic acid.[17] Chalcones isolated from *G. inflata* Bat. have been reported to inhibit leukotriene production and increase cyclic AMP concentrations in human polymorphonuclear neutrophils *in vitro*.[18] Glycyrrhetinic acid derivatives, but not glycyrrhetinic acid, have exhibited inhibitory effects on writhing and vascular permeability tests and on type IV allergy in mice.[19] The dihemiphthalate derivatives were especially active with respect to the two former activities and have previously been found to inhibit lipoxygenase and cyclooxygenase activities, and to prevent formation of gastric ulcer.[19]

Glycyrrhetinic acid is known to inhibit Epstein–Barr virus activation by tumour promotors.[20]

Antimicrobial activity versus *Staphylococcus aureus*, *Mycobacterium smegmatis* and *Candida albicans* has been documented for liquorice and attributed to isoflavonoid constituents (glabridin, glabrol and their derivatives).[2] Antiviral activity has been described for glycyrrhetinic acid, which interacts with virus structures producing different effects according to the viral stage affected.[21] Activity was observed against vaccinia, herpes simplex 1, Newcastle disease and vesicular stomatitis viruses, with no activity demonstrated towards poliovirus 1.[21]

In vitro hepatoprotective activity against CCl_4-induced toxicity has been reported to be greater for glycyrrhetinic acid compared to glycyrrhizin.[22] Glycyrrhetinic acid is thought to act by inhibition of the cytochrome P450 system required for the metabolism of CCl_4 to the highly reactive radical CCl_3.[22] *Glycyrrhiza uralensis* Fisch is used to treat hepatitis B in China, with a success rate reported to be greater than 70%.[23] Other activities documented for *G. uralensis* are anti-inflammatory and anti-allergic, treatment of jaundice, inhibition of fibrosis of the liver, corticosteroid-like immunosuppressing effect and a detoxifying effect.[23]

Screening of several plant extracts for antifertility activity reported liquorice to be ineffective following oral administration to rats in days 1–7 of pregnancy.[24]

Pharmacokinetics The pharmacokinetic profile of glycyrrhizin in rats has been found to be similar to that observed in humans.[25] Glycyrrhizin is primarily (80%) excreted into the bile from the liver against a concentration gradient.[25] This process is saturable and can therefore affect the excretion rate of glycyrrhizin. In addition, enterohepatic recycling occurs with reabsorption of bile-excreted glycyrrhizin from the intestinal tract.[25]

Clinical studies

Carbenoxolone, an ester derivative of glycyrrhetinic acid, has been used in the treatment of gastric and oesophageal ulcers. It is thought to exhibit a mucosal-protecting effect by beneficially interfering with gastric prostanoid synthesis, and increasing mucus production and mucosal blood flow.[26]

Liquorice is thought to exert its mineralocorticoid effect by inhibition of the enzyme 11β-OHSD, which catalyses the conversion of cortisol to the inactive cortisone (*see* Pharmacological Actions, *In vitro* and animal studies). Administration of liquorice to healthy volunteers has resulted in a disturbance of cortisol metabolism and a significant rise in urinary free cortisol, despite there being no change in plasma concentrations. These changes are consistent with this hypothesis, being indicative of 11β-OHSD deficiency.[12] Liquorice has also been found to suppress both plasma renin activity and aldosterone secretion.[27–29]

Subjects consuming 100–200 g liquorice/day have been reported to achieve plasma glycyrrhetinic acid concentrations of 80–480 ng/mL.[12]

Side-effects, Toxicity

Apart from confectionery, liquorice can also be ingested from infusions and by chewing tobaccos. Excessive or prolonged liquorice ingestion has resulted in symptoms typical of primary hyperaldosteronism, namely hypertension, sodium, chloride and water retention, hypokalaemia and weight gain, but also in low levels of plasma renin activity, aldosterone and antidiuretic hormone.[13, 27, 30]

Raised concentrations of atrial natriuretic peptide (ANP), which is secreted in response to atrial stretch and has vasodilating, natriuretic and diuretic properties, have also been observed in healthy subjects following the ingestion of liquorice.[13] Individuals consuming 10–45 g liquorice/day have exhibited raised blood pressure, together with a block of the aldosterone/renin axis and electrocardiogram changes, which resolved one month after withdrawal of liquorice.[31] Individuals consuming vastly differing amounts of liquorice have exhibited similar side-effect symptoms, indicating that the mineralocorticoid effect of liquorice is not dose dependent and is a saturable process.[31]

Hypokalaemic myopathy has also been associated with liquorice ingestion.[32–36] Severe hypokalaemia with rhabdomyolysis has been documented in a male patient following the ingestion of an alcohol-free beverage containing only small amounts of glycyrrhetinic acid (0.35 g/day).[32] The patient had known liver cirrhosis due to alcohol consumption and it was suggested that cirrhotic patients may be more susceptible to the mineralocorticoid side-effects of liquorice.[32] In one case,[34] the myoglobinaemia led to glomerulopathy and tubulopathy but with no clinical evidence of acute renal failure (ARF). The latter was attributed to the volume expansion also caused by the liquorice ingestion.

Rhabdomyolysis without myoglobinuria has been described.[37] In addition, severe congestive heart failure and pulmonary oedema have been reported in a previously healthy man who had ingested 700 g liquorice over eight days.[30] Liquorice extract given orally has been reported to have a similar but longer lasting action to intravenous deoxycortone and it has been noted that sodium chloride and water retention do not have to be accompanied by clinical oedema.[38] Amenorrhoea has been associated with liquorice ingestion (anti-oestrogenic action), with the menstrual cycle re-appearing following the withdrawal of liquorice.[31]

It has been noted that symptoms of hyperaldosteronism often resolve quickly, within a few days to two weeks, following the withdrawal of liquorice, even in individuals who have ingested the substance for many years.[29]

A case has been described where a patient presented with symptoms related to hyperglycaemia and myopathy secondary to liquorice-induced hypokalaemia. An inverse relationship was observed between the concentrations of fasting serum glucose and serum potassium.[39] Interestingly, animal studies have indicated that liquorice may reduce diabetic complications associated with intracellular accumulation of sorbitol.[19]

Contra-indications, Warnings

Numerous instances have been documented where liquorice ingestion has resulted in symptoms of primary hyperaldosteronism, such as water and sodium retention and hypokalaemia. Liquorice should therefore be avoided completely by individuals with an existing cardiovascular-related disorder, and ingested in moderation by other individuals.

Drug interactions None documented. However, the potential for preparations of liquorice to interact with other medicines administered concurrently, particularly those with similar or opposing effects, should be considered. Excessive or prolonged use of liquorice may lead to hypokalaemia and this, therefore, may potentiate the action of cardiac glycosides and interact with antiarrhythmic drugs or with drugs that induce reversion to sinus rhythm (e.g. quinidine), concomitant use of liquorice with other drugs inducing hypokalaemia (e.g. thiazide or loop diuretics, adrenocorticosteroids and stimulant laxatives) may aggravate electrolyte imbalance. There is limited evidence from preclinical studies that constituents of liquorice have oestrogenic and anti-oestrogenic effects, depending on dose.

Pregnancy and lactation In view of the documented pharmacological and toxicological effects, liquorice should not be used during pregnancy and lactation.

Preparations

Proprietary single-ingredient preparations

Brazil: Brefus. *Czech Republic:* Gallentee. *France:* Depiderm; Trio D.

Proprietary multi-ingredient preparations

Argentina: No-Tos Adultos; No-Tos Adultos; No-Tos Infantil; No-Tos Infantil; Urinefrol. *Australia:* Asa Tones; Betaine Digestive Aid; Broncafect; Feminine Herbal Complex; Gingo A; Glycoplex; Glycyrrhiza Complex; Herbal Cold & Flu Relief; Herbal Digestive Formula; Herbal PMS Formula; Hydrastis Complex; Neo-Cleanse; Potassium Iodide and Stramonium Compound; Senega and Ammonia; Verbascum Complex. *Austria:* Gastripan; Heumann's Bronchialtee; Krauter Hustensaft; Laxalpin; Midro Tee; Neoplex; Nesthakchen; Sigman-Haustropfen. *Brazil:* Fontolax; Frutalax; Laxarine; Laxtam; Peitoral Angico Pelotense; Sene Composta; Tamaril; Tamarine; Tamarix; Tussucalman. *Canada:* Bentasil Licorice with Echinacea; Bronchozone; Damiana-Sarsaparilla Formula; Herbal Nerve; Milk Thistle Extract Formula. *Chile:* Naturlax; Neostrata; Pectoral Pasteur. *Czech Republic:* Biotussil; Blasen- und Nierentee; Bronchialtee N; Cajova Smes pri Nachlazeni; Cajova Smes pri Redukcni Diete; Detska Cajova Smes; Detsky Caj s Hermankem; Diabetan; Erkaltungstee; Ipecarin; Magen- und Darmtee N; Naturland Grosser Swedenbitter; Projimava; Pruduskova; Pulmoran; Reduktan; Schlaf-Nerventee N; Species Pectorales Planta; Stoffwechseltee N; Tormentan; Zaludecni Cajova Smes. *France:* Mediflor Tisane Contre la Constipation Passagere No 7; Mediflor Tisane Hepatique No 5; Mediflor Tisane No 4 Diuretique. *Germany:* Gastritol; Heumann Bronchialtee Solubifix T; Heumann Magentee Solu-Vetan; Heweberberol-Tee; Iberogast; Muc-Sabona; Renob Blasen- und Nierentee; Salmiak; Ulcu-Pasc. *Hong Kong:* Mist Expect Stim; Vida Brown Mixture. *India:* Arowash; Diovol Forte DGL; Disogel; N-T-Tus. *Israel:* Gingisan; Gingisan; Lido Tea; Midro-Tea. *Italy:* Cadifen; Cadimint; Dicalmir; Influ-Zinc Gola; Lassatina; Midro; Proctopure; Rabro N; Sciroppo Berta; Tamarine; Tussol. *Malaysia:* Horseradish Plus; Total Man. *Monaco:* Blackoids du Docteur Meur. *Norway:* Solvipect comp; Solvipect. *New Zealand:* Bonningtons Irish Moss. *Portugal:* Midro. *Russia:* Doktor Mom (Доктор Мом); Doktor Mom Herbal Cough Lozenges (Доктор Мом Растительные Пастилки От Кашля); Linkus (Линкас); Original Grosser Bittner Balsam (Оригинальный Большой Бальзам Биттнера); Prostanorm (Простанорм). *South Africa:* Borsdruppels; Chamberlains Cough Remedy Regular; Puma Cough Balsam. *Singapore:* Phytoestrin. *Spain:* Bronpul; Laxomax; Malvaliz; Natusor Astringel; Natusor Gastrolen; Natusor Low Blood Pressure; Pastillas Pectoral Kely; Regamint. *Switzerland:* DAM Antacidum; DemoPectol; DemoTussil; Gem; Iberogast; Kernosan Elixir; Lapidar 10; Makaphyt Gouttes antitussives; Makaphyt Sirop; Pastilles bronchiques S nouvelle formule; Sirop pectoral contre la toux S; Sirop S contre la toux et la bronchite; Strath Gouttes pour l'estomac; Tisane laxative; Tisane pectorale et antitussive; Tisane pectorale pour les enfants. *Thailand:* Brown Mixture; Meloids; Ulgastrin. *UK:* Allens Pine & Honey; Asthma & Catarrh Relief; Chesty Cough Relief; Covonia Mentholated; Culpeper Detox Tea; Honey & Molasses; Jamaican Sarsaparilla; Lane's Sage and Garlic Catarrh Remedy; Lightning Cough Remedy; Napiers Echinacea Tea; Nigroids; Potters Sugar Free Cough Pastilles;

Revitonil; Rob-Bron Tablets; Summertime Tea Blend; Tickly Cough & Sore Throat Relief; Vegetable Cough Remover; Vocalzone.

References

1 Tawata M *et al.* Anti-platelet action of GU-7, a 3-arylcoumarin derivative, purified from *Glycyrrhizae radix*. *Planta Med* 1990; 56: 259–263.
2 Mitscher LA *et al.* Antimicrobial agents from higher plants. Antimicrobial isoflavanoids and related substances from *Glycyrrhiza glabra* L. var. *typica*. *J Nat Prod* 1980; 43: 259–269.
3 Miething H, Speicher-Brinker A. Neolicuroside – A new chalcone glycoside from the roots of *Glycyrrhiza glabra*. *Arch Pharm (Weinheim)* 1989; 322: 141–143.
4 Takino Y *et al.* Quantitative determination of glycyrrhizic acid in liquorice roots and extracts by TLC-densitometry. *Planta Med* 1979; 36: 74–78.
5 Kameoka H, Nakai K. Components of essential oil from the root of *Glycyrrhiza glabra*. *Nippon Nogeikagaku Kaishi [J Ag Chem Soc Japan]* 1987; 61: 1119–1121.
6 Jimenez J *et al.* Flavonoids of *Helianthemum cinereum*. *Fitoterapia* 1989; 60: 189.
7 Chandler RF. Licorice, more than just a flavour. *Can Pharm J* 1985; 118: 421–424.
8 Pizzorno JE, Murray AT. *Glycyrrhiza glabra*. *A Textbook of Natural Medicine*. Seattle, WA: John Bastyr College Publications, 1985 (looseleaf).
9 Tamaya MD *et al.* Possible mechanism of steroid action of the plant herb extracts glycyrrhizin, glycyrrhetinic acid, and paeoniflorin: Inhibition by plant herb extracts of steroid protein binding in the rabbit. *Am J Obstet Gynecol* 1986; 155: 1134–1139.
10 Armanini D *et al.* Binding of agonists and antagonists to mineralocorticoid receptors in human peripheral mononuclear leucocytes. *J Hypertens* 1985; 3 (Suppl. Suppl.3): S157–159.
11 Armanini D *et al.* Affinity of liquorice derivatives for mineralocorticoid and glucocorticoid receptors. *Clin Endocrinol* 1983; 19: 609–612.
12 Stewart PM *et al.* Mineralocorticoid activity of liquorice: 11-beta-hydroxysteroid dehydrogenase deficiency comes of age. *Lancet* 1987; ii: 821–824.
13 Forslund T *et al.* Effects of licorice on plasma atrial natriuretic peptide in healthy volunteers. *J Intern Med* 1989; 225: 95–99.
14 Aida K *et al.* Isoliquiritigenin: A new aldose reductase inhibitor from *Glycyrrhizae radix*. *Planta Med* 1990; 56: 254–258.
15 Yun-ping Z, Jia-qing Z. Oral baicalin and liquid extract of licorice reduce sorbitol levels in red blood cell of diabetic rats. *Chin Med J* 1989; 102: 203–206.
16 Fujita H *et al.* Antiinflammatory effect of glycyrrhizinic acid. Effects of glycyrrhizinic acid against carrageenin-induced edema, UV-erythema and skin reaction sensitised with DCNB. *Pharmacometrics* 1980; 19: 481–484.
17 Amagaya S *et al.* Separation and quantitative analysis of 18α-glycyrrhetinic acid and 18β-glycyrrhetinic acid in *Glycyrrhizae radix* by gas-liquid chromatography. *J Chromatogr* 1985; 320: 430–434.
18 Kimura Y *et al.* Effects of chalcones isolated from licorice roots on leukotriene biosynthesis in human polymorphonuclear neutrophils. *Phytother Res* 1988; 2: 140–145.
19 Inque H *et al.* Pharmacological activities of glycerrhetinic acid derivatives: Analgesic and anti-type IV allergic effects. *Chem Pharm Bull* 1987; 35: 3888–3893.
20 Tokuda H *et al.* Inhibitory effects of ursolic and oleandolic acid on skin tumor promotion by 12-O-tetradecanoylphorbol-13-acetate. *Cancer Lett* 1986; 33: 279–285.
21 Pompei R *et al.* Antiviral activity of glycyrrhizic acid. *Experientia* 1980; 36: 304.
22 Kiso Y *et al.* Mechanism of antihepatotoxic activity of glycyrrhizin, I: Effect on free radical generation and lipid peroxidation. *Planta Med* 1984; 50: 298–302.
23 Chang HM *et al.* *Advances in Chinese Medicinal Materials Research*. Singapore: World Scientific, 1985.
24 Sharma BB *et al.* Antifertility screening of plants. Part I. Effect of ten indigenous plants on early pregnancy in albino rats. *Int J Crude Drug Res* 1983; 21: 183–187.
25 Ichikawa T *et al.* Biliary excretion and enterohepatic cycling of glycyrrhizin in rats. *J Pharm Sci* 1986; 75: 672–675.
26 Guslandi M. Ulcer-healing drugs and endogenous prostaglandins. *Int J Clin Pharmacol Ther Toxicol* 1985; 23: 398–402.
27 Conn J *et al.* Licorice-induced pseudoaldosteronism. Hypertension, hypokalaemia, aldosteronopenia and suppressed plasma renin activity. *JAMA* 1968; 205: 492–496.
28 Epstein MT *et al.* Effect of eating liquorice on the renin-angiotensin aldosterone axis in normal subjects. *BMJ* 1977; 1: 488–490.
29 Mantero F. Exogenous mineralocorticoid-like disorders. *Clin Endocrinol Metab* 1981; 10: 465–478.
30 Chamberlain TJ. Licorice poisoning, pseudoaldosteronism, heart failure. *JAMA* 1970; 213: 1343.
31 Corrocher R *et al.* Pseudoprimary hyperaldosteronism due to liquorice intoxication. *Eur Rev Med Pharmacol Sci* 1983; 5: 467–470.
32 Piette AM *et al.* Hypokaliémie majeure avec rhabdomyolase secondaire à l'ingestion de pastis non alcoolisé. *Ann Med Interne (Paris)* 1984; 135: 296–298.
33 Cibelli G *et al.* Hypokalemic myopathy associated with liquorice ingestion. *Ital J Neurol Sci* 1984; 5: 463–466.
34 Heidermann HT, Kreuzfelder E. Hypokalemic rhabdomyolysis with myoglobinuria due to licorice ingestion and diuretic treatment. *Klin Wochenschr* 1983; 61: 303–305.
35 Ruggeri CS *et al.* L. Carnetina cloruro e KCl nel trattamento di un caso di rabdomiolisi atraumatica senza mioglobinuria da ingestione di liquerizia. *Minn Med* 1985; 76: 725–728.
36 Bannister B *et al.* Cardiac arrest due to liquorice induced hypokalaemia. *BMJ* 1977; 2: 738–739.
37 Maresca MC *et al.* Low blood potassium and rhabdomyolosis. Description of three cases with different aetiologies. *Minerva Med* 1988; 79: 79–81.
38 Molhuysen JA. A liquorice extract with deoxycortone-like action. *Lancet* 1950; ii: 381–386.
39 Jamil A *et al.* Hyperglycaemia related to licorice-induced hypokalaemia. *J Kwt Med Assoc* 1986; 20: 69–71.

Lobelia

Summary and Pharmaceutical Comment

The principal constituent of lobelia is lobeline, an alkaloid with similar pharmacological properties to those of nicotine. Lobelia has previously been used in herbal preparations for the treatment of asthma and bronchitis, and in anti-smoking preparations aimed to lessen nicotine withdrawal symptoms. However, in view of its potent alkaloid constituents, excessive use of lobelia and use during pregnancy and lactation should be avoided.

Species (Family)

Lobelia inflata L. (Campanulaceae)

Synonym(s)

Indian Tobacco

Part(s) Used

Herb

L

Pharmacopoeial and Other Monographs

BHC 1992[(G6)]
BHP 1996[(G9)]
Martindale 35th edition[(G85)]

Legal Category (Licensed Products)

GSL[(G37)]

Constituents

The following is compiled from several sources, including General Reference G6.

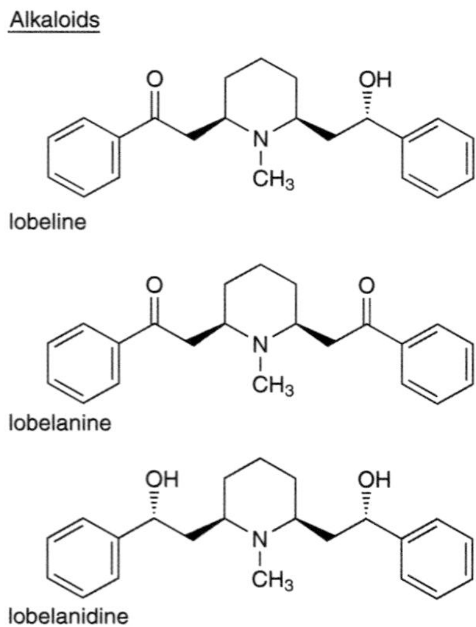

Figure 1 Selected constituents of lobelia.

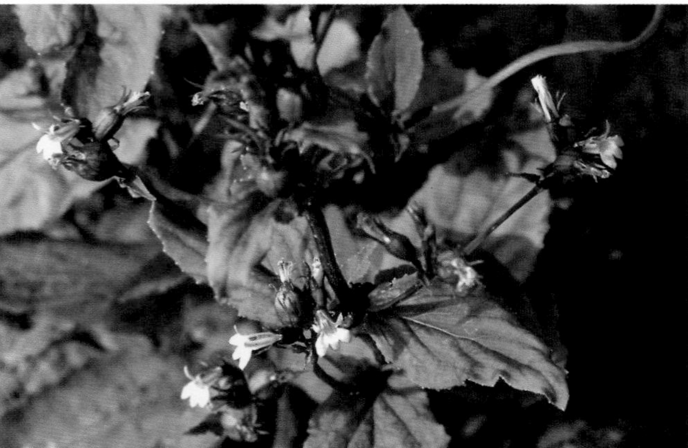

Figure 2 Lobelia (*Lobelia inflata*).

Alkaloids Piperidine-type. 0.48%. Lobeline (major); others include lobelanine, lobelanidine, norlobelanine, lelobanidine, norlelobanidine, norlobelanidine and lobinine.

Other constituents Bitter glycoside (lobelacrin), chelidonic acid, fats, gum, resin and volatile oil.

Food Use

Lobelia is not generally used as a food.

Herbal Use

Lobelia is stated to possess respiratory stimulant, antasthmatic, antispasmodic, expectorant, and emetic properties. Traditionally, it has been used for bronchitic asthma, chronic bronchitis, and specifically for spasmodic asthma with secondary bronchitis. It has also been used topically for myositis and rheumatic nodules.[(G6, G7, G8, G64)]

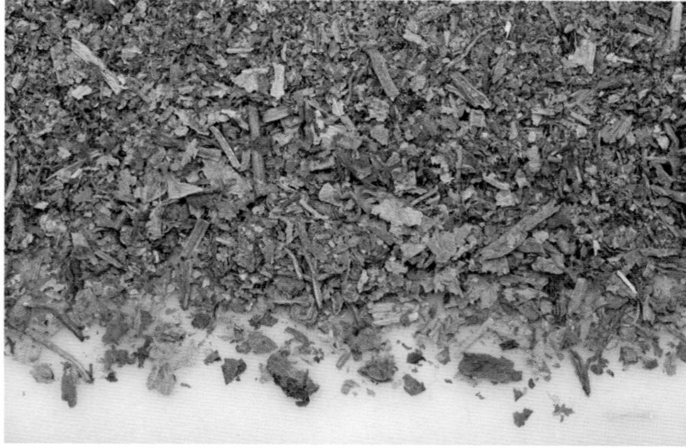

Figure 3 Lobelia – dried drug substance (herb).

Dosage

Dosages for oral administration (adults) for traditional uses recommended in older and contemporary standard herbal and/or pharmaceutical reference texts are given below.

Dried herb 0.2–0.6 g as an infusion or decoction three times daily.[G6, G7]

Liquid extract 0.2–0.6 mL (1 : 1 in 50% alcohol) three times daily.[G6, G7]

Simple Tincture of Lobelia (BPC 1949) 0.6–2.0 mL.

Tincture Lobelia Acid 1–4 mL (1 : 10 in dilute acetic acid) three times daily.[G6, G7]

Pharmacological Actions

The pharmacological activity of lobelia can be attributed to the alkaloid constituents, principally lobeline. Lobeline has peripheral and central effects similar to those of nicotine, but is less potent. Hence, lobeline initially causes CNS stimulation followed by respiratory depression. Lobeline is also reported to possess expectorant properties.

Clinical studies

There is a lack of clinical research assessing the effects of lobelia and rigorous randomised controlled clinical trials are required.

Side-effects, Toxicity

Side-effects of lobeline and lobelia are similar to those of nicotine and include nausea and vomiting, diarrhoea, coughing, tremors and dizziness. Symptoms of overdosage are reported to include profuse diaphoresis, tachycardia, convulsions, hypothermia, hypotension and coma, and may be fatal.[G45]

Contra-indications, Warnings

The pharmacological actions of lobeline are similar to those of nicotine.

Drug interactions None documented. However, the potential for preparations of lobelia to interact with other medicines administered concurrently, particularly those with similar or opposing effects, should be considered. The pharmacological activity of lobeline is similar to that of nicotine.

Pregnancy and lactation Lobelia should not be used during pregnancy or lactation.

Preparations

Proprietary multi-ingredient preparations

UK: Catarrh Tablets.

Marshmallow

Summary and Pharmaceutical Comment

In vitro and animal studies provide some supporting evidence for the use of marshmallow in the treatment of cough, irritation of the throat and gastric inflammation. Antibacterial and anti-inflammatory activities, effects on mucociliary transport, adhesion of polysaccharide to buccal membranes and reduction of cough are reported. However, there is a lack of clinical studies investigating the effects of marshmallow. Although no toxicity data were located, the chemistry of marshmallow and its use in foods indicate that there should not be any reason for concern regarding safety.

Species (Family)

Althaea officinalis L. (Malvaceae)

Synonym(s)

Althaea, *A. taurinensis* DC., *A. kragujevacensis* Panc.

Part(s) Used

Leaf, root

Pharmacopoeial and Other Monographs

BHC 1992(G6)
BHP 1996(G9)
BP 2007(G84)
Complete German Commission E(G3)
ESCOP 2003(G76)
Martindale 35th edition(G85)
Ph Eur 2007(G81)

Legal Category (Licensed Products)

GSL(G37)

Constituents

The following is compiled from several sources, including General References G2, G6 and G52.

Polysaccharides

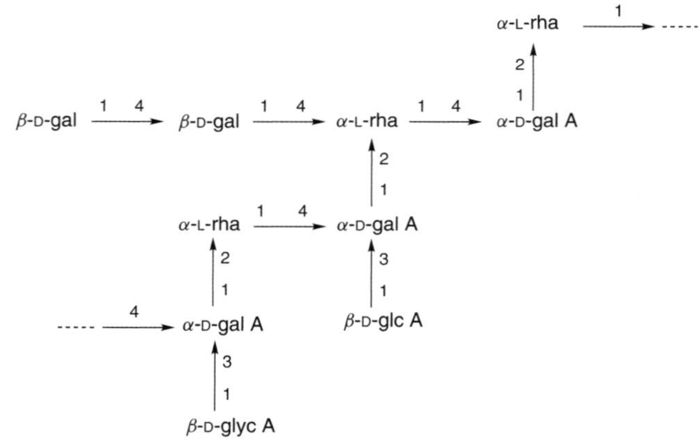

gal = galactose, rha = rhamnose, glyc A = glucuronic acid
gal A = galacturonic acid

Flavonoids

OH HO O R1 R2 OH O

	R1	R2
hypolaetin	OH	OH
isoscutellarein	OH	H

Figure 1 Selected constituents of marshmallow.

Polysaccharides Mucilage polysaccharides (5–10%), consisting of galacturono-rhamnans, arabinans, glucans, arabinogalactans.[1, G52]

Flavonoids Hypolaetin 8-glucoside, isoscutellarein 4′-methylether-8-glucoside-2″-sulfate.[2]

Phenolic acids Caffeic, *p*-coumaric, ferulic, *p*-hydroxybenzoic and syringic.

Other constituents Asparagine 2%, calcium oxalate, coumarins (scopoletin), pectin, starch and tannin.

Food Use

Marshmallow is listed by the Council of Europe as a natural source of food flavouring (category N2). This category indicates that marshmallow can be added to foodstuffs in small quantities, with a possible limitation of an active principle (as yet unspecified) in the final product.[G16] Previously in the USA, marshmallow has been approved for use in foods.[G41]

Herbal Use

Marshmallow is stated to possess demulcent, expectorant, emollient, diuretic, antilithic and vulnerary properties.[G2, G4, G6–G8, G43, G52, G54, G64] Traditionally, it has been used internally for the treatment of respiratory catarrh and cough, peptic ulceration, inflammation of the mouth and pharynx, enteritis, cystitis, urethritis and urinary calculus, and topically for abscesses, boils and varicose and thrombotic ulcers. The German Commission E approved use of root and leaf for irritation of oral and pharyngeal mucosa and associated dry cough and root for mild inflammation of gastric mucosa.[G3] Marshmallow root is used in combination with anise fruit, eucalyptus oil, liquorice and with anise fruit, liquorice and primrose root and with anise fruit and primrose root for catarrh of the upper respiratory tract and resulting dry cough.[G3]

Dosage

Dosages for oral administration (adults) for traditional uses recommended in older and contemporary standard herbal and/or pharmaceutical reference texts are given below.

Dried leaf 2–5 g as an infusion three times daily;[G6, G7] 5 g.[G3]

Leaf, liquid extract 2–5 mL (1 : 1 in 25% alcohol) three times daily.[G6, G7]

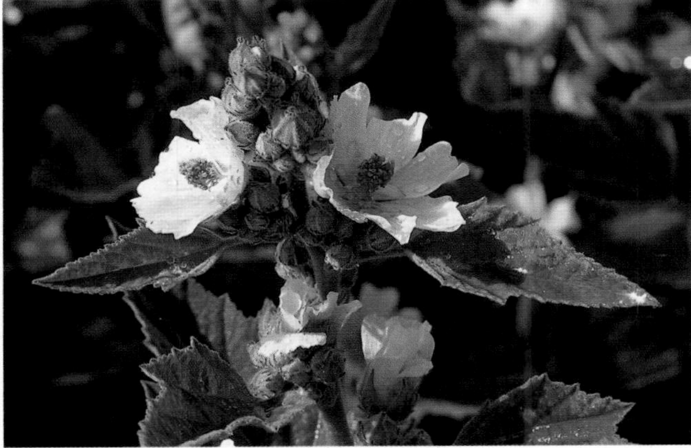

Figure 2 Marshmallow (*Althaea officinalis*).

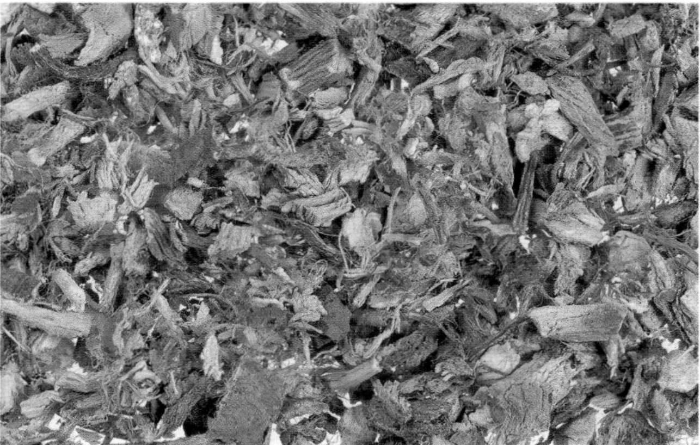

Figure 3 Marshmallow – dried drug substance (root).

Ointment 5% Powdered althaea leaf in usual ointment base three times daily.[G6, G7]

Dried root 2–5 g by cold extraction three times daily;[G6, G7] 6 g.[G3]

Root, liquid extract 2–5 mL (1 : 1 in 25% alcohol) three times daily.[G6, G7]

Syrup of Althaea (BPC 1949) 2–10 mL three times daily.[G6, G7]

Pharmacological Actions

In vitro and animal studies

Antimicrobial activity against *Pseudomonas aeruginosa*, *Proteus vulgaris* and *Staphylococcus aureus* has been documented for marshmallow.[3]

The mucilage has demonstrated considerable hypoglycaemic activity in non-diabetic mice.[4]

Inhibition (17%) of mucociliary transport in ciliated epithelium isolated from frog oesophagus was observed with 200 μL of cold macerate of marshmallow root (6.4 g/140 mL).[G52]

Marshmallow root extract is reported to stimulate phagocytosis, and to release oxygen radicals and leukotrienes from human neutrophils.[G52] In addition, release of cytokines, interleukin 6 and tumour necrosis factor from monocytes occurs, demonstrating potential anti-inflammatory and immunomodulatory effects. In mice, intraperitoneal administration of isolated polysaccharide (10 mg/kg) resulted in activity of macrophages in a carbon clearance test, and was indicative of non-specific immunomodulation.[G52] A lack of anti-inflammatory activity has been observed for marshmallow in the carrageenan-induced rat paw oedema test.[5] The anti-inflammatory effect of an ointment containing 0.05% dexamethasone was enhanced by addition of aqueous extract of marshmallow (20%) as assessed in a rabbit ear irritancy test using UV irradiation or furfuryl alcohol.[G52]

A total extract of root and isolated polysaccharide (100 and 50 mg/kg, respectively) have been tested for their antitussive activity in unanaesthetised cats.[6] The polysaccharide gave a statistically significant decrease in the number of cough efforts from laryngopharyngeal and tracheobronchial areas. The root extract was less effective than the isolated polysaccharide.

A polysaccharide enriched extract showed moderate concentration-dependent adhesive properties in porcine buccal membranes *ex vivo*.[7]

Clinical studies

There is a lack of clinical research assessing the effects of marshmallow and rigorous randomised controlled clinical trials are required.

Side-effects, Toxicity

None documented. However, there is a lack of clinical safety and toxicity data for marshmallow, and further investigation of these aspects is required where therapeutic dosages are greater than the quantities ingested in foods.

Contra-indications, Warnings

Drug interactions None documented. However, the potential for preparations of marshmallow to interact with other medicines administered concurrently, particularly those with similar or opposing effects, should be considered. Marshmallow may delay the absorption of other medicines taken simultaneously.[(G76)] There is limited evidence from preclinical studies that marshmallow has hypoglycaemic activity.

Pregnancy and lactation There are no known problems with the use of marshmallow during pregnancy or lactation. However, amounts ingested should not exceed those used in foods.

Preparations

Proprietary single-ingredient preparations

Canada: Butt-Out. *France:* Primadrill. *Germany:* Phytohustil.

Proprietary multi-ingredient preparations

Australia: Althaea Complex; Cough Relief; Garlic and Horseradish + C Complex; Hydrastis Complex; Potassium Iodide and Stramonium Compound. *Austria:* Heumann's Bronchialtee; Paracodin; The Chambard-Tee; Tuscalman. *Belgium:* Kamfeine. *Brazil:* Asmatiron; Broncofenil; Bronquidex; Brontoss; Expectobron; Expectol; Iodeto de Potassio; Iodeto de Potassio; Iol; Iolin; MM Expectorante; Peitoral Angico Pelotense; Pulmoforte. *Canada:* Original Herb Cough Drops; Swiss Herb Cough Drops. *Chile:* Paltomiel Plus; Pulmagol; Ramistos. *Czech Republic:* Detska Cajova Smes; Detsky Caj s Hermankem; Nontusyl; Pruduskova; Pulmoran; Species Pectorales Planta. *France:* Mediflor Tisane No 4 Diuretique. *Germany:* Heumann Bronchialtee Solubifix T; Tonsilgon. *Italy:* Gastrotuss. *Malaysia:* Horseradish Plus. *Russia:* Linkus (Линкас); Pansoral Teething (Пансорал Первые Зубы); Tonsilgon N (Тонзилгон Н). *South Africa:* Cough Elixir. *Spain:* Bronpul; Llantusil; Malvaliz; Natusor Broncopul; Natusor Farinol; Natusor Gastrolen; Natusor Malvasen; Pazbronquial; Senalsor. *Switzerland:* Malveol; Tisane pectorale et antitussive; Tisane pectorale pour les enfants; Tisane Provencale No 1; Tuscalman. *UK:* Antibron; Asthma & Catarrh Relief; Balm of Gilead; Chest Mixture; Herb and Honey Cough Elixir; Herbelix; Herbheal Ointment; Horehound and Aniseed Cough Mixture; Modern Herbals Cold & Catarrh; Modern Herbals Cold & Congestion; Napiers Uva Ursi Tea; Potter's Catarrh Pastilles; Sinotar; Vegetable Cough Remover. *USA:* Laci Le Beau Super Dieter's Tea.

References

1 Blaschek W, Franz G. A convenient method for the quantitative determination of mucilage polysaccharides in *Althaeae radix*. *Planta Med* 1986; 52 (Suppl. Suppl.): 537.
2 Gudej J. Flavonoids, phenolic acids and coumarins from the roots of *Althaea officinalis*. *Planta Med* 1991; 57: 284–285.
3 Recio MC *et al*. Antimicrobial activity of selected plants employed in the Spanish Mediterranean area Part II. *Phytother Res* 1989; 3: 77–80.
4 Tomodo M *et al*. Hypoglycaemic activity of twenty plant mucilages and three modified products. *Planta Med* 1987; 53: 8–12.
5 Mascolo N *et al*. Biological screening of Italian medicinal plants for anti-inflammatory activity. *Phytother Res* 1987; 1: 28–31.
6 Nosálova G *et al*. Antitussive wirkung des extraktes und der polysaccharide aus eibisch (Althaea officinalis L., var. robusta). *Pharmazie* 1992; 47: 224–226.
7 Schmidgall J *et al*. Evidence for bioadhesive effects of polysaccharides and polysaccharide-containing herbs in an *ex vivo* bioadhesion assay on buccal membranes. *Planta Med* 2000; 66: 48–53.

Maté

Summary and Pharmaceutical Comment

Maté is characterised by the xanthine constituents, which also represent the active principles. The herbal uses of maté can be attributed to the pharmacological actions of caffeine, which are well documented. However, there is a lack of clinical research assessing the efficacy and safety of preparations of maté. Side-effects and warnings associated with other xanthine-containing beverages, such as tea and coffee, are applicable to maté.

Species (Family)

Ilex paraguariensis St. Hil. (Aquifoliaceae)

Synonym(s)

Ilex, Jesuit's Brazil Tea, Paraguay Tea, St Bartholomew's Tea, Yerba Maté

Part(s) Used

Leaf

Pharmacopoeial and Other Monographs

BHP 1996[G9]
Complete German Commission E[G3]
Martindale 35th edition[G85]

Legal Category (Licensed Products)

GSL[G37]

Constituents

The following is compiled from several sources, including General Reference G2.

Alkaloids Xanthine-type. Caffeine 0.2–2.0%, theobromine 0.1–0.2%, theophylline 0.05%.

Flavonoids Kaempferol, quercetin, and their glycosides, including rutin.[1]

Tannins 4–16%.

Terpenoids Ursolic acid (major), β-amyrin, ilexoside A, ilexoside B methyl ester.[2]

Other constituents Choline and trigonellin (amines), amino acids,[1] riboflavin (vitamin B_2), pyridoxine (vitamin B_6), niacin, pantothenic acid, vitamin C and resins.

Other Ilex species Triterpenoid saponins termed ilexsaponins B_1, B_2, and B_3 have been isolated from *Ilex pubescens* Hook. & Arn.[3]

A cyanogenetic glucoside has been isolated from *Ilex aquifolium*.[4]

Purines

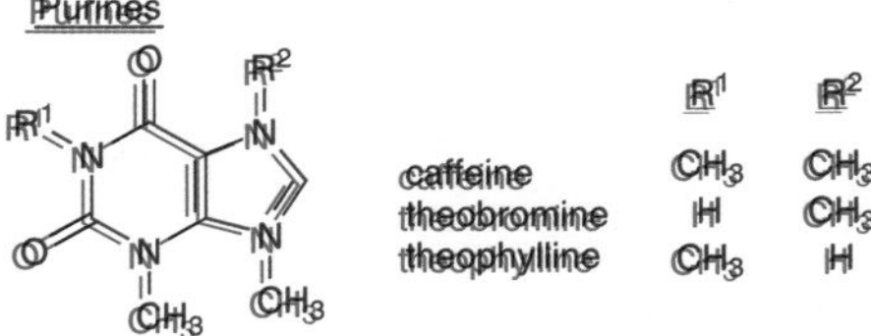

Triterpenes

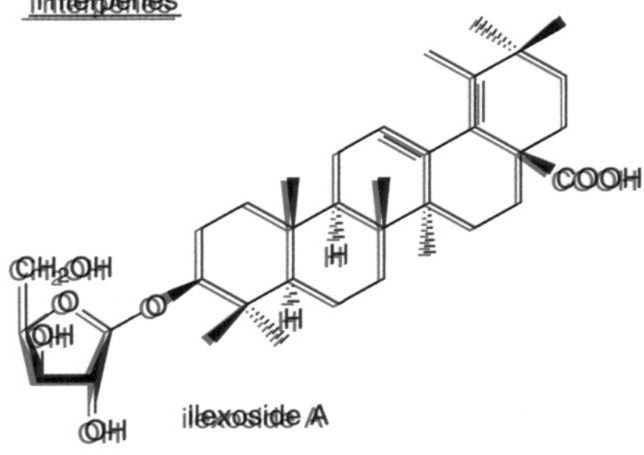

Figure 1 Selected constituents of maté.

Food Use

Maté is listed by the Council of Europe as a natural source of food flavouring (category N2). This category indicates that maté can be added to foodstuffs in small quantities, with a possible limitation of an active principle (as yet unspecified) in the final product.[G16] Maté is commonly consumed as a beverage. It is stated to be less astringent than tea.[G45] Previously, maté has been listed as GRAS (Generally Recognised As Safe).[G65]

Herbal Use

Maté is stated to possess CNS-stimulant, thymoleptic, diuretic, antirheumatic and mild analgesic properties. Traditionally, it has been used for psychogenic headache and fatigue, nervous depression, rheumatic pains, and specifically for headache associated with fatigue.[G2,G7,G8,G64]

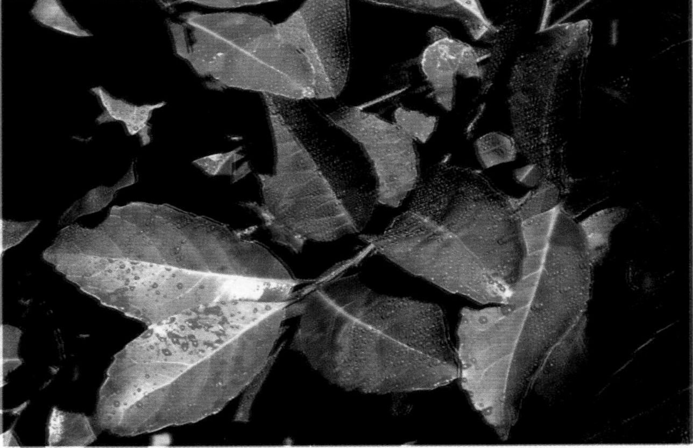

Figure 2 Maté (*Ilex paraguariensis*).

M

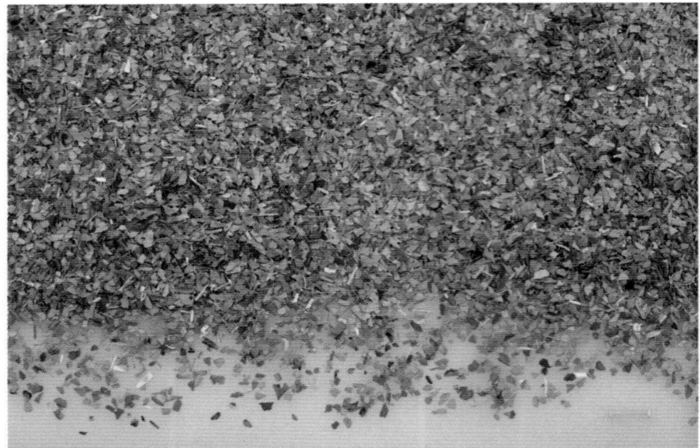

Figure 3 Maté – dried drug substance (leaf).

Dosage

Dosages for oral administration (adults) for traditional uses recommended in standard herbal reference texts are given below.

Dried leaf 2–4 g as an infusion three times daily.[G6, G7]

Liquid extract 2–4 mL (1 : 1 in 25% alcohol) three times daily.[G6, G7]

M

Pharmacological Actions

In vitro and animal studies

In vivo hypotensive activity in rats has been reported for an aqueous extract of *Ilex pubescens* (commonly referred to as maodong qing or MDQ) It was concluded that intravenous administration of MDQ releases histamine.[5]

Clinical studies

There is a lack of clinical research assessing the effects of maté and rigorous randomised controlled clinical trials are required.

The xanthine constituents, in particular caffeine, are the active principles in maté. The pharmacological actions of caffeine are well documented and include stimulation of the CNS, respiration and skeletal muscle, in addition to cardiac stimulation, coronary dilation, smooth muscle relaxation and diuresis.[G41] Reduction of appetite has been documented for maté.[1]

In China, MDQ is used parenterally for the treatment of cardiovascular diseases (hypotensive action).[1]

Side-effects, Toxicity

Side-effects generally associated with xanthine-containing beverages include sleeplessness, anxiety, tremor, palpitations and withdrawal headache.

Veno-occlusive disease of the liver in a young woman has been attributed to the consumption of large quantities of maté over a number of years.[G45] The association between consumption of maté infusions and oesophageal cancer has been investigated in Uruguay, where oesophageal cancer constitutes a major public health problem.[6, 7] Heavy consumption was reported to elevate the relative risk of oesophageal cancer by 6.5 and 34.6 in men and women, respectively.

The fatal dose of caffeine in humans is stated to be 10 g.[G41]

Contra-indications, Warnings

Warnings generally associated with caffeine are applicable, such as restricted intake by individuals with hypertension or a cardiac disorder.

Drug interactions None documented for maté. However, the potential for preparations of maté to interact with other medicines administered concurrently, particularly those with similar or opposing effects, should be considered. Warnings generally associated with caffeine are applicable.

Pregnancy and lactation It is generally recommended that caffeine consumption should be restricted during pregnancy, although conflicting results have been documented concerning the association between birth defects and caffeine consumption. In view of this, excessive consumption of maté during pregnancy should be avoided. Caffeine is excreted in breast milk, but at concentrations too low to represent a hazard to breastfed infants.[G45] As with all xanthine-containing beverages, excessive consumption of maté by breastfeeding mothers should be avoided.

References

1 Ohem N, Holzl J. Some new investigations on *Ilex paraguariensis* – Flavonoids and triterpenes. *Planta Med* 1988; 54: 576.
2 Inada A. Two new triterpenoid glycosides from the leaves of *Ilex chinensis*. *Chem Pharm Bull* 1987; 37: 884–885.
3 Hidaka K *et al*. New triterpene saponins from *Ilex pubescens*. *Chem Pharm Bull* 1987; 35: 524–529.
4 Willems M. Quantification and distribution of a novel cyanogenic glycoside in *Ilex aquifolium*. *Planta Med* 1989; 55: 114.
5 Yang ML, Pang PKT. The vascular effects of *Ilex pubescens*. *Planta Med* 1986; 52: 262–265.
6 Morton JF. The potential carcinogenicity of herbal tea. *Environ Carcino Rev. J Environ Sci Health* 1986; C4: 203–223.
7 Vassallo A *et al*. Esophageal cancer in Uruguay: a case control study. *J Natl Cancer Inst* 1985; 75: 1005–1009.

Meadowsweet

Summary and Pharmaceutical Comment

The chemistry of meadowsweet is characterised by a number of phenolic constituents, including flavonoids, salicylates and tannins. Documented scientific evidence from preclinical studies supports some of the antiseptic, antirheumatic and astringent traditional uses. However, there is a lack of clinical research assessing the efficacy and safety of meadowsweet. No documented toxicity data were located for meadowsweet and, in view of this, excessive use of meadowsweet and use during pregnancy and lactation should be avoided.

Species (Family)

Filipendula ulmaria (L.) Maxim. (Rosaceae)

Synonym(s)

Dropwort, Filipendula, Queen of the Meadow

Part(s) Used

Herb

Pharmacopoeial and Other Monographs

BHC 1992[G6]
BHP 1996[G9]
BP 2007[G84]
Complete German Commission E[G3]
Martindale 35th edition[G85]
Ph Eur 2007[G81]

Legal Category (Licensed Products)

GSL[G37]

Constituents

The following is compiled from several sources, including General References G2 and G6.

Flavonoids Flavonols, flavones, flavanones and chalcone derivatives (e.g. hyperoside[1] and spireoside,[2] kaempferol glucoside[3] and avicularin.[4]

Salicylates Main components of the volatile oil including salicylaldehyde (major, up to 70%), gaultherin, isosalicin, methyl salicylate, monotropitin, salicin, salicylic acid and spirein.[5–8]

Tannins 1% (alcoholic extract), 12.5% (aqueous extract).[5] Hydrolysable type;[9] leaf extracts have also yielded catechols,[1] compounds normally associated with condensed tannins.

Volatile oils Many phenolic components including salicylates (*see above*), benzyl alcohol, benzaldehyde, ethyl benzoate, heliotropin, phenylacetate, vanillin.[4,5]

Other constituents Coumarin (trace),[1] mucilage, carbohydrates and ascorbic acid (vitamin C).

Food Use

Meadowsweet is listed by the Council of Europe as a natural source of food flavouring (category N2). This category indicates that meadowsweet can be added to foodstuffs in small quantities, with a possible limitation of an active principle (as yet unspecified) in the final product.[G16] Previously, meadowsweet has been listed by the Food and Drugs Administration (FDA) as a Herb of Undefined Safety.[G22]

Herbal Use

Meadowsweet is stated to possess stomachic, mild urinary antiseptic, antirheumatic, astringent and antacid properties. Traditionally, it has been used for atonic dyspepsia with heartburn and hyperacidity, acute catarrhal cystitis, rheumatic muscle and joint pains, diarrhoea in children, and specifically for the prophylaxis and treatment of peptic ulcer.[G2,G6,G7,G8,G64]

Dosage

Dosages for oral administration (adults) for traditional uses recommended in standard herbal reference texts are given below.

Dried herb 4–6 g as an infusion three times daily.[G6,G7]

Liquid extract 1.5–6.0 mL (1 : 1 in 25% alcohol) three times daily.[G6,G7]

Tincture 2–4 mL (1 : 5 in 45% alcohol) three times daily.[G6,G7]

Pharmacological Actions

In vitro and animal studies

Lowering of motor activity and rectal temperature, myorelaxation and potentiation of narcotic action have been documented for meadowsweet.[5] In addition, flower extracts have been reported to

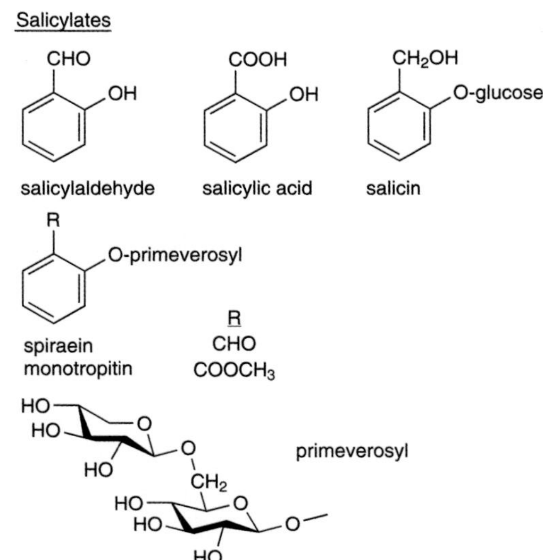

Figure 1 Selected constituents of meadowsweet.

M

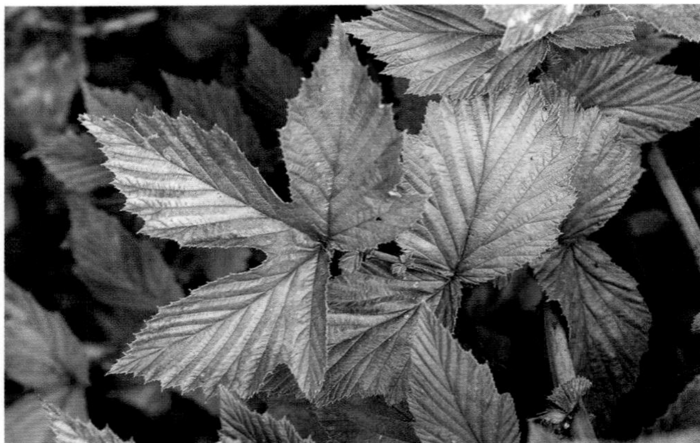

Figure 2 Meadowsweet (*Filipendula ulmaria*).

prolong life expectancy of mice, lower vascular permeability and prevent the development of stomach ulcers in rats and mice.[5, 10, 11] However, meadowsweet has also been reported to potentiate the ulcerogenic properties of histamine in the guinea-pig.[10] The anti-ulcer action documented for meadowsweet is associated with the aqueous extract and greatest activity has been observed with the flowers.[9, 11] Meadowsweet has been reported to increase bronchial tone in the cat[9] and to potentiate the bronchospastic properties of histamine in the guinea-pig.[9] *In vitro*, meadowsweet has been reported to increase intestinal tone in the guinea-pig and uterine tone in the rabbit.[9]

Bacteriostatic activity against *Staphylococcus aureus*, *Staphylococcus epidermidis*, *Escherichia coli*, *Proteus vulgaris* and *Pseudomonas aeruginosa* has been documented for flower extracts.[12]

M

Tannins are generally considered to possess astringent properties and have been reported as constituents of meadowsweet. Meadowsweet is stated to promote uric acid excretion.[G42]

Clinical studies

There is a lack of clinical research assessing the effects of meadowsweet and rigorous randomised controlled clinical trials are required.

Side-effects, Toxicity

None documented. However, there is a lack of clinical safety and toxicity data for meadowsweet and further investigation of these aspects is required.

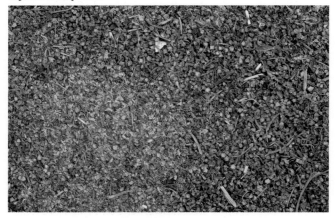

Figure 3 Meadowsweet – dried drug substance (herb).

Contra-indications, Warnings

Salicylate constituents have been documented and therefore the usual precautions recommended for salicylates are relevant for meadowsweet (*see* Willow). Meadowsweet is stated to be used for the treatment of diarrhoea in children, but in view of the salicylate constituents, this is not advisable.

Bronchospastic activity has been documented in preclinical studies and, therefore, it is prudent to advise that meadowsweet should be used with caution by asthmatics.

Aqueous extracts have been reported to contain high tannin concentrations and excessive consumption should therefore be avoided.

Drug interactions None documented. However, the potential for preparations of meadowsweet to interact with other medicines administered concurrently, particularly those with similar or opposing effects, should be considered.

Pregnancy and lactation *In vitro* utero-activity has been documented for meadowsweet. In view of the salicylate constituents and the lack of toxicity data, the use of meadowsweet during pregnancy and lactation should be avoided.

Preparations

Proprietary multi-ingredient preparations

Czech Republic: Antirevmaticky Caj. *France:* Mediflor Tisane Antirhumatismale No 2; Mediflor Tisane No 4 Diuretique; Polypirine. *Italy:* Pik Gel. *Spain:* Dolosul; Natusor Harpagosinol; Natusor Renal. *Switzerland:* Urinex. *UK:* Acidosis; Acidosis; Indigestion Mixture; Napiers Uva Ursi Tea; Roberts Acidosis Tablets. *USA:* Amerigel.

References

1 Genic AY, Ladnaya LY. Phytochemical study of *Filipendula ulmaria* Maxim. and *Filipendula hexapetala* Gilib. of flora of the Lvov region. *Farm Zh (Kiev)* 1980; 1: 50–52.
2 Novikova NN. Use of *Filipendula ulmaria* in medicine. *Tr Perm Farm Inst* 1969; 267–270.
3 Scheer T, Wichtl M. Zum Vorkommen von Kämpferol-4′-O-β-D-glucopyranoside in *Filipendula ulmaria* und *Allium cepa*. *Planta Med* 1987 53: 573–574.
4 Syuzeva ZF, Novikova NN. Flavonoid composition of *Filipendula ulmaria* queen-of-the meadow. *Nauch Tr Perm Farm Inst* 1973; 5: 2–26.
5 Barnaulov OD *et al.* Chemical composition and primary evaluation of the properties of preparations from *Filipendula ulmaria* (L.) Maxim flowers. *Rastit Resur* 1977; 13: 661–669.
6 Saifullina NA, Kozhina IS. Composition of essential oils from flowers of *Filipendula ulmaria*, *F. denudata*, and *F. stepposa*. *Rastit Resur* 1975; 11: 542–544.
7 Thieme H. Isolierung eines neuen phenolischen glykosids aus den blüten von *Filipendula ulmaria* (L.) Maxim. *Pharmazie* 1966; 21: 123.
8 Valle MG *et al.* Das ätherische öl aus *Filipendula ulmaria*. *Planta Med* 1988; 54: 181–182.
9 Barnaulov OD *et al.* Preliminary evaluation of the spasmolytic properties of some natural compounds and galenic preparations. *Rastit Resur* 1978; 14: 573–579.
10 Barnaulov OD, Denisenko PP. Antiulcerogenic action of the decoction from flowers of *Filipendula ulmaria* (L.). *Pharmakol-Toxicol (Moscow)* 1980; 43: 700–705.
11 Yanutsh AY *et al.* A study of the antiulcerative action of the extracts from the supernatant part and roots of *Filipendula ulmaria*. *Farm Zh (Kiev)* 1982; 37: 53–56.
12 Catanicin-Hintz I *et al.* Action of some plant extracts on the bacteria involved in urinary infections. *Clujul-Med* 1983; 56: 381–384.

Melissa

Summary and Pharmaceutical Comment

Randomised clinical trials have suggested that topical lemon balm extract may have some effects on healing cutaneous lesions resulting from HSV-1 virus infection, although further rigorous studies are required to determine whether there is any effect on recurrence of infection. There is some evidence from randomised controlled trials of combination preparations containing lemon balm leaf extract to support the efficacy of such products in individuals with minor sleep disorders, there has been little investigation of the effects of lemon balm extract alone on sleep quality. Further studies are required to determine the effects of preparations of lemon balm leaf extract in individuals with sleep disorders. Supporting evidence for the use of lemon balm for gastrointestinal complaints is limited to *in vitro* work and requires clinical investigation.

Small-scale, short-term studies indicate that oral combination preparations containing lemon balm extract and topical preparations of lemon balm extract are well tolerated. However, there is a lack of research investigating the safety of long-term administration of lemon balm. In view of the lack of toxicity data, oral administration of lemon balm during pregnancy and lactation should be avoided.

Species (Family)

Melissa officinalis L. (Labiatae/Lamiaceae)

Synonym(s)

Balm, *Faucibarba officinalis* (L.) Dulac, Honeyplant, Lemon Balm, *Mutelia officinalis* (L.) Gren. ex Mutel, Sweet Balm, *Thymus melissa* Krause

Part(s) Used

Dried leaves and flowering tops

Pharmacopoeial and Other Monographs

BHP 1996[G9]
BP 2007 (Lemon Balm)[G84]
Complete German Commission E (Lemon Balm)[G3]
ESCOP 2003[G76]
Martindale 35th edition[G85]
Ph Eur 2007[G81]

Legal Category (Licensed Products)

GSL[G37]

Constituents

The following is compiled from several sources, including General References G2 and G52.

Volatile oil 0.06–0.375% v/m.[1, G52] Contains at least 70 components,[G2] including: *monoterpenes* >60%. Mainly aldehydes, including citronellal, geranial, neral; also citronellol, geraniol, nerol, β-ocimene.[2, 3] *Sesquiterpenes* >35%. β-Caryophyllene, germacrene D.

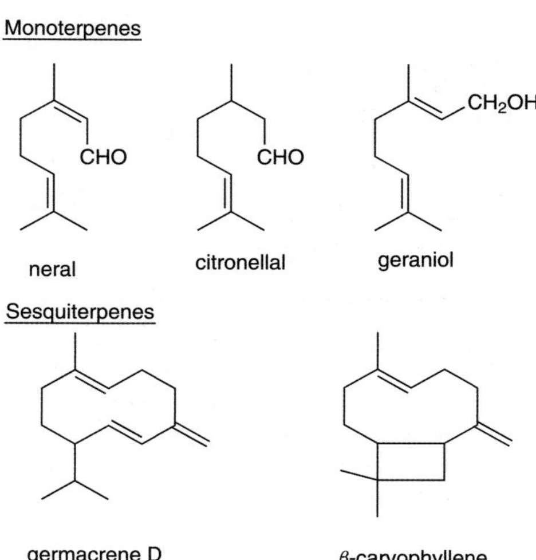

Figure 1 Selected constituents of melissa.

Flavonoids 0.5%. Including glycosides of luteolin (e.g. luteolin 3′-*O*-β-D-glucuronide),[4] quercetin, apigenin and kaempferol.

Polyphenols Protocatechuic acid, hydroxycinnamic acid derivatives,[2] caffeic acid, chlorogenic acid, rosmarinic acid,[2] 2-(3′,4′-dihydroxyphenyl)-1,3-benzodioxole-5-aldehyde.[5]

Food Use

Lemon balm is used to give fragrance to wine, tea and beer. Lemon balm (herb, flowers, flower tips) is listed by the Council of Europe as a natural source of food flavouring (category N2). This category indicates that lemon balm can be added to foodstuffs in small quantities, with a possible limitation of an active principle (as yet unspecified) in the final product.[G16] Previously, lemon balm has been listed as GRAS (Generally Recognised As Safe).[G65]

Herbal Use

Lemon balm has been used traditionally for its sedative, spasmolytic and antibacterial properties.[G54] It is also stated to be a carminative, diaphoretic and a febrifuge,[G64] and has been used for headaches, gastrointestinal disorders, nervousness and rheumatism.[5] Current interest is focused on its use as a sedative, and topically in herpes simplex labialis as a result of infection with herpes simplex virus type 1 (HSV-1). The German Commission E monographs state that lemon balm can be used for nervous sleeping disorders and functional gastrointestinal complaints.[G4]

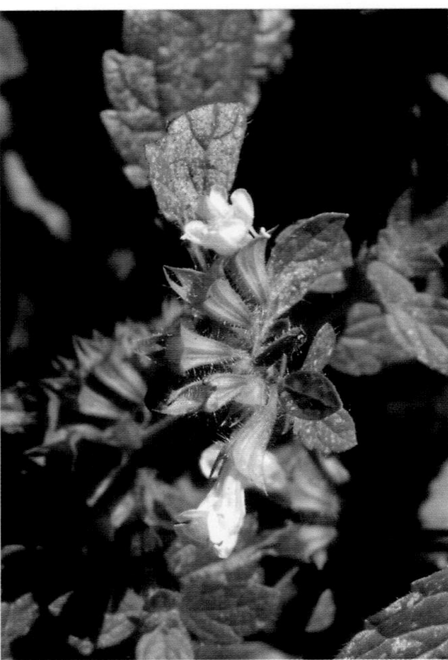

Figure 2 Melissa (*Melissa officinalis*).

Dosage

Dosages for oral administration (adults) for traditional uses recommended in standard herbal reference texts are given below.

Dried herb 1.5–4.5 g as an infusion in 150 mL water several times daily.[G4]

Topical application Cream containing 1% of a lyophilised aqueous extract of dried leaves of *Melissa officinalis* (70 : 1) two to four times daily.[G52]

Pharmacological Actions

In vitro and animal studies

Antiviral activity Aqueous extracts of *Melissa officinalis* have been reported to inhibit the development of several viruses.[6–8, G52] The virucidal effect of several aqueous extracts of *M. officinalis* against HSV-1 has been demonstrated in a rabbit kidney cell line.[9] However, the extracts appeared to have no activity against experimental HSV-1 infection in the eyes of rabbits.[9]

Anti-human immunodeficiency virus type 1 (HIV-1) activity has been reported for an aqueous extract of *M. officinalis* in *in vitro* studies using MT-4 cells; the ED_{50} (50% effective dose for inhibition of HIV-1-induced cytopathogenicity) was found to be 16 μg/mL.[10] Furthermore, the aqueous extract demonstrated potent inhibitory activity (ED_{50} = 62 μg/mL) against HIV-1 replication (KK-1 strain, freshly isolated from a patient with acquired immune deficiency syndrome (AIDS). In other *in vitro* studies, an aqueous extract of *M. officinalis* inhibited giant cell formation in co-cultures of MOLT-4 cells with and without HIV-1 infection, and showed inhibitory activity against HIV-1 reverse transcriptase (ED_{50} = 1.6 μg/mL).[10]

Aqueous extracts of *M. officinalis* have been reported to inhibit protein biosynthesis in a cell-free system from rat liver cells, and it has been suggested that this effect may be due to caffeic acid and a component isolated from the glycoside fraction of the extract.[11] The latter component appears to block the binding of the elongation factor EF-2 to ribosomes, thus terminating peptide elongation.[11]

Antimicrobial activity Antimicrobial activity of essential oil extracted from *M. officinalis* by steam distillation, determined using a micro-atmospheric technique, has been reported against the yeasts *Candida albicans* and *Saccharomyces cerevisiae*, and against *Pseudomonas putida*, *Staphylococcus aureus*, *Micrococcus luteus*, *Mycobacterium smegmatis*, *Proteus vulgaris*, *Shigella sonnei* and *Escherichia coli*.[12]

Other activity In studies in mice, a hydroalcoholic extract of *M. officinalis* leaves administered intraperitoneally significantly reduced behavioural activity in two tests, compared with control, suggesting that the extract has sedative effects.[13] In both tests, the effect was maximum at 25 mg/kg. The same extract demonstrated peripheral analgesic activity by reducing acetic acid-induced writhing and stretching in mice when administered intraperitoneally at doses of 25–1600 mg/kg 30 minutes after intraperitoneal administration of 1.2% acetic acid solution.[13] However, no analgesic effects were observed on heat-induced pain (hotplate test) which suggests a lack of central analgesic activity. In other tests, low doses (3 and 6 mg/kg) of a hydroalcoholic extract of *M. officinalis* leaves administered intraperitoneally induced sleep in mice given an infrahypnotic dose of pentobarbital.[13] By contrast, in the same battery of tests, essential oil obtained from *M. officinalis* by distillation did not demonstrate sedative or sleep-inducing effects.[13]

A 30% alcoholic extract of *M. officinalis* demonstrated an antispasmodic effect on rat duodenum *in vitro*.[14]

Aqueous methanolic extracts of the aerial parts of *M. officinalis* demonstrated inhibition of lipid peroxidation *in vitro* in both enzyme-dependent and enzyme-independent systems.[15] The same tests carried out on the main known phenolic components of *M. officinalis* revealed that rosmarinic acid, caffeic acid, luteolin and luteolin-7-*O*-glucoside were more potent inhibitors of enzyme-dependent lipid peroxidation than enzyme-independent lipid peroxidation.

Clinical studies

Antiviral effects The effects of a topical preparation of a standardised aqueous extract of *M. officinalis* leaves (drug/extract 70 : 1) have been investigated in herpes simplex virus (HSV) infection. In an open, multicentre study, 115 patients with

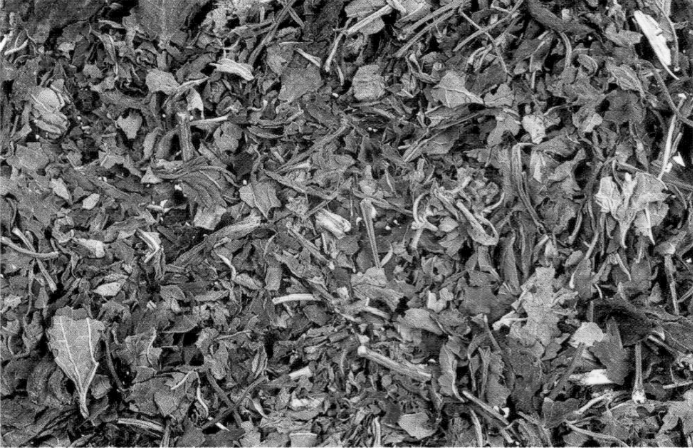

Figure 3 Melissa – dried drug substance (leaf and flowering tops).

HSV infection of the skin or transitional mucosa applied lemon balm leaf extract five times daily for a maximum of 14 days; complete healing of lesions was achieved after eight days of treatment in 96% of participants.[16,17] Subsequently, a randomised, double-blind, placebo-controlled trial involving 116 patients with HSV infection of the skin or transitional mucosa reported statistically significant differences between the treatment (applied locally two to four times daily over 5–10 days) and placebo groups for some (including redness, physician's assessment, patient's assessment), but not all, outcome measures (e.g. extent of scabbing, vesication, pain).[17] Another randomised, double-blind trial that involved 66 patients with an acute episode of recurrent (at least four episodes per year) herpes simplex labialis compared verum cream (applied on the affected area four times daily over five days) with placebo.[18] There was a significant difference in the primary outcome measure – symptom score after two days' treatment – between the two groups ($p = 0.042$). However, further investigation is required to determine if time to recurrence is prolonged.

Sedative effects The acute sedative effects of several plant extracts, including a preparation of *M. officinalis* leaves, were explored in a randomised, double-blind, placebo-controlled, crossover study involving 12 healthy volunteers.[19] *M. officinalis* extract 1200 mg was administered orally as a single dose about two hours before administration of caffeine 100 mg. Melissa extract was one of the extracts tested that showed least effects on increasing tiredness (i.e. it was no different from placebo) as measured using a visual analogue scale score for alertness.

Several other studies have investigated the sedative effects of combination preparations containing extracts of lemon balm and valerian (*Valeriana officinalis*). A randomised, double-blind trial involving healthy volunteers who received Songha Night (*V. officinalis* root extract 120 mg and *M. officinalis* leaf extract 80 mg) three tablets daily taken as one dose 30 minutes before bedtime for 30 days ($n = 66$), or placebo ($n = 32$), found that the proportion of participants reporting an improvement in sleep quality was significantly greater for the treatment group, compared with the placebo group (33.3% versus 9.4%, respectively; $p = 0.04$).[20] However, analysis of visual analogue scale scores revealed only a slight but statistically non-significant improvement in sleep quality in both groups over the treatment period. Another double-blind, placebo-controlled trial involving patients with insomnia who received Euvegal forte (valerian extract 160 mg and lemon balm extract 80 mg) two tablets daily for two weeks reported significant improvements in sleep quality in recipients of the herbal preparation, compared with placebo recipients.[21] A placebo-controlled study involving 'poor sleepers' who received Euvegal forte reported significant improvements in sleep efficiency and in sleep stages three and four in the treatment group, compared with placebo recipients.[22]

Other studies have investigated the sedative effects of combination preparations of extracts of lemon balm, valerian and hops (*Humulus lupulus*). In an open, uncontrolled, multicentre study, 225 individuals who were experiencing nervous agitation and/or difficulties falling asleep and achieving uninterrupted sleep were treated for two weeks with a combination preparation containing extracts of valerian root, hop grains and lemon balm leaves.[23] Significant improvements in the severity and frequency of symptoms were reported, compared with the pretreatment period. Difficulties falling asleep, difficulties sleeping through the night, and nervous agitation were improved in 89%, 80% and 82% of participants, respectively.

Side-effects, Toxicity

Small-scale, short-term (two weeks' duration) studies investigating the sedative effects of oral combination preparations containing lemon balm extract indicate that these preparations are well-tolerated and do not appear to induce a 'hangover effect'. In an open, uncontrolled, multicentre study, 225 individuals who were experiencing nervous agitation and/or difficulties falling asleep and achieving uninterrupted sleep were treated for two weeks with a combination preparation containing extracts of valerian root, hop grains and lemon balm leaves.[23] The tolerability of the preparation was rated as 'good' or 'very good' by 97% of physicians and 96% of patients. In a randomised, double-blind, placebo-controlled trial involving healthy volunteers who received Songha Night (*V. officinalis* root 120 mg and *M. officinalis* leaf extract 80 mg) three tablets daily for 30 days ($n = 66$), or placebo ($n = 32$), the proportion of volunteers reporting adverse events was similar in both groups (around 28%).[20] Sleep disturbances and tiredness were the most common adverse events reported during the study. (Note: the study was designed to assess the effects of the preparation on sleep quality.) No severe adverse events were reported. A randomised, double-blind, placebo-controlled study involving 48 adults assessed the adverse effects of two weeks' treatment with a combination preparation (valerian root extract 95 mg, hops extract 15 mg and lemon balm leaf extract 85 mg) taken alone or with alcohol.[24] Compared with placebo, the herbal combination preparation did not have adverse effects on performance (e.g. concentration, vigilance). Furthermore, co-administration of the combination preparation with alcohol did not have potentiating effects on performance parameters.[24] No serious adverse events were observed during the study.

A randomised, double-blind, placebo-controlled trial of a topical preparation containing 1% dried extract of *M. officinalis* leaves (drug/extract 70 : 1) involving 116 patients with HSV infection of the skin or transitional mucosa reported that there were no statistically significant differences between the treatment and placebo groups with regard to the frequency of adverse effects.[17] Adverse events reported were minor (irritation, burning sensation); there were no reports of allergic contact reactions. However, skin sensitisation may occur with melissa.[G58]

M

Contra-indications, Warnings

None documented.

Drug interactions None documented. However, the potential for preparations of melissa to interact with other medicines administered concurrently, particularly those with similar or opposing effects, should be considered.

Pregnancy and lactation In view of the lack of toxicity data, oral administration of lemon balm during pregnancy and lactation should be avoided. Topical use of lemon balm during pregnancy and lactation is unlikely to be problematic.

Preparations

Proprietary single-ingredient preparations

Austria: Lomaherpan. *Belgium:* Dormiplant. *Chile:* Citromel. *Czech Republic:* Lakinal; Medovka Lekarska; Medunkovy, Medunkova. *Germany:* Gastrovegetalin; Lomaherpan; Me-Sabona; Sedinfant. *Russia:* Novo-Passit (Ново-Пассит). *Switzerland:* Valverde Boutons de fievre creme.

Proprietary multi-ingredient preparations

Argentina: Nervocalm; Valeriana Oligoplex. *Australia:* Natural Deep Sleep. *Austria:* Abdomilon N; Baldracin; Euvekan; Mariazeller; Passedan; Passelyt; Sedogelat; Songha; Species nervinae; The Chambard-Tee; Wechseltee St Severin. *Belgium:* Songha. *Brazil:* Balsamo Branco; Calmapax; Elixir de Passiflora; Passaneuro; Passilex; Sonhare. *Canada:* Herbal Sleep Well. *Chile:* Melipass; Recalm. *Czech Republic:* Alvisan Neo; Baldracin; Blahungstee N; Eugastrin; Euvekan; Fytokliman Planta; Hertz- und Kreislauftee; Hypotonicka; Melaton; Nervova Cajova Smes; Nontusyl; Novo-Passit; Persen; Schlaf-Nerventee N; Songha Night; Species Nervinae Planta; Valofyt Neo. *France:* Biocarde; Dystolise; Elixir Bonjean; Mediflor Tisane Calmante Troubles du Sommeil No 14; Mediflor Tisane Circulation du Sang No 12; Vagostabyl. *Germany:* Abdomilon; Abdomilon N; Baldriparan N Stark; Dormarist; Dr. Scheffler Bergischer Krautertee Nerven- und Beruhigungstee; Euvegal Entspannungs- und Einschlaftropfen; Gutnacht; Gutnacht; Heumann Beruhigungstee Tenerval; Iberogast; Jukunda Melissen-Krautergeist N; Klosterfrau Melisana; Lindofluid N; Me-Sabona plus; Melissengeist; Oxacant-sedativ; Pascosedon; Phytonoctu; Plantival novo; Pronervon Phyto; Schlaf- und Nerventee; Sedacur; Sedariston plus; Stullmaton. *Hungary:* Euvekan. *Israel:* Songha Night. *Italy:* Colimil; Dormiplant; Emmenoiasi; Sedatol; Tisana Kelemata. *Mexico:* Nordimenty; Plantival. *New Zealand:* Botanica Hayfever; Mr Nits. *Portugal:* Erpecalm; Songha. *Russia:* Doppelherz Melissa (Доппельгерц Мелисса); Doppelherz Vitalotonik (Доппельгерц Виталотоник); Persen (Персен). *South Africa:* Melissengeist; Spiritus Contra Tussim Drops. *Spain:* Agua del Carmen; Caramelos Agua del Carmen; Himelan; Jaquesor; Mesatil; Natusor Aerofane; Natusor Jaquesan; Nervikan; Relana; Resolutivo Regium; Solucion Schoum. *Switzerland:* Arterosan Plus; Baldriparan; Cardiaforce; Carmol; Dormiplant; Dragees pour la detente nerveuse; Gastrosan; Hyperiforce comp; Iberogast; Relaxane; Relaxo; Songha Night; Soporin; Tisane calmante pour les enfants; Tisane favorisant l'allaitement; Tisane pour l'estomac; Tisane pour le coeur et la circulation; Tisane pour le sommeil et les nerfs; Tisane pour nourissons et enfants; Valverde Detente dragees; Valviska. *UK:* Boots Alternatives Sleep Well; Boots Sleepeaze Herbal Tablets; Melissa Comp.; Napiers Echinacea Tea; Valerina Day Time; Valerina Day-Time; Valerina Night-Time; Valerina Night-Time.

References

1 Tittel G *et al*. Über die chemische Zusammensetzung von Melissenölen. *Planta Med* 1982; 46: 91–98.

2 Carnat AP *et al*. The aromatic and polyphenolic composition of lemon balm (*Melissa officinalis* L. subsp. officinalis) tea. *Pharm Acta Helv* 1998; 72: 301–305.

3 Sarer E, Kökdil G. Constituents of the essential oil from *Melissa officinalis*. *Planta Med* 1991; 57: 89–90.

4 Heitz A *et al*. Luteolin 3′-glucuronide, the major flavonoid from *Melissa officinalis* subsp. *officinalis*. *Fitoterapia* 2000; 71: 201–202.

5 Tagashira M, Ohtake Y. A new antioxidative 1,3-benzodioxole from *Melissa officinalis*. *Planta Med* 1998; 64: 555–558.

6 Kucera LS, Herrmann ECJr. Antiviral substances in plants of the mint family (Labiatae). I Tannin of *Melissa officinalis*. *Proc Soc Exp Biol Med* 1967; 124: 865–869.

7 Herrmann ECJr, Kucera LS. Antiviral substances in plants of the mint family (Labiatae). II Nontannin polyphenol of *Melissa officinalis*. *Proc Soc Exp Biol Med* 1967; 124: 869–874.

8 May G, Willuhn G. Antivirale Wirkung wässriger Pflanzenextrakte in Gewebekulturen. *Arzneimittelforschung* 1978; 28: 1–7.

9 Dimitrova Z *et al*. Antiherpes effect of *Melissa officinalis* L. extracts. *Acta Microbiol Bulg* 1993; 29: 65–72.

10 Yamasaki K *et al*. Anti-HIV-1 activity of herbs in Labiatae. *Biol Pharm Bull* 1998; 21: 829–833.

11 Chlabicz J, Galasinski W. The components of *Melissa officinalis* L. that influence protein biosynthesis in-vitro. *J Pharm Pharmacol* 1986; 38: 791–794.

12 Larrondo JV *et al*. Antimicrobial activity of essences from labiates. *Microbios* 1995; 82: 171–2.

13 Soulimani R *et al*. Neurotropic action of the hydroalcoholic extract of *Melissa officinalis* in the mouse. *Planta Med* 1991; 57: 105–109.

14 Soulimani R *et al*. Recherche de l'activitébiologique de *Melissa officinalis L.* sur le système nerveux central de la souris in vivo et le duodenum de rat in vitro. *Plantes Méd Phytothér* 1993; 26: 77–85.

15 Hohmann J *et al*. Protective effects of the aerial parts of *Salvia officinalis*, *Melissa officinalis* and *Lavandula angustifolia* and their constituents against enzyme-dependent and enzyme-independent lipid peroxidation. *Planta Med* 1999; 65: 576–578.

16 Wölbling RH, Milbradt R. Klinik und Therapie des Herpes simplex. *Therapiewoche* 1984; 34: 1193–1200.

17 Wölbling RH, Leonhardt K. Local therapy of herpes simplex with dried extract from *Melissa officinalis*. *Phytomedicine* 1994; 1: 25–31.

18 Koytchev R *et al*. Balm mint extract (Lo-701) for topical treatment of recurring Herpes labialis. *Phytomedicine* 1999; 6: 225–230.

19 Schulz H *et al*. The quantitative EEG as a screening instrument to identify sedative effects of single doses of plant extracts in comparison with diazepam. *Phytomedicine* 1998; 5: 449–458.

20 Cerny A, Schmid K. Tolerability and efficacy of valerian/lemon balm in healthy volunteers (a double-blind, placebo-controlled, multicentre study). *Fitoterapia* 1999; 70: 221–228.

21 Dressing H *et al*. Verbesserung der Schlafqualität mit einem hochdosierten Baldrian-Melisse-Präparat. Eine plazebokontrollierte Doppelblindstudie. *Psychopharmakotherapie* 1996; 3: 123–130.

22 Dressing H *et al*. Baldrian-Melisse-Kombinationen versus Benzodiazepin. Bei Schlafstörungen gleichwertig? *Therapiewoche* 1992; 42: 726–736.

23 Orth-Wagner S *et al*. Phytosedativum gegen Schlafstärungen. *Z Phytother* 1995; 16: 147–156.

24 Herberg K-W. Nebenwirkungen pflanzlicher Beruhigungsmittel. *Z Allgemeinmed* 1996; 72: 234–240.

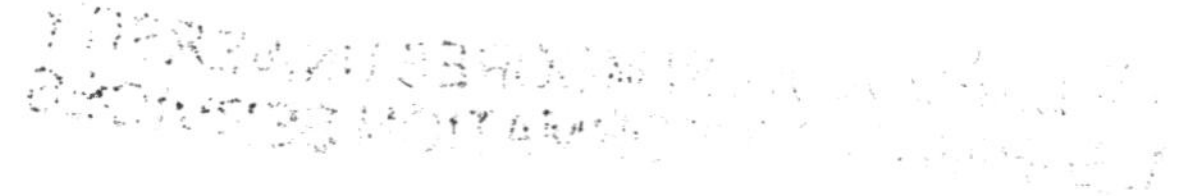

Milk Thistle

Summary and Pharmaceutical Comment

The chemistry of milk thistle is well-documented and there is good evidence that silymarin and its components, particularly silibinin, are responsible for the pharmacological effects.

Documented scientific evidence from *in vitro* and animal studies provides supportive evidence for some of the uses of milk thistle, particularly those relating to hepatoprotective properties.

There have been several controlled clinical trials investigating the effects of milk thistle in a range of liver disorders, including acute viral hepatitis, chronic hepatitis, alcoholic liver disease, cirrhosis and toxic liver damage. The results of these studies are not entirely consistent or conclusive. In addition, some trials have methodological shortcomings, for example the inclusion of patients with different liver disorders, small numbers of patients and failure to control or monitor alcohol intake. Further, well-designed, clinical trials in clearly defined patient groups are required in order to establish the efficacy of milk thistle and its components in different liver disorders. In Germany, milk thistle is approved for the treatment of toxic liver disorders and as a supportive treatment in chronic inflammatory liver disease and hepatic cirrhosis.[G3]

Teas prepared from milk thistle fruits or herb are not commonly used as only a small proportion of silymarin gets into the aqueous extract such that pharmacologically active doses are not attained. For this reason, in Germany teas are recommended only as supportive treatment in functional gall bladder disorders and not for antihepatotoxic effects.[G2] In Germany, milk thistle fruit (3–5 g) as an infusion three or four times daily is also indicated for mild digestive disorders.[G2]

There are some toxicity and safety data for milk thistle which, together with data on the adverse effects reported in clinical trials, provide good evidence for the safety of milk thistle when used at recommended doses in the short term. However, further data on the long-term safety of milk thistle use are required.

Species (Family)

Silybum marianum (L.) Gaertn. (Asteraceae/Compositae)

Synonym(s)

Lady's Thistle, *Mariana lactea* Hill, Marian Thistle, Mediterranean Milk Thistle, St Mary's Thistle.

Part(s) Used

Fruits (often referred to as 'seeds'), herb

Pharmacopoeial and Other Monographs

BHP 1996[G9]
BP 2007[G84]
Complete German Commission E[G3]
Martindale 35th edition[G85]
Ph Eur 2007[G81]
USP29/NF24[G86]

Legal Category (Licensed Products)

Milk thistle is not included in the GSL.[G37]

Constituents

The following is compiled from several sources, including General Reference G2.

Fruit

Flavolignans 1.5–3% silymarin, a mixture containing approximately 50% silibinin (= silybin, silybinin), silichristin and silidianin, as well as silimonin, isosilichristin, isosilibinin, silandrin, silhermin, neosilihermins A and B, 2,3-dehydrosilibinin and tri- to pentamers of silibinin (silybinomers).[1]

Flavonoids Quercetin, taxifolin and dehydrokaempferol.[1]

Lipids 20–30%. Linoleic acid, oleic acid and palmitic acid.

Sterols Cholesterol, campesterol and stigmasterol.

Other constituents Mucilages, sugars (arabinose, rhamnose, xylose, glucose), amines and saponins.[1]

Leaves

Flavonoids Apigenin, luteolin and kaempferol and their glycosides.[1]

Other constituents β-Sitosterol and its glucoside, and a triterpene acetate.[1]

Silymarin is not found in the leaves.

Food Use

Milk thistle is not used in foods.

Herbal Use

Traditionally, milk thistle fruits have been used for disorders of the liver, spleen and gall bladder such as jaundice and gall bladder colic. Milk thistle has also been used for nursing mothers for stimulating milk production, as a bitter tonic, for haemorrhoids, for dyspeptic complaints and as a demulcent in catarrah and pleurisy.[G2, G32, G34, G35, G50, G64] It is stated to possess hepatoprotective, antioxidant and choleretic properties.[1, 2]

Current interest is focused on the hepatoprotective activity of milk thistle and its use in the prophylaxis and treatment of liver damage and disease.

The leaves have also been used for the treatment of liver, spleen and gall bladder disorders and as an antimalarial, emmenagogue and for uterine complaints. Milk thistle leaf preparations are available today, although most research has been conducted with preparations of the fruit since the leaf does not contain the pharmacologically active component silymarin.

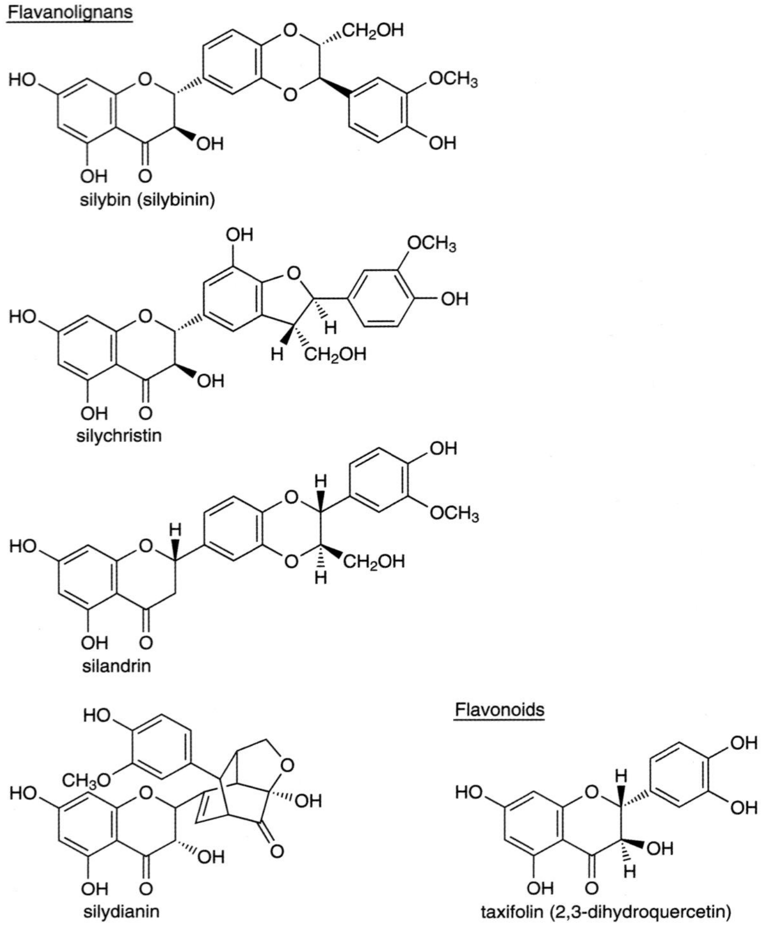

Flavanolignans

silybin (silybinin)

silychristin

silandrin

silydianin

Flavonoids

taxifolin (2,3-dihydroquercetin)

Figure 1 Selected constituents of milk thistle.

Dosage

Dosages for oral administration (adults) for traditional uses recommended in standard herbal reference texts are given below.

Fruit Crude drug 12–15 g daily in divided doses (equivalent to silymarin 200–400 mg daily).[G3]

Herb Approximately 1.5 g of finely chopped material as a tea, two or three cups daily.

The doses of silymarin used in clinical trials have ranged from 280–800 mg/day (equivalent to milk thistle extract 400–1140 mg/day standardised to contain 70% silibinin).[3] For hepatic disorders, doses of up to 140 mg (equivalent to 60 mg silibinin) two or three times daily have been suggested.[G43]

In Germany, the recommended regimen for treatment of *Amanita phalloides* poisoning with a standardised silymarin preparation (Legalon) is a total dose of silibinin (as the disodium dihemisuccinate) (20 mg/kg body weight) over 24 hours, divided into four intravenous infusions each given over a 2-hour period.[G43, G55]

Pharmacological Actions

Several pharmacological activities have been documented for milk thistle fruit, including hepatoprotective, antioxidant, anti-inflammatory, antifibrotic and antitumour properties, as well as inhibition of lipid peroxidation, stimulation of protein biosynthesis and acceleration of liver regeneration. Silymarin (an isomer mixture comprising mainly silibinin, silichristin and silidianin) is the pharmacologically active component of milk thistle fruit; silibinin is the main component of silymarin. There is an extensive literature on the pharmacological effects of silymarin and silibinin, particularly with regard to their hepatoprotective activity which provides supporting evidence for the clinical uses. The pharmacology and clinical efficacy of milk thistle have been reviewed.[1–3, G50, G55] The following represents a summary of selected publications on this subject.

There is a lack of research investigating the pharmacological effects of preparations of milk thistle leaf.[G2, G32, G35]

In vitro and animal studies

Antioxidant activity Silymarin and silibinin (silybin) are antioxidants that react with free radicals (e.g. reactive oxygen species) transforming them into more stable and less reactive compounds.[1, 4–6] Silymarin and silybin have been reported to inihibit lipid peroxidation induced by iron-linked systems in rat liver microsomes[7, 8] and protect against phenylhydrazine-induced lipid peroxidation in rat erythrocytes.[1] Furthermore, in rats, intraperitoneal silymarin has been shown to increase total glutathione in the liver, intestine and stomach and to improve the reduced glutathione to oxidised glutathione ratio.[9] Silymarin has been shown to inhibit copper-induced oxidation of human

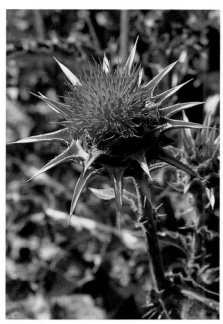

Figure 2 Milk thistle (*Silybum marianum*).

low-density lipoprotein (LDL) *in vitro* in a concentration-dependent manner.[10] Silybin appears to be the constituent of silymarin responsible for the LDL antioxidant effect. In contrast, silichristin and silydianin appeared to act as pro-oxidants, but without significantly reducing the total LDL antioxidant capacity of silymarin.

Free radicals are recognised as having an important role in several pathological processes, including inflammation, necrosis, fibrosis, atherosclerosis, carcinogenesis and ageing and in the hepatotoxic mechanisms of various substances. The antioxidant activity of silymarin is thought to contibute to its hepatoprotective properties.[11, G55]

Hepatoprotective properties *In vitro* studies using isolated hepatocytes have documented the protective activity of silymarin and several of its components against cell damage induced by various cytotoxic substances.[1]

In vivo studies in rats and mice have demonstrated the hepatoprotective activity of silymarin and silybin in acute liver toxicity induced by various toxic agents with different mechanisms of action, including carbon tetrachloride, galactosamine, thioacetamide, ethanol, paracetamol (acetaminophen), thallium, phalloidin and α-amanitin (the main toxic constituents of the mushroom *A. phalloides*).[1] Experimental studies in chronic liver toxicity induced by repeated administration of carbon tetrachloride, heavy metals, thioacetamide and several drugs, including azathioprine and indometacin, have also demonstrated that administration of silymarin and silybin protects against damage.[1] Other studies have reported protective effects of silymarin against liver injury induced by ischaemia[12] and gamma irradiation.[13]

Studies in rabbits fed a high-fat diet for 12 weeks have shown that histopathological alterations were least advanced in animals which also received a silymarin–phospholipid complex.[14] In rats, silymarin inhibited the development of diet-induced hypercholesterolaemia.[15] The hypocholesterolaemic effects of silymarin may be due to the effects of silymarin on lipoprotein metabolism.[16]

The effects of silymarin on biliary bile salt secretion have been seen in studies in rats.[17] Intraperitoneal silymarin (25, 50, 100 and 150 mg/kg/day) for five days induced a dose-dependent increase in bile flow and bile salt secretion. Stimulation of bile salt secretion was mainly accounted for by an increase in the biliary secretion of the hepatoprotective bile salts β-muricholate and ursodeoxycholate.

Nephroprotective properties Silibinin injected into rats prior to administration of cisplatin afforded protection of glomerular and proximal tubular function.[18, 19] Silibinin does not affect the cytotoxic activity of cisplatin.[19] Intraperitoneal silibinin (5 mg/kg) administered to rats 30 minutes before ciclosporin decreased ciclosporin-induced lipid peroxidation but produced no protective effect on the glomerular filtration rate.[20]

Anticancer activity Silybin at concentrations of 0.1–20 μmol/L inhibited the growth of drug-resistant ovarian cancer cells and doxorubicin-resistant breast cancer cells *in vitro*.[21] Furthermore, silybin in the range of 0.1–1.0 μmol/L potentiated the effect of cisplatin and doxorubicin in experimental tumour cell lines. When applied to the skin of SENCAR mice, silymarin gave protection against the effects of the tumour promoters 12-O-tetradecanoylphorbol (TPA) and okaidic acid (OA).[22] Topical application of silymarin prior to that of TPA and OA completely inhibited induction of tumour necrosis factor α (TNFα) mRNA expression in the epidermis. Substantial protection from photocarcinogenesis in mice treated with phorbol ester or 7,12-dimethylbenz(*a*)anthracene has been demonstrated.[23] The antitumour effect is primarily at stage 1 tumour promotion and silymarin acts by inhibiting cyclooxygenase 2 (COX-2) and interleukin 1α (IL-1α).[24] Such effects may involve inhibition of promoter-induced oedema, hyperplasia, the proliferation index and oxidant state.[25]

Treatment of serum-starved human prostate carcinoma DU145 cells with silymarin resulted in significant inhibition of transforming growth factor α (TGFα)-mediated activation of the epidermal growth factor receptor erbB1.[26] There was also a decrease in tyrosine phosphorylation of an immediate downstream target, the adapter protein SHC, together with a decrease in binding to erbB1. In the silymarin-treated cell lines there was a significant induction of the cyclin-dependent kinase inhibitors (CDKIs) Cip1/p21 and Kip/p27 concomitant with a significant decrease in CDK4 expression, but no changes in the levels of CDK2 and CDK6 and their associated cyclins E and D1, respectively. Additional experiments showed that there was a significant inhibition of constitutive tyrosine phosphorylation of both erbB1 and SHC, but

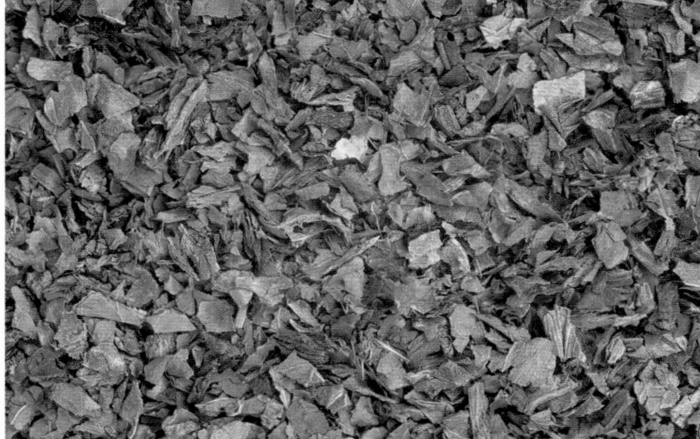

Figure 3 Milk thistle – dried drug substance (leaf).

no changes in their protein levels. The results indicated that silymarin may exert a strong anticarcinogenic effect against prostate cancer and that this effect is likely to involve impairment of the erbB1–SHC-mediated signalling pathway, induction of CDKIs and resultant G_1 arrest.[26]

There was a significant inhibition of mitogen-activated protein kinase (MAPK) ERK activity at lower doses in epidermal A431 cells treated with silymarin, whereas higher doses activated MAPK/JNK1.[27] Silymarin exerted a strong anticarcinogenic effect against human breast carcinoma cells MDA-MB468 with G_1 arrest in cell cycle progression and also induction in protein expression of the CDKI Cip/p21.[28]

The cancer chemoprevention and anticarcinogenic effects of silymarin have been shown to be due to its major constituent silibinin.[29] Silibinin decreases prostate-specific antigen (PSA) in hormone-refractory human prostate carcinoma LNCaP cells and inhibits cell growth via G_1 arrest.[30]

Silibinin was fed orally to SENCAR mice and its tissue distribution investigated.[31] Free silibinin mainly accumulated in the liver, although it was also distributed in other organs. Increases in glutathione-*S*-transferase and quinone reductase activities in the liver, lung, stomach, skin and small bowel were observed. The results demonstrated the bioavailability of and phase II enzyme induction of silibinin in different tissues where silymarin has been shown to be a strong cancer chemopreventive agent.

Anti-inflammatory activity Silymarin administered orally reduced foot-pad abscesses in a dose-dependent manner in the carrageenan rat-paw oedema test (ED_{50} = 62.4 mg/kg).[32] In the xylene-induced inflammation test, topically applied silymarin was comparable with indometacin.[32] Silymarin given intraperitoneally to mice resulted in inhibition of leukocyte accumulation in inflammatory exudates and reduced the neutrophil count.[32] Activation of NF-κB induced by TNF, phorbol ester, okaidic acid and ceramide was blocked by silymarin in a dose-dependent manner.[33] Silymarin also inhibited TNF-induced activation of mitogen-activated protein kinase and *c*-Jun N-terminal kinase.[33] The inhibition of activation of NF-κB and the kinases may provide part of the molecular basis for the anti-inflammatory and anticarcinogenic effects of silymarin.[33] Silymarin potently suppressed both NF-κB–DNA binding activity and its dependent gene expression induced by okaidic acid in the hepatoma cell line Hep G2.[34] In addition, silymarin inhibits COX-2 and IL-1α.[24]

Gastric ulcer protective effects Oral administration of silymarin to rats prevented gastric ulceration induced by cold-restraint stress.[35] Gastric secretion volume and acidity were not affected, but histamine concentration was significantly decreased. It was suggested that the anti-ulcerogenic effect of silymarin may be related to inhibition of enzymic peroxidation by the lipoxygenase pathway.[35] The protective effect of silymarin on gastric injury induced in rats by ischaemia–reperfusion and its effects on mucosal myeloperoxidase has been compared with that of allopurinol.[36] The mean ulcer indexes (4.75, 4.50 and 3.63 ui, respectively) of rats treated with 25, 50 and 100 mg/kg silymarin were significantly lower than in control rats, although allopurinol was considerably more potent (2.3 ui; 100 mg/kg).[36]

Other effects Silymarin has been shown to prevent alloxan-induced diabetes mellitus in rats, possibly due to its antioxidant activity and increases in plasma and pancreatic glutathione concentrations.[37]

It has been reported that *Silybum marianum* and silymarin beneficially affect skin elasticity. A phospholipid–silymarin complex (Silymarin–Phytosome) evaluated for its topical effects against croton oil dermatitis in mice and UV-induced erythema in humans showed reduction of oedema and inhibition of myeloperoxidase activity.[38] A standardised extract of *S. marianum* significantly inhibited porcine elastase *in vitro*.[39] An 80% ethanol extract of *S. marianum* aerial parts showed activity against *Bacillus subtilis*, *Staphylococcus aureus*, *Streptococcus haemolyticus*, *Escherichia coli*, *Klebsiella pneumoniae*, *Proteus mirabilis*, *Pseudomonas aeruginosa* and *Salmonella typhi*.[40]

Clinical studies

Clinical trials with milk thistle preparations have focused on their use in alcoholic liver disease, cirrhosis and acute viral and chronic hepatitis. However, several trials have included patients with liver disease of different aetiology, e.g. alcoholic and non-alcoholic cirrhosis. There is also interest in the use of silymarin in toxin- and drug-induced hepatitis, for example following ingestion of the death cap mushroom *A. phalloides*.

A randomised, double-blind, placebo-controlled, multicentre trial involving 200 alcoholic patients with histologically or laparoscopically proven liver cirrhosis investigated the effects of administration of silymarin (150 mg) three times daily.[41] The results indicated that silymarin had no effect on survival and the clinical course in these patients: 125 patients (silymarin $n = 57$ and placebo $n = 68$) completed the two-year study period, during which 29 died ($n = 15$ and 14 for silymarin and placebo, respectively; no statistically significant difference).

In a randomised, double-blind, placebo-controlled trial, patients with alcoholic ($n = 91$) or non-alcoholic ($n = 79$) cirrhosis received silymarin (140 mg) three times daily or placebo for two years.[42] The four-year survival rate was significantly higher in silymarin-treated patients than in placebo recipients (58% versus 39%, respectively, $p = 0.036$). Subgroup analysis indicated that the effect of silymarin on mortality was more pronounced in those patients with alcoholic cirrhosis.

Another randomised, double-blind, placebo-controlled trial carried out over four years reported a significantly higher survival rate in patients with alcoholic cirrhosis treated with silymarin (420 mg) daily compared with placebo recipients, although the effect in patients with non-alcoholic cirrhosis was less marked.[43]

Other controlled trials have also investigated the effects of silymarin in patients with alcohol-related liver damage. Several of these,[44,45] but not all,[46] reported statistically significant benefits with silymarin, e.g. on serum transaminases, compared with placebo.[1] In a randomised controlled trial, 60 patients with diabetes caused by alcoholic liver cirrhosis received silymarin (600 mg/day) or no silymarin treatment for six months.[47] At the end of the study period, the mean values for fasting blood glucose, daily blood glucose, daily glycosuria, glycosylated haemoglobin, daily insulin requirement, malondialdehyde and glucagon-stimulated C peptide were significantly lower in silymarin-treated patients than in those who did not receive silymarin treatment.

A pilot study involving 20 patients with chronic active hepatitis randomised to receive a silybin–phosphatidylcholine complex preparation (IdB1016; Silipide) (240 mg) twice daily or placebo for seven days reported significant reductions in the mean serum concentrations of aspartate aminotransferase (AST), alanine aminotransferase (ALT), γ-glutamyltranspeptidase (GGT) and total bilirubin in silybin complex-treated patients compared with values in placebo recipients.[48] The same preparation has been reported to reduce serum concentrations of liver enzymes (AST and ALT) in 65 patients with chronic persistent hepatitis in a randomised placebo-controlled trial.[49]

A Cochrane systematic review of trials assessing milk thistle preparations for the treatment of alcoholic and/or hepatitis B or C virus induced liver disease included 13 randomised trials involving a total of 915 patients.[50] The methodological quality of included trials was considered to be low: only 23% reported an adequate method for concealment of treatment allocation and only 46% were adequately double-blinded. When all trials were considered, mortality due to liver disease was found to be significantly reduced in the milk thistle group compared with controls (relative risk (95% confidence interval) 0.50 (0.29 to 0.88)), but not when data from only high-quality trials were assessed (0.57 (0.28 to 1.19)). There were no statistically significant differences for milk thistle, compared with placebo or no treatment controls, with respect to all-cause mortality, complications of liver disease and liver histology.[50]

The hepatoprotective effects of silymarin in 222 *de novo* tacrine-treated patients with mild to moderate dementia of the Alzheimer type were investigated in a randomised, double-blind (for silymarin), placebo-controlled, multicentre, 12-week trial.[51] Patients received tacrine plus silymarin (420 mg/day) (n = 110) or tacrine plus placebo (n = 112); silymarin (and placebo) were initiated one week before tacrine (40 mg/day for six weeks then 80 mg/day for six weeks). An intention-to-treat analysis indicated that there was no difference in serum ALT concentrations between the two groups, but that silymarin-treated patients experienced significantly fewer gastrointestinal and cholinergic side-effects without any impact on cognitive status than did placebo recipients.[51]

The effects of silymarin in preventing psychotropic drug-induced hepatic damage have been investigated in a randomised, double-blind, placebo-controlled trial.[52] Sixty women aged 40–60 years who had been taking phenothiazines or butyrophenones for at least five years and who had AST and ALT activity twice normal values were randomised to continued treatment with psychotropic agents or suspension of treatment and to silymarin (800 mg/day) or placebo for 90 days. The findings indicated that treatment with silymarin reduced the lipoperoxidative hepatic damage associated with prolonged administration of butyrophenones and phenothiazines and that the protective effect was greater when treatment with these psychotropic agents was suspended for three months.[52]

There have been numerous case reports, many of which report favourable outcomes, on the therapeutic use of silymarin and silibinin, usually given in combination with standard treatment, in poisoning caused by ingestion of the death cap mushroom *A. phalloides*, although there are no controlled trials in this indication.[1, 52–55, G55] Silibinin is usually given intravenously and case reports have indicated that early administration appears to be important.[56, 57]

Pharmacokinetics Studies of the pharmacokinetics of silymarin and its components and of a silibinin–phosphatidylcholine complex preparation (IdB 1016; Silipide) in both healthy volunteers and patients with cirrhosis and those who have undergone cholecystectomy have been reviewed.[1, G50, G55] Approximately 20–50% of silymarin is absorbed following oral administration and approximately 80% of the dose, whether administered orally or intravenously, is excreted in the bile.[58] Studies in healthy volunteers have reported an elimination half-life of approximately six hours following administration of single doses of silymarin corresponding to approximately 240 mg silibinin.[59, 60] Other studies have compared the pharmacokinetics of different silymarin preparations and shown statistically significant differences in bioavailability.[61, 62]

The bioavailability of a silybin–phosphatidylcholine complex preparation (IdB 1016) has been shown to be several times greater than that of silymarin in single-dose studies involving healthy volunteers[63] and patients with hepatic cirrhosis.[64]

Side-effects, Toxicity

Clinical data

Clinical safety and toxicity data for milk thistle are limited and further investigation of these aspects is required.

No adverse events were noted in a pharmacokinetic study involving healthy male volunteers following single oral doses of silymarin corresponding to up to 254 mg silibinin.[60]

Clinical trials involving patients with liver disorders of various origin and who received oral silymarin at doses of up to 600–800 mg/day for up to six months have reported that no adverse effects were observed.[42, 47, 52]

Data from drug monitoring studies involving more than 3500 patients, including one study involving 2637 patients with various types of chronic liver disease treated with silymarin (Legalon) (560 mg/day) for eight weeks, have indicated that the frequency of adverse effects with silymarin is approximately 1%. Adverse effects are mainly transient, non-serious, gastrointestinal complaints.[4, 65, G55] It is stated that silymarin may occasionally produce a mild laxative effect.[G3]

A case report from Australia described a reaction associated with a preparation of milk thistle. The symptoms included episodes of severe sweating, abdominal cramping, nausea, vomiting, diarrhoea and weakness and these were verified by rechallenge.[66] Another report described a case of anaphylactic shock in a 54-year-old man with immediate-type allergy to kiwi fruit.[67] He experienced facial oedema, swelling of the oral mucosa, bronchospasm, respiratory distress and decreased blood pressure after taking a preparation of milk thistle; a skin-prick test of an extract of milk thistle fruit elicited an immediate-type reaction.

Preclinical data

The acute toxicity of oral and intravenous silymarin and silibinin has been investigated in various animal species (mice, rats, rabbits and dogs).[1] Oral silymarin administered to mice and dogs at doses of 20 and 1 g/kg, respectively, did not cause adverse effects or mortality. Long-term oral administration of silymarin (100 mg/kg/day) to rats for 16 or 22 weeks did not reveal any adverse effects.

Contra-indications, Warnings

None documented. In view of the lack of long-term safety data, excessive use of milk thistle should be avoided (except where its use may help to prevent toxicity caused by other substances).

Milk thistle is contra-indicated for individuals with hypersensitivity to species of Asteraceae.

Drug interactions None documented. However, the potential for preparations of milk thistle to interact with other medicines administered concurrently, particularly those with similar or opposing effects, should be considered.

Pregnancy and lactation In view of the lack of toxicity data, use of milk thistle preparations during pregnancy and lactation should be avoided.

Preparations

Proprietary single-ingredient preparations

Australia: Bioglan Liver-Vite; Herbal Liver Formula; Prol; Silymarin Phytosome. *Austria:* Apihepar; Ardeyhepan; Eurixor; Helixor; Iscador; Isorel; Legalon; Silyhexal. *Belgium:* Legalon. *Brazil:* Legalon; Siliver. *Czech Republic:* Lagosa; Nat Cubetu Benediktu; Nat Jmeli. *France:* Legalon. *Germany:* Abnobaviscum; Alepa; Ardeyhepan; Cefalektin; Cefasliymarin; durasilymarin; Eurixor; Helixor; Hepa-Loges; HepaBesch S; Hepar-Pasc; Hepatos; Heplant; Hypercircin; Iscador; Lagosa; Legalon; Lektinol; Mariendistel Curarina; Mistel Curarina; Mistel-Krautertabletten; Misteltropfen Hofmanns; Misteltropfen; Phytohepar; Salus Mistel-Tropfen; Silibene; Silicur; Silimarit; Silmar; Silvaysan; Viscysat. *Hungary:* Hegrimarin; Legalon; Silegon. *Italy:* Legalon; Silimarin. *Portugal:* Legalon. *Switzerland:* Iscador; Legalon.

Proprietary multi-ingredient preparations

Argentina: Quelodin F. *Australia:* Antioxidant Forte Tablets; Bupleurum Complex; Bupleurum Compound; Calmo; Digest; Extralife Liva-Care; Herbal Cleanse; Lifesystem Herbal Formula 7 Liver Tonic; Liver Tonic Herbal Formula 6; Livstim; Livton Complex; Pacifenity; Silybum Complex; St Mary's Thistle Plus. *Austria:* Hepabene; Rutiviscal; Wechseltee St Severin. *Canada:* Milk Thistle Extract Formula; Milk Thistle. *Czech Republic:* Alvisan Neo; Hepabene; Hypotonicka; Naturland Grosser Swedenbitter; Ungolen. *France:* Mediflor Tisane Circulation du Sang No 12. *Germany:* Antihypertonicum S; Bilisan Duo; Cholhepan N; Cholosom-Tee; Gallexier; Heumann Verdauungstee Solu-Lipar; Iberogast; Ilja Rogoff. *Hungary:* Hepabene. *Italy:* Epagest; Venoplus. *Portugal:* Cholagutt. *Russia:* Hepabene (Гепабене); Herbion Drops for the Heart (Гербион Сердечные Капли). *Singapore:* Hepatofalk Planta. *Switzerland:* Demonatur Gouttes pour le foie et la bile; Iberogast; Tisane hepatique et biliaire. *USA:* Liver Formula.

M

References

1 Morazzoni P, Bombardelli E. *Silybum marianum* (*Carduus marianus*). *Fitoterapia* 1995; 66: 3–42.
2 Awang D. Milk thistle. *Can Pharm J* 1993; 403–404, 422.
3 Pepping J. Milk thistle: *Silybum marianum*. *Am J Health-Syst Pharm* 1999; 56: 1195–1197.
4 Leng-Peschlow E. Properties and medical use of flavolignans (silymarin) from *Silybum marianum*. *Phytother Res* 1996; 10: S25–26.
5 Pascual C *et al*. Effect of silymarin and silybinin on oxygen radicals. *Drug Dev Res* 1993; 29: 73–77.
6 Mira L *et al*. Scavenging of reactive oxygen species by silibinin dihemisuccinate. *Biochem Pharmacol* 1994; 48: 753–759.
7 Bindoli A *et al*. Inhibitory action of silymarin of lipid peroxide formation in rat liver mitochondria and microsomes. *Biochem Pharmacol* 1977; 26: 2405–2409.
8 Valenzuela A *et al*. Antioxidant properties of the flavonoids silybin and (+)-cyanidanol-3: comparison with butylated hydroxyanisole and butylated hydroxytoluene. *Planta Med* 1986; 19: 438–440.
9 Valenzuela A *et al*. Selectivity of silymarin on the increase of the glutathione content in different tissues of the rat. *Planta Med* 1989; 55: 420–422.
10 Skottova N *et al*. Activities of silymarin and its flavolignans upon low density lipoprotein oxidizability *in vitro*. *Phytother Res* 1999; 13: 535–537.
11 Valenzuela A, Garrido A. Biochemical basis of the pharmacological action of the flavonoid silymarin and its structural isomer silibinin. *Biol Res* 1994; 27: 105–112.
12 Wu CG *et al*. Protective effect of silymarin on rat liver injury induced by ischaemia. *Virchows Arch B Cell Pathol Mol Pathol* 1993; 64: 259–263.
13 Kropacova K *et al*. Protective and therapeutic effect of silymarin on the development of latent liver damage. *Radiat Biol Radioecol* 1998; 38: 411–415.
14 Drozdzik M *et al*. Effect of silymarinphospholipid complex on the liver in rabbits maintained on a high-fat diet. *Phytother Res* 1996; 10: 406–409.
15 Krecman V *et al*. Silymarin inhibits the development of diet-induced hypercholesterolemia in rats. *Planta Med* 1998; 64: 138–142.
16 Skottova N, Krecman V. Silymarin a potential hypocholesterolaemic drug. *Physiol Res* 1998; 47: 1–7.
17 Crocenzi FA *et al*. Effect of silymarin on biliary bile salt secretion in the rat. *Biochem Pharmacol* 2000; 59: 1015–1022.
18 Gaedeke J *et al*. Cisplatin nephrotoxicity and protection by silibinin. *Nephrol Dial Transplant* 1996; 11: 55–62.
19 Bokemeyer C *et al*. Silibinin protects against cisplatin-induced nephrotoxicity without compromising cisplatin or ifosfamide anti-tumour activity. *Br J Cancer* 1996; 74: 2036–2041.
20 Zima T *et al*. The effect of silibinin on experimental cyclosporine nephrotoxicity. *Renal Failure* 1998; 20: 471–479.
21 Scambia G *et al*. Antiproliferative effects of silybin on gynaecological malignancies: synergism with cisplatin and doxorubicin. *Eur J Cancer* 1996; 32A: 877–882.
22 Zi X *et al*. Novel cancer chemopreventative effects of a flavonoid constituent silymarin: inhibition of mRNA expression of an endogenous tumour promoter TNFalpha. *Biochem Biophys Res Commun* 1997; 239: 334–339.
23 Katiyar SK *et al*. Protective effects of silymarin against photocarcinogenesis in a mouse skin model. *J Natl Cancer Inst* 1997; 89: 556–566.
24 Zhao J *et al*. Significant inhibition by the flavonoid antioxidant silymarin against 12-*O*-tetradecanoylphorbol 13-acetate caused modulation of anti oxidant and inflammatory enzymes and cyclooxygenase 2 and interleukin-1 alpha expression in SENCAR mouse epidermis: implications in the prevention of stage I tumour promotion. *Mol Carcinogen* 1999; 26: 321–333.
25 Lahiri-Chatterjee M *et al*. A flavonoid antioxidant, silymarin, affords exceptionally high protection against tumour promotion in the SENCAR mouse skin tumorigenic model. *Cancer Res* 1999; 59: 622–632.
26 Zi X *et al*. A flavonoid antioxidant, silymarin, inhibits activation of erbB1 signaling and induces cyclin-dependent kinase inhibitors, G_1 arrest and anticarcinogenic effects in human prostate carcinoma DU145 cells. *Cancer Res* 1998; 58: 1920–1929.
27 Zi X, Agarwal R. Modulation of mitogen-activated protein kinase activation and cell cycle regulators by the potent skin cancer preventative agent silymarin. *Biochem Biophys Res Commun* 1999; 263: 528–536.
28 Zi X *et al*. Anticarcinogenic effect of a flavonoid antioxidant, silymarin, in human breast cancer cells MDA-MB468: induction of G_1 arrest through an increase in Cip1/p21 concomitant with a decrease in kinase activity of cyclin-dependent kinases and associated cyclins. *Clin Cancer Res* 1998; 4: 1055–1064.
29 Bhatia N *et al*. Inhibition of human carcinoma cell growth and DNA synthesis by silibinin, an active constituent of milk thistle: comparison with silymarin. *Cancer Lett* 1999; 147: 77–84.
30 Zi X *et al*. Silibinin decreases prostate-specific antigen with cell growth inhibition via G_1 arrest, leading to differentiation of prostate carcinoma cells: implications for prostate cancer intervention. *Proc Natl Acad Sci USA* 1999; 96: 7490–7495.
31 Zhao J, Agarwal R. Tissue distribution of silibinin, the major active constituent of silymarin, in mice and its association with enhancement of phase II enzymes: implications in cancer chemoprevention. *Carcinogenesis* 1999; 20: 2101–2108.

32 De La Puerta R *et al*. Effect of silymarin on different acute inflammation models and in leukocyte migration. *J Pharm Pharmacol* 1996; 48: 968–970.
33 Manna SK *et al*. Silymarin suppresses TNF-induced activation of NF-kappaB, *c*-Jun N-terminal kinase and apoptosis. *J Immunol* 1999; 163: 6800–6809.
34 Saliou C *et al*. Selective inhibition of NF-kappaB activation by the flavonoid hepatoprotector silymarin in HepG2. *FEBS Lett* 1998; 440: 8–12.
35 De La Lastra C *et al*. Gastric antiulcer activity of silymarin, a lipoxygenase inhibitor, on rats. *J Pharm Pharmacol* 1992; 44: 929–931.
36 De La Lastra C *et al*. Gastroprotection induced by silymarin, the hepatoprotective principle of *Silybum marianum* in ischaemia–reperfusion mucosal injury: role of neutrophils. *Planta Med* 1995; 61: 116–119.
37 Soto CP *et al*. Prevention of alloxan-induced diabetes mellitus in the rat by silymarin. *Comp Biochem Physiol* 1998; 119C: 125–129.
38 Bombardelli E *et al*. Ageing skin: protective effect of silymarin–Phytosome®. *Fitoterapia* 1991; 62: 115–122.
39 Benaiges A *et al*. Study of the refirming effect of a plant complex. *Int J Cosmet Sci* 1998; 20: 223–233.
40 Izzo AA *et al*. Biological screening of Italian medicinal plants for antibacterial activity. *Phytother Res* 1995; 9: 281–286.
41 Pares A *et al*. Effects of silymarin in alcoholic patients with cirrhosis of the liver: results of a controlled, double-blind, randomized and multicenter trial. *J Hepatol* 1998; 28: 615–621.
42 Ferenci P *et al*. Randomized controlled trial of silymarin treatment in patients with cirrhosis of the liver. *J Hepatol* 1989; 9: 105–113.
43 Benda L *et al*. The influence of therapy with silymarin on the survival rate of patients with liver cirrhosis. *Wien Klin Wschr* 1980; 92: 678–683.
44 Salmi H, Sarna S. Effect of silymarin on the chemical, functional and morphological alterations of the liver. *Scand J Gastroenterol* 1982; 17: 517–521.
45 Feher J *et al*. Hepatoprotective activity of silymarin Legalon® therapy in patients with chronic alcoholic liver disease. *Orv Hetil* 1989; 130: 2723–2727.
46 Trinchet JC *et al*. Traitement de l'hépatite alcoolique par la silymarine. Une étude comparative en double insu chez 116 malades. *Gastroenterol Clin Biol* 1989; 13: 120–124.
47 Velussi M *et al*. Silymarin reduces hyperinsulinaemia, malondialdehyde levels, and daily insulin need in cirrhotic diabetic patients. *Curr Ther Res* 1993; 53: 533–545.
48 Buzzelli G *et al*. A pilot study on the liver protective effect of silybin–phosphatidylcholine complex (IdB1016) in chronic active hepatitis. *Int J Clin Pharmacol Ther Toxicol* 1993; 31: 456–460.
49 Marcelli R *et al*. Cited by Morazzoni P *et al*. *Silybum marianum* (*Carduus marianus*). *Fitoterapia* 1995; 66: 3–42. *Eur Bull Drug Res* 1992; 1: 131–135.
50 Rambaldi A *et al*. Milk thistle for alcoholic and/or hepatitis B or C virus liver diseases (review). Cochrane Database of Systematic Reviews, 2005, Issue 2. Art. No.: CD003620.
51 Allain H *et al*. Aminotransferase levels and silymarin in *de novo* tacrine-treated patients with Alzheimer's disease. *Dementia Geriat Cogn Disord* 1999; 10: 181–185.
52 Palasciano G *et al*. The effect of silymarin on plasma levels of malon-dialdehyde in patients receiving long-term treatment with psychotropic drugs. *Curr Ther Res* 1994; 55: 537–545.
53 Klein AS *et al*. *Amanita* poisoning: treatment and the role of liver transplantation. *Am J Med* 1989; 86: 187–193.
54 Floersheim GL *et al*. Die Klinische Knollenblatterpilzverg; Ftung: prognostische faktoren und therapeutische massnahmen. *Schweiz Med Wochenschr* 1982; 112: 1164–1177.
55 Carducci R *et al*. Silibinin and acute poisoning with *Amanita phalloides*. *Minerva Anestesiol* 1996; 62: 187–193.
56 Hruby K *et al*. Pharmacotherapy of *Amanita phalloides* poisoning using silybin. *Wien Klin Wochenschr* 1983; 95: 225–231.
57 Hruby K *et al*. Chemotherapy of *Amanita phalloides* poisoning with intravenous silibinin. *Hum Toxicol* 1983; 2: 183–190.
58 Mennicke WH. Zur biologischen Verfügbarkeit und Verstoffwechselung von Silybin. *Dtsch Apoth Ztg* 1975; 115: 1205–1206.
59 Lorenz D *et al*. Pharmacokinetic studies with silymarin in human serum and bile. *Meth Find Exp Clin Pharmacol* 1984; 6: 655–661.
60 Weyhenmeyer R *et al*. Study on the dose-linearity of the pharmacokinetics of silibinin diastereomers using a new stereospecific assay. *Int J Clin Pharmacol Ther Toxicol* 1992; 30: 134–138.
61 Cho J-Y *et al*. Pharmacokinetic evaluation of two formulations containing silymarin: Legalon 140™ cap and Silymarin™. *J Korean Soc Clin Pharmacol Ther* 1998; 6: 119–127.
62 Schulz H-U *et al*. Untersuchungen zum Freisetzungsverhalten und zur Bioäquivalenz von Silymarin–Präparaten. *Arzneimittelforschung* 1995; 45: 61–64.
63 Barzaghi N *et al*. Pharmacokinetic studies on IdB 1016, a silybin–phosphatidylcholine complex, in healthy human volunteers. *Eur J Drug Metab Pharmacokinet* 1990; 15: 333–338.
64 Orlando R *et al*. Silybin kinetics in patients with liver cirrhosis: a comparative study of silybin–phosphatidylcholine complex and silymarin. *Med Sci Res* 1990; 18: 861–863.
65 Albrecht M, Fredrick H. Therapy of toxic liver pathologies with Legalon. *Z Klin Med* 1992; 47: 87–92.
66 Anon. An adverse reaction of the herbal medication milk thistle (*Silybum marianum*). Adverse Drug Reactions Advisory Committee. *Med J Aust* 1999; 170: 218–219.
67 Geier J *et al*. Anaphylactic shock due to an extract of *Silybum marianum* in a patient with immediate-type allergy to kiwi fruit. *Allergologie* 1990; 13: 387–388.

Mistletoe

Summary and Pharmaceutical Comment

The chemistry of mistletoe is well-documented (*see* Constituents). The profile of constituents is, to some extent, thought to be dependent on the host plant on which mistletoe is a parasite. The lectin and viscotoxin constituents are considered to be the main active principles, although there is some evidence that certain activities, e.g. cytotoxicity, can be modulated by other constituents. Mistletoe is reputed to be a cardiac depressant, although cardioactive constituents are not generally recognised as constituents of mistletoe; however, this may depend on the host plant on which mistletoe has grown.

Scientific investigation into the effects of mistletoe has centred primarily on the pharmacological and toxicological properties of mistletoe extracts and the lectin and viscotoxin constituents. Preclinical research has focused on the cytotoxic and immunomodulatory activities, and provides a large body of supporting evidence with regard to clinical use of mistletoe in cancer and other conditions involving the immune system.

The results of clinical trials of various commercial mistletoe preparations and purified components have, however, been less convincing. Furthermore, different mistletoe preparations vary markedly in their qualitative and quantitative composition. Hence, results regarding efficacy (and safety) need to be considered for each individual product.[G56]

Numerous clinical studies of mistletoe preparations have been conducted, although few used rigorous randomised controlled clinical trial methodology. Several systematic reviews of clinical trials of mistletoe preparations involving patients with cancer have concluded that there is insufficient evidence from well-designed clinical trials that mistletoe preparations, or their isolated components, are effective in the treatment of cancer or as adjunctive treatments in cancer. Further research using rigorous clinical trial methodology to test the effects of well-characterised mistletoe extracts is warranted.

Reviews of clinical trials which have provided an assessment of the safety of mistletoe, generally have reported mistletoe preparations to be well tolerated. The most frequently reported adverse events in trials using lectin-standardised mistletoe preparations are local reactions, such as urticaria and/or erythema at the injection site, which usually resolve within 48 hours.

The toxic nature of the mistletoe constituents (e.g. lectins, viscotoxins) indicates that mistletoe is unsuitable for self-medication. Mistletoe berries are poisonous and, in the UK, sale/supply is restricted to pharmacies only and by or under the supervision of a pharmacist.

Species (Family)

Viscum album L. (Loranthaceae)

Synonym(s)

Viscum

Part(s) Used

Leaf, fruit (berry), twig

Pharmacopoeial and Other Monographs

BHMA 2003[G66]
BHP 1996[G9]
Complete German Commission E[G3]
Martindale 35th edition[G85]

Legal Category (Licensed Products)

Mistletoe is not included in the GSL.[G37]

Constituents

The following is compiled from several sources, including References 1 and 2 and General Reference G2.

Acids Fatty acids (C_{12}–C_{22}), 80% oleic and palmitic, myrisitic;[3] phenolic acids, e.g. caffeic, *p*-coumaric, gentisic, *p*-hydroxybenzoic, *p*-hydroxyphenylacetic, protocatechuic, vanillic;[3,4] anisic, quinic and shikimic.[3,4]

Alkaloids It has been suggested that alkaloids can be passed on from hosts to parasitic plants such as mistletoe (e.g. nicotine alkaloids have been isolated from mistletoe growing on Solanaceae shrubs).[5]

Amines Acetylcholine, choline, β-phenylethylamine, histamine, propionylcholine and tyramine.[6]

Flavonoids Chalcones, e.g. 2′-hydroxy-4′, 6′-dimethoxy-chalcone-4-*O*-glucoside, 2′-hydroxy-3, 4′, 6′-trimethoxychalcone-4-*O*-glucoside, 2′-hydroxy-4′,6′-dimethoxychalcone-4-*O*-(apiosyl-1→2)-glucoside.[1,7]

Flavanones, e.g. (2*R*)-5,7-dimethoxyflavanone-4′-*O*-glucoside, (2*S*)-3′, 5, 7-trimethoxyflavanone-4′-*O*-glucoside, homoeriodictyol (4′,5,7-trihydroxy-5′-methoxyflavanone.[1,7]

Flavones, e.g. quercetin, isorhamnetin, sakuranetin, rhamnazin (3,4′,5-trihydroxy-3′,7-dimethoxyflavone; quercetin 3′,7-dimethyl ether) and its glycoside rhamnazin-3,4′-di-*O*-glucoside and other quercetin methyl ethers.[1,7]

Lectins Lectins are heterodimeric glycoproteins (mol. wt between 55 kDa and 63 kDa),[1] which belong to a group of type 2 ribosome-inactivating proteins (RIPs) and are structurally similar to ricin. They are composed of two distinct subunits, one B-subunit (B-chain, the galactose-binding site; 34 kDa) and one toxophoric A-subunit (A-chain, the cytotoxic-binding site, RNA-*N*-glycosidase; 29 kDa). The structure of the B-chain of mistletoe lectins is based on 264 amino acids. Seven cysteine residues and three *N*-linked carbohydrate chains are included. Mistletoe lectins (*V. album* agglutinin-1, viscumin (mol. wt 60 000)) are galactoside-specific plant lectins (63 kDa). Three different mistletoe lectins have been isolated: ML-1 (main component; broad range of affinity for α/β-linked galactopyranosyl residues), ML-2 (affinity for D-galactose and *N*-acetyl-D-galactosamine) and ML-3 (affinity for *N*-acetyl-D-galactosamine). The chitin-binding lectin (chitin-binding-agglutinin, visalb-CBA or visalb-CBL), which is distinct from ML-1, ML-2 and ML-3, is a homodimer lectin with two identical subunits (10.8 kDa). Its amino acid composition is similar to that of other chitin-binding hololectins.(1) Reported yields of ML-1, ML-2 and ML-3 from leaves and stems are 3–170 mg/100 g dry weight, 0.1–35 mg/100 g dry weight, and 0–67 mg/100 g dry weight, respectively.(1)

ML-1, ML-2 and ML-3 have been isolated from Iscador Qu Special and Iscador M Special. Iscador P contains almost no mistletoe lectins (R Dierdorf, personal communication, September 2003).(8)

Terpenoids An acyclic monoterpene glucoside, 2,6-dimethylocta-2,7-diene-1,6-diol-6-O-[6′-β-D-apiofuranosyl]-β-D-glucopyranoside, has been isolated from leaves and stems.(9) Phytosterols, including β-sitosterol, stigmasterol and glycosides, together with pentacyclic triterpenes β-amyrin and its acetate, betulinic acid, oleandrin and oleanolic acid are present.(2, 10)

Viscotoxins Viscotoxins (mol. wt 5 kDa) have been isolated from leaf homogenates. Viscotoxins are amphipathic, strongly basic polypeptides that are highly enriched with cysteine residues; they belong to the family of α- and β-thionins.(1) Viscotoxins consist of 46 amino acid residues with three disulphide bonds, which stabilise the conformation of the molecule. Several different viscotoxins have been isolated, the main ones being viscotoxins A2, A3 and B.

Other constituents Lignans Syringaresinol 4,4′-O-diglucoside (eleutheroside E).(1)

Phenylpropanoids Syringenin-4′-O-glucoside (syringin), syringenin-4′-O-apiosyl-1→2-glucoside (syringoside).(1)

Polyalcohols 1-D-1-O-Methyl-*muco*-inositol (a derivative of O-methyl-inositol),(G2) mannitol, pinitol, quebrachitol and viscumitol.(1)

Polysaccharides Mainly a methylester of 1→4α-galacturonic acid in the leaves and rhamnogalacturans in the berries. Pectin (mol. wt 42 kDa), arabinogalactan (mol. wt 110 kDa) are present in leaves, and a rhamnogalacturan (mol. wt 700 kDa) is found in the berries. The berries contain acidic (mol. wt 1340 kDa) and neutral (mol. wt 30 kDa) polysaccharides. The acidic polysaccharides interact with ML-1. Simple sugars and tannins are also present.(1)

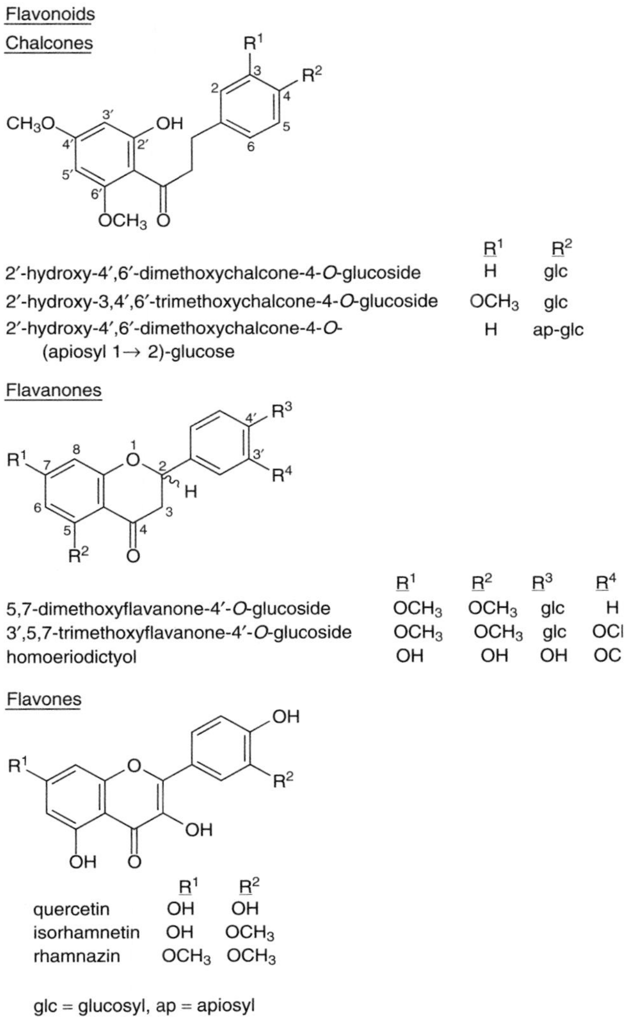

Flavonoids

Chalcones

	R1	R2
2′-hydroxy-4′,6′-dimethoxychalcone-4-O-glucoside	H	glc
2′-hydroxy-3,4′,6′-trimethoxychalcone-4-O-glucoside	OCH_3	glc
2′-hydroxy-4′,6′-dimethoxychalcone-4-O-(apiosyl 1→ 2)-glucose	H	ap-glc

Flavanones

	R1	R2	R3	R4
5,7-dimethoxyflavanone-4′-O-glucoside	OCH_3	OCH_3	glc	H
3′,5,7-trimethoxyflavanone-4′-O-glucoside	OCH_3	OCH_3	glc	OCI
homoeriodictyol	OH	OH	OH	OC

Flavones

	R1	R2
quercetin	OH	OH
isorhamnetin	OH	OCH_3
rhamnazin	OCH_3	OCH_3

glc = glucosyl, ap = apiosyl

Figure 1 Selected constituents of mistletoe.

Terpenoids

2,6-dimethylocta-2,7-diene-1,6-diol-6-O-(6-O-β-D-apiofuranosyl)-β-D-glucopyranoside

Lignans

syringaresinol-4,4′-O-diglucoside (eleutheroside E)

Phenylpropanoids

syringenin

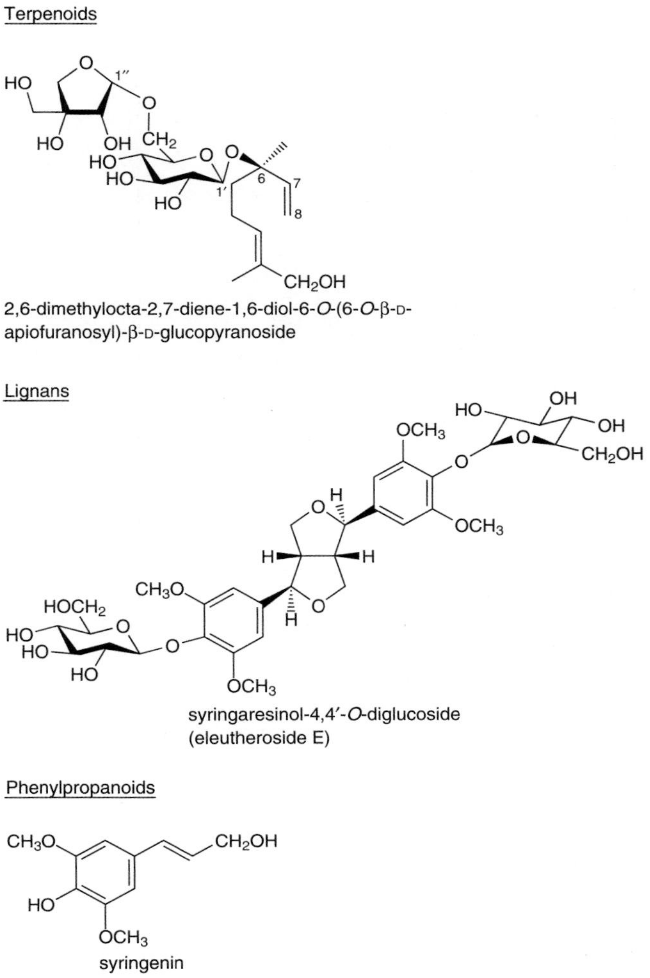

Figure 2 Selected constituents of mistletoe.

Food Use

Mistletoe is not generally used as a food. The branches and berries of mistletoe are listed by the Council of Europe as natural sources of food flavouring (category N3).[G16] This category indicates that mistletoe may be added to foodstuffs in the traditionally accepted manner, although there is insufficient information available for an adequate assessment of potential toxicity.

Herbal Use

Mistletoe is stated to possess hypotensive, cardiac-depressant and sedative properties. Traditionally, it has been used for high blood pressure, arteriosclerosis, nervous tachycardia, hypertensive headache, chorea and hysteria.[G2, G7, G66, G69]

Modern use of mistletoe preparations is focused on use as a treatment and as an adjuvant treatment in cancer. Clinical studies of mistletoe preparations have assessed mistletoe preparations as a treatment, or as an adjunctive treatment, in patients with different types of cancers. A small number of other clinical trials have been conducted involving patients with chronic hepatitis C infection, human immunodeficiency virus (HIV) infection and respiratory infections. (*see* Pharmacological Actions, Clinical studies).

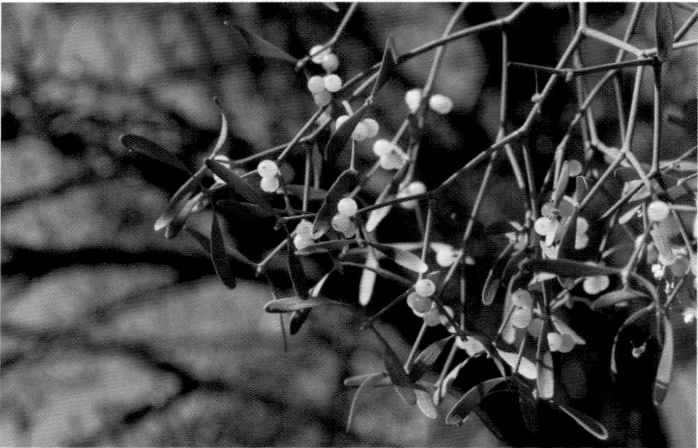

Figure 3 Mistletoe (*Viscum album*).

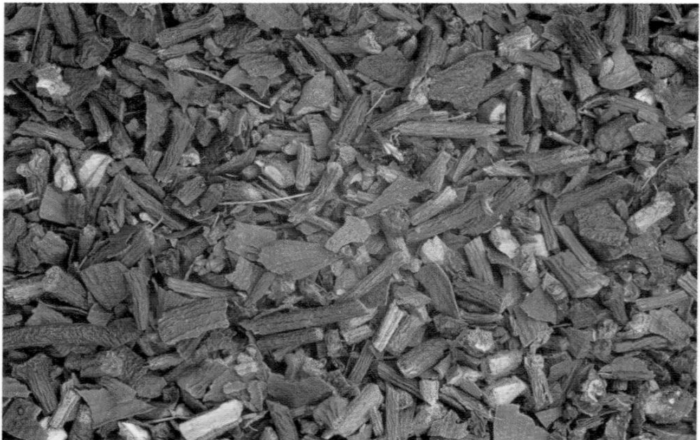

Figure 4 Mistletoe – dried drug substance (twig).

Dosage

Dosages for oral administration (adults) recommended in standard herbal reference texts for the traditional uses are given below.

Dried leaves 2–6 g as an infusion three times daily.[G7]

Liquid extract 1–3 mL (1 : 1 in 25% alcohol) three times daily.[G7]

Tincture 0.5 mL (1 : 5 in 45% alcohol) three times daily.[G7]

Infusion 40–120 mL (1 : 20 in cold water) daily.[G7]

Soft extract 0.3–0.6 mL (1 : 8 infusion or tincture) three times daily.[G7]

The administration of mistletoe preparations as adjunctive treatments in cancer is mostly by subcutaneous injection, and the manufacturer's recommendations for the specific mistletoe preparations should be followed. Dosages used in clinical trials assessing different mistletoe preparations, therefore, vary widely and are often complex; dosage regimens also vary depending on the type of cancer being treated. Trials involving ML-1 standardised mistletoe preparations usually describe the dose of mistletoe extract in terms of the equivalent amount of ML-1. For example, in a trial involving patients with head and neck squamous cell carcinoma, an ML-1 standardised mistletoe extract (Eurixor) equivalent to ML-1 1 ng/kg body weight twice weekly was given by subcutaneous injection over a 60-week period in treatment cycles of 12 weeks followed by a break in treatment after every four weeks.[11]

Pharmacological Actions

There is a vast scientific literature relating to the biochemical and pharmacological effects of mistletoe and its constituents, particularly the lectin and viscotoxin constituents, which are believed to be the active principles.[12] There is also a substantial literature on clinical investigations with mistletoe extracts and purified components, and at least one scientific meeting focused solely on research into mistletoe in cancer therapy.[13]

In vitro and animal studies

Preclinical research has focused on investigating the cytotoxic and immunomodulatory activities of mistletoe and its constituents, although other effects, such as agglutinating and hypotensive properties have also been documented. These activities have been summarised in several comprehensive reviews.[5, 12, 14–18] A brief summary of some of the scientific literature on the properties of mistletoe and its constituents is given below. Evaluation, interpretation and comparison of preclinical studies is not straightforward as studies have investigated the effects of different types of mistletoe extracts and commercial products, some of which are not characterised or their composition is not adequately described in reports of studies; a number of other studies have used purified mistletoe lectins and/or viscotoxins.

Cytotoxic and anticancer activities The lectin and, to a lesser extent, viscotoxin constituents of mistletoe are the main cytotoxic components.[12] Cytotoxic activity *in vitro* has been documented for mistletoe extracts and for purified mistletoe lectins and viscotoxins. In one study, aqueous extracts (ABNOBAviscum) of mistletoe sourced from two host trees and purified mistletoe lectins II and III inhibited cell growth for several tumour cell lines, including murine B cell hybridomas, P815 (murine mastocytoma), EL-4 (murine thymoma), MOLT-4 (human T cell acute lymphoblastic leukaemia) and U937 (human histiocytoma).[19] For example, the mistletoe extract sourced from apple trees at a dilution of 1 : 10 (corresponding to aqueous extract 0.15 mg/mL) resulted in 98% inhibition of the growth of the MOLT-4 tumour cell line. The effects of another mistletoe extract (Isorel M), also obtained from mistletoe grown on apple trees, on normal and tumour cell growth were compared with those of its low and high molecular weight components and mistletoe lectins *in vitro* using melanoma B16 cell cultures. At the highest concentration tested (2 μg/mL), all preparations significantly inhibited [^{3}H]thymidine incorporation into melanoma cells, compared with control.[20] However, separately, the low and high molecular weight components achieved less inhibition than the total mistletoe extract, suggesting that the constituents of both fractions are needed for optimal activity.

In another *in vitro* study, mistletoe lectin I and purified viscotoxins (ratio of viscotoxins A2 : A3 : B was 1:1.6:0.6) showed cytotoxic activity against MOLT-4 cells as well as Yoshida sarcoma cells and K562 human myeloid cells in a concentration-dependent manner.[21] Mistletoe lectins I, II and III showed cytotoxic activity against sensitive and resistant human colon cancer cell lines in a concentration-dependent manner *in vitro*.[22]

The mechanism of growth arrest demonstrated with mistletoe extracts in *in vitro* studies using human and murine tumour cell lines was shown to be due to the induction by mistletoe constituents of programmed cell death (apoptosis).[19] Induction of apoptosis by mistletoe extracts (various Iscador preparations) has also been demonstrated in endothelial cells.[23] The apoptosis-inducing properties and hence cytotoxicity of *V. album* extracts depend on the content of active compounds, mainly the mistletoe lectins, the content of which in turn is dependent on factors such as the host tree and the manufacturing process.[24,25] Furthermore, other compounds present in mistletoe extract may modulate the cytotoxic activity.

It has recently been reported following *in vitro* studies in hepatocarcinoma cells that mistletoe lectin II from Korean mistletoe induces apoptosis by inhibiting telomerase, an enzyme that maintains protein–nucleic acid complexes (telomeres) at the ends of chromosomes.[26] This effect appeared to be mediated via a pathway independent of p53.

Antitumour activity in animal models has been demonstrated for several different commercial preparations of mistletoe extract, and for mistletoe lectins. In one study, mice bearing a hind-limb melanoma B16F10 tumour were given a single dose (100 mg/kg body weight, intraperitoneally) of a mistletoe extract (Isorel M) obtained from mistletoe growing on apple trees. Compared with a control group (which received a saline injection), mice treated with mistletoe showed a statistically significant reduction in tumour volume measured two days after mistletoe administration.[27] Inhibition of tumour growth was documented for an aqueous mistletoe extract (Lektinol, containing mistletoe lectins 405 μg/mL), administered intraperitoneally or subcutaneously at doses equivalent to mistletoe lectins 30 and 300 ng/mL/kg per day for up to four weeks, in mice with Renca (renal cell carcinoma), C8 colon 38 carcinoma and F9 testicular carcinoma, when compared with control.[28] No such inhibitory effect was observed in mice with Lewis lung carcinoma and B16 melanoma under the same conditions.

Anticarcinogenic activities have been described for a bacterially fermented mistletoe extract (Iscador M; mistletoe grown on apple trees).[29] Methylcholanthrene-induced sarcoma formation was inhibited in mice treated with Iscador M (1.66 mg twice weekly for 15 weeks, intraperitoneally), compared with a control group. In separate experiments, mistletoe was reported to markedly inhibit the development of lung metastases when co-administered with metastatic B16F10 melanoma cells through the lateral tail vein;[29] however, the results from this experiment were not subjected to statistical testing. Antimetastatic activity has also been documented for other commercial mistletoe preparations (e.g. Lektinol, Helixor) standardised for mistletoe lectin content in other *in vivo* studies (mice).[30–32]

Immunomodulatory activity Certain types of immune cells, such as natural killer (NK) cells, can lyse tumour cells; this can occur with or without activation by cytokines.[12] Extracts of mistletoe have been shown to enhance the cytolytic activity of NK cells in studies using human peripheral blood mononuclear cells and a human cancer cell line (K562 leukaemia).[33] Several other studies have described the enhancing effects of mistletoe extracts and their isolated components on natural killer activity of peripheral blood mononuclear cells *in vitro* and *in vivo*.[17]

Components of mistletoe have also been reported to induce the proliferation of human peripheral blood mononuclear cells *in vitro*.[9,34] In one study, of six mistletoe extracts tested, an extract (Iscador P) derived from mistletoe grown on pine trees induced the strongest proliferative response on peripheral blood mononuclear cells from non-treated individuals.[9] This extract is almost devoid of lectins, suggesting that a non-lectin-associated antigen from this extract is responsible for the observed effects.

Stimulation of cytokine release (e.g. interleukin 1 (IL-1), IL-2, IL-6, IL-12, tumour necrosis factor α (TNFα)) by mistletoe extracts or mistletoe lectins has been demonstrated in various experimental studies *in vitro*.[12,35–37]

Immunostimulant activity in mice, demonstrated for example by an increase in the phagocytic activity of peritoneal macrophages, has been documented for mistletoe lectin 1 and for mistletoe extracts standardised for mistletoe lectin 1 content.[12] *In vivo* immunostimulant activity in mice (humoral and cellular), demonstrated by an enhancement of delayed hypersensitivity and antibody formation to sheep red blood cells, has been documented for the crude plant juice, Iscador and for a polysaccharide fraction isolated from the berries.[38] Activity was attributed to stimulation of the monophagocytic system and to induction of inflammation. The results indicated that the immunostimulant property of mistletoe is not solely attributable to the polysaccharides found in the berries (plant juice also active) or to the lactobacilli content of the fermented plant juice (crude extract also active). Non-specific immunological effects with mistletoe extracts are reported to be dependent on the frequency and quantity of the applied extract.[39]

Agglutinating activity Agglutinating activity that is preferential towards tumour cells over erythrocytes has been exhibited by Iscador and by a lectin fraction.[40–42] The lectins have been shown to bind to a number of cells including erythrocytes (non-specific to blood type),[43,44] lymphocytes, leukocytes, macrophages, glycoproteins and plasma proteins.[44,45] Binding has been found to be stereospecific towards units containing a D-galactose molecule,[42,45,46] although D-galactose units with unmodified hydroxyl groups at C_2, C_3 and C_4 inhibit erythrocyte agglutination.[47] Tyrosine residues are also thought to be involved in the agglutination process.[46] Plasma proteins compete for the lectin receptor site and, therefore, decrease the agglutination of erythrocytes and tumour cells.[48] Unlike many other sugars, lactose units have also been found to inhibit erythrocyte agglutination.[47]

Mistletoe lectins have been reported to prevent viscotoxin- and allergen-stimulated histamine release from human leukocytes.[49]

Hypotensive effect The hypotensive effect documented for mistletoe has been attributed to various biologically active constituents such as acetylcholine, histamine, gamma aminobutyric acid (GABA), tyramine and flavones.[G24] The exact nature of the hypotensive effect of mistletoe seems unclear: it has been reported that activity is mainly due to an inhibitory action on the excitability of the vasomotor centre in the medulla oblongata.[50] However, it has also been stated that the hypotensive action of mistletoe is mainly of a reflex character, exerting a normalising effect on both hypertensive and hypotensive states.[50] The effect of different mistletoe plant parts and host plant on the hypotensive activity has been studied with highest activity reported for mistletoe leaves parasitising on willow.[50]

Antimicrobial activity Extracts of the *V. album* subspecies *album*, *abietis*, *austriacum* and *pallasiana* have been tested for activity against *Mycobacterium tuberculosis* H37A *in vitro*. Ether extracts of the *V. album* subspecies *album*, *abietis* and *austriacum* and petroleum ether extracts of the subspecies *abietis* and *austriacum* were active against *M. tuberculosis* (minimum inhibitory concentration, MIC: 200 μg/mL for each).[51] From these results, it is not possible to determine whether polar or non-polar compounds are responsible for the observed antimycobacterial activity.

Clinical studies

Numerous clinical studies of mistletoe preparations have been carried out, mostly in the area of oncology, although few used rigorous randomised controlled clinical trial methodology and meet today's good clinical practice standards for the conduct of clinical trials. Collectively, the results of these studies are difficult to interpret as they involved patients with different types of cancer, who were or were not receiving different types of conventional cancer treatment (surgery, radiotherapy and/or cancer chemotherapy), and investigated the effects of different mistletoe preparations which vary markedly in their qualitative and quantitative composition. Hence, results regarding efficacy (and safety) need to be considered for each individual product.[G56]

Nevertheless, several narrative reviews and systematic reviews of clinical trials of mistletoe preparations involving patients with cancer have been published. In short, there is insufficient evidence from well-designed clinical trials that mistletoe preparations, or their isolated components, are effective in the treatment of cancer or as adjunctive treatments in cancer. Although a small number of reasonably well-designed trials have reported statistically significant results for mistletoe, compared with controls, at present, there is insufficient evidence to support the use of any specific mistletoe preparation in the treatment of any specific type of cancer. Further research using rigorous clinical trial methodology to test the effects of well-characterised mistletoe extracts is warranted. A summary of the clinical trial evidence relating to mistletoe preparations is given below.

Pharmacokinetics There is a lack of clinical pharmacokinetic data for the constituents of mistletoe preparations.

Therapeutic effects Cancer A systematic review of prospective, controlled clinical trials of mistletoe preparations in the treatment of cancers included 23 studies, of which 16 involved random allocation to treatment, two involved quasi-randomisation and the remaining five were non-randomised studies; three of the studies were nested within an epidemiological cohort study.[52] In total, the trials involved over 3500 patients with different types of cancer (and at different stages), including breast (n = 4 studies), lung (4), colorectal (3), melanoma (2), stomach, kidney, bladder, glioma, and head and neck (1 each); several trials studied more than one cancer type. Most trials tested the anthroposophical mistletoe preparations Iscador and Helixor (n = 14 and 3, respectively), whereas in six the intervention was Eurixor. In most trials, the mistletoe intervention was administered in addition to conventional treatment (cancer chemotherapy, radiotherapy, corticosteroids and/or surgery) and compared with conventional treatment alone; other trials involved a no-treatment control group, or compared the mistletoe preparation directly with conventional treatment. Only two studies included a placebo control group, and blinding of the intervention was not undertaken in any of the trials (reliable blinding is hard to achieve as parenteral administration of mistletoe can cause local skin reactions at the injection site).[52] An assessment of the methodological quality of the included clinical trials revealed that many of the studies had methodological limitations to their design and/or analysis and that most did not meet contemporary standards in these respects.

The results of this group of clinical trials need to be considered critically because of the poor methodological quality of the studies. Furthermore, the heterogeneity of the studies precluded a quantitative assessment of effect size.[52] Of the 23 trials, 12 recorded statistically significant results in favour of the mistletoe intervention, compared with control, in at least one clinically relevant outcome measure (e.g. mean/median survival time, five-/six-year survival rate). Of the five trials that incorporated a quality-of-life outcome measure, three reported statistically significant results in favour of mistletoe, compared with control, one reported no effect and one result was omitted from the original publication of the study. Three other trials reported statistically significant results for mistletoe, compared with control, in reducing the frequency of adverse effects of concomitantly administered conventional cancer treatments. In summary, although several trials reported positive results for certain mistletoe preparations, the data are inconclusive because of the studies' methodological limitations, and further research using well-designed and properly conducted trials is necessary.[52]

Another systematic review of prospective controlled clinical trials of mistletoe preparations involving patients with cancer employed stricter inclusion/exclusion criteria: only randomised trials were considered. The review included 10 studies, eight of which were included in the systematic review[52] described above; the other two studies were available only as a conference abstract and unpublished data from a manufacturer of a mistletoe preparation, which prevented their thorough critical analysis.[53] Of the eight trials for which a full assessment of methodological quality was possible, the best five scored 3 points from a maximum of 5; as with the previous review,[53] a quantitative analysis of data from the included studies was not possible because of the heterogeneity of the trials. From this review, it was concluded that the evidence does not provide strong support for the efficacy of mistletoe preparations as a treatment for cancer, or as supportive therapy in cancer.[53]

The two reviews[52, 53] described above have superseded a previous systematic review[54] of controlled clinical trials of mistletoe preparations in cancer, although there is little difference in the respective conclusions of the more recent and older reviews. The earlier review included 11 controlled trials, only one of which was judged to be of high methodological quality, although even this did not involve masking (blinding) of the intervention. This trial was the only study included in the review that did not show a beneficial effect on outcome for a mistletoe preparation. The review concluded that mistletoe extracts could not be recommended in the treatment of patients with cancer, except in the setting of clinical trials.(54)

One other review (which does not fully describe the methods used so must be described as non-systematic) included only those trials which had evaluated the effects of well-characterised mistletoe extracts standardised for their content of mistletoe lectins I, II and III. The conclusions of the review concur with those of systematic reviews in that mistletoe preparations do not have an established place in oncology and that further rigorous clinical trials are necessary.(55) This review did not involve a formal assessment of the methodological quality of included studies, but did highlight that two trials(11, 56) only were conducted using contemporary rigorous clinical trial methodology and in accordance with the principles of good clinical practice. These two studies were included in the two recent systematic reviews(52, 53) described above, but at the time, data from one study(56) were available only in promotional literature produced by a manufacturer of a mistletoe preparation.

One of these studies was a randomised controlled trial of an ML-1 standardised mistletoe extract (Eurixor) involving 477 patients with head and neck squamous cell carcinoma. Participants were stratified into two groups – surgery only, or surgery followed by radiotherapy groups – and randomised to receive additional treatment with the mistletoe extract.(11) The dosage regimen for mistletoe extract was equivalent to ML-1 1 ng/kg body weight twice weekly by subcutaneous injection over a 60-week period in treatment cycles of 12 weeks followed by a break in treatment after every four weeks. Mistletoe treatment was commenced 1–4 days before surgery in 72% of participants; the remainder (for whom early administration was not possible) first received mistletoe shortly after undergoing surgery.

In total, 200 (42%) of the 477 participants experienced a relapse during the follow-up period (median four years for surviving participants); there was no statistically significant difference between the mistletoe and control groups in incidence of relapse and in the development of metastases and second primary tumours.(11) In an intention-to-treat analysis, there was no statistically significant difference between the two groups in disease-free survival, the primary efficacy parameter (adjusted hazard ratio, 95% confidence interval (CI): 0.959, 0.725–1.268). There were also no statistically significant differences between the treatment and control groups in secondary outcome measures (immune parameters, quality-of-life score) assessed at different time points throughout the study. The conclusion of the study was that the ML-1 standardised mistletoe extract tested (Eurixor) is not effective as an adjuvant treatment for patients with head and neck cancer.(11)

The second of these studies (now published as an abstract so full details are still not available) was a randomised, double-blind, multicentre trial involving 272 patients with breast cancer who had undergone surgery and were receiving treatment with cyclophosphamide, methotrexate and 5-fluorouracil. In addition, they received one of three doses of mistletoe extract (Lektinol) equivalent to 5, 15 or 35 ng ML-1, or placebo, twice weekly by subcutaneous injection for 15 weeks. This was the first study to incorporate double-blinding into the study design, although it is not clear from the published information how this was achieved and whether or not a check on the success of blinding was carried out. Participants who received the intermediate dose of mistletoe extract had statistically significant improvements in quality-of-life scores, compared with those in the placebo group; this result was not observed with the lower and higher doses of mistletoe extract.(56)

This result is difficult to interpret from a dose–response perspective. However, the assumption that the optimal dose of a herbal medicine is the highest tolerated dose has been challenged previously, particularly since some herbal medicines, including mistletoe, appear to act at least in part through immunostimulatory or immunomodulatory mechanisms.(57) This view is borne out by the results of the present study(56) since the apparently effective dose of mistletoe extract (equivalent to ML-1 15 ng, twice weekly) was not the highest dose tested (mistletoe extract equivalent to ML-1 35 ng, twice weekly). Furthermore, the effective dose was much lower than that administered in a previous study(11) (equivalent to ML-1 1 ng/kg body weight, albeit of a different ML-1 standardised mistletoe extract) which found no effect for mistletoe extract, compared with control, on quality of life. The hypothesis that high doses of mistletoe extract adversely affect quality of life requires testing.

The results of another prospective randomised controlled trial, which have now been published in more detail since systematic reviews(52, 53) were conducted, have echoed previous findings that mistletoe extract (in this case, Iscador M) is not effective as an adjuvant treatment in cancer. Patients involved in this study had either high-risk stage II (thickness > 3 mm) or stage III (regional lymph node metastases) melanoma without distant metastases.(58) The study, carried out by the German Cancer Society (DKG), at present is published only as a joint report with another randomised controlled trial set up by the European Organisation for Research and Treatment of Cancer (EORTC) to assess the value of low doses of the recombinant interferons (rIFNs) rIFN-$\alpha 2\beta$ and rIFN-γ; the DKG study contributed patients randomised to the rIFNs and control groups. With respect to mistletoe, the report provides analysis only for the Iscador M group versus the control group, and not for Iscador M versus rIFNs.

The DKG study randomised 407 patients to receive Iscador M in escalating doses as recommended (n = 102), rIFN-$\alpha 2\beta$ 1 MU subcutaneously every other day (n = 101), rIFN-γ 0.2 mg subcutaneously every other day (n = 102), or control (n = 102), for one year, or until tumour progression. The Iscador M regimen was as follows: escalating doses from 0.01 to 1.0 mg/mL (volume administered not stated) every other day over two weeks, resumed after three treatment-free days for 14 doses of 20 mg/mL every other day, followed by seven treatment-free days, and repeated over one year (or until tumour progression).(58)

In an intention-to-treat analysis, there was no statistically significant difference between the mistletoe group and the control group with respect to the primary end-point of the study, the disease-free interval, and duration of survival (estimated hazard ratio (95% CI): 1.32 (0.93–1.87), p = 0.12 and 1.21 (0.84–1.75), p = 0.31 for disease-free interval and survival, respectively). Thus, adjuvant treatment with Iscador M in patients with melanoma did not lead to a more favourable outcome, when compared with control.(58) The findings raised the hypothesis that mistletoe treatment potentially may have an adverse effect in patients with melanoma by stimulating melanoma cell proliferation.

Another prospective, randomised, controlled, multicentre trial, conducted in China, compared the effects of a mistletoe preparation (Helixor A) with those of a polysaccharide biological response modifier (Lentinan; 4 mg by intramuscular injection, daily) on quality of life in 233 patients with breast (n = 68), ovarian (n = 71) and non-small-cell lung cancer (n = 94) who also received conventional cancer chemotherapy.[59] Participants randomised to the mistletoe group received escalating doses, administered three times weekly by subcutaneous injection and starting with 1 mg up to a maximum of 200 mg (although it is not stated in a report of the study, this probably refers to the amount of mistletoe extract, rather than the mistletoe lectin content). The duration of treatment for standard and adjuvant therapy was not stated in a report of the trial.

A statistically significant improvement in the Karnofsky Performance Index (which measures physical condition) was reported for the mistletoe group, compared with the placebo group (proportion of participants reporting an improvement: 50.4% and 32.4% for Helixor A and Lentinan, respectively; p = 0.002).[59] However, it is not known to what extent the lack of blinding of treatment allocation could have influenced the results and, in view of this and other methodological limitations (e.g. no sample size calculation), the results of this trial cannot be considered conclusive.

A new instrument has been developed to measure specifically the quality of life of patients with cancer treated with mistletoe preparations in the clinical trial setting.[60]

M

Effects on immunological parameters Immunomodulatory effects do not necessarily translate into clinical efficacy, and the influence of some immune parameters, for example, interleukin-1 and -6, may be to stimulate the growth of certain types of tumour cells.[15] Other factors, such as resistance to changes in immune parameters, can occur in advanced stages in some types of cancer, thus the responses of different tumour types towards immunomodulatory effects need to be considered separately.

Many studies involving patients with cancer have investigated the effects of mistletoe preparations on immune parameters, such as lymphocytes, natural killer cells and cytokines. Most, but not all, of these studies describe effects for different mistletoe preparations. The results of several studies have been summarised in a non-systematic, yet comprehensive, review of clinical trials of well-characterised, lectin-standardised mistletoe extracts in patients with different types of cancer.[55]

The two most methodologically rigorous randomised controlled trials (*see* Therapeutic effects, Cancer), which assessed the effects of mistletoe extracts on immune parameters (as well as on clinical outcome measures), reported conflicting results. In a randomised controlled trial involving 477 patients with head and neck squamous cell carcinoma who received an ML-1 standardised mistletoe extract (Eurixor) in addition to conventional treatment, there were no statistically significant differences between the treatment and control groups in blood concentrations of the following lymphocyte subsets when assessed at different time points throughout the study: CD3+, CD4+, CD8+, CD19+, CD16+53+3+, CD16+53+3, CD25+ and CD3+DR.[11] In contrast, a randomised, double-blind, multicentre trial involving 272 patients with breast cancer who received mistletoe extract (Lektinol) equivalent to 5, 15 or 35 ng ML-1, or placebo, in addition to conventional treatment found a statistically significant increase in blood concentrations of CD4+ cells in the mistletoe group, compared with the placebo group.[56]

Other studies discussed in the review had methodological flaws and their results cannot be considered definitive. In one of these studies – a randomised, controlled trial involving 35 patients with malignant stage III/IV glioma – statistically significant increases in peripheral blood CD3+, CD4+ and CD8+ cell counts were observed after three months' treatment with mistletoe extract (Eurixor) equivalent to 1 ng/kg body weight twice weekly, compared with values for the control group.[61] Another trial, in which 47 patients with advanced breast cancer were randomised to receive mistletoe extract (Eurixor) equivalent to 0.5 or 1 ng/kg body weight twice weekly by subcutaneous injection for eight weeks followed by a four-week break, for at least two cycles, reported increases in plasma β-endorphin concentrations and enhanced activity of natural killer cells and T-lymphocytes, compared with pretreatment values.[62] This trial supported the findings of an earlier similar study,[63] which also reported increased *in vitro* release of cytokines (IL-2, IFN-γ and TNFα) by mononuclear cells from patients with breast cancer treated with mistletoe extract (Eurixor).

Other preliminary studies have described the production of anti-ML-1 antibodies in patients with cancer who were treated with mistletoe extracts.[64–67] The antibodies produced were typically of the immunoglobulin G type, although in some instances, antibodies of the immunoglobulin E and other types were produced.[65] There is some evidence that the antibody response differs depending on the type of mistletoe preparation administered (i.e. the profile of antigens within the extract).[65] In association with this work, *in vitro* studies showed that anti-ML-1 antibodies neutralised the cytotoxic effect of mistletoe lectins on peripheral blood mononuclear cells,[64,65] and tumour cell lines.[68]

In a small (n = 14), uncontrolled study, an increase in the incorporation of [^{3}H]thymidine into the DNA of unstimulated lymphocytes, as a marker for DNA repair, was observed in patients with breast cancer who received mistletoe extract (Iscador M; single intravenous infusion then, after two days, subcutaneous injections daily for seven days).[69] The effect was greatest on days 7–9 of treatment when values were 2.7 times higher than pretreatment values. This finding raised several hypotheses which require further testing.

Mistletoe preparations have also been documented to induce immunological responses in healthy volunteers. In a randomised, double-blind, placebo-controlled study involving 48 healthy volunteers, Iscador Q (in increasing doses twice weekly by subcutaneous injection, over 12 weeks), but not Iscador P (in increasing doses twice weekly by subcutaneous injection over 12 weeks), induced eosinophilia after five weeks' treatment which persisted until the end of treatment (week 12), when compared with placebo.[70] At the end of the study, anti-ML-1 antibodies were detected in all 16 volunteers in the Iscador Q group, but in less than half those exposed to Iscador P, whereas anti-viscotoxin A2 immunoglobulin G antibodies were found in all mistletoe-exposed participants.[71] In a preliminary study involving healthy volunteers who received Iscador Q by subcutaneous injection, significant increases in the microcirculation were observed, both local to the injection site and in other target tissues investigated (e.g. gingival, rectal). Increased transmigration of white blood cells was also noted both locally and in other target tissues, a phenomenon which is believed to be important in the immunological response.[72]

In other studies, T-lymphocytes were obtained from blood samples from patients with cancer who had received subcutaneous injections three times weekly of aqueous mistletoe extracts prepared from mistletoe grown on apple and pine trees to examine their response to subsequent incubation with the mistletoe extracts *in vitro*.[73,74] Proliferation of T-lymphocytes from mistletoe-treated patients occurred, but was not observed for T-lymphocytes obtained from untreated control subjects. Further investigation revealed that the responding cells were the CD4+ T-cell subset.[73,74] A small uncontrolled study described increases in the release of cytokines, such as TNFα and IL-6, measured in the supernatants of cultured peripheral blood mononuclear cells obtained from patients with breast cancer who were treated with mistletoe extract (ABNOBA-Viscum, 0.2 mg fresh plant material/30 kg body weight by subcutaneous injection twice weekly for 16 weeks).[66]

Other conditions Clinical investigation of the effects of mistletoe preparations in conditions other than cancer is limited. Several preliminary investigations in patients with chronic hepatitis C infection,[75] respiratory infections[76,77] and HIV infection[78] have been undertaken. Some of these studies have reported improvements in clinical outcomes and immunological parameters in mistletoe recipients, compared with pretreatment values or with placebo or other control group values. However, due to the methodological limitations of these studies, the results are inconclusive.

Side-effects, Toxicity

Clinical data

Clinical safety and toxicity data for mistletoe are limited and further investigation of these aspects is required. Many clinical trials have not provided an assessment of safety or have reported little information on safety aspects, and there is a paucity of well-designed postmarketing surveillance studies of mistletoe preparations.

The UK Medicines and Healthcare products Regulatory Agency's (MHRA) national spontaneous reporting scheme for suspected adverse drug reactions has received a total of four reports of suspected adverse drug reactions (ADRs) associated with Iscador preparations up to 2004.[79] These reports described 12 suspected ADRs, including hepatitis and abnormal liver function (two reports), myalgia, dizziness, wheezing, cough, hoarseness, abdominal pain, pyrexia, urticaria (one report) and a suspected interaction (one report).[79] The MHRA has received one further suspected ADR report of arteritis associated with a multi-ingredient product containing mistletoe (no further details available at the time of writing). Causality in these cases has not been established.

Reviews of clinical trials which have provided an assessment of the safety of mistletoe, generally have reported mistletoe preparations to be well tolerated.[52,55] The most frequently reported adverse events in trials using ML-standardised mistletoe preparations were local reactions, such as urticaria and/or erythema, at the injection site which usually resolved within 48 hours.[55] The frequency of occurrence of such reactions in patients with cancer who received mistletoe preparations by injection has been described as being up to 48%.[55]

This information, however, comes mostly from small-scale clinical trials involving patients with different types of cancer who were also receiving various different conventional treatments (surgery, radiotherapy and/or cancer chemotherapeutic agents) in addition to mistletoe preparations. Furthermore, studies have assessed the effects of different types of mistletoe preparations, which vary both qualitatively and quantitatively in their composition, administered according to different dosage regimens. Against this background, the safety of each individual mistletoe preparation needs to be considered.

In a randomised controlled trial involving 477 patients with head and neck squamous cell carcinoma receiving conventional treatment, an ML-1 standardised mistletoe extract (Eurixor) was administered in doses equivalent to ML-1 1 ng/kg body weight twice weekly by subcutaneous injection over a 60-week period in treatment cycles of 12 weeks followed by a break in treatment after every four weeks; the control group did not receive any additional treatment.[11] In total, 43% of mistletoe recipients developed local and/or systemic adverse events at the onset of mistletoe treatment, although this fell to around 8% by week 32 or later of treatment. The most common local reactions occurring at the onset of treatment were rubor, prurigo and indurations (hard spots); vesiculation was observed in 1–3% of mistletoe recipients over the treatment period. Other reactions (melalgia, fever, sleeplessness, tiredness, cold or heat sensations and sneezing) occurred in 1–4% of the mistletoe group. In total, around 18% of mistletoe recipients refused further injections during the study (after a median of 12 weeks) because of adverse events believed to be induced by mistletoe.[11]

In a randomised controlled trial involving 407 patients with melanoma who received mistletoe extract (Iscador M in escalating doses as recommended), rIFN-$\alpha 2\beta$, rIFN-γ, or control, for one year or until tumour progression, study withdrawals due to anorexia, malaise, depressive moods, fever and inflammation at the injection site occurred in 4.9%, 4.6% and 7.8% of the mistletoe-, rIFN-$\alpha 2\beta$- and rIFN-γ recipients, respectively.[58] Apart from the statement that no organ toxicity was observed during the study, no further information on safety aspects was provided.

Several small, non-randomised, controlled studies have assessed the tolerability of mistletoe preparations in immunocompromised HIV-positive and healthy individuals. In two studies in which participants received mistletoe extracts (Iscador Qu FrF or Iscador Qu Special) by subcutaneous injection twice weekly in increasing doses for up to 68 weeks, erythema at the injection site occurred in all but one participant.[80,81]

Other adverse events rated to be possibly or probably associated with mistletoe extract (Iscador Qu FrF) were headache, fatigue, fever and inflammation; diarrhoea and nausea occurred in small numbers of participants, but were not thought to be associated with mistletoe treatment.[80,81] Significant increases in serum urea nitrogen and creatinine concentrations were observed for HIV-positive participants after mistletoe treatment, compared with baseline values (statistical comparisons with the control group were not undertaken), but concentrations remained within the normal range; no other statistically significant changes in biochemical parameters, including liver function test values, were seen.

Aspects of the local skin reaction that occurs following subcutaneous injection of mistletoe extracts (Iscador QFrF or Qu Special) have been described following studies involving healthy volunteers.[82,83] The reaction appears to involve a subepidermal lymphomonocytic infiltrate, induced by mistletoe extract, at the injection site.

Hepatitis has been documented in a woman who had ingested a herbal preparation containing kelp, motherwort, scullcap and mistletoe.[84] Mistletoe was assumed by the authors of the report to be the causal factor since it was the only ingredient of the remedy known to contain toxic constituents (although these had not previously been linked with hepatotoxicity).[84] No other instances of hepatotoxicity have been associated with mistletoe ingestion and, since the case report was published, hepatitis has been documented with scullcap (*see* Scullcap).

V. album should not be confused with American mistletoe (*Phoradendron leucarpum*, *P. serotinum*, *P. flavescens*). The safety of American mistletoe has been reviewed.[G21, 85–87]

Anaphylactic reactions There are isolated reports of anaphylactic reactions occurring in individuals who have received parenteral treatment with mistletoe extracts. One report described three such cases involving patients who were already undergoing treatment with mistletoe, but did not provide full details of the mistletoe preparations administered, the reactions and outcomes, and did not undertake a causality assessment.[88] One case involved a non-atopic, 44-year-old man who was admitted to an intensive care unit with hypotension, urticaria and loss of consciousness which had developed within five minutes of an injection of *V. album* L. (Quercus) 10 mg (route of injection not specified). The man was treated with intravenous fluids and corticosteroids. A similar case involved a 70-year-old non-atopic woman after receiving her 25th dose (0.1 mg) of mistletoe extract; one month later, she displayed a positive result (which included generalised pruritus, pharyngeal oedema and malaise) following an intradermal challenge with *V. album* at one-tenth dilution.[88] The third case involved a 42-year-old man with multiple sclerosis who received a maintenance dose of *V. album* (Quercus) 10 mg and who immediately developed pruritus, oedema, asthma and hypotension.

Preclinical data

Data from an *in vitro* study involving human melanoma cell lines indicate that clinically relevant low concentrations of mistletoe lectin may stimulate tumour cell proliferation.[89] In contrast, other *in vitro* experiments did not demonstrate that an aqueous mistletoe extract (containing galactoside-specific mistletoe lectin 265 μg/mL) stimulated tumour cell proliferation.[90]

Toxicity in animals has been documented for mistletoe lectins and viscotoxins. Intravenous administration of viscotoxin to cats (35 μg/kg) resulted in a negative inotropic effect on cardiac muscle, reflex bradycardia and hypotension.[91] Viscotoxins A3 and B have also caused muscle contracture and progressive depolarisation in isolated smooth, skeletal and cardiac muscle preparations (rabbit, frog).[92] The mode of action was thought to involve the displacement of calcium from cell membrane-bound sites. The viscotoxins precipitate histamine release from human leukocytes in an irritant manner without destroying the cells.[49] Viscotoxin is toxic on parenteral administration and an LD_{50} value (mice, intraperitoneal injection) has been estimated as 0.7 mg/kg.[93]

Mistletoe lectins inhibit protein synthesis in both cells and cell-free systems.[94] In common with other known toxic lectins (e.g. ricin), mistletoe lectins bind to plasma proteins, are specific towards D-galactose, possess some cytotoxic activity and have caused macroscopic lesions in rats (e.g. ascites, congested intestine, pancreatic haemorrhages).[38] An LD_{50} (mice) value for mistletoe lectin fraction is reported as 80 μg/kg compared with 3 μg/kg for ricin.[94]

Documented LD_{50} values (mice, intraperitoneal injection) are greater than 2.25 mg for the polysaccharide fraction from the berries, 32 mg for the crude plant juice, and 276 mg for Iscador.[38]

Contra-indications, Warnings

Mistletoe is contra-indicated in cases of known allergy to mistletoe preparations, acute inflammatory conditions and high fever, and chronic progressive conditions, such as tuberculosis.[G56] Increases in body temperature can occur following mistletoe injection.

Drug interactions In view of the documented pharmacological activities of mistletoe, whether or not there is potential for clinically important interactions between mistletoe and other medicines with similar or opposing effects, such as existing cardiac, immunosuppressant, hypo/hypertensive, antidepressant and anticoagulant/coagulant therapies, should be considered.

Pregnancy and lactation The use of mistletoe is contra-indicated in pregnancy and breastfeeding in view of the toxic constituents.

References

1 Pfüller U. Chemical constituents of European mistletoe (*Viscum album* L.) isolation and characterisation of the main relevant ingredients: lectins, viscotoxins, oligo-/polysaccharides, flavonoids, alkaloids. In: Büssing A, ed. *Mistletoe. The Genus Viscum.* Amsterdam: Harwood Academic Press, 2000: 101–122.

2 Fukunaga T *et al.* Studies on the constituents of the European mistletoe, *Viscum album* L. *Chem Pharm Bull* 1987; 35: 3292–3297.

3 Krzaczek T. Pharmacobotanical studies of the subspecies *Viscum album* L. IV. *Ann Univ Mariae Curie-Sklodowska, Sect D* 1977; 32: 281–291.

4 Becker H, Exner J. Comparative studies of flavonoids and phenylcarboxylic acids of mistletoes from different host trees. *Z Pflanzenphysiol* 1980; 97: 417–428.

5 Khwaja TA *et al.* Recent studies on the anticancer activities of mistletoe (*Viscum album*) and its alkaloids. *Oncology* 1986; 43: 42–50.

6 Graziano MN *et al.* Isolation of tyramine from five Argentine species of Loranthaceae. *Lloydia* 1967; 30: 242–244.

7 Khwaja TA *et al.* Isolation of biologically active alkaloids from Korean mistletoe *Viscum album*, coloratum. *Experientia* 1980; 36: 599–600.

8 Stein GM, Berg PA. Non-lectin component in a fermented extract from *Viscum album* L. grown on pines induces proliferation of lymphocytes from healthy and allergic individuals *in vitro*. *Eur J Clin Pharmacol* 1994; 47: 33–38.

9 Deliorman D *et al.* A new acyclic monoterpene glucoside from *Viscum album* ssp *album*. *Fitoterapia* 2002; 72: S101.

10 Krzaczek T. Pharmacobotanical studies of the subspecies *Viscum album* L. III. Terpenes and sterols. *Ann Univ Mariae Curie-Sklodowska, Sect D* 1977; 32: 125–134.

11 Steuer-Vogt MK *et al.* The effect of an adjuvant mistletoe treatment programme in resected head and neck cancer patients: a randomised controlled clinical trial. *Eur J Cancer* 2001; 37: 23–31.

12 Mengs U *et al.* Mistletoe extracts standardized to mistletoe lectins in oncology: review on current status of preclinical research. *Anticancer Res* 2002; 22: 1399–1408.

13 Die Mistel in der Tumortherapie. Grundlagenforschung und klinik. In: Proceedings of the 3rd Mistletoe Symposium, Nonnweiler-Otzenhausen, Germany, 2003. Nonnweiler-Otzenhausen: Europäisches Bildungszentrum Otzenhausen, 2003.

14 Mansky PJ. Mistletoe and cancer: controversies and perspectives. *Semin Oncol* 2002; 29: 589–594.

15 Gabius H-J *et al.* From ill-defined extracts to the immunomodulatory lectin: will there be a reason for oncological application of mistletoe? *Planta Med* 1994; 60: 2–7.

16 Bocci V. Mistletoe (*Viscum album*) lectins as cytokine inducers and immunoadjuvant in tumor therapy. A review. *J Biol Reg Homeostatic Agents* 1993; 7: 1–6.
17 Schink M. Mistletoe therapy for human cancer: the role of the natural killer cells. *Anti-Cancer Drugs* 1997; 8 (Suppl. Suppl.1): S47–S51.
18 Büssing A. Biological and pharmacological properties of *Viscum album* L. From tissue flask to man. In: Büssing A, ed. *Mistletoe. The Genus Viscum*. Amsterdam: Harwood Academic Press, 2000: 128–182.
19 Janssen O *et al. In vitro* effects of mistletoe extracts and mistletoe lectins. Cytotoxicity towards tumor cells due to the induction of programmed cell death (apoptosis). *Arzneim Forsch/Drug Res* 1993; 43: 1221–1227.
20 Žarković N *et al.* Comparison of the effects of high and low concentrations of the separated *Viscum album* L. lectins and of the plain mistletoe plant preparation (Isorel) on the growth of normal and tumor cells *in vitro*. *Periodicum Biologorum* 1995; 97: 61–67.
21 Urech K *et al.* Comparative study on the cytotoxic effect of viscotoxin and mistletoe lectin on tumour cells in culture. *Phytother Res* 1995; 9: 49–55.
22 Valentiner U *et al.* The cytotoxic effect of mistletoe lectins I, II and III on sensitive and multidrug resistant human colon cancer cell lines *in vitro*. *Toxicology* 2002; 171: 187–199.
23 Van Huyen J-PD *et al.* Induction of apoptosis of endothelial cells by *Viscum album*: a role for anti-tumoral properties of mistletoe lectins. *Mol Med* 2002; 8: 600–606.
24 Büssing A *et al.* Differences in the apoptosis-inducing properties of *Viscum album* L. extracts. *Anti-Cancer Drugs* 1997; 8 (Suppl. Suppl.1): S9–S14.
25 Büssing A, Schietzel M. Apoptosis-inducing properties of *Viscum album* L. extracts from different host trees correlate with their content of toxic mistletoe lectins. *Anticancer Res* 1999; 19: 23–28.
26 Li S-S. Mistletoe lectins: telomerase inhibitors in alternative cancer therapy. *Drug Discovery Today* 2002; 7: 896–897.
27 Žarković N *et al.* The *Viscum album* preparation Isorel inhibits the growth of melanoma B16F10 by influencing the tumour-host relationship. *Anticancer Drugs* 1997; Suppl. Suppl.1: S17–S22.
28 Burger AM *et al.* Anticancer activity of an aqueous mistletoe extract (AME) in syngeneic murine tumor models. *Anticancer Res* 2001; 21: 1965–1968.
29 Kuttan G *et al.* Anticarcinogenic and antimetastatic activity of Iscador. *Anticancer Drugs* 1997; Suppl. Suppl.1: S15–S16.
30 Weber K *et al.* Effects of a standardized mistletoe preparation on metastatic B16 melanoma colonization in murine lungs. *Arzneim Forsch/Drug Res* 1998; 48: 497–502.
31 Braun JM *et al.* Standardized mistletoe extract augments immune response and down-regulates local and metastatic tumor growth in murine models. *Anticancer Res* 2002; 22: 4187–4190.
32 Braun JM *et al.* Application of standardized mistletoe extracts augment immune response and down regulates metastatic organ colonization in murine models. *Cancer Lett* 2001; 170: 25–31.
33 Mueller EA *et al.* Biochemical characterization of a component in extracts of *Viscum album* enhancing human NK cytotoxicity. *Immunopharmacology* 1989; 17: 11–18.
34 Hostanska K *et al.* A plant lectin derived from *Viscum album* induces cytokine gene expression and protein production in cultures of human peripheral blood mononuclear cells. *Nat Immun* 1995; 14: 295–304.
35 Braun JM *et al.* Cytokine release of whole blood from adult female donors challenged with mistletoe lectin-1 standardised mistletoe extract and *E. coli* endotoxin or phytohaemagglutinin (PHA). *Anticancer Res* 2003; 23: 1349–1352.
36 Ribéreau-Gayon G *et al.* Modulation of cytotoxicity and enhancement of cytokine release by Viscum album L. extracts or mistletoe lectins. *Anti-Cancer Drugs* 1997; 8 (Suppl. Suppl.1): S3–S8.
37 Joller PW *et al.* Stimulation of cytokine production via a special standardized mistletoe preparation in an in vitro human skin bioassay. *Arzneim Forsch/Drug Res* 1996; 46: 649–653.
38 Bloksma N *et al.* Stimulation of humoral and cellular immunity by *Viscum* preparations. *Planta Med* 1982; 46: 221–227.
39 Coeugniet EG, Elek E. Immunomodulation with *Viscum album* and *Echinacea purpurea* extracts. *Onkologie* 1987; 10: 27–33.
40 Luther P, Mehnert WH. Zum serologischen Verhalten einiger handelsüblicher Präparate aus *Viscum album* L., insbesondere des Iscador, in bezug aug menschliche Blutzellen und Aszites-Tumorzellen von Mäusen. *Acta Biol Med Ger* 1974; 33: 351–357.
41 Luther P *et al.* Isolation and characterization of mistletoe extracts. II. Action of agglutinating and cytotoxic fractions on mouse ascites tumor cells. *Acta Biol Med Ger* 1977; 36: 119–125.
42 Luther P *et al.* Reaktionen einiger antikörperähnlicher Substanzen aus Insekten (Protektine) und Pflanzen (Lektine) mit Aszites-Tumorzellen. *Acta Biol Med Ger* 1973; 31: K11–K18.
43 Ziska P *et al.* The lectin from *Viscum album* L. purification by biospecific affinity chromatography. *Experientia* 1978; 34: 123–124.
44 Franz H *et al.* Isolation and properties of three lectins from mistletoe (*Viscum album* L.). *Biochem J* 1981; 195: 481–484.
45 Luther P *et al.* The lectin from *Viscum album* L. – isolation, characterization, properties and structure. *Int J Biochem* 1980; 11: 429–435.
46 Ziska P *et al.* Chemical modification studies on the D-galactopyranosyl binding lectin from the mistletoe *Viscum album* L. *Acta Biol Med Ger* 1979; 38: 1361–1363.
47 Ziska P, Franz H. Studies on the interaction of the mistletoe lectin I with carbohydrates. *Experientia* 1981; 37: 219.
48 Franz H *et al.* Isolation and characterization of mistletoe extracts. I. Affinity chromatography of mistletoe crude extract on insolubilized plasma proteins. *Acta Biol Med Ger* 1976; 36: 113–117.
49 Luther P *et al.* Allergy and lectins: interaction between IgE-mediated histamine release and glycoproteins from *Viscum album* L. (mistletoe). *Acta Biol Med Ger* 1978; 37: 1623–1628.
50 Petkov V. Plants with hypotensive, antiatheromatous and coronarodilatating action. *Am J Chin Med* 1979; 7: 197–236.
51 Deliorman D *et al.* Evaluation of antimycobacterial activity of *Viscum album* subspecies. *Pharmaceutical Biol* 2001; 39: 381–383.
52 Kienle GS *et al.* Mistletoe in cancer. A systematic review on controlled clinical trials. *Eur J Med Res* 2003; 8: 109–119.
53 Ernst E *et al.* Mistletoe for cancer? A systematic review of randomised clinical trials. *Int J Cancer* 2003; 107: 262–267.
54 Kleijnen J, Knipschild P. Mistletoe treatment for cancer. Review of controlled trials in humans. *Phytomedicine* 1994; 1: 255–260.
55 Stauder H, Kreuser E-D. Mistletoe extracts standardised in terms of mistletoe lectins (ML 1) in oncology: current state of clinical research. *Onkologie* 2002; 25: 374–380.
56 Wetzel D, Schäfer M. Results of a randomised placebo-controlled multicentre study with PS76A2 (standardised mistletoe preparation) in patients with breast cancer receiving adjuvant chemotherapy [abstract]. *Phytomedicine* 2000; II(Suppl): 34.
57 Vickers A. Botanical medicines for the treatment of cancer: rationale, overview of current data, and methodological considerations for phase I and II trials. *Cancer Invest* 2002; 29: 1069–1979.
58 Kleeberg UR *et al.* for the EORTC Melanoma Group in cooperation with the German Cancer Society (DKG). Final results of the EORTC 18871/DKG 80–1 randomised phase III trial: rIFN-α2β versus rIFN-γ versus Iscador M® versus observation after surgery in melanoma patients with either high-risk primary (thickness > 3 mm) or regional lymph node metastasis. *Eur J Cancer* 2004; 40: 390–402.
59 Piao BK *et al.* Impact of complementary mistletoe extract treatment on quality of life in breast, ovarian and non-small cell lung cancer patients. A prospective randomized controlled clinical trial. *Anticancer Res* 2004; 24: 303–310.
60 Kirchberger I *et al.* Development and validation of an instrument to measure the effects of a mistletoe preparation on quality of life of cancer patients: the Life Quality Lection-53 (LQL-53) Questionnaire. *Qual Life Res* 2004; 13: 463–479.
61 Lenartz D *et al.* Immunoprotective activity of the galactoside-specific lectin from mistletoe after destructive therapy in glioma patients. *Anticancer Res* 1996; 16: 3799–3802.
62 Heiny B-M *et al.* Correlation of immune cell activities and β-endorphin release in breast carcinoma patients treated with galactoside-specific lectin standardized mistletoe extract. *Anticancer Res* 1998; 18: 583–586.
63 Heiny B-M, Beuth J. Mistletoe extract standardized for the galactoside-specific lectin (ML-1) induces β-endorphin release and immunopotentiation in breast cancer patients. *Anticancer Res* 1994; 14: 1339–1342.
64 Stettin A *et al.* Anti-mistletoe lectin antibodies are produced in patients during therapy with an aqueous mistletoe extract derived

from *Viscum album* L. and neutralize lectin-induced cytotoxicity *in vitro*. *Klin Wochenschr* 1990; 68: 896–900.
65 Stein GM *et al*. Induction of anti-mistletoe lectin antibodies in relation to different mistletoe extracts. *Anti-Cancer Drugs* 1997; 8 (Suppl. Suppl.1): S57–S59.
66 Stein GM *et al*. Modulation of the cellular and humoral immune responses of tumor patients by mistletoe therapy. *Eur J Med Res* 1998; 3: 194–202.
67 Stein GM *et al*. Recognition of different antigens of mistletoe extracts by anti-mistletoe lectin antibodies. *Cancer Lett* 1999; 135: 165–170.
68 Tonevitsky AG *et al*. Hybridoma cells producing antibodies against A-chain of mistletoe lectin are resistant to this toxin. *Immunol Lett* 1995; 46: 5–8.
69 Kovacs E *et al*. Improvement of DNA repair in lymphocytes of breast cancer patients treated with *Viscum album* extract (Iscador). *Eur J Cancer* 1991; 27: 1672–1676.
70 Huber R *et al*. Effects of a lectin- and a viscotoxin-rich mistletoe preparation on clinical and hematologic parameters: a placebo-controlled evaluation in healthy subjects. *J Altern Comp Med* 2002; 8: 857–866.
71 Klein R *et al*. *In vivo*-induction of antibodies to mistletoe lectin-1 and viscotoxin by exposure to aqueous mistletoe extracts: a randomised double-blinded placebo-controlled phase I study in healthy individuals. *Eur J Med Res* 2002; 7: 155–163.
72 Klopp R *et al*. Changes in immunological characteristics of white blood cells after administration of standardized mistletoe extract. *In Vivo* 2001; 15: 447–458.
73 Fischer S *et al*. Oligoclonal in vitro response of CD4 T cells to vesicles of mistletoe extracts in mistletoe-treated cancer patients. *Cancer Immunol Immunother* 1997; 44: 150–156.
74 Fischer S *et al*. Stimulation of the specific immune system by mistletoe extracts. *Anti-Cancer Drugs* 1997; 8 (Suppl. Suppl.1): S33–S37.
75 Huber R *et al*. Effects of a mistletoe preparations with defined lectin content on chronic hepatitis C: an individually controlled cohort study. *Eur J Med Res* 2001; 6: 399–405.
76 Chernyshov VP *et al*. Immunomodulatory actions of *Viscum album* (Iscador) in children with recurrent respiratory disease as a result of the Chernobyl nuclear accident. *Comp Ther Med* 1997; 5: 141–146.
77 Chernyshov VP *et al*. Immunomodulatory and clinical effects of *Viscum album* (Iscador M and Iscador P) in children with recurrent respiratory infections as a result of the Chernobyl nuclear accident. *Am J Therapeut* 2000; 7: 195–203.
78 Stoss M, Gorter RW. No evidence of IFN-γ increase in the serum of HIV-positive and healthy subjects after subcutaneous injection of a non-fermented *Viscum album* L. extract. *Nat Immun* 1998; 16: 157–164.
79 Medicines and Healthcare products Regulatory Agency. Adverse Drug Reactions On-line Information Tracking (ADROIT) database (accessed 26 July 2004).
80 Van Wely M *et al*. Toxicity of a standardized mistletoe extract in immunocompromised and healthy individuals. *Am J Therapeut* 1999; 6: 37–43.
81 Gorter RW *et al*. Tolerability of an extract of European mistletoe among immunocompromised and healthy individuals. *Altern Ther* 1999; 5: 37–48.
82 Gorter RW *et al*. Subcutaneous infiltrates induced by injection of mistletoe extracts (Iscador). *Am J Therapeut* 1998; 5: 181–187.
83 Stoss M *et al*. Decrease of activated lympocytes four and nine hours after a subcutaneous injection of a *Viscum album* L. extract in healthy volunteers. *Nat Immun* 1998; 16: 185–197.
84 Harvey J, Colin-Jones DG. Mistletoe hepatitis. *BMJ* 1981; 282: 186–187.
85 Hall AH *et al*. Assessing mistletoe toxicity. *Ann Emerg Med* 1986; 15: 1320–1323.
86 Spiller HA *et al*. Retrospective study of mistletoe ingestion. *Clin Toxicol* 1996; 34: 405–408.
87 Krenzelok EP *et al*. American mistletoe exposures. *Am J Emerg Med* 1997; 15: 516–520.
88 Hutt N *et al*. Anaphylactic reactions after therapeutic injection of mistletoe (*Viscum album* L.). *Allergol Immunol* 2001; 29: 201–203.
89 Gabius H-J *et al*. Evidence for stimulation of tumor proliferation in cell lines and histotypic cultures by clinically relevant low doses of the galactoside-binding mistletoe lectin, a component of proprietary extracts. *Cancer Invest* 2001; 19: 114–126.
90 Burger AM *et al*. No evidence of stimulation of human tumor cell proliferation by a standardized aqueous mistletoe extract *in vitro*. *Anticancer Res* 2003; 23: 3801–3806.
91 Rosell S, Samuelsson G. Effect of mistletoe viscotoxin and phoratoxin on blood circulation. *Toxicon* 1966; 4: 107–110.
92 Andersson K-E, Jöhannsson M. Effects of viscotoxin on rabbit heart and aorta, and on frog skeletal muscle. *Eur J Pharmacol* 1973; 23: 223–231.
93 Samuelsson G. Screening of plants of the family Loranthaceae for toxic proteins. *Acta Pharm Suec* 1966; 3: 353–362.
94 Stirpe F *et al*. Inhibition of protein synthesis by a toxic lectin from *Viscum album* L. (mistletoe). *Biochem J* 1980; 190: 843–845.

Motherwort

Summary and Pharmaceutical Comment

The common name motherwort may be applied to one of many *Leonurus* species. *L. cardiaca* is the typical European species utilised, whereas *Leonurus japonicus* Houtt is commonly used in traditional Chinese medicine. Other species referred to as motherwort include *Leonurus sibirious* and *L. heterophyllus*. The chemistry of *L. cardiaca* is well studied although the presence of the uterotonic principle leonurine has been disputed. Cardioactivity *in vitro* has been reported for motherwort (*L. cardiaca*), although the clinical relevance of this is not clear. There is a lack of clinical research assessing the efficacy and safety of motherwort, and any symptoms of cardiac disorder are not suitable for self-diagnosis and treatment with a herbal remedy. In view of the lack of toxicity data, excessive use of motherwort and use during pregnancy and lactation should be avoided.

Species (Family)

Leonurus cardiaca L. (Labiatae/Lamiaceae)

Synonym(s)

Leonurus

Part(s) Used

Herb

Pharmacopoeial and Other Monographs

BHC 1992[G6]
BHP 1996[G9]
BP 2007[G84]
Complete German Commission E[G3]
Martindale 35th edition[G85]
Ph Eur 2007[G81]

Legal Category (Licensed Products)

GSL[G37]

Constituents

The following is compiled from several sources, including General Reference G6.

Alkaloids 0.35%. Stachydrine (a pyrrolidine-type alkaloid), betonicine and turicin (stereoisomers of 4-hydroxystachydrine), leonurine 0.0068% (a guanidine derivative),[1] leonuridin, leonurinine. The presence of leonurine in *L. cardiaca* has been disputed, although it has been documented for other *Leonurus* species.

Flavonoids Glycosides of apigenin, kaempferol, and quercetin (e.g. hyperoside, kaempferol-3-D-glucoside, genkwanin, quinqueloside, quercitrin and rutin).[2,3]

Iridoids Ajugol, ajugoside, galiridoside, leonuride and three or four more unidentified glycosides.[4]

Tannins 2–8%. Type not specified. Pseudotannins (e.g. pyrogallol, catechins).

Terpenoids Volatile oil 0.05%, resin, wax, ursolic acid, leocardin (a labdane diterpene)[5] as an epimeric mixture, and a diterpene lactone similar to marrubiin.[2] Cardiac glycosides (bufadienolide/bufanolide type) have been documented although their presence in motherwort has not been confirmed.

Other constituents Citric acid, malic acid, oleic acid, bitter principles,[6,7] carbohydrates 2.89%, choline and a phenolic glycoside (caffeic acid 4-rutinoside).[8]

A *Cad*-specific lectin has been isolated from the seeds.[9]

Food Use

Motherwort is not used in foods. Previously, motherwort has been listed by the Food and Drugs Administration (FDA) as a Herb of Undefined Safety.[G22]

Herbal Use

Motherwort is stated to possess sedative and antispasmodic properties. Traditionally, it has been used for cardiac debility, simple tachycardia, effort syndrome, amenorrhoea, and specifically for cardiac symptoms associated with neurosis.[G6,G7,G8,G64]

Alkaloids

stachydrine

betonicine

leonurine

Iridoids

leonuride

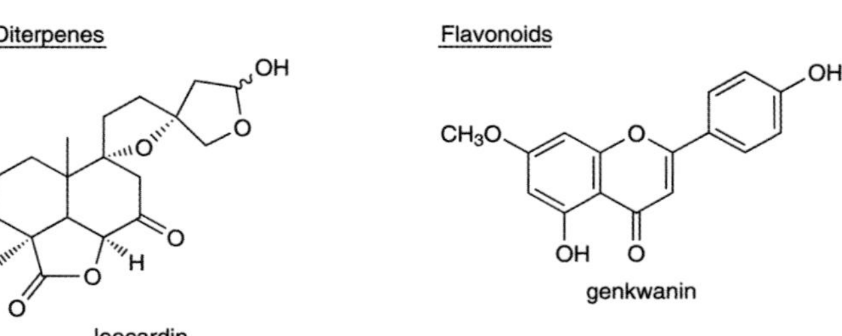

Figure 1 Selected constituents of motherwort.

Dosage

Dosages for oral administration (adults) for traditional uses recommended in standard herbal reference texts are given below.

Dried herb 2–4 g as an infusion three times daily.[G6, G7]

Liquid extract 2–4 mL (1 : 1 in 25% alcohol) three times daily.[G6, G7]

Tincture 2–6 mL (1 : 5 in 45% alcohol) three times daily.[G6, G7]

Pharmacological Actions

In vitro and animal studies

The uterotonic principle in motherwort is unclear, although leonurine is reported to be the utero-active constituent in various *Leonurus* species. In addition, oxytocic activity documented for *L. cardiaca* has been attributed to another alkaloid constituent, stachydrine.[G30] Uterotonic activity has been reported for leonurine in various *in vitro* preparations including human myometrial strips and isolated rat uterus.[10, 11]

In vitro cardioactivity has been documented for motherwort.[12] An alcoholic extract was found to have a direct inhibitory effect on myocardial cells: antagonistic action towards calcium chloride (provided that the extract was administered before calcium chloride), and towards both α- and β-adrenoceptor stimulation was observed. No significant effect on the cardiac activity of the isolated guinea-pig heart was noted for caffeic acid 4-rutinoside.[8]

Ursolic acid has been reported to possess antiviral, tumour-inhibitory and cytotoxic activities.[13, 14] Ursolic acid was found to inhibit the Epstein–Barr virus *in vitro* and to inhibit tumour production by 12-*O*-tetradeconoyl phorbol (TPA) in mouse skin, with activity comparable to that of retinoic acid, a known tumour-promoter inhibitor.[14] *In vitro* cytotoxicity was documented in lymphocytic leukaemia (P-388, L-1210), human lung carcinoma (A-549), KB cells, human colon (HCT-8) and mammary tumour (MCF-7).[13]

Clinical studies

There is a lack of clinical research assessing the effects of motherwort and rigorous randomised controlled clinical trials are required.

Side-effects, Toxicity

Clinical data

There is a lack of clinical safety and toxicity data for motherwort and further investigation of these aspects is required.

It has been stated that the leaves of motherwort may cause contact dermatitis and that the lemon-scented oil may result in photosensitisation.[G51]

Preclinical data

No documented toxicity studies were located. Cytotoxic activities have been reported for ursolic acid (*see* Pharmacological Actions, *In vitro* and animal studies).

M

Contra-indications, Warnings

Sensitive individuals may experience an allergic reaction.

Drug interactions None documented. However, the potential for preparations of motherwort to interact with other medicines administered concurrently, particularly those with similar or opposing effects, should be considered.

Pregnancy and lactation Motherwort is reputed to affect the menstrual cycle.[G22] In view of the lack of toxicity data and the documented *in vitro* uterotonic activity,[G30] the use of motherwort during pregnancy and lactation should be avoided.

Preparations

Proprietary multi-ingredient preparations

Australia: Pacifenity; Valerian. *Austria:* Thyreogutt. *France:* Biocarde. *Germany:* Biovital Aktiv; Biovital Classic; Mutellon; Oxacant-sedativ. *Hungary:* Biovital; Biovital. *Switzerland:* Tisane pour le coeur et la circulation. *UK:* Fenneherb Prementaid; Menopause Relief; Modern Herbals Stress; Period Pain Relief; Prementaid; Quiet Life; Roberts Alchemilla Compound Tablets; SuNerven; Wellwoman.

References

1 Gulubov AZ. Structure of alkaloids from *Leonurus cardiaca*. *Nauch Tr Vissh Predagog Inst Plovdiv Mat Fiz Khim Biol* 1970; 8: 129–132.
2 Scott JH *et al*. Components of *Leonurus cardiaca*. *Sci Pharm* 1973; 41: 149–155.
3 Kartnig T *et al*. Flavonoid-O-glycosides from the herbs of *Leonurus cardiaca*. *J Nat Prod* 1985; 48: 494–507.
4 Buzogany K, Cucu V. Comparative study between the species of *Leonurus quinquelobatus*. Part II Iridoids. *Clujul Med* 1983; 56: 385–388.
5 Malakov P *et al*. The structure of leocardin, two epimers of a diterpenoid from *Leonurus cardiaca*. *Phytochemistry* 1985; 24: 2341–2343.
6 Brieskorn CH, Hofmann R. Labiatenbitterstoffe: Ein clerodanderivat aus *Leonurus cardiaca* L. *Tetrahedron Lett* 1979; 27: 2511–2512.
7 Brieskorn CH, Broschek W. Bitter principles and furanoid compounds of *L. cardiaca*. *Pharm Acta Helv* 1972; 47: 123–132.
8 Tschesche R *et al*. Caffeic acid 4-rutinoside from *Leonurus cardiaca*. *Phytochemistry* 1980; 19: 2783.
9 Bird GWG, Wingham J. Anti-Cad lectin from the seeds of *Leonurus cardiaca*. *Clin Lab Haematol* 1979; 1: 57–59.
10 Yeung HW *et al*. The structure and biological effect of leonurine – a uterotonic principle from the Chineses drug, I-mu Ts'ao. *Planta Med* 1977; 31: 51–56.
11 Kong YC *et al*. Isolation of the uterotonic principle from *Leonorus artemisia*, the Chinese motherwort. *Am J Chin Med* 1976; 4: 373–382.
12 Yanxing X. The inhibitory effect of motherwort extract on pulsating myocardial cells in vitro. *J Trad Chin Med* 1983; 3: 185–188.
13 Kuo-Hsiung L *et al*. The cytotoxic principles of *Prunella vulgaris*, *Psychotria serpens*, and *Hyptis capitata*: Ursolic acid and related derivatives. *Planta Med* 1988; 54: 308.
14 Tokuda H *et al*. Inhibitory effects of ursolic and oleanolic acid on skin tumor promotion by 12-O-tetradecanoylphorbol-13-acetate. *Cancer Lett* 1986; 33: 279–285.

Myrrh

Summary and Pharmaceutical Comment

The volatile oil, gum and resin components of myrrh are well documented. The anti-inflammatory and antipyretic activities documented in animals support some of the traditional uses. Phenol components of the volatile oil may account for the antimicrobial properties of myrrh, although no documented studies were located. Lipid-lowering properties via a stimulant action on the thyroid gland have been documented for *C. mukul* both in animals and, to a limited extent, in humans. However, robust clinical research assessing the efficacy and safety of myrrh is lacking. In view of the lack of toxicity data, excessive use of myrrh and use during pregnancy and lactation should be avoided.

Species (Family)

Commiphora myrrha (Nees) Engl. (Burseraceae)

Synonym(s)

African Myrrh, Arabian Myrrh, Balsamodendron Myrrha, *Balsamodendron myrrha* (Nees), Bitter Myrrh, Commiphora, *Commiphora molmol* (Engl.) Engl., *C. coriacea* Engl., *C. cuspidata* Chiov., *C. habessinica* (O. Berg) Engl. var. *grossedentata* Chiov., *C. myrrha* (Nees) Engl. var. *molmol* Engl., *C. playfairii* (Oliv.) Engl. var. *benadirensis* Chiov., *C. rivae* Engl., Diddin, Didin, Male Myrrh, Malmal, Mohmol, Molmol, Murr, Myrrh, Somali Myrrh, Yemen Myrrh

Part(s) Used

Oleo-gum-resin

Pharmacopoeial and Other Monographs

BHC 1992[(G6)]
BHP 1996[(G9)]
BP 2007[(G84)]
Complete German Commission E[(G3)]
ESCOP 2006[(G76)]
Martindale 35th edition[(G85)]
Ph Eur 2007[(G81)]
USP29/NF24[(G86)]

Legal Category (Licensed Products)

GSL[(G37)]

Constituents

The following is compiled from several sources, including General References G2, G6 and G52.

Carbohydrates Up to 60% gum yielding arabinose, galactose, xylose, and 4-O-methylglucuronic acid following hydrolysis.

Resins Up to 40% (average 20%) consisting of α-, β- and γ-commiphoric acids, commiphorinic acid, α- and β-heerabomyrrhols, heeraboresene and commiferin.

Steroids Campesterol, cholesterol and β-sitosterol.

Terpenoids α-Amyrin. Furanosesquiterpenes, including furaneudesma-1,3-diene (major), furaneudesma-1,4-diene-6-one, lindestrine, curzerenone, furanodiene, 2-methoxyfuranodiene and 4,5-dihydrofuranodiene-6-one.[(1, G52)]

Volatile oils 1.5–17%. Main constituents are furanosesquiterpenes. Dipentene, cadinene, heerabolene, limonene, pinene, eugenol, *m*-cresol, cinnamaldehyde, cuminaldehyde, cumic alcohol and others.

Food Use

Myrrh is listed by the Council of Europe as a natural source of food flavouring (category N2). This category indicates that myrrh can be added to foodstuffs in small quantities, with a possible limitation of an active principle (as yet unspecified) in the final product.[(G16)] Previously, in the USA, myrrh has been permitted for use in alcoholic beverages.[(G65)]

Herbal Use

Myrrh is stated to possess antimicrobial, astringent, carminative, expectorant, anticatarrhal, antiseptic and vulnerary properties. Traditionally, it has been used for aphthous ulcers, pharyngitis, respiratory catarrh, common cold, furunculosis, wounds and abrasions, and specifically for mouth ulcers, gingivitis and pharyngitis.[(G2, G4, G6–G8, G43, G52, G64)] The German Commission E approved topical use for mild inflammation of the oral and pharyngeal mucosa.[(G3)]

Dosage

Dosages for oral administration (adults) for traditional uses recommended in older pharmaceutical reference texts are given below.

Myrrh Tincture (BPC 1973) 2.5–5.0 mL; in a glass of water several times daily as a gargle or a mouthwash. For skin, undiluted or diluted.[(G52)]

Tincture Myrrh Co (Thompsons) (1 part Capsicum Tincture BPC 1973 to 4 parts Myrrh Tincture BPC 1973) 1.0– 2.5 mL.

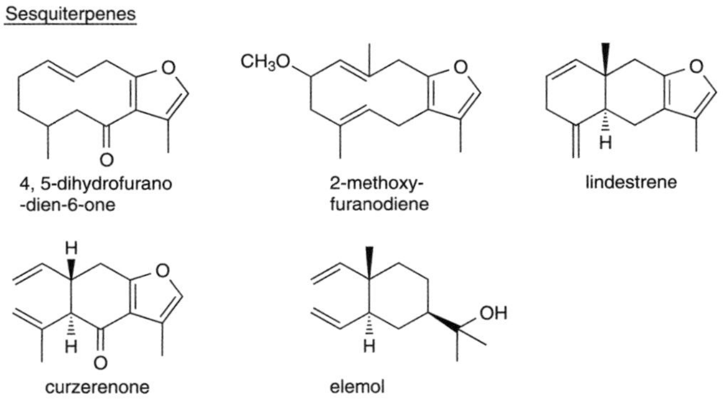

Figure 1 Selected constituents of myrrh.

M

Pharmacological Actions

In vitro and animal studies

Anti-inflammatory activity Anti-inflammatory (carrageenan-induced inflammation and cotton pellet granuloma)[2] and antipyretic activities in mice[2,3] have been documented for *C. molmol*.

Hypoglycaemic activity Hypoglycaemic activity in both normal and diabetic rats has been reported for a myrrh extract.[4,5] Together with an aloe gum extract, myrrh was found to be an active component of a multi-plant extract that exhibited antidiabetic activity. The mode of action was thought to involve a decrease in gluconeogenesis and an increase in peripheral utilisation of glucose in diabetic rats.

Myrrh is stated to have astringent properties on mucous membranes[G45] and to have antimicrobial activities *in vitro*.[G41]

Anti-inflammatory activity Anti-inflammatory activities have been reported for an Indian plant, *Commiphora mukul*, commonly known as guggulipid. Anti-inflammatory activity was described for a crystalline steroidal fraction of guggulipid in both acute (carrageenan-induced rat paw oedema test) and chronic (adjuvant arthritis) models of inflammation.[6]

Lipid-lowering effects A ketosteroid has been identified as the active hypocholesterolaemic principle in guggulipid.[7] In some animal species, thyroid suppression is required as well as cholesterol administration in order to achieve experimental hypercholesterolaemia. Results of studies in chicks administered a thyroid suppressant and cholesterol indicated that guggulipid prevents endogenous hypercholesterolaemia via stimulation of the thyroid gland.[7] When fed to rabbits, guggulipid has been found to reverse the decrease in catecholamine concentrations and dopamine-β-decarboxylase activity that are associated with hyperlipidaemia.[8]

Stimulation of phagocytosis Stimulation of phagocytosis has been documented in mice innoculated with *Escherichia coli* and given with extracts of myrrh by intraperitoneal injecton.[G52]

Cytoprotective activity An aqueous suspension of myrrh administered to rats at oral doses of 250–1000 mg/kg gave significant and dose-dependent protection to gastric mucosa against various ulcerogenic agents.[G52]

Analgesic activity In mice, powdered myrrh (1 mg/kg, orally) had significant analgesic activity in the hotplate test.[G52] Isolated furanoeudesma-1,3-dione (50 mg/kg, orally) was significantly more effective than control ($p < 0.01$) in the mouse writhing test, and the effective dose was reversed by naloxone (1 mg/kg).[G52]

Anti-tumour and cytotoxic activities In mice with Ehrlich solid tumours, an aqueous suspension of myrrh (250 or 500 mg/kg, orally) produced significant decreases in tumour weight ($p < 0.05$) after 25 days.[G52] Aqueous suspension of myrrh increased survival time in mice with Ehrlich ascite tumours.

Clinical studies

There is a lack of clinical research assessing the effects of myrrh and rigorous randomised controlled clinical trials are required.

Guggulipid has been reported to lower the concentration of total serum lipids, serum cholesterol, serum triglycerides, serum phospholipids and β-lipoproteins in 20 patients.[9] This effect was reported to be comparable to that of two other known lipid-lowering drugs also used in the study.

Side-effects, Toxicity

There is a lack of clinical safety and toxicity data for myrrh and further investigation of these aspects is required.

No reported side-effects were located for *C. molmol* or *C. abyssinica*. Hiccup,[9] diarrhoea,[7] restlessness and apprehension,[9] were documented as side-effects for guggulipid when administered to 20 patients.[9] Myrrh has been reported to be non-irritating, non-sensitising and non-phototoxic to human and animal skins.[G41]

Contra-indications, Warnings

Drug interactions None documented. However, the potential for preparations of myrrh to interact with other medicines administered concurrently, particularly those with similar or opposing effects, should be considered. There is limited evidence from preclinical studies that myrrh has hypoglycaemic activity.

Pregnancy and lactation In view of the lack of safety information, use of myrrh during pregnancy and lactation should be avoided.

Preparations

Proprietary single-ingredient preparations

Germany: Inspirol P.

Proprietary multi-ingredient preparations

Argentina: Parodontax Fluor. *Australia:* Eczema Relief. *Austria:* Brady's-Magentropfen; Dentinox; Original Schwedenbitter; Paradenton; Parodontax; Parodontax. *Brazil:* Paratonico; Parodontax. *Canada:* Chase Coldsorex; Cold Sore Lotion. *Chile:* Astrijesan. *Czech Republic:* Dr Theiss Rheuma Creme; Dr Theiss Schweden Krauter; Dr Theiss Schwedenbitter. *Denmark:* Dolodent. *Germany:* Ad-Muc; Mint-Lysoform; Myrrhinil-Intest; Repha-Os. *Hong Kong:* Ad-Muc. *Italy:* Gengivario. *Russia:* Original Grosser Bittner Balsam (Оригинальный Большой Бальзам Биттнера). *South Africa:* Helmontskruie; Lewensessens. *Spain:* Buco Regis. *Switzerland:* Pommade au Baume; Sanogencive. *UK:* Golden Seal Indigestion Tablets; Herbal Indigestion Naturtabs; HRI Golden Seal Digestive; Indigestion and Flatulence; Napiers Digestion Tablets; Nervous Dyspepsia Tablets; Vocalzone; Wind & Dyspepsia Relief. *Venezuela:* One Drop Spray.

References

1 Brieskorn CH, Noble P. Constituents of the essential oil of myrrh. II: Sesquiterpenes and furanosesquiterpenes. *Planta Med* 1982; 44: 87–90.
2 Tariq M *et al*. Anti-inflammatory activity of *Commiphora molmol*. *Agents Actions* 1986; 17: 381–382.
3 Mohsin A *et al*. Analgesic, antipyretic activity and phytochemical screening of some plants used in traditional Arab system of medicine. *Fitoterapia* 1989; 60: 174–177.
4 Al-Awadi FM, Gumaa KA. Studies on the activity of individual plants of an antidiabetic plant mixture. *Acta Diabetol Lat* 1987; 24: 37–41.
5 Al-Awadi FM *et al*. On the mechanism of the hypoglycaemic effect of a plant extract. *Diabetologia* 1985; 28: 432–434.

M

6 Arora RB *et al*. Anti-inflammatory studies on a crystalline steroid isolated from *Commiphora mukul*. *Indian J Med Res* 1972; 60: 929–931.
7 Tripathi SN *et al*. Effect of a keto-steroid of *Commifora mukul* L. on hypercholesterolemia and hyperlipidemia induced by neomercazole and cholesterol mixture in chicks. *Indian J Exp Biol* 1975; 13: 15–18.
8 Srivastava M *et al*. Effect of hypocholesterolemic agents of plant origin on catecholamine biosynthesis in normal and cholesterol fed rabbits. *J Biosci* 1984; 6: 277–282.
9 Malhotra SC, Ahuja MMS. Comparative hypolipidaemic effectiveness of gum guggulu (*Commiphora mukul*) fraction 'A', ethyl-*p*-chlorophenoxyisobutyrate and Ciba-13437-Su. *Indian J Med Res* 1971; 59: 1621–1632.

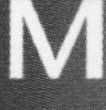

Nettle

Summary and Pharmaceutical Comment

The chemistry of nettle is well documented. Limited pharmacological data are available to support the traditional herbal uses although hypoglycaemic activity *in vivo* has been reported. There is very limited evidence from clinical trials to support the diuretic and anti-inflammatory effects of nettle, and for the effects of nettle in relief of symptoms of allergic rhinitis. Clinical evidence exists to support the efficacy of root extracts in the treatment of benign prostatic hyperplasia. However, further well-designed clinical trials of nettle involving large numbers of patients are required to establish the benefits. Irritant properties have been documented for nettle, and excessive use and use during pregnancy and lactation should be avoided.

Species (Family)

Urtica dioica L. (Urticaceae)

Synonym(s)

Stinging Nettle, Urtica

Part(s) Used

Herb

Pharmacopoeial and Other Monographs

BHC 1992[G6]
BHP 1996[G9]
BP 2007[G84]
Complete German Commission E[G3]
ESCOP 2003[G76]
Martindale 35th edition[G85]
Ph Eur 2007[G81]
USP29/NF24[G86]

Legal Category (Licensed Products)

GSL[G37]

Constituents

The following is compiled from several sources, including General References G6 and G52.

Acids Carbonic, caffeic, caffeoylmalic, chlorogenic, formic, silicic, citric, fumaric, glyceric, malic, oxalic, phosphoric, quinic, succinic, threonic and threono-1,4-lactone.[1]

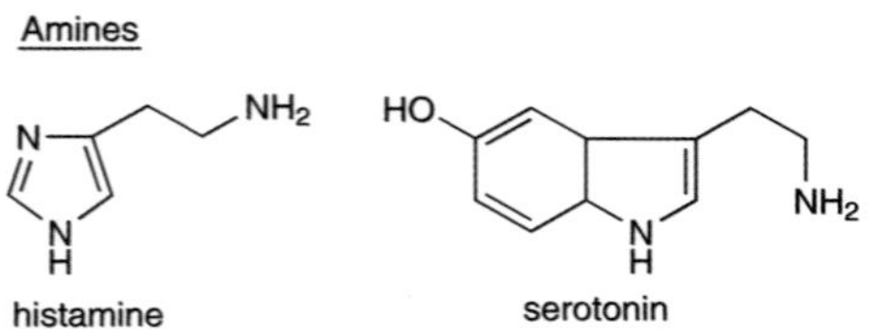

Amines

histamine serotonin

Figure 1 Selected constituents of nettle.

Amines Acetylcholine, betaine, choline, lecithin, histamine, serotonin[2] and a glycoprotein.[3]

Flavonoids Flavonol glycosides (e.g. isorhamnetin, kaempferol, quercetin).[4]

Inorganics Up to 20% minerals, including calcium, potassium and silicon.

Lignans Several lignans, including (−)-secoisolariciresinol.

Other constituents Choline acetyltransferase,[5] scopoletin,[4] β-sitosterol and tannin

Other plant parts The rhizome contains lectin (*Urtica dioica* agglutinin) composed of six isolectins,[6,7] coumarin (scopoletin), triterpenes (β-sitosterol, its glucoside, and six stearyl derivatives),[8,9] two phenylpropane derivatives, and six lignans.[10]

Food Use

Nettle (herbs and leaves) is listed by the Council of Europe as a natural source of food flavouring (category 1) (*see* Appendix 3).[G17] Nettle is used in soups and herbal teas. Previously, in the USA, nettle has been listed by the Food and Drugs Administration (FDA) as a Herb of Undefined Safety.[G22]

Herbal Use

Nettle is stated to possess antihaemorrhagic and hypoglycaemic properties. Traditionally, it has been used for uterine haemorrhage, cutaneous eruption, infantile and psychogenic eczema, epistaxis, melaena and specifically for nervous eczema.[G2, G4, G6–G8, G32, G43, G50, G52, G54, G64] The German Commission E approved internal use of nettle leaf as supportive therapy for rheumatic ailments and as irrigation therapy for inflammatory disease of the lower urinary tract and prevention of kidney gravel; internal and external use for rheumatic ailments.[G3] The root is approved for difficulty in urination from benign prostatic hyperplasia.[G3]

Dosage

Dosages for oral administration (adults) for traditional uses recommended in standard herbal reference texts are given below.

Dried herb 2–4 g as an infusion three times daily;[G6, G7] 8–12 g daily;[G3] fresh juice 10–15 mL three times daily.[G52]

Liquid extract 3–4 mL (1 : 1 in 25% alcohol) three times daily.[G6, G7]

Tincture 2–6 mL (1 : 5 in 45% alcohol) three times daily.[G6, G7]

Pharmacological Actions

In vitro and animal studies

The pharmacological properties of nettle have been reviewed.[G50, G52, G56] Information from these reviews and other sources is summarised below.

Anti-inflammatory activity An aqueous ethanol extract and isolated caffeoylmalic acid partially inhibited the biosynthesis of

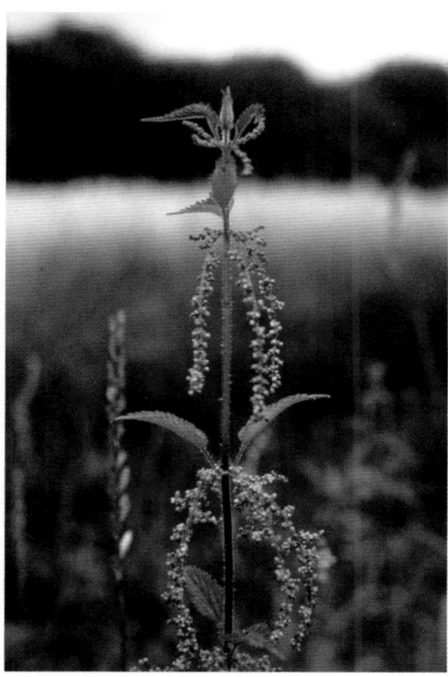

Figure 2 Nettle (*Urtica dioica*).

arachidonic acid *in vitro*.[G52] Nettle extract (0.1 mg/mL) and isolated acid (1 mg/mL) inhibited 5-lipoxygenase-derived biosynthesis of leukotriene B_4 by 20.8% and 68.2%, respectively, and inhibited synthesis of cyclooxygenase-derived prostaglandins (IC_{50} 92 μg/mL and 38 μg/mL, respectively). The same extract significantly reduced tumour-necrosis-factor-α (TNFα) and interleukin 1β (IL-1β) concentrations after lipopolysaccharide (LPS)-stimulated secretion of these proinflammatory cytokines in human blood.[G52] An aqueous ethanol extract (0.25 mg/mL) inhibited platelet-activating factor (PAF)-induced exocytosis of elastase from human neutrophils by 93%, but failed to inhibit biosynthesis of prostaglandins from [^{14}C]arachidonic acid.[G52]

In vitro addition of a commercial preparation of nettle leaf (IDS-23) to whole human blood resulted in an inhibition of LPS-stimulated TNFα and IL-1β secretion, correlating with drug ingestion. The same preparation inhibited phytohaemogglutinin-stimulated production of T helper cell 1 (Th1)-specific interleukin-2 (IL-2) and interferon-γ (IFNγ) in culture in a dose-dependent manner up to 50% and 74%, respectively.[11] By contrast, T helper cell 2 (Th2)-specific interleukin-4 (IL-4) production was stimulated. The results suggested that the nettle leaf extract acts by mediating a switch in T helper cell-derived cytokine patterns and may inhibit the inflammatory cascade in autoimmune diseases such as rheumatoid arthritis.[11] The transcription factor NF-κB is elevated in several chronic inflammatory diseases and is responsible for the enhanced expression of some proinflammatory gene products. A nettle leaf extract (IDS 23) potently inhibited NF-κB activation in a number of cells, including human T cells, macrophages, epithelial cells and mouse L929 fibrosarcoma cells *in vitro*.[12] It was proposed that part of the anti-inflammatory effects of nettle may be due to its inhibitory effect on NF-κB activity.

Benign prostatic hyperplasia activity Several lignans and their metabolites reduce binding activity of human sex hormone-binding globulin (SHBG) *in vitro*. Lignans from nettle are competitive inhibitors of the interaction between SHBG and 5α-dihydrotestosterone.[G50] An aqueous extract of nettle root led to a concentration-dependent (0.6–10 mg/mL) inhibition of SHBG interaction with its receptor on human prostatic membranes. A 20% methanol extract of root inhibited binding capacity of SHBG after preincubation in human serum.[G50]

Subfractions of an aqueous methanol extract of nettle root inhibited cellular proliferation in benign prostatic hyperplasia (BPH) tissue. A root extract had a specific and concentration-dependent inhibition of human leukocyte elastase (HLE) activity *in vitro*. (HLE is an important marker in clinically silent genitourinary tract infection and inflammation.) Root extracts inhibited alternative and classic complementary pathways and significantly inhibited prostate growth in mice with induced BPH (by 51%, compared with control; $p < 0.003$).[G50]

Other activities CNS-depressant activity has been documented for nettle. It has been shown to produce a reduction in spontaneous activity in rats and mice,[13, 14] inhibition of drug-induced convulsions, and a lowering of body temperature in rats.[13] Nettle has been reported to have no effect on the blood pressure of mice,[14] whereas in cats it has produced a marked hypotensive effect and bradycardia.[15] Atropine was reported to have no effect on these latter actions and a mode of action via α-adrenoceptors was suggested.[15]

Nettle is stated to contain both hypoglycaemic and hyperglycaemic principles.[16] The hypoglycaemic component has been termed 'urticin' and nettle has been reported to lower the blood sugar concentration in hyperglycaemic rabbits.[16]

An 80% ethanolic and an aqueous extract of nettle administered to mice at a dose of 25 mg/kg orally prior to glucose load, led to hypoglycaemia effects.[17] No diuretic or ion excretion effects were observed in rats after oral administration of an aqueous extract of nettle (1 g/kg).[14, 18] Dried nettle had a potassium ion to sodium ion ratio of 63 : 1, whereas an aqueous decoction had a corresponding ratio of 448 : 1.[19] It was suggested that the high potassium ion concentration in aqueous decoctions may contribute to their diuretic activity.

Utero-activity has been documented for nettle in pregnant and non-pregnant mice; betaine and serotonin were stated to be the active constituents.[20] A nettle extract was reported to be devoid of antifertility activity following oral administration to mice (250 mg/kg).[21] Analgesic activity in mice has been documented.[14] Administration of an aqueous extract (1200 mg/kg) to mice showed resistance to stimulation in the hotplate test at 55°C with a 190% increase in reaction time.[14] Conversely, no analgesic activity was noted in the hotplate test on rats given an ethanolic

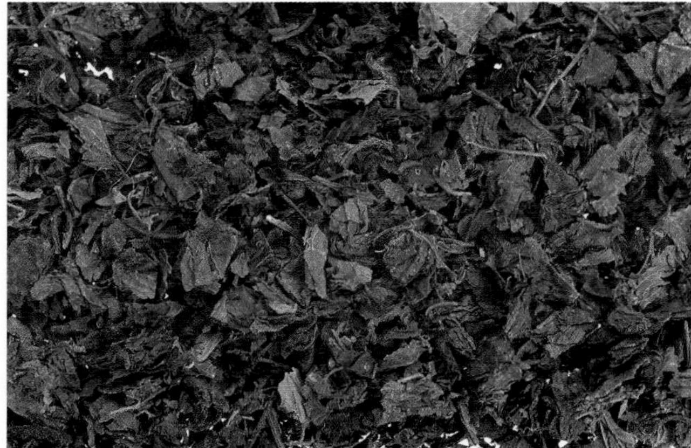

Figure 3 Nettle – dried drug substance (leaf).

extract, but the same extract did reduce the writhing response to phenylquinone after oral (1 g/kg) and intraperitoneal (500 mg/kg) treatment.[18]

The isolectins isolated from the rhizome are reported to cause non-specific agglutination of erythrocytes, to induce the synthesis of interferon by human lymphocytes,[6,7] and have carbohydrate-binding properties.[6,7]

An extract of nettle at a concentration of 1.2 mg/mL has been reported to be active against L-1210 leukaemic cells in mice.[22]

Clinical studies

Diuretic effect In an open, uncontrolled study, 32 patients with myocardial or chronic venous insufficiency were treated with 15 mL of nettle juice three times daily for two weeks.[G52] A significant increase in daily volume of urine was observed throughout the study, the volume by day two being 9.2% ($p < 0.0005$) higher than the baseline value in patients with myocardial insufficiency and 23.9% higher than the baseline value ($p < 0.0005$) in those with chronic venous insufficiency. It has been proposed that the diuretic activity of aqueous extracts of nettle may be attributed to the high potassium content.[19] The reputed diuretic effects of nettle require further investigation.

Arthritis and rheumatism An open, uncontrolled multicentre study involving 152 patients with various, mainly degenerative, rheumatic conditions reported that 70% of participants experienced symptom relief by the end of the three-week treatment period.[G52] In an open, randomised pilot study involving 37 patients with acute arthritis, diclofenac 50 mg plus stewed nettle herb 50 g was compared with diclofenac 200 mg.[23] Assessment was based on the decrease in elevated acute phase C-reactive protein serum concentrations, and clinical signs of acute arthritis. Clinical improvement was observed in both groups to a similar extent. On the basis of the findings, it was suggested that nettle herb administration may enhance the effectiveness of diclofenac in rheumatic conditions. However, this requires further investigation.

In a randomised, double-blind, crossover study, 27 patients with osteoarthritis pain at the base of the thumb and index finger, received stinging nettle leaf (applied for 30 seconds daily for one week to the painful area) or white dead nettle (*Lamium album*) as placebo, followed by a five-week wash-out period before crossing to the other arm of the study.[24] The results indicated that reductions in visual analogue scale scores for pain and in a health assessment questionnaire score for disability were significantly better for the stinging nettle group, compared with the placebo group ($p = 0.026$ and $p = 0.0027$ for pain and disability, respectively).

Benign prostatic hyperplasia A small number of clinical studies has assessed the effectiveness of nettle preparations in the treatment of symptoms of benign prostatic hyperplasia (BPH).

Several uncontrolled trials have reported improvements in urological symptoms, compared with baseline values, following administration of nettle root extract (5 : 1) 600–1200 mg daily for three weeks to 20 months.[G50] Large observational studies involving patients with BPH who received nettle root extract for two to three months have reported improvements in various symptoms, such as urinary frequency, urinary flow and nocturia.[G50] These studies provide justification for further, rigorous investigation of the effects of nettle in BPH.

A placebo-controlled trial involving 79 patients with BPH assessed the effects of nettle root extract 600 mg daily for six to eight weeks. Compared with placebo, nettle root extract administration resulted in greater improvements in urinary flow and urine volume and residual volume.[G50] Another placebo-controlled trial of nettle root extract 600 mg daily for nine weeks in men with BPH ($n = 50$) reported a significant decrease in SHBG concentrations and significant improvement in micturition volume and maximum urinary flow.[G50]

Rhinitis A randomised, double-blind, placebo-controlled study assessed the effects of a freeze-dried preparation of nettle herb in individuals with allergic rhinitis.[25] Participants received nettle herb 600 mg, or placebo, at the onset of symptoms over a one-week period. Assessment was based on daily symptom diaries and global responses recorded at follow-up visits after one week of therapy. Nettle herb was rated more highly than placebo in the global assessment, but was rated less highly on the basis of data from the symptom diaries. It was concluded that there should be further investigation with a larger sample size and involving a longer treatment period.

Side-effects, Toxicity

Clinical data

There is a lack of clinical safety and toxicity data for nettle and further investigation of these aspects is required.

Postmarketing surveillance studies involving a total of almost 2000 patients with rheumatoid arthritis treated for three weeks with nettle leaf extract (IDS-23) administered as an adjuvant to non-steroidal anti-inflammatory drugs (NSAIDs), or as monotherapy, have reported that the extract was well-tolerated.[26,27]

Consumption of nettle tea has caused gastric irritation, a burning sensation of the skin, oedema and oliguria.[G22] The leaves are extremely irritant in view of their acetylcholine- and histamine-containing glandular hairs.

Preclinical data

An LD_{50} in mice following intraperitoneal administration of nettle has been reported as 3.625 g/kg.[12] The LD_{50} for intravenous infusion of nettle leaf in mice has been documented as 1.92 g/kg, and the LD_{50} for chronic administration in rats has been stated as 1.31 g/kg.[G50] An ethanolic extract of nettle (plant part unspecified) showed low toxicity in rats and mice after oral and intraperitoneal administration at doses equivalent to 2 g/kg.[18]

Contra-indications, Warnings

Gastrointestinal irritation has been documented following consumption of nettle tea.

Drug interactions None documented. However, the potential for preparations of nettle to interact with other medicines administered concurrently, particularly those with similar or opposing effects, should be considered. There is limited evidence from preclinical studies that nettle preparations have hypoglycaemic, hypotensive and CNS depressant effects.

Pregnancy and lactation Nettle is reputed to be an abortifacient and to affect the menstrual cycle.[G30] Utero-activity has been documented in animal studies. In view of this and other documented pharmacological activities, the use of nettle during pregnancy and lactation should be avoided.

Preparations

Proprietary single-ingredient preparations

Austria: Uro-POS. *Czech Republic:* Koprivovy Caj, Koprivova Nat; Zihlava. *Germany:* Arthrodynat N; Asendra; Azuprostat Urtica; Bazoton; Flexal Brennessel; Hox Alpha; Natu-lind; Natu-prosta; Pro-Sabona Uno; Prosta-Truw; Prostaforton; Prostagalen; Prostaherb N; Prostamed Urtica; Prostata; Prostawern; Rheuma-Hek; Rheuma-Stada; Uro-POS; Urtivit; utk. *Switzerland:* Valverde Prostate capsules.

Proprietary multi-ingredient preparations

Australia: Cough Relief; Extralife Flow-Care; Infant Tonic; Irontona; Urapro; Vitatona. *Austria:* Anaemodoron; Berggeist; Menodoron; Mentopin; Prostagutt; Prostatonin. *Brazil:* Prostem Plus. *Canada:* Allercept; Ultra Quercitin. *Czech Republic:* Abfuhr-Heilkrautertee; Diabeticka Cajova Smes-Megadiabetin; Nephrosal; Perospir; Prostakan Forte; Prostatonin; Pulmoran; Species Urologicae Planta; Stoffwechseltee N. *France:* Fitacnol. *Germany:* Combudoron; Prostagutt forte; Vollmers praparierter gruner N; Winar. *Italy:* Biothymus DS; Prostaplant. *Malaysia:* Cleansa Plus. *Mexico:* Prosgutt. *Russia:* Herbion Urtica (Гербион Уртика). *South Africa:* Combudoron; Enzian Anaemodoron Drops; Menodoron. *Spain:* Natusor Artilane. *Switzerland:* Combudoron; Prostagutt-F; Prostatonin; The a l'avoine sauvage de Vollmer; Tisane Diuretique; Tisane pour les problemes de prostate. *UK:* Culpeper Detox Tea; Napiers Echinacea Tea; Summertime Tea Blend. *USA:* Prostate Health.

References

1 Bakke ILF *et al* Water-soluble acids from *Urtica dioica* L. *Medd Nor Farm Selsk* 1978; 40: 181–188.

2 Adamski R, Bieganska J. Studies on substances present in *Urtica dioica* L. leaves II. Analysis for protein amino acids and nitrogen containing non-protein amino acids. *Herba Pol* 1984; 30: 17–26.

3 Andersen S, Wold JK. Water-soluble glycoprotein from *Urtica dioica* leaves. *Phytochemistry* 1978; 17: 1875–1877.

4 Chaurasia N, Wichtl M. Flavonolglykoside aus *Urtica dioica. Planta Med* 1987; 53: 432–434.

5 Barlow RB, Dixon ROD. Choline aceytltransferase in the nettle *Urtica dioica* L. *Biochem J* 1973; 132: 15–18.

6 Shibuya N *et al*. Carbohydrates binding properties of the stinging nettle (*Urtica dioica*) rhizome lectin. *Arch Biochem Biophys* 1986; 249: 215–224.

7 Damme EJM *et al*. The *Urtica dioica* agglutinin is a complex mixture of isolectins. *Plant Physiol* 1988; 86: 598–601.

8 Chaurasia N, Wichtl M. Scopoletin, 3-β-sitosterin und 3-β-D-glucosid aus Brennesselwurzel (*Urticae radix*). *Dtsch Apothek Zeitung* 1986; 126: 81–83.

9 Chaurasia N, Wichtl M. Sterols and steryl glycosides from *Urtica dioica. J Nat Prod* 1987; 50: 881–885.

10 Chaurasia N, Wichtl M. Phenylpropane und lignane aus der wurzel von *Urtica dioica* L. *Dtsch Apothek Zeitung* 1986; 126: 1559–1563.

11 Klingelhoefer S *et al*. Antirheumatic effect of IDS 23, a stinging nettle leaf extract, on *in vivo* expression of T helper cytokines. *J Rheumatol* 1999; 26: 2517–2522.

12 Riehemann K *et al*. Plant extracts from stinging nettle (*Urtica dioica*), an antirheumatic remedy, inhibit the proinflammatory transcription factor NF-κB. *FEBS Lett* 1999; 442: 89–94.

13 Broncano J *et al*. Estudio de diferentes preparados de *Urtica dioica* L sobre SNC. *An R Acad Farm* 1987; 53: 284–291.

14 Lasheras B *et al*. Étude pharmacologique préliminaire de *Prunus spinosa* L. Amelanchier ovalis medikus *Juniperus communis* L. et *Urtica dioica* L. *Plant Méd Phytothér* 1986; 20: 219–226.

15 Broncano FJ *et al*. Étude de l'effet sur le centre cardiovasculaire de quelques préparations de l'*Urtica dioica* L. *Planta Med* 1983; 17: 222–229.

16 Oliver-Bever B, Zahland GR. Plants with oral hypoglycaemic activity. *Q J Crude Drug Res* 1979; 17: 139–196.

17 Neef H *et al*. Hypoglycaemic activity of selected European plants. *Phytother Res* 1995; 9: 45–48.

18 Tita B *et al*. *Urtica dioica* L.: Pharmacological effect of ethanol extract. *Pharmacol Res* 1993; 27: 21–22.

19 Szentmihályi K *et al*. Potassium-sodium ratio for the characterization of medicinal plants extracts with diuretic activity. *Phytother Res* 1998; 12: 163–166.

20 Broncano FJ *et al*. Estudio de efecto sobre musculatura lisa uterina de distintos preparados de las hojas de *Urtica dioica* L. *An R Acad Farm* 1987; 53: 69–76.

21 Sharma BB *et al*. Antifertility screening of plants. Part I. Effect of ten indigenous plants on early pregnancy in albino rats. *Int J Crude Drug Res* 1983; 21: 183–187.

22 Ilarionova M *et al*. Cytotoxic effect on leukemic cells of the essential oils from rosemary, wild geranium and nettle and concret of royal bulgarian rose. *Anticancer Res* 1992; 12: 1915.

23 Chrubasik S *et al*. Evidence for antirheumatic effectiveness of herba *Urtica dioicae* in acute arthritis: a pilot study. *Phytomedicine* 1997; 4: 105–108.

24 Randall C *et al*. Randomized controlled trial of nettle sting for treatment of base-of-thumb pain. *J R Soc Med* 2000; 93: 305–309.

25 Mittman P. Randomized, double-blind study of freeze-dried *Urtica dioica* in the treatment of allergic rhinitis. *Planta Med* 1990; 56: 44–47.

26 Sommer R-G, Sinner B. Kennen sie den neuen zytokinanatagonisten? *Therapiewoche* 1996; 1: 44–49.

27 Ramm S, Hansen C. Brennesselblätter-extrakt bei arthrose und rheumatoider arthritis-Multizentrische anwendungsbeobachtung mit rheuma-hek. *Therapiewoche* 1996; 28: 1575–1578.

Parsley

Summary and Pharmaceutical Comment

Parsley is commonly consumed as part of the diet. The pharmacological and toxicological properties of parsley are primarily associated with the volatile oil, particularly the apiole, myristicin and furanocoumarin constituents. Most of the reported uses of parsley are probably due to the volatile oil; no documented information was located regarding antirheumatic and antimicrobial properties. There is a lack of clinical research assessing the efficacy and safety of parsley. Parsley should not be consumed in doses that greatly exceed the amounts used in foods, as excessive ingestion may result in apiole and myristicin toxicity.

Species (Family)

Petroselinum crispum (Mill.) Hill (Apiaceae/Umbelliferae)

Synonym(s)

Apium petroselinum L., *Carum petroselinum* (L.) Benth., *Petroselinum sativum* Hoffm., *P. peregrinum* (L.) Lag., *P. hortense* auct., *P. vulgare* Lag.

Part(s) Used

Leaf, root, seed

Pharmacopoeial and Other Monographs

BHC 1992[G6]
BHP 1996[G9]
Complete German Commission E[G3]
Martindale 35th edition[G85]

Legal Category (Licensed Products)

GSL[G37]

Constituents

The following is compiled from several sources, including General References G2 and G6.

Flavonoids Glycosides of apigenin, luteolin (e.g. apiin, luteolin-7-apiosyl-glucoside, apigenin-7-glucoside (leaf only), luteolin-7-diglucoside (leaf only)).

Furanocoumarins Bergapten and oxypeucedanin as major constituents (up to 0.02% and 0.01% respectively); also 8-methoxypsoralen, imperatorin, isoimperatorin, isopimpinellin, psoralen, xanthotoxin (up to 0.003%).[1]

Volatile oils 2–7% in seed, 0.05% in leaf. The seed contains apiole, myristicin, tetramethoxyallylbenzene, various terpene aldehydes, ketones, and alcohols. The leaf contains myristicin (up to 85%), apiole, 1,3,8-*p*-menthatriene, 1-methyl-4-isopropenylbenzene, methyl disulfide, monoterpenes (e.g. α- and β-pinene, β-myrcene, β-ocimene, β-phellandrene, *p*-terpinene, α-terpineol), sesquiterpenes (e.g. α-copaene, carotol, caryophyllene).

Other constituents Fixed oil, oleo-resin, proteins, carbohydrates, and vitamins (especially vitamins A and C).

A detailed vitamin and mineral analysis is given elsewhere.[G22]

Food Use

Parsley is listed by the Council of Europe as natural source of food flavouring (category N2). This category indicates that parsley can be added to foodstuffs in small quantities, with a possible limitation of an active principle (as yet unspecified) in the final product.[G16] Parsley is commonly used in foods. Previously, parsley has been listed as GRAS (Generally Recognised As Safe).[G65]

Herbal Use

Parsley is stated to possess carminative, antispasmodic, diuretic, emmenagogue, expectorant, antirheumatic and antimicrobial properties. Traditionally, it has been used for flatulent dyspepsia, colic, cystitis, dysuria, bronchitic cough in the elderly, dysmenorrhoea, functional amenorrhoea, myalgia and specifically for flatulent dyspepsia with intestinal colic.[G2, G6, G7, G8, G64]

Dosage

Dosages for oral administration (adults) for traditional uses recommended in standard herbal reference texts are given below.

Leaf/root 2–4 g as an infusion.

Seed 1–2 g.

Dried root 2–4 g or by infusion three times daily.[G6, G7]

Liquid extract 2–4 mL (1 : 1 in 25% alcohol) three times daily.[G6, G7]

Pharmacological Actions

In vitro and animal studies

Parsley extract (0.25–1.0 mL/kg, by intravenous injection) has been reported to lower the blood pressure of cats by more than 40%,[2] and to decrease both respiratory movements and blood pressure in anaesthetised dogs.[3] Parsley exhibits a tonic effect on both intestinal and uterine muscle.[3] This uterine effect has been attributed to the apiole content,[G30] but has also been observed with apiole-free aqueous extracts.[3] An aqueous extract of parsley has been documented to contain an antithiamine substance which was unaffected by cooking or contact with gastric juice.[3] Myristicin and apiole are both effective insecticides.[4]

Parsley seed oil has been reported to stimulate hepatic regeneration in a rat model.[5]

Clinical studies

There is a lack of clinical research assessing the effects of parsley and rigorous randomised clinical trials are required.

Myristicin is the hallucinogenic principle present in nutmeg seed. It has been hypothesised that myristicin is converted in the body to amfetamine, to which it is structurally related.[4]

P

Phenylpropanoids

apiole myristicin allyltetra-methoxybenzene

Furanocoumarins

oxypeucedanin

	R^1	R^2
psoralen	H	H
bergapten	OCH_3	H
8-methoxypsoralen	H	OCH_3
imperatorin	H	isopentenyl
isopimpinellin	OCH_3	OCH_3

Figure 1 Selected constituents of parsley.

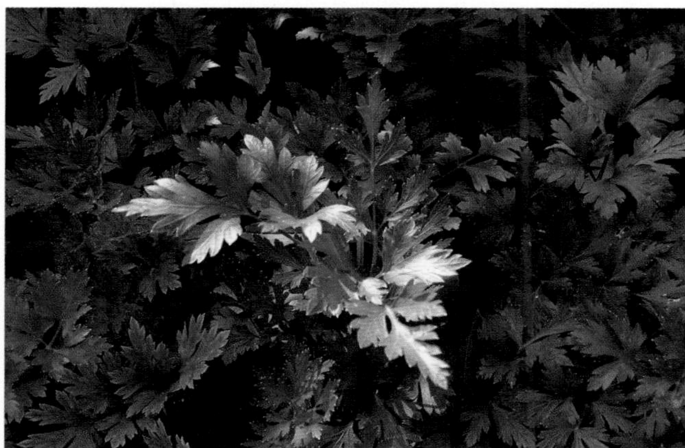

Figure 2 Parsley (*Petroselinum crispum*).

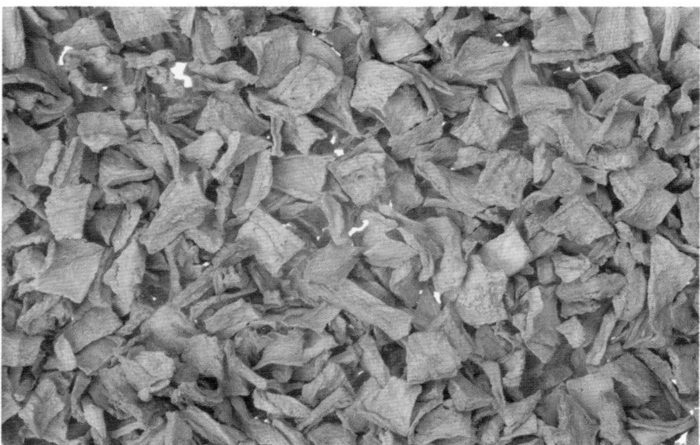

Figure 3 Parsley – dried drug substance (root).

Myristicin has a structural similarity with sympathomimetic amines and it is thought that it may compete for monoamine oxidase enzymes, thereby exhibiting a monoamine oxidase inhibitor (MAOI)-like action.[6] However, this requires confirmation. Parsley oil has been included in the diet of pregnant women and is reported to increase diuresis, and plasma protein and plasma calcium concentrations.[4]

The diuretic effect associated with the consumption of parsley may be attributable to the pharmacological activities of myristicin (sympathomimetic action) and apiole (irritant effect).

Side-effects, Toxicity

There is a lack of clinical safety and toxicity data for parsley and further investigation of these aspects is required. The suggestion that myristicin, a constituent of parsley, has MAOI-like activity requires confirmation.

Chronic and excessive consumption of fresh parsley (170 g daily for 30 years) has been associated with generalised itching and pigmentation of the lower legs in a 70-year-old woman.[6] The symptoms were attributed to excessive ingestion of parsley in the presence of chronic liver disease. The aetiology of the chronic hepatitis was unknown, but considered possibly related to the chronic exposure to the psoralen constituents in parsley.[6] Apiole and myristicin are also documented to be hepatotoxic.

The ingestion of approximately 10 g apiole has been reported to cause acute haemolytic anaemia, thrombocytopenia purpura, nephrosis and hepatic dysfunction. However, ingestion of 10 g of apiole would require a dose of more than 200 g parsley. The amount of apiole ingested as a result of normal dietary consumption of parsley is not hazardous. Myristicin has been documented to cause giddiness, deafness, hypotension, decrease in pulse rate, and paralysis, followed by fatty degeneration of the liver and kidney.[G22] In addition, myristicin is known to possess hallucinogenic properties. However, when compared to nutmeg, parsley contains a relatively low concentration of myristicin (less than 0.05% in parsley leaf, about 0.4–0.89% in nutmeg); parsley seed is potentially hazardous in view of its higher volatile oil content (about 2–7%) which contains apiole and myristicin.

Parsley contains phototoxic furanocoumarins (*see* Celery). However, photodermatitis resulting from the oral ingestion of parsley is thought to be unlikely. The ingestion of 50 g parsley provides negligible amounts of bergapten (0.5–0.8 g).[7] The concentration of oxypeucedanin provided was not mentioned. However, a photoactive reaction from topical contact with parsley is possible.

Apiole is an irritant component of the volatile oil and may cause irritation of the kidneys during excretion.

Parsley seed oil has been reported to stimulate hepatic regeneration.[4] Myristicin and apiole are documented to have a similar chemical structure and acute toxicity to safrole, which is known to be carcinogenic and hepatotoxic (*see* Sassafras).[4] The carcinogenic potential of apiole and myristicin has not been evaluated.[4]

LD_{50} (mice, intravenous injection) values for apiole and myristicin have been documented as 50 mg/kg and 200 mg/kg body weight, respectively.[4]

Contra-indications, Warnings

Parsley should not be ingested in excessive amounts in view of the documented toxicities of apiole and myristicin. Parsley may cause a photoactive reaction, especially following external contact, and may aggravate existing renal disease.

Drug interactions None documented. However, the potential for preparations of parsley to interact with other medicines administered concurrently, particularly those with similar or opposing effects, should be considered.

Pregnancy and lactation Parsley is reputed to affect the menstrual cycle.[G7] Utero-activity has been documented in humans and animals,[G30] and parsley is stated to be contra-indicated during pregnancy.[G49, G58] Myristicin has been reported to cross the placenta and can lead to foetal tachycardia.[8] In view of this, parsley should not be taken during pregnancy and lactation in doses that greatly exceed the amounts used in foods.

Preparations

Proprietary multi-ingredient preparations

Australia: Extralife Fluid-Care; Medinat PMT-Eze; Odourless Garlic; Uva-Ursi Plus. *Canada:* Herbal Diuretic; Herbal Throat. *Czech Republic:* Species Diureticae Planta; Species Urologicae Planta; Urologicka Cajova Smes. *Germany:* Asparagus-P; nephro-loges. *Malaysia:* Total Man. *Russia:* Herbion Urological Drops (Гербион Урологические Капли). *UK:* Athera; Fre-bre; Höfels One-A-Day Garlic with Parsley; Mixed Vegetable Tablets; Modern Herbals Menopause. *USA:* Natural Herbal Water Tablets; PMS Control.

References

1 Chaudhary SK *et al*. Oxypeucedanin, a major furocoumarin in parsley, *Petroselinum crispum*. *Planta Med* 1986; 52: 462–464.
2 Petkov V. Plants with hypotensive, antiatheromatous and coronarodilatating action. *Am J Chin Med* 1979; 7: 197–236.
3 Opdyke DLJ. Parsley seed oil. *Food Cosmet Toxicol* 1975; 13 (Suppl. Suppl.): 897–898.
4 Buchanan RL. Toxicity of spices containing methylenedioxybenzene derivatives: A review. *J Food Safety* 1978; 1: 275–293.
5 Gershbein LL. Regeneration of rat liver in the presence of essential oils and their components. *Food Cosmet Toxicol* 1977; 15: 171–181.
6 Cootes P. Clinical curio: liver disease and parsley. *BMJ* 1982; 285: 1719.
7 Zaynoun S *et al*. The bergapten content of garden parsley and its significance in causing cutaneous photosensitization. *Clin Exp Dermatol* 1985; 10: 328–331.
8 Lavy G. Nutmeg intoxication in pregnancy. *J Reprod Med* 1987; 32: 63–64.

Parsley Piert

Summary and Pharmaceutical Comment

Little chemical information is available on parsley piert. No scientific evidence was found to justify the herbal uses. There is a lack of clinical research assessing the efficacy and safety of parsley piert. In view of the lack of toxicity data, excessive use of parsley piert and use during pregnancy and lactation should be avoided.

Species (Family)

Aphanes arvensis L. (Rosaceae)

Synonym(s)

Alchemilla arvensis Scop., Aphanes

Part(s) Used

Herb

Pharmacopoeial and Other Monographs

BHP 1983[G7]
Martindale 35th edition[G85]

Legal Category (Licensed Products)

GSL[G37]

Constituents

The following is compiled from several sources, including General Reference G7.

Limited information is available. Parsley piert is stated to contain an astringent principle.[G6]

Food Use

Parsley piert is not used in foods.

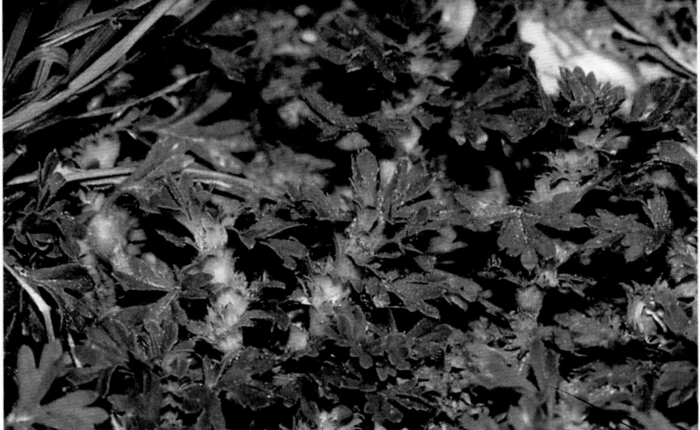

Figure 1 Parsley piert (*Aphanes arvensis*).

Herbal Use

Parsley piert is stated to possess diuretic and demulcent properties, and to dissolve urinary deposits. Traditionally, it has been used for kidney and bladder calculi, dysuria, strangury, oedema of renal and hepatic origin, and specifically for renal calculus.[G7, G64]

Dosage

Dosages for oral administration (adults) for traditional uses recommended in standard herbal reference texts are given below.

Dried herb 2–4 g as an infusion three times daily.[G7]

Liquid extract 2–4 mL (1 : 1 in 25% alcohol) three times daily.[G7]

Tincture 2–10 mL (1 : 5 in 45% alcohol) three times daily.[G7]

Pharmacological Actions

None documented.

Clinical studies

There is a lack of clinical research assessing the effects of parsley piert and rigorous randomised clinical trials are required.

Side-effects, Toxicity

None documented. However, there is a lack of clinical safety and toxicity data for parsley piert and further investigation of these aspects is required.

Contra-indications, Warnings

None documented.

Drug interactions None documented. However, the potential for preparations of parsley piert to interact with other medicines administered concurrently should be considered.

Pregnancy and lactation In view of the lack of phytochemical, pharmacological, and toxicity information, the use of parsley piert during pregnancy and lactation should be avoided.

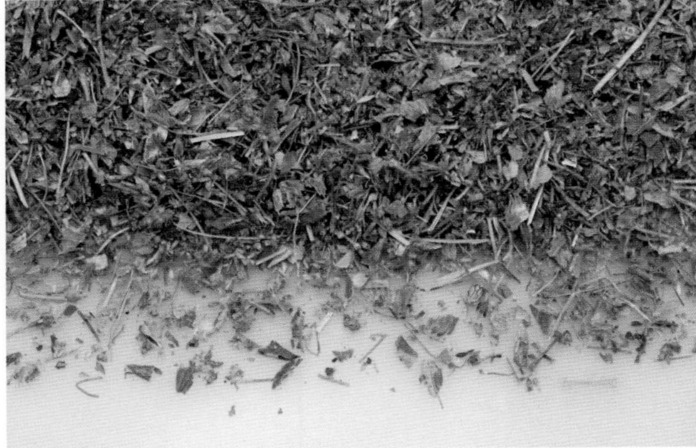

Figure 2 Parsley piert – dried drug substance (herb).

Preparations

Proprietary single-ingredient preparations

Czech Republic: Kontryhelova Nat.

Proprietary multi-ingredient preparations

Australia: Profluid; Protemp. *Canada:* Swiss Herb Cough Drops. *Czech Republic:* Fytokliman Planta; Gynastan. *France:* Gonaxine. *UK:* Backache Relief; Buchu Backache Compound Tablets; Diuretabs; HRI Water Balance; Roberts Black Willow Compound Tablets; Watershed.

Passionflower

Summary and Pharmaceutical Comment

The chemistry of *Passiflora incarnata* is well-documented. The active constituents have not been clearly identified, although the flavonoid and possibly the alkaloid constituents are considered to be important in this respect.

Several pharmacological properties, including anxiolytic, sedative, anticonvulsant and anti-inflammatory effects, have been described for preparations of *P. incarnata* following preclinical studies, providing supporting evidence for some of the traditional uses. However, well-designed clinical trials of *P. incarnata* preparations are lacking and further studies are required to determine their clinical efficacy and effectiveness. The few clinical trials available generally have investigated the effects of proprietary products containing *P. incarnata*, in some cases in combination with other herbal ingredients, in patients with anxiety disorders. Further investigation of the efficacy and effectiveness of *P. incarnata* preparations is required.

Trials of monopreparations of *P. incarnata* have involved relatively small numbers of participants (less than 70 per trial) and been of short duration (up to four weeks). Information on the safety and toxicity of *P. incarnata* preparations is limited and, in view of this, excessive use (higher than recommended dosages and/or for long periods of time) and use during pregnancy and lactation should be avoided.

Species (Family)

Passiflora incarnata L. (Passifloraceae)

Synonym(s)

Apricot Vine, Grenadille, Maypop, Passiflora, Passion Vine

Part(s) Used

Herb

Pharmacopoeial and Other Monographs

BHC 1992[(G6)]
BHMA 2003[(G66)]
BHP 1996[(G9)]
BP 2007[(G84)]
Complete German Commission E[(G3)]
ESCOP 2003[(G76)]
Martindale 35th edition[(G85)]
Ph Eur 2007[(G81)]

Legal Category (Licensed Products)

GSL[(G37)]

Constituents

Alkaloids Indole alkaloids of the β-carboline type, including harman, harmol, harmine, harmalol and harmaline. The alkaloids are minor constituents and may be present in ppm or even not detectable in some samples of plant material. The yields of harman and harmine in the aerial parts of greenhouse grown plants have been reported as 0.012% and 0.007%, respectively, while the yields in field grown plants were 0.005% and not detectable, respectively.[(1–3)]

Flavonoids Pharmacopoeial standard not less than 1.5% expressed as vitexin.[(G81, G84)] Aglycones apigenin, chrysin (5,7-hydroxyflavone), luteolin, quercetin and kaempferol. C-glycosides of apigenin (e.g. vitexin, isovitexin, schaftoside, isoschaftoside) and of luteolin (e.g. orientin, iso-orientin)[(4)] and related

Flavonoid C–glycosides

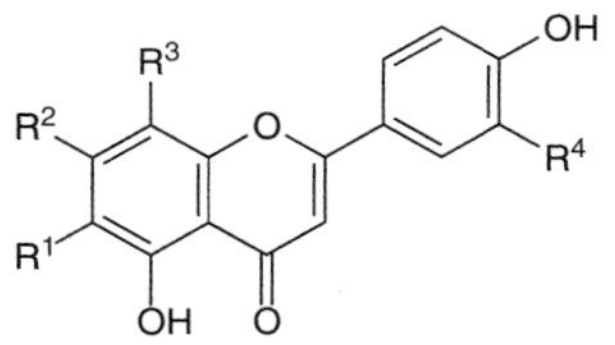

	R^1	R^2	R^3	R^4
vitexin	H	OH	glc	H
isovitexin	glc	OH	H	H
orientin	H	OH	glc	OH
isoorientin	glc	OH	H	OH
schaftoside	glc	OH	ara	H
isoschaftoside	ara	OH	glc	H
swertisin	glc	OCH_3	H	H
vicenin-2	glc	OH	glc	H
lucenin-2	glc	OH	glc	OH
isovitexin-2″-*O*-glucoside	soph	OH	H	H
isoorientin-2″-*O*-glucoside	soph	OH	H	OH

ara = α–L–arabinopyranosyl
glc = β–D–glucopyranosyl
soph = sophorosyl (sophorose = glucose $\xrightarrow{1\ 2}$ glucose)

Alkaloids

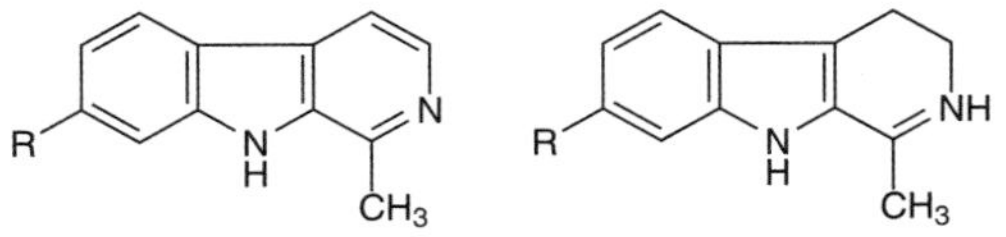

	R
harman	H
harmol	OH
harmine	OCH_3

	R
harmalol	OH
harmaline	OCH_3

Cyanogenic glucosides: gynocardin

γ– Benzopyrans: maltol

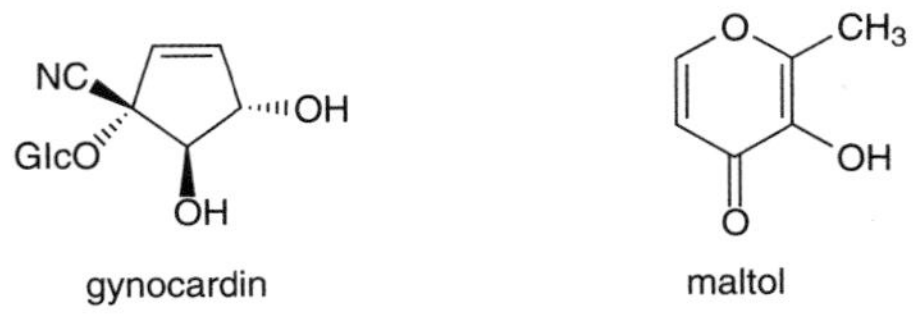

Figure 1 Selected constituents of passionflower.

flavonoids. There is considerable variation, qualitatively and quantitatively; in the flavonoid composition depending on the source of plant material.[5,6,G76] The four major C-glycosidic flavonoids have been identified as schaftoside, isoschaftoside, isovitexin-2″-O-glucopyranoside and iso-orientin-2″-O-glucopyranoside on the basis of mass spectral and [^{13}C] NMR data.[7]

Other constituents Cyanogenic glycoside gynocardin,[8,9] γ-benzopyrones maltol and ethylmaltol,[10] polyacetylene passicol,[11] essential oil (hexanol, benzylalcohol, linalool, 2-phenylethyl alcohol, 2-hydroxybenzoic acid methyl ester, carvone (major), transanethole, eugenol, isoeugenol, β-ionone, α-bergamolol, phytol),[12] amino acids, fatty acids (e.g. linoleic, linolenic, myristic, palmitic, oleic acids), formic and butyric acids, sterols (e.g. stigmasterol, sitosterol), sugars (e.g. raffinose, sucrose, glucose, fructose).

Other plant parts Coumarins (scopoletin and umbelliferone) are found in the root.

Other *Passiflora* species

Passiflora edulis Sims, source of edible passionflower fruit, contains numerous glycosides including flavonoids (e.g. luteolin-6-C-chinovoside, luteolin-6-C-fucoside),[13]cyanogenic glycosides (e.g. passibiflorin, epipassibiflorin, passicapsin, passicoriacin, epipassicoriacin, cyanogenic-β-rutinoside, epitetraphyllin B, amygdalin, prunasin,[9,13] triterpenoid glycosides (e.g.passiflorine) and salicylate glycosides. Also present are the β-carboline alkaloids harman, harmine, harmaline and harmalol,[14] phenols, carotenes and γ-lactones.

Cyanogenic glycosides are present in species of Passifloraceae including species of *Passiflora*.[15] When the genus was reviewed in 2002 for the presence of cyanogenic glycosides, only 33 species (7%) of some 460 species had been investigated chemically for these constituents.[9] Four structurally different types of glycosides have been identified and their occurrence related to the subgeneric classification of this large genus. In a subsequent review of the chemical constituents of *Passiflora*, it was claimed that only 46 of the 500 species of the genus had been investigated chemically.[13] Flavonoids and cyanogenic glycosides are present in many of the species. Low concentrations (ppm) of harman-type alkaloids were detected in 53 of 104 samples, representing 91 species of *Passiflora* analysed by HPLC. The highest concentration detected of total alkaloids in any species was 6.35 ppm.[16]

Quality of plant material and commercial products

Flavonoids The presence of complex mixtures and varying composition of flavonoids, both qualitatively and quantitatively; in *P. incarnata* herb and its preparations has led to a number of analytical investigations.[4,6] The C-glycosides are readily separated by HPLC and the major ones characterised by MS,[17] MS-[^{13}C]-NMR,[7] and MS-2D-NMR.[18] HPLC separation of C-glycosides provides a 'fingerprint' for the C-glycosides and analyses of 14 different commercial samples of *P. incarnata* revealed considerable qualitative and quantitative differences.[19] Vitexin and orientin were absent from some samples but detected in others at concentrations of 0.05–0.25%. Swertisin was the major C-glycoside in two samples whilst it was absent in others, isovitexin was the major compound in five samples, isovitexin-2″-O-glucoside was the major compound in four samples with schaftoside and isoschaftoside being major in the three other samples. Interpretation of HPLC analytical results was simplified by acid hydrolysis resulting in the loss of O-glycosides but not C-glycosyl flavonoids. HPLC was used to compare the flavonoid content of six different species of *Passiflora* grown under identical conditions.[20] The highest concentration of isovitexin was found in *P. incarnata* leaves. Accelerated solvent extraction and HPLC analysis were used to investigate the presence of schaftoside, isoschaftoside, orientin, iso-orientin, vitexin and isovitexin in 115 samples of *Passiflora* species obtained from the Americas, Europe and Australia.[21] There was a wide diversity in the number and concentration of the flavonoid C-glycosides. The methodology was claimed to be suitable for the analysis of phytochemical preparations containing *P. incarnata*.

High performance thin layer chromatography (HPTLC) and densitometry have been used for the quantitative determination of total flavonoids and of orientin and iso-orientin in the leaves of four species of *Passiflora*.[22] The results were compared with those of HPLC-UV analyses. Although HPTLC proved to be a reliable and fast method for 'fingerprinting' *P. incarnata*, HPLC proved to be more useful for quantitative determination of the flavonoids. These methods were used to examine 11 commercial samples of *Passiflora* leaf.

Capillary zone electrophoresis (CZE) has been used for the separation and resolution of 14 flavonoid glycosides from *P. incarnata*.[23] The technique was applied to 18 different commercial samples and demonstrated the great variability in qualitative composition. Four C-glycoside flavonoid patterns of *P. incarnata* were defined: high isovitexin content; high swertisin content; high isovitexin-2″-O-glucoside content; four flavonoids present, namely isovitexin, isoschaftoside, schaftoside and iso-orientin. CZE has also been used to separate and quantify 13 flavonoids from 10 different commercial samples of *P. incarnata* herb.[24] There were differences in the amount of individual flavonoids present and the total flavonoid content was 0.37–3.75%.

HPLC analysis of 12 liquid and 14 solid pharmaceutical preparations of *P. incarnata* revealed that the flavonoid content ranged from 0.31–5.81 mg/g and 2.56–2.68 mg/100 mg extract, respectively. HPLC-DAD and HPLC-MS have been applied to study the stability of flavonoids in tinctures of *P. incarnata*.[25] The shelf-life of a 60% v/v tincture was determined as being six months.

Alkaloids Reversed phase HPLC was used to screen 17 different samples of *P. incarnata* herb for the presence of alkaloids.[1] Only one sample yielded a possible harman content of approximately 0.1 ppm. A sample of Japanese *P. incarnata* herb was quantified by reversed-phase HPLC for the presence of harmol, harman and harmine. The amounts present were determined as being 410, 126 and 30.8 ng/g dry weight, respectively.[26] HPLC analysis of nine different samples of *P. incarnata* herb available in Australia resulted in a range of concentrations for harman (not detected to 0.112 μg/g) and harmine (not detected to 0.271 μg/g); harmol was not detected.[27] Reversed phase HPLC with photodiode array detection was used to determine the harman alkaloid content of 104 samples (91 species) of *Passiflora*.[16] One sample of *P. incarnata* contained harmalol, harmol, harman, harmaline and harmine (0.05, 0.09, 0.11, 0.20 and 0.23 ppm, respectively).

Food Use

Passionflower is listed by the Council of Europe as a natural source of food flavouring (category N3). This category indicates that passionflower can be added to foodstuffs in the traditionally accepted manner, but that there is insufficient information

P

available for an adequate assessment of potential toxicity.[G16] Previously in the USA, passionflower has been permitted for use in food.[G65]

Herbal Use

Passionflower is stated to possess sedative, hypnotic, antispasmodic and anodyne properties.[G69] Traditionally, it has been used for neuralgia, generalised seizures, hysteria, nervous tachycardia, spasmodic asthma, and specifically for insomnia.[G7] The German Commission E approved internal use for nervous restlessness.[G3] Passionflower is used in combination with valerian root and lemon balm for conditions of unrest, difficulty in falling asleep due to nervousness.[G3] Passionflower is used extensively in homeopathy.

Dosage

Dosages for oral administration (adults) recommended in older standard herbal reference texts for the traditional uses are given below.

For restlessness and resulting irritability and insomnia, and nervous tension 0.5–1 g of dried plant equivalent three times daily;[G49] 4–8 g herb daily.[G3]

Modern standard herbal reference texts recommend the following dosages for oral administration (adults).

For tenseness, restlessness and irritability with difficulty falling asleep: 0.5–2 g of drug three to four times daily; 2.5 g of drug as an infusion three to four times daily; 1–4 mL of tincture (1 : 8) three to four times daily.[G76]

There has been insufficient clinical investigation of *P. incarnata* preparations to describe dosages typically used in clinical trials.

Pharmacological Actions

In vitro and animal studies

Preclinical studies have focused on investigating the anxiolytic and sedative properties of preparations of *Passiflora incarnata*, although other activities, such as anticonvulsant, anti-inflammatory, anti-addictive and aphrodisiac effects, have also been explored.[13] There are conflicting reports on which of the constituents of *P. incarnata* are responsible for the documented pharmacological effects; the alkaloids and flavonoids are considered to be important for activity, although the alkaloids are not detected in some samples of *P. incarnata* material. A tri-substituted benzoflavone moiety has been associated with various activities.[13]

A mechanism of action for *P. incarnata* has not clearly been established.[13] In radioligand receptor binding studies, extracts of *P. incarnata* aerial parts (containing 3% or 9% flavonoids) at concentrations of 10–1000 μg/mL did not interact with benzodiazepine, dopaminergic and histaminergic binding sites.[28] Two flavonoid constituents of *P. incarnata*, isovitexin-2"-*O*-glucoside and iso-orientin-2"-*O*-glucoside, at concentrations up to 30 μmol/L also failed to inhibit the interaction of ligands with the benzodiazepine receptor binding site. *In vitro* experiments utilising rat CNS receptors have shown that a multi-herb product (containing hydroalcoholic extracts of *P. incarnata* stalks and leaves and *Valeriana officinalis* roots, aqueous extracts of *Crataegus oxyacantha* flowers and *Ballota foetida*, and dried seed powder of *Paullinia cupana* and *Cola nitida*) as well as *P. incarnata* extract alone, inhibited the binding of ligands to central, but not peripheral, benzodiazepine receptors (IC_{50} 37.1 and 601.4 μg/mL for the multi-herb extract and *P. incarnata* extract, respectively).[29] The multi-herb extract and *P. incarnata* extract also inhibited the binding of ligands to alpha-2 adrenoceptors, but had no such effect on binding of ligands to serotonergic 5-HT_1 and 5-HT_2 and dopaminergic DA_1 and DA_2 receptors.

Anxiolytic activity Several studies have explored the anxiolytic properties of *P. incarnata* preparations in experimental models. In a battery of experiments in mice, a hydroalcoholic extract (10% w/v) of the fresh aerial parts of *P. incarnata* collected in Italy was administered intraperitoneally at doses ranging from 3 to 800 mg/kg (doses expressed in terms of dry plant material) body weight 30 minutes before tests.[30] Compared with controls, animals treated with *P. incarnata* extract displayed increased activity in the staircase test (at doses of 400 and 800 mg/kg body weight) and increased time spent in the light compartment in the light/dark avoidance test (at a dose of 400 mg/kg body weight). These results were indicative of anxiolytic, rather than sedative effects. Mixtures comprising different quantities of maltol plus different quantities of indole alkaloids or flavonoids found in *P. incarnata*, also administered intraperitoneally, had no effect on behavioural activity in the staircase test, suggesting that these compounds are not responsible for activity.[30]

Anxiolytic activity has also been documented for *P. incarnata* following studies using the elevated plus-maze model, an experimental test used to observe anxiolytic behaviour; less

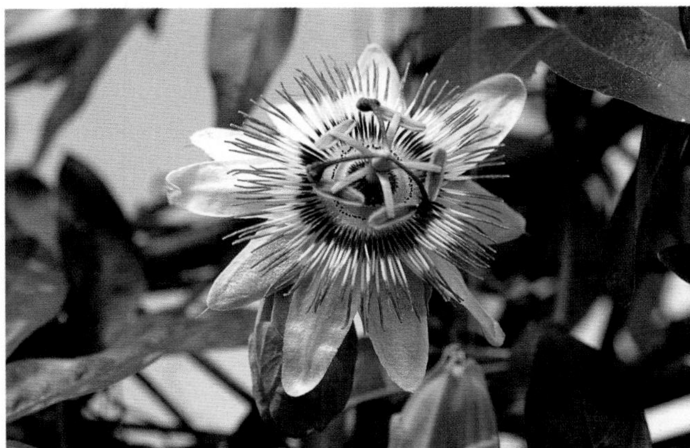

Figure 2 Passionflower (*Passiflora incarnata*).

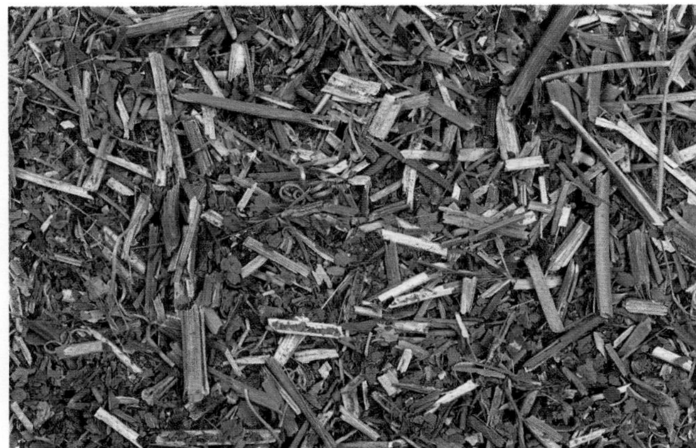

Figure 3 Passionflower – dried drug substance (herb).

anxious animals spend more time in the 'open' arms of the plus maze. In mice, a methanol extract of the aerial parts of *P. incarnata* was significantly more effective than control in increasing the amount of time animals spent in the open arms of the model ($p < 0.001$) when administered orally at doses ranging from 75 to 200 mg/kg body weight. By contrast, a methanol extract of the aerial parts of *P. edulis*, a related species with which *P. incarnata* has been confused, was virtually devoid of activity in this test.[31]

Subsequent work using different extracts of carefully separated plant parts of *P. incarnata* found that methanol extracts of the respective plant parts showed the greatest anxiolytic activity in mice in an experiment involving the elevated plus-maze model.[32] It was concluded that methanol extracts of the leaves/petioles and the stems/tendrils achieved greater anxiolytic activity than did extracts of the flowers/buds, the whole plant and the roots, although statistical tests for intergroup differences were not carried out. Selection of the entire aerial parts excluding the flowers may be the optimum approach to achieving a maximal anxiolytic effect.[32] Further investigations, utilising bioactivity-guided fractionation and chromatographic techniques, indicated that a subfraction of a methanol extract of the aerial parts of *P. incarnata* showed the greatest anxiolytic activity in mice in the elevated plus-maze model. Anxiolytic activity of this subfraction at a dose of 10 mg/kg body weight orally was comparable to that of diazepam 2 mg/kg body weight orally.[33] The subfraction comprised β-sitosterol and a compound reported to be a benzoflavone derivative.

In a study involving mice, animals received ethanol 2 g/kg twice daily orally and a benzoflavone fraction (obtained from a methanol extract of the aerial parts of *P. incarnata*) 10, 20 or 50 mg/kg orally, or control, twice daily for six days. The anxiogenic profile of the animals was assessed on day seven after treatment with alcohol with or without the benzoflavone fraction had ceased. Compared with control, treated animals showed reductions in hyperanxiety due to alcohol cessation, as assessed by mean duration of time spent in the open arms of the elevated plus-maze model ($p < 0.001$).[34]

P

Chrysin, a flavonoid found in *P. incarnata*, has been reported to have anxiolytic activity following a series of experiments carried out in rats. Compared with control, chrysin 1 mg/kg administered intraperitoneally significantly increased the length of time spent in the light compartment in the light/dark test of anxiety ($p < 0.05$). The anxiolytic effect of chrysin was inhibited by pre-treatment of animals with the benzodiazepine receptor antagonist flumazenil (3 mg/kg, intraperitoneally).[35]

Sedative activity Sedative effects for preparations of *P. incarnata* have also been documented following several studies.

An aqueous extract (10% w/v) of the fresh aerial parts of *P. incarnata* collected in Italy exhibited sedative effects in three tests when administered at doses of 400 and 800 mg/kg body weight.[30] Treatment with flumazenil (a benzodiazepine receptor antagonist) 10 mg/kg body weight before administration of *P. incarnata* aqueous extract 400 mg/kg body weight did not influence the sedative activity observed in the staircase test. A methanol extract of the leaves of *P. incarnata* administered at doses of 100, 200, 300 and 400 mg/kg body weight intraperitoneally to mice one hour before intraperitoneal administration of pentobarbital sodium 25 mg/kg body weight significantly prolonged the pentobarbital-induced sleeping time (time elapsed between loss and recovery of the righting reflex), compared with control ($p < 0.05$ for all doses).[36] A similar result was obtained with a multifraction dry extract of the whole aerial parts (leaves, stems and flowers) of *P. incarnata* administered orally at a dose of 60 mg/kg body weight.[37]

An aqueous ethanolic extract of *P. incarnata* fresh aerial parts administered intraperitoneally at a dose of 160 mg/kg body weight to rats prolonged sleeping time induced by pentobarbital (50-4000 mg/kg) and reduced spontaneous locomotor activity.[38] In mice, a 70% ethanol extract of *P. incarnata* herb (1000 mg/kg, intraperitoneally) administered 10 minutes prior to sodium pentobarbitol (40 mg/kg, intraperitoneally) resulted in a significant prolongation (40%) of sleeping time,[39] although a p value was not provided. When given by gastric tube one hour prior to amfetamine (5 mg/kg, subcutaneous), the same extract at a dose of 500 mg/kg body weight caused a significant reduction in hypermotility.

CNS sedation, prolongation of hexobarbitone-induced sleeping time (at high doses) and a reduction in spontaneous motor activity (at low doses) have been documented for maltol and ethylmaltol in mice.[10, 40] Subsequent research documenting similar activities in mice was unable to attribute the observed activities to either flavonoid or alkaloid components present in the extract tested.[38] However, maltol is reportedly an artefact and not a relevant constituent.[41]

There are conflicting reports on the role of the flavonoid chrysin (5,7-dihydroxyflavone) in the sedative effects of *P. incarnata* preparations. In the pentobarbital-induced sleeping test in mice, there was a significant prolongation in sleeping time in chrysin-treated animals, compared with controls (p value not stated) although the dose required to achieve this effect (30 mg/kg) was higher than that reported to be found in extracts of *P. incarnata*.[42] In a study in rats, chrysin (50 mg/kg body weight intraperitoneally) did not have any significant effect on the pentobarbital-induced sleeping time (time elapsed between loss and return of righting reflex.[35] Chrysin and another flavonoid found in *P. incarnata*, apigenin, displayed sedative activity as determined by reductions in locomotor behaviour when administered intraperitoneally to rats at doses of 25–100 mg/kg body weight. This activity was not influenced by prior administration of the benzodiazepine receptor antagonist flumazenil (3 mg/kg intraperitoneally).[35]

An aqueous ethanolic extract of *P. incarnata* fresh aerial parts administered intraperitoneally at a dose of 160 mg/kg body weight to rats raised the threshold to nociceptive stimuli in tail flick and hotplate tests.[38] A methanol extract of the leaves of *P. incarnata* administered at doses of 100, 200, 300 and 400 mg/kg body weight intraperitoneally to mice one hour before intraperitoneal administration of acetic acid (0.6% v/v) 10 mL/kg body weight significantly reduced the number of writhings in treated animals, compared with controls ($p < 0.05$ for all doses).[36]

Anticonvulsant activity A methanol extract of the leaves of *P. incarnata* administered at doses of 100, 200, 300 and 400 mg/kg body weight intraperitoneally to mice one hour before intraperitoneal administration of the convulsant agent pentylenetetrazole 50 mg/kg body weight significantly delayed the onset of convulsions and increased survival time in treated animals, compared with controls ($p < 0.05$ for all doses).[36] A similar result was obtained with a multi-fraction dry extract of the whole aerial parts (leaves, stems and flowers) of *P. incarnata* administered orally at a dose of 60 mg/kg body weight ($p < 0.01$ for treated animals versus controls).[37]

Anticonvulsant activity (at high doses) has been documented for maltol and ethyl maltol in mice.[10, 40]

Anti-addictive activities Reports from several preclinical studies have documented that the tri-substituted benzoflavone moiety found in *P. incarnata* reverses tolerance and dependence to several substances,[43] including the cannabinoid delta-9 tetrahydrocannabinol (THC),[44] diazepam,[45] ethanol,[34] morphine[46] and nicotine.[47] These studies have typically involved oral administration to mice of the benzoflavone moiety at a dose of 10 or 20 mg/kg body weight (10–100 mg/kg in the case of morphine) concomitantly with the addictive substance (THC and morphine: 10 mg/kg body weight orally twice daily; diazepam 20 mg/kg body weight orally; nicotine 2 mg/kg body weight subcutaneously four times daily; ethanol 2 g/kg body weight orally twice daily) for up to 21 days.

Aphrodisiac activity A methanol extract of *P. incarnata* leaves administered to male mice at oral doses of 75, 100 and 150 mg/kg body weight significantly increased the number of mounts on non-oestrus female mice, compared with control.[48] The greatest mounting activity was seen during the assessment period covering 105 to 120 minutes post administration, and for mice given the 100 mg/kg body weight dose, compared with control (mean (standard deviation) number of mounts: 15.67 (1.21) and 1.0 (1.09), respectively; $p < 0.001$). The extract tested was reported to contain *P. incarnata* flavonoids and glycosides, but was free of alkaloids. In another preclinical study, in which a benzoflavone moiety isolated from a methanol extract of the aerial parts of *P. incarnata* was administered orally to male rats at a dose of 10 mg/kg body weight, a significant increase in mounting behaviour was observed in the treated group, compared with the control group at each of three assessment periods ($p < 0.05$ versus control).[49] Sperm count was also significantly higher in treated rats, compared with rats in the control group, as was the proportion of female rats (with whom male rats were given the opportunity to mate) who became pregnant (6/15 versus 14/15 for control and treated rats, respectively; p value not reported). Further controlled experiments have described restoration of THC-induced decline in sexual function in male rats given THC and the benzoflavone moiety concurrently.[50] Prevention of ethanol- and nicotine-induced changes in parameters of sexual function has also been reported in male rats treated with the benzoflavone moiety, compared with control.[51]

Other activities A methanol extract of the leaves of *P. incarnata* significantly reduced the extent of carrageenan-induced paw oedema in mice when administered intraperitoneally one hour before injection into paws of carrageenan 0.1 mL.[36] Anti-inflammatory activity was greatest in animals treated with *P. incarnata* extract 400 mg/kg body weight ($p < 0.05$ versus control). An ethanolic extract of *P. incarnata* flowering and fruiting tops administered orally to rats one hour prior to injection of carrageenan into rat paws at doses of 75–500 mg/kg body weight reduced oedema in a dose-dependent manner, with significant reductions in oedema in treated rats, compared with control rats, observed with doses of 125 mg/kg and above.[52] Significant effects in other experimental models of inflammation, including dextran-induced pleurisy and cotton pellet-induced granuloma, were also documented for the *P. incarnata* extract.

Antitussive activity has been documented for a methanol extract of *P. incarnata* leaves. In mice, *P. incarnata* leaf extract administered orally at doses of 100 or 200 mg/kg body weight significantly reduced sulphur dioxide induced cough (39.4% and 65% reduction in frequency of cough for the lower and higher doses, respectively, compared with control; $p < 0.01$).[53] In an experimental model of asthma, a methanol extract of *P. incarnata* leaves administered orally to guinea pigs at doses of 50, 100 and 200 mg/kg body weight significantly reduced acetylcholine induced bronchospasm at the two highest doses, compared with control ($p < 0.05$).[54]

An ethanol extract of *P. incarnata* (whole plant) significantly inhibited phorbol-ester-promoted Epstein–Barr virus early antigen (EBV-EA) activation *in vitro*.[55] This assay is used to identify potential cancer chemopreventive substances. An ethanol extract of *P. incarnata* aerial parts had no calcium antagonist activity in *in vitro* experiments involving inhibition of aortic contractions induced by potassium ion depolarisation.[56] Passicol exhibits antimicrobial activity towards a wide variety of moulds, yeasts and bacteria.[11] Group A haemolytic streptococci are more susceptible than are *Staphylococcus aureus*, with *Candida albicans* of intermediate susceptibility.[11]

Pharmacokinetics Hard gelatin capsules containing different preparations of 'Passiflora' (likely *P. incarnata*) material have different dissolution profiles *in vitro*.[57] Dissolution profiles for capsules containing 100 mg freeze-dried extract of *P. incarnata* or 164.8 mg of a commercial dried purified extract of *P. incarnata* (Passoflo2-LMF) showed that the release of flavonoids from both preparations was almost 100% after ten minutes, whereas flavonoid release from capsules containing 410.6 mg *P. incarnata* powder was only around 50% after the same amount of time.

Clinical studies

Pharmacokinetics No information relating to the clinical pharmacokinetics of *P. incarnata* preparations was found.

Therapeutics Clinical investigation of *P. incarnata* preparations is limited. The few clinical trials available generally have investigated the effects of proprietary products containing *P. incarnata*, in some cases in combination with other herbal ingredients, in patients with anxiety disorders. Further investigation of the efficacy and effectiveness of *P. incarnata* preparations is required.

In a randomised, double-blind study, 36 patients with generalised anxiety disorder received *P. incarnata* extract (Passipay; Iran) 45 drops daily (no further details of preparation provided), or oxazepam 30 mg daily, for four weeks. At the end of the study, participants in both groups showed significant reductions in anxiety scores (assessed using the Hamilton Anxiety Rating Scale), compared with baseline values ($p < 0.001$ for both), and there were no statistically significant differences between the two groups.[58] However, this was a small study, a sample size calculation does not appear to have been carried out, and it is possible that the study was not large enough to detect a difference between the two treatments. In addition, the study did not include a placebo arm, so it is also possible that the effects in both groups could be explained as a placebo response.

Another randomised, double-blind trial compared the effects of *P. incarnata* extract 20 drops three times daily (no further details of preparation provided) plus clonidine 0.8 mg daily (maximum dose) with clonidine alone on the opiate withdrawal syndrome in 65 men addicted to opiates. At the end of the two-week study, participants in both groups experienced significant reductions in total symptom scores (both physical and mental symptoms), compared with baseline values ($p < 0.05$) for both.[59] The reduction in total score in the *P. incarnata* plus clonidine was greater than that observed with clonidine alone ($p = 0.011$). This study also has methodological limitations, including an apparent lack of a sample size calculation.

Two further studies have explored the effects of a combination herbal preparation (Euphytose) containing dry extracts of *P. incarnata* (40 mg), *Valeriana officinalis* (50 mg), *Crataegus oxyacantha* (10 mg) and *Ballota foetida* (10 mg) as well as powdered *Paullinia cupana* (15 mg) and *Cola nitida* (15 mg) (plant part(s) for each not stated). In a randomised, double-blind, multi-centre study in a general practice setting, 182 patients diagnosed with adjustment disorder with anxious mood received Euphytose two tablets three times daily, or placebo, for 28 days.[60] At the end of the study, the mean Hamilton anxiety scale score (the primary outcome variable) was reported to be significantly lower for the treatment group, compared with the placebo group, although the p value given for this was $\leqslant 0.05$. A significantly greater proportion of participants in the treatment group was classified as 'responders' (participants with Hamilton anxiety scale score $<$ 10 at the end of the study: 42.9% and 25.3% for the treatment and placebo groups, respectively; $p = 0.012$).[60] Although this was a reasonably good-sized study, a formal sample size calculation was not reported. Other methodological limitations are that details of the method of randomisation were not provided, there was no description of the formulation of the placebo preparation, a check for the success of blinding does not appear to have been carried out, and although the two groups were reported to be similar at baseline, baseline data on age, sex and other characteristics were not provided in a report of the study.

A randomised, double-blind, placebo-controlled study involving healthy volunteers assessed the psychometric effects of Euphytose. Sixty participants received the herbal preparation, or placebo, twice daily for 14 days and underwent a battery of psychometric tests, including the number-symbol pair test, the reaction choice test and the flicker-fusion test. There were no statistically significant differences between the treatment and placebo groups on assessments on days three, seven and 14 of the study.[61]

A protocol for a Cochrane systematic review of studies assessing the effectiveness of 'passiflora' or 'passionflower' in the treatment of any generalised anxiety disorder has been published.[62] The protocol does not state that the review will be limited to preparations of *P. incarnata*, yet it is important to consider phytochemical differences between species (and between different manufacturers' products) which could result in different clinical outcomes.

P

Side-effects, Toxicity

Cyanogenic glycosides have been documented for related *Passiflora* species.

Clinical data

There are only limited clinical data on safety aspects of *P. incarnata* preparations. No post-marketing surveillance-type studies were identified, and there is only a small number of clinical trials of *P. incarnata*.

In a randomised, double-blind study in which 36 patients with generalised anxiety disorder received *P. incarnata* extract (Passipay; Iran) 45 drops daily (no further details of preparation provided), or oxazepam 30 mg daily, for four weeks, no statistically significant differences in the overall frequency of adverse effects was observed between the two groups ($p = 0.831$).[58] Impairment of job performance occurred more frequently in the oxazepam group, although this only just reached statistical significance ($p = 0.049$). There were no statistically significant differences in the frequencies of other adverse effects assessed, such as dizziness, drowsiness and confusion ($p > 0.1$ for all). A report of another randomised, double-blind trial involving the same preparation of *P. incarnata*[59] did not provide adverse event data.

In a randomised, double-blind, multi-centre study in a general practice setting, 182 patients diagnosed with adjustment disorder with anxious mood received Euphytose (a combination herbal preparation containing *P. incarnata* dry extract as well as five other herbal ingredients) two tablets three times daily, or placebo, for 28 days.[60] Four adverse events (dry mouth, headache, constipation, drowsiness) judged probably related to treatment occurred in the Euphytose group, and eight occurred in the placebo group.

Several case reports describe suspected adverse reactions associated with the ingestion of preparations of *P. incarnata*. In Australia, a 34-year-old woman developed severe nausea and vomiting within 24 to 48 hours of first taking three tablets of a herbal preparation, Sedacalm (containing *P. incarnata* 500 mg per tablet; no further details of preparation provided). The woman also developed a prolonged QT_c interval and experienced episodes of non-sustained ventricular tachycardia, and was admitted to hospital for cardiac monitoring and treatment with intravenous fluids.[63] She stopped taking the herbal preparation after two days, and within one week all symptoms had resolved. A sample of the product had a similar chromatographic profile to that of a sample from another batch of the same product and to a sample of *P. incarnata*, and digoxin and digitoxin were not detected.[63] No further details of this analysis were provided.

Another report describes a 77-year-old man with rheumatoid arthritis who was a participant in a clinical trial of a gel containing a NSAID for treatment of wrist synovitis.[64] The man had already been taking diclofenac and cyclopenthiazide for five years and, over the previous three weeks, had taken two tablets of a herbal preparation (Naturest) containing 'passionflower' extract on alternate nights for insomnia. After six applications of the gel, the man developed a pruritic erythematous rash on areas of his chest, and continued to develop blisters, papules and purpura on several areas of his body despite ceasing use of the gel; this clinical picture was suggestive of a hypersensitivity vasculitis.[64] Subsequently, it was revealed that the man had been randomised to the placebo gel group, thus removing suspicion from the gel product as the causative agent. In addition, because of the temporal relationship between use of the herbal product and the onset of the reaction, the herbal product was suspected as being associated with the reaction. However, causality in this case has not been established.

Two further cases describe hepatotoxic reactions associated with the use of herbal combination preparations containing *P. incarnata*,[65–67] although in both cases, *P. incarnata* was not the main suspected herbal ingredient. One case involved a 43-year-old woman who developed jaundice, nausea and vomiting, hepatitis and markedly raised liver function test values in association with use of a product reported to contain passionflower as well as seven other herbal ingredients, including skullcap, black cohosh and valerian.[65] The duration of administration of the herbal product, and the time to onset of symptoms were not known. A second case describes a 56-year-old woman who developed acute hepatic failure and who died.[66] The woman had taken a preparation labelled as containing kava (*Piper methysticum*), *P. incarnata* and *Scutellaria lateriflora*, although analysis of the product failed to identify *S. lateriflora* as an ingredient but did reveal an unidentified compound (no further details provided).

The World Health Organization's Uppsala Monitoring Centre (WHO-UMC; Collaborating Centre for International Drug Monitoring) receives summary reports of suspected adverse drug reactions from national pharmacovigilance centres of over 70 countries worldwide, including the UK. At the end of July 2005, the WHO-UMC's Vigisearch database contained a total of 16 reports, describing a total of 39 adverse reactions, for products reported to contain *P. incarnata* only as the active ingredient (*see* Table 1).[68] This number includes at least one of the case reports[64] described in details above. Reports originated from seven different countries, although most reports ($n = 8$) came from the UK. In 11 of the 16 reports, *P. incarnata* was the sole suspected drug, and in four of these cases, the patient concerned was taking other medicines. The database contains at least four further reports describing a total of 11 adverse reactions associated with herbal combination products containing *P. incarnata* in addition to other herbal ingredients.

Preclinical data

Preclinical toxicity for *P. incarnata* preparations are also limited. In mice, the acute toxicity threshold of an aqueous ethanolic extract of *P. incarnata* fresh aerial parts administered intraperitoneally was greater than 900 mg/kg body weight.[38] Also in mice, a dose of 250 mg/kg body weight of a hydrochloric acid soluble fraction of *P. incarnata* extract caused decreases in spontaneous activity, respiratory rate and heart rate.[10] The same fraction at a dose of 1000 mg/kg body weight caused tremor-like symptoms and death. LD_{50} values for maltol and ethylmaltol in mice after subcutaneous administration were 820 and 910 mg/kg body weight, respectively.[10]

In rats, a benzoflavone moiety isolated from a methanol extract of the aerial parts of *P. incarnata*, administered orally to male rats at a dose of 10 mg/kg body weight, was associated with a significantly higher sperm count in treated rats, compared with rats in the control group.[49] The proportion of female rats (with whom male rats were given the opportunity to mate) who became pregnant was also significantly higher in treated rats, compared with rats in the control group (6/15 versus 14/15 for control and treated rats, respectively; p value not reported).

Table 1 Summary of spontaneous reports ($n = 16$) of suspected adverse drug reactions associated with single-ingredient *Passiflora incarnata* preparations held in the Vigisearch database of the World Health Organization's Uppsala Monitoring Centre for the period up to end of July 2005[68, a]

System organ class. Adverse drug reaction name (number)	Total
Body as a whole – general disorders. Abdomen enlarged (1); malaise (1); pallor (1); withdrawal syndrome (1)	4
Cardiovascular disorders, general. Hypotension (1)	1
Central and peripheral nervous system disorders. Dizziness (1); headache (2); hypoaesthesia (1); hypokinesia (1); tremor (1); vertigo (1)	7
Gastrointestinal system disorders. Abdominal pain (1); diarrhoea (2); haemorrhage intra-abdominal (1); nausea (3); vomiting (1)	8
Heart rate and rhythm disorders. Tachycardia (1)	1
Liver–biliary . Hepatitis (2); hepatitis, cholestatic (1); jaundice (2)	5
Platelet, bleeding and clotting disorders. Prothrombin decreased (1); purpura (1)	2
Psychiatric. Agitation (1); mental deficiency (1); psychosis (1); paranoid reaction (1); sleep disorder (1); somnolence (1)	6
Red blood cell disorders. Pancytopenia (1)	1
Respiratory . Laryngitis (1); throat tightness (1)	2
Skin. Pruritus (1); rash erythematous (1)	2
Total number of suspected adverse drug reactions	39

[a]Caveat statement. These data were obtained from the Vigisearch database held by the WHO Collaborating Centre for International Drug Monitoring, Uppsala, Sweden. The information is not homogeneous at least with respect to origin or likelihood that the pharmaceutical product caused the adverse reaction. Any information included in this report does not represent the opinion of the World Health Organization

Contra-indications, Warnings

None documented, although it is possible that use of doses (*see* Dosage) of passionflower higher than those recommended may cause sedation to a greater extent than intended. In view of the lack of safety data, use of *P. incarnata* extracts at dosages higher than those recommended and/or for longer periods should be avoided.

Drug interactions No interactions have been documented for *P. incarnata*. However, in view of the documented pharmacological effects, whether or not there is potential for clinically important interactions with other medicines with similar or opposing effects and used concurrently should be considered.

Pregnancy and lactation No clinical data regarding the use of passionflower during pregnancy or lactation were identified. A hydroalcoholic extract of *P. incarnata* aerial parts (400–1600 μg/mL) was reported to potentiate the rhythmic spasms induced by potassium chloride (10 mmol/L) when added to isolated rat uterus suspended in Tyrode's solution.[69] The highest concentration of *P. incarnata* extract also increased spontaneous contractions, and reduced the response of the tissue to acetylcholine, when compared with control ($p < 0.05$).

In view of the lack of information on the use of *P. incarnata* during pregnancy and lactation, its use should be avoided during these periods.

P

Preparations

Proprietary single-ingredient preparations

Argentina: Sedante Noche. *Austria:* Passiflorin. *Germany:* Passiflora Curarina. *Russia:* Novo-Passit (Ново-Пассит). *Switzerland:* Passelyt. *UK:* Modern Herbals Sleep Aid; Natracalm; Naturest; Nodoff; Phytocalm. *Venezuela:* Floral Pas.

Proprietary multi-ingredient preparations

Argentina: Armonil; Nervocalm; Passacanthine; SDN 200; Sedante Dia; Serenil; Sigmasedan; Yerba Diet. *Australia:* Calmo; Euphorbia Complex; Executive B; Extralife Sleep-Care; Goodnight Formula; Herbal Anxiety Formula; Humulus Compound; Infant Calm; Lifesystem Herbal Plus Formula 2 Valerian; Multi-Vitamin Day & Night; Natural Deep Sleep; Nervatona Plus; Pacifenity; Passiflora Complex; Passionflower Plus; Proesten; Prosed-X; Relaxaplex; Valerian Plus Herbal Plus Formula 12. *Austria:* Nervenruh; Passedan; Passelyt; Sedogelat; Wechseltee St Severin. *Belgium:* Sedinal; Seneuval. *Brazil:* A Saude da Mulher; Benzomel; Bronquiogem; Calman;

Calmapax; Calmazin; Calmiplan; Composto Emagrecedor; Elixir de Passiflora; Emagrevit; Floriny; Gotas Nican; Pasalix; Passaneuro; Passaneuro; Passi Catha; Passicalm; Passiflora Composta; Passiflorine; Passilex; Sedalin; Serenus; Sominex; Vagostesyl. *Canada:* Herbal Sleep Aid; Herbal Sleep Well. *Chile:* Armonyl; Recalm. *Czech Republic:* Bio-Strath; Novo-Passit; Visinal. *France:* Biocarde; Euphytose; Mediflor Tisane Calmante Troubles du Sommeil No 14; Natudor; Neuroflorine; Nocvalene; Panxeol; Passiflorine; Passinevryl; Sedatif Tiber; Sympaneurol; Sympavagol. *Germany:* Biosedon; Dormo-Sern; Dormoverlan; Dr. Scheffler Bergischer Krautertee Nerven- und Beruhigungstee; Gutnacht; Gutnacht; Kytta-Sedativum; Moradorm S; Nervendragees; Nervinfant N; Nervoregin forte; Neurapas; Passin; Phytonoctu; Pronervon Phyto; Tornix; Valeriana mild; Vivinox Day. *Israel:* Calmanervin; Calmanervin; Nerven-Dragees; Passiflora Compound; Passiflora. *Italy:* Anevrasi; Biocalm; Dormil; Fitosonno; Noctis; Parvisedil; Passiflorine; Reve; Sedatol; Sedatol; Sedofit; Sedopuer F. *Malaysia:* Cleansa Plus. *Mexico:* Ifupasil; Pasinordin. *Monaco:* Neuropax. *Portugal:* Neurocardol; Valesono. *South Africa:* Avena Sativa Comp; Biral. *Spain:* Passiflorine; Sedasor; Sedonat; Valdispert Complex. *Switzerland:* Circulan; Dragees antirhumatismales; Dragees pour la detente nerveuse; Dragees pour le coeur et les nerfs; Phytomed Cardio; Relaxane; Relaxo; Soporin; Strath Gouttes pour le coeur; Strath Gouttes pour le nerfs et contre l'insomnie; Tisane antirhumatismale; Tisane calmante pour les enfants; Valverde Coeur; Valverde Detente dragees. *UK:* Anased; Avena Sativa Comp; Bio-Strath Valerian Formula; Daily Tension & Strain Relief; Fenneherb Sweetdreams; Gerard House Serenity; Herbal Pain Relief; HRI Night; Kalms Sleep; Modern Herbals Stress; Nighttime Herb; Nodoff; Nytol Herbal; PMT Formula; Quiet Life; Quiet Nite; Quiet Tyme; Relax B+; Sleepezy; Slumber; Sominex Herbal; SuNerven. *USA:* Calming Aid. *Venezuela:* Cratex; Equaliv; Eufytose; Lupassin; Pasidor; Pasifluidina; Passiflorum; Rendetil.

P

References

1 Rehwald A *et al.* Trace analysis of harman alkaloids in *Passiflora incarnata* by reversed-phase high performance liquid chromatography. *Phytochem Anal* 1995; 6: 96–100.
2 Lohdefink J, Kating H. Zur Frage des Vorkommens von Harmanalkaloiden in Passiflora-Arten. *Planta Med* 1974; 25: 101–104.
3 Lutomski J, Nourcka B. Simple carboline alkaloids. VI. Comparative chemical evaluation of alkaloid fractions from different sources. *Herba Polon* 1968; 14: 235–238.
4 Schmidt PC, Ortega GG. Passionsblumenkraut. Bestimmung des Gesamtflavonoidgehaltes von Passiflorae herba. *Deutsche Apotheker Zeitung* 1993; 47(25): 17–26.
5 Schilcher H. Zur Kenntnis der Flavon-C-Glykoside in Passiflora incarnata L. *Z Naturforsch* 1968; 23b: 1393.
6 Meier B. Passiflorae herba – pharmazeutische Qualität. *Z Phytother* 1995; 16: 90–99.
7 QM Li *et al.* Mass spectral characterisation of C-glycosidic flavonoids isolated from a medicinal plant (*Passiflora incarnata*). *J Chromatog* 1991; 562: 435–446.
8 Spencer KC, Seigler DS. Gynocardin from Passiflora. *Planta Med* 1984; 50: 356–357.
9 Jaroszewski JW *et al.* Cyanohydrin glycosides of *Passiflora*: distribution pattern, a saturated cyclopentane derivative from *P. guatemalensis*, and formation of pseudocyanogenic α-hydroxyamides as isolation artefacts. *Phytochemistry* 2002; 59: 501–511.
10 Aoyagi N *et al.* Studies on *Passiflora incarnata* dry extract. I. Isolation of maltol and pharmacological action of maltol and ethyl maltol. *Chem Pharm Bull* 1974; 22: 1008–1013.
11 Nicholls JM *et al.* Passicol, an antibacterial and antifungal agent produced by *Passiflora* plant species: qualitative and quantitative range of activity. *Antimicrob Agents Chemother* 1973; 3: 110–117.
12 Buchbauer G, Jirovetz L. Volatile constituents of the essential oil of *Passiflora incarnata*. *J Essent Oil Res* 1992; 4: 329–334.
13 Dhawan K *et al.* *Passiflora*: a review update. *J Ethnopharmacol* 2004; 94: 1–23.
14 Lutomski J *et al.* Pharmacochemical investigation of the raw materials from *Passiflora* genus. *Planta Med* 1975; 27: 112–121.
15 Olafsdottir ES *et al.* Cyanohydrin glycosides of Passifloraceae. *Phytochemistry* 1989; 28(1): 127–132.
16 Abourashed EA *et al.* High-speed extraction and HPLC fingerprinting of medicinal plants – II. Application of harman alkaloids of genus Passiflora. *Pharmaceutical Biol* 2003; 41(2): 100–106.
17 Raffaelli A *et al.* Mass spectrometric characterization of flavonoids in extracts from *Passiflora incarnata*. *J Chromatog A* 1997; 777: 223–231.
18 Chimichi S *et al.* Isolation and characterization of an unknown flavonoid in dry extracts from *Passiflora incarnata*. *Nat Prod Letts* 1998; 11: 225–232.
19 Rehwald A *et al.* Qualitative and quantitative reversed-phase high-performance liquid chromatography of flavonoids in *Passiflora incarnata* L. *Pharm Acta Helv* 1994; 69: 153–158.
20 Menghini A *et al.* Flavonoid contents in Passiflora spp. *Pharmacol Res* 1993; 27 (Suppl. Suppl.1): 13–14.
21 Abourashed EA *et al.* High-speed extraction and HPLC fingerprinting of medicinal plants – I. Application to *Passiflora flavonoids*. *Pharmaceut Biol* 2002; 40(2): 81–91.
22 Pereira CAM *et al.* A HPTLC densitometric determination of flavonoids from *Passiflora alata*, *P. edulis*, *P. incarnata* and *P. caerulea* and comparison with HPLC method. *Phytochemical Anal* 2004; 15: 241–248.
23 Voirin B *et al.* Separation of flavone C-glycosides and qualitative analysis of *Passiflora incarnata* L. by capillary zone electrophoresis. *Phytochemical Anal* 2000; 11: 90–98.
24 Marchart E *et al.* Quantification of the flavonoid glycosides in *Passiflora incarnata* by capillary electrophoresis. *Planta Med* 2003; 69: 452–456.
25 Bilia AR *et al.* Stability of the constituents of calendula, milk thistle and passionflower tinctures by LC-DAD and LC-MS. *J Pharm Biomed Anal* 2002; 30: 613–624.
26 Tsuchiya H *et al.* Beta-carboline alkaloids in crude drugs. *Chem Pharm Bull* 1999; 47(3): 440–443.
27 Grice ID *et al.* Identification and simultaneous analysis of harmane, harmine, harmol, isovitexin, and vitexin in *Passiflora incarnata* extracts with a novel HPLC method. *J Liq Chrom Rel Technol* 2001; 24(16): 2513–2523.
28 Burkard W *et al.* Receptor binding studies in the CNS with extracts of *Passiflora incarnata*. *Pharm Pharmacol Lett* 1997; 7: 25–26.
29 Valli M *et al.* Euphytose®, an association of plant extracts with anxiolytic activity: investigation of its mechanism of action by an *in vitro* binding study. *Phytotherapy Res* 1991; 5: 241–244.
30 Soulimani R *et al.* Behavioural effects of *Passiflora incarnata* L. and its indole alkaloid and flavonoid derivatives and maltol in the mouse. *J Ethnopharmacol* 1997; 57: 11–20.
31 Dhawan K *et al.* Comparative biological activity study on *Passiflora incarnata* and *P. edulis*. *Fitoterapia* 2001; 72: 698–702.
32 Dhawan K *et al.* Anxiolytic activity of aerial and underground parts of *Passiflora incarnata*. *Fitoterapia* 2001; 72: 922–926.
33 Dhawan K *et al.* Anti-anxiety studies on extracts of *Passiflora incarnata* Linneaus. *J Ethnopharmacol* 2001; 78: 165–170.
34 Dhawan K *et al.* Suppression of alcohol-cessation-oriented hyper-anxiety by the benzoflavone moiety of *Passiflora incarnata* Linneaus in mice. *J Ethnopharmacol* 2002; 81: 239–244.
35 Zanoli P *et al.* Behavioral characterisation of the flavonoids apigenin and chrysin. *Fitoterapia* 2000; 71: S117–S123.
36 Dhawan K *et al.* Evaluation of central nervous system effects of *Passiflora incarnata* in experimental animals. *Pharm Biol* 2003; 41(2): 87–91.
37 Speroni E *et al.* Sedative effects of crude extract of *Passiflora incarnata* after oral administration. *Phytotherapy Res* 1996; 10: S92–S94.
38 Speroni E, Minghetti A. Neuropharmacological activity of extracts from *Passiflora incarnata*. *Planta Med* 1988; 54: 488–491.

39 Capasso A, Pinto A. Experimental investigations of the synergistic-sedative effect of passiflora and kava. *Acta Ther* 1995; 21: 127–140.

40 Kimura R *et al.* Central depressant effects of maltol analogs in mice. *Chem Pharm Bull* 1980; 28: 2570–2579.

41 Meier B. *Passiflora incarnata* L.-Passionsblume-Portrait einer Arzneipflanze. *Z Phytother* 1995; 16: 115–126.

42 Speroni E *et al.* Role of chrysin in the sedative effects of *Passiflora incarnata* L. *Phytotherapy Res* 1996; 10: S98–S100.

43 Dhawan K. Drug/substance reversal effects of a novel tri-substituted benzoflavone moiety (BZF) isolated from *Passiflora incarnata* Linn.—a brief perspective. *Addiction Biology* 2003; 8: 379–386.

44 Dhawan K *et al.* Reversal of cannabinoids (Δ^9-THC) by the benzoflavone moiety from methanol extract of *Passiflora incarnata* Linneaus in mice: a possible therapy for cannabinoid addiction. *J Pharm Pharmacol* 2002; 54: 875–881.

45 Dhawan K *et al.* Attenuation of benzodiazepine dependence in mice by a tri-substituted benzoflavone moiety of *Passiflora incarnata* Linneaus: a non-habit forming anxiolytic. *J Pharm Pharmaceut Sci* 2003; 6(2): 215–222.

46 Dhawan K *et al.* Reversal of morphine tolerance and dependence by *Passiflora incarnata* — a traditional medicine to combat morphine addiction. *Pharmaceutical Biology* 2002; 40(8): 576–580.

47 Dhawan K *et al.* Nicotine reversal effects of the benzoflavone moiety from *Passiflora incarnata* Linneaus in mice. *Addiction Biology* 2002; 7: 435–441.

48 Dhawan K *et al.* Aphrodisiac activity of methanol extract of leaves of *Passiflora incarnata* Linn. in mice. *Phytotherapy Research* 2003; 17: 401–403.

49 Dhawan K *et al.* Beneficial effects of chrysin and benzoflavone on virility in 2-year-old male rats. *J Med Food* 2002; 5(1): 43–48.

50 Dhawan K, Sharma A. Restoration of chronic- Δ^9-THC-induced decline in sexuality in male rats by a novel benzoflavone moiety from *Passiflora incarnata* Linn. *Br J Pharmacol* 2003; 138: 117–120.

51 Dhawan K, Sharma A. Prevention of chronic alcohol and nicotine-induced azospermia, sterility and decreased libido, by a novel tri-substituted benzoflavone moiety from *Passiflora incarnata* Linneaus in healthy male rats. *Life Sciences* 2002; 71: 3059–3069.

52 Borrelli F *et al.* Anti-inflammatory activity of *Passiflora incarnata* L. in rats. *Phytotherapy Research* 1996; 10 (Suppl. Suppl.): S104–S106.

53 Dhawan K, Sharma A. Antitussive activity of the methanol extract of *Passiflora incarnata* leaves. *Fitoterapia* 2002; 73: 397–399.

54 Dhawan K *et al.* Antiasthmatic activity of the methanol extract of leaves of *Passiflora incarnata*. *Phytotherapy Research* 2003; 17: 821–822.12916087

55 Kapadia GJ *et al.* Inhibitory effect of herbal remedies on 12-O-tetradecanoylphorbol-13-acetate-promoted Epstein-Barr virus early antigen activation. *Pharmacol Res* 2002; 45(3): 213–220.

56 Rauwald HW *et al.* Screening of nine vasoactive medicinal plants for their possible calcium antagonistic activity. Strategy of selection and isolation for the active principles of *Olea europaea* and *Peucedanum ostruthium*. *Phytotherapy Research* 1994; 8: 135–140.

57 Taglioli V *et al.* Evaluation of the dissolution behaviour of some commercial herbal drugs and their preparations. *Pharmazie* 2001; 56: 868–870.

58 Akhondzadeh S *et al.* Passionflower in the treatment of generalized anxiety: a pilot double-blind randomized controlled trial with oxazepam. *J Clin Pharm Ther* 2001; 26: 363–367.

59 Akhondzadeh S *et al.* Passionflower in the treatment of opiates withdrawal: a double-blind randomized controlled trial. *J Clin Pharm Ther* 2001; 26: 369–373.

60 Bourin M *et al.* A combination of plant extracts in the treatment of outpatients with adjustment disorder with anxious mood: controlled study versus placebo. *Fundament Clin Pharmacol* 1997; 11: 127–132.

61 Bourin M. Étude des effets d'Euphytose® sur les performances psychométriques du volontaire sain. *Psychologie Medicale* 1994; 26 (14): 1471–1478.

62 Miyasaka LS *et al.* Passiflora for anxiety disorder (protocol). The Cochrane Database of Systematic Reviews, 2003, Issue 4. Art. No.: CD004518.

63 Fisher AA *et al.* Toxicity of *Passiflora incarnata* L. *Clin Toxicol* 2000; 38(1): 63–66.

64 Smith GW *et al.* Vasculitis associated with herbal preparation containing *Passiflora* extract. *Br J Rheumatol* 1993; 32(1): 87–88.

65 Whiting PW *et al.* Black cohosh and other herbal remedies associated with acute hepatitis. *Med J Aus* 2002; 177: 432–435.

66 Gow PJ *et al.* Fatal fulminant hepatic failure induced by a natural therapy containing kava. *Med J Aus* 2003; 178: 442–443.

67 Thomsen M *et al.* Fatal fulminant hepatic failure induced by a natural therapy containing kava. *Med J Aus* 2004; 180: 198–199.

68 Uppsala Monitoring Centre. Vigibase, WHO Adverse Reactions database (accessed 25 July, 2005)

69 Sadraei H *et al.* Effects of Zataria multiflora and Carum carvi essential oils and hydroalcoholic extracts of *Passiflora incarnata*, *Berberis integerrima* and *Crocus sativus* on rat isolated uterus contractions. *Int J Aromather* 2003; 13(2/3): 121–127.

Pennyroyal

Summary and Pharmaceutical Comment

Interest in pennyroyal has focused on the toxicity associated with the volatile oil. No documented reports of the pharmacological actions exhibited by the herb were located. In view of its potential toxicity, pennyroyal oil is not suitable for internal or external use.

Species (Family)

**Mentha pulegium* L. (Labiatae/Lamiceae)
†*Hedeoma pulegioides* (L.) Pers.

Synonym(s)

**Pulegium vulgare* Mill., *P. parviflorum* (Req.) Samp. pro parte
†*Melissa pulegioides* L., Squaw Mint

Part(s) Used

Herb

Pharmacopoeial and Other Monographs

BHP 1983[G7]
Martindale 35th edition[G85]

Legal Category (Licensed Products)

Pennyroyal is not included in the GSL.[G37]

P

Constituents

The following is compiled from several sources, including General References G22, G48 and G58.

Volatile oils 1–2%. Pulegone is the principal component (60–90%); others include menthone, *iso*-menthone, 3-octanol, piperitenone and *trans-iso*-pulegone.

Food Use

Pennyroyal is not commonly used in foods. It is listed by the Council of Europe as a natural source of food flavouring (category N3).[G16] This category indicates that there is insufficient information available for an adequate assessment of toxicity (*but see* Side-effects, Toxicity). Previously, in the USA, pennyroyal has been permitted for use in foods.[G65]

Herbal Use

Pennyroyal is stated to possess carminative, antispasmodic, diaphoretic and emmenagogue properties, and has been used topically as a refrigerant, antiseptic and insect repellent. Traditionally, it has been used for flatulent dyspepsia, intestinal colic, common cold, delayed menstruation, and topically for cutaneous eruptions, formication and gout.[G7]

Dosage

Dosages for oral administration (adults) for traditional uses recommended in standard herbal reference texts are given below. Pennyroyal oil is not suitable for internal or external use.

Herb 1–4 g as an infusion three times daily.[G7]

Liquid extract 1–4 mL (1 : 1 in 45% alcohol) three times daily.[G7]

Pharmacological Actions

None documented.

Clinical studies

There is a lack of clinical research assessing the effects of pennyroyal.

Side-effects, Toxicity

Clinical data

The toxicity of pennyroyal oil is well recognised and human fatalities following its ingestion as an abortifacient have been reported.[1–3] Symptoms reported following ingestion of the oil include abdominal pain, nausea, vomiting, diarrhoea, lethargy and agitation, pyrexia, raised blood pressure and pulse rate, and generalised urticarial rash. Generally, doses required for an abortifacient effect are also toxic and fatalities have involved both nephrotoxicity and hepatotoxicity.[2–4] Doses of one ounce and 30 mL[1–3] have proved fatal, whereas individuals have recovered following unsuccessful abortion attempts involving the ingestion of 7.5 mL oil.[3] The mechanism of hepatotoxicity for pennyroyal is not known.[2] A direct hepatoxic action has been suggested for the ketone component, pulegone.[2] Alternatively, metabolic conversion of pulegone to a reactive intermediate, a furan or epoxide, has been proposed.[2]

Preclinical data

Acute LD_{50} values for pennyroyal oil are documented as 0.4 g/kg (oral, rats) and 4.2 g/kg (dermal, rabbits).[4] The oil is non- or moderately irritating, non-sensitising and non-phototoxic.[4] Acute LD_{50} values documented for pulegone, the principal oil component, are, not suprisingly, similar to those for the oil: 0.47 g/kg (oral, rats), 3.09 g/kg (dermal, rabbits).[5] Steroid (pregnenolone-16α-carbonitrile) treatment has reduced hepatotoxicity

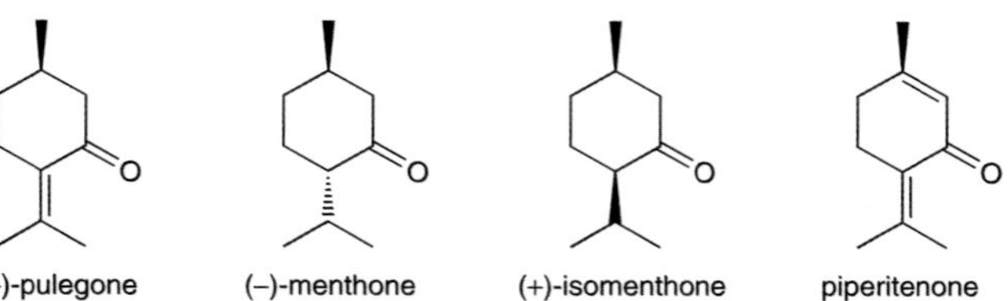

Figure 1 Selected constituents of pennyroyal.

observed in female rats fed pulegone, whereas triamcinolone has increased it.[5] Toxicity of pulegone is unaffected by partial hepatectomy or ligation of the common bile duct, while partial nephrectomy intensified toxicity.[5]

Contra-indications, Warnings

Pennyroyal oil is irritant and instances of hepatotoxicity and nephrotoxicity have been documented following its ingestion. Both the internal and external use of pennyroyal oil are contra-indicated.[G58]

Pregnancy and lactation Pennyroyal is contra-indicated in pregnancy.[G7] Traditionally, it has been employed as an abortifacient; fatalities have resulted from the doses of oil required to exert an abortifacient effect.

References

1 Vallance WB. Pennyroyal poisoning. A fatal case. *Lancet* 1955; ii: 850–851.
2 Sullivan JB *et al*. Pennyroyal oil poisoning and hepatotoxicity. *JAMA* 1979; 242: 2873.
3 Gunby P. Plant known for centuries still causes problems today. *JAMA* 1979; 241: 2246–2247.
4 Opdyke DLJ. Pennyroyal oil european. *Food Cosmet Toxicol* 1974; 12: 949–950.
5 Opdyke DLJ. Fragrance raw materials monographs: d-pulegone. *Food Cosmet Toxicol* 1978; 16: 867–868.

Pilewort

Summary and Pharmaceutical Comment

Limited information is available on the chemistry of pilewort. Little scientific information was located to justify the herbal uses, although antihaemorrhoidal activity has been documented for the saponin constituents in preclinical investigations. There is a lack of clinical research assessing the efficacy and safety of pilewort. In view of the toxic and irritant properties stated for protoanemonin, the excessive use of pilewort and use during pregnancy and lactation should be avoided.

Species (Family)

Ranunculus ficaria L. (Ranunculaceae)

Synonym(s)

Ficaria, *Ficaria ranunculoides* Roth, *F. degenii* Hervier, *F. nudicaulis* A. Kern., *F. verna* Huds., *F. vulgaris* A. St.-Hil., Lesser Celandine, Ranunculus

Part(s) Used

Herb

Pharmacopoeial and Other Monographs

BHP 1996[G9]
Martindale 35th edition[G85]

Legal Category (Licensed Products)

GSL[G37]

Constituents

The following is compiled from several sources, including General References G40 and G42.

Lactones Anemonin (dimer), protoanemonin (precursor to anemonin).

Triterpenoids Glycosides based on the sapogenins hederagenin and oleanolic acid, with arabinose, glucose and rhamnose, as sugar moieties.[1]

Other constituents Tannin and ascorbic acid (vitamin C).

Food Use

Pilewort is not used in foods.

Herbal Use

Pilewort is stated to possess astringent and demulcent properties. Traditionally, it has been used for haemorrhoids, and specifically for internal or prolapsed piles with or without haemorrhage, by topical application as an ointment or a suppository.[G7, G64]

Dosage

Dosages for oral administration (adults) for traditional uses recommended in older and contemporary standard herbal and/or pharmaceutical reference texts are given below. Another source states that pilewort is not suitable for internal use.[G49]

Dried herb 2–5 g as an infusion three times daily.[G7]

Liquid extract 2–5 mL (1 : 1 in 25% alcohol) three times daily.[G7]

Pilewort Ointment (BPC 1934) 30% fresh herb in benzoinated lard.

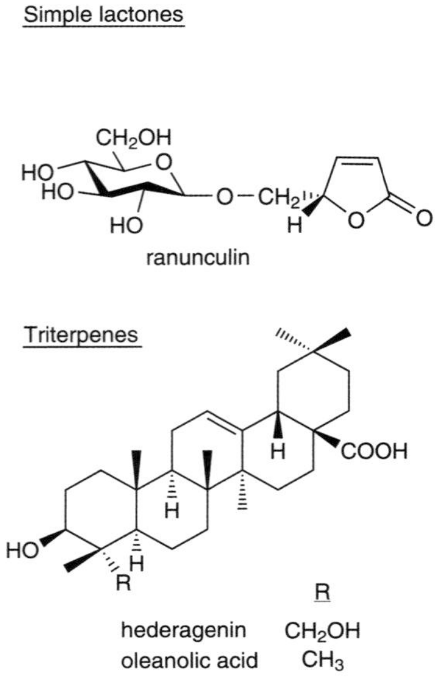

Figure 1 Selected constituents of pilewort.

Pharmacological Actions

In vitro and animal studies

Local antihaemorrhoidal activity has been documented for the saponin constituents.[1] Antibacterial and antifungal properties have been documented for both anemonin and protoanemonin, although anemonin is reported to exhibit much weaker activity.[G33, G48]

The reported presence of tannin constituents[G42] supports the reputed astringent activity of pilewort, although no pharmacological studies were located.

Clinical studies

There is a lack of clinical research assessing the effects of pilewort and rigorous randomised clinical trials are required.

Side-effects, Toxicity

There is a lack of clinical safety and toxicity data for pilewort and further investigation of these aspects is required.

The sap of pilewort is stated to be irritant.[G51] Protoanemonin is stated to be an acrid skin irritant, although it is readily converted into the inactive dimer anemonin.[G33] Protoanemonin is stated to have a marked ability to combine with sulfhydryl (-SH) groups and it is thought that the toxic subdermal properties of protoanemonin may depend on the inactivation of enzymes containing -SH groups.[G33] An LD_{50} value (mice, intraperitoneal injection) for anemonin has been reported as 150 mg/kg body weight.[G48]

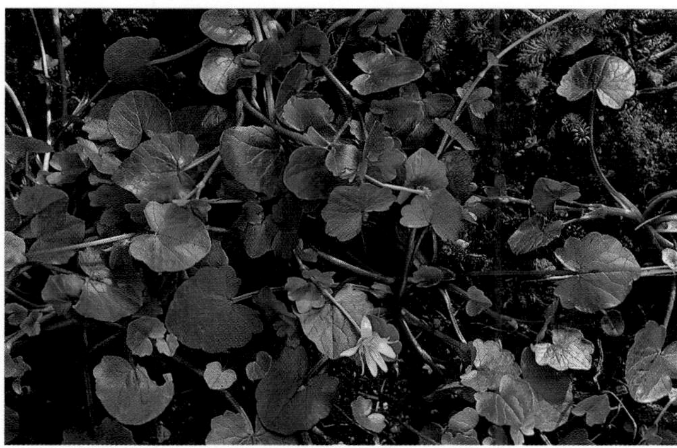

Figure 2 Pilewort (*Ranunculus ficaria*).

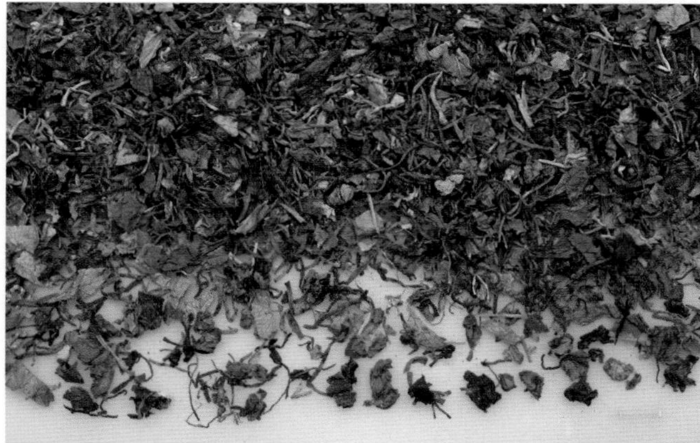

Figure 3 Pilewort – dried drug substance (herb).

Contra-indications, Warnings

Pilewort is not recommended for internal consumption.[G49] Topical use of pilewort may cause irritant skin reactions.

Pregnancy and lactation The safety of pilewort has not been established. In view of this, the use of pilewort during pregnancy and lactation should be avoided.

Preparations

Proprietary multi-ingredient preparations

Argentina: Confortel. *Czech Republic:* Avenoc. *France:* Apaisance; Hemorrogel. *UK:* Piletabs; Roberts Anti-Irritant Ointment.

P

Reference

1 Texier O *et al.* A triterpenoid saponin from *Ficaria ranunculoides* tubers. *Phytochemistry* 1984; 23: 2903–2905.

Plantain

Summary and Pharmaceutical Comment

The constituents of plantain are well-documented and the reputed antihaemorrhagic properties may be attributable to the tannin constituents. In addition, bronchospastic activity has been documented in preclinical and preliminary clinical studies. The toxicity of plantain is reported to be low, but excessive ingestion should be avoided.

Species (Family)

Plantago major L. (Plantaginaceae)

Synonym(s)

Common Plantain, General Plantain, Greater Plantain, *Plantago asiatica* auct. eur. pro parte, non L.

Part(s) Used

Leaf

Pharmacopoeial and Other Monographs

BHP 1996[G9]
BP 2007[G84]
Complete German Commission E[G3]
Martindale 35th edition[G85]

Legal Category (Licensed Products)

Plantain is not included in the GSL.[G37]

Constituents

The following is compiled from several sources, including General References G2, G40, G51 and G62.

Acids Benzoic acid, caffeic acid, chlorogenic acid, cinnamic acid, *p*-coumaric acid, ferulic acid, fumaric acid, gentisic acid, *p*-hydroxybenzoic acid, neochlorogenic acid, salicylic acid, syringic acid, ursolic acid, vanillic acid;[1,2] oleanolic acid and ascorbic acid.

Alkaloids Trace (unspecified),[3,4] boschniakine and the methyl ester of boschniakinic acid[5]

Amino acids DL-α-Alanine, asparagine, L-histidine, DL-lysine, DL-leucine, serine and tryptophan.[6]

Carbohydrates L-Fructose, D-glucose, planteose, saccharose, stachyose, *d*-xylose, sorbitol, tyrosol, mucilage and gum.[7]

Flavonoids Apigenin, baicalein, scutellarein, baicalin, homoplantaginin, nepitrin, luteolin, hispidulin and plantagoside.[8–10]

Iridoids Aucubin, aucubin derivatives, plantarenaloside, aucuboside and melitoside.[5,11,12]

Tannins 4%. Unspecified.

Other constituents Choline, allantoin, invertin and emulsin (enzymes), fat 10–20%, resin, saponins, steroids[13] and thioglucoside.

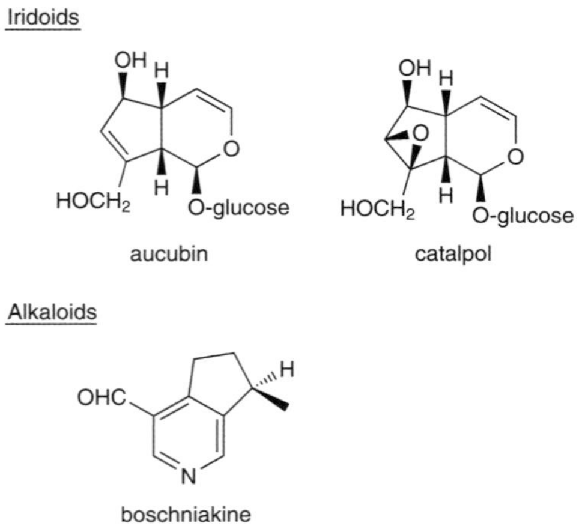

Iridoids

OH H
HOCH$_2$ H O-glucose
aucubin

OH H
HOCH$_2$ H O-glucose
catalpol

Alkaloids

OHC H N
boschniakine

Figure 1 Selected constituents of plantain.

Food Use

Plantain leaf is not used in foods. A related species, *Plantago lanceolata* L., is listed by the Council of Europe as a natural source of food flavouring (category N2). This category indicates that *P. lanceolata* can be added to foodstuffs in small quantities, with a possible limitation of an active constituent (as yet unspecified) in the final product.[G16] Previously, plantain has been listed by the Food and Drugs Administration (FDA) as a Herb of Undefined Safety.[G22]

Herbal Use

Plantain is stated to possess diuretic and antihaemorrhagic properties. Traditionally, it has been used for cystitis with haematuria, and specifically for haemorrhoids with bleeding and irritation.[G2,G7,G42,G64]

Dosage

Dosages for oral administration (adults) for traditional uses recommended in standard herbal reference texts are given below.

Dried leaf 2–4 g as an infusion three times daily.[G7]

Liquid extract 2–4 mL (1 : 1 in 25% alcohol) three times daily.[G7]

Tincture 2–4 mL (1 : 5 in 45% alcohol) three times daily.[G7]

Pharmacological Actions

In vitro and animal studies

An aqueous extract has been reported to possess bronchodilatory activity in guinea-pigs. It was more effective against acetylcholine-induced contraction, than towards constriction induced by histamine or serotonin.[14] The bronchodilatory activity of plantain in guinea-pigs has been reported to be less active and of shorter duration compared to salbutamol or atropine.[15]

Hypotensive activity in normotensive, anaesthetised dogs has been documented; 125 mg/kg extract was found to decrease arterial blood pressure by 20–40 mmHg.[16]

An aqueous extract, reported to contain flavonoids, saponins, steroids and alkaloids, was shown to possess anti-inflammatory activity in the rat using various models of inflammation, and a strengthening of capillary vessels has also been documented.[13] However, an extract was found to exhibit minimal (11%) inhibition of carrageenan-induced rat paw oedema.[17] Leaf extracts in hexane have shown potent wound-healing activity in rabbits; the effect was primarily attributed to C_{26}–C_{30} alcohols present in the extract.[18] Both the anti-inflammatory and wound-healing activities of plantain have been attributed to the high content of chlorogenic and neochlorogenic acids.[2]

Aucubin and a haemolytic saponin fraction have exhibited antibiotic activity towards *Micrococcus flavus* and *Staphylococcus aureus* (aucubin only).[19] Antibacterial activity towards *Bacillus subtilis* has been documented for the fresh plant juice, which was also found to lack activity towards Gram-positive organisms and fungi.[20] A negative response to cytotoxic, antitumour and antiviral activity was also reported for the plant juice.[20]

A mild laxative action has been reported in mice administered iridoid glycosides, including aucubin.[21] Plantain seed is sometimes used as a substitute for ispaghula (a bulk laxative).[G45]

Plantain has been documented to lower concentrations of total plasma lipids, cholesterol, β-lipoproteins and triglycerides in rabbits with experimental atherosclerosis.[22] Plantain has been reported to be useful in lowering plasma cholesterol concentrations.[23]

A tonus-raising effect on isolated guinea-pig and rabbit uterus tissue has been documented for an aqueous extract.[24]

Aucubin has been stated to be the active principle responsible for a hepatoprotective effect documented for plantain.[25]

Clinical studies

Clinical research assessing the effects of plantain is limited and rigorous randomised clinical trials are required.

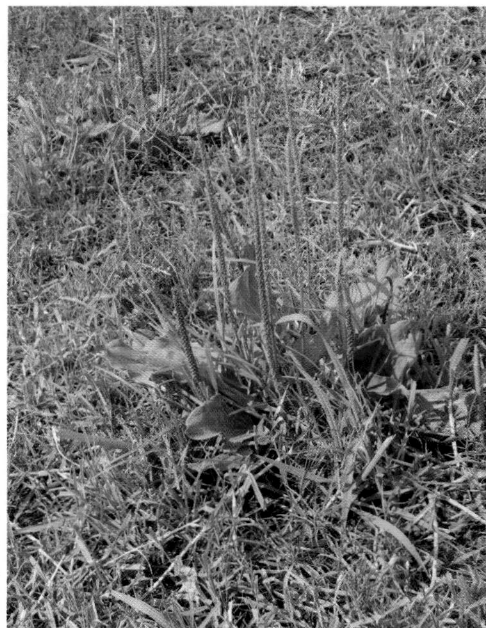

Figure 2 Plantain (*Plantago major*).

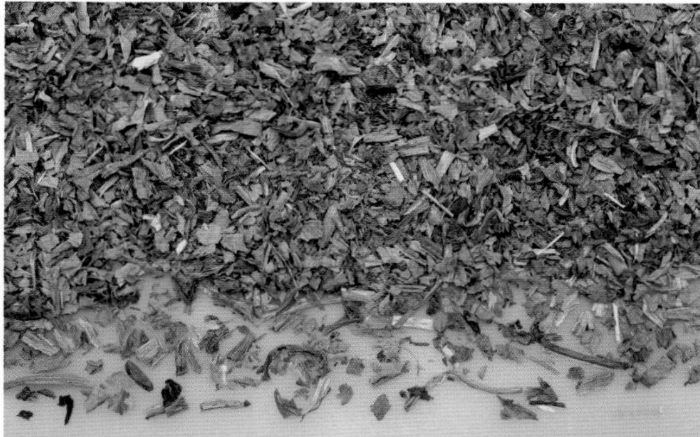

Figure 3 Plantain – dried drug substance (leaf).

Plantain has been reported to be effective in the treatment of chronic bronchitis of a spastic or non-spastic nature.[14, 26, 27] A pronounced improvement in both subjective and objective symptoms of the common cold following treatment with plantain has also been reported.[28] Plantain, in combination with agrimony, German chamomile, peppermint and St. John's wort, has been documented to provide pain relief in patients with chronic gastroduodenitis.[29] Following treatment, previously diagnosed erosions and haemorrhagic mucous changes were stated to have disappeared. However, the methodological limitations of these studies preclude definitive conclusions.

Side-effects, Toxicity

Clinical data

There is a lack of clinical safety and toxicity data for plantain and further investigation of these aspects is required.

Allergic contact dermatitis to plantain has been reported.[G51] The green parts of the plant are thought to yield a mustard oil-type of thioglucoside, which releases an irritant principle (isothiocyanate) upon enzymatic hydrolysis.[G51] The seed may also cause sensitisation and dermatitis.

Preclinical data

Plantain is reported to be of low toxicity with LD_{50} values in the rat documented as 1 g/kg (intraperitoneal injection) and greater than 4 g/kg (by mouth).[15]

Contra-indications, Warnings

Plantain may cause a contact allergic reaction; it induces the formation of IgE antibodies, which may cross-react to psyllium.[30] Excessive doses may exert a laxative effect and a hypotensive effect.

Drug interactions None documented. However, the potential for preparations of plantain to interact with other medicines administered concurrently, particularly those with similar or opposing effects, should be considered.

Pregnancy and lactation *In vitro* uterotonic activity has been documented for plantain. In view of this, and the lack of information on safety, use of plantain should be avoided during pregnancy and lactation.

Preparations

Proprietary single-ingredient preparations

France: Sensivision au plantain.

Proprietary multi-ingredient preparations

France: Ephydrol. *Portugal:* Erpecalm. *Switzerland:* Kernosan Elixir; Pastilles pectorales Demo N; Pectoral N; Tisane pectorale et antitussive; Tisane pectorale pour les enfants. *UK:* Napiers Breathe Easy Tea.

References

1 Andrzejewska-Golec E, Swiatek K. Chemotaxonomic studies on the genus *Plantago* II. Analysis of phenolic acid fraction. *Herba Pol* 1986; 32: 19–31.

2 Maksyutina NP. Hydroxycinnamic acids of *Plantago major* and *Pl. lanceolata*. *Khim Prirodn Soedin* 1971; 7: 795.

3 Smolenski SJ *et al*. Alkaloid screening. IV. *Lloydia* 1974; 37: 30–61.

4 Pailer M, Haschke-Hofmeister E. Inhaltsstoffe aus *Plantago major*. *Planta Med* 1969; 17: 139–145.

5 Popov S *et al*. Cyclopentanoid monoterpenes from *Plantago* species. *Izv Khim* 1981; 14: 175–180.

6 Maksyutin GV. Amino acids in *Plantago* (plantain) *major* leaves and *Matricaria recutita* inflorescences. *Rastit Resur* 1972; 8: 110–112.

7 Tomoda M *et al*. Plant mucilages. XXIX. Isolation and characterization of a mucous polysaccharide, plantago-mucilage A, from the seeds of *Plantago major* var. *asiatica*. *Chem Pharm Bull* 1981; 29: 2877–2884.

8 Lebedev-Kosov VI. Flavonoids of *Plantago major*. *Khim Prirodn Soedin* 1976; 12: 730.

9 Lebedev-Kosov VI *et al*. Flavonoids of *Plantago major*. *Khim Prirodn Soedin* 1977; 13: 223.

10 Endo T *et al*. The glycosides of *Plantago major* var. japonica Nakai. A new flavone glycoside, plantagoside. *Chem Pharm Bull* 1981; 29: 1000–1004.

11 Oshio H, Inouye H. Two new iridoid glucosides of *Plantago asiatica*. *Planta Med* 1982; 44: 204–206.

12 Andrzejewska-Golec E, Swiatek K. Chemotaxonomic studies on the genus *Plantago* I. Analysis of the iridoid fraction. *Herba Pol* 1984; 30: 9–16.

13 Lambev I *et al*. Study of the anti-inflammatory and capillary restorative activity of a dispersed substance from *Plantago major* L. *Probl Vatr Med* 1981; 9: 162–169.

14 Koichev A *et al*. Pharmacologic-clinical study of a preparation from *Plantago major*. *Probl Pneumol Ftiziatr* 1983; 11: 68–74.

15 Marcov M *et al*. Pharmacologic study of the influence of the disperse substance extracted from *Plantago major* on bronchial smooth muscles. *Probl Vatr Med* 1980; 8: 132–139.

16 Kyi KK *et al*. Hypotensive property of *Plantago major* Linn. *J Life Sci* 1971; 4: 167–171.

17 Mascolo N *et al*. Biological screening of Italian medicinal plants for anti-inflammatory activity. *Phytother Res* 1987: 1: 28–31.

18 Mironov VA *et al*. Physiologically active alcohols of *Plantago major*. *Khim-Farm Zh* 1983; 17: 1321–1325.

19 Tarle D. Antibiotic effect of aucubin, saponins and extract of plantain leaf – herba or folium *Plantaginis lanceolata*. *Farm Glas* 1981; 37: 351–354.

20 Lin Y-C *et al*. Search for biologically active substances in Taiwan medicinal plants I. Screening for anti-tumor and anti-microbial substances. *Chin J Microbiol* 1972; 5: 76–78.

21 Inouye H *et al*. Purgative activities of iridoid glycosides. *Planta Med* 1974; 25: 285–288.

22 Maksyutina NP *et al*. Chemical composition and hypocholesterolemic action of some drugs from *Plantago major* leaves. Part I. Polyphenolic compounds. *Farm Zh (Kiev)* 1978; 4: 56–61.

23 Ikram M. Medicinal plants as hypocholesterolemic agents. *J Pak Med Assoc* 1980; 30: 278–279.

24 Shipochliev T. Extracts from a group of medicinal plants enhancing the uterine tonus. *Vet Med Nauki* 1981; 18: 94–98.

25 Chang I-M, Yun (Choi) HS. Plants with liver-protective activities: pharmacology and toxicology of aucubin. In: Chang HM *et al*., eds. *Advances in Chinese Medical Material Research*. Singapore: World Scientific, 1985: 269.

26 Koichev A. Complex evaluation of the therapeutic effect of a preparation from *Plantago major* in chronic bronchitis. *Probl Vatr Med* 1983; 11: 61–69.

27 Matev M *et al*. Clinical trial of *Plantago major* preparation in the treatment of chronic bronchitis. *Vatr Boles* 1982; 21: 133–137.

28 Koichev A. Study on the therapeutic effect of different doses from the preparation *Plantago major* in cold. *Prob Vatr Med* 1982; 10: 117–124.

29 Chakarski I *et al*. Clinical study of a herb combination consisting of *Agrimonia eupatoria*, *Hipericum perforatum*, *Plantago major*, *Mentha piperita*, *Matricaria chamomila* for the treatment of patients with gastroduodenitis. *Probl Vatr Med* 1982; 10: 78–84.

30 Rosenberg S *et al*. Serum IgE antibodies to psyllium in individuals allergic to psyllium and English plantain. *Ann Allergy* 1982; 48: 294–298.

Pleurisy Root

Summary and Pharmaceutical Comment

The chemistry of pleurisy root is poorly documented, but phytochemical studies on pleurisy root and related *Asclepias* species have identified many cardiac glycoside constituents. No scientific evidence was found to justify the herbal uses. There is a lack of clinical research assessing the efficacy and safety of pleurisy root. In view of the potential toxicity of pleurisy root, excessive use and use during pregnancy and lactation should be avoided.

Species (Family)

Asclepias tuberosa L. (Asclepiadaceae)

Synonym(s)

Asclepias, Butterfly Weed

Part(s) Used

Root

Pharmacopoeial and Other Monographs

BHP 1983[G7]
Martindale 35th edition[G85]

Legal Category (Licensed Products)

GSL[G37]

Constituents

Little chemical information is available for pleurisy root. Cardiac glycosides of the cardenolide type (e.g. afroside, asclepin, calactin, calotropin, gomphoside, syriogenin, syrioside, uscharidin, uscharin and uzarigenin) have been documented for many *Asclepias* species,[1–4] including *A. tuberosa*.[5] Concentrations of cardiac glycosides are reported to vary between *Asclepias* species[1] and individual plant parts,[4] in descending order of latex, stem, leaf and root.[6]

No other data regarding constituents of the root were located.

Other plant parts Constituents documented for the herb include flavonols (e.g. kaempferol and quercetin) and flavonol glycosides (e.g. rutin and isorhamnetin), amino acids, caffeic acid, chlorogenic acid, choline, carbohydrates (e.g. glucose, fructose and sucrose), β-sitosterol, triterpenes (e.g. α-amyrin and β-amyrin, lupeol, friedelin, viburnitol), volatile oil and resin.[7,8,G48]

Food Use

Pleurisy root is not used in foods.

Herbal Use

Pleurisy root is stated to possess diaphoretic, expectorant, antispasmodic and carminative properties. It has been used for bronchitis, pneumonitis, influenza, and specifically for pleurisy.[G7,G42,G64]

Dosage

Dosages for oral administration (adults) for traditional uses recommended in standard herbal reference texts are given below.

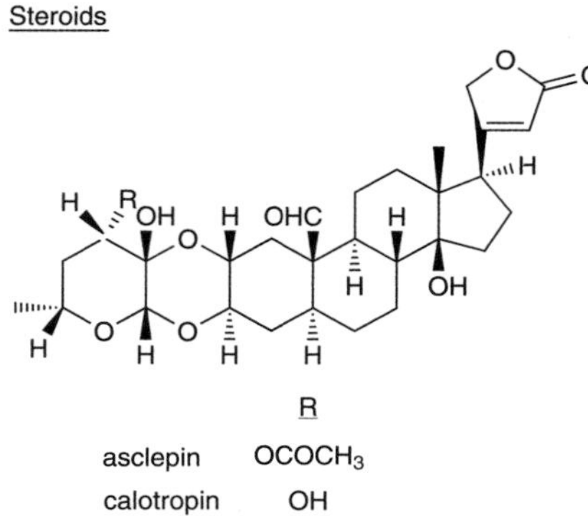

Figure 1 Selected constituents of pleurisy root.

Dried root 1–4 g as an infusion three times daily.[G7]

Liquid extract 1–4 mL (1:1 in 45% alcohol) three times daily.[G7]

Tincture 1–5 mL (1 : 10 in 45% alcohol) three times daily.[G7]

Pharmacological Actions

In vitro and animal studies

Low doses of extracts of *Asclepias* species including *A. tuberosa* have been documented to cause uterine contractions (*in vivo*) and to exhibit oestrogenic effects.[5,9,10,G30] No effect was observed on blood pressure or respiration (*in vivo*), or on the isolated heart (frog, turtle).[9]

Various activities have been reported for related *Asclepias* species. A positive inotropic action (*in vivo* and *in vitro*) has been

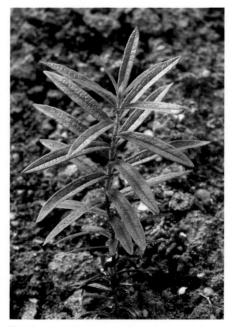

Figure 2 Pleurisy root (*Asclepias tuberosa*).

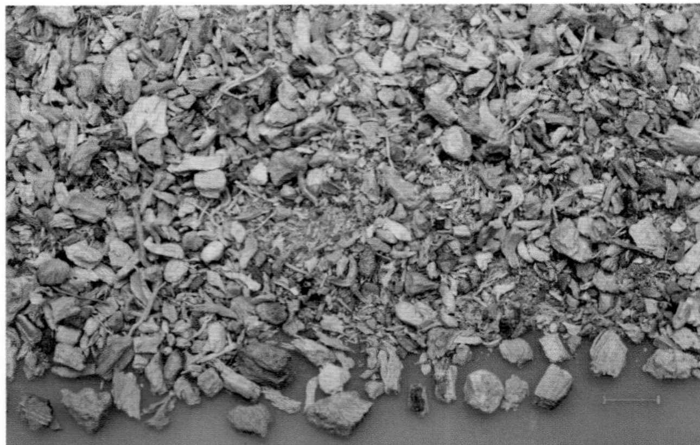

Figure 3 Pleurisy root – dried drug substance (root).

reported for asclepin (*Asclepias curassavica*), which was found to be more potent, longer acting and with a wider safety margin when compared with other cardiac glycosides (including digoxin).[11–13] Asclepin was also reported to exhibit a more powerful activity towards weak cardiac muscle.[13] Plant extracts of *A. curassavica*, *Asclepias engelmanniana* and *Asclepias glaucescens* have exhibited a stimulatory effect on the mammalian CNS, causing an increase in serotonin and noradrenaline concentrations.[14] Antitumour/cytotoxic activities have been documented for *A. albicans* and were attributed to various cardenolide constituents.[15]

Clinical studies

There is a lack of clinical research assessing the effects of pleurisy root and rigorous randomised clinical trials are required.

Side-effects, Toxicity

Clinical data

There is a lack of clinical safety and toxicity data for pleurisy root and further investigation of these aspects is required.

Pleurisy root and other *Asclepias* species have been documented to cause dermatitis; the milky latex is reported to be irritant.[G51] Large doses may cause nausea, vomiting and diarrhoea.[G7, G42]

Preclinical data

Various *Asclepias* species, including *A. tuberosa,* are known to be toxic to livestock, with cardenolides implicated as the toxic constituents.[1, 5] Toxic effects on the lungs, gastrointestinal tract, kidneys, brain and spinal cord have been observed in rats and rabbits following intravenous administration of an alcoholic extract.[10]

Toxicity studies involving related *Asclepias* species have also been documented. The cardenolide fraction of *Asclepias eriocarpa* is reported to contain toxic principles. The whole plant, plant extracts, an isolated and purified cardenolide (labriformin) and digoxin were all found to show qualitatively similar signs of toxicity and gross pathology in sheep and guinea-pigs.[16] LD_{50} values (mice, intraperitoneal injection) for cardenolides obtained from *A. curassavica* and *A. eriocarpa* were all estimated at less than 50 mg/kg body weight. Asclepin (*A. curassavica*) was reported to be safe following a three-month toxicity study in rats, using doses of 0.8, 8 and 20 mg/kg (route unspecified).[13] Asclepin has also been documented to have a wider margin of safety than digoxin[11–13] (*see In vitro* and animal studies).

Studies in cats have reported asclepin to be less cumulative compared to digoxin.[13]

Contra-indications, Warnings

Drug interactions None documented. However, the potential for preparations of pleurisy root to interact with other medicines administered concurrently, particularly those with similar or opposing effects, should be considered. Cardiac glycosides (*see* Constituents) have been documented as constituents of pleurisy root.

Pregnancy and lactation Uterotonic activity (*in vivo*) has been reported for pleurisy root.[5, G30] In view of this and the potential toxicity of pleurisy root, it should be avoided during pregnancy or lactation.

Preparations

Proprietary multi-ingredient preparations

Australia: Broncafect; Verbascum Complex. *UK:* Antibron; Chest Mixture; Horehound and Aniseed Cough Mixture; Vegetable Cough Remover.

References

1 Seiber JN *et al*. New cardiac glycosides (cardenolides) from *Asclepias* species. Proceedings of the Australia/USA Poisonous Plants Symposium. Plant Toxicol 1985: 427–437.
2 Radford DJ *et al*. Naturally occurring cardiac glycosides. *Med J Aust* 1986; 144: P540–544.
3 Jolad SD *et al*. Cardenolides and a lignan from *Asclepias subulata*. *Phytochemistry* 1986; 25: 2581–2590.
4 Seiber JN *et al*. Cardenolides in the latex and leaves of seven *Asclepias* species and *Calotropis procera*. *Phytochemistry* 1982; 21: 2343–2348.
5 Conway GA, Slocumb JC. Plants used as abortifacients and emmenagogues by Spanish New Mexicans. *J Ethnopharmacol* 1979; 1: 241–261.
6 Duffey SS, Scudder GGE. Cardiac glycosides in North American Asclepiadaceae, a basis for unpalatability in brightly coloured Hemiptera and Coleoptera. *J Insect Physiol* 1972; 18: 63–78.
7 Nelson CJ *et al*. Seasonal and intraplant variation of cardenolide content in the California milkweed *Asclepias eriocarpa* and implications for plant defense. *J Chem Ecol* 1981; 7: 981–1010.
8 Pagani F. Plant constituents of *Asclepias tuberosa* (Asclepiadaceae). *Boll Chim Farm* 1975; 114: 450–456.
9 Costello CH, Butler CL. The estrogenic and uterine-stimulating activity of *Asclepias tuberosa*. *J Am Pharm Assoc Sci Educ* 1949; 39: 233–237.
10 Hassan WE, Reed HL. Studies on species of *Asclepias* VI. Toxicology, pathology and pharmacology. *J Am Pharm Assoc Sci Educ* 1952; 41: 298–300.
11 Patnaik GK, Dhawan BN. Pharmacological investigations on asclepin – a new cardenolide from *Asclepius curassavica*. Part I. Cardiotonic activity and acute toxicity. *Arzneimittelforschung* 1978; 28: 1095–1099.
12 Patnaik GK, Koehler E. Comparative studies on the inotropic and toxic effects of asclepin, g-strophanthin, digoxin and digitoxin. *Arzneimittelforschung* 1978; 28: 1368–1372.
13 Dhawan BN, Patnaik GK. Investigation on some new cardioactive glycosides. *Indian Drugs* 1985; 22: 285–290.
14 Del Pilar Alvarez Pellitero M. Pharmacological action of medicinal plants in the nervous system. *An Inst Farmacol Espan* 1971; 20: 299–387.
15 Koike K *et al*. Potential anticancer agents. V. Cardiac glycosides of *Asclepias albicans* (Asclepiadaceae). *Chem Pharm Bull* 1980; 28: 401–405.
16 Benson JM *et al*. Comparative toxicology of cardiac glycosides from the milkweed *Asclepias eriocarpa*. *Toxicol Appl Pharmacol* 1977; 41: 131–132.

P

Pokeroot

Summary and Pharmaceutical Comment

There is limited chemical information available for pokeroot. Apart from its traditional use as a herbal remedy, pokeroot is also known to possess molluscicidal properties. Anti-inflammatory activity documented in animal studies supports the traditional use of pokeroot in rheumatism. However, there is a lack of clinical research assessing the efficacy and safety of pokeroot. Pokeroot is recognised as a toxic plant. The effects of pokeroot intoxication arise from the ingestion of any or all plant parts, liquid preparations of plant extracts such as herbal teas, or through skin contact with the plant. The main toxic agents are the pokeweed mitogen (lectins) and the glycoside saponins. The toxic properties of these two classes of compounds, mitogenic and irritant respectively, are well recognised. In view of this, excessive use of pokeroot and use during pregnancy and lactation should be avoided.

Species (Family)

Phytolacca americana L. (Phytolaccaceae)

Synonym(s)

Phytolacca dodecandra L., Pocan, Pokeberry, Pokeweed, Red Plant

Part(s) Used

Root

Pharmacopoeial and Other Monographs

BHP 1996[G9]
Martindale 35th edition[G85]

Legal Category (Licensed Products)

GSL [G37]

Constituents

The following is compiled from several sources, including General References G22, G48 and G64.

Alkaloids Betalain-type. Betanidine, betanine, isobetanine, isobetanidine, isoprebetanine, phytolaccine and prebetanine.

Lectins Pokeweed mitogen (PWM) consisting of five glycoproteins Pa^{-1} to Pa^{-5}.

Saponins Triterpenes – phytolaccosides A-1, D_2, and O,[1–3] aglycones include phytolaccagenin, jaligonic acid, phytolaccagenic acid, aesculentic acid,[2,4–6] acinosolic acid methyl ester;[5] monodesmosidic and bidesmosidic compounds with oleanolic acid and phytolaccagenic acids as aglycone in *P. dodecandra*.[7]

Other constituents Isoamericanin A (neo-lignan),[8]PAP (pokeweed antiviral protein)[9], α-spinasterol,[5], histamine and gamma aminobutyric acid (GABA).[10]

Betalain alkaloids

RO
HO
H
$COO^{\ominus}$
$N^{\oplus}$
H
HOOC
N
H
COOH

	R
betanidin	H
betanin	glucose

Triterpenes

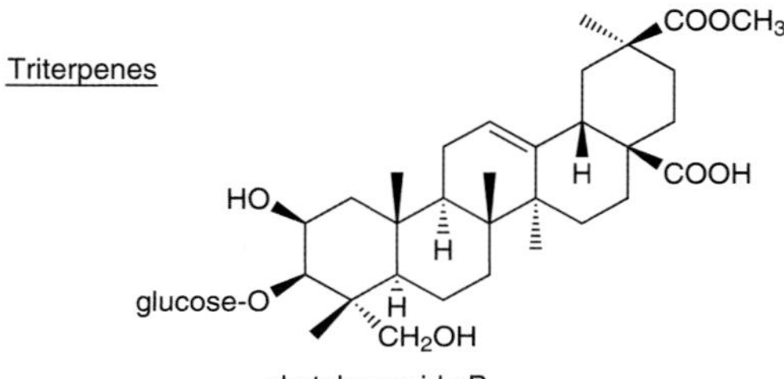

Figure 1 Selected constituents of pokeroot.

Food Use

Pokeroot is not commonly used in foods. Previously, in the USA, the Herb Trade Association has recommended that pokeroot should not be sold as a herbal beverage or food.[11]

Herbal Use

Pokeroot is stated to possess antirheumatic, anticatarrhal, mild anodyne, emetic, purgative, parasiticidal and fungicidal properties. Traditionally, it has been used for rheumatism, respiratory catarrh, tonsillitis, laryngitis, adenitis, mumps, skin infections

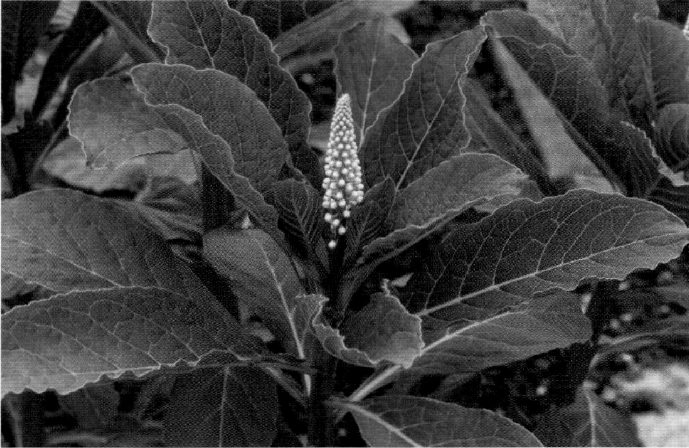

Figure 2 Pokeroot (*Phytolacca americana*).

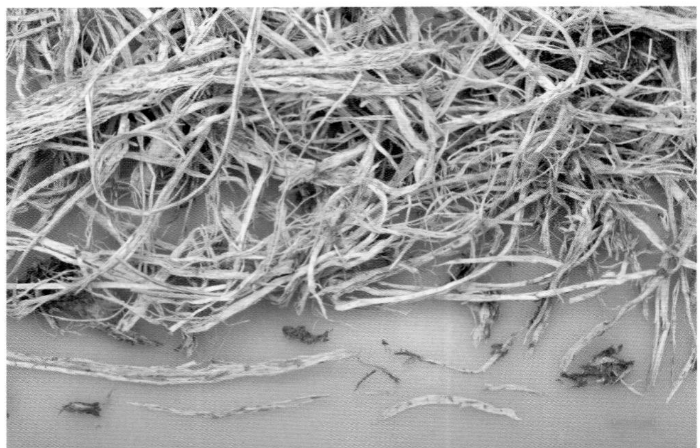

Figure 3 Pokeroot – dried drug substance (root).

(e.g. scabies, tinea, sycosis, acne), mammary abscesses and mastitis.[G7, G64]

Dosage

Dosages for oral administration (adults) for traditional uses recommended in standard herbal reference texts are given below.

Dried root 0.06–0.3 g as an decoction three times daily.[G7]

Liquid extract 0.1–0.5 mL (1:1 in 45% alcohol) three times daily.[G7]

Pharmacological Actions

In vitro and animal studies

Anti-inflammatory activity has been documented for saponin fractions isolated from *P. americana*.[2, 12] Activity comparable to or greater than that of cortisone acetate was observed in the carageenan rat paw oedema test when the extract was administered by intraperitoneal injection. The major aglycone, phytolaccagenin, was reported to exhibit greater activity than glycyrrhetic acid and oleanolic acid, which are both known to be effective in acute inflammation. Oral administration required a six-fold increase in dose for comparable activity.[12] Potency of the saponin extract was reduced to one-eighth of that of cortisone when tested against chronic inflammation (granuloma pouch method).[12] The ED_{50} for saponin and phytolaccagenin fractions against carrageenan-induced oedema in the rat (intraperitoneal injection) has been determined as 15.1 and 26 mg/kg respectively.[12]

Isoamericanin A (a neo-lignan) isolated from the seeds of *P. americana* has been reported to increase prostaglandin I_2 (PGI_2) production from the rat aorta by up to about 150% at a concentration of 10^{-5} and to elicit a moderate inductive effect on the *in vivo* release of PGI_2.[8]

Hypotensive properties have been described for a pokeroot extract with the activity attributed to histamine and GABA.[10]

A diuretic effect has been described in rats administered pokeroot extract orally at a dose of 500 mg/kg.[13] The effect was reported to be significantly greater than that observed in the saline-treated group of rats, but less than in the furosemide-treated (150 mg/kg) group.

In vitro contraction of the guinea-pig ileum has been described for pokeroot extracts.[14] Activity was attributed to a single active constituent that proved to be heat resistant.

The properties of pokeweed antiviral protein have been reviewed.[15]

Molluscicidal activity against schistosomiasis-transmitting snails and spermicidal activity have been documented for saponin components obtained from the fruits of the related species, *P. dodecandra*.[7, 16, 17] An enzyme located in the seeds has been found to be necessary for molluscicidal activity of *P. dodecandra*.[18] Crushing the seeds to release the enzyme is critical for activity. The enzyme is inactivated by heat or alcohol and a cold water extraction of the finely ground fruits was found to provide the greatest molluscicidal activity. The saponin-containing extract of *P. dodecandra* is commonly referred to as 'Endod'.[19] Fruits of *P. americana* also possess molluscicidal properties.[G44]

Abortifacient activity in mice has been exhibited by a related species *P. acinosa* Roxb. with activity strongest in the seed and weakest in the leaf. Activity in the various extracts was destroyed by heat and pepsin suggesting a protein to be the active principle.[20]

Side-effects, Toxicity

Clinical data

Haematological aberrations have been observed in human peripheral blood following oral ingestion of the berries or exposure of broken skin/conjunctival membrane to the berry juice.[21–23] Analysis of peripheral blood revealed plasmacytoid cells, dividing cells and mature plasmacytes. Eosinophilia was also noted. The mitogenic principles in pokeroot, lectins, are reported to be a mixture of agglutinating and non-agglutinating glycoproteins affecting both T cell and B cell lymphocytes.[24] Pokeroot leaf extracts have been reported to be agglutinating, but lacking in mitogenic activity.[25]

A 43-year-old woman suffered the following symptoms 30 minutes after drinking a cup of herbal tea prepared from half a teaspoon of powdered pokeroot: nausea, vomiting, cramping, generalised abdominal pain followed by profound watery diarrhoea, weakness, haematemesis and bloody diarrhoea, hypotension and tachycardia.[26] Chewing the root for the relief of a sore throat and cough has resulted in severe abdominal cramps, protracted vomiting and profuse watery diarrhoea.[27] Additional symptoms of poisoning that have been documented for pokeroot include difficulty with breathing, spasms, severe convulsions and death.[28]

The clinical symptoms of pokeroot poisoning have been reviewed.[27]

All parts of the pokeroot plant are considered as potentially toxic, with the root generally recognised as the most toxic part.[27] Toxicity is reported to increase with plant maturity although the young green berries are more toxic compared to the more mature red fruits.[27]

Preclinical data

High doses of saponin extracts have produced thymolytic effects in rats.[12]

LD_{50} values for the saponin fraction (intraperitoneal injection) have been determined as 181 mg/kg in mice and 208 mg/kg in rats.[12] In contrast, no deaths were observed in rats administered phytolaccagenin intraperitoneal injection up to a dose of 2 g/kg.[12] Oral doses of saponin up to 1.5 g/kg did not produce any mortalities in treated rats.[12]

The mutagenic potential of *P. americana* and *P. dodecandra* fruit extracts has been tested using *Salmonella typhimurium* strain TM677.[19] No activity was found for any of the extracts tested.

Contra-indications, Warnings

Fresh pokeroot is poisonous and the dried root emetic and cathartic.[G42] The toxic effects documented following the ingestion of pokeroot make it unsuitable for internal ingestion. In addition, external contact with the berry juice should be avoided: systemic symptoms of toxicity have occurred following exposure of broken skin and conjunctival membranes to the juice.

In 1979, the American Herb Trade Association declared that pokeroot should no longer be sold as a herbal beverage or food.[11] It further recommended that all packages containing pokeroot carry an appropriate warning regarding the potential toxicity of pokeroot when taken internally. In the UK, manufacturers of licensed medicinal products are permitted to include pokeroot provided that the dose is restricted and that suitable evidence is given to demonstrate the absence of the toxic protein constituents.

Drug interactions None documented. However, the potential for preparations of pokeroot to interact with other medicines administered concurrently, particularly those with similar or opposing effects, should be considered.

Pregnancy and lactation Pokeroot is reputed to affect the menstrual cycle and is documented to exhibit uterine stimulant activity in animals.[G30] In view of this and the documented toxic effects, pokeroot should not be used during pregnancy and lactation.

Preparations

Proprietary multi-ingredient preparations

UK: Catarrh Tablets; Psorasolv.

References

1 Woo WS *et al.* Triterpenoid saponins from the roots of *Phytolacca americana. Planta Med* 1978; 34: 87–92.
2 Woo WS *et al.* Constituents of *Phytolacca* species. (I) Anti-inflammatory saponins. *Korean J Pharmacog* 1976; 7: 47–50.
3 Kang SK, Woo WS. Two new saponins from *Phytolacca americana. Planta Med* 1987; 53: 338–340.
4 Kang S, Woo WS. Triterpenes from the berries of *Phytolacca americana. J Nat Prod* 1980; 43: 510–513.
5 Woo WS *et al.* Constituents of *Phytolacca* species (II). Comparative examination on constituents of the roots of *Phytolacca americana, P. esculenta* and *P. insularis. Korean J Pharmacog* 1975; 7: 51–54.
6 Woo WS, Kang SS. The structure of Phytolaccoside G. *Pharm Soc Korea* 1977; 21: 159–162.
7 Dorsaz A-C, Hostettmann K. Further saponins from *Phytolacca dodecandra* l'Herit. *Helv Chim Acta* 1986; 69: 2038–2047.
8 Hasegawa T *et al.* Structure of isoamericanin A, a prostaglandin I_2 inducer, isolated from the seeds of *Phytolacca americana* L. *Chem Lett* 1987; 2: 329–332.
9 Ready MP *et al.* Extracellular localization of pokeweed antiviral protein. *Proc Natl Acad Sci USA* 1986; 83: 5033–5056.
10 Funayama S, Hikino H. Hypotensive principles of *Phytolacca* roots. *J Nat Prod* 1979; 42: 672–674.
11 Tyler VE *et al.* Poke root. In: *Pharmacognosy*, 8th edn. Philadelphia: Lea and Febiger, 1981: 493–494.
12 Woo WS, Shin KH. Antiinflammatory action of *Phytolacca* saponin. *J Pharm Soc Korea* 1976; 20: 149–155.
13 Anokbonggo WW. Diuretic effect of an extract from the roots of *Phytolacca dodecandra* l'Herit in the rat. *Biochem Biol* 1975; 11: 275–277.
14 Anokbonggo WW. Extraction of pharmacologically active constituents of the roots of *Phytolacca dodecandra. Planta Med* 1975; 28: 69–75.
15 Irvin JD. Pokeweed antiviral protein. *Pharmac Ther* 1983; 21: 371–387.
16 Adewunmi CO, Marzuis VO. Comparative evaluation of the molluscicidal properties of aridan (*Tetrapleura tetrapleura*) laplapa pupa (*Jatropha gossypyfolia*) endod (*Phytolacca dodecandra*) and bayluscide. *Fitoterapia* 1987; 58: 325–328.
17 Dorsaz A-C, Hostettmann K. Further saponins from *Phytolacca dodecandra*: their molluscicidal and spermicidal properties. *Planta Med* 1986; 52: 557–558.
18 Parkhurst RM *et al.* The molluscicidal activity of *Phytolacca dodecandra*. I. Location of the activating esterase. *Biochem Biophys Res Commun* 1989; 158: 436–439.
19 Pezzuto JM *et al.* Evaluation of the mutagenic potential of endod (*Phytolacca dodecandra*), a molluscicide of potential value for the control of schistosomiasis. *Toxicol Lett* 1984; 22: 15–20.
20 Yeung HW *et al.* Abortifacient activity in leaves, roots and seeds of *Phytolacca acinosa. J Ethnopharmacol* 1987; 21: 31–35.
21 Barker BE *et al.* Haematological effects of pokeweed. *Lancet* 1967; i: 437.
22 Barker BE *et al.* Peripheral blood plasmacytosis following systemic exposure to *Phytolacca americana* (pokeweed). *Pediatrics* 1966; 38: 490–493.
23 Barker BE *et al.* Mitogenic activity in *Phytolacca americana* (pokeweed). *Lancet* 1965; i: 170.
24 McPherson A. Pokeweed and other lymphocyte mitogens. In: Kinghorn AD, ed. *Toxic Plants.* New York: Columbia University Press, 1979: 84–102.
25 Downing HJ *et al.* Plant agglutinins and mitosis. *Nature* 1968; 217: 655.
26 Lewis WH, Smith PR. Pokeroot herbal tea poisoning. *JAMA* 1979; 242: 2759–2760.
27 Roberge R *et al.* The root of evil – poke weed intoxication. *Ann Emerg Med* 1986; 15: 470–473.
28 Hardin JW, Arena JM. *Human Poisoning from Native and Cultivated Plants*, 2nd edn. Durham: Duke University Press, 1974: 69–73.

Poplar

Summary and Pharmaceutical Comment

The chemistry of poplar is characterised by the phenolic glycoside components, which support some of the reputed herbal uses. However, there is a lack of clinical research assessing the efficacy and safety of poplar. The usual precautions associated with other salicylate-containing drugs are applicable to poplar. In view of the lack of information, the use of poplar during pregnancy and lactation should be avoided.

Species (Family)

Populus tremuloides Michx. (Salicaceae)

Synonym(s)

Aspen, Populus Alba, Quaking Aspen, White Poplar

Part(s) Used

Bark

Pharmacopoeial and Other Monographs

BHP 1996[(G9)]
Complete German Commission E[(G3)]
Martindale 35th edition[(G85)]

Legal Category (Licensed Products)

GSL[(G37)]

Constituents

The following is compiled from several sources, including General References G6, G39 and G40.

Glycosides Salicin (about 2.4%), salicortin, salireposide and various benzoate derivatives including populin (salicin-6-benzoate), tremuloidin (salicin-2-benzoate) and tremulacin (salicortin-2-benzoate).

Other constituents Tannins (unspecified), triterpenes including α-amyrin and β-amyrin, carbohydrates including glucose, fructose and various trisaccharides, fats, waxes.

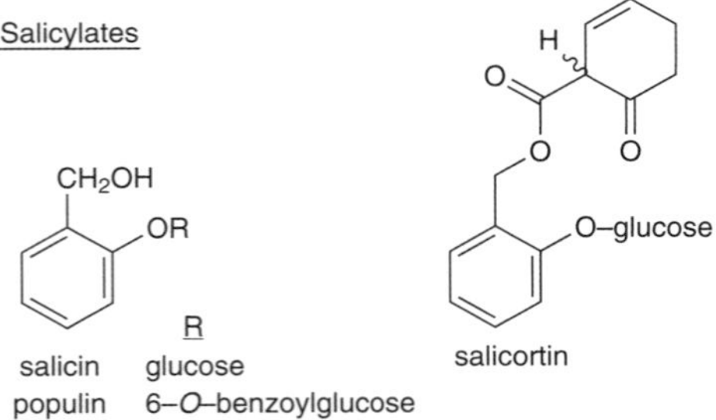

Figure 1 Selected constituents of poplar.

Food Use

Poplar is listed by the Council of Europe as a natural source of food flavouring (category N2). This category indicates that poplar can be added to foodstuffs in small quantities, with a possible limitation of an active principle (as yet unspecified) in the final product.[(G16)] Previously, in the USA, poplar has been permitted for use in foods.[(G65)]

Herbal Use

Poplar is stated to possess antirheumatic, anti-inflammatory, antiseptic, astringent, anodyne and cholagogue properties. Traditionally, it has been used for muscular and arthrodial rheumatism, cystitis, diarrhoea, anorexia with stomach or liver disorders, common cold, and specifically for rheumatoid arthritis.[(G6, G7, G64)]

The buds of *Populus tremula* (European white poplar, aspen) and *Populus nigra* (black poplar) are used, reputedly as expectorant and circulatory stimulant remedies, for upper respiratory tract infections and rheumatic conditions.[(G49)]

Dosage

Dosages for oral administration (adults) for traditional uses recommended in standard herbal reference texts are given below.

Dried bark 1–4 g as a decoction three times daily.[(G6, G7)]

Liquid extract 1–4 mL (1 : 1 in 25% alcohol) three times daily.[(G6, G7)]

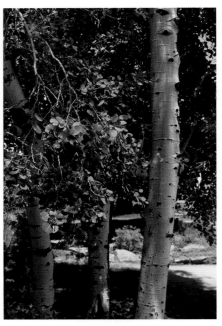

Figure 2 Poplar (*Populus tremuloides*).

P

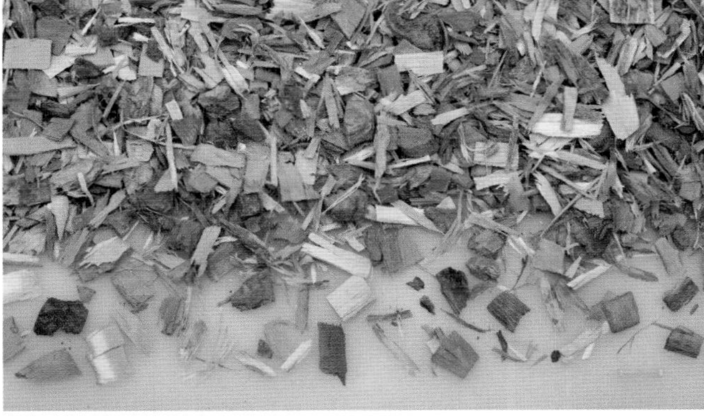

Figure 3 Poplar – dried drug substance (bark).

Pharmacological Actions

In vitro and animal studies

None documented for poplar. *See* Willow for the pharmacological actions associated with salicylates.

Clinical studies

There is a lack of clinical research assessing the effects of poplar and rigorous randomised clinical trials are required. The pharmacological actions of salicylates in humans are well documented and are applicable to poplar. Salicin is a prodrug that is metabolised to saligenin in the gastrointestinal tract and to salicylic acid following absorption.

Side-effects, Toxicity

None documented. However, there is a lack of clinical safety and toxicity data for poplar and further investigation of these aspects is required. *See* Willow for side-effects and toxicity associated with salicylates.

Contra-indications, Warnings

See Willow for contra-indications and warnings associated with salicylates.

Drug interactions None documented. However, the potential for preparations of poplar to interact with other medicines administered concurrently, particularly those with similar or opposing effects, should be considered. The concurrent administration of poplar with other salicylate-containing medicines should be avoided. Drug interactions listed for salicylates are also applicable to poplar and include oral anticoagulants, methotrexate, metoclopramide, phenytoin, probenecid, spironolactone and valproate (*see* Willow for more information on drug interactions with salicylates).

Pregnancy and lactation The safety of poplar taken during pregnancy has not been established (*see* Willow for contra-indications and warnings regarding the use of salicylates during pregnancy and lactation). Use of poplar during pregnancy and lactation should be avoided.

Preparations

Proprietary multi-ingredient preparations

UK: Tabritis Tablets.

Prickly Ash, Northern

Summary and Pharmaceutical Comment

Northern prickly ash contains similar alkaloid constituents to the southern species but varies with respect to other documented components. No pharmacological studies documented specifically for northern prickly ash were located. However, activities have been reported for individual alkaloid constituents and the monograph for southern prickly ash should be consulted. There is limited scientific evidence from preclinical studies to support the traditional herbal uses. Also, there is a lack of robust clinical research assessing the efficacy and safety of northern prickly ash. In view of the pharmacologically active constituents and potential toxicity associated with the alkaloids, excessive use of northern prickly ash and use during pregnancy and lactation should be avoided.

Species (Family)

Zanthoxylum americana Mill. (Rutaceae)

Synonym(s)

Toothache Bark, Toothache-tree, Xanthoxylum, Zanthoxylum

Part(s) Used

Bark, berry

Pharmacopoeial and Other Monographs

BHP 1983[G7]
Martindale 35th edition[G85]

Legal Category (Licensed Products)

Northern prickly ash is not included in the GSL.[G37]

Constituents

The following is compiled from several sources, including General Reference G6.

Alkaloids Isoquinoline-type. Lauriflorine and nitidine (major constituents), candicine, chelerythrine, magnoflorine and tembetarine.

Coumarins Xanthyletin, xanthoxyletin, alloxanthoxyletin and 8-(3,3-dimethylallyl)alloxanthoxyletin.

Other constituents Resins, tannins and acrid volatile oil.

Other plant parts Two furoquinoline alkaloids (γ-fagarine and skimmianine) have been isolated from the leaves.

Food Use

Prickly ash is listed by the Council of Europe as a natural source of food flavouring (category N3). This category indicates that prickly ash can be added to foodstuffs in the traditionally accepted manner, but that there is insufficient information available for an adequate assessment of potential toxicity.[G16] Previously, in the USA, prickly ash has been listed as GRAS (Generally Recognised As Safe).[G65]

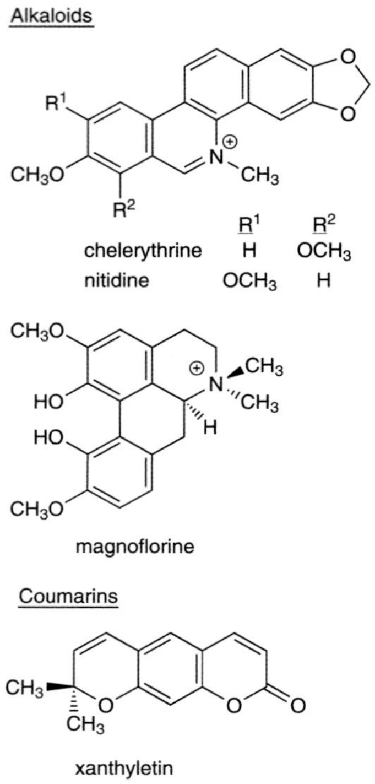

Alkaloids

	R^1	R^2
chelerythrine	H	OCH_3
nitidine	OCH_3	H

magnoflorine

Coumarins

xanthyletin

Figure 1 Selected constituents of northern prickly ash.

Herbal Use

Prickly ash is stated to possess circulatory stimulant, diaphoretic, antirheumatic, carminative and sialagogue properties. Traditionally, it has been used for cramps, intermittent claudication, Raynaud's syndrome, chronic rheumatic conditions, and specifically for peripheral circulatory insufficiency associated with rheumatic symptoms. The berries are stated to be therapeutically more active in circulatory disorders.[G6, G7, G64]

Dosage

Dosages for oral administration (adults) for traditional uses recommended in standard herbal reference texts are given below.

Dried bark 1–3 g as a decoction three times daily.[G6, G7]

Bark, liquid extract 1–3 mL (1 : 1 in 45% alcohol) three times daily.[G6, G7]

Bark, tincture 2–5 mL (1 : 5 in 45% alcohol) three times daily.[G6, G7]

Dried berry 0.5–1.5 g.[G6, G7]

Berry, liquid extract 0.5–1.5 mL (1 : 1 in 45% alcohol).[G6, G7]

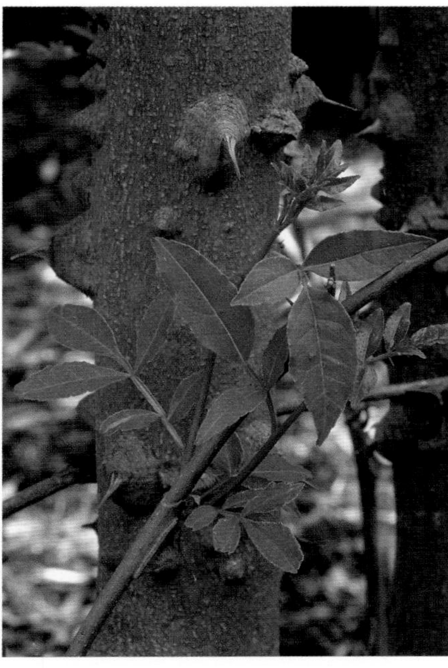

Figure 2 Northern prickly ash (*Zanthoxylum americana*).

Pharmacological Actions

In vitro and animal studies

None documented for northern prickly ash. *See* Prickly Ash, Southern for activities of alkaloid constituents (e.g. chelerythrine and nitidine).

Clinical studies

There is a lack of clinical research assessing the effects of northern prickly ash and rigorous randomised clinical trials are required.

Side-effects, Toxicity

There is a lack of clinical safety and toxicity data for northern prickly ash and further investigation of these aspects is required.

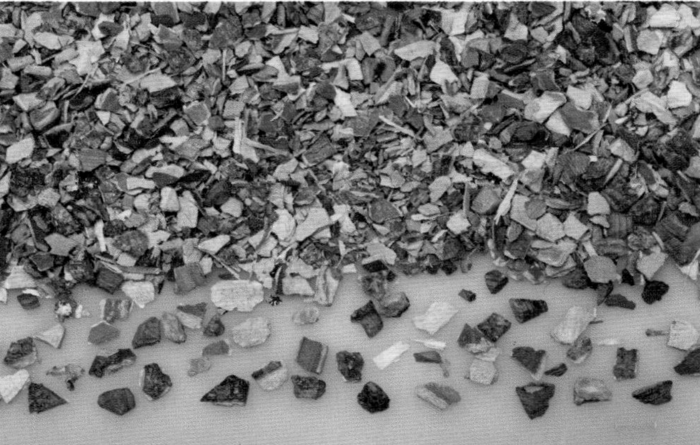

Figure 3 Northern prickly ash – dried drug substance (bark).

The alkaloid constituents are potentially toxic (*see* Prickly Ash, Southern).

Contra-indications, Warnings

Drug interactions None documented. However, the potential for preparations of northern prickly ash to interact with other medicines administered concurrently, particularly those with similar or opposing effects, should be considered. Coumarin constituents detected so far in northern prickly ash do not possess the minimum structural requirements[G87] for anticoagulant activity.

Pregnancy and lactation The safety of northern prickly ash has not been established. In view of the pharmacologically active constituents the use of northern prickly ash during pregnancy and lactation should be avoided.

Preparations

Proprietary multi-ingredient preparations

UK: Tabritis Tablets.

Prickly Ash, Southern

Summary and Pharmaceutical Comment

The chemistry of southern prickly ash is well documented and particularly characterised by the alkaloid constituents. Limited pharmacological information has been documented for southern prickly ash, although several properties have been described for individual constituents. Few data have been documented that support the herbal uses. Further, there is a lack of robust clinical research assessing the efficacy and safety of southern prickly ash. Limited toxicity data are available; some benzophenanthridine alkaloids are associated with cytotoxicity. In view of this, excessive use of prickly ash and use during pregnancy and lactation should be avoided. Northern prickly ash has been used for similar herbal uses but has a different chemical composition compared to the Southern species (*see* Prickly Ash, Northern).

Species (Family)

Zanthoxylum clava-herculis L. (Rutaceae)

Synonym(s)

Hercules-club, Toothache Bark, Xanthoxylum, Zanthoxylum

Part(s) Used

Bark, berry

Pharmacopoeial and Other Monographs

BHC 1992[G6]
BHP 1996[G9]
Martindale 35th edition[G85]

Legal Category (Licensed Products)

GSL[G37]

Constituents

The following is compiled from several sources, including General Reference G6.

Alkaloids Isoquinoline-type. Chelerythrine and magnoflorine (major constituents), candicine, lauriflorine, nitidine, *N*-acetylanonaine[1] and tembetarine.

Amides Cinnamamide, herculin and neoherculin.

Lignans (−)-Asarinin, (−)-sesamin, γ,γ-dimethylallyl ether of (−)-pluviatilol.[1]

Other constituents Resins, tannins and an acrid volatile oil (about 3.3%).

Food Use

Southern prickly ash is listed by the Council of Europe as a natural source of food flavouring (category N3). This category indicates that prickly ash can be added to foodstuffs in the traditionally accepted manner, but that there is insufficient information available for an adequate assessment of potential toxicity.[G16]

Herbal Use

Southern prickly ash is stated to possess circulatory stimulant, diaphoretic, antirheumatic, carminative and sialogogue properties. Traditionally, it has been used for cramps, intermittent claudication, Raynaud's syndrome, chronic rheumatic conditions, and specifically for peripheral circulatory insufficiency associated with rheumatic symptoms. The berries are stated to be therapeutically more active in circulatory disorders.[G6, G7, G8, G64]

Dosage

Dosages for oral administration (adults) for traditional uses recommended in standard herbal reference texts are given below.

Dried bark 1–3 g as a decoction three times daily.[G6, G7]

Bark, liquid extract 1–3 mL (1 : 1 in 45% alcohol) three times daily.[G6, G7]

Bark, tincture 2–5 mL (1 : 5 in 45% alcohol) three times daily.[G6, G7]

Dried berry 0.5–1.5 g.[G6, G7]

Berry, liquid extract 0.5–1.5 mL (1 : 1 in 45% alcohol).[G6, G7]

Pharmacological Actions

In vitro and animal studies

Southern prickly ash has been reported to act as a reversible neuromuscular blocking agent. Activity was associated with a neutral fraction of the bark that was thought to act primarily by blockade of endplate receptors.[2]

Various activities have been documented for the benzophenanthridine alkaloids (e.g. chelerythrine, nitidine) present in southern prickly ash. Hypotensive properties in mice have been documented for nitidine chloride, a single dose of 2 mg/kg body weight lowered the blood pressure by 20% within 90 minutes and persisted for six hours.[3] Nitidine was also found to antagonise the effects of angiotensin-induced hypertension.[3] Antileukaemic activity has been documented for nitidine, although preclinical toxicity prevented further investigations.[4, 5]

Anti-inflammatory activity in rats has been documented for chelerythrine (10 mg/kg by mouth) comparable to that achieved with indometacin (5 mg/kg by mouth).[6] Chelerythrine has also been reported to potentiate the analgesic effect of morphine, prolong barbiturate-induced sleep, and cause temporary hypertension followed by hypotension in cats, mice and rabbits.[7]

Significant antimicrobial activity towards Gram-positive bacteria and *Candida albicans* has been documented for chelerythrine, although conflicting activities have been reported regarding Gram-negative bacteria.[6] Chelerythrine has been shown to interact with Na^+K^+ ATPase and to inhibit hepatic L-alanine and L-aspartate aminotransferases in the rat, while nitidine has been reported to inhibit tRNA methyltransferase and catechol-*O*-methyltransferase.[5]

The lignan component, asarinin, has been reported to possess antitubercular activity.[G41] Neoherculin is reported to possess insecticidal and sialogogic properties.[1]

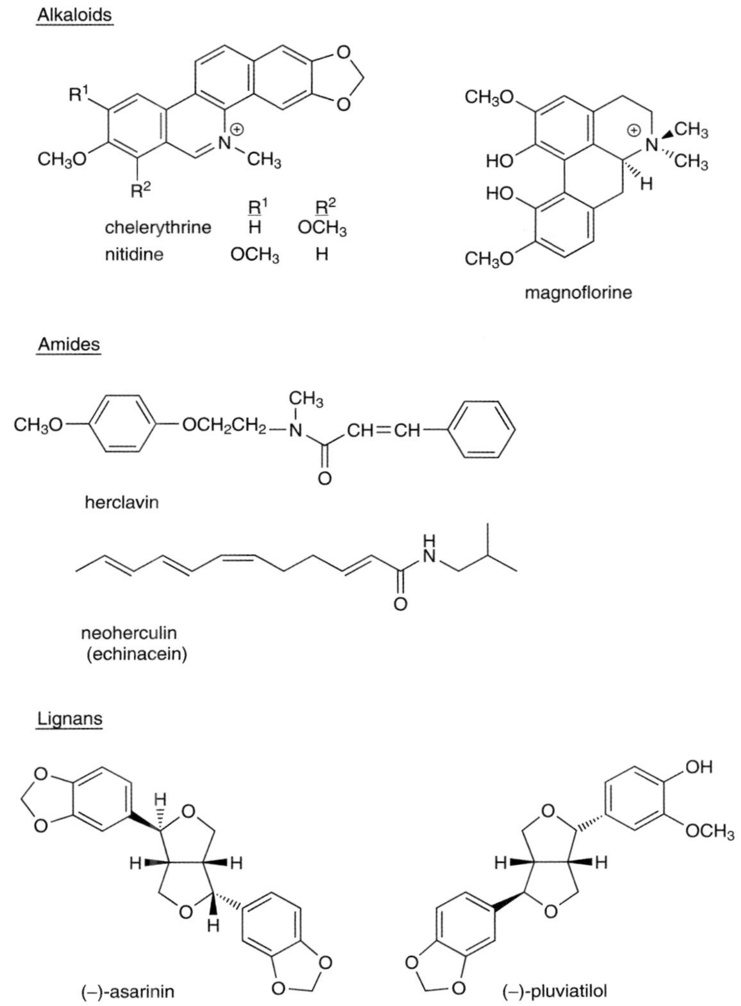

Alkaloids

	R^1	R^2
chelerythrine	H	OCH_3
nitidine	OCH_3	H

magnoflorine

Amides

herclavin

neoherculin (echinacein)

Lignans

(–)-asarinin

(–)-pluviatilol

Figure 1 Selected constituents of southern prickly ash.

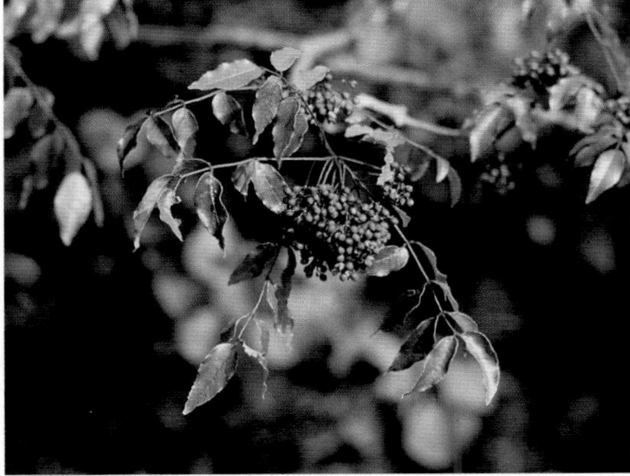

Figure 2 Southern prickly ash (*Zanthoxylum clava-herculis*).

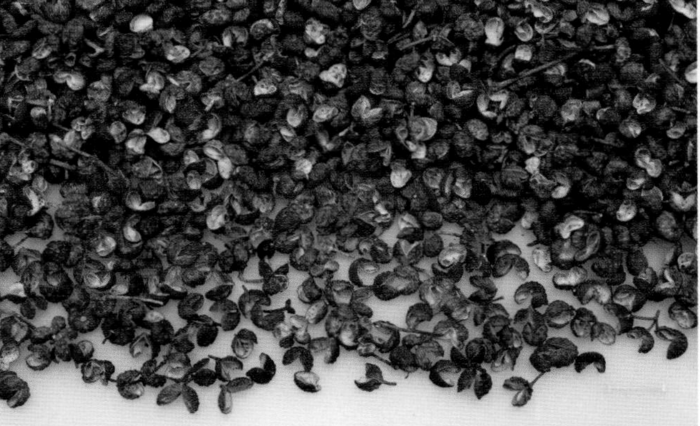

Figure 3 Southern prickly ash – dried drug substance (berry).

Side-effects, Toxicity

Clinical data

No toxicity documented. However, there is a lack of clinical safety and toxicity data for southern prickly ash and further investigation of these aspects is required.

Preclinical data

Ingestion of southern prickly ash by cattle, chicken and fish has proved lethal. This was attributed to the neuromuscular blocking properties of the bark.[2] Neoherculin is reported to be the major ichthyotoxic principle in an extract of southern prickly ash bark.

The acute and chronic toxicity of chelerythrine in mice is reported to be low.[4] LD_{50} values were stated as 18.5 mg/kg body weight (intravenous injection) and 95 mg/kg (subcutaneous injection). Oral administration of 10 mg/kg for three days followed by 5 mg/kg for seven days produced no adverse effects.

Contra-indications, Warnings

None documented. The alkaloid constituents in southern prickly ash are potentially toxic.

Drug interactions None documented. However, the potential for preparations of southern prickly ash to interact with other medicines administered concurrently, particularly those with similar or opposing effects, should be considered. Chelerythrine has been reported to interact with Na^+K^+ ATPase. However the clinical relevance of this with respect to prickly ash is unknown. Hypotensive and sedative activities have been documented in animals. Both chelerythrine and nitidine have been reported to inhibit various hepatic enzymes (*see* Pharmacological Actions, *In vitro* and animal studies).

Pregnancy and lactation The safety of southern prickly ash has not been established. In view of this and the pharmacologically active compounds, the use of southern prickly ash during pregnancy and lactation should be avoided.

References

1 Rao KV, Davies R. The ichthyotoxic principles of *Zanthoxylum clava-herculis*. *J Nat Prod* 1986; 49: 340–342.
2 Bowen JM, Cole RJ. Neuromuscular blocking properties of southern prickly ash toxin. *Fedn Proc* 1981; 40: 696.
3 Addae-Mensah I *et al*. Structure and anti-hypertensive properties of nitidine chloride from *Fagara* species. *Planta Med* 1986; 52 (Suppl. Suppl.): 58.
4 Krane BD *et al*. The benzophenanthridine alkaloids. *J Nat Prod* 1984; 47: 1–43.
5 Simánek V. Benzophenanthridine alkaloids. In: Brossi A, ed. *The Alkaloids*, vol 26. New York: Academic Press, 1985: 185–240.
6 Lenfield J *et al*. Antiinflammatory activity of quaternary benzophenanthridine alkaloids from *Chelidonium majus*. *Planta Med* 1981; 43: 161–165.
7 Preininger V. In: Manske RHF, ed. *The Alkaloids*, vol 15. New York: Academic Press, 1975: 242.

P

Pulsatilla

Summary and Pharmaceutical Comment

Pulsatilla is widely used in both herbal and homeopathic preparations, although little documented chemical and pharmacological information is available to assess its effects. There is a lack of robust clinical research assessing the efficacy and safety of pulsatilla. The fresh plant is known to be irritant; it contains a toxic principle (protoanemonin) and should not be ingested. The dried plant material is not considered to be toxic, but allergic reactions have been documented. In view of this and the lack of safety information, the use of pulsatilla during pregnancy and lactation should be avoided.

Species (Family)

**Pulsatilla vulgaris* Mill. (Ranunculaceae)
†*Pulsatilla pratensis* (L.) Mill.
‡*Pulsatilla patens* (L.) Mill.

Synonym(s)

**Anemone pulsatilla* L., *Pulsatilla ucrainica* (Ugr.) E.D. Wissjul, Pasque Flower
†*Anemone pratensis* L., *Pulsatilla nigricans* Störck, Small Pasque Flower
‡*Anemone patens* (L.) Mill.

Part(s) Used

Herb

Pharmacopoeial and Other Monographs

BHC 1992[(G6)]
BHP 1996[(G9)]
Martindale 35th edition[(G85)]

Legal Category (Licensed Products)

GSL[(G37)]

Constituents

The following is compiled from several sources, including General Reference G6.

Flavonoids Delphinidin and pelargonidin glycosides.

Saponins Hederagenin (as the aglycone).

Volatile oils Ranunculin (a glycoside); enzymatic hydrolysis yields the unstable lactone protoanemonin which readily dimerises to anemonin.

Other constituents Carbohydrates (e.g. arabinose, fructose, galactose, glucose, rhamnose), triterpenes (e.g. β-amyrin) and β-sitosterol.

Food Use

Pulsatilla is not used in foods.

Herbal Use

Pulsatilla is stated to possess sedative, analgesic, antispasmodic and bactericidal properties. Traditionally, it has been used for dysmenorrhoea, orchitis, ovaralgia, epididymitis, tension headache, hyperactive states, insomnia, boils, skin eruptions associated with bacterial infection, asthma and pulmonary disease, earache, and specifically for painful conditions of the male or female reproductive system.[(G6, G7, G8, G64)] Pulsatilla is widely used in homeopathic preparations as well as in herbal medicine.

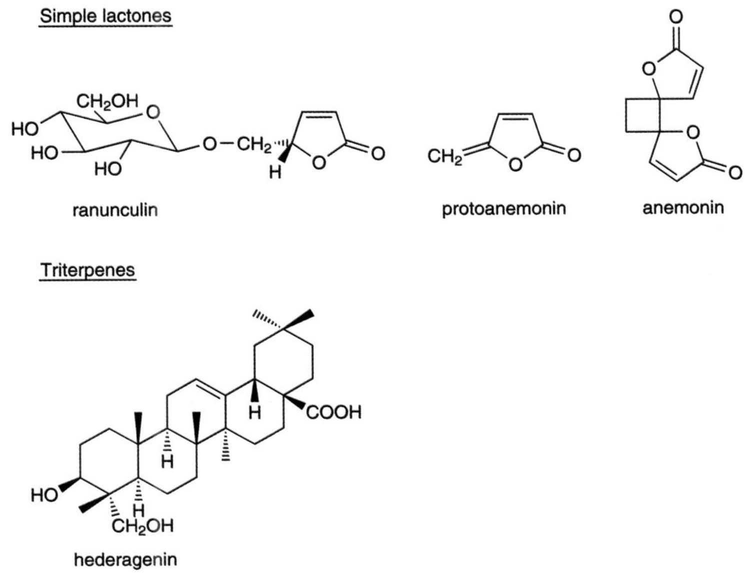

Figure 1 Selected constituents of pulsatilla.

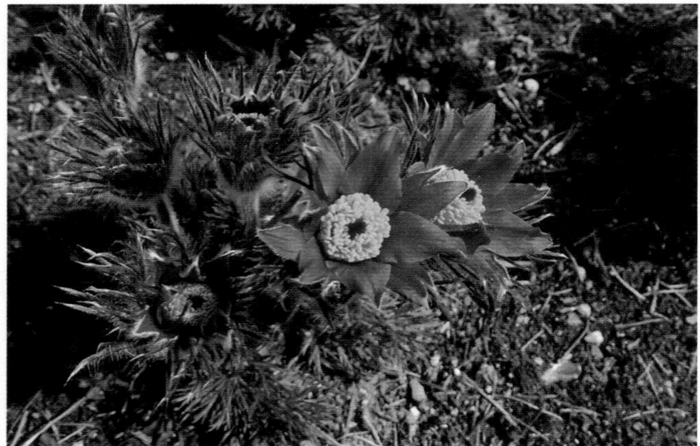

Figure 2 Pulsatilla (*Pulsatilla vulgaris*).

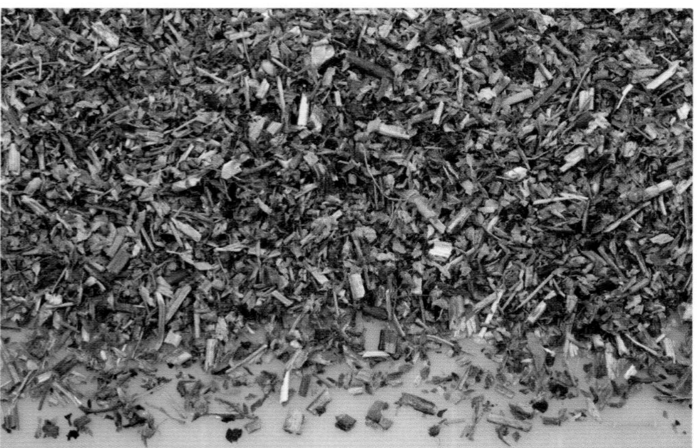

Figure 3 Pulsatilla – dried drug substance (herb).

Dosage

Dosages for oral administration (adults) for traditional uses recommended in standard herbal reference texts are given below.

Dried herb 0.12–0.3 g as an infusion or decoction three times daily.[G6, G7]

Liquid extract 0.12–0.3 mL (1 : 1 in 25% alcohol) three times daily.[G6, G7]

Tincture 0.3–1.0 mL (1 : 10 in 40% alcohol) three times daily.[G6, G7]

Pharmacological Actions

In vitro and animal studies

Utero-activity (stimulant and depressant) has been documented for pulsatilla.[1, 2, G30] *In vivo* sedative and antipyretic properties in rodents have been documented for anemonin and protoanemonin.[3]

Cytotoxicity (KB tumour system) has been reported for anemonin.[G22]

Clinical studies

There is a lack of clinical research assessing the effects of pulsatilla and rigorous randomised clinical trials are required.

Side-effects, Toxicity

Clinical data

There is a lack of clinical safety and toxicity data for pulsatilla and further investigation of these aspects is required.

Fresh pulsatilla is poisonous because of the toxic volatile oil component, protoanemonin. Protoanemonin rapidly degrades to the non-toxic anemonin. Inhalation of vapour from the volatile oil may cause irritation of the nasal mucosa and conjunctiva.[G51] Allergic reactions to pulsatilla have been documented and patch tests have produced vesicular reactions with hyperpigmentation.[G51]

Preclinical data

Cytotoxicity has been documented for anemonin (*see* Pharmacological Actions, *In vitro* and animal studies).

Contra-indications, Warnings

Fresh pulsatilla is poisonous and should not be ingested. External contact with the fresh plant should be avoided. The toxic principle, protoanemonin, rapidly degrades to the non-toxic anemonin during drying of the plant material. Individuals may experience an allergic reaction to pulsatilla, especially those with an existing hypersensitivity.

Drug interactions None documented. However, the potential for preparations of pulsatilla to interact with other medicines administered concurrently, particularly those with similar or opposing effects, should be considered. There is limited evidence from preclinical studies that certain constituents of pulsatilla (e.g. anemonin) have sedative activity. The clinical relevance of this is not known.

Pregnancy and lactation Pulsatilla is reputed to affect the menstrual cycle.[G22] Utero-activity has been documented for pulsatilla (*see* Pharmacological Actions, *In vitro* and animal studies). In view of this, the use of pulsatilla during pregnancy and lactation should be avoided.

Preparations

Proprietary multi-ingredient preparations

Australia: Bioglan Cirflo; Calmo; Lifesystem Herbal Formula 4 Women's Formula; Proflo; Women's Formula Herbal Formula 3. *Brazil:* Eviprostat. *Czech Republic:* Cicaderma. *France:* Hepatoum; Histo-Fluine P. *Germany:* Eviprostat N. *Japan:* Eviprostat. *South Africa:* Cough Elixir. *Singapore:* Eviprostat. *UK:* Anased; Calmanite Tablets; Fenneherb Prementaid; Menopause Relief; Napiers Back Ache Tea; Napiers Monthly Calm Tea; Nytol Herbal; Period Pain Relief; Prementaid; Roberts Alchemilla Compound Tablets. *USA:* Eye Support Formula.

References

1 Pilcher JM *et al*. The action of the so-called female remedies on the excised uterus of the guinea-pig. *Arch Intern Med* 1916; 18: 557–583.

2 Pilcher JM *et al*. The action of 'female remedies' on intact uteri of animals. *Surg Gynecol Obstet* 1918; 18: 97–99.

3 Martin ML *et al*. Pharmacological effects of lactones isolated from *Pulsatilla alpina* subsp. *apiifolia*. *J Ethnopharmacol* 1988; 24: 185–191.

Quassia

Summary and Pharmaceutical Comment

The chemistry of quassia is well-studied and is characterised by bitter terpenoids (quassinoids) and β-carboline indole alkaloids. Limited data have been documented to justify the traditional herbal uses although the bitter principles support the use of quassia as an appetite stimulant in anorexia. However, there is a lack of robust clinical research assessing the efficacy and safety of quassia. In view of the documented cytotoxic activities and limited toxicological data, quassia should not be taken in amounts greatly exceeding those used in foods. The use of quassia during pregnancy and lactation should be avoided.

Species (Family)

**Picrasma excelsa* (Sw.) Planch. (Simaroubaceae)
†*Quassia amara* L.

Synonym(s)

Bitterwood, Picrasma
**Aeschrion excelsa* (Sw.) Kuntze, Jamaican Quassia, *Quassia excelsa* Sw., *Simarouba excelsa* (Sw.) DC.
†Surinam Quassia

Part(s) Used

Stem wood

Pharmacopoeial and Other Monographs

BHC 1992[G6]
BHP 1996[G9]
Martindale 35th edition[G85]

Legal Category (Licensed Products)

GSL[G37]

Constituents

The following is compiled from several sources, including General References G2 and G6.

Alkaloids Indole-type. Canthin-6-one, 5-methoxycanthin-6-one, 4-methoxy-5-hydroxycanthin-6-one, *N*-methoxy-1-vinyl-β-carboline.[1,2]

Terpenoids Isoquassin (picrasmin) in *P. excelsa*, quassin 0.2%, quassinol, quassimarin,[3] 18-hydroxyquassin, neoquassin, a dihydronorneoquassin[4] and simalikalactone D in *Q. amara*.

Coumarins Scopoletin.[1]

Other constituents β-Sitosterol, β-sitostenone; thiamine 1.8% (in *P. excelsa*).

Nortriterpenes

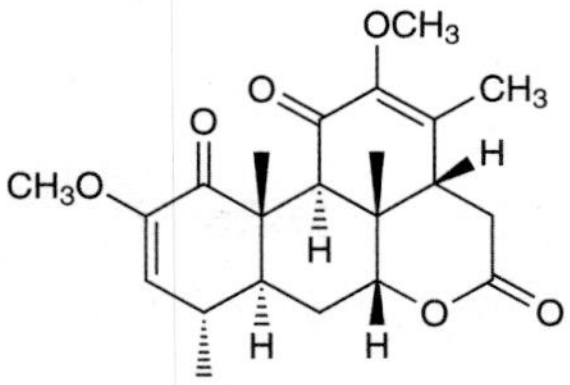

quassin

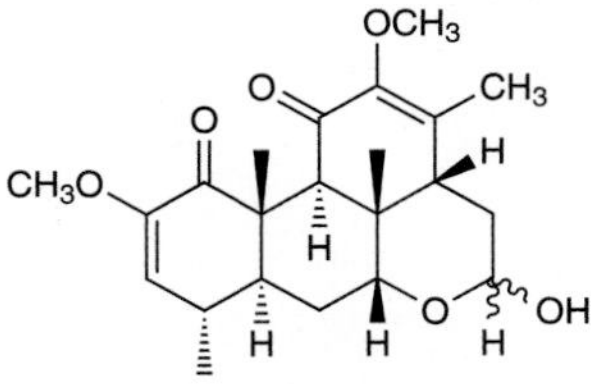

neoquassin

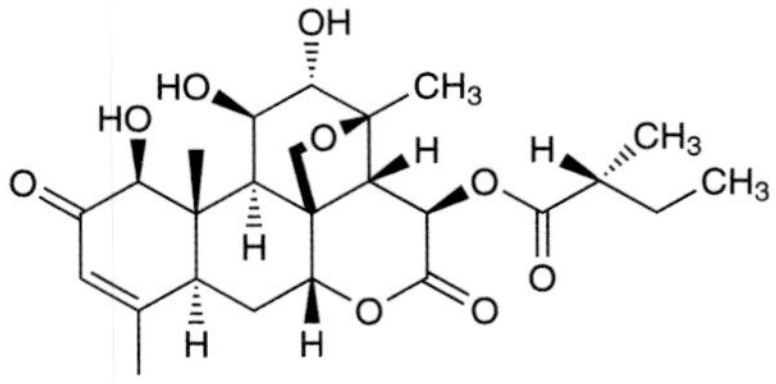

similikilactone D

Alkaloids

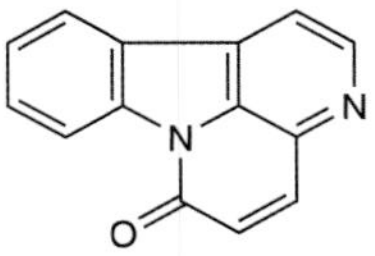

canthin-6-one

Coumarins

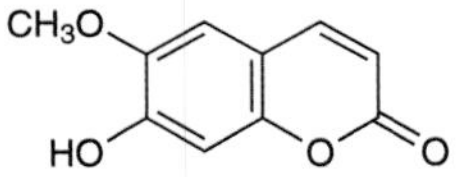

scopoletin

Figure 1 Selected constituents of quassia.

Food Use

Quassia is listed by the Council of Europe as a natural source of food flavouring (category N2). This category indicates that quassia can be added to foodstuffs in small quantities, although the concentration of quassin must not exceed 5 mg/kg; a concentration of 50 mg/kg is permitted in alcoholic beverages and 10 mg/kg in pastilles and lozenges.[G16] Previously, quassia has been regarded by the Food and Drugs Administration (FDA) as GRAS (Generally Regarded As Safe).

Herbal Use

Quassia is stated to possess bitter, orexigenic, sialogogue, gastric stimulant and anthelmintic properties. Traditionally, it has been used for anorexia, dyspepsia, nematode infestation (by oral or rectal administration), pediculosis (by topical application), and specifically for atonic dyspepsia with loss of appetite.[G2, G6, G7, G8, G64]

Dosage

Dosages for oral administration (adults) for traditional uses recommended in older and contemporary standard herbal and pharmaceutical reference texts are given below.

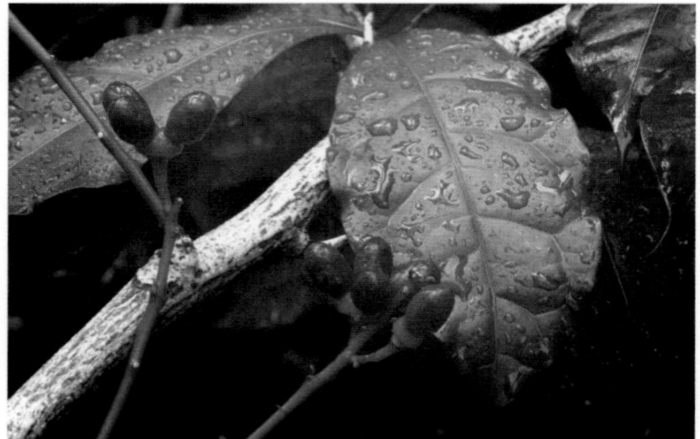

Figure 2 Quassia (*Picrasma excelsa*).

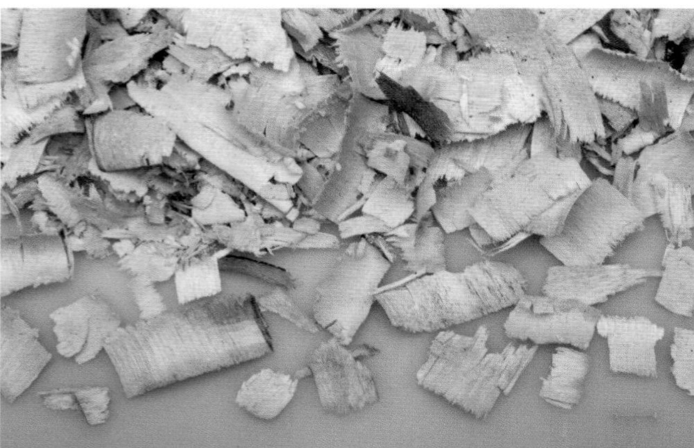

Figure 3 Quassia – dried drug substance (stem wood).

Dried wood 0.3–0.6 g by cold infusion three times daily.[G6, G7]

Concentrated Quassia Infusion (BPC 1959) 2–4 mL. Quassia Infusion is prepared by diluting one volume of Concentrated Quassia Infusion to eight volumes with water.

Tincture of Quassia (BP 1948) 2–4 mL.

Enema 150 mL per rectum (infusion with cold water, 1 in 20) on three successive mornings together with 16 g magnesium sulfate by mouth.

Pharmacological Actions

In vitro and animal studies

The β-carboline alkaloids have exhibited positive inotropic activity *in vitro*.[1] Canthin-6-one is reported to possess antibacterial and antifungal activity. Cytotoxic and amoebicidal activities (assessed against guinea-pig keratinocyte and *Entamoeba histolytica* test systems, respectively) have been documented for canthin-6-one and quassin (*P. excelsa*).[5] However, later studies have disputed any amoebicidal action. Quassin is reported to be inactive against P388 leukaemia and 9KB test systems. Significant antitumour activity in mice against the P388 lymphatic leukaemia and *in vitro* against human carcinoma of the nasopharynx (KB) has been documented.[3] Quassimarin and simalikalactone were both isolated from the active extract.

Clinical studies

There is a lack of clinical research assessing the effects of quassia and rigorous randomised controlled clinical trials are required.

The effective treatment of 454 patients with headlice has been documented for quassia tincture.[6] Quassia has been used as an enema to expel threadworms.[G44]

Side-effects, Toxicity

Clinical data

There is a lack of clinical and preclinical safety and toxicity data for quassia and further investigation of these aspects is required.

No side-effects have been reported in 454 patients who used quassia tincture as a scalp lotion to treat headlice.[6] Large doses of quassia may irritate the stomach and cause vomiting.[G6]

Contra-indications, Warnings

Large doses of quassia are emetic.

Drug interactions None documented. However, the potential for preparations of quassia to interact with other medicines administered concurrently, particularly those with similar or opposing effects, should be considered. There is limited evidence from preclinical studies that certain constituents of quassia have cardiac effects, however, the clinical relevance of this is not clear. Coumarin constituents detected so far in quassia do not possess the minimum structural requirements for anticoagulant activity.

Pregnancy and lactation In view of the reported cytotoxic and emetic activities, the use of quassia during pregnancy and lactation should be avoided.

Preparations

Proprietary single-ingredient preparations

Argentina: Cuassicum Prevent 2 en 1.

Proprietary multi-ingredient preparations

Argentina: Cuassicum; Uze Active; Yalu. *France:* Quintonine. *Italy:* Dekar 2. *South Africa:* Essens Amara of Groen Amara; Versterkdruppels. *Switzerland:* Stomacine. *UK:* Sanderson's Throat Specific.

References

1 Wagner H *et al*. New constituents of *Picrasma excelsa*, I. *Planta Med* 1979; 36: 113–118.

2 Wagner H, Nestler T. *N*-Methoxy-1-vinyl-β-carbolin, ein neues Alkaloid aus *Picrasma excelsa* (Swartz) Planchon. *Tetrahedron Lett* 1978; 31: 2777–2778.

3 Kupchan SM, Streelman DR. Quassimarin, a new antileukemic quassinoid from *Quassia amara*. *J Org Chem* 1976; 41: 3481–3482.

4 Grandolini G *et al*. A new neoquassin derivative from *Quassia amara*. *Phytochemistry* 1987; 26: 3085–3087.

5 Harris A, Phillipson JD. Cytotoxic and amoebicidal compounds from *Picrasma excelsa* (Jamaican Quassia). *J Pharm Pharmacol* 1982; 34: 43P.

6 Jensen O *et al*. Pediculosis capitis treated with quassia tincture. *Acta Dermat Venereol (Stockholm)* 1978; 58: 557–559.

Queen's Delight

Summary and Pharmaceutical Comment

The Euphorbiaceae plant family is characterised by the diterpene esters. These compounds, known as phorbol, ingenane or daphnane esters depending on their skeleton type, have been investigated as constituents of genera such as *Euphorbia* and *Croton*, and some of them have been found to be co-carcinogenic and highly irritant to mucous membranes.(G33) No scientific evidence was found to justify the reputed herbal uses. In view of the lack of data on pharmacological effects, efficacy and safety, and the potential toxicity of queen's delight, the appropriateness of medicinal use of queen's delight should be considered; and excessive use, at least, and use during pregnancy and lactation should be avoided.

Species (Family)

Stillingia sylvatica L. (Euphorbiaceae)

Synonym(s)

Ditrysinia sylvatica (L.) Raf., *Excoecaria sylvatica* (L.) Baill., Queen's Root, *Sapium sylvaticum* (L.) Torr., Stillingia, *Stillingia sylvatica* var. *genuina* Müll. Arg, Yaw Root

Part(s) Used

Root

Pharmacopoeial and Other Monographs

BHP 1996(G9)

Legal Category (Licensed Products)

GSL(G37)

Constituents

Terpenoids Gnidilatin, a daphnane diterpene.(1) Eight compounds, termed stillingia factors S_1–S_8, have been isolated and identified as daphnane-type and tigliane-type esters carrying saturated, polyunsaturated or hydroxylated fatty acids.(2)

Other constituents Volatile oil 3–4%, fixed oil, acrid resin (sylvacrol), resinic acid, stillingine (a glycoside) and tannin.

Other plant parts Hydrocyanic acid (leaf and stem).(2)

Food Use

Queen's delight is not used in foods.

Herbal Use

Queen's delight is stated to possess sialogogue, expectorant, diaphoretic, dermatological, astringent, antispasmodic and, in large doses, cathartic properties. Traditionally, it has been used for bronchitis, laryngitis, laryngismus stridulus, cutaneous eruptions, haemorrhoids, constipation and specifically for exudative skin eruption with irritation and lymphatic involvement, and laryngismus stridulus.(G7, G64)

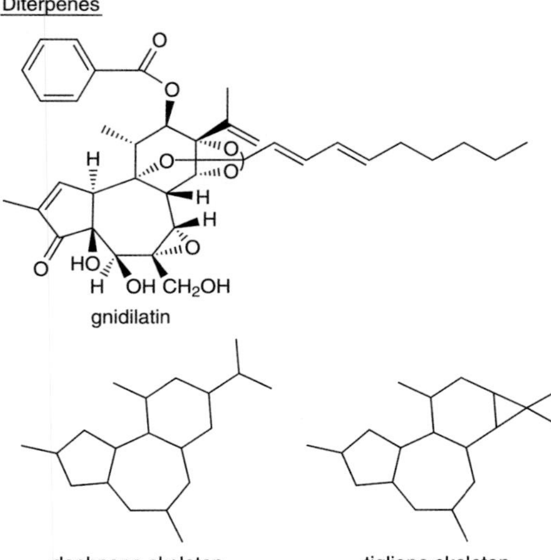

Figure 1 Selected constituents of queen's delight.

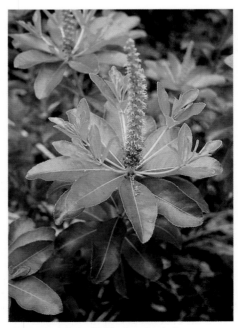

Figure 2 Queen's delight (*Stillingia sylvatica*).

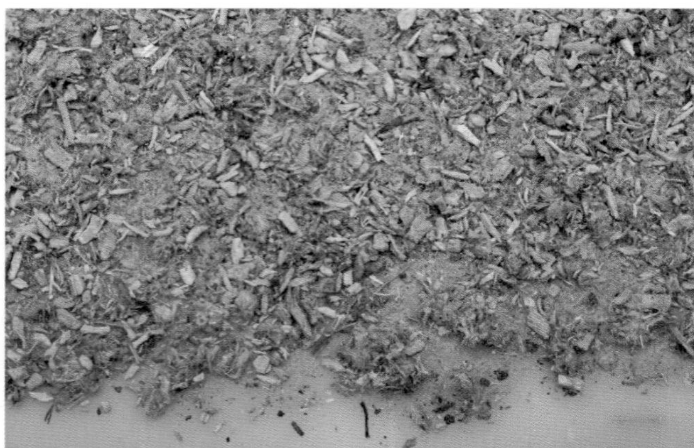

Figure 3 Queen's delight – dried drug substance (root).

Dosage

Dosages for oral administration (adults) recommended in standard herbal reference texts are given below.

Dried root 1–2 g as a decoction three times daily.[G7]

Liquid extract 0.5–2.0 mL (1 : 1 in 25% alcohol) three times daily.[G7]

Tincture 1–4 mL (1 : 5 in 45% alcohol) three times daily.[G7]

Pharmacological Actions

None documented.

Clinical studies

There is a lack of clinical research assessing the effects of queen's delight and rigorous randomised controlled clinical trials are required.

Side-effects, Toxicity

Clinical data

There is a lack of clinical safety and toxicity data for queen's delight and further investigation of these aspects is required.

Overdose of queen's delight is reported to cause vertigo, burning sensation of the mouth, throat and gastrointestinal tract, diarrhoea, nausea and vomiting, dysuria, aches and pains, pruritus and skin eruptions, cough, depression, fatigue and perspiration.[G22] The diterpene esters are toxic irritant principles known to cause swelling and inflammation of the skin and mucous membranes.[2, G33]

Preclinical data

The leaves and stem are documented to be toxic to sheep because of the hydrocyanic acid content.[3]

Contra-indications, Warnings

In view of the irritant nature of the diterpene esters, queen's delight may cause irritation to the mucous membranes. In view of the lack of data on pharmacological effects, efficacy and safety, and the potential toxicity of queen's delight, whether or not queen's delight is appropriate for medicinal use should be considered.

Pregnancy and lactation In view of the irritant and potentially toxic constituents, the use of queen's delight during pregnancy and lactation should be avoided.

References

1 *Dictionary of Natural Products*. Chapman & Hall, 1982–2005.

2 Adolf W, Hecker E. New irritant diterpene-esters from roots of *Stillingia sylvatica* L. (Euphorbiaceae). *Tetrahedron Lett* 1980; 21: 2887–2890.

3 Lewis WH, Elvin-Lewis MPF. *Medical Botany*. New York: Wiley Interscience, 1977.

Raspberry

Summary and Pharmaceutical Comment

Limited phytochemical information is available for raspberry leaf. The presence of tannin constituents supports some of the reputed traditional uses, although it is unsuitable to use as a herbal remedy to treat eye infections, such as conjunctivitis. Raspberry leaf is widely recommended to be taken during pregnancy to help facilitate easier parturition. However, evidence from rigorous randomised controlled clinical trials to support the efficacy of preparations of raspberry leaf to facilitate parturition is lacking; the sole clinical trial reported a lack of effect for a raspberry leaf preparation on several outcome variables. Further investigation to assess the effects of well-characterised raspberry leaf preparations in well-designed randomised controlled trials involving sufficient numbers of participants is required. There is limited evidence from *in vitro* studies that raspberry leaf has effects on uterine tissue.

There are only limited data on safety aspects of raspberry leaf preparations, including when taken during pregnancy. In view of this, raspberry leaf should not be taken during pregnancy unless under medical supervision. Raspberry leaf preparations should be avoided during breastfeeding. Use of raspberry leaf preparations at doses higher than those recommended and/or for excessive periods should be avoided until further information is available on their safety with long-term use. In view of the documented pharmacological actions of raspberry leaf preparations, the potential for interactions with other medicines administered concurrently, particularly those with similar or opposing effects, should be considered.

Species (Family)

Rubus idaeus L. (Rosaceae)

Synonym(s)

Rubus

Part(s) Used

Leaf

Pharmacopoeial and Other Monographs

BHP 1996[G9]
Martindale 35th edition[G85]

Legal Category (Licensed Products)

GSL[G37]

Constituents

Flavonoids Total flavonoid content in dried leaves 0.46–1.05%[1] and up to 5%.[2] Derivatives of kaempferol and quercetin,[1] including quercetin-3-O-β-D-glucoside,[3] quercetin- and kaempferol-3-O-β-D-galactosides, kaempferol-3-O-β-L-arabinopyranoside and kaempferol-3-O-β-D-(6′-*p*-coumaroyl)-glucoside (tiliroside).[4]

Polyphenols Gallo- and ellagi-tannins 2.06-6.89%[1] and up to 10%.[5]

Other constituents Volatile components, e.g. E-2-hexenal and Z-3-hexenol, glycosides of C_{13}-norisoprenoids, vitamin C.[G75]

Other parts of the plant Berries contain anthocyanins, hydrolysable tannins, sanquin H6, a dimeric ellagitannin, lambertianin (a tetrameric ellagitannin), triterpenoids α- and β-amyrin, stigmasterol, campesterol, cycloartenol, cholesterol,[6] and raspberry ketone.[7]

Related species Mono-, sesqui-, di- and tri-terpenoids are present in several species, and five labdane-type diterpenes have been isolated from *R. suavissimus*.[8]

Food Use

Both the leaf and fruit are listed by the Council of Europe as natural sources of food flavouring (categories N2 and N1, respectively). Category N2 allows the addition of the leaf to foodstuffs in small quantities, with a possible limitation of an active principle (as yet unspecified) in the final product. Category N1 indicates that no restrictions apply to the fruit.[G16] Raspberry fruit is commonly used in foods.

Herbal Use

Raspberry is stated to possess astringent and *partus praeparator* properties. Traditionally, it has been used for diarrhoea, pregnancy, stomatitis, tonsillitis (as a mouthwash), conjunctivitis

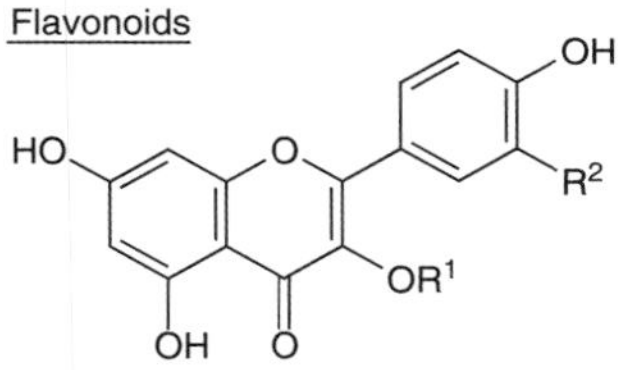

	R¹	R²
quercetin	H	OH
quercetin-3-*O*-β-D-galactoside	gal	OH
kaempferol	H	H
kaempferol-3-*O*-β-D-galactoside	gal	H
kaempferol-3-*O*-β-L-arabinoside	ara	H

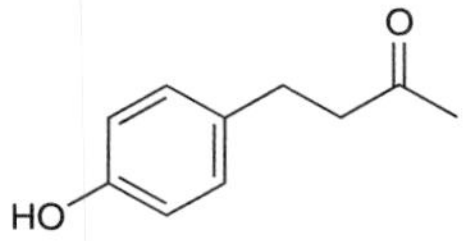

gal = galactoside, ara = arabinoside

Figure 1 Selected constituents of raspberry.

R

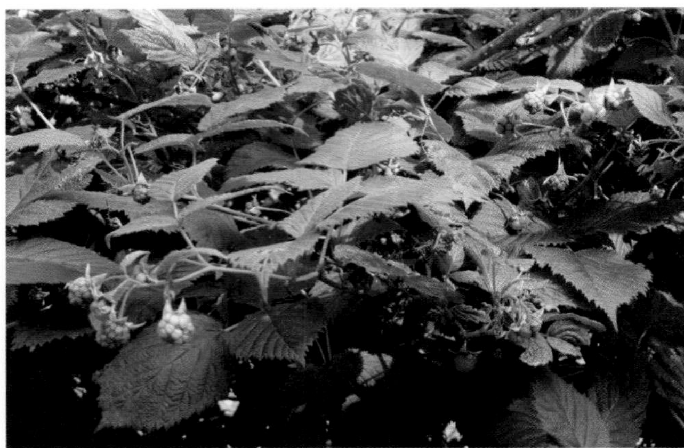

Figure 2 Raspberry (*Rubus idaeus*).

(as an eye lotion), and specifically to facilitate parturition.(G2, G7, G64) Modern interest is focused on the use of raspberry leaf to stimulate and facilitate labour and to shorten its duration.

Dosage

Dosages for oral administration (adults) for traditional uses recommended in standard herbal reference texts are given below.

Dried leaf 4–8 g as an infusion three times daily.(G7)

Liquid extract 4–8 mL (1 : 1 in 25% alcohol) three times daily.(G7)

Pharmacological Actions

There is only a limited amount of basic and clinical research exploring the effects of raspberry leaf preparations.

In vitro and animal studies

A conference abstract published in the older literature describes utero-activity for a raspberry leaf infusion (1 g dried leaves infused with 15 ml of saline for 10 minutes at 95°C, then filtered) when applied to rat and human uterine tissue. The extract had little or no effect on the uterine strips from non-pregnant rats, but inhibited contractions of those from pregnant rats.(9) Similarly, the extract had no effect on strips from non-pregnant human uteri, but initiated contractions in strips from human uteri obtained at 10–16 weeks of pregnancy. The intrinsic rhythm of the uterine tissue in which a pharmacological effect was observed (pregnant rat and human uteri) was reported to become more regular, with contractions, in most cases, less frequent.(9) No data are provided in a report of these experiments, and no statistical analyses appear to have been carried out; replication of this work is necessary in order to confirm or refute the findings.

A methanol extract of fresh, dried *R. idaeus* leaves relaxed transmurally stimulated guinea-pig ileum *in vitro*, whereas no response was seen with exposure of the system to extracts prepared with less polar solvents (*n*-hexane and ethyl acetate).(10) Subsequent methanol extraction and bioassay-guided fractionation revealed activity associated with fractions eluted with trichloromethane/methanol (95 : 5) and trichloromethane/methanol (50 : 50). The two most active fractions relaxed transmurally stimulated guinea-pig ileum in a concentration-dependent manner.

Aqueous extracts of raspberry leaves have been reported to contain a number of active constituents, including a smooth muscle stimulant, an anticholinesterase, and an antispasmodic that antagonised the stimulant actions of the two previous fractions. The smooth muscle stimulant fraction was more potent towards uterine muscle.(11)

Flavonoids isolated from 70% ethanol extracts of the leaves from four varieties of raspberry (species not stated) collected in Russia have antioxidant activity *in vitro*, as assessed in a system involving measurement of the rate of oxygen absorption during initiated oxidation of isopropylbenzene.(2)

Hypoglycaemic activity has been documented for extracts of the leaves of a related species, *Rubus fructicosus* L., in both non-diabetic and diabetic (glucose-induced and alloxan-induced) rabbits.(12) The reduction in blood glucose concentrations, compared with controls, was greatest in glucose-induced diabetic rabbits. In addition, blood insulin concentrations increased significantly, compared with baseline values, following administration of an ethyl ether extract of *R. fructicosus* leaf to hyperglycaemic rabbits.(12) However, confirmation of these findings using more robust experimental methods is required. *In vitro* antiviral activity documented for raspberry fruit extract has been attributed to the phenolic constituents, in particular to tannic acid.(13)

Tannins are known to possess astringent properties.

Clinical studies

The effects of a raspberry leaf preparation on labour, birth and the post-partum period were investigated in a randomised, double-blind, placebo-controlled trial involving 240 low-risk, nulliparous women. Participants received tablets containing 1.2 g raspberry leaf extract, one tablet twice daily, taken from 32 weeks' gestation until the onset of labour (regular contractions).(14)

In total, 192 women (n = 96 per group) completed the study; the 48 withdrawals were evenly distributed across the two groups. There were no statistically significant differences between the two groups with respect to the length of gestation (p = 0.51), likelihood of medical augmentation of labour (p = 0.91), need for pethidine (meperidine) (p value not stated), need for artificial rupture of membranes (p = 0.35), time spent in first, third (p value not stated) and second stages of labour (p = 0.28), proportion of normal vaginal births (62.4% and 50.6% for the raspberry leaf and placebo groups, respectively; p = 0.19) and emergency caesarean section rate (p value not stated). There were also no statistically significant differences between the two groups with respect to safety outcomes in labour, including blood loss > 600 mL (p = 0.86), neonatal birth weight (p = 0.46), Apgar score

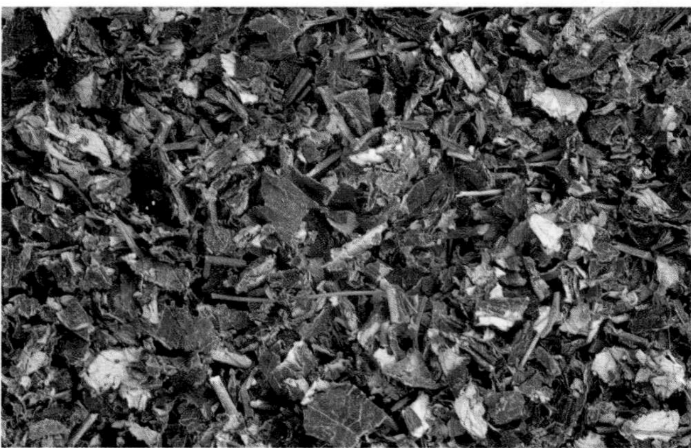

Figure 3 Raspberry – dried drug substance (leaf).

at five minutes ($p = 0.11$) and occurrence of meconium-stained fluid (p value not stated).[14] However, a higher proportion of women in the raspberry leaf group developed pre-eclampsia (4.2% and 2.1% in the raspberry and placebo groups, respectively), and a higher proportion of babies admitted to special care units was born to mothers from the raspberry leaf group than to those from the placebo group (p values not stated). Several of the above parameters showed a tendency (although not statistically significant at $p < 0.05$) for more favourable outcomes in the raspberry leaf group and, on this basis, further research investigating other dosage regimens may be worth while.[14]

Side-effects, Toxicity

Clinical data

There is only a limited amount of information on the safety and toxicity of raspberry leaf preparations and further investigation of these aspects is required. In a randomised, double-blind, placebo-controlled trial, 240 low-risk, nulliparous women received tablets containing 1.2 g raspberry leaf extract, one tablet twice daily, taken from 32 weeks' gestation until the onset of labour (regular contractions); 192 women, 96 in each group completed the study.[14] A higher number of adverse events was reported by raspberry leaf recipients than by placebo recipients (31 and 24, for the raspberry leaf and placebo groups, respectively, corresponding to 32.3% and 25.0% of women in each group, respectively), although no statistical analysis for this comparison was reported. No congenital abnormalities were reported for either group. Also, there were no statistically significant differences between the two groups with respect to several safety outcomes in labour (*see* Pharmacological Actions, Clinical studies). This study provides only very limited information on the safety of raspberry leaf when taken during pregnancy (weeks 32 to labour onset) as clinical trials are designed primarily to assess efficacy, not safety, and have the statistical power only to detect common, acute adverse effects.

Contra-indications, Warnings

As excessive ingestion of tannins is not recommended, raspberry leaf tea should not be used for prolonged periods.

Drug interactions None documented. In view of the pharmacological actions described for raspberry leaf, the potential for preparations of raspberry leaf to interfere with other medicines administered concurrently, particularly those with similar or opposing effects, should be considered.

Pregnancy and lactation Preparations of raspberry leaf have been used traditionally during labour to help ease parturition. However, there is limited and conflicting scientific evidence that raspberry leaf has effects on uterine contractions. A preliminary report published in the older literature describes inhibition of contractions of tissue obtained from the uteri of pregnant rats and initiation of contractions in uterine strips obtained from pregnant women at 10–16 weeks of pregnancy following application of a raspberry leaf infusion *in vitro*. These findings require confirmation. Furthermore, a randomised, double-blind, placebo-controlled trial found no statistically significant differences in labour outcomes for raspberry leaf extract 1.2 g twice daily taken from 32 weeks' gestation to labour onset, when compared with placebo. Hence, at present, as there is a lack of evidence to support the efficacy of preparations of raspberry leaf during late pregnancy to assist parturition, and in view of the lack of safety data, preparations of raspberry leaf should not be used during pregnancy and labour. If raspberry leaf is taken during these periods, this should only be under medical supervision.

There is a lack of information on the use of raspberry leaf during breastfeeding. Until information is available, raspberry leaf preparations should be avoided during breastfeeding.

Preparations

Proprietary multi-ingredient preparations

France: IgeE. *UK:* Fenneherb Monthly. *USA:* Women's Menopause Formula.

References

1 Gudej J, Tomczyk M. Determination of flavonoids, tannins and ellagic acid in leaves from Rubus L. species. *Arch Pharm Res* 2004; 27: 1114–1119.
2 Nikitina VS *et al.* Flavonoids from raspberry and blackberry leaves and their antioxidant activities. *Pharm Chem J* 2000; 34: 596–598.
3 Khabibullaeva LA, Khalmatov KK. Phytochemical study of raspberry leaves. *Mater Yubileinoi Resp Nauchn Konf Farm Posvyashch* 1972; Sept: 101–102.
4 Gudej J. Kaempferol and quercetin glycosides from *Rubus idaeus* L. leaves. *Acta Polon Pharm* 2003; 60: 313–316.
5 Cygan F-C. Die Himbeere – *Rubus idaeus* L. Portrait einer Arzneipflanze. *Z Phytother* 1995; 16: 366–374.
6 Puupponen-Pimia R *et al.* Bioactive berry compounds – novel tools against human pathogens. *Appl Microbiol Biotech* 2005; 67: 8–18.
7 Morimoto C *et al.* Anti-obese action of raspberry ketone. *Life Sci* 2005; 77: 194–204.
8 Patel AV *et al.* Therapeutic constituents and actions of Rubus species. *Curr Med Chem* 2004; 11: 1501–1512.
9 Bamford DS *et al.* Raspberry leaf tea: a new aspect to an old problem. *Br J Pharmacol* 1970; 40: 161–162.
10 Rojas-Vera J *et al.* Relaxant activity of raspberry (*Rubus idaeus*) leaf extract in guinea-pig ileum *in vitro*. *Phytotherapy Res* 2002; 16: 665–668.
11 Beckett AH *et al.* The active constituents of raspberry leaves. A preliminary investigation. *J Pharm Pharmacol* 1954; 6: 785–796.
12 Alonso R *et al.* A preliminary study of hypoglycaemic activity of *Rubus fruticosus*. *Planta Med* 1980; 40 (Suppl. Suppl.): 102–106.
13 Konowalchuk JK, Speirs JI. Antiviral activity of fruit extracts. *J Food Sci* 1976; 41: 1013–1017.
14 Simpson M *et al.* Raspberry leaf in pregnancy: its safety and efficacy in labor. *J Midwifery Women's Health* 2001; 46(2): 51–59.

Red Clover

Summary and Pharmaceutical Comment

The chemistry of red clover is well documented. Limited information is available on the pharmacological properties and no documented scientific evidence was found to justify the herbal uses. Robust clinical research assessing the efficacy and safety of red clover is limited. Reported oestrogenic side-effects in grazing animals have been attributed to the isoflavone constituents. Few toxicity data are available for red clover. In view of this and the isoflavone and coumarin components, excessive use and use during pregnancy and lactation should be avoided.

Species (Family)

Trifolium pratense L. (Leguminosae)

Synonym(s)

Cow Clover, Meadow Clover, Purple Clover, Trefoil, *Trifolium borysthenicum* Gruner, *T. bracteatum* Schousb., *T. lenkoranicum* (Grossh.) Rosk., *T. pratense* L. var. *lenkoranicum* Grossh., *T. ukrainicum* Opp.

Part(s) Used

Flowerhead

Pharmacopoeial and Other Monographs

BHC 1992[G6]
BHP 1996[G9]
Martindale 35th edition[G85]

Legal Category (Licensed Products)

GSL[G37]

Constituents

The following is compiled from several sources, including General Reference G6.

Carbohydrates Arabinose, glucose, glucuronic acid, rhamnose, xylose (following hydrolysis of saponin glycosides); polysaccharide (a galactoglucomannan).

Coumarins Coumarin, medicagol.

Isoflavonoids

	R
formononetin	CH_3
daidzein	H

	R
biochanin A	CH_3
genistein	H

Figure 1 Selected constituents of red clover.

Isoflavonoids Biochanin A, daidzein, formononetin, genistein, pratensin, trifoside, calycosine galactoside[1] and pectolinarin.

Flavonoids Isorhamnetin, kaempferol, quercetin, and their glycosides.[2]

Saponins Soyasapogenols B–F (C–F artefacts) and carbohydrates (*see above*) yielded by acid hydrolysis.[3]

Other constituents Coumaric acid, phaseolic acid, salicylic acid, *trans*- and *cis*-clovamide (L-dopa conjugated with *trans*- and *cis*-caffeic acids), resin, volatile oil (containing furfural),[4] fats, vitamins and minerals. Cyanogenetic glycosides have been documented for a related species, *Trifolium repens*.[G33]

Food Use

Red clover is listed by the Council of Europe as a natural source of food flavouring (category N2). This category indicates that it can be added to foodstuffs in small quantities, with a possible limitation of an active principle (as yet unspecified) in the final product.[G16] Previously, red clover has been listed as GRAS (Generally Recognised As Safe).[G65]

Herbal Use

Red clover is stated to act as a dermatological agent, and to possess mildly antispasmodic and expectorant properties. Tannins are known to possess astringent properties. Traditionally red clover has been used for chronic skin disease, whooping cough, and specifically for eczema and psoriasis.[G6, G7, G8, G64]

Dosage

Dosages for oral administration (adults) for traditional uses recommended in standard herbal reference texts are given below.

Dried flowerhead 4 g as an infusion three times daily.[G6, G7]

Liquid extract 1.5–3.0 mL (1 : 1 in 25% alcohol) three times daily.[G6, G7]

Tincture 1–2 mL (1 : 10 in 45% alcohol) three times daily.[G6, G7]

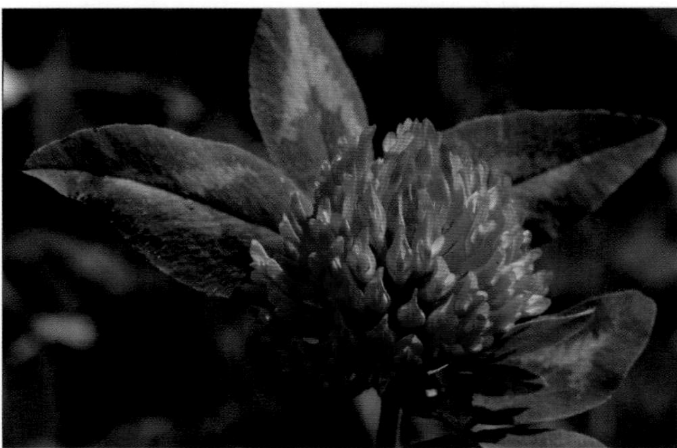

Figure 2 Red clover (*Trifolium pratense*).

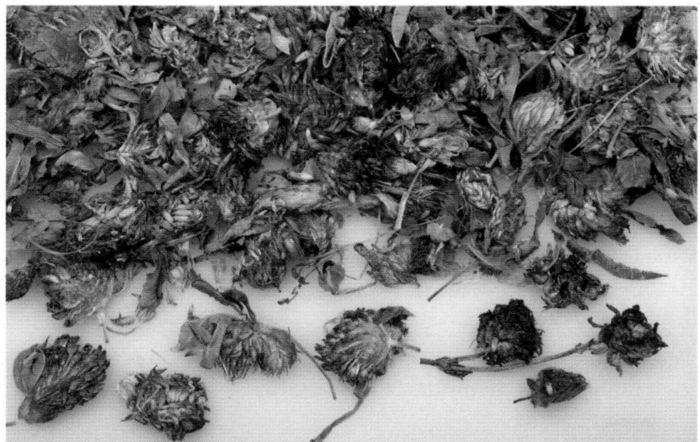

Figure 3 Red clover – dried drug substance (flowerhead).

Pharmacological Actions

In vitro and animal studies

Biochanin A, formononetin and genistein (isoflavones) are known to possess oestrogenic properties.[5] The saponin constituents are reported to lack any haemolytic or fungistatic activity.[3] A possible chemoprotective effect has been documented for biochanin A, which has been reported to inhibit carcinogenic activity in cell culture.[6]

Clinical studies

A systematic review of randomised clinical trials assessing the efficacy of products containing *T. pratense* isoflavones in reducing the frequency of hot flushes in menopausal women identified 17 articles of which five were suitable for inclusion into a meta-analysis.[7] The five studies assessed the effects of *T. pratense* isoflavones administered in doses ranging from 40–82 mg daily. Meta-analysis of data from these trials indicated that the frequency of hot flushes was lower for red clover, compared with placebo (weighted mean difference (95% confidence interval): −1.5 (−2.94 to 0.03); $p = 0.05$). The clinical relevance, if any, of this finding is unclear. Another systematic review, which assessed the efficacy of phytoestrogens for treatment of menopausal symptoms, also included five trials that examined the effects of red clover extracts on frequency of hot flushes for red clover preparations, compared with control groups (weighted mean difference (95% confidence interval): −0.60 (−1.71 to 0.51)).[8]

Side-effects, Toxicity

Clinical data

There is a lack of clinical and toxicity data for red clover and further investigation of these aspects is required.

Urticarial reactions have been documented.[G51]

Preclinical data

Infertility and growth disorders have been reported in grazing animals.[G33] These effects have been attributed to the oestrogenic isoflavone constituents, in particular to formononetin.[5]

Contra-indications, Warnings

In view of the oestrogenic constituents, excessive ingestion should be avoided.

Drug interactions None documented. However, the potential for preparations of red clover to interact with other medicines administered concurrently, particularly those with similar or opposing effects, should be considered. There is evidence that constituents of red clover have oestrogenic effects and the possibility that this could interfere with the activity of hormonal therapies taken concurrently should be considered.

Pregnancy and lactation In view of the oestrogenic components the use of red clover during pregnancy and lactation should be avoided.

Preparations

Proprietary single-ingredient preparations

Australia: Promensil; Trinovin. *Brazil:* Climadil. *UK:* Menoflavon.

Proprietary multi-ingredient preparations

Australia: Bioglan Mens Super Soy/Clover; Bioglan Soy Power Plus; Lifechange Menopause Formula; Trifolium Complex. *Canada:* Natural HRT. *Malaysia:* Cleansa Plus. *USA:* Women's Menopause Formula.

References

1 Saxena VK, Jain AK. A new isoflavone glycoside from *Trifolium pratense*. *Fitoterapia* 1987; 58: 262–263.
2 Jain AK, Saxena VK. Isolation and characterisation of 3-methoxyquercetin 7-O-β-D-glucopyranoside from *Trifolium pratense*. *Natl Acad Sci Lett* 9: 379–380.
3 Olesek WA, Jurzysta M. Isolation, chemical characterization and biological activity of red clover (*Trifolium pratense* L.) root saponins. *Acta Soc Bot Pol* 1986; 55: 247–252.
4 Opdyke DLJ. Furfural. *Food Cosmet Toxicol* 1978; 16: 759–764.
5 Kelly RW *et al*. Formononetin content of 'Grasslands Pawera' red clover and its oestrogenic activity to sheep. *NZ J Exp Agric* 1979; 7: 131–134.
6 Cassady JM *et al*. Use of a mammalian cell culture benzo(*a*)pyrene metabolism assay for the detection of potential anticarcinogens from natural products: inhibition of metabolism by biochanin A, an isoflavone from *Trifolium pratense* L. *Cancer Res* 1988; 48: 6257–6261.
7 Coon JT, *et al*. *Trifolium pratense* isoflavones in the treatment of menopausal hot flushes: a systematic review and meta-analysis. *Phytomedicine* 2007; 14(2–3): 158–159.
8 Krebs EE, *et al*. Phytoestrogens for treatment of menopausal symptoms: a systematic review. *Obstet Gynecol* 2004; 104(4): 824–836.

Rhodiola

Summary and Pharmaceutical Comment

The chemistry of *Rhodiola rosea* root and rhizome is well documented. The precise chemical constituents responsible for the documented pharmacological activities are not fully understood, although tyrosol and salidroside (rhodioloside) and the phenylpropanoid glycoside constituents (rosin, rosavin, rosarin) (*see* Constituents) are believed to be important for certain activities.

Over 200 other *Rhodiola* species have been described, and several of these are used as local medicines in China. Certain constituents of *R. rosea* have also been reported for other *Rhodiola* species. For example, salidroside has been documented for extracts of *R. crenulata*, *R. quadrifida* and *R. sachalinensis* root.

A substantial body of research investigating the pharmacological and clinical properties of *R. rosea* has been undertaken, although much of this work has been published in the Russian scientific literature, making it difficult to access. A limited number of reports of *in vitro* and animal studies published in the English scientific literature have described certain adaptogenic and other effects, such as antitumour and antimetastatic activities, for extracts of *R. rosea*, although further investigation is required to confirm these findings. Well-designed clinical trials of *R. rosea* root/rhizome extracts published in the English (or other European language) scientific literature are lacking. To date, clinical investigations are limited to a small number of single-dose or short-term trials (lasting less than three weeks) involving small numbers of healthy volunteers.

In view of the lack of safety and toxicity data, excessive use (higher than recommended dosages and/or for long periods of time) of *R. rosea* should be avoided.

Pharmacists and other healthcare professionals should be aware that herbal products containing rhodiola are readily available over the internet and from retail outlets; such products are often promoted as being beneficial in supporting mental and physical performance, emotional balance, cardiovascular health, resistance to infection, male sexual function and in increasing ability to cope with stressful situations. There are no licensed rhodiola products available in the UK, so the quality of commercially available products is not assured.

Species (Family)

Rhodiola rosea L. (Crassulaceae)

Synonym(s)

Arctic root, Golden root, Hong Jing Tian, Rhodiola, Rodiola, Rose root, *Sedum rosea* (L.) Scop., *Sedum roseum* Scop.

Rhodiola rosea and several other *Rhodiola* species are used as local medicines in China.[1]

Part(s) Used

Rhizome and root

Pharmacopoeial and Other Monographs

None

Legal category (Licensed Products)

Rhodiola is not on the GSL. There are no licensed products containing rhodiola available in the UK.

Constituents

Flavonoids Herbacetin, gossypetin, kaempferol and their glycosides rhodionin, rhodionidin, rhodiolgin, rhodiolgidin, rhodalin, rhodalidin, rhodiosin and kaempferol-7-*O*-α-L-rhamnopyranoside.[2]

Phenylethanoids Hydroxyphenylethyl tyrosol (*p*-tyrosol) and its glycoside salidroside (rhodioloside; *p*-hydroxyphenylethyl-*O*-β-D-glucopyranoside).[3]

Phenylpropanoids Rosin (cinnamyl-*O*-β-D-glucopyranoside), rosarin (cinnamyl-(6′-*O*-α-L-arabinofuranosyl)-*O*-β-D-glucopyranoside), rosavin (cinnamyl-(6′-*O*-α-L-arabinopyranosyl)-*O*-β-D-glucopyranoside),[4] sachaliside 1 (4-hydroxy-cinnamyl-*O*-β-D-glucopyranoside), vimalin (4-methoxy-cinnamyl-*O*-β-D-glucopyranoside), cinnamyl-(6′-*O*-β-xylopyranosyl)-*O*-β-glucopyranoside, 4-methoxy-cinnamyl-(6′-*O*-α-arabinopyranosyl)-*O*-β-glucopyranoside[4] and cinnamyl alcohol.[2]

Volatile oils 0.05% (1% has been documented for Russian material) of dry weight of crude rhizome, containing monoterpene hydrocarbons, monoterpene alcohols and straight-chain aliphatic alcohols as major components; major compounds (>3%) include geraniol, 1,4-*p*-menthadien-7-ol, limonene, α-pinene (monoterpenes), and decanol and dodecanol (aliphatic alcohols).[5] The monoterpenes rosiridol[2] and rosiridin[6] are also present.

Other constituents Picein ((4-*O*-β-D-glucopyranosyl)-acetophenone), benzyl-*O*-β-D-glucopyranoside,[4] sterols (β-sitosterol, daucosterol),[2] tannins,[7] gallic acid and its esters.[8]

Quality

As with other herbal medicines, there can be qualitative and quantitative variation in the profile of constituents present in crude rhodiola material and in marketed products. Content of salidroside and tyrosol in samples of *R. rosea* root obtained from different outlets in the Yanbian area of China has been reported to vary up to ten-fold (range: 1.3–11.1 and 0.3–2.2 mg/g for salidroside and tyrosol, respectively).[9]

Standardisation of commercial extracts of *R. rosea* may be for content of 'salidrosides' and 'rosavins', although the precise composition of these groups may not always be stated.[6] For example, one commercial product available in the UK is described as containing 3% 'rosavins', 1% 'salidrosides' and 24% polyphenols per 100 mg capsule of rhodiola. Several other rhodiola products are stated to contain 1% 'salidrozid' and 40% polyphenols. The quality of these products is not assured as they are not licensed products.

Phenylethanoids

	R
tyrosol	H
salidroside	(glucosyl)

Phenylpropanoids

	R^1	R^2
rosin	H	H
rosarin	(arabinofuranosyl)	H
rosavin	(arabinopyranosyl)	H
sachaliside	H	OH
4-methoxy-cinnamyl-*O*-*β*-D-glucopyranoside	H	OCH_3
cinnamyl-(6′-*O*-*β*-xylopyranosyl)-*O*-*β*-D-glucopyranoside	(xylopyranosyl)	H
4-methoxy-cinnamyl-(6′-*O*-*α*-arabinosyl) *O*-*β*-D-glucopyranoside	(arabinopyranosyl)	OCH_3

Figure 1 Selected constituents of rhodiola.

An extract of *R. rosea* (SHR-5) tested in clinical trials was standardised for salidroside content (170 mg[10] or 185 mg[11] extract provided approximately 4.5 mg salidroside).[10, 11]

Analysis of 19 samples of dried rhizome from 10 *Rhodiola* species other than *R. rosea*, obtained in the east of Qinghai province in China, found that all species contained salidroside, although only five species had a content greater than 0.3%.[12] Five species also contained lotaustralin, a cyanoglucoside which is toxic to humans following oral administration.

Food Use

Rhodiola root and rhizome are not used in foods, although the aerial parts of *R. rosea* are used as a food ingredient.[10]

Herbal Use

Rhodiola has a long history of use as a medicinal plant in several traditional systems. It is reported to have been used as a 'brain tonic', to treat headache and lung disorders,[10] and to eliminate fatigue and improve work capacity.[13] It is also stated to have stimulant properties, and to prevent stress.[10]

Modern interest in rhodiola is focused on its adaptogenic properties. (Adaptogens increase an organism's resistance to physical, chemical and biological stressors, and have a normalising influence on bodily systems.)

Other glycosides

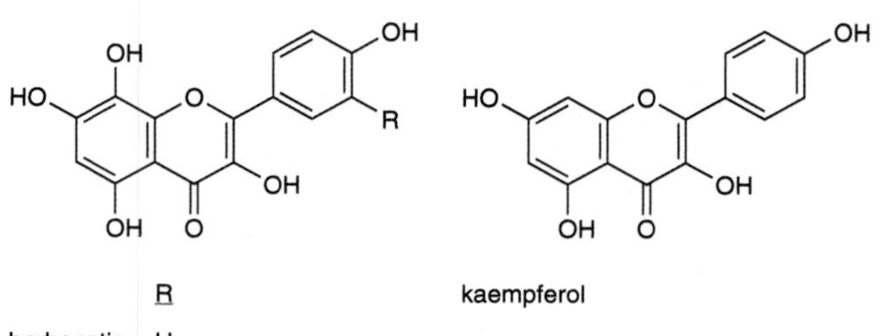

Flavonoids

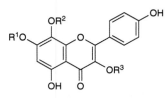

	R
herbacetin	H
gossypetin	OH

kaempferol

	R^1	R^2	R^3
rhodalin	H	xylose	H
rhodionin	xylose	H	H
rhodalidin	H	xylose	glucose
rhodiosin	glucose$^{1\rightarrow3}$rhamnose	H	H
rhodionidin	rhamnose	glucose	H

Figure 2 Selected constituents of rhodiola.

Monoterpenes

geraniol

	R
rosiridol	H
rosiridin	Glucose

limonene

α-pinene

Figure 3 Selected constituents of rhodiola.

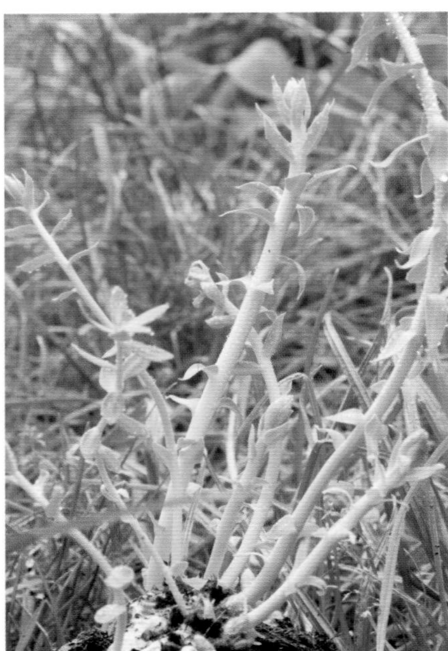

Figure 4 Rhodiola (*Rhodiola rosea*).

Dosage

Authoritative guidance on dosages of *R. rosea* preparations for adults and children hitherto is lacking. Given the intended uses of *R. rosea*, it is not suitable for use in children.

In clinical trials involving young adults, dosages used have ranged from *R. rosea* root extract (SHR-5) 50 mg twice daily (salidroside content not stated)[14] to 170 mg daily (equivalent to approximately 4.5 mg salidroside) for two weeks.[10] In another study investigating the effects of *R. rosea* on fatigue and stress, participants took a single dose of two or three capsules (total daily doses of 370 mg and 555 mg *R. rosea* extract, respectively).[11]

Other dosages have been suggested, although data supporting these regimens are not available. For example, for long-term use as an adaptogen (up to four months) daily doses of *R. rosea* extract standardised for 1% rosavin of 360–600 mg (equivalent to 3.6–6 mg rosavin daily), initiated several weeks before an anticipated period of increased stress and continued for its duration, have been stated.[15] For use as an adaptogen in acute stressful situations, such as taking an examination, a dose three times that suggested for longer term administration, taken as a single dose (i.e. 1080–1800 mg *R. rosea* extract standardised for 1% rosavin, equivalent to 10.8–18 mg rosavin), has been advised.[15]

Pharmacological Actions

A substantial body of research investigating the pharmacological and clinical properties of *R. rosea* has been undertaken, although much of this work has been published in the Russian scientific literature, making it difficult to access. The following represents a summary of some of this literature, together with that published in English. Where papers published in Russian or Ukrainian are cited, information has been taken from the English abstract and/or previous authoritative reviews only, thus the data and methods have not been scrutinised here. The information is included here to guide the interested reader to the original literature, and should not be taken as confirmation of the effects described.

Several activities, including various adaptogenic effects, as well as anti-arrhythmic, cardioprotective, antimutagenic and antitumour properties, have been described for *R. rosea* following preclinical and/or clinical studies. Several of these more specific activities are often considered as part of the overall profile of adaptogenic activity of *R. rosea*. The precise chemical constituents responsible for the documented pharmacological activities of *R. rosea* root and rhizome are not fully understood, although tyrosol and salidroside (rhodioloside) and the cinnamyl (phenylpropanoid) glycoside constituents (rosin, rosavin, rosarin) (*see* Constituents) are believed to be important for certain activities.[3,4,16]

In vitro and animal studies

Adaptogenic effects Several adaptogenic properties have been described for *R. rosea* extracts following preclinical studies.

The effects of *R. rosea* extract on erythropoiesis and granulocytopoiesis following paradoxical sleep deprivation (which leads to behavioural disorders and changes in haematopoiesis, for example, suppression of bone marrow erythropoiesis and activation of granulocytopoiesis) have been explored in experiments in mice.[17,18] In one study, mice were given *R. rosea* extract (no further details given) 1 ml/kg once daily by gastric lavage for five days before sleep deprivation.[17] Measurement of peripheral blood reticulocytes over days 1–7 following treatment indicated that *R. rosea*, compared with control, stimulated erythropoiesis during the early stage (days 1–3) but inhibited accumulation of erythroid cells in the bone marrow during days 4–7. In contrast, in a similar experiment using the same dosage regimen, administration of *R. rosea* before sleep deprivation did not modulate granulocytopoiesis as demonstrated by bone marrow content of neutrophilic granulocytes.[18]

A protective effect against various stress conditions was shown for an aqueous extract of *R. rosea* (SHR-5; containing rosavin 3.6%, salidroside 1.6% and *p*-tyrosol <0.1%) when applied to preparations of three-day-old larvae of the freshwater snail *Lymnaea stagnalis* before they were exposed to stressors.[19] Preincubation of larvae with increasing concentrations of *R. rosea* extract (ranging from 4.05 to 40.5 μg/mL) for 20 hours resulted in a concentration-dependent protective effect against exposure to lethal heat shock (43°C for 4 minutes) for concentrations above 4.05 μg/mL. A protective effect of *R. rosea* was also demonstrated against other stressors (menadione, copper and cadmium) although the effect was less marked than against lethal heat shock. Further investigations, involving incubation of larvae with

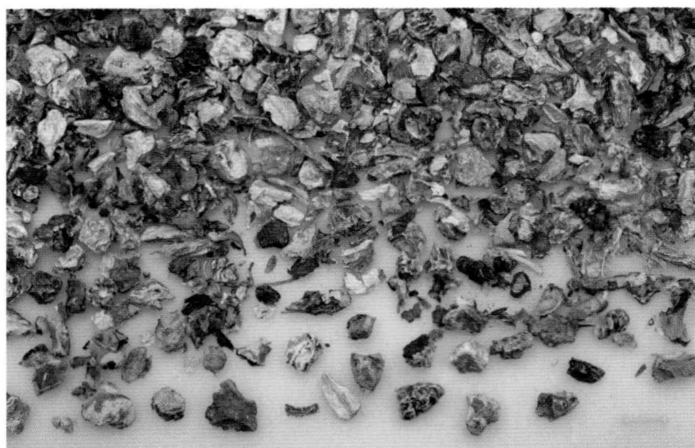

Figure 5 Rhodiola – dried drug substance (rhizome).

R. rosea extract at a concentration of 40.5 µg/mL for 20 hours, ruled out induction of the synthesis of heat shock proteins by *R. rosea* extract as a possible mechanism of action for its protective effect against stressors.[19]

Cognitive effects The effects of a 40% ethanol extract of *R. rosea* root on learning and memory were investigated in rats in a battery of tests, including those involving passive avoidance and active avoidance with negative or positive reinforcement.[13] The results of these studies were conflicting. A single oral dose of *R. rosea* root extract of 0.1 mL given 30 minutes before maze training significantly facilitated learning and improved memory at 24 hours after administration ($p < 0.01$ compared with control), whereas doses of 0.02 and 1 mL had no demonstrable effect. In other tests using the staircase method (which trains animals to retrieve food from the top stair), oral administration of *R. rosea* extract 0.1 mL daily for 10 days before training resulted in a significantly greater proportion of trained rats, compared with control (92.3% versus 61.5%, respectively; $p < 0.05$). However, in other tests (including passive avoidance and active avoidance with negative reinforcement methods), this dosage regimen of *R. rosea* root extract had no significant effects on learning and memory.[13] Oral administration of a 40% ethanol extract of *R. rosea* rhizome 0.1 mL daily for 10 days before training also had no effect on electroconvulsive shock-impaired learning and memory in rats.[20]

The CNS depressant effects of a 50% ethanol extract (said to be of *Sedum rosea*; plant part not stated) at doses of 10, 30 and 100 mg/kg body weight intraperitoneally were investigated in mice.[21] Animals were given a single dose of sodium pentobarbital (50 mg/kg body weight, intraperitoneally) 30 minutes after *S. rosea*, and the narcosis time (time between loss and recovery of the righting reflex; the righting reflex is any one of the neuromuscular responses that restore the body to its upright position when it has been displaced) was measured by a blinded observer. It was reported that *S. rosea* extract potentiated the effects of pentobarbital, since the time to recovery of the righting reflex was significantly longer for treated mice than for controls. However, this finding is questionable since numerical data and a precise *p*-value were not reported (the *p*-value was given as $p \leqslant 0.05$).

Antitumour activities Antitumour and antimetastatic effects have been reported for an extract of *R. rosea* (no further details given) following *in vivo* experiments. In one study, mice transplanted with Ehrlich adenocarcinoma were treated with *R. rosea* extract 0.5 mL/kg body weight orally daily from day 4 post-transplantation until day 13 or 15 post-transplantation when the animals were sacrificed.[22] It was reported that tumour growth was significantly inhibited in treated mice, compared with controls. However, the findings of this study are questionable since the *p*-value given for this finding was $p = 0.05$, and the number of animals involved in the experiment was not stated. A similar experiment involved rats transplanted with metastasising Pliss lymphosarcoma and treated with *R. rosea* extract according to the same regimen. In this study, the extent of metastasis in treated rats was reported to be 50% that in control animals ($p < 0.01$) and the mass of metastases was significantly less than that in control animals (mean (standard deviation): 142.5 (23.0) and 203.3 (27.0), for treated and control groups, respectively; $p < 0.05$).[22] However, again, the sample size for this study was not stated.

In another *in vivo* study, an extract of *R. rosea* root was tested for its effects on the haematotoxicity of cyclophosphamide in mice transplanted with Ehrlich ascites tumour and Lewis lung carcinoma. After transplantation, mice were treated with cyclophosphamide (100 mg/kg body weight), *R. rosea* root extract (0.5 mL/kg orally on days 2–8 following transplantation), or both substances.[23] Cyclophosphamide, but not *R. rosea* extract, reduced the numbers of leukocytes and myelokaryocytes to 40–50%, compared with control ($p < 0.05$); when the two substances were given in combination, the numbers of leukocytes and myelokaryocytes were reported to increase by 30% and 16–18%, respectively, although only the change in the former parameter was reported to be statistically significant ($p < 0.05$). *R. rosea* extract was also reported to have no effect on the colony-forming activity of myelokaryocytes, whereas cyclophosphamide inhibited the proliferation of these cells. In mice given a combination of the two substances, no inhibition of colony-forming activity was observed; this was stated to be statistically significant, compared with values for mice treated with cyclophosphamide alone, although no *p*-value was given.[23]

Antimutagenic activities Antimutagenic activity has been described for extracts of *R. rosea*. Ethanol extracts (20% and 40%) of *R. rosea* were reported to counteract gene mutations induced by various chemical mutagens in the Ames test (*Salmonella typhimurium*).[24] In another *in vitro* experiment, *R. rosea* extract (no further details given) was reported to reduce the yield of bone marrow cells with chromosome aberrations induced *in vivo* (mice) by cyclophosphamide. It is postulated in abstracts of the Russian and Ukrainian literature that *R. rosea* acts as an antimutagen by increasing the efficiency of intracellular DNA repair mechanisms.[25] Since this information is taken from abstracts, confirmation is required.

Cardiovascular activities Inotropic, anti-arrhythmic and other cardioprotective activities have been described in abstracts of papers published in Russian for *R. rosea* extracts. *R. rosea* extract (no further details given), administered orally, was reported to have an anti-arrhythmic effect in epinephrine (adrenaline)-induced arrhythmia in rat heart,[26] and to prevent the reperfusion-induced decrease in contraction amplitude in isolated perfused rat heart.[27] Since both these effects were reversed by naloxone administered by intravenous infusion, the authors postulated that the observed cardioprotective effects of *R. rosea* extract may be related to stimulation of the endogenous opioid system. This information is taken only from abstracts, so confirmation is required.

Clinical studies

Mental performance Several clinical trials, with reports published in the English scientific literature, have investigated the effects of preparations containing a dry extract of *R. rosea* rhizome (SHR-5; Swedish Herbal Institute) on stress-induced fatigue and on mental work capacity.

In a randomised, double-blind, placebo-controlled, parallel-group trial, 40 healthy male Indian medical students took tablets containing *R. rosea* dry extract 50 mg, orally twice daily, or placebo, for 20 days during an examination period.[14] At the end of the study, statistically significant improvements in self-assessed mental fatigue, self-assessed general well-being and in one of the psychomotor tests (accuracy of movement versus speed in a maze test) were reported for the treated group, compared with the placebo group ($p < 0.01$, 0.05 and 0.01, respectively). Statistically non-significant differences were reported in several other tests, including another psychomotor test (tapping test) and two mental capacity tests. The findings of the study are limited since no predefined primary outcome measure was stated, the sample size was small, and the method of randomisation of participants was not adequately described. It was stated in a report of the study that students who received *R. rosea* extract achieved a higher average mark in the examinations than did placebo recipients (3.47 and 3.20, respectively) and that this indicated the 'usefulness' of *R. rosea*.[14] However, this is a post-hoc outcome measure and was not subjected to statistical testing, therefore the conclusion is not necessarily valid.

A similar study, using a randomised, double-blind, placebo-controlled, crossover design, assessed the effects of *R. rosea* dry extract 170 mg (containing approximately 4.5 mg salidroside) daily for 14 days on mental performance among 56 healthy Armenian physicians aged 24–35 years undertaking night duty.[10] Participants underwent a battery of tests before and after the 14-day treatment period, at the end of the 14-day wash-out period and after crossing over to the other study arm for 14 days. It was reported that participants who received *R. rosea* during the first 14-day period experienced statistically significant improvements in tests for fatigue, compared with placebo recipients, but that there was no difference between the two groups at the end of the crossover period.[10] The investigators use this as evidence of the beneficial effects of *R. rosea* extract, but this analysis and, therefore, the conclusion is flawed since it takes no account of the second treatment period. Crossover studies are used as a means of increasing the statistical power of a study without increasing the sample size, so ignoring the second treatment period in effect halves the sample size of the study.

As the two studies described above had used doses of *R. rosea* that were considered to be low, a subsequent randomised, double-blind, placebo-controlled, parallel-group study assessed the effects of two different doses of *R. rosea* extract on capacity for mental work against a background of fatigue. In this study, 121 healthy male cadets aged 19–21 years received two (n = 41) or three (n = 20) capsules containing *R. rosea* extract (SHR-5, 185 mg contains 4.5 mg salidroside); equivalent to a total of 370 mg (9 mg salidroside) and 555 mg extract (13.5 mg salidroside), respectively, or placebo (n = 40), as a single dose; a further 20 participants were allocated to a no-treatment control group.[11] Participants underwent a battery of tests at 5 pm before undertaking night duties, and took their allocated study medication at 4 am the next morning, 1 hour before assessment in the test battery a second time.

Participants who received higher dose *R. rosea* extract performed significantly better than did placebo recipients in all five measures of capacity for mental work in the test battery (scanning for pre-assigned symbols, number of errors in this test, recall of digit sequences, arrangement of numbers in a grid and number of errors in this test; $p < 0.05$ in each test). Statistically significant improvements with lower dose *R. rosea* extract, compared with placebo, were observed in only two of the five tests ($p < 0.01$ for each). Both doses of *R. rosea* extract, compared with placebo, were reported to achieve significantly better scores on an Antifatigue Index (mean (standard deviation): 1.04 (0.29), 1.02 (0.21) and 0.90 (0.32) for lower and higher dose *R. rosea* extract and placebo, respectively; $p < 0.0001$ for dose of *R. rosea* extract versus placebo).[11]

This study, however, has several methodological flaws. For example, a formal sample size calculation was not carried out, the study had no predefined primary outcome measure, and in the analysis, no adjustment appears to have been made for multiple statistical tests. Further, although the study was said to include random allocation to treatment, the randomisation process as described in a report of the study is inadequate and, additionally, the no-treatment control group was not randomly allocated at all but simply comprised the last 20 cadets to be enrolled into the study.

Other conditions In a double-blind, placebo-controlled, cross-over study designed to assess the effects of *R. rosea* on hypoxia and oxidative stress, 15 healthy volunteers aged 20–33 years received capsules each containing *R. rosea* 447 mg (no further details given), four daily for seven days, or placebo, before undergoing hypoxic exposure (to simulate conditions at an elevation of 4600 m).[28] (The study also assessed the effects of a supplement claimed to contain dissolved oxygen, although these results are not reported here.) Fourteen participants completed the study. There were no statistically significant differences between *R. rosea* and placebo recipients in any of the outcome measures, including arterial capillary blood oxygen (concentration – PcO_2), blood oxyhaemoglobin saturation as assessed using a pulse oximeter on an index finger, and serum lipid peroxide and urine malondialdehyde concentrations (as markers of oxidative stress).[28] However, given the small sample size for this study, further investigation into the effects of *R. rosea* preparations in hypoxia is warranted.

Preliminary studies conducted in China and involving men living and working at high altitude have compared the effects of a multiherbal product containing the related species *Rhodiola kirilowii* (Regel) Maxim. with those of acetazolamide.[29,30]

Side-effects, Toxicity

Clinical data

There is a lack of reliable, accessible information relating to the safety and toxicity of preparations of *R. rosea*. Data from clinical trials of *R. rosea* are extremely limited, and no postmarketing surveillance or other pharmacoepidemiological studies have been identified.

Clinical trials involving small numbers of healthy young (<35 years) volunteers who received *R. rosea* extract (SHR-5) 100 mg for 20 days,[14] or 170 mg for 14 days[10] (*see* Pharmacological Actions, Clinical studies for further details), have reported that no adverse effects or events were observed during the studies.[10,14] Another study in which healthy young (19–21 years) volunteers received *R. rosea* extract (SHR-5) 370 mg (containing 9 mg salidroside) or 555 mg (containing 13.5 mg salidroside) as a single dose also reported that no adverse effects or events were observed.[11]

Preclinical data

In vitro experiments have investigated the effects of incubation of three-day-old larvae of the freshwater snail *Lymnaea stagnalis* with different concentrations of an aqueous extract of *R. rosea* (SHR-5; containing rosavin 3.6%, salidroside 1.6% and *p*-tyrosol <0.1%) for 24 hours. At a concentration of *R. rosea* extract of 1.35 mg/mL, all larvae were killed; at 405 μg/mL, around 80% were killed.[19] With a longer period of exposure (up to four days), *R. rosea* extract 81.2 μg/mL did not induce death of exposed larvae, but their development appeared to be retarded: specimens hatched later and were smaller than control specimens, yet no deformations or other abnormalities were observed. Exposure of larvae to *R. rosea* 40.5 μg/mL for up to four days was not associated with any slowing down of growth or development.

Abstracts of papers published in Russian or Ukrainian have described antimutagenic activity for *R. rosea* extracts, although confirmation of these data is required. Antimutagenic activity has been reported for ethanol extracts (20% and 40%) of *R. rosea* in the Ames test (*Salmonella typhimurium*).[24] A reduction in the yield of bone marrow cells with chromosome aberrations induced *in vivo* (mice) by cyclophosphamide has also been described for an extract of *R. rosea*.[25]

Contra-indications, Warnings

None documented. In view of the lack of safety data, use of *R. rosea* extracts at dosages higher than those recommended (*see* Dosage) and/or for longer periods should be avoided.

Drug interactions No interactions have been documented for *R. rosea*. However, in view of the documented pharmacological effects, whether or not there is potential for clinically important interactions with other medicines with similar or opposing effects should be considered.

Pregnancy and lactation The safety of *R. rosea* has not been established. In view of the lack of information on the use of *R. rosea* during pregnancy and lactation, its use should be avoided during these periods.

References

1 Yoshikawa M *et al*. Bioactive constituents of Chinese natural medicines. II. *Rhodiolae radix*. (1). Chemical structures and antiallergic activity of rhodiocyanosides A and B from the underground part of *Rhodiola quadrifida* (Pall.) Fisch et Mey. (Crassulaceae). *Chem Pharm Bull* 1996; 44: 2086–2091.

2 Tolonen A. Analysis of secondary metabolites in plant and cell culture tissue of *Hypericum perforatum* L. and *Rhodiola rosea* L. Oulu, Finland: University of Oulu, 2003; (PhD thesis). Available at http://herkules.oulu.fi/isbn9514271610/index.html?lang=en (accessed 16 July 2004).

3 Ssaratikov SA *et al*. [Rhodioloside, a new glycoside from *Rhodiola rosea* and its pharmacological properties]. *Pharmazie* 1968; 23: 392–395 [German].

4 Tolonen A *et al*. Phenylpropanoid glycosides from *Rhodiola rosea*. *Chem Pharm Bull* 2003; 51: 467–470.

5 Rohloff J. Volatiles from rhizomes of *Rhodiola rosea* L. *Phytochemistry* 2002; 59: 955–661.

6 Ganzera M *et al*. Analysis of the marker compounds of *Rhodiola rosea* L. (golden root) by reversed phase high performance liquid chromatography. *Chem Pharm Bull* 2001; 49: 465–467.

7 Nekratova NA *et al*. [Changes of quantitative contents of salidroside and tannins in underground organs of *Rhodiola rosea* L. in its natural habitats in Altai]. *Rastit Resur* 1992; 28: 40–48 [Russian].

8 Dubichev AG *et al*. [HPLC study of the composition of *Rhodiola rosea* rhizomes]. *Khim Prir Soedin* 1991; 2: 188–193 [Russian].

9 Linh PT *et al*. Quantitiative determination of salidroside and tyrosol from the underground part of *Rhodiola rosea* by high performance liquid chromatography. *Arch Pharm Res* 2000; 23: 349–352.

10 Darbinyan V *et al*. *Rhodiola rosea* in stress induced fatigue – a double blind cross-over study of a standardized extract SHR-5 with a repeated low-dose regimen on the mental performance of healthy physicians during night duty. *Phytomedicine* 2000; 7: 365–371.

11 Shetsov VA *et al*. A randomized trial of two different doses of a SHR-5 *Rhodiola rosea* extract versus placebo and control of capacity for mental work. *Phytomedicine* 2003; 10: 95–105.

12 Kang S, Wang J. [Comparative study of the constituents from 10 rhodiola plants]. *Zhong Yao Cai* 1997; 20: 616–618 [Chinese].

13 Petkov VD *et al*. Effects of alcohol aqueous extract from *Rhodiola rosea* L. roots on learning and memory. *Acta Physiol Pharmacol Bulg* 1986; 12: 3–15.

14 Spasov AA *et al*. A double-blind, placebo-controlled pilot study of the stimulating and adaptogenic effect of *Rhodiola rosea* SHR-5 extract on the fatigue of students caused by stress during an examination period with a repeated low-dose regimen. *Phytomedicine* 2000; 7: 85–89.

15 Anon. *Rhodiola rosea*. *Altern Med Rev* 2002; 7: 421–423.

16 Sokolov S *et al*. [Studies of neurotropic activity of new compounds isolated from *Rhodiola rosea* L.]. *Khim Farm Zh* 1985; 19: 1367–1371 [Russian].

17 Provalova NV *et al*. Mechanisms underling the effects of adaptogens on erythropoiesis during paradoxical sleep deprivation. *Bull Exp Biol Med* 2002; 133: 428–432.

18 Provalova NV *et al*. Effects of adaptogens on granulocytopoiesis during paradoxical sleep deprivation. *Bull Exp Biol Med* 2002; 3: 261–264.

19 Boon-Niermeijer EK *et al*. Phyto-adaptogens protect against environmental stress-induced death of embryos from the freshwater snail *Lymnaea stagnalis*. *Phytomedicine* 2000; 7: 389–399.

20 Lazarova MB *et al*. Effects of meclofenoxate and extr. *Rhodiolae roseae* L. on electroconvulsive shock-impaired learning and memory in rats. *Meth Find Exp Clin Pharmacol* 1986; 8: 547–552.

21 Ahumada F *et al*. Effect of certain adaptogenic plant extracts on drug-induced narcosis in female and male mice. *Phytother Res* 1991; 5: 29–31.

22 Udintsev SN, Shakhov VP. The role of humoral factors of regenerating liver in the development of experimental tumors and the effect of *Rhodiola rosea* extract on this process. *Neoplasma* 1991; 38: 323–331.

23 Udintsev SN, Schakhov VP. Decrease of cyclophosphamide haematotoxicity by *Rhodiola rosea* root extract in mice with Ehrlich and Lewis transplantable tumours. *Eur J Cancer* 1991; 27: 1182.

24 Duhan OM *et al*. [The antimutagenic activity of biomass extracts from the cultured cells of medicinal plants in the Ames test]. *Tsitol Genet* 1999; 33: 19–25.

25 Salikhova RA *et al*. [Effect of *Rhodiola rosea* on the yield of mutation alterations and DNA repair in bone marrow cells]. *Patol Fiziol Eksp Ter* 1997; 4: 22–22 [Russian].

26 Maimeskulova LA *et al*. [The participation of the mu-, delta- and kappa-opioid receptors in the realization of the anti-arrhythmia effect of *Rhodiola rosea*]. *Eksp Klin Farmakol* 1997; 60: 38–39.

27 Lishmanov IuB *et al*. [Contribution of the opioid system to realization of inotropic effects of *Rhodiola rosea* extracts in ischemic and reperfusion heart damage *in vitro*]. *Eksp Klin Farmakol* 1997; 60: 34–36.

28 Wing SL *et al*. Lack of effect of rhodiola or oxygenated water supplementation on hypoxemia and oxidative stress. *Wilderness Environ Med* 2003; 14: 9–16.

29 Ha Z *et al*. [The effect of rhodiola and acetazolamide on the sleep architecture and blood oxygen saturation in men living at high altitude]. *Chin J Tuberc Respir Dis* 2002; 25: 527–530 [Chinese].

30 Ma Y *et al*. [Effect of rhodiola and acetazolamide in improving hypoxia at high altitude]. *Chin Ment Health J* 2001; 15: 117–118 [Chinese].

Rhubarb

Summary and Pharmaceutical Comment

The chemistry of rhubarb is characterised by the anthraquinone derivatives. The laxative action of these compounds is well recognised and justifies the use of rhubarb as a laxative. As with all anthraquinone-containing preparations, the use of non-standardised products should be avoided because their pharmacological effect will be variable and unpredictable. *See* Senna for information on side-effects, toxicity, contra-indications and warnings, including drug interactions and use in pregnancy and lactation, for anthraquinone-containing preparations.

Species (Family)

**Rheum officinale* Baill.
†*R. palmatum* L. (Polygonaceae)

Synonym(s)

*Yao Yong Da Huang
†*R. potaninii* Losinsk., *R. qinlingense* Y.K. Yang *et al.*, *R. tanguticum* (maxim. ex Regel) Maxim., Zhang Ye Da Huang

Part(s) Used

Rhizome, root

Pharmacopoeial and Other Monographs

BHC 1992(G6)
BHP 1996(G9)
BP 2007(G84)
Complete German Commission E(G3)
ESCOP 2003(G76)
Martindale 35th edition(G85)
Ph Eur 2007(G81)
WHO volume 1 1999(G63)

Legal Category (Licensed Products)

GSL(G37)

Constituents

The following is compiled from several sources, including General References G2, G6 and G59.

Hydroxyanthracenes Primarily anthraquinone *O*-glycosides (anthraglycosides) of aloe-emodin, emodin, chrysophanol and physcion; dianthrone glycosides of rhein (sennosides A and B) and their oxalates; heterodianthrones including palmidin A (aloe-emodin, emodin), palmidin B (aloe-emodin, chrysophanol), palmidin C (chrysophanol, emodin), sennidin C (rhein, aloe-emodin), rheidin B (rhein, chrysophanol), and reidin C (rhein, physcion); free anthraquinones mainly aloe-emodin, chrysophanol, emodin, physcion and rhein.

Tannins Hydrolysable and condensed including glucogallin, free gallic acid, (−)-epicatechin gallate and catechin.

Other constituents Calcium oxalate, fatty acids, rutin, resins, starch (about 16%), stilbene glycosides, carbohydrates, volatile oil (trace) with more than 100 components.

Anthraquinone aglycones

	R^1	R^2
rhein	COOH	H
aloe-emodin	CH_2OH	H
chrysophanol	CH_3	H
emodin	CH_3	OH
physcion	CH_3	OCH_3

Dianthrone aglycones

Homodianthrones	R^1	R^2	R^3	R^4
aloe-emodin dianthrone	CH_2OH	H	CH_2OH	H
chrysophanol dianthrone	CH_3	H	CH_3	H
emodin dianthrone	CH_3	OH	CH_3	OH
physcion dianthrone	CH_3	OCH_3	CH_3	OCH_3
sennidin A,B	COOH	H	COOH	H
Heterodianthrones				
palmidin A	CH_3	OH	CH_2OH	H
palmidin B	CH_3	H	CH_2OH	H
palmidin C	CH_3	H	CH_3	OH
palmidin D	CH_3	H	CH_3	OCH_3
rheidin A	CH_3	OH	COOH	H
rheidin B	CH_3	H	COOH	H
rheidin C	CH_3	OCH_3	COOH	H
sennidin C,D	CH_2OH	H	COOH	H

Figure 1 Selected constituents of rhubarb.

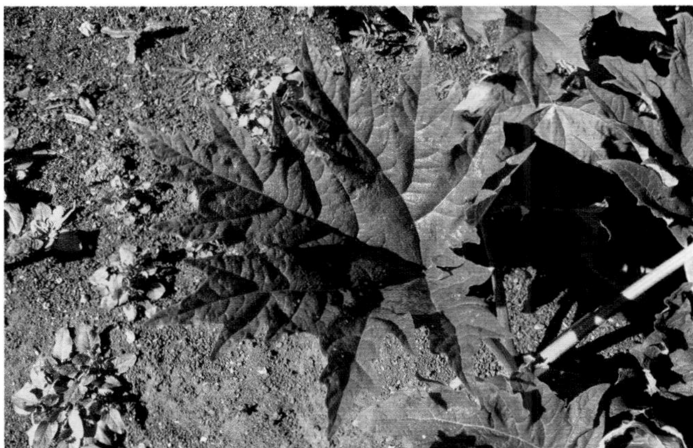

Figure 2 Rhubarb (*Rheum officinale*).

Food Use

Rhubarb is listed by the Council of Europe as a natural source of food flavouring (category N2). This category indicates that it can be added to foodstuffs in small quantities, with a possible limitation of an active principle (as yet unspecified) in the final product.[G16] Rhubarb stems are commonly eaten as a food. Previously, rhubarb has been listed as GRAS (Generally Recognised As Safe).[G65]

Herbal Use

Rhubarb has been used traditionally both as a laxative and an antidiarrhoeal agent.[G2, G6, G8, G64]

Dosage

Rhizome/root 0.2–1.0 g.

Pharmacological Actions

The laxative action of anthraquinone derivatives is well recognised (*see* Senna). Rhubarb also contains tannins, which exert an astringent action. At low doses, rhubarb is stated to act as an antidiarrhoeal because of the tannin components, whereas at higher doses it exerts a cathartic action.[G42]

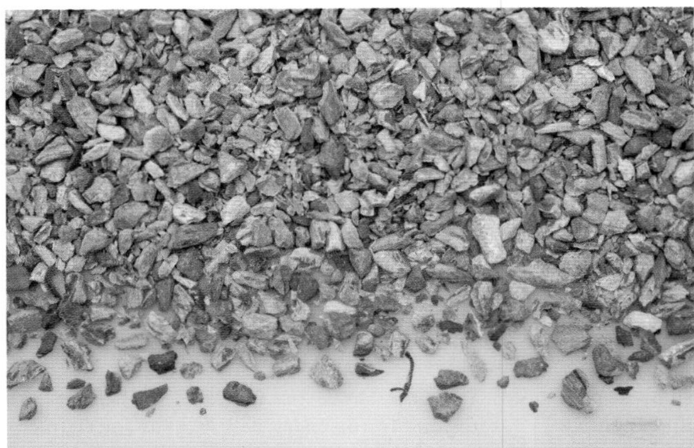

Figure 3 Rhubarb – dried drug substance (rhizome).

Side-effects, Toxicity

See Senna for side-effects and toxicity associated with anthraquinone-containing drugs. Rhubarb leaves are toxic because of the oxalic acid content and should not be ingested. A case of anaphylaxis following rhubarb ingestion has been documented.[G51]

Contra-indications, Warnings

See Senna for contra-indications and warnings associated with anthraquinone-containing drugs.[G20] The astringent effect of rhubarb may exacerbate, rather than relieve, symptoms of constipation.[1] It has been stated that rhubarb should be avoided by individuals suffering from arthritis, kidney disease or urinary problems.[G42]

Drug interactions *See* Senna for information on drug interactions associated with anthraquinone-containing drugs.

Pregnancy and lactation It is stated that rhubarb should be avoided during pregnancy.[G42] *See* Senna for contra-indications and warnings regarding the use of stimulant laxatives during pregnancy and lactation.

Preparations

Proprietary single-ingredient preparations

Czech Republic: Bukosan.

Proprietary multi-ingredient preparations

Argentina: LX-30; Oralsone Topic; Parodium; Pyralvex. *Australia:* Betaine Digestive Aid; Neo-Cleanse; Pyralvex; SM-33 Adult Formula. *Austria:* Eucarbon; Eucarbon Herbal; Novocholin; Pyralvex; Sabatif; Silberne. *Belgium:* Pyralvex. *Brazil:* Bilifel; Bisuisan; Boldopeptan; Eparema; Regulador Xavier N-2. *Canada:* Herbal Laxative; Herbalax. *Czech Republic:* Cynarosan; Dr Theiss Rheuma Creme; Dr Theiss Schweden Krauter; Dr Theiss Schwedenbitter; Species Cholagogae Planta; Zlucnikova Cajova Smes. *France:* Parodium; Pyralvex; Resource Rhubagil. *Germany:* Abdomilon. *Greece:* Pyralvex. *Hong Kong:* Hepatofalk; Pyralvex. *Hungary:* Bolus Laxans. *Ireland:* Pyralvex. *Israel:* Davilla; Encypalmed; Eucarbon; Novicarbon. *Italy:* Amaro Medicinale; Caramelle alle Erbe Digestive; Colax; Critichol; Digelax; Dis-Cinil Complex; Eparema-Levul; Eparema; Eucarbon; Eupatol; Lactolas; Lassatina; Lassativi Vetegali; Magisbile; Mepalax; Neoform; Puntualax; Pyralvex; Stimolfit. *Netherlands:* Pyralvex. *Portugal:* Pyralvex. *Russia:* Parodium (Пародиум). *South Africa:* Helmontskruie; Lewensessens; Moultons Herbal Extract; Pyralvex; Wonderkroonessens. *Singapore:* Pyralvex. *Spain:* Crislaxo; Laxante Bescansa Aloico; Menabil Complex; Pyralvex; Solucion Schoum. *Switzerland:* Padma-Lax; Padmed Laxan; Pyralvex; Schweden-Mixtur H nouvelle formulation. *Thailand:* Pyralvex. *UK:* Acidosis; Digestive; Fam-Lax Senna; Fam-Lax; Golden Seal Indigestion Tablets; Herbal Laxative Tablets; HRI Golden Seal Digestive; Indian Brandee; Jacksons Herbal Laxative; Nervous Dyspepsia Tablets; Pegina; Pyralvex; Rhuaka; Stomach Mixture; Wind & Dyspepsia Relief. *Venezuela:* Orafilm; Pinvex; Pyralvex.

Reference

1 Rohrback JA. Some uses of rhubarb in veterinary medicine. *Herbalist* 1983; 1: 239–241.

Rosemary

Summary and Pharmaceutical Comment

In addition to the well-known culinary uses of rosemary, various medicinal properties are also associated with the herb. Documented antibacterial, anti-inflammatory and spasmolytic actions, which support the traditional uses of the herb, are attributable to the essential oil. Anticomplement and antioxidant activities documented for rosmarinic acid have stimulated interest in a potential preventative use against endotoxin shock and adult respiratory distress syndrome. However, these effects and other activities documented for rosemary and/or its constituents following preclinical studies require confirmation in robust clinical studies. Rosemary should not be used by epileptic patients, or used during pregnancy and lactation, in doses greatly exceeding amounts used in food.

Species (Family)

Rosmarinus officinalis L. (Labiatae/Lamiaceae)

Synonym(s)

Rosmarinus laxiflorus Noë ex Lange

Part(s) Used

Leaf, twig

Pharmacopoeial and Other Monographs

BP 2007[(G84)]
BHP 1996[(G9)]
Complete German Commission E[(G3)]
ESCOP 2003[(G76)]
Martindale 35th edition[(G85)]
Ph Eur 2007[(G81)]

Legal Category (Licensed Products)

GSL[(G37)]

Constituents

The following is compiled from several sources, including General References G2, G41, G52 and G58.

Flavonoids Include diosmetin, diosmin, genkwanin and derivatives, luteolin and derivatives, hispidulin, nepetin, nepitrin and apigenin.

Phenols Caffeic, chlorogenic, labiatic, neochlorogenic and rosmarinic acids.

Volatile oil 1–25%. Components vary according to chemotype. Composed mainly of monoterpene hydrocarbons including α- and β-pinenes, camphene and limonene, together with 1,8-cineole, borneol, camphor (20–50% of the oil), linalool, verbinol, terpineol, 3-octanone and isobornyl acetate.

Flavonoids

	R^1	R^2	R^3
genkwanin	H	OH	CH_3
luteolin	OH	OH	H
diosmetin	OH	OCH_3	H

Phenylpropanoids

rosmarinic acid

Monoterpenes

1,8-cineole

	R
borneol	H
bornyl-acetate	$COCH_3$

camphor

Diterpenes

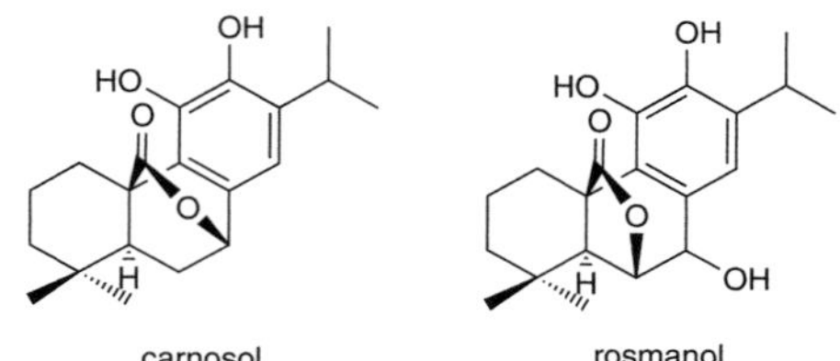

Figure 1 Selected constituents of rosemary.

Terpenoids Carnosol, carnosolic acid, rosmanol (diterpenes);[(1)] oleanolic and ursolic acids (triterpenes).

Food Use

Rosemary herb and oil are commonly used as flavouring agents in foods. Rosemary is listed by the Council of Europe as a source of natural food flavouring (category N2). This category indicates that rosemary can be added to foodstuffs in small quantities, with a possible limitation of an active principle (as yet unspecified) in the final product.[(G16)] Previously, rosemary has been listed as GRAS (Generally Recognised As Safe).[(G65)]

Herbal Use

Rosemary is stated to act as a carminative, spasmolytic, thymoleptic, sedative, diuretic and antimicrobial.[(G7)] Topically, rubefacient, mild analgesic and parasiticide properties are documented.[(G7)] Traditionally rosemary is indicated for flatulent dyspepsia, headache, and topically for myalgia, sciatica, and intercostal neuralgia. The German Commission E approved

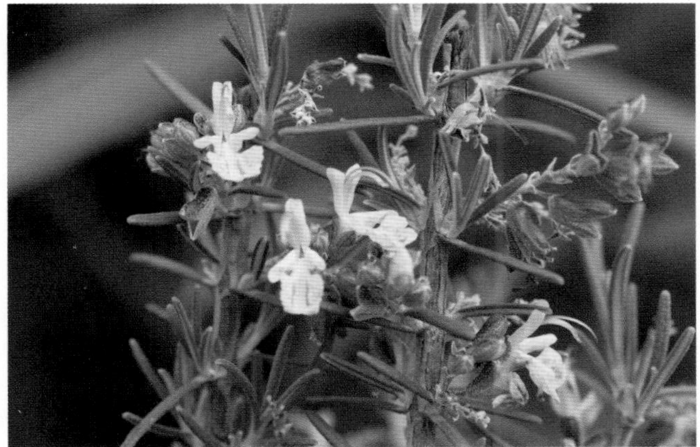

Figure 2 Rosemary (*Rosmarinus officinalis*).

internal use for dyspeptic complaints and external use as supporting therapy for rheumatic diseases and circulatory problems.(G3)

Dosage

Dosages for oral administration (adults) for traditional uses recommended in standard herbal reference texts are given below.

Dried leaf/twig 2–4 g as an infusion three times daily;(G7) 4–6 g daily; external use 50 g for one bath.(G3)

Liquid extract 2–4 mL (1 : 1 in 45% alcohol) three times daily.(G7)

Pharmacological Actions

In vitro and animal studies

Antimicrobial activity Antibacterial and antifungal activities *in vitro* have been reported for rosemary oil.(2, G41, G52) Rosemary herb is an effective antimicrobial agent against *Staphylococcus aureus* in meat and against a wide range of bacteria in laboratory media.(1) Antimicrobial activity has been documented for the oil towards moulds, and Gram-positive and Gram-negative bacteria(1) including *S. aureus*, *S. albus*, *Vibrio cholerae*, *Escherichia coli* and corynebacteria.(3) Carnosol and ursolic acid have inhibited a range of food spoilage microbes (*S. aureus*, *E. coli*, *Lactobacillus brevis*, *Pseudomonas fluorescens*, *Rhodotorula glutinis* and *Kluyveromyces bulgaricus*). Activity was comparable to that of known antioxidants – butylated hydroxyanisole (BHA) and butylated hydroxytoluene (BHT) – and correlated with the respective antioxidant properties of the two compounds (carnosol > ursolic acid).(1)

Antiviral activity A dried 95% ethanol extract of rosemary (2–100 μg/mL) inhibited *in vitro* formation of herpes simplex virus type 2 plaques from 2–100% in a concentration-dependent manner. Carnosolic acid had activity against human immunodeficiency virus type 1 (HIV-1) protease (IC_{50} value 0.08 μg/mL) when assayed against HIV-1 replication (IC_{90} value 0.32 μg/mL).(4, 5) Carnosolic acid was cytotoxic to lymphocytes with a TC_{90} on H9 lymphocytes of 0.36 μg/mL.

Antitumour activity An extract of rosemary (precipitate from aqueous phase of 70% alcohol extract) inhibited KB cells by 87% when applied at a concentration of 50 μg/mL.(G52) The volatile oil (1.2–300 μg/mL) was reported to be toxic to L-1210 leukaemia cells.(6) Topical administration of a methanol extract five minutes prior to application of carcinogens to the dorsal surface of CD-1 mice reduced the irritation and promotion of tumours. Application of rosemary extract (1.2 mg and 3.6 mg) prior to [^{3}H]-benzo(*a*)pyrene reduced the formation of metabolite–DNA adducts by 30% and 54%, respectively.(7) In rats, dietary supplementation with 1% rosemary extract for 21 weeks reduced the development of dimethylbenz(*a*)anthracene mammary carcinoma in the treated group, compared with the control group (40% versus 75%, respectively).(8)

Antispasmodic and anticonvulsant activities Rosemary oil, 1,8-cineole, and bornyl acetate have exerted a spasmolytic action in both smooth muscle (guinea-pig ileum) and cardiac muscle (guinea-pig atria) preparations, with the latter more sensitive.(9) In smooth muscle this spasmolytic effect has been attributed to antagonism of acetylcholine,(10) with borneol considered the most active component of the oil.(10) The spasmolytic action of rosemary oil is preceded by a contractile action, which is attributed to the pinene components.(10) α-Pinenes and β-pinenes have exhibited a spasmogenic activity towards smooth muscle, with no effect on cardiac muscle.(9)

Spasmolytic action *in vivo* (guinea-pigs) has been demonstrated by rosemary oil (administered intravenously) via a relaxant action on Oddi's sphincter contracted by morphine. Activity increased with incremental doses of oil until an optimum dose was reached (25 mg/kg) at which the unblocking effect was immediate.(11) Further increases in dose reintroduced a delayed response time.(11) Smooth muscle-stimulant and analgesic actions have been documented for a rosmaricine derivative.(G41)

The volatile oil of rosemary inhibited contractions of rabbit tracheal smooth muscle induced by acetylcholine, and inhibited contraction of guinea-pig tracheal smooth muscle induced by histamine.(12) The oil also inhibited contractions in both preparations induced by high potassium concentrations. Contractions of rabbit and guinea-pig tracheal smooth muscle induced by acetylcholine and histamine, respectively, were inhibited by rosemary oil in calcium ion-free solution. It was suggested that the oil has calcium antagonist activity.(12) A 30% ethanol extract of rosemary produced a spasmolytic effect on guinea-pig ileum, as demonstrated by measuring the increase in the ED_{50} of acetylcholine (4.9 μg/L after addition of 2.5 mL extract and 25.1 μg/L after addition of 10 mL extract).(G52) An increase in the ED_{50} for histamine from 8.1 μg/L to 44.6 μg/L, respectively, was noted for the same doses of extract.

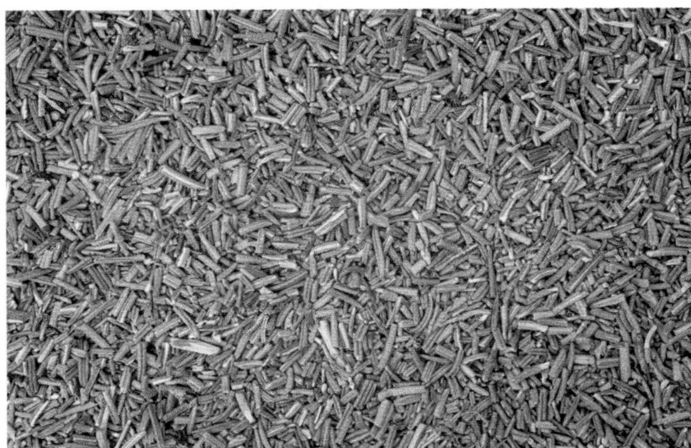

Figure 3 Rosemary – dried drug substance (leaf).

Noradrenaline (norephinephrine)- and potassium ion-induced contractions of rabbit aortic rings were significantly reduced by rosemary oil 0.48 mg/mL and 0.64 mg/mL, respectively. It was proposed that action was by a direct vascular smooth muscle effect.[13]

Anti-inflammatory activity Complement activation and subsequent triggering of the arachidonic acid cascade are thought to play an important role in the early phase of shock. An intact complement system is required for the formation of vasoactive prostanoids (prostacyclin, thromboxane A_2), arterial hypotension and thrombocytopenia.[14] The effect of rosmarinic acid on endotoxin-induced haemodynamic and haematological changes has been studied in a rabbit model of circulatory shock.[14,15] Rosmarinic acid (20 mg/kg, intravenous) was found to suppress the endotoxin-induced activation of complement, formation of prostacyclin, hypotension, thrombocytopenia, and the release of thromboxane A_2.[14] Unlike non-steroidal anti-inflammatory drugs (NSAIDs), the mode of action by which rosmarinic acid suppresses prostaglandin formation does not involve interference with cyclooxygenase activity or prostacyclin synthetase.[15] Activity has been attributed to inhibition of complement factor C3 conversion to activated complement components, which mediate the inflammatory process.[15] Rosmarinic acid has inhibited carrageenan-induced rat paw oedema, and passive cutaneous anaphylaxis, also in rats (ID_{50} 1 mg/kg, intravenously; 10 mg/kg, intramuscularly).[16]

Topical application of rosmarinic acid (5%) to rhesus monkeys reduced gingival plaque indices when compared with placebo.[G52] A methanol extract of herb (3.6 mg) applied topically to CD-1 mice twice daily for four days inhibited skin inflammation and hyperplasia caused by 12-*O*-tetradecanoylphorbol-13-acetate (TPA).[G52] A similar extract inhibited both TPA- and arachidonic acid-induced inflammation as well as TPA-induced hyperplasia.[7]

Anti-hepatotoxic activity A lyophilised aqueous extract of rosemary significantly reduced hepatotoxicity of *t*-butylperoxide to rat hepatocytes *in vitro*, significantly decreasing malonaldehyde formation, release of lactic acid dehydrogenase and aspartate aminotransferase.[17] Pretreatment of rats with an aqueous extract (1 mg of lyophilisate equivalent to 7 mg young shoots) 30 minutes prior to exposure to carbon tetrachloride, resulted in a 72% decrease in plasma glutamic-pyruvic transaminase.[18] Rosemary extract supplementation in the diet of rats enhanced the activity of GSH-transferase and NAD(P)H-quinone reductase.[G52]

Cholagogic activity A lyophilised ethanolic extract (1 mg) of young shoots at doses of 0.1, 1.0 and 2.0 g/kg was injected into the jugular vein of common bile duct-cannulated Sprague–Dawley rats infused with sodium taurocholate.[18] A significant, rapid increase in bile flow (114%) was achieved with maximum effect in 30 minutes. The extract of young shoots was significantly more active in stimulating bile flow than a similar extract of whole plant. A rapid increase in bile secretion was observed (138% in 40 minutes) in cannulated guinea-pigs given an aqueous–ethanol extract (15%).[G52]

Antioxidant activity Several extracts and constituents of rosemary have been shown to have antioxidant activity.[G52] An antioxidant action, demonstrated by inhibition of chemiluminescence and hydrogen peroxide generation from human granulocytes, has been reported for rosmarinic acid.[15]

Lipophilic and hydrophobic fractions of rosemary showed activity which was attributed to the diterpenes carnosol, carnosolic acid and rosmanol inhibiting superoxide anion production in the xanthine/xanthine oxidase system.[19] These diterpenes at concentrations of 3–30 μmol/L also completely inhibit mitochondrial and microsomal lipid peroxidation induced by NADPH or NADPH oxidation.[19]

The complement-inhibiting and antioxidant properties of rosmarinic acid are not thought to adversely affect the chemotaxic, phagocytic and enzymatic properties of polymorphonuclear leukocytes.[20]

Other activities A hyperglycaemic effect was observed in glucose-loaded rats treated with a solution of rosemary oil (925 mg/kg, intramuscular).[21] In rabbits with alloxan-induced diabetes given rosemary oil (25 mg/kg, intramuscular) six hours after fasting, plasma glucose concentrations increased by 17% six hours later.

Pretreatment with rosmarinic acid (20 mg/kg and 10 mg/kg, intravenously) has been reported to inhibit the development of adult respiratory distress syndrome (ARDS) in a rabbit model.[20] This action can be attributed to both the antioxidant and anticomplement activities of rosmarinic acid.[20]

The ability to reduce capillary permeability has been described for diosmin.[G41] Activity reportedly exceeds that exhibited by rutin.[G41]

An increase in locomotor activity has been observed in mice following either inhalation or oral administration of rosemary oil.[22] The increase in activity paralleled a dose-related increase in the serum 1,8-cineole concentration. Biphasic elimination of 1,8-cineole from the blood was observed ($t_{1/2}$ = 6 minutes, $t_{1/2}$ = 45 minutes).[22]

In rats, antigonadotrophic activity has been documented for oxidation products of rosmarinic acid administered intramuscularly.[23] Activity was determined by suppression of pregnant mares' serum-induced increase in ovarian and uterine weights. Concentrations of 10^{-7} mol/L of the flavonoids nepitrin and nepetin inhibited aldose-reductase activity in homogenised rat eye lenses by 31%.[G52]

Clinical studies

There is a lack of clinical research assessing the effects of rosemary and rigorous randomised clinical trials are required.

Side-effects, Toxicity

Clinical data

There is a lack of clinical safety and toxicity data for rosemary and further investigation of these aspects is required.

Rosemary oil is stated to be non-irritating and non-sensitising when applied to human skin,[G58] but moderately irritating when applied undiluted to rabbit skin.[G41] Bath preparations, cosmetics and toiletries containing rosemary oil may cause erythema and dermatitis in hypersensitive individuals.[G51] Photosensitivity has been associated with the oil.[G51]

Preclinical data

Rosmarinic acid exhibits low toxicity (an LD_{50} in mice is stated as 561 mg/kg for intravenous administration) and is rapidly eliminated from the circulation ($t_{1/2}$ = 9 minutes following intravenous administration).[16] Transient cardiovascular actions become pronounced at intravenous doses exceeding 50 mg/kg.[16] Acute LD_{50} values quoted include 5 mL/kg (rat, oral) and >10 mL/kg (rabbit, dermal).[3]

Diosmin is reportedly less toxic than rutin.(G41) No mortality was seen in Wistar rats and Swiss mice given single intraperitoneal doses of 2 g/kg of aqueous alcoholic rosemary extract (15%).(G52)

Contra-indications, Warnings

Topical preparations containing rosemary oil should be used with caution by hypersensitive individuals. Rosemary oil contains 20–50% camphor; orally, camphor readily causes epileptiform convulsions if taken in sufficient quantity.(G58)

Drug interactions None documented. However, the potential for preparations of rosemary to interact with other medicines administered concurrently, particularly those with similar or opposing effects, should be considered. There is limited evidence from preclinical studies that rosemary oil has hyperglycaemic activity. The clinical relevance of this, if any, is not clear.

Pregnancy and lactation Rosemary is reputed to be an abortifacient(G30) and to affect the menstrual cycle (emmenagogue).(G48) In view of this, rosemary should not be ingested during pregnancy and lactation in amounts greatly exceeding those normally encountered in foods.

Preparations

Proprietary single-ingredient preparations

Brazil: Alrinte.

Proprietary multi-ingredient preparations

Argentina: Acnetrol; Acnetrol; Sequals G. *Australia:* Avena Complex; Garlic Allium Complex; Vitanox. *Austria:* Euka. *Chile:* Rhus Opodeldoc. *Czech Republic:* Hertz- und Kreislauftee; Naturland Grosser Swedenbitter. *France:* Depuratum; Hepax; Mediflor Tisane Contre la Constipation Passagere No 7; Mediflor Tisane Digestive No 3; Mediflor Tisane Hepatique No 5; Romarene; Romarinex. *Germany:* Canephron; Melissengeist. *Russia:* Canephron N (Канефрон Н). *Spain:* Linimento Naion; Mesatil; Natusor Hepavesical; Natusor Low Blood Pressure; Natusor Sinulan; Resolutivo Regium. *Switzerland:* Phytomed Cardio. *UK:* Supa-Tonic Tablets; Wood Sap Ointment.

References

1 Collin MA, Charles HP. Antimicrobial activity of carnosol and ursolic acid: two anti-oxidant constituents of *Rosmarinus officinalis* L. *Food Microbiol* 1987; 4: 311–315.

2 Panizzi L *et al*. Composition and antimicrobial properties of essential oils of four Mediterranean Lamiaceae. *J Ethnopharmacol* 1993; 39: 167–170.

3 Opdyke DLJ. Rosemary oil. *Food Cosmet Toxicol* 1974; 12: 977–978.

4 Pariš A *et al*. Inhibitory effect of carnosolic acid on HIV-1 protease in cell-free assays. *J Nat Prod* 1993; 56: 1426–1430.

5 Pukl M *et al*. Inhibitory effect of carnosolic acid on HIV-1 protease. *Planta Med* 1992; 58: A632.

6 Ilarionova M *et al*. Cytotoxic effect on leukemic cells of the essential oils from rosemary, wild geranium and nettle and concret of royal bulgarian rose. *Anticancer Res* 1992; 12: 1915.

7 Huang M-T *et al*. Inhibition of skin tumorigenesis by rosemary and its constituents carnosol and ursolic acid. *Cancer Res* 1994; 54: 701–708.

8 Singletary K. Inhibition of DMBA-induced mammary tumorigenesis by rosemary extract. *FASEB J* 1991; 5: 5A927.

9 Hof S, Ammon HPT. Negative inotropic action of rosemary oil, 1,8-cineole, and bornyl acetate. *Planta Med* 1989; 55: 106–107.

10 Taddei I *et al*. Spasmolytic activity of peppermint, sage and rosemary essences and their major constituents. *Fitoterapia* 1988; 59: 463–468.

11 Giachetti D *et al*. Pharmacological activity of essential oils on Oddi's sphincter. *Planta Med* 1988; 389–392.

12 Aqel MB. Relaxant effect of the volatile oil of *Rosmarinus officinalis* on tracheal smooth muscle. *J Ethnopharmacol* 1991; 33: 57–62.

13 Aqel MB. A vascular smooth muscle relaxant effect of *Rosmarinus officinalis*. *Int J Pharmacog* 1992; 30: 281–288.

14 Bult H *et al*. Modification of endotoxin-induced haemodynamic and haematological changes in the rabbit by methylprednisolone, F(ab′)2 fragments and rosmarinic acid. *Br J Pharmacol* 1985; 84: 317–327.

15 Rampart M *et al*. Complement-dependent stimulation of prostacyclin biosynthesis: inhibition by rosmarinic acid. *Biochem Pharmacol* 1986; 35: 1397–1400.

16 Parnham MJ, Kesselring K. Rosmarinic acid. *Drugs Future* 1985; 10: 756–757.

17 Joyeux M *et al*. Screening of antiradical, antilipoperoxidant and hepatoprotective effects of nine plants extracts used in Caribbean folk medicine. *Phytother Res* 1995; 9: 228–230.

18 Hoefler C *et al*. Comparative choleretic and hepatoprotective properties of young sprouts and total plant extracts of *Rosmarinus officinalis* in rats. *J Ethnopharmacol* 1987; 19: 133–143.

19 Haraguchi H *et al*. Inhibition of lipid peroxidation and superoxide generation by diterpenoids from *Rosmarinus officinalis*. *Planta Med* 1995; 61: 333–336.

20 Nuytinck JKS *et al*. Inhibition of experimentally induced microvascular injury by rosmarinic acid. *Agents Actions* 1985; 17: 373–374.

21 Al-Hader AA *et al*. Hyperglycemic and insulin release inhibitory effects of *Rosmarinus officinalis*. *J Ethnopharmacol* 1994; 43: 217–221.

22 Kovar KA *et al*. Blood levels of 1,8-cineole and locomotor activity of mice after inhalation and oral administration of rosemary oil. *Planta Med* 1987; 315–318.

23 Gumbinger HG *et al*. Formation of compounds with antigonadotropic activity from inactive phenolic precursors. *Contraception* 1981; 23: 661–665.

Sage

Summary and Pharmaceutical Comment

The characteristic components of sage (*Salvia officinalis*) to which its traditional uses can be attributed are the volatile oil and tannins. The oil of a related species *Salvia lavandulifolia* is being investigated for symptomatic treatment of Alzheimer's disease. However, at present, there is a lack of well-designed clinical studies investigating the reputed effects of sage. Sage oil contains high concentrations of thujone, a toxic ketone, and should not be ingested. Sage is commonly used as a culinary herb and presents no hazard when ingested in amounts normally encountered in foods. However, extracts of the herb should be used with caution and should not be ingested in large amounts or over prolonged periods.

Sage should not be used during pregnancy and lactation.

Species (Family)

**Salvia officinalis* L. (Labiatae/Lamiaceae)
S. lavandulifolia Vahl

Synonym(s)

*Dalmatian Sage, Garden Sage, True Sage

Part(s) Used

Leaf

Pharmacopoeial and Other Monographs

BHP 1996[(G9)]
BP 2007[(G84)]
Complete German Commission E[(G3)]
ESCOP 2003[(G76)]
Martindale 35th edition[(G85)]
Ph Eur 2007[(G81)]

Legal Category (Licensed Products)

GSL[(G37)]

Constituents

The following is compiled from several sources, including Reference 1 and General References G2, G52, G58 and G62.

Acids Phenolic – caffeic, chlorogenic, ellagic, ferulic, gallic and rosmarinic.[(2)]

Flavonoids 5-Methoxysalvigenin.

Terpenes Monoterpene glycosides. Diterpenes, abietanes including carnosic acid and derivatives, e.g. carnasol. Triterpenes, oleanolic acid and derivatives.

Tannins 3–8%. Hydrolysable and condensed.[(2, 3)]

Volatile oil 1–2.8%. Pharmacopoeial standard not less than 1.0% cut herb.[(G81, G84)] Major components are α- and β-thujones (35–50%, mainly α). Others include 1,8-cineole, borneol, camphor, caryophyllene, linalyl acetate and various terpenes.[(4, 5)]

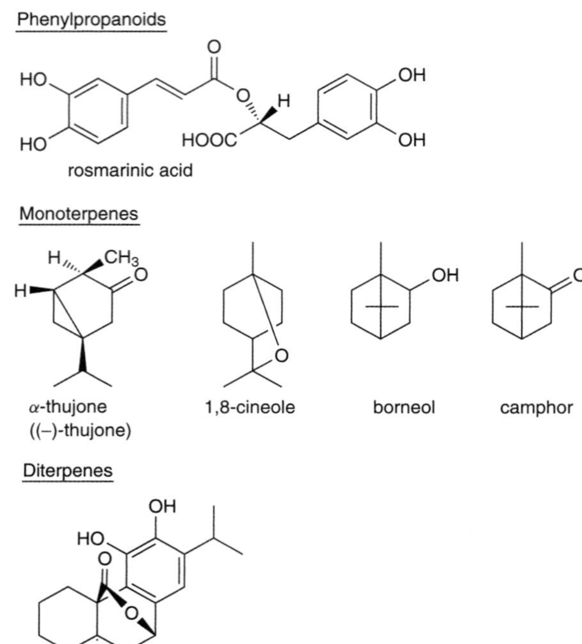

Figure 1 Selected constituents of sage.

It has been noted that commercial sage may be substituted with *Salvia triloba*.[(1)] In contrast to *S. officinalis*, the principal volatile oil component of *S. triloba* is 1,8-cineole, with α-thujone only accounting for 1–5%.[(1)] Compared with *S. officinalis*, the volatile oil yield of various *Salvia* species is lower, with lower total ketone content and higher total alcohol content.[(6)]

Food Use

Sage is commonly used as a culinary herb. It is listed by the Council of Europe as a natural source of food flavouring (category N2).[(G16)] This category indicates that sage can be added to foodstuffs providing the concentration of thujones (α and β) present in the final product does not exceed 0.5 mg/kg, with the exceptions of alcoholic beverages (10 mg/kg), bitters (35 mg/kg), food containing sage (25 mg/kg) and sage stuffing (250 mg/kg).[(G16)] Previously, sage has been listed as GRAS (Generally Recognised As Safe).[(G65)]

Herbal Use

Sage is stated to possess carminative, antispasmodic, antiseptic, astringent and antihidrotic properties. Traditionally, it has been used to treat flatulent dyspepsia, pharyngitis, uvulitis, stomatitis, gingivitis, glossitis (internally or as a gargle/mouthwash), hyperhidrosis, and galactorrhoea.[(G2, G4, G7, G32, G43, G52, G54, G64)] The herbals of Gerard, Culpeper and Hill credit sage with the ability to enhance memory.[(7)] The German Commission E approved internal use for dyspeptic symptoms and excessive

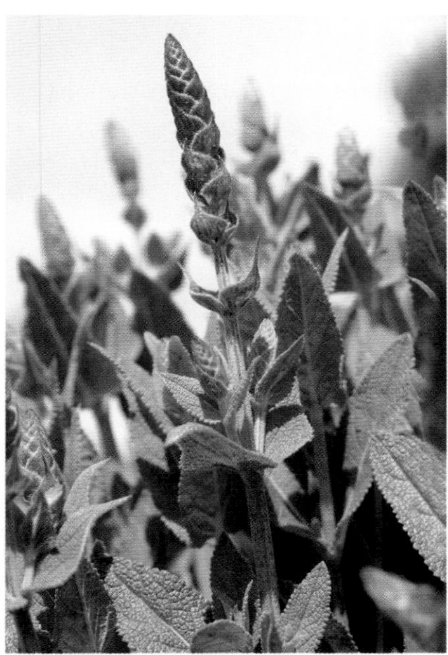

Figure 2 Sage (*Salvia officinalis*).

perspiration, and external use for inflammation of mucous membranes of mouth and throat.(G3)

Dosage

Dosages for oral administration (adults) for traditional uses recommended in standard herbal reference texts are given below.

Leaf 1–4 g as an infusion three times daily;(G7) 4–6 g daily. (G3)

Liquid extract 1–4 mL (1:1 in 45% alcohol) three times daily.(G7)

Gargles, rinses 2.5 g/100 mL water.(G3)

Pharmacological Actions

In vitro and animal studies

Hypotensive activity in anaesthetised cats, CNS-depressant action (prolonged barbiturate sleep) in anaesthetised mice, and an antispasmodic action *in vitro* (guinea-pig ileum) have been reported for a sage extract(8) and for the essential oil.(9)

Antispasmodic activity Inhibition of contractions induced by acetylcholine, histamine, serotonin and barium chloride by 60–80% has been noted for a total sage extract, with lesser activity exhibited by a total flavonoid extract.(8) An initial spasmogenic action exhibited by low doses of sage oil has been attributed to the pinene content.(9) Antispasmodic activity *in vivo* (guinea-pigs) has been reported for sage oil administered intravenously, which released contraction of Oddi's sphincter induced by intravenous morphine.(5)

Anticholinesterase activity Early herbals claim that sage enhances the memory.(7) The anticholinesterase activity of several *Salvia* species and their constituents have been investigated in the search for new drugs for the treatment of Alzheimer's disease. The inhibition of anticholinesterase *in vitro* by an ethanolic extract of *S. officinalis* (2.5 mg/mL) was 68%, and by oils of *S. officinalis* and *S. lavandulifolia* (0.1 μg/mL) was 52% and 63%, respectively.(10) The IC_{50} value of *S. lavandulifolia* oil is reportedly 0.03 μg/mL.(11) The monoterpenes 1,8-cineole and α-pinene from the oil have been identified as the inhibitors of acetylcholinesterase with IC_{50} values of 0.67 and 0.63 mmol/L, respectively.(11) Rats given *S. lavandulifolia* oil (20 μL or 50 μL for five days) were sacrificed, and acetylcholinesterase activity assessed for striatum, cortex and hippocampus of brain left hemisphere.(12) At the lower dose, there was a decrease in acetylcholinesterase activity in the striatum, but not in the hippocampus or cortex of treated rats. At the higher dose, there was a decrease in striatal acetylcholinesterase activity. It was concluded that the oil inhibited acetylcholinesterase in selective areas of the brain.

Hypoglycaemic activity Hypoglycaemic activity *in vivo* (rabbits) has been reported for *S. lavandulifolia.*(13) and for mixed phytotherapy preparations containing various *Salvia* species, including *S. officinalis.*(14) Activity in normoglycaemic, hypoglycaemic and in alloxan-diabetic rabbits was observed, although no change in insulin concentrations was noted.(13)

Antimicrobial and antiviral activity Antimicrobial activity of the volatile oil has been attributed to the thujone content.(4) Antimicrobial activity *in vitro* was noted against *Escherichia coli*, *Shigella sonnei*, *Salmonella* species, *Klebsiella ozanae* (Gram-negative), *Bacillus subtilis* (Gram-positive), and against various fungi (*Candida albicans*, *C. krusei*, *C. pseudotropicalis*, *Torulopsis glabrata*, *Cryptococcus neoformans*).(15) No activity was observed versus *Pseudomonas aeruginosa.*(4) Microencapsulation of sage oil into gelatin-acacia capsules introduced a lagtime with respect to antibacterial activity and inhibited antifungal activity.(4) Diterpene constituents of *S. officinalis* are reported to be active against vesicular stomatitis virus.(G52)

Other activities An aqueous ethanolic extract of sage (50%) strongly inhibited collagenolytic activity of *Porphyromonas gingivitis.*(G52) In addition to anticholinesterase activity, other biological activities have relevance in the treatment of Alzheimer's disease. In this context, *S. lavandulifolia* and its individual constituents have been assessed for antioxidant, anti-inflammatory and oestrogenic activities.(11) An ethanolic extract of dried herb (5 mg/mL) and the monoterpenes α- and β-pinene and 1,8-cineole (0.1 mol/L) inhibited bovine brain liposome peroxidate activity. Anti-inflammatory activity was demonstrated by weak inhibition of thromboxane B_2 and leukotriene B_4 synthesis, and possible oestrogenic activity of sage oil (0.01 mg/mL) and geraniol (0.1–2 mmol/L), demonstrated by induction of β-galactosidase in yeast cells.

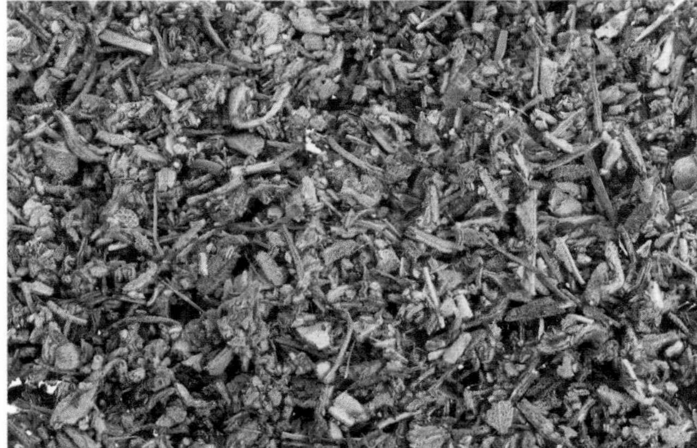

Figure 3 Sage – dried drug substance (leaf).

Clinical studies

Clinical research assessing the effects of sage is limited and rigorous randomised controlled clinical trials are required.

Excessive sweat induced by pilocarpine was inhibited by a dialysate of an aqueous extract of fresh sage.[G52] In an open study, 40 patients were given dried aqueous extract of sage (440 mg, equivalent to 2.6 g herbs) and 40 were given infusion of sage (4.5 g herb daily). Reduction of sweat (less than 50%) was achieved in both groups of patients with idiopathic hyperhidrosis.[G52] It should be noted, however, that this study did not include a control group and, therefore, the observed effects cannot be attributed to sage with any certainty.

A double-blind, placebo-controlled, crossover study involving 20 healthy volunteers compared the effects of 50 μL, 100 μL and 150 μL of *S. lavandulifolia* oil and sunflower oil.[12] Cognitive assessment indicated improvements in both immediate and delayed word recall scores, coupled with decrements in accuracy and speed of attention, with sage oil 50 μL. At this dose, self-related alertness at 2.5 hours and calmness at four hours and six hours were reported to be reduced.

Side-effects, Toxicity

Clinical data

There is a lack of clinical safety and toxicity data for sage and further investigation of these aspects is required.

A case of human poisoning has been documented following ingestion of sage oil for acne.[16] Convulsant activity in humans (and animals) has been documented for sage oil.[17, 18]

Sage oil is reported to be a moderate skin irritant[19] and is not recommended for use in aromatherapy.[G58]

Preclinical data

In rats, the subclinical, clinical and lethal doses for convulsant action of sage oil are estimated as 0.3, 0.5, and 3.2 g/kg.[17] This toxicity has been attributed to the ketone terpenoids in the volatile oil, namely camphor and thujone. Acute LD_{50} values for sage oil are documented as 2.6 g/kg in rats for oral administration and 5 g/kg in rabbits for intradermal administration.[19] *S. officinalis* has no mutagenic or DNA-damaging activity in either the Ames test or *Bacillus* rec-assay.[G52]

S

Contra-indications, Warnings

Sage oil is toxic (due to the thujone content) and should not be ingested. *S. lavandulifolia* oil has a much lower content of thujone than does *S. officinalis* oil.[12] In view of the toxicity of the essential oil, sage extracts should be used with caution and not ingested in large amounts.

Drug interactions None documented. However, the potential for preparations of sage to interact with other medicines administered concurrently, particularly those with similar or opposing effects, should be considered. There is limited evidence from preclinical studies that sage has hypoglycaemic activity. Sage oil has a high content of thujones, which are convulsants.

Pregnancy and lactation Sage is contra-indicated during pregnancy. Traditionally, it is reputed to be an abortifacient and to affect the menstrual cycle.[G30] The volatile oil contains a high proportion of α- and β-thujones, which are known to be abortifacient and emmenagogic. Sage should not be used during lactation.

Preparations

Proprietary single-ingredient preparations

Austria: Salvysat. *Czech Republic:* Caj ze Salveje; Florsalmin; List Salveje Lekarske; Nat Salveje Lekarske; Salvejova Nat. *Germany:* Aperisan; Salbei Curarina; Salvysat; Sweatosan N; Viru-Salvysat. *Italy:* Saugella Dermoliquido.

Proprietary multi-ingredient preparations

Argentina: Acnetrol; Parodontax Fluor; Sigmafem; Sigmafen Free; Tereonsit. *Australia:* Feminine Herbal Complex. *Austria:* Cional; Dynexan; Mentopin; Paradenton. *Canada:* Original Herb Cough Drops. *Chile:* Eciclean. *Czech Republic:* Diabetan; Diabeticka Cajova Smes-Megadiabetin; Pulmoran; Stomatosan; Tormentan. *France:* Bolcitol; Gonaxine; Saugella; Tisane Hepatique de Hoerdt. *Germany:* Amara-Tropfen; Melissengeist; Parodontal. *Israel:* Baby Paste + Chamomile; Kamilotract. *Italy:* Donalg; Saugella Attiva; Saugella Dermolatte; Saugella Fitothym; Saugella Salviettine; Saugella Solido ph 3.5. *South Africa:* Amara; Dynexan. *Spain:* Diabesor; Menstrunat; Natusor Farinol; Natusor Low Blood Pressure. *Switzerland:* Strath Gouttes pour les muqueuses; Tisane pectorale et antitussive; Wala Echinacea. *Venezuela:* One Drop Spray. *UK:* Lane's Sage and Garlic Catarrh Remedy; Menopace Plus; Napiers Echinacea Tea.

References

1 Tucker AO *et al*. Botanical aspects of commercial sage. *Econ Bot* 1980; 34: 16–19.
2 Petri G *et al*. Tannins and other polyphenolic compounds in the genus *Salvia*. *Planta Med* 1988: 54: 575.
3 Murko D *et al*. Tannins of *Salvia officinalis* and their changes during storage. *Planta Med* 1974; 25: 295–300.
4 Jalsenjak V *et al*. Microcapsules of sage oil: Essential oils content and antimicrobial activity. *Pharmazie* 1987; 42: 419–420.
5 Giachetti D *et al*. Pharmacological activity of essential oils on Oddi's sphincter. *Planta Med* 1988: 54: 389–392.
6 Ivanic R, Savin K. A comparative analysis of essential oils from several wild species of *Salvia*. *Planta Med* 1976; 30: 25–31.
7 Perry EK *et al*. Medicinal plants and Alzheimer's disease: integrating ethnobotanical and contemporary scientific evidence. *J Alt Complement Med* 1998; 4: 419–428.
8 Todorov S *et al*. Experimental pharmacological study of three species from genus *Salvia*. *Acta Physiol Pharmacol Bulg* 1984; 10: 13–20.
9 Taddei I *et al*. Spasmolytic activity of peppermint, sage and rosemary essences and their major constituents. *Fitoterapia* 1988; 59: 463–468.
10 Perry N *et al*. European herbs with cholinergic activities: potential in dementia therapy. *Int J Geriat Psychiat* 1996; 11: 1063–1069.
11 Perry NSL *et al*. *In-vitro* inhibition of human erythrocyte acetylcholinesterase by *Salvia lavandulaefolia* essential oil and constituent terpenes. *J Pharm Pharmacol* 2000; 52: 895–902.
12 Houghton PJ. *Personal communication.*
13 Jimenez J *et al*. Hypoglycaemic activity of *Salvia lavandulifolia*. *Planta Med* 1986: 52: 260–262.
14 Cabo J *et al*. Accion hipoglucemiante de preparados fitoterapicos que contienen especies del genero salvia. *Ars Pharmac* 1985; 26: 239–249.
15 Recio MC *et al*. Antimicrobial activity of selected plants employed in the Spanish Mediterranean area. Part II. *Phytother Res* 1989; 3: 77.
16 Centini F *et al*. A case of sage oil poisoning. *Zacchia* 1987; 60: 263–174.
17 Millet Y. Experimental study of the toxic convulsant properties of commercial preparations of essences of sage and hyssop. *Electroencephal Clin Neurophysiol* 1980; 49: 102P.
18 Millet Y *et al*. Toxicity of some essential plant oils – clinical and experimental study. *Clin Toxicol* 1981; 18: 1485–1498.
19 Opdyke DLJ. Sage oil Dalmatian. *Food Cosmet Toxicol* 1974; 12: 987–988.

Sarsaparilla

Summary and Pharmaceutical Comment

Phytochemical studies on sarsaparilla have focused on the nature of the steroidal saponin constituents, with limited information available regarding additional constituents. No documented scientific evidence from preclinical studies was found to justify the herbal uses. Also, there is a lack of robust clinical research assessing the efficacy and safety of sarsaparilla. No toxicity data were located, although large doses may be irritant to the gastrointestinal mucosa and should, therefore, be avoided.

There are no known problems with the use of sarsaparilla during pregnancy and lactation but, as a precaution, amounts ingested should not exceed those usually found in foods.

Species (Family)

**Smilax regelii* Killip & C.V. Morton (*Smilacaceae*)
†*S. purhampuy* Ruiz

Synonym(s)

**Smilax ornata* Hook
†*S. febrifuga* Kunth, *S. febrifuga* var. *aequatoris* A. DC

Part(s) Used

Rhizome, root

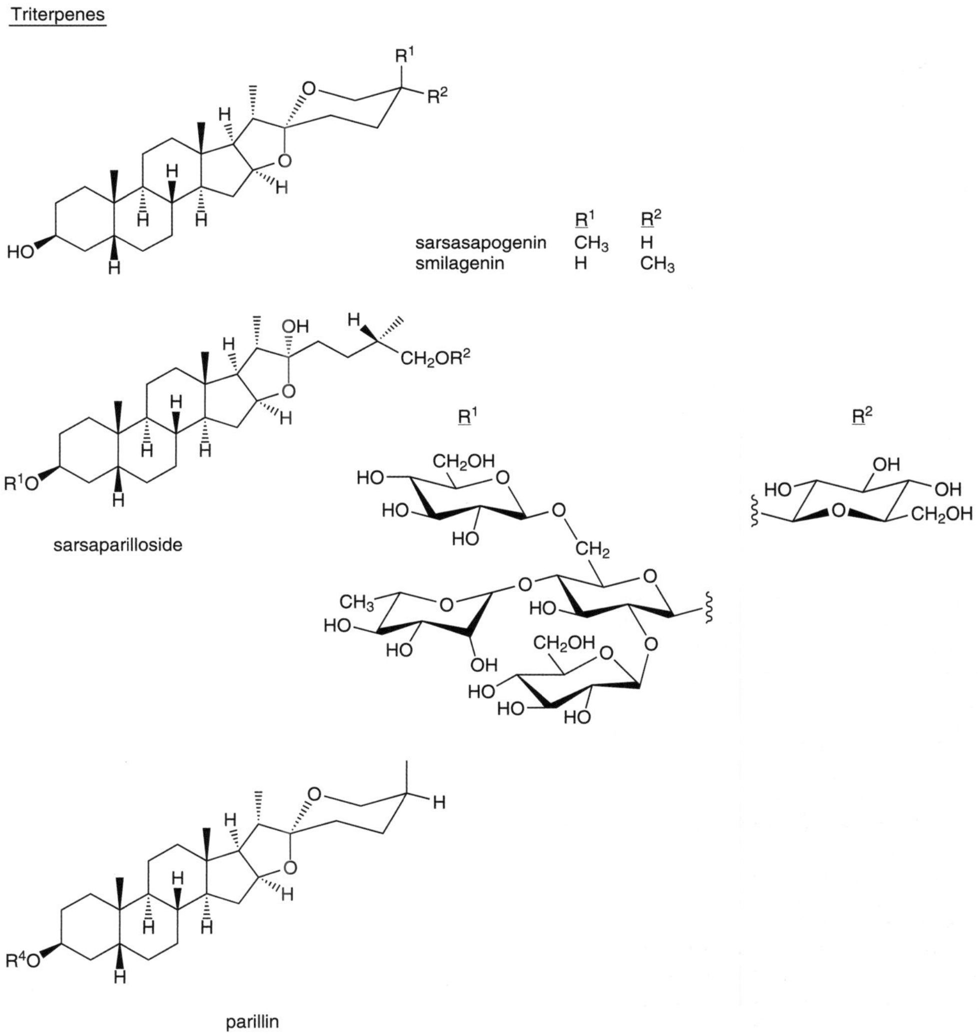

Triterpenes

	R^1	R^2
sarsasapogenin	CH_3	H
smilagenin	H	CH_3

sarsaparilloside

parillin

Figure 1 Selected constituents of sarsaparilla.

Pharmacopoeial and Other Monographs

BHC 1992[G6]
BHP 1996[G9]
Martindale 35th edition[G85]

Legal Category (Licensed Products)

GSL[G37]

Constituents

The following is compiled from several sources, including General Reference G6.

Saponins About 2%. Sarsasapogenin (parigenin), smilagenin, diosgenin, tigogenin, asperagenin, laxogenin from various species,[1] sarsasaponin (parillin), smilasaponin (smilacin) and sarsaparilloside.

Other constituents Caffeoylshikimic acid, ferulic acid, shikimic acid, kaempferol, quercetin, phytosterols (e.g. β-sitosterol, stigmasterol, pollinastanol), resin, starch, volatile oil (trace) and cetyl alcohol.

Food Use

Sarsaparilla is listed by the Council of Europe as a natural source of food flavouring (category N4). This category indicates that the use of sarsaparilla as a flavouring agent is recognised but that there is insufficient information available to further classify it into categories N1, N2 or N3.[G16] Sarsaparilla has been used as a vehicle and flavouring agent for medicaments,[G45] and is widely employed in the manufacture of non-alcoholic beverages.[G59] Previously, sarsaparilla has been listed as GRAS (Generally Recognised As Safe).

Herbal Use

Sarsaparilla is stated to possess antirheumatic, antiseptic and antipruritic properties. Traditionally, it has been used for psoriasis and other cutaneous conditions, chronic rheumatism, rheumatoid arthritis, as an adjunct to other treatments for leprosy, and specifically for psoriasis.[G6, G7, G8, G64]

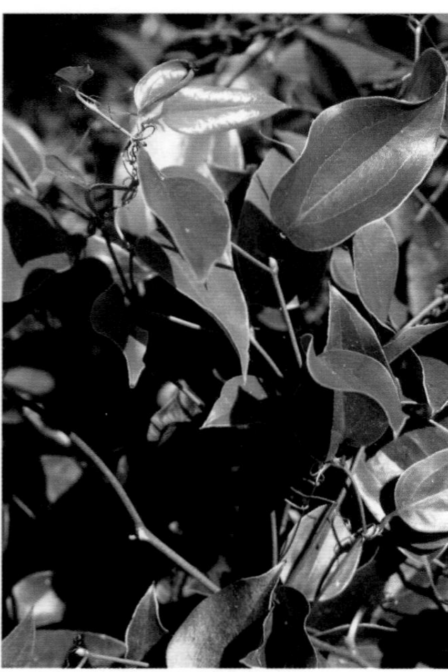

Figure 2 Sarsaparilla (*Smilax regelii*).

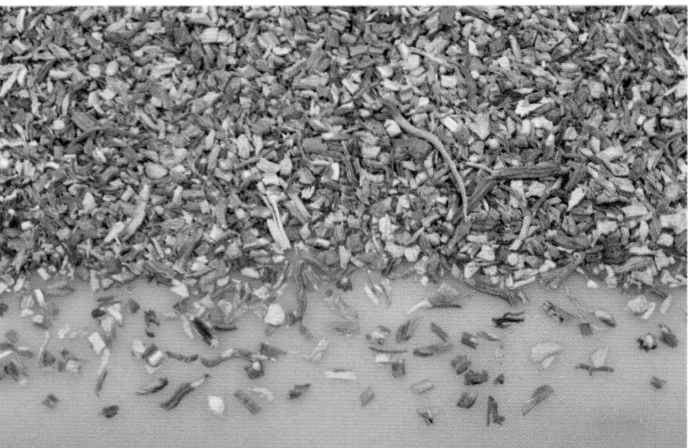

Figure 3 Sarsaparilla – dried drug substance (root).

Dosage

Dosages for oral administration (adults) for traditional uses recommended in standard herbal reference texts are given below.

Dried root 1–4 g as a decoction three times daily.[G6]

Pharmacological Actions

In vitro and animal studies

Anti-inflammatory[2] and hepatoprotective[3] effects have been described following studies in rats.

Clinical studies

There is a lack of clinical research assessing the effects of sarsaparilla and rigorous randomised clinical trials are required. The following observations and uses require assessment in well-designed clinical studies.

Improvement of appetite and digestion[4] as well as a diuretic[4, 5] action have been reported. Limited clinical data utilising extracts indicate improvement in psoriasis;[6] the extract has also been used as an adjuvant for the treatment of leprosy.[7]

Side-effects, Toxicity

None documented for sarsaparilla. However, there is a lack of clinical safety and toxicity data for sarsaparilla and further investigation of these aspects is required. Large doses of saponins are reported to cause gastrointestinal irritation resulting in diarrhoea and vomiting. Although haemolytic activity has been documented for the saponins,[G62] they are not harmful when taken by mouth and are only highly toxic if injected into the bloodstream.[G59]

Contra-indications, Warnings

None documented for sarsaparilla. In view of the possible irritant nature of the saponin constituents, excessive ingestion should be avoided.

Drug interactions None documented. However, the potential for preparations of sarsaparilla to interact with other medicines administered concurrently, particularly those with similar or opposing effects, should be considered.

Pregnancy and lactation There are no known problems with the use of sarsaparilla during pregnancy and lactation. However, in view of the possible irritant nature of the saponin components, excessive ingestion (amounts greater than those found in foods) should be avoided.

Preparations

Proprietary multi-ingredient preparations

Argentina: Urinefrol. *Australia:* Dermaco; Herbal Cleanse; Proesten. *Brazil:* Elixir de Inhame; Elixir de Marinheiro. *Canada:* Damiana-Sarsaparilla Formula. *Italy:* Tisana Kelemata. *Malaysia:* Cleansa Plus; Total Man. *UK:* Gerard House Reumalex; HRI Clear Complexion; Jamaican Sarsaparilla; Napiers Skin Tablets; Skin Eruptions Mixture.

References

1 Sharma SC *et al.* Über Saponine von *Smilax parvifolia* Wall. *Pharmazie* 1980; 35: 646.
2 Ageel AM *et al.* Experimental studies on antirheumatic crude drugs used in Saudi traditional medicine. *Drugs Exp Clin Res* 1989; 15: 369–372.
3 Rafatullah S *et al.* Hepatoprotective and safety evaluation studies on sarsaparilla. *Int J Pharmacog* 1991; 29: 296–301.
4 Harnischfeger G, Stolze H. Smilax species – Sarsaparille. In: *Bewahrte Pflanzendrogen in Wissenschaft und Medizin.* Bad Homburg/Melsungen: Notamed Verlag., 1983: 216–225.
5 Hobbs C. Sarsaparilla – a literature review. *Herbalgram* 1988; 17: 1, 10–15.
6 Thermon FM. The treatment of psoriasis with a sarsaparilla compound. *N Engl J Med* 1942; 227: 128–133.
7 Rollier R. Treatment of lepromatous leprosy by a combination of DDS and sarsaparilla (*Smilax ornata*). *Int J Leprosy* 1959; 27: 328–340.

Sassafras

Summary and Pharmaceutical Comment

In addition to its traditional herbal use for treating dermatological and rheumatic ailments, sassafras also used to be a common flavouring ingredient in beverages, in particular root beer. However, animal studies have revealed the carcinogenic and hepatotoxic potential of safrole, the major component of sassafras volatile oil. Consequently, the use of safrole is no longer permitted in foods and sassafras is not permitted as an ingredient in licensed medicinal products.

Antiseptic and diuretic properties claimed for sassafras are probably attributable to the volatile oil, although no documented studies were found supporting the antirheumatic claims. Sassafras should not be used as a herbal remedy, either internally or externally.

Species (Family)

Sassafras albidum (Nutt.) Nees (Lauraceae)

Synonym(s)

Ague Tree, Cinnamon Wood, Saloop, *Sassafras sassfras* (L.) Karst., *S. albidum* var. *molle* (Raf.) Fern., Saxifrax

Part(s) Used

Inner root bark

Pharmacopoeial and Other Monographs

BHP 1983[G7]
Martindale 35th edition[G85]

Legal Category (Licensed Products)

Sassafras is not permitted for use in medicinal products.

Constituents

The following is compiled from several sources, including General Reference G2.

Alkaloids Isoquinoline-type about 0.02%. Boldine, isoboldine, norboldine, cinnamolaurine, norcinnamolaurine and reticuline.

Volatile oils 5–9%. Safrole as major component (80–90%), others include anethole, apiole, asarone, camphor, caryophyllene, coniferaldehyde, copaene, elemicin, eugenol, 5-methoxyeugenol, menthone, myristicin, α-pinene, α- and β-phellandrene, piperonylacrolein and thujone.

Other constituents Gum, mucilage, lignans (sesamin, desmethoxyaschantin), resin, sitosterol, starch, tannins and wax.

Food Use

Sassafras oil was formerly used as flavouring agent in beverages including root beer.[G58] However, in the 1960s safrole, the major component of the volatile oil, was reported to be carcinogenic.[G58] The use of safrole in foods is now banned, and its use in

Phenylpropanoids

safrole

Alkaloids

R^1O R^2O $N-CH_3$ CH_3O OH

	R^1	R^2
boldine	H	CH_3
isoboldine	CH_3	H

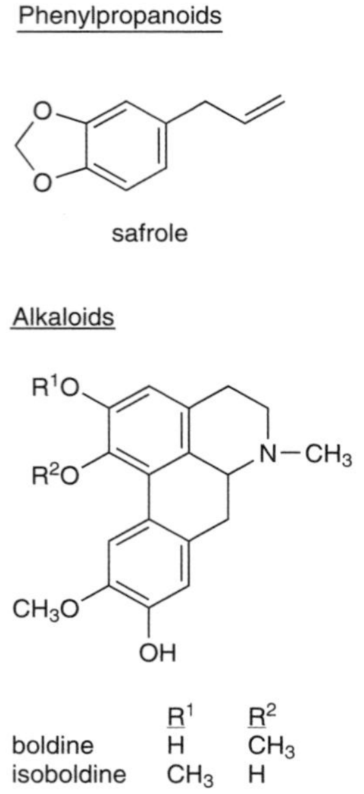

Figure 1 Selected constituents of sassafras.

toilet preparations controlled.[G45] Previously, in the USA, safrole-free sassafras extract, leaf and leaf extract have been approved for food use. In 1976, the US Food and Drugs Administration (FDA) banned interstate marketing of sassafras for sassafras tea.[G22]

Herbal Use

Sassafras is stated to possess carminative, diaphoretic, diuretic, dermatologic and antirheumatic properties. Traditionally, it has been used for cutaneous eruptions, gout and rheumatic pains.[G2, G7, G64]

Dosage

Dosages for oral administration (adults) for traditional uses recommended in standard herbal reference texts are given below. However, sassafras is no longer recommended for internal or external use.

Bark 2–4 g as an infusion three times daily.[G7]

Liquid extract 2–4 mL (1 : 1 in 25% alcohol) three times daily.[G7]

Pharmacological Actions

Studies have concentrated on investigating the toxicity associated with the bark. However, aqueous and alcoholic extracts have been reported to elicit ataxia, hypersensitivity to touch, CNS depression and hypothermia in mice.[1] Both inhibition and induction of hepatic microsomal enzymes have been documented for safrole.[2, 3] Enzyme-inducing activity was found to be a transient phenomenon, with activity falling after the onset of hepatic toxicity (*see* Side-effects, Toxicity).[2] Safrole is reported to induce both cytochrome P488 and P450 activities. Sassafras oil has been used as a topical antiseptic, pediculicide and carminative.[4]

S

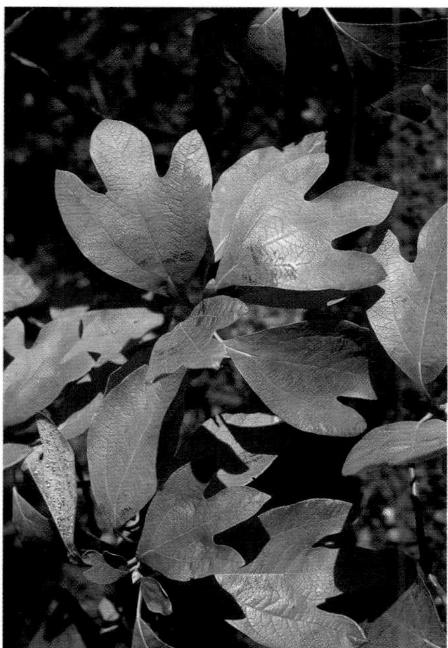

Figure 2 Sassafras (*Sassafras albidum*).

Side-effects, Toxicity

Clinical data

The toxicity of sassafras is attributable to the volatile oil, and in particular to the safrole content. It is estimated that a few drops of sassafras oil are sufficient to kill a toddler and as little as one teaspoonful has proved fatal in an adult.[5] Symptoms of poisoning are described as vomiting, stupor and collapse. High doses may cause spasm followed by paralysis.[G58] Large amounts of the oil are reported to be psychoactive with the hallucinogenic effects lasting for several days.[G22] One of the components of the oil is myristicin, the hallucinogenic principle in nutmeg. Sassafras has traditionally been used as an ingredient of beverages. To put the potential toxicity of sassafras into perspective, the following estimation has been made.[1] Extrapolation of results from animal toxicity studies indicate that 0.66 mg/kg may prove hazardous in humans.[1] By comparison, a cup of sassafras tea, prepared from a 2.5 g teabag, may provide up to 200 mg safrole, representing approximately 3 mg/kg.[1]

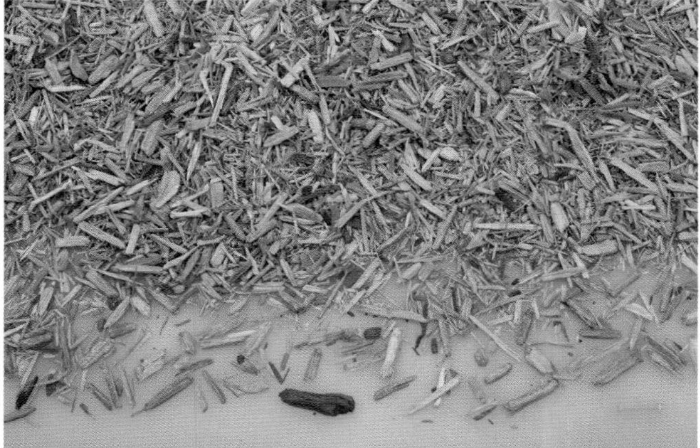

Figure 3 Sassafras – dried drug substance (inner root bark).

Preclinical data

Safrole, the principal component of the volatile oil, was first recognised to be a hepatocarcinogen in the 1960s[6] and many animal studies have been documented concerning this toxicity.[7] Both benign and malignant tumours have developed in laboratory animals, depending on the dose of safrole administered.[2]

Both human and animal studies have shown that safrole gives rise to a large number of metabolites.[8] A sulfate ester (formed via a hydroxylated metabolite) has been established as the ultimate carcinogen for safrole with tumour incidence paralleling the rate of conversion to the ester.[9] Induction of cytochrome P450 activity has been associated with mutagenic and carcinogenic activity of the inducing agent.[10] The inducing effect of safrole on certain metabolising enzymes is thought to play a role in the carcinogenic activity of safrole. The liver has a high level of cytochrome P450 activity and is therefore susceptible to induction.[10]

Acute oral LD_{50} values for safrole have been reported as 1.95 g/kg (rats) and 2.35 g/kg (mice).[2] Major symptoms of toxicity are stated as ataxia, depression, diarrhoea, followed by death within four hours to seven days.[11] Rats fed safrole in their diet at concentrations of 0.25, 0.5 and 1.0% exhibited reduction in growth, stomach and testicular atrophy, liver necrosis, biliary proliferation and primary hepatomas.[G22] Animals have also developed tumours when fed safrole-free extracts.[G22]

Conflicting results have been reported from studies investigating the mutagenicity of safrole, using the Ames test and DNA repair test.[12, 13] Purity of the safrole, test system employed, type of metabolic activation mix, and toxicity of the test system have been suggested as reasons for the observed variations.[12]

Contra-indications, Warnings

Sassafras should not be used internally or externally. Safrole, the major component in the volatile oil of sassafras, is hepatotoxic and even safrole-free extracts of sassafras have been reported to produce tumours in animals. Sassafras essential oil is contra-indicated in internal and external use.[G58] Sassafras has been reported to inhibit and induce microsomal enzymes.

Pregnancy and lactation Sassafras is contra-indicated during pregnancy and lactation. The oil is reported to be abortifacient.[5]

References

1 Segelman AB *et al*. Sassafras and herb tea. Potential health hazards. *JAMA* 1976; 238: 477.
2 Opdyke DLJ. Safrole. *Food Cosmet Toxicol* 1974; 12: 983–986.
3 Jaffe H *et al*. *In vivo* inhibition of mouse liver microsomal hydroxylating systems by methylenedioxyphenyl insecticidal synergists and related compounds. *Life Sci* 1968; 7: 1051–1062.
4 International Agency for Research on Cancer. *IARC Monographs on the Evaluation of Carcinogenic Risk of Chemicals to Man. Some Naturally Occurring Substances, vol 10*. Geneva: WHO, 1976.
5 Craig JO. Poisoning by the volatile oils in childhood. *Arch Dis Child* 1953; 28: 475–483.
6 Homburger F, Boger E. The carcinogenicity of essential oils, flavors, and spices: A review. *Cancer Res* 1968; 28: 2372–2374.
7 Opdyke DLJ. Sassafras oil. *Food Cosmet Toxicol* 1982; 20: 825–826.
8 Ioannides C *et al*. Safrole: its metabolism, carcinogenicity and interactions with cytochrome P-450. *Food Cosmet Toxicol* 1981; 19: 657–666.
9 Bock KW, Schirmer G. Species differences of glucuronidation and sulfation in relation to hepatocarcinogenesis. *Arch Toxicol* 1987; 10 (Suppl. Suppl.): 125–135.

10 Iwasaki K *et al*. Induction of cytochrome P-448 activity as exemplified by the *O*-deethylation of ethoxyresorufin. Effects of dose, sex, tissue and animal species. *Biochem Pharmacol* 1986; 35: 3879–3884.

11 Jenner PM *et al*. Food flavourings and compounds of related structure. I. Acute oral toxicity. *Food Cosmet Toxicol* 1964; 2: 327–343.

12 Sekizawa J, Shibamoto T. Genotoxicity of safrole-related chemicals in microbial test systems. *Mutat Res* 1982; 101: 127–140.

13 Swanson AB *et al*. The mutagenicities of safrole, estragole, eugenol, *trans*-anethole, and some of their known or possible metabolites for *Salmonella typhimurium* mutants. *Mutat Res* 1979; 60: 143–153.

Saw Palmetto

Summary and Pharmaceutical Comment

The chemistry of saw palmetto is well-documented. Several pharmacological activities have been described for saw palmetto *in vitro* and *in vivo* (animals). Some of these properties, such as inhibition of 5-α-reductase activity, inhibition of androgen binding and spasmolytic activity, are thought to explain, at least in part, the effects of saw palmetto in benign prostatic hyperplasia (BPH). However, some experimental and clinical studies report conflicting results, particularly with regard to the inhibition of 5-α-reductase activity and α-adrenoceptor blocking activity by saw palmetto extracts. Thus, the mechanism(s) of action of saw palmetto extracts in BPH remain unclear. This is not surprising, given that, at present, the exact cause of BPH is unknown. In addition to the effects of saw palmetto in experimental models of BPH, immunostimulant and anti-inflammatory activities have been documented in laboratory studies.

BPH is not an indication suitable for self-diagnosis and self-treatment, and over-the-counter use of saw palmetto extract for BPH should be under medical supervision.

Collectively, evidence from clinical trials of saw palmetto products indicates that preparations containing saw palmetto improve urinary symptoms and flow measures in men with BPH and that improvement is similar to that achieved with finasteride.

Data from randomised clinical trials and post-marketing surveillance studies indicate that, generally, saw palmetto is well-tolerated; typically, adverse events reported are mild and relate mainly to gastrointestinal symptoms. Use of saw palmetto preparations at doses higher than those recommended for therapeutic effects should be avoided; further information is required on the safety of saw palmetto with long-term use (more than one year). There is a lack of information of the safety of saw palmetto when taken by women (e.g. for acne). In view of the documented pharmacological actions of saw palmetto preparations, the potential for interactions with other medicines administered concurrently, particularly those with similar or opposing effects, should be considered. Studies have assessed the effects of combination preparations containing saw palmetto, as well as different manufacturers' products (which vary qualitatively and quantitatively in their phytochemical composition); at least eight studies involved one particular saw palmetto product. These points should be taken into account when considering the evidence to support the efficacy and safety of individual products. PC-SPES, a combination preparation containing saw palmetto fruit extract and seven other herbal ingredients, has been found to be adulterated with diethylstilbestrol, indometacin (indomethacin), warfarin and ethinylestradiol.

Species (Family)

Serenoa repens (W. Bart.) Small (Arecaceae/Palmae)

Synonym(s)

Sabal, *Sabal serrulata* (Michx.) Schult. f., Serenoa, *Serenoa serrulata* (Michx.) Hook. f. ex B.D. Jacks

Part(s) Used

Fruit

Pharmacopoeial and Other Monographs

BHP 1996[G9]
BHMA 2003[G66]
BP 2007[G84]
BPC 1934[G10]
Complete German Commission E[G3]
ESCOP 2003[G76]
Martindale 35th edition[G85]
Ph Eur 2007[G81]
USP29/NF24[G86]

Legal Category (Licensed Products)

GSL[G37]

Constituents

Carbohydrates Invert sugar 28.2%, mannitol, high molecular weight polysaccharides (e.g. MW 100 000) with galactose, arabinose and uronic acid[1] identified as main sugar components for one.

Fixed oils 26.7%. Many free fatty acids and their glycerides. Monoacylglycerides (1-monolaurin, 1-monomyristicin).[2] Oleic acid (unsaturated) and capric acid, caproic acid, caprylic acid, lauric acid, myristic acid, palmitic acid and stearic acid (saturated).

Steroids β-Sitosterol, campesterol, stigmasterol and other compounds.[3–5]

Other constituents Flavonoids (e.g. rutin, isoquercitrin, kaempferol),[5] pigment (carotene), resin, tannin and volatile oil 1.5%.

Most commercial preparations of saw palmetto contain lipophilic extracts.[G56]

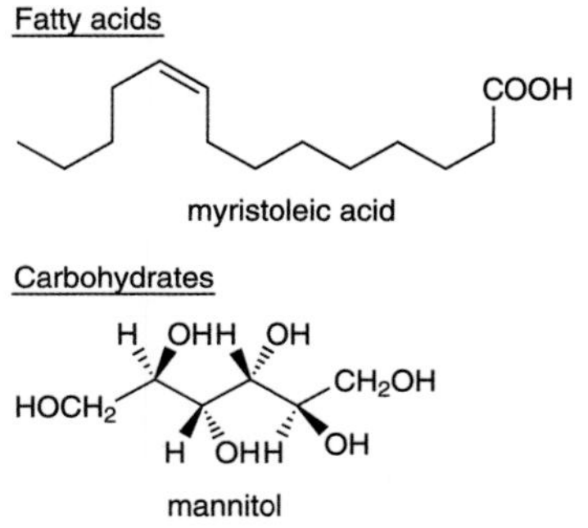

Figure 1 Selected constituents of saw palmetto.

S

Quality of plant material and commercial products

As with other herbal medicinal products, there is variation in the qualitative and quantitative composition of saw palmetto crude plant material and commercial preparations of saw palmetto fruit. Analysis of 14 saw palmetto products marketed in Europe and the USA for content of specific groups of constituents using liquid and gas chromatography revealed substantial variations in the concentrations of constituents present in different products.[6] Free fatty acid content ranged from 40.7% (in one product which contained 50% olive oil) to 80.7%, content of methyl and ethyl esters ranged from 1.5% (in one product which contained 50% olive oil) to 16.7%, long-chain esters from 0.7% to 1.4% and glycerides from 6.8% to 52.2% (in one product which contained 50% olive oil). Although it is clear that there are variations between products, data from this analytical study are difficult to interpret as values for actual content of the respective constituents were not reported.

Food Use

Saw palmetto is not used in foods. Previously, saw palmetto has been listed by the Food and Drugs Administration (FDA) as a Herb of Undefined Safety.[G41]

Herbal Use

Saw palmetto is stated to possess diuretic, urinary antiseptic, endocrinological and anabolic properties. Traditionally, it has been used for chronic or subacute cystitis, catarrh of the genitourinary tract, testicular atrophy, sex hormone disorders and specifically for prostatic enlargement.[G7, G32, G64] Modern interest in saw palmetto is focused on its use in the treatment of symptoms of benign prostatic hyperplasia (BPH).

Dosage

Dosages for oral administration (adults) for traditional uses recommended in older standard herbal reference texts are given below.

Dried fruit 0.5–1.0 g as a decoction three times daily.[G7]

Extract 320 mg lipophilic ingredients extracted with lipophilic solvents (hexane or ethanol 90% v/v).[G3]

Clinical trials have assessed the effects of lipophilic extracts (containing lipids and sterols) of saw palmetto usually at a dosage of 160 mg twice daily.

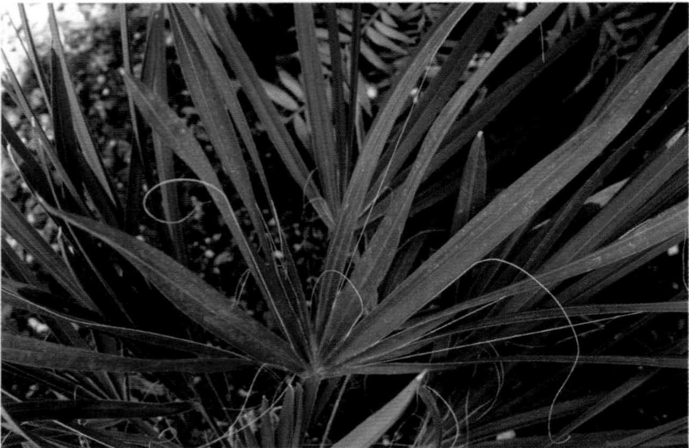

Figure 2 Saw palmetto (*Serenoa repens*).

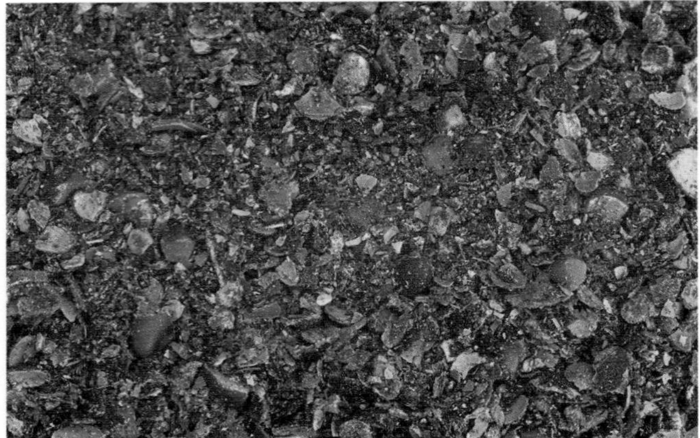

Figure 3 Saw palmetto – dried drug substance (fruit).

Pharmacological Actions

In vitro and animal studies

Several pharmacological activities have been documented for saw palmetto *in vitro* and *in vivo* (animals). Several of these properties, such as inhibition of 5-α-reductase activity, inhibition of androgen binding and spasmolytic activity, are thought to explain, at least in part, the effects of saw palmetto in BPH. However, the clinical significance of the *in vitro* inhibition of 5-α-reductase activity by saw palmetto has not been clearly established (*see* Clinical studies).

5-α-Reductase is the enzyme that catalyses the conversion of testosterone to 5-α-dihydrotestosterone (DHT) in androgen target tissues, including the prostate. DHT is more potent than testosterone, and is thought to be implicated in the development of BPH. There is evidence that 5-α-reductase activity is higher in cells obtained from BPH tissue than from normal prostate tissue.

A lipidic (liposterolic) extract of saw palmetto was found to inhibit 5-α-reductase-mediated conversion of testosterone to dihydrotestosterone, and 3-ketosteroid reductase-mediated conversion of dihydrotestosterone to an androgen derivative.[5] Other *in vitro* studies have shown that an ethanolic extract of saw palmetto (IDS-89) inhibited 5-α-reductase activity in the epithelium and stroma of human BPH tissue in a concentration-dependent manner.[7] The IC_{50} was around 2.2 mg/mL. This study also demonstrated that the inhibitory effect of IDS-89 was mainly due to the fatty acid constituents of a saponifiable subfraction of the extract, as non-saponifiable and hydrophilic subfractions showed little or no inhibition of 5-α-reductase activity. Inhibition of 5-α-reductase by a liposterolic extract of saw palmetto has also been documented in porcine prostatic microsomes.[8]

There are at least two isoenzymes of 5-α-reductase (5-α-reductase types I and II), and several studies have documented that a liposterolic extract (Permixon) of saw palmetto inhibits both isoenzymes in prostate epithelial cells[9, 10] and fibroblast cells.[10] Several other studies have documented inhibition of 5-α-reductase activity by liposterolic extracts of saw palmetto *in vitro*.[5, G50] Permixon was reported to inhibit 5-α-reductase activity without affecting the secretion of prostate-specific antigen (PSA) by epithelial cells, suggesting that use of saw palmetto extract should not interfere with PSA measurements for prostate-cancer screening.[9]

Anti-androgenic activity has been documented for a hexane liposterolic extract (Permixon) of saw palmetto. *In vitro* studies in rat prostate tissue and human foreskin fibroblasts indicated that this extract competitively inhibited the binding of dihydrotestosterone to cytosolic and nuclear androgen receptor sites.[11,12] By contrast, an alcoholic extract of saw palmetto appeared to be without androgen receptor-binding activity.[13]

Liposterolic extracts of saw palmetto have also been investigated in animal models of BPH. A liposterolic extract (Permixon) of saw palmetto 50 mg/kg body weight administered for 30 days to castrated rats with estradiol/testosterone-induced prostate enlargement resulted in significant reductions in the wet weight of the dorsal region of the prostate, compared with control.[14] Another study in rats compared the effects of a liposterolic extract of saw palmetto with those of the 5-α-reductase inhibitor finasteride in rat prostate hyperplasia induced by hyperprolactinaemia.[15] It was reported that the liposterolic extract of saw palmetto inhibited rat prostate hyperplasia in the lateral lobe induced by hyperprolactinaemia, and that finasteride did not antagonise the action of prolactin. By contrast, a study in dogs with BPH reported a lack of effect for saw palmetto extract on prostatic weight, prostatic volume, prostatic histologic scores, prostatic ultrasonographs and serum testosterone concentrations.[16] In the study, 20 dogs with BPH, determined by raised prostatic volume and prostatic volume per kilogram body weight, received saw palmetto extract (type of extract not specified) 1500 mg daily in meatballs ($n = 8$), 300 mg daily in meatballs ($n = 6$) or unmedicated meatballs ($n = 6$), for 91 days. Dogs included in this study did not have clinical signs of BPH (i.e. decreased urinary flow and residual urine volume) that often occur in human males with BPH. Dogs did not appear to be randomly assigned to treatment, and the mean prostatic volume in the control group was higher than that in the active treatment groups before treatment, although it was stated that this was not statistically significant. Assessments and data analysis were carried out by blinded investigators.

Spasmolytic activity and effects on the micturition reflex have also been documented for saw palmetto extract, although the contribution of these effects to effects in men with BPH is unclear. In anaesthetised, saline-infused rats, mean micturition interval, micturition volume and bladder capacity were significantly increased, and maximum micturition pressure was significantly decreased, compared with baseline values ($p < 0.05$ for each), in animals that received intraduodenal administration of saw palmetto extract (Permixon) at a dose of 60 mg/kg body weight, but not 6 mg/kg body weight.[17] In anaesthetised rats infused with 0.1% acetic acid, mean micturition interval, micturition volume and bladder capacity were significantly increased, compared with baseline values ($p < 0.05$ for each), in animals that received intraduodenal administration of saw palmetto extract (Permixon) at a dose of 12 or 20 mg/kg body weight. However, p values for statistical tests comparing saw palmetto-treated rats with vehicle-treated rats (control group) are not reported for these sets of experiments. In rats given saw palmetto extract 6 mg/kg body weight orally for 14 days, total mean micturition volume was increased significantly, compared with baseline values, for days 9 to 14 ($p < 0.05$); however, a comparison with a parallel control group was not reported. Further experiments using rat bladder and prostate tissues showed that saw palmetto extract (10 to 300 μg/mL) competitively inhibited the binding of [N-methyl-^{3}H]-scopolamine methyl chloride (IC_{50} 46 μg/mL in bladder tissue) and [^{3}H]-prazosin (IC_{50} 183 μg/mL in prostate tissue) in a concentration-dependent manner.[17]

An ethanolic lipidic extract was reported to produce a concentration-dependent relaxation of rat uterus tonic contraction induced by vanadate (EC_{50} 11.41 μg/mL).[18] Further investigation suggested that a mechanism for the observed effect could be interference with intracellular calcium mobilisation, possibly mediated via cyclic AMP. Other *in vitro* studies demonstrated that a lipophilic ethanolic extract of saw palmetto 0.3–0.75 mg/mL reduced norepinephrine (noradrenaline)-induced contractions in rat deferential duct. Further study indicated that the relaxant effect of saw palmetto extract results from either α-adrenoceptor blockade or from calcium-blocking activity.[19]

Cytotoxic and related activities In a study using human prostate tissue, a liposterolic extract of saw palmetto (Permixon) 30 μg/mL significantly inhibited basic fibroblast growth factor-induced proliferation of human prostate cell cultures, compared with control, although the extract did not affect basal prostate cell proliferation.[20] An unsaponified fraction of the extract also markedly inhibited basic fibroblast growth factor-induced cell proliferation, but had only a minimal effect on basal cell proliferation. In a study using stromal and epithelial tissue from normal prostate and from patients with BPH, cell numbers and proliferative indices were found to be higher in BPH tissue than in tissue from normal prostates.[21] In tissue from patients with BPH who had been treated with a liposterolic extract of saw palmetto (Permixon), there was significant induction of apoptosis and inhibition of cell proliferation, compared with tissue from patients with BPH who had not received saw palmetto extract. In another *in vitro* study, incubation with Permixon 10 μg/mL also increased the apoptotic index for prostate epithelial cells by 35%.[10]

Other *in vitro* studies have explored the effects of saw palmetto extract and its constituents on human prostatic cancer cells and other tumour cell lines. An extract of saw palmetto fruit, prepared by supercritical fluid extraction with carbon dioxide, induced cell death in LNCaP cells (a hormonal therapy-resistant prostatic cancer cell line) in a concentration-dependent manner.[22] This confirms the findings of previous studies demonstrating the effect of a liposterolic extract of saw palmetto (Permixon) on the mortality rate of LNCaP cells: increased mortality was observed with saw palmetto extract 50 μg/mL, compared with control.[23] Further investigation identified myristoleic acid as a component of saw palmetto extract that caused cell death. The EC_{50} for both the extract and myristoleic acid was around 100 μg/mL.[22] Following incubation of LNCaP cells with saw palmetto extract 130 μg/mL or myristoleic acid 100 μg/mL, the proportions of apoptotic and necrotic cells were 16.5% and 46.8%, respectively, for the extract, and 8.8% and 81.8%, respectively, for myristoleic acid. An extract of saw palmetto obtained by supercritical extraction with carbon dioxide inhibited the invasion of PC-3 cells (derived from human adenocarcinoma of the prostate) into Matrigel *in vitro* in a concentration-dependent manner at concentrations in the range 1–10 μg/mL.[24] However, LNCaP cells and SKRC-1 cells (derived from human renal carcinoma) were unaffected by the extract. The extract was also shown to inhibit the activity of urokinase-type plasminogen activator, a protease enzyme that is necessary for tumour-cell invasion into basement membranes. The monoacylglycerides 1-monolaurin and 1-monomyristicin isolated from saw palmetto demonstrated *in vitro* activity against renal (A-498) and pancreatic (PACA-2) human tumour cells (EC_{50} for 1-monolaurin: 3.77 μg/mL and 2.33 μg/mL, respectively; EC_{50} for 1-monomyristicin: 3.58 μg/mL and 1.87 μg/mL, respectively).[2] However, only borderline cytotoxicity was observed against PC-3 cells (EC_{50} for 1-monomyristicin: 8.84 μg/mL).[2]

PC-SPES, a combination preparation containing saw palmetto fruit extract and seven other herbal ingredients, has cytotoxic and pro-apoptotic activity *in vitro* in prostate carcinoma cells,[25] and in drug-sensitive (H69) and drug-resistant (H69V) human small-cell lung carcinoma cells.[26] Batches of PC-SPES have, however, been found to be adulterated with diethylstilbestrol, indometacin and/or warfarin, and cytotoxic activity in prostate carcinoma cells has been attributed to these contaminants.[25] In contrast, in experiments involving H69 and H69V cells, the cytotoxic activity of the contaminants was insufficient to account for the cytotoxicity of PC-SPES.[26] Adding contaminants to a 'less' contaminated batch of PC-SPES did not alter the cytotoxic activity of the herbal preparation in H69 and H69V cells. None of the contaminants displayed apoptotic activity at concentrations found as contaminants and higher, whereas both contaminated and 'less contaminated' batches of PC-SPES exhibited pro-apoptotic activity in these small-cell lung carcinoma cell lines.[25]

Other activities *In vivo* oestrogenic activity in the rat has also been documented for an alcoholic extract.[27] Activity was attributed to the high content of β-sitosterol, a known oestrogenic agent, present in saw palmetto.

In vivo anti-oedema activity in the rat has been documented for a hexane extract of saw palmetto, acting by inhibition of histamine-induced increase in capillary permeability.[28] Low doses of an aqueous extract were effective in carrageenan-induced paw oedema and pellet tests in the rat, although the extract was not found to influence the proliferative stage of inflammation.[1,29] The observed anti-inflammatory activity was attributed to a high molecular weight polysaccharide (approximately 100 000). Polysaccharides possessing immunostimulating activity have also been documented for saw palmetto and were stated to contain a high content of glucuronic acid.[1,29]

An extract (SG-291) prepared from saw palmetto fruits by supercritical fluid extraction with carbon dioxide was reported to inhibit both cyclooxygenase and 5-lipoxygenase *in vitro* (IC_{50} 28.1 μg/mL and 18.0 μg/mL, respectively).[30] Further study indicated that the component(s) of saw palmetto extract that inhibits these enzymes must be within the acidic lipophilic fraction. Subsequent studies have documented that a liposterolic extract of saw palmetto (Permixon) significantly inhibited the production of 5-lipoxygenase metabolites, including leukotriene B_4, by human polymorphonuclear neutrophils at concentrations of saw palmetto extract of 5 μg/mL and above.[31]

S

Clinical studies

Pharmacokinetics Some data on the pharmacokinetics of saw palmetto extracts in healthy male volunteers (n = 12) come from an open, randomised, single-dose bioequivalence study of a 320-mg capsule of a liposterolic extract of saw palmetto compared with two capsules of saw palmetto extract 160 mg as the reference preparation.[32] The plasma concentration–time curves were reported to be almost identical for both preparations. The maximum concentration (C_{max}) for saw palmetto extract 320-mg capsule and 2 × 160-mg capsules was 2.54–2.61 μg/mL and 2.57–2.67 μg/mL, respectively, and time to C_{max} (T_{max}) was 1.58 and 1.5 hours for the 320-mg capsule and 2 × 160-mg capsules, respectively. Another study explored the bioavailability and pharmacokinetic profile of a rectal formulation of saw palmetto extract 640 mg in healthy male volunteers (n = 12).[33] The mean maximum plasma concentration of the second component of saw palmetto was almost 2.6 μg/mL at around three hours after drug administration.

Pharmacodynamics The inhibitory effects of saw palmetto extract on 5-α-reductase activity documented *in vitro* (*see* Pharmacological Actions, *In vitro* and animal studies) have been confirmed in some studies in humans, and refuted by others.

In one study, 25 men with symptomatic, established BPH were randomised to receive either a liposterolic extract of saw palmetto (Permixon) 320 mg/day for three months (n = 10), or no treatment (n = 15).[34] At the end of the treatment period, analysis of samples of BPH tissue, obtained by suprapubic prostatectomy, showed that dihydrotestosterone concentrations were significantly reduced and that testosterone concentrations were significantly higher in the treatment group, compared with the control group ($p < 0.001$ for both). A significant reduction in concentrations of epidermal growth factor in total BPH tissue was also observed in the treatment group, compared with the control group ($p < 0.01$). The reported biochemical effects were most evident in BPH tissue from the periurethral region.

In another study, biopsy specimens of the prostate were taken from 44 men with symptomatic BPH participating in a randomised, placebo-controlled trial of a herbal combination preparation containing saw palmetto lipoidal extract 106 mg together with nettle root extract, pumpkin seed oil, lemon bioflavonoid extract and vitamin A.[35,36] There were no statistically significant differences in median tissue dihydrotestosterone and testosterone concentrations between the treatment and placebo groups at baseline. At the end of the study, mean tissue dihydrotestosterone concentrations decreased significantly in the treatment group, compared with baseline values ($p = 0.005$), whereas there was no significant change in dihydrotestosterone concentrations in the placebo group. However, in a separate analysis, it was reported that the median change in tissue dihydrotestosterone concentrations for the treatment group (1.38 ng/g) did not differ significantly from the corresponding change in the placebo group (0.87 ng/g). The findings of this study should be interpreted cautiously as it is possible there are other explanations for the observed effect.

Another randomised, double-blind trial involving 18 men with BPH compared saw palmetto extract (IDS-89; Strogen) 640 mg three times daily (i.e. six times the normal dose) for three months with placebo.[37] This high dose of saw palmetto extract achieved only a moderate decrease in 5-α-reductase activity.

An open, randomised, placebo-controlled study involving 32 healthy male volunteers compared the effects of a liposterolic extract of saw palmetto (Permixon) 80 mg twice daily for seven days with those of finasteride 5 mg daily for seven days on inhibition of 5-α-reductase activity.[38] Serum dihydrotestosterone concentrations were reported to decrease significantly with finasteride, compared with baseline values, but no significant changes were observed for the saw palmetto and placebo groups. Thus, this study did not support a mechanism of action for saw palmetto in BPH by inhibition of 5-α-reductase activity.

In addition, in a double-blind, placebo-controlled, four-way, crossover study in which 12 healthy male volunteers received three different saw palmetto extract preparations (Prostagutt uno, Prostess uno, Talso uno; 320 mg daily for eight days each, separated by wash-out phases of at least two weeks), none of the study medications showed signs of α_1-adrenoceptor subtype occupancy as determined by a radioreceptor assay.[39]

Effects of saw palmetto fruit extract on certain cytokines have also been described. In an open, randomised, multicentre study, 30 men with BPH received a liposterolic extract of *Serenoa repens* (Permixon) 160 mg twice daily for three months before undergoing surgery, or to no treatment for three weeks before undergoing surgery.[40] It was stated that at the end of the three-month treatment period, prostatic tissue concentrations of the cytokines TNF-α and interleukin-1β were significantly lower in Permixon recipients, compared with participants in the no-treatment control group (p = 0.012 and 0.004, respectively). No significant differences were observed, however, in concentrations of IL-6, TGF (transforming growth factor) or EGF (epidermal growth factor).

The effects of a combination preparation containing 106 mg of a lipoidal extract of saw palmetto, as well as nettle root extract, pumpkin seed oil, lemon bioflavonoid extract and vitamin A, were assessed in a randomised, double-blind, placebo-controlled trial involving 40 men with symptomatic BPH.[41] At the end of the six-month study, 23/60 and 25/60 nuclear morphometric descriptors (NMDs) for nuclei of 200 randomly selected epithelial cells were altered, compared with baseline characteristics, in prostatic tissue from men in the treatment group and placebo groups, respectively. A statistically significant multivariate change from baseline in NMDs was apparent for the treatment group but not the placebo group. These preliminary data may reflect effects such as alterations in gene expression, but this and the contribution of the saw palmetto extract, require testing in further studies.[41]

Therapeutic effects Numerous clinical studies have investigated the effects of saw palmetto extracts in men with BPH.

A systematic review and meta-analysis included 21 randomised controlled clinical trials (18 of which were double-blind) of saw palmetto extracts involving a total of 3139 men with BPH.[42] This work is an update of a previous Cochrane systematic review.[43] The updated review included 12 studies which compared saw palmetto extracts alone with placebo, four comparing saw palmetto extracts in combination with other herbals with placebo, two comparing saw palmetto extracts alone with an active control, one comparing saw palmetto extracts in combination with other herbals with an active control, one comparing saw palmetto extract with another herb and with placebo, and one comparing oral saw palmetto extract with a rectal formulation of saw palmetto extract. The mean duration of the included studies was 13 weeks (range 4–48 weeks).

Compared with placebo, saw palmetto extracts were associated with a decrease in urinary symptom scores (weighted mean difference (WMD), 95% confidence interval (CI): −1.41, −2.52 to −0.30; one trial), nocturia (WMD, 95% CI: −0.76, −1.21 to −0.32; ten trials) and residual volume (WMD, 95% CI: −22.95, −42.33 to −3.56; six trials), and improvements in peak urine flow (WMD, 95% CI: 1.86, 0.60 to 3.12; nine trials), mean urine flow (WMD, 95% CI: 2.23, 1.18 to 3.27; four trials) and physician and self-rating of urinary symptoms (weighted risk ratio, 95% CI: 1.72, 1.11 to 2.66; three trials and 1.76, 1.21 to 2.54; six trials, respectively).[42] Saw palmetto extracts had no effect, however, on prostate size.

Compared with finasteride, saw palmetto extracts (mono- and combination preparations) achieved similar improvements in urinary symptom scores, frequency of nocturia, peak urine flow, mean urine flow and residual volume, but not prostate size.

The conclusions of the review were that there is evidence that preparations containing saw palmetto improve urinary symptoms and flow measures in men with BPH and that improvement is similar to that achieved with finasteride. However, the review included trials which assessed the effects of preparations containing saw palmetto alone and in combination with other herbal ingredients, as well as saw palmetto preparations produced by different manufacturers, which vary qualitatively and quantitatively in their phytochemical composition (although at least eight studies involved one particular saw palmetto product). The results of the trials discussed above cannot necessarily be transferred to other saw palmetto products unless they are pharmaceutically and bioequivalent.

Another systematic review and meta-analysis included only trials involving a particular saw palmetto extract (Permixon) in men with BPH. The review included 14 randomised controlled trials (several of which were included in the Cochrane review[42] described above), of which nine were placebo-controlled, four compared Permixon with standard drugs (finasteride, tamsulosin, prazosin, alfuzosin) and one compared two doses of Permixon; the remaining three were open, uncontrolled studies. The meta-analysis found similar results to that of the Cochrane review: compared with placebo, Permixon resulted in a significant improvement in peak flow rate and a reduction in nocturia, and a five-point reduction in International Prostate Symptom Scale (IPSS) score.[44] Data from an unpublished study included in the meta-analysis have recently been published.[45,46]

A randomised, double-blind, placebo-controlled trial involving 100 men with BPH published since the Cochrane review found no statistically significant effects for a carbon dioxide extract of *S. repens* 320 mg daily on symptoms of BPH as assessed using IPSS scores, peak urinary flow rate and the International Index of Erectile Function questionnaire.[47] A sample size calculation was used in determining the size of the study, so it seems unlikely that the trial did not have sufficient statistical power to detect a difference between groups. This finding is in contrast to findings from previous studies, and warrants further investigation, particularly with respect to the phytochemical composition of the extract relative to that of other preparations for which significant effects on symptoms of BPH have been described. Another randomised, double-blind, placebo-controlled trial not included in the Cochrane review assessed the effects of a combination preparation containing saw palmetto complex (standardised for 40–50% free fatty acids and β-sitosterol 43%), cernitin (a pollen mixture comprising rye, timothy and corn) and vitamin E two 'pills' daily (equivalent to total daily doses of saw palmetto and β-sitosterol 286 mg, cernitin 378 mg, vitamin E 100 IU and β-sitosterol) for 90 days in 144 men with symptoms of BPH. At the end of the study, statistically significant differences were reported for the treatment group, compared with placebo, in nocturia, urinary frequency and total American Urological Association symptom score.[48]

Several other clinical studies of saw palmetto extracts in BPH have been conducted although these did not meet the inclusion criteria for the Cochrane review.

In a study involving 75 men with mild/moderate BPH according to their International Prostate Symptom Score (IPSS), participants received a liposterolic extract of saw palmetto (Permixon) 160 mg twice daily for nine weeks (n = 57).[49] A control group (n = 18) did not receive any medical treatment for BPH, and there was no random allocation to treatment, although it was stated that baseline parameters were comparable between the two groups. It was reported that, at the end of the study, IPSS and quality-of-life scores, compared with baseline values, significantly improved in Permixon-treated men (p < 0.001). There were no significant differences in these parameters, compared with baseline values, for the control group.

Two randomised studies involving men with symptomatic BPH have compared the effects of different regimens of saw palmetto extract.[50,51] A multi-centre, randomised, single-blind trial involving 132 men with BPH compared the effects of saw palmetto extract (Prostaserene) 320 mg once daily with 160 mg twice daily for one year.[50] Another study compared a liposterolic extract of saw palmetto (Permixon) 320 mg daily with 160 mg twice daily for three months in 100 men with symptomatic BPH.[51] For each regimen, both studies reported significant improvements in the mean IPSS, maximum and mean urinary flow rates and residual urine volume, at the end of the studies, compared with baseline values. However, as these studies did not include a placebo-control group, the possibility that the observed effects are placebo effects cannot be excluded.

Several open, uncontrolled studies of saw palmetto extracts (alone or in combination with other herbs), several of which were drug-monitoring studies which also assessed effectiveness, have reported improvements in symptoms of BPH at the end of treatment, compared with baseline values.[52–56] Doses assessed in these studies were usually 160 mg two or three times daily for up to three years. These studies are discussed in more detail later (*see* Side-effects, Toxicity).

A small number of studies have explored the effects of saw palmetto extracts in disorders other than BPH. In a single-blind, controlled trial, 64 men with USA National Institutues of Health category III prostatitis (chronic pelvic pain syndrome) were randomised to receive saw palmetto extract 325 mg daily (not further specified), or finasteride 5 mg daily, for one year.[57] At the end of the study, the proportion of participants with a statistically significant improvement in Chronic Prostatitis Symptom Index score was higher for finasteride, compared with placebo (65% versus 24%; $p < 0.02$).

The effects of a softgel capsule preparation containing saw palmetto extract 200 mg (standardised for 85–95% liposterolic content) and β-sitosterol 50 mg in the treatment of androgenetic alopecia (which affects men and women) were assessed in a randomised, double-blind, placebo-controlled pilot trial.[58] In the study, 26 men aged 23 to 64 years with mild-to-moderate androgenetic alopecia received one softgel capsule, or placebo, twice daily for up to 21 weeks (precise duration of treatment not stated). Overall, 19 men completed the study and, for these, investigator-assessed hair growth was deemed to be improved in a greater proportion of those who received the active treatment, compared with those who received placebo (60% versus 11%), although no statistical tests were undertaken. With respect to participants' self-assessment of their hair condition, none of the active treatment recipients thought their condition had deteriorated, compared with 33% of placebo recipients. The hypothesis that saw palmetto extract (with β-sitosterol) is beneficial in androgenetic alopecia requires testing in well-designed randomised controlled trials.

Saw palmetto is one of the eight herbal ingredients contained in a commercial preparation known as PC-SPES; the other herbal ingredients were stated as being chrysanthemum, isatis, licorice, *Ganoderma lucidum*, *Panax pseudoginseng*, *Rabdosia rubescens* and *Scutellaria* (scullcap). The combination preparation has been investigated for oestrogenic activity, and for its potential effects in the treatment of hormone-sensitive prostate cancer.[59] In a randomised, controlled, crossover trial, 90 men with androgen-independent prostate cancer received three capsules of PC-SPES three times daily, or diethylstilbestrol 3 mg once daily. Participants crossed to the other arm of the study on reaching clinical or prostate-specific antigen progression. The median times to progression for PC-SPES and diethylstilboestrol were 5.5 and 2.9 months, respectively.[60] However, the study was terminated prematurely because PC-SPES was withdrawn from the market after being found to be contaminated with diethylstilbesterol and ethinylestradiol. Other contaminants, including warfarin and indometacin have also been reported.[25,26]

Side-effects, Toxicity

Clinical data

A systematic review and meta-analysis included 21 randomised controlled clinical trials (18 of which were double-blind) of saw palmetto extracts involving a total of 3139 men with BPH (*see* Clinical studies, Therapeutic effects).[42] Of these,12 studies compared saw palmetto extracts alone with placebo; the mean duration of all included studies was 13 weeks (range 4–48 weeks). The review found that the frequency and type of adverse events reported for saw palmetto extracts were similar to those reported for placebo. There were no statistically significant differences between participant withdrawal rates for saw palmetto, placebo and finasteride (8.9, 7.1 and 9.0%, respectively; $p = 0.17$ for saw palmetto versus placebo and $p = 1.0$ for saw palmetto versus finasteride), and in the frequency of gastrointestinal adverse events (1.3, 0.9, 1.5%, respectively; $p > 0.5$ for saw palmetto versus finasteride). Impotence was reported more frequently by finasteride recipients than by saw palmetto recipients, or placebo recipients (4.9, 1.1 and 0.7%, respectively; $p < 0.001$ for saw palmetto versus finasteride and $p= 0.58$ for saw palmetto versus placebo).[42] Clinical trials, however, are designed primarily to assess efficacy, not safety, and have the statistical power only to detect common acute adverse effects.

Several post-marketing surveillance type studies involving over 4000 men with BPH have assessed the safety and tolerability of different saw palmetto extracts taken at recommended doses and have also found preparations to be well-tolerated. Studies conducted to date have, however, assessed the effects of several different preparations of saw palmetto extract; these are likely to vary qualitatively and quantitatively in their pharmaceutical quality, and the implications of this for safety of specific products should be considered. Some studies have monitored the effects of longer term treatment (one to three years) with saw palmetto preparations, but further well-designed post-marketing surveillance studies are necessary to assess the safety of use of saw palmetto fruit extracts in men with BPH for even longer periods. To date, almost all clinical studies of saw palmetto fruit products have involved men only, so there is a lack of information on the safety of saw palmetto fruit preparations when used by women (for example, for androgenetic alopecia and other conditions such as acne).

In a drug-monitoring study involving 1334 men with BPH, the tolerability of saw palmetto extract 160 mg twice daily for 12 weeks was reported to be 'good' or 'excellent' by more than 95% of participants.[55] This is similar to a finding from a three-year prospective, uncontrolled study involving 435 men with BPH, in which the tolerability of saw palmetto extract (IDS-89) 160 mg twice daily was classified as 'good' or 'very good' by both physicians and patients for 98% of participants.[54] A total of 46 adverse events was reported in 34 patients. Of these, 30% were gastrointestinal disturbances. The withdrawal rate from the study was 1.8%, mostly because of digestive disturbances ($n = 3$) and tumours ($n = 3$). Non-serious adverse effects (4.95–6.63%), mainly minor gastrointestinal effects, such as gastralgia, nausea, diarrhoea, constipation and anorexia, as well as vertigo, headache, dry mouth and pruritus, were reported in an open study involving 413 men with BPH who received saw palmetto extract 160 mg twice daily for three months.[53] An observational study involving

2080 patients with BPH who received a combination of saw palmetto extract (WS-1473) and nettle root extract (WS-1031) reported that the tolerability of the preparation was classified by physicians to be 'good' or 'very good' for the majority of participants.[56] Mild adverse effects were reported in 15 patients (0.72%).

Studies assessing the equivalence of two different regimens of saw palmetto extract (320 mg once daily and 160 mg twice daily) report that adverse events occurred with a similar frequency in both groups.[50,51] Most events were deemed to be unrelated or unlikely to be related to treatment with saw palmetto extract.

In a small obervational study involving 155 men with BPH who received a lipidosterolic extract of saw palmetto (Permixon) 160 mg twice daily for two years, 10 adverse events (including four cardiovascular events; not further specified), none of which were considered to be related to saw palmetto, were reported by nine participants (5.8%).[61] However, the study did not involve sufficient numbers of participants to have the statistical power to detect rare adverse effects.

An isolated report describes a 53-year-old white man with a meningioma who experienced a bleeding episode during resection of the tumour.[62] The man lost around two litres of blood before the haemorrhage was stopped using standard treatments. Laboratory values for prothrombin time and activated partial thromboplastin time were reported to be within normal ranges, although the bleeding time when measured after surgery was found to be 21 minutes (normal range reported to be 2–10 minutes). The bleeding normalised over the next five days. The patient stated that he had not taken non-steroidal anti-inflammatory agents before undergoing surgery, but said he had been taking saw palmetto for BPH. The authors of the report stated that the prolonged bleeding time was 'probably' due to cyclooxygenase inhibition caused by saw palmetto and affecting platelets. However, this case relies on the patient's self-report of saw palmetto use, no details of the saw palmetto product implicated were provided in a report of the case, and no analysis of the product was undertaken. Causality has not been established.

The World Health Organization's Uppsala Monitoring Centre (WHO-UMC; Collaborating Centre for International Drug Monitoring) receives summary reports of suspected adverse drug reactions from national pharmacovigilance centres of over 70 countries worldwide. To the end of the year 2005, the WHO-UMC's Vigisearch database contained a total of 187 reports, describing a total of 313 adverse reactions, for products reported to contain *S. repens* only as the active ingredient (*see* Table 1).[63] This number may include the case reports described above. Reports originated from several different countries.

Toxicity Incubation of high concentrations of saw palmetto extract (Permixon) 9.0 mg/mL for 48 hours inhibited sperm motility, compared with control.[64] Cytotoxic activity has been described for saw palmetto fruit extracts and certain individual constituents *in vitro* (*see* Pharmacological Actions, *In vitro* and animal studies).

Contra-indications, Warnings

None specified. BPH, the main intended use for saw palmetto, is not suitable for self-treatment.

Drug interactions In view of the reported anti-androgen and oestrogenic activities, the possibility that saw palmetto extracts could affect concurrent hormonal therapy, including the oral contraceptive pill and hormone replacement therapy, should be considered. Drug interaction studies involving small numbers of healthy volunteers who received saw palmetto extracts have indicated that 14 or 28 days' oral administration of saw palmetto extract 320 mg daily (equivalent to 396 mg non-esterified fatty acids and 6.3 mg β-sitosterol daily,[65] or 277 mg non-esterified fatty acids daily[66]) did not influence the activity of the cytochrome P450 enzymes CYP2D6, and CYP 3A4,[65,66] and also CYP1A2 and CYP2E1.[66]

Table 1 Summary of spontaneous reports (n = 187) of suspected adverse drug reactions associated with single-ingredient *Serenoa repens* preparations held in the Vigisearch database of the World Health Organization's Uppsala Monitoring Centre for the period up to end of 2005[63,a,b]

System organ class. **Adverse drug reaction name (number)**	**Total**
Application site disorders	1
Body as a whole – general disorders. Including asthenia (5)	22
Cardiovascular disorders, general. Including hypertension (4)	6
Central and peripheral nervous system disorders. Including dizziness (3); headache (4); paraesthesia (3)	19
Endocrine disorders. Including gynaecomastia (9)	10
Gastrointestinal system disorders. Including abdominal pain (11); diarrhoea (9); dyspepsia (18); eructation (3); flatulence (4); nausea (11); vomiting (8)	76
Heart rate and rhythm disorders. Including atrial fibrillation (3); tachycardia (3)	15
Liver and biliary system disorders. Including hepatitis, cholestatic (4)	15
Metabolic and nutritional disorders. Including alkaline phosphatase increased (3); weight decrease (3)	9
Musculo-skeletal system disorders.	2
Myoendopericardial and valve disorders	1
Neoplasm	1
Platelet, bleeding and clotting disorders.	8
Psychiatric disorders. Including confusion (3); impotence (11); libido decreased (8)	33
Red blood cell disorders.	4
Reproductive disorders, female and male. Including testis disorder (3)	7
Respiratory system disorders. Including dyspnoea (4)	7
Skin and appendages disorders. Including eczema (3); pruritus (6); rash (3); rash, erythematous (3); rash, psoriaform (5); urticaria (5)	37
Special senses other, disorders.	2
Urinary system disorders. Including urinary retention (4)	18
Vascular (extracardiac) disorders.	3
White cell and res disorders. Including granulocytopenia (3)	6
Other reactions described using terms not included in database	11
Total number of suspected adverse drug reactions	313

[a]Specific reactions described where n = 3 or more
[b]Caveat statement. These data were obtained from the Vigisearch database held by the WHO Collaborating Centre for International Drug Monitoring, Uppsala, Sweden. The information is not homogeneous at least with respect to origin or likelihood that the pharmaceutical product caused the adverse reaction. Any information included in this report does not represent the opinion of the World Health Organization

S

Pregnancy and lactation The safety of saw palmetto has not been established. In view of the lack of toxicity data and the documented hormonal activity, the use of saw palmetto during pregnancy and lactation should be avoided.

Preparations

Proprietary single-ingredient preparations

Argentina: Beltrax Uno; Permicaps; Permixon. *Australia:* Bioglan Pro-Guard; Prosta. *Austria:* Permixon; Prosta-Urgenin. *Belgium:* Prosta-Urgenin; Prostaserene. *Brazil:* Prostalium; Prostatal; Renopen. *Chile:* Prostafort. *Czech Republic:* Capistan; Prostakan Mono; Prostamol Uno. *Denmark:* Spalda Sabal. *France:* Permixon. *Germany:* Azuprostat Sabal; Eviprostat-S; Hyperprost Uno; Normurol; Planturol; Prosta-Urgenin; Prosta Urgenin Uno; Prostagutt mono; Prostagutt uno; Prostaplant; Prostess; Remiprostan uno; Sabacur uno; Sabal; Sabal uno; Sabalvit; Sabonal Uno; Sita; Steiprostat; Strogen; Talso. *Greece:* Libeprosta. *Hungary:* Prostakan; Prostamol Uno; Strogen Uno. *Israel:* Permixon. *Italy:* Permixon; Prosteren; Rilaprost; Saba; Serpens. *Mexico:* Permixon; Prostasan; Prostex; Urogutt. *Portugal:* Permixon; Prostiva. *Russia:* Permixon (Пермиксон); Prostamol Uno (Простамол Уно). *Spain:* Permixon; Sereprostat. *Switzerland:* Permixon; Prosta-Urgenine; ProstaMed; Prostasan; SabCaps. *Thailand:* Permixon. *UK:* Sabalin; Sabalin. *Venezuela:* Permixon.

Proprietary multi-ingredient preparations

Argentina: Anastim con RTH; Argeal; Catiz Plus; Keracnyl; Keracnyl; Normoprost Plus; PR21; Sabal; Ultracal. *Australia:* Bioglan Mens Super Soy/Clover; Extralife Flow-Care; Lifechange Mens Complex with Saw Palmetto; Serenoa Complex; Urapro; Urgenin; Urinase. *Austria:* Prostagutt; Spasmo-Urgenin; Urgenin. *Belgium:* Urgenin. *Canada:* Damiana-Sarsaparilla Formula; Prostate Ease; Prostease; ProstGard. *Czech Republic:* Prostakan Forte. *France:* Argeal; Kelual DS; Keracnyl; Keracnyl; Sabal. *Germany:* Cefasabal; Granu Fink Prosta; Nephroselect M; Prostagutt forte. *Hong Kong:* Phyto-Ease; Prostease; Urgenin. *Israel:* Urgenin. *Italy:* Biothymus M Urto; Prostaplant. *Malaysia:* Total Man. *Mexico:* Prosgutt. *Portugal:* Efluvium Anti-caspa; Efluvium Anti-seborreico; Spasmo-Urgenin. *Singapore:* Palmetto Plus. *Spain:* Neo Urgenin; Spasmo-Urgenin; Urgenin. *Switzerland:* Granu Fink Prosta; Prosta-Caps Chassot N; Prostagutt-F. *Thailand:* Spasmo-Urgenin. *UK:* Antiglan; Daily Fatigue Relief; Damiana and Kola Tablets; Elixir Damiana and Saw Palmetto; Prostaid; Regina Royal Concorde; Roberts Black Willow Compound Tablets; Strength; Strength Tablets; Supa-Tonic Tablets. *USA:* ProstatExcell; Prostate Health.

References

1 Wagner H, Flachsbarth H. A new antiphlogistic principle from *Sabal serrulata*, I. *Planta Med* 1981; 41: 244–251.
2 Shimada H *et al.* Biologically active acylglycerides from the berries of saw palmetto (*Serenoa repens*). *J Nat Prod* 1997; 60: 417–418.
3 Schöpflin G *et al.* β-Sitosterin als möglicher Wirkstoff der Sabalfrüchte. *Planta Med* 1966; 14: 402–407.
4 Hänsel R *et al.* Eine Dünnschichtchromatographische Untersuchung der Sabalfrüchte. *Planta Med* 1964; 12: 169–172.
5 Bombardelli E, Morazzoni P. *Serenoa repens* (Bartram) J.K. Small. *Fitoterapia* 1997; 68: 99–113.
6 Habib FK, Wyllie MG. Not all brands are created equal: a comparison of selected components of different brands of *Serenoa repens* extract. *Prostate Canc Prostatic Dis* 2004; 7: 195–200.
7 Weisser H *et al.* Effects of the Sabal serrulata extract IDS 89 and its subfractions on 5-α-reductase activity in human benign prostatic hyperplasia. *Prostate* 1996; 28: 300–306.
8 Palin M-F *et al.* Inhibitory effects of *Serenoa repens* on the kinetic of pig prostatic microsomal 5α-reductase activity. *Endocrine* 1998; 9: 65–69.
9 Bayne CW *et al. Serenoa repens* (Permixon®): a 5α-reductase types I and II inhibitor – new evidence in a coculture model of BPH. *Prostate* 1999; 40: 232–241.
10 Bayne CW *et al.* The selectivity and specificity of the actions of the lipido-sterolic extract of Serenoa repens (Permixon®) on the prostate. *J Urol* 2000; 164: 876–881.
11 Carilla E *et al.* Binding of permixon, a new treatment for prostatic benign hyperplasia, to the cytosolic androgen receptor in the rat prostate. *J Steroid Biochem* 1984; 20: 521–523.
12 Sultan C *et al.* Inhibition of androgen metabolism and binding by a liposterolic extract of '*Serenoa repens* B' in human foreskin fibroblasts. *J Steroid Biochem* 1984; 20: 515–519.
13 Düker E-M *et al.* Inhibition of 5-α-reductase activity by extracts from Sabal serrulata. *Planta Med* 1989; 55: 587.
14 Paubert-Braquet M *et al.* Effect of *Serenoa repens* extract (Permixon®) on estradiol/testosterone-induced experimental prostate enlargement in the rat. *Pharmacol Res* 1996; 34: 171–179.
15 Van Coppenolle F *et al.* Pharmacological effects of the lipidosterolic extract of *Serenoa repens* (Permixon®) on rat prostate hyperplasia induced by hyperprolactinaemia: comparison with finasteride. *Prostate* 2000; 43: 49–58.
16 Barsanti JA *et al.* Effects of an extract of *Serenoa repens* on dogs with hyperplasia of the prostate gland. *Am J Vet Res* 2000; 61: 880–885.
17 Oki T *et al.* Effects of saw palmetto extract on micturition reflex of rats and its autonomic receptor binding activity. *J Urol* 2005; 173: 1395–1399.
18 Gutiérrez M *et al.* Spasmolytic activity of a lipidic extract from *Sabal serrulata* fruits: further study of the mechanisms underlying this activity. *Planta Med* 1996; 62: 507–511.
19 Odenthal KP. Phytotherapy of benign prostatic hyperplasia (BPH) with *Cucurbita*, *Hypoxis*, *Pygeum*, *Urtica* and *Sabal serrulata* (*Serenoa repens*). *Phytother Res* 1996; 10: S141–S143.
20 Paubert-Braquet M *et al.* Effect of the lipidosterolic extract of *Serenoa repens* (Permixon®) and its major components on basic fibroblast growth factor-induced proliferation of cultures of human prostate biopsies. *Eur Urol* 1998; 33: 340–347.
21 Vachero F *et al.* Induction of apoptosis and inhibition of cell proliferation by the lipidosterolic extract of *Serenoa repens* (LSEr, Permixon®) in benign prostatic hyperplasia. *Prostate* 2000; 45: 259–266.
22 Iguchi K *et al.* Myristoleic acid, a cytotoxic component in the extract from *Serenoa repens*, induces apoptosis and necrosis in human prostatic LNCaP cells. *Prostate* 2001; 47: 59–65.
23 Ravenna L *et al.* Effects of the lipidosterolic extract of *Serenoa repens* (Permixon®) on human prostatic cell lines. *Prostate* 1996; 29: 219–230.
24 Ishii K *et al.* Extract from *Serenoa repens* suppresses the invasion activity of human urological cancer cells by inhibiting urokinase-type plasminogen activator. *Biol Pharm Bull* 2001; 24: 188–190.
25 Sovak M *et al.* Herbal composition PC-SPES for management of prostate cancer: identification of active principles. *J Nat Canc Inst* 2002; 94: 1275–1281.
26 Sadava D, Winesburg J. Contaminants of PC-SPES are not responsible for cytotoxicity in human small-cell lung carcinomas. *Cancer Lett* 2005; 220(2): 171–175.
27 Elghamry MI, Hänsel R. Activity and isolated phytoestrogen of shrub palmetto fruits (*Serenoa repens* Small), a new estrogenic plant. *Experientia* 1969; 25: 828–829.
28 Stenger A *et al.* Pharmacology and biochemistry of hexane extract of *Serenoa repens*. *Gazz Med Fr* 1982; 89: 2041–2048.
29 Wagner H *et al.* A new antiphlogistic principle from *Sabal serrulata* II. *Planta Med* 1981; 41: 252–258.
30 Breu W *et al.* Antiphlogistic activity of an extract from Sabal serrulata fruits prepared by supercritical carbon dioxide: *in vitro* inhibition of

S

cyclooxygenase and 5-lipoxygenase metabolism. *Arzneimittelforschung* 1992; 42: 547–551.
31 Paubert-Braquet M *et al.* Effect of the lipidic lipidosterolic extract of *Serenoa repens* (Permixon®) on the ionophore A23187-stimulated production of leukotriene B_4 (LTB_4) from human polymorphonuclear neutrophils. *Prostaglandins Leukot Essent Fatty Acids* 1997; 57: 299–304.
32 De Bernardi di Valserra M *et al. Serenoa repens* capsules: a bioequivalence study. *Acta Toxicol Ther* 1994; 15: 21–39.
33 De Bernardi di Valserra M, Tripodi AS. Rectal bioavailability and pharmacokinetics in healthy volunteers of *Serenoa repens* new formulation. *Arch Med Intern* 1994; 46: 77–86.
34 Di Silverio F *et al.* Effects of long-term treatment with *Serenoa repens* (Permixon®) on the concentrations and regional distribution of androgens and epidermal growth factor in benign prostatic hyperplasia. *Prostate* 1998; 37: 77–83.
35 Marks LS *et al.* Tissue effects of saw palmetto and finasteride: use of biopsy cores for in situ quantification of prostatic androgens. *Urology* 2001; 57: 999–1005.
36 Marks LS *et al.* Effects of a saw palmetto herbal blend in men with symptomatic benign prostatic hyperplasia. *J Urol* 2000; 163: 1451–1456.
37 Weisser H *et al.* Enzyme activities in tissue of human benign prostatic hyperplasia after three months' treatment with the *Sabal serrulata* extract IDS 89 (Strogen®) or placebo. *Eur Urol* 1997; 31: 97–101.
38 Strauch G *et al.* Comparison of finasteride (Proscar®) and *Serenoa repens* (Permixon®) in the inhibition of 5-alpha-reductase in healthy male volunteers. *Eur Urol* 1994; 26: 247–252.
39 Goepel M *et al.* Do saw palmetto extracts block human α_1-adrenoceptor subtypes *in vivo*? *Prostate* 2001; 46: 226–232.
40 Vela Navarrete R *et al.* BPH and inflammation: pharmacological effects of Permixon on histological and molecular inflammatory markers. Results of a double-blind pilot clinical assay. *European Urol* 2003; 44: 549–555.
41 Veltri RW *et al.* Saw palmetto alters nuclear measurements reflecting DNA content in men symptomatic BPH: evidence for a possible molecular mechanism. *Urology* 2002; 60: 617–622.
42 Wilt T *et al.* Serenoa repens for benign prostatic hyperplasia (review). The Cochrane Database of Systematic Reviews, 2002, Issue 3. Art. No.: CD001423.
43 Wilt TJ *et al. Serenoa repens* for treatment of benign prostatic hyperplasia. In: *The Cochrane Library*, Issue 3, 2001. Oxford: Update Software.
44 Boyle P *et al.* Updated meta-analysis of clinical trials of *Serenoa repens* extract in the treatment of symptomatic benign prostatic hyperplasia. *BJU International* 2004; 93: 751–756.
45 Debruyne F *et al.* Comparison of a phytotherapeutic agent (Permixon) with an α-blocker (tamsulosin) in the treatment of benign prostatic hyperplasia: a 1-year randomized international study. *European Urol* 2002; 41: 497–507.
46 Debruyne F *et al.* Evaluation of the clinical benefit of Permixon and tamsulosin in severe BPH patients – PERMAL study subset analysis. *European Urol* 2004; 45: 773–780.
47 Willetts KE *et al. Serenoa repens* extract for benign prostate hyperplasia: a randomized controlled trial. *BJU International* 2003; 92: 267–270.
48 Preuss HG *et al.* Randomized trial of a combination of natural products (cernitin, saw palmetto, β-sitosterol, vitamin E) on symptoms of benign prostatic hyperplasia (BPH). *Int Urol Nephrol* 2001; 33: 217–225.
49 Al-Shukri SH *et al.* Early urodynamic effects of the lipido-sterolic extract of *Serenoa repens* (Permixon®) in patients with lower urinary tract symptoms due to benign prostatic hyperplasia. *Prostate Cancer Prostatic Dis* 2000; 3: 195–199.
50 Braeckman J *et al.* Efficacy and safety of the extract of *Serenoa repens* in the treatment of benign prostatic hyperplasia: therapeutic equivalence between twice and once daily dosage forms. *Phytother Res* 1997; 11: 558–563.
51 Stepanov VN *et al.* Efficacy and tolerability of the lipidosterolic extract of *Serenoa repens* (Permixon®) in benign prostatic hyperplasia: a double-blind comparison of two dosage regimens. *Adv Ther* 1999; 16: 231–241.
52 Gerber GS *et al.* Saw palmetto (*Serenoa repens*) in men with lower urinary tract symptoms: effects on urodynamic parameters and voiding symptoms. *Urology* 1998; 51: 1003–1007.
53 Braeckman J *et al.* Efficacy and safety of the extract of *Serenoa repens* in the treatment of benign prostatic hyperplasia: an open multicentre study. *Eur J Clin Res* 1997; 9: 47–57.
54 Bach D, Ebeling L. Long-term drug treatment of benign prostatic hyperplasia – results of a prospective 3-year multicenter study using Sabal extract IDS 89. *Phytomedicine* 1996; 3: 105–111.
55 Vahlensieck W *et al.* Benigne Prostatahyperplasie – Behandlung mit Sabalfrucht-Extrakt. *Fort schritte Ther* 1993; 18: 45–48.
56 Schneider H-J *et al.* Behandlung der benignen Prostatahyperplasie. *Fortschritte Ther* 1995; 3: 37–40.
57 Kaplan SA *et al.* A prospective, 1-year trial using saw palmetto versus finasteride in the treatment of category III prostatitis/chronic pelvic pain syndrome. *J Urol* 2004; 171: 284–288.
58 Prager N *et al.* A randomized, double-blind, placebo-controlled trial to determine the effectiveness of botanically derived inhibitors of 5-α-reductase in the treatment of androgenetic alopecia. *J Alt Comp Med* 2002; 8: 143–152.
59 DiPaola RS *et al.* Clinical and biological activity of an estrogenic herbal combination (PC-SPES) in prostate cancer. *N Engl J Med* 1998; 339: 785–791.
60 Oh WK *et al.* Prospective, multicenter, randomized phase II trial of the herbal supplement, PC-SPES, and diethylstilboestrol in patients with androgen-independent prostate cancer. *J Clin Oncol* 2004; 22(18): 3705–3712.
61 Pytel YA *et al.* Long-term clinical and biologic effects of the lipidosterolic extract of *Serenoa repens* in patients with symptomatic benign prostatic hyperplasia. *Adv Ther* 2002; 19: 297–306.
62 Cheema P *et al.* Intraoperative haemorrhage associated with the use of saw palmetto herb: a case report and review of literature. *J Int Med* 2001; 250: 167–169.
63 Uppsala Monitoring Centre. Vigibase, WHO Adverse Reactions database (accessed 6 January, 2006).
64 Ondrizek RR *et al.* Inhibition of human sperm motility by specific herbs used in alternative medicine. *J Assist Reprod Genet* 1999; 16: 87–91.
65 Markowitz JS *et al.* Multiple doses of saw palmetto (*Serenoa repens*) did not alter cytochrome P450 2D6 and 3A4 activity in normal volunteers. *Clin Pharmacol Ther* 2003; 74: 536–542.
66 Gurley BJ *et al. In vivo* assessment of botanical supplementation of human cytochrome P450 phenotypes: *Citrus aurantium*, *Echinacea purpurea*, milk thistle and saw palmetto. *Clin Pharmacol Ther* 2004; 76: 428–440.

Scullcap

Summary and Pharmaceutical Comment

Limited information has been documented regarding the chemistry of scullcap. Most of the pharmacological activities reported for other *Scutellaria* species have been attributed to the flavonoid constituents. Despite the traditional uses of scullcap as a sedative and anticonvulsant, there are no documented scientific data to support these uses. Commercial scullcap is commonly recognised to be adulterated with *Teucrium* species, notably *Teucrium canadense*. Herbal preparations stated to contain scullcap may therefore contain a *Teucrium* species. Few pharmacological studies have been undertaken for *Teucrium* species. Hepatitis has been associated with germander (*Teucrium chamaedrys*). Hepatotoxicity has resulted in humans taking commercially available remedies in the UK which are stated to contain scullcap. In view of the possibility of contamination, and the lack of pharmacological information, it would seem advisable to avoid ingestion of scullcap.

Species (Family)

**Scutellaria lateriflora* L.
†*S. baicalensis* Georgi (Labiatae/Lamiaceae)

Synonym(s)

*Helmet Flower, Hoodwort, Quaker Bonnet, Scutellaria, Skullcap
†*S. lanceolaria* Miq., *S. macrantha* Fisch., Huang Qin

Part(s) Used

Herb

Pharmacopoeial and Other Monographs

BHP 1996[G9]
Martindale 35th edition[G85]

Legal Category (Licensed Products)

GSL[G37]

Constituents

The following is compiled from several sources, including General References G20 and G60.

Limited information has been documented regarding the constituents of *S. lateriflora* and *S. baicalensis*.

Flavonoids Apigenin, hispidulin, luteolin, scutellarein, scutellarin (bitter glycoside).

Iridoids Catalpol.

Volatile oils Limonene, terpineol (monoterpenes); *d*-cadinene, caryophyllene, *trans*-β-farnesene, β-humulene (sesquiterpenes).

Other constituents Lignin, resin and tannin. *S. baicalensis* is reported to contain baicalein, baicalin, chrysin, oroxylin A, skullcapflavone II and wogonin.[1–3]

Other* Scutellaria *species The related species *S. galericulata* is stated to contain apigenin, baicalein, baicalin, apigenin-7-glucoside and galeroside (baicalein-β-L-rhamnofuranoside).[4]

Food Use

Scullcap is not used in foods. Previously, scullcap has been listed by the Food and Drugs Administration (FDA) as a Herb of Undefined Safety.[G22]

Herbal Use

Scullcap is stated to possess anticonvulsant and sedative properties.[G34, G64] Traditionally, it has been used for epilepsy, chorea, hysteria, nervous tension states, and specifically for grand mal epilepsy.[G7] In Chinese herbal medicine, the roots of *S. baicalensis* Georgi have been used traditionally as a remedy for inflammation, suppurative dermatitis, allergic diseases, hyperlipidaemia and atherosclerosis.

Dosage

Dosages for oral administration (adults) for traditional uses recommended in standard herbal reference texts are given below.

Dried herb 1–2 g as an infusion three times daily.[G7]

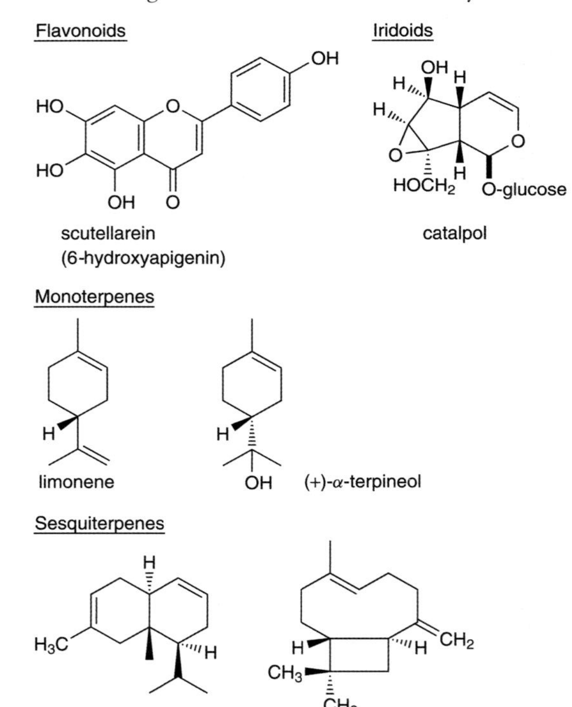

Figure 1 Selected constituents of scullcap.

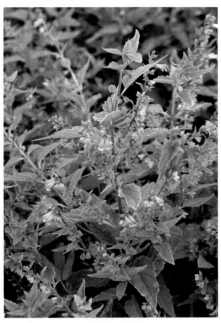

Figure 2 Scullcap (*Scutellaria lateriflora*).

Liquid extract 2–4 mL (1 : 1 in 25% alcohol) three times daily.[G7]

Tincture 1–2 mL (1:5 in 45% alcohol) three times daily.[G7]

Pharmacological Actions

In vitro and animal studies

Many investigations have been undertaken to study the pharmacological actions of *S. baicalensis* root. Documented actions have primarily been attributed to the various flavonoid constituents and include: *in vitro* inhibition of mast cell histamine release comparable to disodium cromoglicate for some flavonoids;[1] *in vitro* cytotoxicity of scullcap flavone II;[5] *in vivo* and *in vitro* inhibition of lipid peroxidation;[6–8] *in vitro* inhibition of lipoxygenase and cyclooxygenase pathways;[9] hypocholesterolaemic activity in rats.[10] This *in vivo* effect has been linked to *in vitro* actions documented for various flavonoids, including prevention of ethanol-induced hyperlipidaemia,[11] catecholamine-induced lipolysis[10, 11] and lipogenesis in adipose tissue;[10, 11] there is no pronounced effect on blood pressure in cats and rabbits.[12] In addition, the latter study found no CNS-depressant and no antispasmodic activity. However, it did find marked antibacterial activity against various Gram-positive bacteria (e.g. *Bacillus subtilis*, *Escherichia coli*, *Sarcina lutea* and *Staphylococcus aureus*).[13]

Clinical studies

There is a lack of clinical research assessing the effects of scullcap and rigorous randomised clinical trials are required.

Clinical investigation of scutellarin, a constituent of *S. lateriflora*, involving 634 cases of cerebral thrombosis, cerebral embolism, and paralysis caused by stroke has been undertaken. An overall effective rate of more than 88% was reported following intramuscular, intravenous or oral administration.[14] However, information from case series provides only a low level of clinical evidence and the observed effects cannot be attributed definitively to scutellarin.

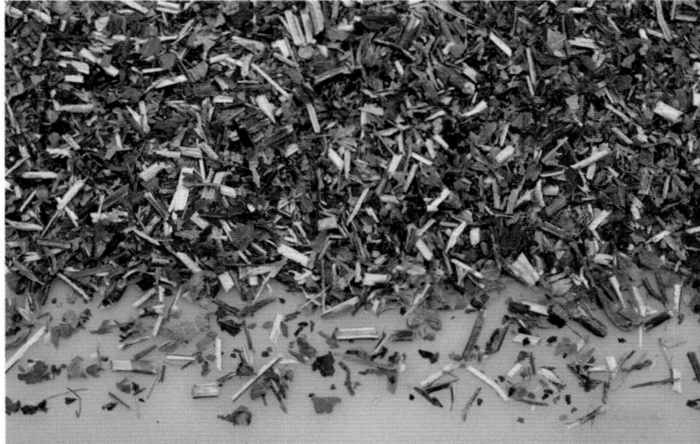

Figure 3 Scullcap – dried drug substance (herb).

Side-effects, Toxicity

There is a lack of clinical safety and toxicity data for scullcap and further investigation of these aspects is required.

Symptoms caused by overdosage of scullcap tincture include giddiness, stupor, confusion and seizures.[G20] Hepatotoxic reactions have been reported after ingestion of preparations stated to contain scullcap;[15, G20] however, adulteration of scullcap herb by *Teucrium* species is recognised and several cases of hepatitis have been associated with germander (*Teucrium chamaedrys*).[16]

Contra-indications, Warnings

None documented. In view of the possible hepatotoxicity associated with scullcap preparations adulterated with germander, its use is best avoided.

Drug interactions None documented. However, the potential for preparations of scullcap to interact with other medicines administered concurrently, particularly those with similar or opposing effects, should be considered.

Pregnancy and lactation Scullcap is stated to have been used traditionally to eliminate a mother's afterbirth and to promote menstruation.[G22] Limited information is known regarding the pharmacological activity and toxicity of scullcap. In view of this and concerns over hepatotoxicity of adulterated preparations, scullcap should not be taken during pregnancy and lactation.

S

Preparations

Proprietary multi-ingredient preparations

Australia: Albizia Complex; Andrographis Compound; Calmo; Euphrasia Compound; Feminine Herbal Complex; Goodnight Formula; Nevaton; Pacifenity; Passiflora Complex; Passionflower Plus; Relaxaplex; Valerian. *Canada:* Herbal Nerve. *UK:* Fenneherb Newrelax; Herbal Indigestion Naturtabs; HRI Calm Life; Inflamol; Napiers Tension Tablets; Newrelax; Nodoff; Quiet Days; Quiet Tyme; Scullcap & Gentian Tablets; Sleepezy; St Johns wort Compound; Stressless; Vegetable Cough Remover; Wellwoman.

References

1 Kubo M *et al*. *Scutellariae radix*. X. Inhibitory effects of various flavonoids on histamine release from rat peritoneal mast cells *in vitro*. *Chem Pharm Bull* 1984; 32: 5051–5054.
2 Tomimori T *et al*. Studies on the constituents of Scutellarian species. *Yakugaku Zasshi* 1985; 105: 148–155.
3 Tomimori T *et al*. Studies on the constituents of *Scutellaria* species. VI. On the flavonoid constituents of the root of *Scutellaria baicalensis* Georgi (5). Quantitative analysis of flavonoids in Scutellaria roots by high-performance liquid chromatography. *Yakugaku Zasshi* 1985; 105: 148–155.
4 Popova TP *et al*. Chemical composition and medicinal properties of *Scutellaria galericulata*. *Farm Zh (Kiev)* 1972; 27: 58–61.
5 Ryn SH *et al*. The cytotoxic principle of *Scutellariae radix* against L1210 cell. *Planta Med* 1985; 51: 355.
6 Kimura Y *et al*. Studies on *Scutellariae radix*; IX. New component inhibiting lipid peroxidation in rat liver. *Planta Med* 1984; 50: 290–295.
7 Kimura Y *et al*. Studies on *Scutellariae radix*. IV. Effects on lipid peroxidation in rat liver. *Chem Pharm Bull* 1981; 29: 2610–2617.
8 Kimura Y *et al*. Studies on *Scutellariae radix*. VI. Effects of flavanone compounds on lipid peroxidation in rat liver. *Chem Pharm Bull* 1982; 30: 1792–1795.
9 Kimura Y *et al*. Studies on *Scutellariae radix*. XIII. Effects of various flavonoids on arachidonate metabolism in leukocytes. *Planta Med* 1985; 51: 132–136.
10 Kimura Y *et al*. Studies on *Scutellariae radix*. III. Effects on lipid metabolism in serum, liver and fat cells of rats. *Chem Pharm Bull* 1981; 29: 2308–2312.
11 Kimura Y *et al*. Studies on *Scutellariae radix*. V. Effects on ethanol-induced hyperlipidemia and lipolysis in isolated fat cells. *Chem Pharm Bull* 1982; 30: 219–222.
12 Kurnakov BA. Pharmacology of skullcap. *Farmakol i Toksikol* 1957; 20: 79–80.
13 Kubo M *et al*. Studies on *Scutellariae radix*. Part II: The antibacterial substance. *Planta Med* 1981; 43: 194–201.
14 Peigen X, Keji C. Recent advances in clinical studies of Chinese medicinal herbs. 1. Drugs affecting the cardiovascular system. *Phytother Res* 1987; 1: 53–57.
15 Perharic L *et al*. Toxicological problems resulting from exposure to traditional remedies and food supplements. *Drug Safety* 1994; 11: 284–294.
16 Larrey D *et al*. Hepatitis after germander (*Teucrium chamaedrys*) administration: another instance of herbal medicine toxicity. *Am Coll Physicians* 1992; 117: 129–132.

Senega

Summary and Pharmaceutical Comment

The chemistry and pharmacology of senega has been extensively investigated but only limited clinical data are available. The activity of the saponins in animals supports the herbal use for bronchitis. In view of the lack of toxicity data and uncertainty regarding the risk associated with chronic ingestion of haemolytic saponins, excessive use of senega, and use during pregnancy and lactation should be avoided.

Species (Family)

Polygala senega L. (Polygalaceae) and other closely related *Polygala* species cultivated in western Canada and Japan.

Synonym(s)

Northern Senega (Canada), Polygala, *Polygala senega* var. *latifolia*, Rattlesnake Root, Senega Root, Senega Snakeroot, Snake Root

Part(s) Used

Root, rootstock

Pharmacopoeial and Other Monographs

BHC 1992[(G6)]
BHP 1996[(G9)]
BP 2007[(G84)]
Complete German Commission E[(G3)]
ESCOP 2003[(G76)]
Martindale 35th edition[(G85)]
Ph Eur 2007[(G81)]

Legal Category (Licensed Products)

GSL[(G37)]

Constituents

See Reference 1 and General References G2, G6, G20, G52, G59 and G62.

Acids Salicylic acid and its methyl ester 0.1–0.2%; hydroxycinnamic acids (e.g. caffeic acid, ferulic acid, sinapic acid) free or esterified with saponins.[(2)]

Carbohydrates Arabinose, fructose, glucose, melibiose, raffinose, saccharose, stachyose, sucrose; 1,5-anhydro-D-glucitol and other D-glucitol derivatives;[(3, 4)] trisaccharides; mucilage, pectin. A series of oligosaccharide esters, senegoses A–O, containing acetic, benzoic, *trans*- and *cis*-ferulic acid moieties linked to glucose and fructose.[(5, 6)] Five acylated sucrose glycosides, tenuifolisides A–E, have been isolated from *P. tenuifolia*.[(7, 8)] The esterifying acids are 3,4,5-trimethoxycinnamic, *p*-hydroxybenzoic, sinapic and ferulic.

Terpenoids A complex mixture of bidesmosidic triterpene saponins (6–10%) based on the aglycone presenegin. The total saponin mixture may be referred to as senegin. The saponins of *P. senega* var. *latifolia* are 3-glucosides of presenegin with tetra-, penta- or hexa-glucosyl groups linked at C-28 and including 4″-methoxycinnamoyl or 3″,4″-dimethoxycinnamoylfucosyl resulting in *E*- and *Z*-cinnamoyl isomers of each saponin.[(9–11)] Senegins I–IV were the first saponins to be characterised and were *E*-isomers.[(12, 13)] *P. tenuifolia* contains similar saponins named onjisaponins A–G.[(14, 15)]

Xanthones A number of xanthones have been isolated from *P. tenuifolia* including 4-C-[β-D-apiofuranosyl-(1→6)-β-D-glucopyranosyl]-1,3,6-trihydroxy-7-methoxyxanthone.[(8)]

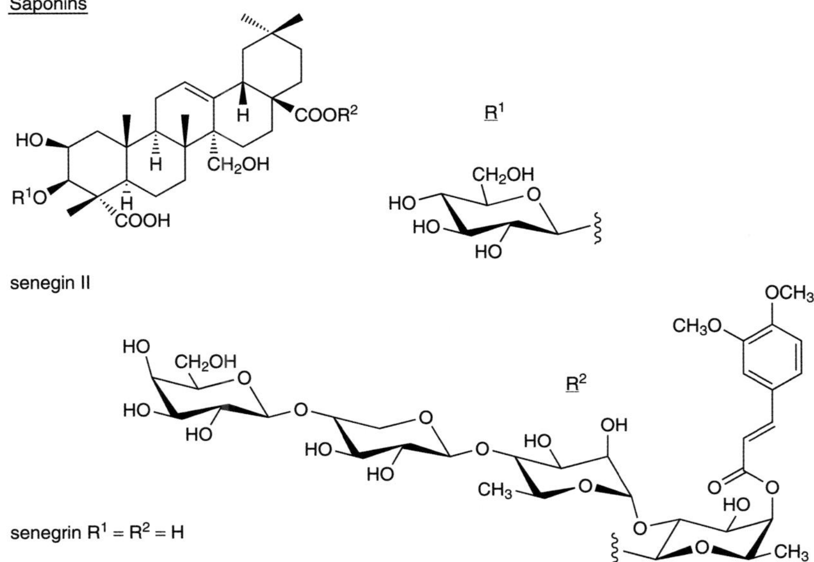

Figure 1 Selected constituents of senega.

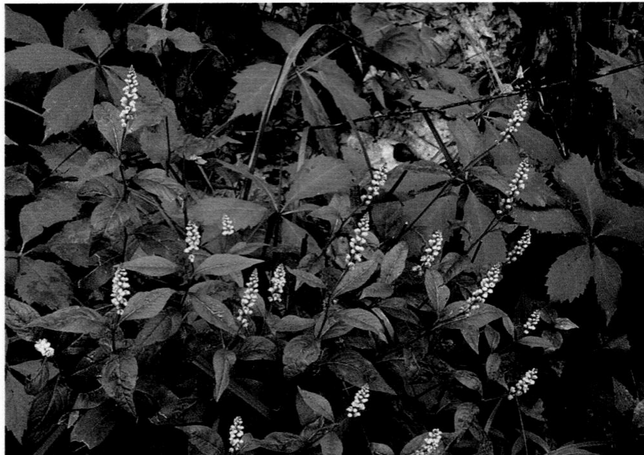

Figure 2 Senega (*Polygala senega*).

Other constituents Fat, resin, sterols and valeric acid ester.

Other* Polygala *species *Polygala paniculata* contains coumarins (aurapten, murrangatin, phebalosin and 7-methoxy-8-(1,4-dihydroxy-3-methyl-2-butenyl) coumarin,[16] pyranocoumarin).[17] *Polygala chamaebuxus* (European species) contains hydroxycinnamic acid esters involving acetic, ferulic and sinapic acids as the ester moieties, saponins, tenuifolin (prosapogenin), rutin (flavonoid glycoside), coniferin and syringen (phenolic glycosides).[2]

Other European species (e.g. *Polygala alpestris*, *Polygala comosa*, *Polygala vayredae*) contain complex mixtures of bidesmosidic saponins, tenuifolin (prosapogenin), hydroxycinnimic acid esters similar to those reported for *P. chamaebuxus*.[18] *Polygala triphylla* contains B-ring oxygen-free trioxygenated- and glucosyloxy-xanthones.[19] *Polygala polygama* contains podophyllotoxin and demethylpodophyllotoxin (lignans).[20]

Food Use

Senega is listed by the Council of Europe as a natural source of food flavouring (category N2). This category indicates that senega can be added to foodstuffs in small quantities, with a possible limitation of an active principle (as yet unspecified) in the final product.[G16]

S

Herbal Use

Senega is stated to possess expectorant, diaphoretic, sialogogue and emetic properties. Traditionally, it has been used for bronchitic asthma, chronic bronchitis, as a gargle for pharyngitis, and specifically for chronic bronchitis.

Dosage

Dosages for oral administration (adults) for traditional uses recommended in older and contemporary standard herbal and pharmaceutical reference texts are given below.

Dried root 0.5–1.0 g as an infusion three times daily.[G6, G7]

Senega Liquid Extract (BPC 1968) 0.3–1.0 mL.

Senega Tincture (BPC 1968) 2.5–5.0 mL.

Pharmacological Actions

In vitro and animal studies

Mucosal secretion Polygalic acid and senegin are stated to be irritant to the gastrointestinal mucosa, and to cause a reflex secretion of mucus in the bronchioles.[1, G6, G44, G52] A fluid extract of senega increased respiratory tract fluid secretion in guinea-pig, cat and dog, but not in rabbit.[G52]

CNS-depressant activity CNS-depressant properties in mice (e.g. reduction in spontaneous activity, inhibition of amfetamine stimulation, potentiation of barbiturate-induced sleeping time, and decrease in rectal temperature) have been documented for *Polygala microphylla*.[21] Similar properties have been reported for *Polygala tenuifolia* and have been attributed to the saponin constituents. A methanolic extract of *P. tenuifolia*, various fractions and pure onjisaponins B, F and G prolonged hexobarbital sleeping time in mice.[G52] Onjisaponin F produced sleep times in mice of 33 and 35 minutes for doses of 5 and 20 mg/kg, respectively, compared with 24 minutes for control and 42 minutes for chlorpromazine hydrochloride (2 mg/kg).

Inhibition of alcohol absorption *E,Z*-senegin II and *E,Z*-senagasaponins a and b from *P. senega* var. *latifolia* have potent inhibitory effects on alcohol absorption in rats. *E,Z*-senegasaponins a or b (100 mg/kg) administered orally to rats 1 hour after 20% aqueous ethanol (5 mL/kg, orally) reduced blood alcohol concentrations after 1 hour from 0.5 mg/mL to 0.02 mg/mL.[10] Under similar test conditions, *E,Z*-senegin II administration led to a blood ethanol concentration of 0.09 mg/mL.

Hypoglycaemic activity Senegin II and *E,Z*-senegasaponins a and b have significant hypoglycaemic effects in rodents.[22] Senegin II (2.5 mg/kg, intraperitoneally) reduced blood glucose concentrations in normal mice from 220 mg/dL to 131 mg/dL 4 hours after administration and also significantly lowered blood glucose concentrations in KK-Ay mice from 434 mg/dL to 142 mg/dL under similar test conditions ($p < 0.001$, compared with control, for both studies). In glucose tolerance tests in rats, administration of *E,Z*-senegasaponins a and b (100 mg/kg, orally) resulted in glucose concentrations of 107–123 mg/mL after 30 minutes compared with 156 mg/mL in control animals ($p < 0.01$).[11]

Hypolipidaemic activity Seven hours after administration of an *n*-butanol fraction of a methanolic extract of *P. senega* var. *latifolia* containing senegin II (5 mg/kg, intraperitoneally), the mean

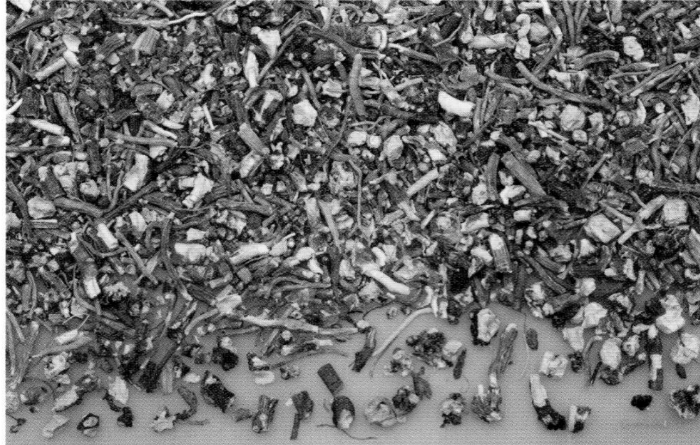

Figure 3 Senega – dried drug substance (root).

(standard deviation) blood triglyceride concentration was 65 (9) mg/100 mL, compared with 152 (17) mg/mL in control animals ($p < 0.05$).[23] The blood triglyceride concentration in cholesterol-fed mice was also significantly reduced ($p < 0.05$) under the similar test conditions. Pure senegin II at a dose of 5 mg/kg was also reported to lower blood triglyceride concentrations in mice.[23]

Other activities Guinea-pig serum taken two hours after administration of lyophilised aqueous extract of *P. tenuifolia* (600 mg, intraperitoneally) inhibited the growth of herpes simplex virus type 1 (HSV-1) in Vero cells.[G52] An unspecified senegin from *P. senega* produced a 34% inhibition of influenza virus (A2/Japan 305) at a concentration of 12.5 μg/mL.[G52] An ethanolic extract of *P. senega* has been reported to inhibit growth of a range of fungi.[G52]

Polygala erioptera and *P. paniculata* have exhibited molluscicidal activity, and *P. paniculata* is reported to possess antifungal activity.[17] A butanol extract of *P. tanuifolia* containing onjisaponins (100 μg/mL) inhibited cyclic adenosine monophosphate (cAMP) diesterase by 73%.[G52] Isolated onjisaponins E, F and G inhibited cAMP phosphodiasterase, with IC_{50} values of 3.1, 2.9, and 3.7×10^{-5} mol/L, respectively, being similar in action to papaverine. A total saponin concentration of *P. senega* var. *latifolia* increased rat plasma concentrations of adrenocorticotrophic hormone (ACTH), corticosterone and glucose 30 minutes after intraperitoneal administration (25 mg/kg). Single doses of a dried methanol (50%) extract of *P. senega* var. *latifolia* and *P. tanuifolia* administered orally (2 g/kg) to rats produced 62% and 100% inhibition, respectively, of congestive oedema.[G52] Under the same conditions, furosemide 100 mg/kg produced 100% inhibition of congestive oedema.

Clinical studies

There is a lack of clinical research assessing the effects of senega and rigorous randomised clinical trials are required. The following observations and uses require assessment in well-designed clinical studies.

A fluid extract of senega root was reported to reduce the viscosity of sputum in patients with bronchiectasis.[G52] A French patent has stated that a triterpenic acid extracted from senega possesses anti-inflammatory activity and is effective against graft rejection, eczema, psoriasis and multiple sclerosis.[24] These reports provide only a low level of clinical evidence and the observed effects cannot be attributed definitively to senega or its constituents.

Side-effects, Toxicity

There is a lack of clinical safety and toxicity data for senega and further investigation of these aspects is required.

Saponins are generally regarded as irritant to the gastrointestinal mucosa, and irritant properties have been documented for senega and other *Polygala* species.[G51] Large doses of senega are reported to cause vomiting and purging.[G60]

The haemolytic index (HI) of senega saponins is stated to be between 2500 and 4500.[G62] Haemolytic saponins are toxic to mammals when administered intravenously, but have a low toxicity when given orally because they do not cross the gastrointestinal mucosa.[25] Contact with damaged mucosal areas may cause a problem. Toxicity associated with chronic exposure of the gastrointestinal mucosa to haemolytic saponins has not been established. It has been stated that the suitability of saponins for nutritional and pharmacological use requires further investigation: free saponins in the gastrointestinal tract may interact with the mucosal cells, causing a transient increase in the permeability of the small intestine to intraluminal solutes and inhibiting active nutrient absorption.[25] This action may consequently facilitate the entry of antigens and biologically active food peptides into the blood circulation, with adverse systemic effects.[25] Aqueous and methanol extracts of *P. senega* and *P. tenuifolia* were negative in the rec-assay with *Bacillus subtilis* and in the reversion assay with Ames strains TA98 and TA100 of *Salmonella typhimurium*.[G52] A mixture of senegins given to rats (i.p.) gave an LD_{50} value of 3 mg/kg and inhibited the growth of Walker carcinoma in rats with an ED_{50} value of 1.5 mg/kg.[G52]

Cytotoxic lignans have been documented as constituents of a related species, *P. polygama*.[10]

Contra-indications, Warnings

Senega may exacerbate existing gastrointestinal inflammation and excessive doses may cause vomiting. There is limited evidence from preclinical studies that constituents of senega have hypoglycaemic activity. The clinical relevance of this is not clear although, until further information is available, senega should not be used by patients with diabetes.

Drug interactions None documented. However, the potential for preparations of senega to interact with other medicines administered concurrently, particularly those with similar or opposing effects, should be considered. There is limited evidence from preclinical studies that certain constituents of senega have hypoglycaemic activity. The clinical relevance of this, if any, is not clear; however, until further information is available, it is recommended that senega should not be used by patients receiving hypoglycaemic agents.

Pregnancy and lactation Limited information is available on the chemistry, pharmacology and toxicity of senega. In view of this, and the potential irritant properties of senega, its use during pregnancy and lactation should be avoided.

Preparations

Proprietary multi-ingredient preparations

Argentina: Antitos; Hebert Caramelos; Ixana; Ixana; No-Tos Adultos; No-Tos Adultos; No-Tos Infantil; Pectobron. *Australia:* Senagar; Senega and Ammonia. *Austria:* Eicebaer; Tussimont. *Belgium:* Tux. *Brazil:* Expectomel; Pectal. *Canada:* Bronchial; Bronchozone; Sirop Cocillana Codeine; Wampole Bronchial Cough Syrup. *Czech Republic:* Stodal. *France:* Neo-Codion. *Hong Kong:* Coci-Fedra; Cocillana Christo; Cocillana Compound; Cocillana Compound; Mefedra-N; Mist Expect Stim. *Portugal:* Stodal. *Russia:* Neo-Codion Babies (Нео-Кодион Для Младенцев). *South Africa:* Borstol Cough Remedy. *Spain:* Broncovital; Pastillas Pectoral Kely; Pulmofasa. *Sweden:* Cocillana-Etyfin. *Switzerland:* Hederix; Makaphyt Gouttes antitussives; Makaphyt Sirop; Pectocalmine; Pectoral N; Phol-Tux. *UK:* Antibron; Chest Mixture; Chesty Cough Relief; Tickly Cough & Sore Throat Relief. *Venezuela:* Acetoben.

References

1 Briggs CJ. Senega Snakeroot – A traditional Canadian herbal medicine. *Can Pharm J* 1988; 121: 199–201.

S

2 Hamburger M, Hostettmann K. Hydroxycinnamic acid esters from *Polygala chamaebuxus*. *Phytochemistry* 1985; 24: 1793–1797.
3 Takiura K *et al*. Studies on oligosaccharides. XIII. Oligosaccharides in *Polygala senega* and structures of glycosyl-1,5-anhydro-D-glucitols. *Yakugaku Zasshi* 1974; 94: 998–1003.
4 Takiura K *et al*. Studies on oligosaccharides XVI. New trisaccharides found in *Senega radix*. *Yakugaku Zasshi* 1975; 95: 166–169.
5 Saitoh H *et al*. Senegoses A–E, oligosaccharide multi-esters from *Polygala senega* var. latifolia Torr. *et* Gray. *Chem Pharm Bull* 1993; 41: 1127–1131.
6 Saitoh H *et al*. Senegoses F–I, oligosaccharide multi-esters from the roots of *Polygala senega* var. latifolia Torr. *et* Gray. *Chem Pharm Bull* 1993; 41: 2125–2128.
7 Ikeya Y *et al*. Four new phenolic glycosides from *Polygala tenuifolia*. *Chem Pharm Bull* 1991; 39: 2600–2605.
8 Ikeya Y *et al*. Xanthone C-glycoside and acylated sugar from *Polygala tenuifolia*. *Chem Pharm Bull* 1994; 42: 2305–2308.
9 Yoshikawa M *et al*. *E*-Senegasaponins a and b, *Z*-senegasaponins a and b, *Z*-senegins II and III, new type inhibitors of ethanol absorption in rats from senegae radix, the roots of *Polygala senega* L. var *latifolia* Torrey et Gray. *Chem Pharm Bull* 1995; 43: 350–352.
10 Yoshikawa M *et al*. Bioactive saponins and glycosides. I. Senegae radix. (1): *E*-senegasaponins a and b and *Z*-senegasaponins a and b, their inhibitory effect on alcohol absorption and hypoglycemic activity. *Chem Pharm Bull* 1995; 43: 2115–2122.
11 Yoshikawa M *et al*. Bioactive saponins and glycosides. II. Senegae radix. (2): Chemical structures, hypoglycemic activity, and ethanol absorption-inhibitory effect of *E*-senegasaponin c, *Z*-senegasaponins c, and *Z*-senegins II, III, and IV. *Chem Pharm Bull* 1996; 44: 1305–1313.
12 Tsukitani Y *et al*. Studies on the constituents of Senegae radix. II. The structure of senegin-II, a saponin from *Polygala senega* Linne var. *latifolia* Torry et Gray. *Chem Pharm Bull* 1973; 21: 791–799.
13 Tsukitani Y, Shoji J. Studies on the constituents of Senegae radix III. The structures of senegin-III and -IV, saponins from *Polygala senega* Linne var. latifolia Torry et Gray. *Chem Bull Pharm* 1973; 21: 1564–1574.
14 Sakuma S, Shoji J. Studies on the constituents of the root of *Polygala tenuifolia* Willdenow. I. Isolation of saponins and the structures of onjisaponins g and f. *Chem Pharm Bull* 1981; 29: 2431–2441.
15 Sakuma S, Shoji J. Studies on the constituents of the root of *Polygala tenuifolia* Willdenow. II. On the structures of onjisaponins a, b and e. *Chem Pharm Bull* 1982; 30: 810–821.
16 Hamburger M *et al*. Coumarins from *Polygala paniculata*. *Planta Med* 1985; 51: 215–217.
17 Hamburger M *et al*. A new pyranocoumarin diester from *Polygala paniculata* L. *Helv Chim Acta* 1984; 67: 1729–1733.
18 Hamburger M, Hostettmann K. Glycosidic constituents of some European *Polygala* species. *J Nat Prod* 1986; May–June: 557.
19 Ghosal S *et al*. 1,2,3-Trioxygenated glucosyloxy xanthones. *Phytochemistry* 1981; 20: 489–492.
20 Hokanson GC. Podophyllotoxin and 4-demethylpodophyllotoxin from *Polygala polygama* (Polygalaceae). *Lloydia* 1978; 41: 497–498.
21 Carretero ME *et al*. Études pharmacodynamiques préliminaires de *Polygala microphylla* (L.), sur le système nerveux central. *Plant Méd Phytothér* 1986; 20: 148–154.
22 Kako M *et al*. Effect of senegin-II on blood glucose in normal and NIDDM mice. *Biol Pharm Bull* 1995; 18 (Suppl. Suppl.8): 1159–1161.
23 Masuda H *et al*. Intraperitoneal administration of senegae radix extract and its main component, senegin-II, affects lipid metabolism in normal and hyperlipidemic mice. *Biol Pharm Bull* 1996; 19: 315–317.
24 Tubery P. Antiinflammatory triterpenic alcohol acids. *Fr Demande Patent* 2,202,683.
25 Johnson IT *et al*. Influence of saponins on gut permeability and active nutrient transport in vitro. *J Nutr* 1986; 116: 2270–2277.

Senna

Summary and Pharmaceutical Comment

The chemistry of senna is characterised by the hydroxyanthracene derivatives. The laxative action of these compounds is well recognised and supports the herbal use of senna as a laxative for the treatment of constipation. However, the use of non-standardised hydroxyanthracene-containing preparations should be avoided since their pharmacological effect will be variable and unpredictable. The sennoside content of many licensed senna products is standardised and generally calculated as sennoside B. The use of senna during pregnancy and lactation should be avoided.

Species (Family)

Senna alexandrina Mill. (Leguminosae)

Synonym(s)

Alexandrian Senna, *Cassia acutifolia* Delile, *C. angustifolia* M. Vahl, *C. alexandrina* (Garsault) Thell., *C. senna* L., Indian Senna, Khartoum Senna, *Senna acutifolia* (Delile) Batka, *S. alexandrina* Garsault, *S. angustifolia* (Vahl) Batka, Tinnevelly Senna

Part(s) Used

Fruit (pod), leaf

Pharmacopoeial and Other Monographs

BHC 1992[(G6)]
BHP 1996[(G9)]
BP 2007[(G84)]
Complete German Commission E[(G3)]
EMEA HMPC Community Herbal Monograph[(1)]
ESCOP 2003[(G76)]
Martindale 35th edition[(G85)]
Ph Eur 2007[(G81)]
USP29/NF24[(G86)]
WHO volume 1 1999[(G63)]

Legal Category (Licensed Products)

GSL[(G37)]

Constituents

The following is compiled from several sources, including General References G2,G6, G7, G20 and G52.

Hydroxyanthracenes Pharmacopoeial standards not less than 2.5% for leaf and 2.2% for *C. angustifolia* fruit.[(G81, G84)] Dianthrone glycosides (1.5–3% leaf; 2–5% fruit), primarily sennosides A and B (rhein dianthrones) with sennosides C and D (rhein aloe-emodin heterodianthrones), aloe-emodin dianthrone. Sennosides A and B yield sennidin A and B respectively. Free anthraquinones including aloe-emodin, chrysophanol and rhein with their glycosides.

Carbohydrates Polysaccharides (about 2.5%)[(2)] including mucilage (arabinose, galactose, galacturonic acid, rhamnose) and a galactomannan (galactose, mannose);[(3)] free sugars (e.g. fructose, glucose, pinitol, sucrose).

Flavonoids Flavonols, including isorhamnetin and kaempferol.

Glycosides 6-Hydroxymusizin and tinnevellin glycosides.

Other constituents Chrysophanic acid, salicylic acid, saponin, resin, volatile oil (trace).

Food Use

Senna is listed by the Council of Europe as a natural source of food flavouring. Previously, senna has been listed as GRAS (Generally Recognised As Safe).

Herbal Use

Senna is stated to possess cathartic properties (leaf greater than fruit) and has been used traditionally for constipation.[(G2, G4, G6–G8, G32, G43, G52, G54, G56, G64)] The German Commission E approved use for constipation.[(G3)] Senna is also used in combination with ispaghula for constipation.[(G3)] The EMEA Committee on Herbal Medicinal Products (HMPC) has adopted community herbal monographs for senna leaf and senna fruit with indications for short-term use in cases of occasional constipation.[(3)]

Dosage

Dosages for oral administration (adults) for traditional uses recommended in older and contemporary standard herbal and pharmaceutical reference texts are given below.

Dried pods 3–6 pods (Alexandrian) or 4–12 pods (Tinnevelly) steeped in 150 mL warm water for 6–12 hours;[(G6, G7)] 0.6–0.2 g (equivalent to 20–30 mg hydroxyanthracene glycosides calculated as sennosides B).[(G52)]

Hydroxyanthracene glycosides

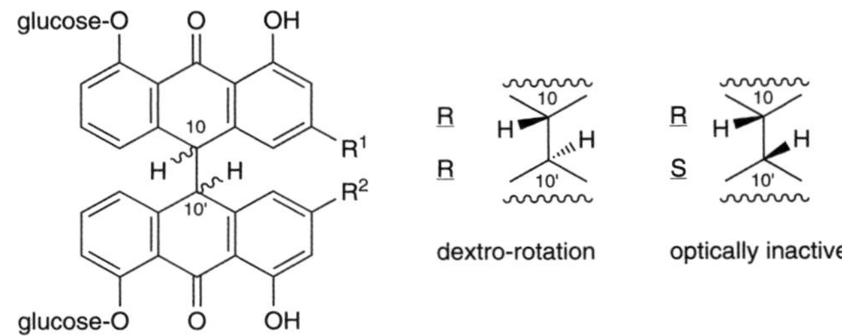

	R^1	R^2	Isomeric form
sennoside A	COOH	COOH	(+), *trans*
sennoside B	COOH	COOH	*meso, cis*
sennoside C	COOH	CH_2OH	(+), *trans*
sennoside D	COOH	CH_2OH	*meso, cis*

Figure 1 Selected constituents of senna.

Dried leaflets 0.5–2.0 g[G6, G7] (equivalent to 20–30 mg hydroxyanthracene glycosides calculated as sennoside B).[G52]

Leaf, liquid extract 0.5–2.0 mL (1 : 1 in 25% alcohol).[G6, G7]

Senna Liquid Extract (BPC 1973) 0.5–2.0 mL.

Herbal drug preparations Equivalent to 15–30 mg hydroxyanthracene derivatives (calculated as sennoside B) to be taken at night.[1]

Pharmacological Actions

The cathartic action of hydroxyanthracene-containing drugs is well recognised and such preparations have been used as laxatives for many years. However, there is still some uncertainty as to the exact mode of action of the hydroxyanthracenes. It is thought that hydroxyanthracene glycosides are absorbed from the gastrointestinal tract, the aglycones liberated during metabolism and excreted into the colon resulting in stimulation and an increase in peristalsis. However, it has also been suggested that the purgative action of senna is due to the action of intestinal bacteria.[4] Using human intestinal flora, it was found that sennoside A is reduced to 8-glucosyl rheinanthrone, hydrolysed to rheinanthrone and oxidised to sennidin A. The active principle causing peristaltic movements of the large intestine was thought to be rheinanthrone.[4]

In vitro and animal studies

Sennosides A and B, and their natural metabolites sennidins A and B, have been reported to act specifically on the large intestine in the rat with the acceleration of colonic transport the major component of their laxative effect.[5] Sennosides A and B have also been reported to induce fluid secretion exclusively in the colon, following oral administration of the glycosides to rats.[6]

It has been suggested that the laxative action of the sennosides involves prostaglandins. Indometacin has been found to partly inhibit the action of sennosides A and B, although a bolus injection of prostaglandins into the caecal lumen was stated neither to influence transit time nor to induce diarrhoea.[5] Pretreatment of mice with indometacin and a prostaglandin E (PGE) antagonist has been documented to prevent diarrhoea caused by intracaecal administration of rhein, which stimulates the production of PGE-like material specifically in the colon.[7] Indometacin was found to depress the large intestinal propulsive activity of rhein, but did not suppress PGE_2-induced diarrhoea. The authors suggest that the action of rhein is mediated by prostaglandin biosynthesis and release.[7]

Antihepatotoxic activity has been documented for naphtho-α-pyrone and naphtho-γ-pyrone glycosides, and for the hydroxyanthracene glycosides isolated from a related species *Cassia tora*.[8] Greatest activity was documented for the naphtho-γ-pyrone glycosides.

Significant inhibitory activity in mice against leukaemia P388 has been documented for aloe-emodin.[G41]

Clinical studies

In a randomised, controlled trial, 91 patients with terminal cancer received senna 12 mg daily, or lactulose, for 27 days.[9] At the end of the study, no differences were found between the two groups in defecation-free intervals, or in days with defecation. The general health of each group was also reported to be similar.

A randomised, double-blind, double-dummy, multicentre, controlled, crossover study involving 77 hospitalised elderly patients with a history of chronic constipation compared the effects of a senna–fibre combination (senna 12.4%, ispaghula 54.2%, 10 mL daily) and lactulose (15 mL twice daily) for two 14-day periods with a three- to five-day wash-out period.[10] Assessments included stool frequency and consistency, ease of evacuation, adverse effects and costs of treatment. The senna–fibre combination was reported to be significantly more effective than lactulose.[10]

Commercial preparations containing senna and ispaghula have been reported to be equally effective for the treatment of constipation in small clinical studies involving elderly hospitalised patients and/or residents in nursing homes.[11]

Side-effects, Toxicity

Clinical data

Senna may cause mild abdominal discomfort such as colic or cramps. Prolonged use or overdosage can result in diarrhoea with excessive loss of potassium, albuminuria and haematuria.[G3] Potassium deficiency may lead to disorders of the heart and muscular weakness especially with concurrent use of cardiac glycosides, diuretics or corticosteroids. An atonic non-functioning colon may also develop.[G45] Excessive use and abuse of senna has been associated with finger clubbing and with the development of cachexia and reduced serum globulin concentrations.[12]

Preclinical data

Sennosides A and B are reported to be most potent with respect to laxative action, but to be the least toxic compared with other hydroxyanthracene fractions in senna. Similarly, fractions with a low laxative activity (e.g. rhein-8-glucoside) are reported to have the highest acute toxicity.[13] LD_{50} values in mice following intravenous injection of sennosides A and B and of rhein-8-glycoside are reported to be 4.1 g/kg and 400 g/kg, respectively.[13] The acute oral toxicity of all senna fractions in mice has been reported to be greater than 5 g/kg, although all of the animals were stated to have died by the following week. The toxicity of total senna extracts is greater than that of the individual sennosides and it has been proposed that the laxative and toxic components of senna could be separated.[7]

In vitro carcinogenicity testing has reported certain anthraquinones, including aloe-emodin, to be active in more than one strain of *Salmonella typhimurium*.[14] Aglycones were documented to exhibit genotoxic activity in a mammalian cell assay.[14]

Sensitising properties have been documented for emodin (*see* Aloes).[G51]

The EMEA HMPC Community Herbal Monographs for senna include the following information.[1] There are no new, systematic preclinical tests for senna leaf or preparations thereof. Most data refer to extracts of senna fruit containing 1.4–3.5% of hydroxyanthacenes, corresponding to 0.9–2.35% of potential rhein, 0.05–0.15% potential aloe-emodin and 0.001–0.006% of potential emodin, or to isolated active constituents, e.g. rhein or sennosides A and B. The acute toxicity of senna fruit and specified extracts thereof, as well as of sennosides in rats and mice was low after oral treatment. As a result of investigations with parenteral application in mice, extracts are supposed to possess a higher toxicity than purified glucosides, possibly due to the content of aglycones.

Sennosides displayed no specific toxicity when tested at doses up to 500 g/kg in dogs for four weeks and up to 100 g/kg in rats for six months. Data for herbal drug preparations are not available.

There was no evidence of any embryolethal, teratogenic or fetotoxic actions in rats or rabbits after oral treatment with sennosides. Furthermore, there was no effect on the postnatal development of young rats, on rearing behaviour of dams or on male and female fertility in rats. Data on herbal drug preparations are not available.

An extract and aloe-emodin were mutagenic in *in vitro* tests; sennosides A and B and rhein gave negative results. *In vivo* examinations of a defined extract of senna pods were negative. A specified senna extract given orally for two years was not carcinogenic in male or female rats. The extract investigated contained approximately 40.8% of hydroxyanthracenes from which 35% were sennosides, corresponding to about 25.2% of potential rhein, 2.3% of potential aloe-emodin and 0.007% of potential emodin, and 142 ppm free aloe-emodin and 9 ppm free emodin.

Contra-indications, Warnings

It is recommended that senna should not be given to patients with intestinal obstruction and stenosis, atony, inflammatory colon diseases (e.g. Crohn's disease, ulcerative colitis), appendicitis, with undiagnosed abdominal symptoms; severe dehydration states with water and electrolyte depletion. Prolonged use should be avoided.[1, G20, G45, G52]

The EMEA HMPC Community Herbal Monographs for senna include the following information.[1]

As with all laxatives, senna should not be given when any undiagnosed acute or persistent abdominal symptoms are present. If laxatives are needed every day the cause of the constipation should be investigated. Long-term use of laxatives should be avoided. Use for more than two weeks requires medical supervision. Chronic use may cause pigmentation of the colon (pseudomelanosis coli) which is harmless and reversible after drug discontinuation.

Abuse, with diarrhoea and consequent fluid and electrolyte losses, may cause dependence, with possible need for increased dosages, disturbance of water and electrolyte (mainly hypokalaemia) balance, atonic colon with impaired function. Intake of anthranoid containing laxatives exceeding short-term use may result in an aggravation of constipation.

Hypokalaemia can result in cardiac and neuromuscular dysfunction, especially if cardiac glycosides, diuretics or corticosteroids are also taken. Chronic use may result in albuminuria and haematuria.

In chronic constipation, stimulant laxatives are not an acceptable alternative to a changed diet.

Interaction with other medicaments and other forms of interaction Hypokalaemia (resulting from long-term use of senna) may potentiate the action of cardiac glycosides and interacts with antiarrhythmic drugs, with drugs which induce reversion to sinus rhythm (e.g. quinidine). Concomitant use with other drugs inducing hypokalaemia (e.g. thiazide diuretics, adreno corticosteroids and liquorice root) may enhance electrolyte imbalance. Abdominal spasms and pain may occur, in particular in patients with irritable colon.[1]

Anthraquinones cause discoloration of the urine which may interfere with diagnostic tests.[G45]

Pregnancy and lactation Non-standardised hydoxyanthracene containing laxative preparations should not be taken during pregnancy or lactation since their pharmacological action is unpredictable. Although hydroxyanthracene derivatives may be excreted in the breast milk, following normal dosage their concentration is usually insufficient to affect the nursing infant.[G45]

The EMEA HMPC Community Herbal Monographs for senna include the following information.[1]

Pregnancy Not recommended during pregnancy. There are no reports of undesirable or damaging effects during pregnancy and on the fetus when used at the recommended dosage schedule. However, experimental data concerning a genotoxic risk of several anthranoids (e.g. emodine and physcione) and senna are not counterbalanced by sufficient studies to eliminate a possible risk.[1]

Lactation Breastfeeding is not recommended as there are insufficient data on the excretion of metabolites in breast milk. Excretion of active principles in breast milk has not been investigated. However, small amounts of active metabolites (e.g. rhein) from other anthranoids are known to be excreted in breast milk. A laxative effect in breastfed babies has not been reported.[1]

Preparations

Proprietary single-ingredient preparations

Argentina: Ciruela Fibra; Laxiruela Ciruela Fibra. *Australia:* Bekunis Herbal Tea; Bekunis Instant. *Austria:* Bekunis; Colonorm; Darmol; X-Prep. *Belgium:* Darlin; Fuca; Midro; Prunasine; Transix. *Brazil:* Senan. *Canada:* Experience; GNC Herbal Laxative; Sennaprep; Sennatab; Senokot; X-Prep. *Chile:* Cholax; Naturlax. *Czech Republic:* Caj z Listu Senny; List Senny; Regulax; Sennove Lusky; Sennovy List; Tisasen; X-Prep. *Finland:* Exprep; Pursennid; Sennapur. *France:* Senokot. *Germany:* Abfuhrtee N; Bekunis Instant; Bekunis-Krautertee N; Bekunis Plantaardig; Bekunis Senna; Depuran; Heverto; Liquidepur; Midro Abfuhr; Midro Tee; Neda Fruchtewurfel; Ramend; Regulax N; Styptysat. *Greece:* X-Prep. *Hong Kong:* Senokot. *Israel:* Bekunis; Florilax; Jungborn; Laxikal Forte. *Italy:* Falquilax; Tisana Kelemata; X-Prep. *Mexico:* Arsen; Bekunis; Ciruelax Comp; Ciruelax TE; Lagenbach; X-Prep. *Netherlands:* Sennocol. *Norway:* Senokot; X-Prep. *Portugal:* X-Prep. *South Africa:* Depuran; Gal; Hamburg Tea; Sennalax; Soflax. *Singapore:* Senokot. *Spain:* Laxante Bescansa Normal; Laxante Olan; Laxante Salud; Takata. *Sweden:* Pursennid. *Switzerland:* Bekunis; Darmol; Demodon Neo; Fuca N; Grains de Vals Nouvelle formule; Midro; Tisane laxative H nouvelle formulation; X-Prep. *United Arab Emirates:* Laxal. *UK:* Ex-Lax; Nylax with Senna; Senokot; Sure-Lax. *USA:* Agarol Extra; Agarol with Sennosides; Black-Draught; Dosaflex; Ex-Lax; Fletchers Castoria; Maximum Relief Ex-Lax; Senna-Gen; Senokot; Senokotxtra; X-Prep.

Proprietary multi-ingredient preparations

Argentina: Agiolax; Cirulaxia; Gelax; Kronolax; LX-30; Rapilax Fibras. *Australia:* Agiolax; Neo-Cleanse; Peritone; Prolax; Soflax. *Austria:* Abfuhrtee St Severin; Agiolax; Carilax; Entschlackender Abfuhrtee EF-EM-ES; Eucarbon; Eucarbon Herbal; Frugelletten; Laxalpin; Laxolind; Mag Kottas Krauterexpress Abfuhrtee; Mag Kottas May-Cur-Tee; Menodoron; Midro Tee; Neda Fruchtewurfel; Planta Lax; Sabatif; The Chambard-Tee. *Belgium:* Agiolax; Tux. *Brazil:*

Agiolax; Circanetten; Estomafitino; Fitolax; Florlax; Fontlax; Frutalax; Laxarine; Laxtam; Plantax; Sene Composta; Tamaril; Tamarine; Tamarine; Tamarix; Varicell. *Canada:* Cholasyn II; Constipation; Doulax; Ex-Lax Gentle Strength; Herbal Laxative; Herbalax; Laxaco; Mucinum; Prodiem Plus; Senna-S; Senokot-S. *Chile:* Bilaxil; Naturlax; Tamarine. *Czech Republic:* Abfuhr-Heilkrautertee; Dr Theiss Rheuma Creme; Dr Theiss Schweden Krauter; Dr Theiss Schwedenbitter; Projimava; Reduktan. *Denmark:* Figen. *Finland:* Agiolax. *France:* Agiolax; Grains de Vals; Herbesan; Histo-Fluine P; Ideolaxyl; Mediflor Tisane Contre la Constipation Passagere No 7; Mediflor Tisane Hepatique No 5; Modane; Mucinum a l'Extrait de Cascara; Tamarine. *Germany:* Agiolax; Alasenn; Ramend Krauter. *Hong Kong:* Agiolax; Mucinum Cascara. *Hungary:* Bolus Laxans. *Israel:* Agiolax; Eucarbon; Jungborn; Lido Tea; Midro-Tea; Novicarbon. *Italy:* Agiolax; Colax; Confetti Lassativi CM; Cuscutine; Eucarbon; Fibrolax Complex; Lactolas; Lassatina; Midro; Ortisan; Stimolfit; Tamarine; Tisana Kelemata. *Mexico:* Agiolax; Ciruelax Jalea; Jarabe de Manzanas; Laxacaps. *Netherlands:* Agiolax; Prunacolon; Prunasine. *Norway:* Agiolax. *Portugal:* Agiolax; Midro; Xarope de Macas Rainetas. *South Africa:* Agiolax; Clairo; Menodoron. *Spain:* Agiolax; Bekunis Complex; Crislaxo; Jarabe Manceau; Laxante Sanatorium; Laxomax; Natusor Malvasen; Proctosor; Pruina; Senalsor. *Sweden:* Agiolax. *Switzerland:* Agiolax; Dragees aux figues avec du sene; Fruttasan; Lapidar 10; Linoforce; LinoMed; Phyto-Laxia; Phytolaxin; Schweden-Mixtur H nouvelle formulation; Tisane laxative; Tisane Provencale No 1; Valverde Constipation dragees; Valverde Constipation sirop. *Thailand:* Agiolax; Circanetten. *UK:* Antitis; Athera; Boots Alternatives Laxative; Califig; Cleansing Herbs; Compound Laxative Syrup of Figs; Constipation Tablets; Dual-Lax Extra Strong; Dual-Lax Normal Strength; Fam-Lax Senna; Fibre Plus; Jacksons Herbal Laxative; Kas-Bah; Laxative Tablets; Lion Cleansing Herbs; Lustys Herbalene; Manevac; Modern Herbals Laxative; Modern Herbals Menopause; Natural Herb Tablets; Out-of-Sorts; Pripsen; Rhuaka; Sciargo; Skin Cleansing; Tabritis. *USA:* Laci Le Beau Super Dieter's Tea; Perdiem; Senokot-S; X-Prep Bowel Evacuant Kit-1. *Venezuela:* Agiolax; Fibralax.

References

1 European Medicines Agency. Committee on Herbal Medicinal Products (HMPC). Community Herbal Monograph on *Cassia senna* L., fructus and *Cassia angustifolia* Vahl, fructus. London, 7 September 2006. Doc Ref. EMEA/HMPC/51871/2006; European Medicines Agency. Committee on Herbal Medicinal Products (HMPC). Community Herbal Monograph on *Cassia senna* L. and *Cassia angustifolia* Vahl, folium. London, 7 September 2006. Doc Ref. EMEA/HMPC/51869/2006.

2 Müller BM *et al.* Isolation and structural investigation of a polysaccharide from *Cassia angusti folia* leaves. *Planta Med* 1989; 55: 99.

3 Alam N, Gupta PC. Structure of a water-soluble polysaccharide from the seeds of *Cassia angustifolia*. *Planta Med* 1986; 52: 308–310.

4 Kobashi K *et al.* Metabolism of sennosides by human intestinal bacteria. *Planta Med* 1980; 40: 225–236.

5 Leng-Peschlow E. Acceleration of large intestine transit time in rats by sennosides and related compounds. *J Pharm Pharmacol* 1986; 38: 369–373.

6 Leng-Peschlow E. Dual effect orally administered sennosides on large intestine transit and fluid absorption in the rat. *J Pharm Pharmacol* 1986; 38: 606–610.

7 Yagi T *et al.* Involvement of prostaglandin E-like material in the purgative action of rhein anthrone, the intraluminal active metabolite of sennosides A and B in mice. *J Pharm Pharmacol* 1988; 40: 27–30.

8 Wong SM *et al.* Isolation and structural elucidation of new antihepatotoxic naphtho-gamma-pyrone glycosides, naphtho-α-pyrone glycoside and anthraquinone glycosides from the seeds of *Cassia tora*. *Planta Med* 1989; 55: 112.

9 Agra Y *et al.* Efficacy of senna versus lactulose in terminal cancer patients treated with opioids. *J Pain Symptom Management* 1998; 15: 1–7.

10 Passmore AP *et al.* Chronic constipation in long stay elderly patients: a comparison of lactulose and a senna-fibre combination. *BMJ* 1993; 307: 769–771.

11 Petticrew M *et al.* Epidemiology of constipation in the general adult population. *Health Technol Assess* 1997; 1: 1–52.

12 Senna *Lawrence Review of Natural Products*. Levittown, Pennsylvania: Pharmaceutical Information Associates Ltd, 1989.

13 Hietala P *et al.* Laxative potency and acute toxicity of some anthraquinone derivatives, senna extracts and fractions of senna extracts. *Pharmacol Toxicol* 1987; 61: 153–156.

14 Westendorf J *et al.* Possible carcinogenicity of anthraquinone-containing medical plants. *Planta Med* 1988; 54: 562.

S

Shepherd's Purse

Summary and Pharmaceutical Comment

The chemistry of shepherd's purse is well documented. Several actions affecting the circulatory system have been observed in animal studies, although these actions do not relate to the traditional herbal uses. There is a lack of robust clinical research assessing the efficacy and safety of shepherd's purse. Limited toxicity data are available. In view of this together with the demonstrated pharmacological activity of the herb, excessive use of shepherd's purse and use during pregnancy and lactation should be avoided.

Species (Family)

Capsella bursa-pastoris (L.) Medik (Brassicaceae/Cruciferae)

Synonym(s)

Capsella

Part(s) Used

Herb

Pharmacopoeial and Other Monographs

BHP 1996[(G9)]
Complete German Commission E[(G3)]
Martindale 35th edition[(G85)]

Legal Category (Licensed Products)

GSL[(G37)]

Constituents

The following is compiled from several sources, including General References G2 and G7.

Amines Acetylcholine, choline, amino acids 2.33% (major component proline), histamine, tyramine and unidentified crystalline alkaloids.[(1)]

Flavonoids Quercetin, diosmetin, luteolin, hesperetin and their glycosides (e.g. rutin, diosmin, hesperidin).[(2)]

Volatile oils 0.02%. Camphor (major); at least 74 components identified.[(3, 4)]

Other constituents Carotenoids, fumaric acid, sinigrin (mustard oil glucoside), ascorbic acid (vitamin C) and vitamin K.[(4, 5, G2)]

Food Use

Shepherd's purse is not used in foods.

Herbal Use

Shepherd's purse is stated to possess antihaemorrhagic and urinary antiseptic properties. Traditionally, it has been used for menorrhagia, haematemesis, haematuria, diarrhoea and acute catarrhal cystitis.[(G2, G7, G64)]

Dosage

Dosages for oral administration (adults) for traditional uses recommended in standard herbal reference texts are given below.

Dried herb 1–4 g as an infusion three times daily[(G7)]

Liquid extract 1–4 mL (1 : 1 in 25% alcohol) three times daily.[(G7)]

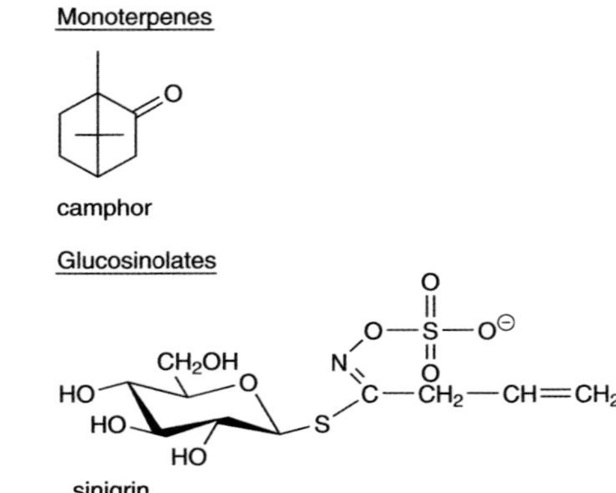

Figure 1 Selected constituents of shepherd's purse.

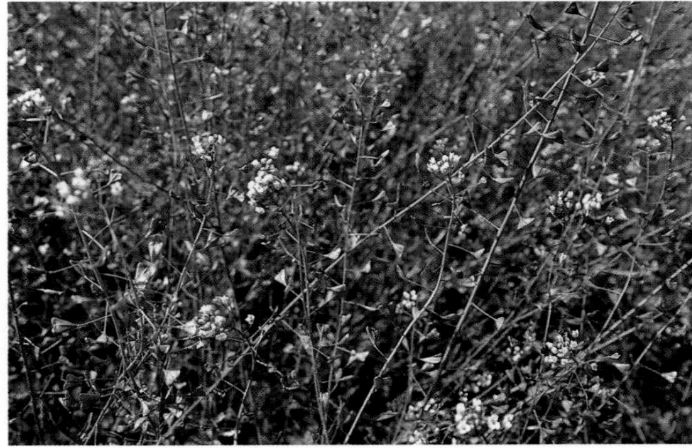

Figure 2 Shepherd's purse (*Capsella bursa-pastoris*).

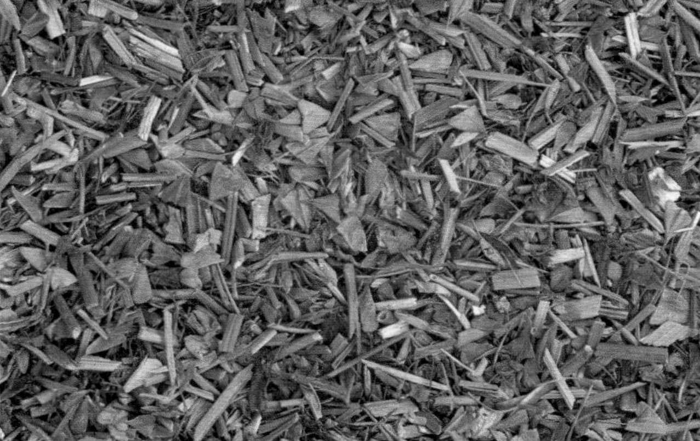

Figure 3 Shepherd's purse – dried drug substance (herb).

S

Pharmacological Actions

In vitro and animal studies

A variety of actions has been documented for an ethanolic extract of shepherd's purse in various animal models.[6–9] Anti-inflammatory activity has been exhibited versus carrageenan-induced and dextran-induced rat paw oedema.[7] A reduction in capillary permeability in the guinea-pig, induced by histamine and serotonin, has also been observed,[7] and flavonoid components isolated from shepherd's purse have been reported to reduce blood vessel permeability in mice.[2] Anti-ulcer activity has been documented in rats following intraperitoneal injection. The extract did not affect gastric secretion, but accelerated recovery from stress-induced ulcers.[7] A hypotensive effect observed in cats, dogs, rabbits and rats, following intravenous injection, was inhibited by a β-adrenoceptor blocker but not by atropine, thus dismissing earlier reports that this action was attributable to cholinergic compounds present in shepherd's purse.[8,9]

Diuresis has been reported in mice, following oral or intraperitoneal administration of shepherd's purse. The mode of action was stated to involve an increase in the glomerular filtration rate.[7]

Documented cardiac actions include increased coronary blood flow in dogs following intra-arterial administration, and a slight inhibitory effect on ouabain-induced ventricular fibrillation in the rat following intraperitoneal injection, together with a negative chronotropic effect.[9] Studies on the isolated heart have reported negative chronotropic and inotropic actions in the guinea-pig and rabbit and coronary vasodilatation.[9]

A CNS-depressant action in mice has been demonstrated (potentiation of barbiturate-induced sleeping time).[9]

Weak antibacterial activity, mainly towards Gram-positive organisms, has been reported.[10]

Antineoplastic activity in rats has been documented for fumaric acid, which prevented the development of hepatic neoplasms when co-administered with the carcinogen 3-MeDAB.[11]

Shepherd's purse seeds are stated to possess rubefacient and vesicant properties because of their isothiocyanate-yielding components.[G51]

In vitro studies have documented stimulatory action in various smooth muscle tissues. Induced contractions of the small intestine in the guinea-pig were reported to be unaffected by atropine and diphenhydramine, but were inhibited by papaverine.[8,9] Induced utero-activity in the rat, equivalent to the effect of oxytocin 0.1 i.u., was unaffected by atropine, but inhibited by competitive inhibitors of oxytocin.[8] Two unidentified alkaloid components of shepherd's purse have also been stated to elicit a physiological activity on the uterus.[1] Induced tracheal contractions in the guinea-pig were unaffected by adrenaline, which did inhibit acetylcholine-induced contractions.[9] These studies concluded that the active substance (s) in shepherd's purse responsible for the observed actions on smooth muscle were neither acetylcholine nor histamine.[8,9]

Clinical studies

There is a lack of clinical research assessing the effects of shepherd's purse and rigorous randomised clinical trials are required.

Side-effects, Toxicity

Clinical data

There is a lack of clinical safety and toxicity data for shepherd's purse and further investigation of these aspects is required.

Preclinical data

Shepherd's purse extracts have been reported to exhibit low toxicity in mice. LD_{50} values reported are 1.5 g/kg body weight (mice, intraperitoneal injection) and 31.5 g/kg (mice, subcutaneous injection).[9] Signs of toxicity were described as sedation, enlargement of pupils, paralysis of hind limbs, difficulty in respiration, and death by respiratory paralysis.[9] Following hydrolysis, the constituent sinigrin yields allyl isothiocyanate which is an extremely powerful irritant and produces blisters on the skin.[G41] Isothiocyanates have been implicated in endemic goitre (hypothyroidism with thyroid enlargement) and have been reported to produce goitre in experimental animals.[G41]

Contra-indications, Warnings

Drug interactions None documented. However, the potential for preparations of shepherd's purse to interact with other medicines administered concurrently, particularly those with similar or opposing effects, should be considered. There is limited evidence from preclinical studies that shepherd's purse and/or certain isolated constituents have hypotensive, diuretic and cardiac activities and effects on thyroid fuction.

Pregnancy and lactation Shepherd's purse is reputed to act as an abortifacient and to affect the menstrual cycle, and tyramine is documented as a utero-active constituent.[G30] In view of this, the reported oxytocin-like activity and the general lack of safety data, the use of shepherd's purse during pregnancy and lactation should be avoided.

Preparations

Proprietary multi-ingredient preparations

UK: Fenneherb Cystaid.

References

1 Kuroda K, Kaku T. Pharmacological and chemical studies on the alcohol extract of *Capsella bursa-pastoris*. *Life Sci* 1969; 8: 151–155.
2 Jurisson S. Flavonoid substances of *Capsella bursa pastoris*. *Farmatsiya (Moscow)* 1973; 22: 34–35.
3 Miyazawa M *et al*. The constituents of the essential oils from *Capsella bursa-pastoris* Medik. *Yakugaku Zasshi* 1979; 99: 1041–1043.
4 Park RJ. The occurrence of mustard oil glucosides in *Lepidium hyssopifolium*, *L. bonariense*, and *Capsella bursa pastoris*. *Aust J Chem* 1967; 20: 2799–2801.
5 Jurisson S. Vitamin content of shepherd's purse. *Farmatsiya (Moscow)* 1976; 25: 66–67.
6 Kuroda K, Takagi K. Studies on *Capsella bursa pastoris*. I. General pharmacology of ethanol extract of the herb. *Arch Int Pharmacodyn Ther* 1969; 178: 382–391.
7 Kuroda K, Takagi K. Studies on capsella bursa pastoris. II. Diuretic, anti-inflammatory and anti-ulcer action of ethanol extracts of the herb. *Arch Int Pharmacodyn Ther* 1969; 178: 392–399.
8 Kuroda K, Takagi K. Physiologically active substance in *Capsella bursa-pastoris*. *Nature* 1968; 220: 707–708.
9 Jurisson S. Determination of active substances of *Capsella bursa pastoris*. *Tartu Riiliku Ulikooli Toim* 1971; 270: 71–79.
10 Moskalenko SA. Preliminary screening of far-eastern ethnomedicinal plants for antibacterial activity. *J Ethnopharmacol* 1986; 15: 231–259.
11 Kuroda K. Neoplasm inhibitor from *Capsella bursa pastoris*. *Japan Kokai* 1977; 41: 207.

Skunk Cabbage

Summary and Pharmaceutical Comment

There is only limited information available on the constituents, pharmacological activities and safety of skunk cabbage (even though citings as early as 1817 reported its irritant properties). No documented evidence was found to justify the herbal uses. In view of the lack of data, the appropriateness of medicinal use of skunk cabbage should be considered. In view of the documented irritant properties, excessive use, at least, should be avoided. Skunk cabbage should not be used during pregnancy and breastfeeding. The potential for skunk cabbage preparations to interact with other medicines should be considered.

Species (Family)

Symplocarpus foetidus (L.) Salisb. ex W. Barton (Araceae)

Synonym(s)

Dracontium foetidum L., Skunkweed

Part(s) Used

Rhizome, root

Pharmacopoeial and Other Monographs

BHP 1983[G7]
Martindale 35th edition[G85]

Legal Category (Licensed Products)

GSL[G37]

Constituents

Reported constituents include starch, gum-sugar, fixed and volatile oils, resin, tannin, an acrid principle and iron.[G22, G64]

Other plant parts Large amounts of alkaloids (unspecified), phenolic compounds and glycosides have been isolated from all plant parts of skunk cabbage.[1] The leaves are reported to contain hydroxytryptamine.[G22] The flower contains the anthocyanins cyanidin-3-monoglucoside, cyanidin-3-rutinoside and peonidin-3-rutinoside.[2]

Food Use

Skunk cabbage is not used in foods.

Herbal Use

Skunk cabbage is stated to possess expectorant, antispasmodic and mild sedative properties. Traditionally, it has been used for bronchitis, whooping cough, asthma and specifically for bronchitic asthma.[G7, G64]

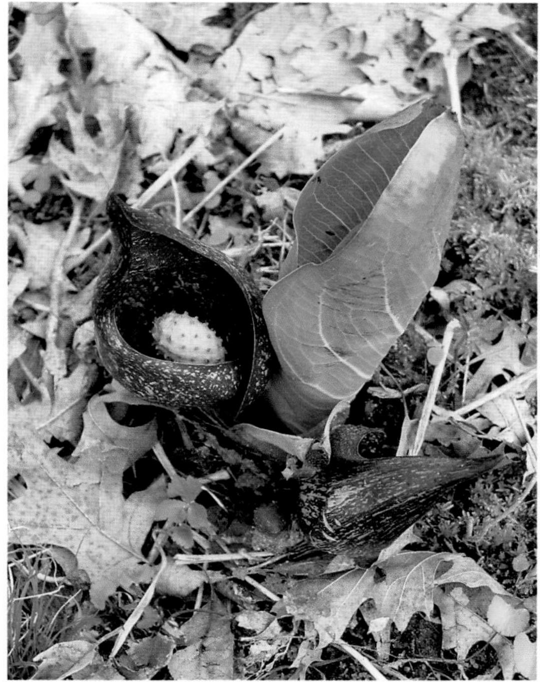

Figure 1 Skunk cabbage (*Symplocarpus foetidus*).

Dosage

Dosages for oral administration (adults) for traditional uses recommended in standard herbal reference texts are given below.

Powdered rhizome/root 0.5–1.0 g in honey or as an infusion or decoction three times daily.[G7]

Liquid extract 0.5–1.0 mL (1 : 1 in 25% alcohol) three times daily.[G7]

Tincture 2–4 mL (1 : 10 in 45% alcohol) three times daily.[G7]

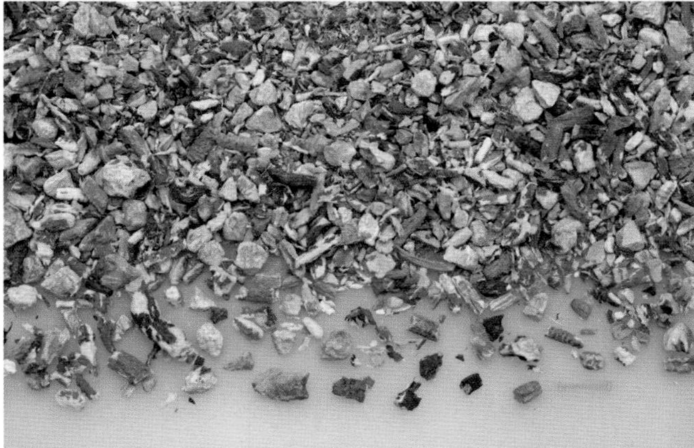

Figure 2 Skunk cabbage – dried drug substance (rhizome).

Pharmacological Actions

In vitro and animal studies

None documented for the rhizome/root. There is a preliminary report of bacteriostatic activity for ethanol extracts of skunk cabbage (plant parts not specified), although data on minimum inhibitory concentrations were not provided. The leaf extract has haemolytic properties,[(G23)] although the scientific basis for this statement is not clear.

Clinical studies

There is a lack of clinical research assessing the effects of skunk cabbage and rigorous randomised clinical trials are required.

Side-effects, Toxicity

There is a lack of clinical safety and toxicity data for skunk cabbage and further investigation of these aspects is required.

The root is reported to be bitter and acrid, with a disagreeable odour. Severe itching and inflammation of the skin has been documented.[(G51)] No published toxicity studies were located.

Contra-indications, Warnings

It has been stated that the fresh plant can cause blistering.[(G42)] In view of the acrid principle thought to be present in both the dried and fresh root,[(G51)] skunk cabbage should be used with caution.

Drug interactions None documented. In view of the lack of information on the constituents of skunk cabbage and their pharmacological activities, the potential for skunk cabbage preparations to interact with other medicines used concurrently should be considered.

Pregnancy and lactation Skunk cabbage is reputed to affect the menstrual cycle[(G22)] although the scientific basis for this statement is not clear. In view of the lack of phytochemical, pharmacological, and toxicological information, and the irritant properties, the use of skunk cabbage during pregnancy and lactation should be avoided.

Preparations

Proprietary multi-ingredient preparations

UK: Horehound and Aniseed Cough Mixture; Vegetable Cough Remover.

References

1 Konyukhov VP *et al*. Dynamics of the accumulation of biologically active agents in *Lysichitum camtsochatcense* and *Symplocarpus foetidus*. *Uch Zap Khabarovsk Gos Pedagog Inst* 1970; 26: 59–62.
2 Chang N *et al*. Anthocyanins in *Symplocarpus foetidus* (L.) Nutt. (Araceae). *Bot J Linn Soc* 1970; 63: 95–96.

S

Slippery Elm

Summary and Pharmaceutical Comment

The primary constituent in slippery elm is mucilage, thereby justifying the herbal use of the remedy as a demulcent, emollient and antitussive. There is, however, a lack of documented scientific evidence to support the use of slippery elm. The mucilage component of slippery elm is unlikely to cause toxicity, although slippery elm has other constituents, not all of which are documented. The use of slippery elm as a food flavouring agent has not been recommended because of insufficient information to assess potential toxicity. In view of the lack of information, the appropriateness of medicinal use of slippery elm should be considered. Excessive use, at least, should be avoided. Slippery elm should not be used during pregnancy and breastfeeding. The potential for slippery elm preparations to interact with other medicines should be considered. The supply of whole bark is controlled by regulations.

Species (Family)

Ulmus rubra Muhl. (Ulmaceae)

Synonym(s)

Ulmus fulva Mich.

Part(s) Used

Bark (inner)

Pharmacopoeial and Other Monographs

BHC 1992[G6]
BHP 1996[G9]
Martindale 35th edition[G85]

Legal Category (Licensed Products)

GSL.[G37] Whole (unpowdered) slippery elm is controlled by regulations.[1]

Constituents

The following is compiled from several sources, including General References G6 and G59.

Carbohydrates Mucilage (major constituent) consisting of hexoses, pentoses, methylpentoses, at least two polyuronides, and yielding on hydrolysis galactose, glucose and fructose (trace), galacturonic acid, L-rhamnose and D-galactose.[2]

Other constituents Tannins 3.0–6.5% (type unspecified), phytosterols (β-sitosterol, citrostadienol, dolichol), sesquiterpenes, calcium oxalate and cholesterol.

Food Use

Slippery elm is listed by the Council of Europe as a natural source of food flavouring (category N3). This category indicates that there is insufficient information available to make an adequate assessment of potential toxicity.[G16]

Herbal Use

Slippery elm is stated to possess demulcent, emollient, nutrient and antitussive properties. Traditionally, it has been used for inflammation or ulceration of the stomach or duodenum, convalescence, colitis, diarrhoea and locally for abcesses, boils and ulcers (as a poultice).[G6, G7, G8, G64]

Dosage

Dosages for oral administration (adults) for traditional uses recommended in standard herbal reference texts are given below.

Powdered bark 4–16 mL (1 : 8 as a decoction) three times daily.[G6, G7]

Powdered bark 4 g in 500 mL boiling water as a nutritional supplement three times daily.[G6, G7]

Coarse powdered bark With boiling water as a poultice.[G6, G7]

Liquid extract 5 mL (1 : 1 in 60% alcohol) three times daily.[G6, G7]

Pharmacological Actions

In vitro and animal studies

There is a lack of information on the pharmacological properties of slippery elm. Mucilages are known to have demulcent and emollient properties. Mucilage is the principal constituent of slippery elm. Tannins are known to possess astringent properties.

Clinical studies

There is a lack of clinical research assessing the effects of slippery elm and rigorous randomised clinical trials are required.

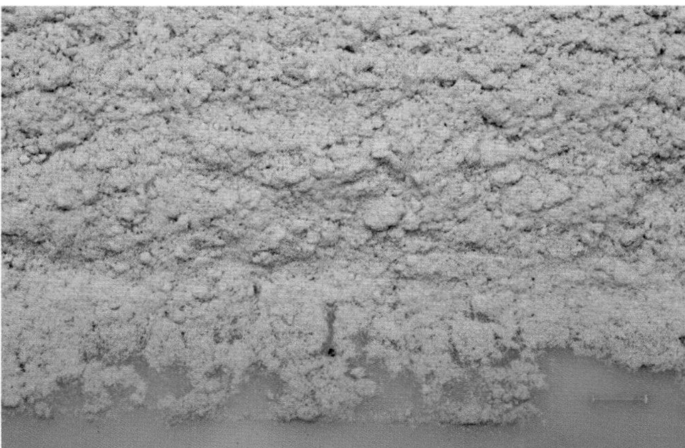

Figure 1 Slippery elm – dried drug substance (powdered bark).

Side-effects, Toxicity

None documented. However, there is a lack of clinical and preclinical safety and toxicity data for slippery elm and further investigation of these aspects is required.

Contra-indications, Warnings

Drug interactions None documented. In view of the lack of information on the constituents of slippery elm and their pharmacological activities, the potential for slippery elm preparations to interact with other medicines administered concurrently should be considered.

Pregnancy and lactation Whole bark has been used to procure abortions. In view of this and the lack of information on the pharmacological properties of slippery elm, it should not be used during pregnancy and breastfeeding.

Preparations

Proprietary multi-ingredient preparations

Australia: Bioglan Psylli-Mucil Plus; Cal Alkyline; Digestive Aid; Herbal Cleanse; PC Regulax; Travelaide. *Canada:* Herbal Throat. *UK:* Modern Herbals Pile; Pileabs; Slippery Elm Skin Soap; Slippery Elm Stomach Tablets; Wood Sap Ointment. *USA:* Laci Le Beau Throat Care.

References

1 The Medicines (Retail Sale or Supply of Herbal Medicines) Order 1977, SI 2130.

2 Tamayo C *et al*. The chemistry and biological activity of herbs used in Flor-Essence™ herbal tonic and Essiac™. *Phytotherapy Res* 2000; 14: 1–14.

Squill

Summary and Pharmaceutical Comment

Squill is characterised by its cardiac glycoside components and unusual flavonoid constituents. The reputed actions of squill as an expectorant, emetic and cathartic can be attributed to the cardioactive components and squill has been used as an expectorant for many years. However, in view of the documented cardioactive and emetic properties of the aglycones, excessive use and use during pregnancy and lactation should be avoided. Red squill is primarily used as a rodenticide.

Species (Family)

Drimia maritima (L.) Stearn (Asparagaceae)

Synonym(s)

Scilla, Sea Onion, Urginea, *Urginea maritima* (L.) Baker, *Urginea scilla* Steinh., White Squill

Part(s) Used

Bulb (red and white varieties)

Pharmacopoeial and Other Monographs

BHC 1992[(G6)]
BHP 1996[(G9)]
BP 2007[(G84)]
Complete German Commission E[(G3)]
Martindale 35th edition[(G85)]

Legal Category (Licensed Products)

GSL[(G37)]

Constituents

See References 1 and 2 and General References G6 and G62.

Cardiac glycosides Scillaren A and proscillaridin A (major constituents); others include glucoscillaren A, scillaridin A, scillicyanoside, scilliglaucoside, scilliphaeoside, scillicoeloside, scillazuroside and scillicryptoside. Scillaren B represents a mixture of the squill glycosides.

Flavonoids Apigenin, dihydroquercetin, isovitexin, iso-orientin, luteolin, orientin, quercetin, taxifolin and vitexin.

Other constituents Stigmasterol, tannin, volatile and fixed oils.

Food Use

The Food Additives and Contaminants Committee (FACC) recommended that squill be prohibited as a food flavouring.[(G45)]

Herbal Use

Squill is stated to possess expectorant, cathartic, emetic, cardioactive and diuretic properties. Traditionally, it has been used for chronic bronchitis, asthma with bronchitis, whooping cough, and specifically for chronic bronchitis with scanty sputum.[(G6, G7, G8, G64)]

Dosage

Dosages for oral administration (adults) for traditional uses recommended in older and contemporary standard herbal and pharmaceutical reference texts are given below.

Dried bulb 60–200 mg as an infusion three times daily.[(G6, G7)]

Squill Liquid Extract (BPC 1973) 0.06–0.2 mL.

Squill Tincture (BPC 1973) 0.3–2.0 mL.

Squill Vinegar (BPC 1973) 0.6–2.0 mL.

Pharmacological Actions

The aglycone components of the cardiac glycoside constituents possess digitalis-like cardiotonic properties.[(G41)] However, the squill aglycones are poorly absorbed from the gastrointestinal tract and are less potent than digitalis cardiac glycosides.[(1, 2)]

Expectorant, emetic and diuretic properties have been documented for white squill.[(G41)] Squill is reported to induce vomiting by both a central action and local gastric irritation.[(1, 2)] Subemetic or near-emetic doses of squill appear to exhibit an expectorant effect, causing an increase in the flow of gastric secretions.[(1, 2)]

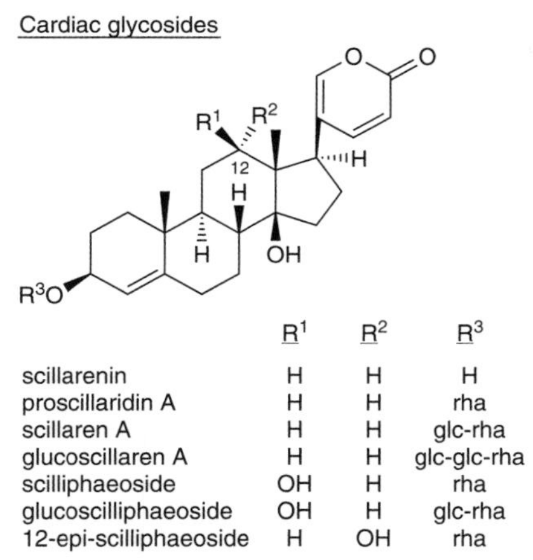

	R1	R2	R3
scillarenin	H	H	H
proscillaridin A	H	H	rha
scillaren A	H	H	glc-rha
glucoscillaren A	H	H	glc-glc-rha
scilliphaeoside	OH	H	rha
glucoscilliphaeoside	OH	H	glc-rha
12-epi-scilliphaeoside	H	OH	rha

glc = glucosyl, rha = rhamnosyl

O
O
H
CHO H
OCOCH3
H OH
O-glucosyl

	R
scilliglaucoside	H
scillicyanoside	$OCOCH_3$

Figure 1 Selected constituents of squill.

S

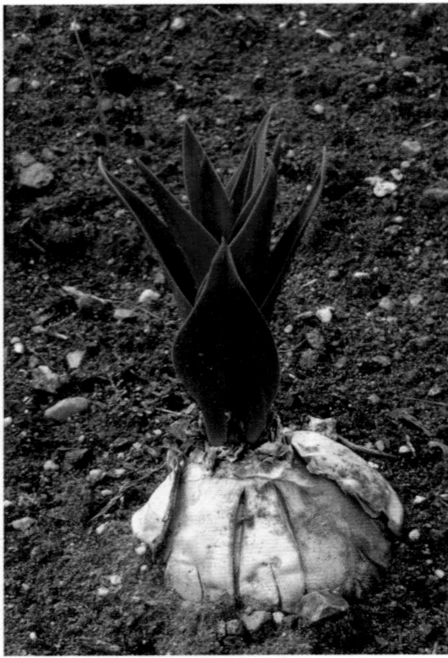

Figure 2 Squill (*Drimia maritima*).

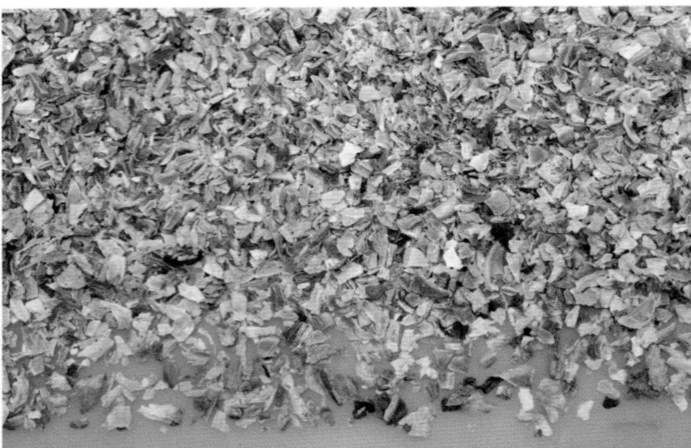

Figure 3 Squill – dried drug substance (bulb).

Antiseborrhoeic properties have been documented for methanol extracts of red squill which have been employed as hair tonics for the treatment of chronic seborrhoea and dandruff.[G41]

Squill extracts have been reported to exhibit peripheral vasodilatation and bradycardia in anaesthetised rabbits.[1,2]

Side-effects, Toxicity

Clinical data

Excessive use of squill is potentially toxic because of the cardiotonic constituents. However, squill is also a gastric irritant and large doses will stimulate a vomiting reflex.

Preclinical data

Red squill is toxic to rats and is mainly used as a rodenticide, causing death by a centrally induced convulsant action.[1,2] A squill soft mass (crude extract) has been stated to be toxic in guinea-pigs at a dose of 270 mg/kg body weight. A fatal dose for Indian squill (*Urginea indica* Kunth.) is documented as 36 mg/kg.

Contra-indications, Warnings

Squill may cause gastric irritation and should be avoided by individuals with a cardiac disorder. In view of the cardiotonic constituents, precautions applied to digoxin therapy should be considered for squill.

Drug interactions None documented. However, the potential for preparations of squill to interact with other medicines administered concurrently, particularly those with similar or opposing effects, should be considered. Squill contains cardiac glycosides, and interactions listed for digoxin should be considered for squill.

Pregnancy and lactation Squill is reputed to be an abortifacient and to affect the menstrual cycle.[G30] In addition, cardioactive and gastrointestinal irritant properties have been documented. The use of squill during pregnancy and lactation should be avoided.

References

1 Court WE. Squill – energetic diuretic. *Pharm J* 1985; 235: 194–197.
2 Anon. *Squill: Lawrence Review of Natural Products*. Levittown, Pennsylvania: Pharmaceutical Information Associates Ltd, 1989.

S

St John's Wort

Summary and Pharmaceutical Comment

The chemical composition of St John's wort has been well studied. Documented pharmacological activities provide supporting evidence for several of the traditional uses stated for St John's wort. Many pharmacological activities appear to be attributable to hypericin, hyperforin and/or the flavonoid constituents; hypericin is also reported to be responsible for the photosensitive reactions that have been documented for St John's wort. With regard to the antidepressant effects of St John's wort, hyperforin rather than hypericin, as originally thought, has emerged as one of the major constituents responsible for antidepressant activity. However, further research is required in order to determine which other constituents contribute to the antidepressant effect.

There are now over forty clinical trials of *H. perforatum* preparations involving patients with different types of depression, although a rigorous systematic review and meta-analysis found that overall the evidence is inconsistent and complex. *H. perforatum* preparations and standard antidepressant agents appear to show similar effects, whereas *H. perforatum* preparations have only small benefits over placebo in patients with major depression; in older studies in patients with mild-to-moderate depression, *H. perforatum* preparations appear to be of more benefit than placebo. A previous systematic review/meta-analysis, for which inclusion criteria for trials were slightly less strict, found evidence from randomised, controlled trials that St John's wort preparations were more efficacious than placebo in the treatment of mild-to-moderately severe depression.

An important point is that there is heterogeneity not only among the trials and their results, but also among the different manufacturers' products tested. Products are not necessarily equally effective, and the results of the analyses above should not be extrapolated to other *H. perforatum* preparations, which may differ considerably in their pharmaceutical quality. These comments also imply that the need for dose adjustment should be considered for patients changing from one St John's wort product to another.

Clinical safety data from randomised controlled trials, systematic reviews and meta-analyses of trials, and post-marketing surveillance and other observational studies, indicate that certain St John's wort extracts are well-tolerated when taken at recommended doses for shorter periods of time (around eight weeks). Certain St John's wort preparations do appear to have a more favourable safety profile, at least with short-term use, than standard antidepressants, particularly older antidepressant agents, a factor that may be important in patients continuing to take medication. Data from the small number of longer-term (one year) studies support the tolerability of certain St John's wort extracts, although further investigation of long-term use is warranted. Adverse events/effects reported are generally mild and most commonly gastrointestinal symptoms. These observations, however, are based on data collected in the settings of formal randomised or observational studies, and usually where *H. perforatum* has been prescribed under the supervision of a physician. The safety of St John's wort products taken as self-treatment without supervision by a healthcare professional requires further study.

The risk of photosensitive reactions following oral ingestion of St John's wort preparations appears to be low, since serum and skin concentrations of hypericin (the photosensitising constituent) after oral administration of recommended doses are below 100 ng/mL, although caution is advised as it is possible that there may be unusual absorption of hypericin in some individuals and in fair-skinned individuals and after extended periods of solar irradiation, there may be increased susceptibility to the photosensitising properties of hypericin. Likewise, the phototoxic potential of topical application of *H. perforatum* preparations appears to be low, although caution is necessary, particularly as hypericin may penetrate more highly through broken or lesional skin, and there may be increased susceptibility to the photosensitising properties of hypericin in fair-skinned individuals and after extended periods of solar irradiation.

There are important pharmacokinetic interactions between St John's wort preparations and certain other medicines, leading to a loss of or reduction in the therapeutic effect of those medicines, and potential for important pharmacodynamic interactions, which could lead to enhancement or antagonism of pharmacological effects, depending on the activities of the co-administered medicines. Drugs that may be affected by pharmacokinetic interactions include certain anticonvulsants, ciclosporin, digoxin, indinavir (and other HIV protease inhibitors), oral contraceptives, theophylline and warfarin, and by pharmacodynamic interactions, triptans and selective serotonin reuptake inhibitors. Advice is that patients taking these medicines should stop taking St John's wort preparations, generally after seeking professional advice, as dose adjustment may be necessary.

There is evidence that pharmacokinetic interactions arise through induction, by constituents of St John's wort preparations, of the cytochrome P450 (CYP) drug-metabolising enzyme CYP3A4 (and possibly certain other CYP enzymes), and through effects on P-glycoprotein (a transport protein). As CYP3A4 is involved in the metabolism of many drugs, and as P-glycoprotein is involved widely in drug transport, it is possible that St John's wort preparations interact with other medicines in addition to those already identified.

In view of the lack of toxicity data, St John's wort preparations should not be used during pregnancy and lactation.

Pharmacists and other healthcare professionals should be mindful that patients at all levels of health care may self-treat with herbal and other non-prescription medicines, and that use is not necessarily disclosed to healthcare professionals. St John's wort products may be used in addition to, or instead of, standard antidepressants and other conventional medicines. The prevalence of concurrent use of St John's wort products and antidepressant medicines may be particularly high among certain subgroups of patients with depression: a cross-sectional survey involving members of a depression self-help group reported that over 50% were using St John's wort and that, among these individuals, the concurrent use of St John's wort and conventional antidepressants was 29% (*see* Side-effects, Toxicity, Clinical data).

Species (Family)

Hypericum perforatum L. (Guttiferae/Clusiaceae)

Synonym(s)

Hypericum, *Hypericum veronense* Schrank, *H. noeanum* Boiss., Millepertuis

Part(s) Used

Herb

Pharmacopoeial and Other Monographs

American Herbal Pharmacopoeia[G1]
BHMA 2003[G66]
BHP 1996[G9]
BP 2007[G84]
Complete German Commission E[G3]
ESCOP 2003 [G76]
Martindale 35th edition[G85]
Ph Eur 2007[G81]
USP29/NF24[G86]
WHO volume 2 (2002)[G70]

Legal Category (Licensed Products)

GSL (for external use only)[G37]

Constituents

See also References 1 and 2 and General References G1 and G2.

Anthraquinone derivatives (naphthodianthrones) Hypericin, pseudohypericin and isohypericin; protohypericin and protopseudohypericin (biosynthetic precursors of hypericin and pseudohypericin, respectively) are present in fresh material. Cyclopseudohypericin is also stated to be present. The hypericin content (approximately 0.1–0.15%) includes both hypericin and pseudohypericin[3] and is sometimes referred to as 'total hypericins'.

Flavonoids Flavonols (e.g. kaempferol, quercetin), flavones (e.g. luteolin) and glycosides (e.g. hyperoside, isoquercitrin, quercitrin, rutin), biflavonoids including biapigenin (a flavone) and amentoflavone (a biapigenin derivative)[4,5] and catechins (flavonoids often associated with condensed tannins).[6,7] The concentrations of rutin, hyperoside and isoquercitrin have been reported as 1.6, 0.9 and 0.3%, respectively.[8]

Prenylated phloroglucinols Hyperforin (2.0–4.5%) and adhyperforin (0.2–1.9%).[6,9,10,G1]

Tannins 8–9%. Type not specified. Proanthocyanidins (condensed type) have been reported.[G2]

Other phenols Caffeic, chlorogenic, *p*-coumaric, ferulic, *p*-hydroxybenzoic and vanillic acids.

Volatile oils 0.05–0.9%. Major component (not less than 30%) is methyl-2-octane (saturated hydrocarbon); others include *n*-nonane and traces of methyl-2-decane and *n*-undecane (saturated hydrocarbons),[11] α- and β-pinene, α-terpineol, geraniol, and traces of myrcene and limonene (monoterpenes), caryophyllene and humulene (sesquiterpenes).[12,13]

Other constituents Acids (isovalerianic, nicotinic, myristic, palmitic, stearic), carotenoids, choline, nicotinamide, pectin, β-sitosterol, straight-chain saturated hydrocarbons (C_{16}, C_{30})[11,14] and alcohols (C_{24}, C_{26}, C_{28}).[11,14]

Quality of plant material and commercial products

According to the British and European Pharmacopoeias, St John's wort herb consists of the whole or cut dried flowering tops of *H. perforatum*, harvested during flowering time, and contains not less than 0.08% of total hypericins, expressed as hypericin, calculated with reference to the dried drug.[G81,G84] Detailed descriptions of *H. perforatum* herb for use in botanical, microscopic and macroscopic identification have been published, along with qualitative and quantitative methods for the assessment of *H. perforatum* herb raw material.[G1]

As with other herbal medicinal products, there is variation in the qualitative and quantitative composition of commercial St John's wort preparations. In the USA, analysis of 21 St John's wort products (18 of which claimed to contain only standardised extracts and three of which were combinations of extracts and crude plant material) found that seven products did not meet at least one of the quality criteria assessed: four products had a hypericin content ranging from 77% to 85% of that stated on their labels or, if not stated on the label, of the minimum acceptable concentration permitted in the analysis; one of the two products claiming to contain hyperforin contained only 21.7% of the stated amount; five products contained cadmium exceeding acceptable concentrations in the analysis, and two of these products contained more than twice the permitted concentration of cadmium.[15] Overall, five of the 18 products labelled with hypericin and/or hyperforin concentrations, and five of the seven products labelled as being produced from 'aerial parts', failed the analysis. Another analytical study which investigated eight St John's wort products marketed in the USA found that their hyperforin content varied from 0.01–1.89%, and that only two products contained more than one percent hyperforin, the minimum concentration suggested to be required for antidepressant effects.[16] Similarly, hypericin content varied from 0.03–0.29% and, for several products, the actual content ranged from 57–130% of that stated on the label.

Analysis (using a liquid chromatographic method with fluorescent detection) of 54 commercially available St John's wort products purchased in the USA and Canada found that only two of the products had a total naphthodianthrone concentration (hypericin and pseudohypericin) within 10% of that stated on the label.[17] Overall, total naphthodianthrone content for tablets and capsules, respectively, ranged from 0–108.6% and from 31.3–80.2% of the amount stated on the label. The naphthodianthrone content of products formulated as tinctures ranged from 0–118.6 μg/mL.

Isolated hyperforin is susceptible to oxidation, although the hyperforin content of dried herb and preparations containing extracts of *H. perforatum* appears to be more stable.[18] Degradation products for hyperforin include deoxyfurohyperforin A,[19] furohyperforin, furoadhyperforin and furohyperforin A and other oxygenated hyperforin analogues.[20,21]

A fast high-performance liquid chromatographic (HPLC) method with photodiode array detection has been developed for the determination of six of the naphthodianthrone (including hypericin) and phloroglucinol (including hyperforin) compounds in *H. perforatum* extracts.[22] The method allows quantitative determination of concentrations as low as 2 μg/mL and 0.5 μg/mL for hyperforin and hypericin, respectively, while detection limits for these compounds were 0.1 and 0.02 μg/mL, respectively.

Variation in St John's wort products is not limited to product composition, but as with other herbal medicinal products also applies to the dissolution profiles of products which might be considered to be pharmaceutically equivalent. *In vitro* dissolution tests using biorelevant conditions (i.e. simulated gastric fluid and similar substances as the dissolution media) were used to determine the dissolution profiles of five St John's wort products purchased in Germany. All products were ethanol or methanol extracts of St John's wort, formulated as tablets or capsules and contained 300–612 mg extract per unit dosage form.[23] In simulated gastric fluid without pepsin, and under conditions simulating the fasted state in the proximal small intestine, dissolution of hyperforin was 'not detected' and 'poor', respectively. Dissolution of hyperforin improved under conditions simulating postprandial conditions in the proximal small intestine for some products (e.g. 90% release within two hours), but was relatively poor for other products (e.g. <50% release within two hours). Dissolution of hypericins into simulated gastric fluid was also not detected; results for dissolution of hypericins into other media were either not available or were deemed to be unreliable. Dissolution of the flavonoid compounds tested (rutin, hyperoside, isoquercitrin and quercitrin) was good into all media tested, although there were variations between products in the release of rutin.[23] These results indicate that these St John's wort products cannot be considered interchangeable; the implication being that the need for dose adjustment should be considered for patients changing from one St John's wort product to another.

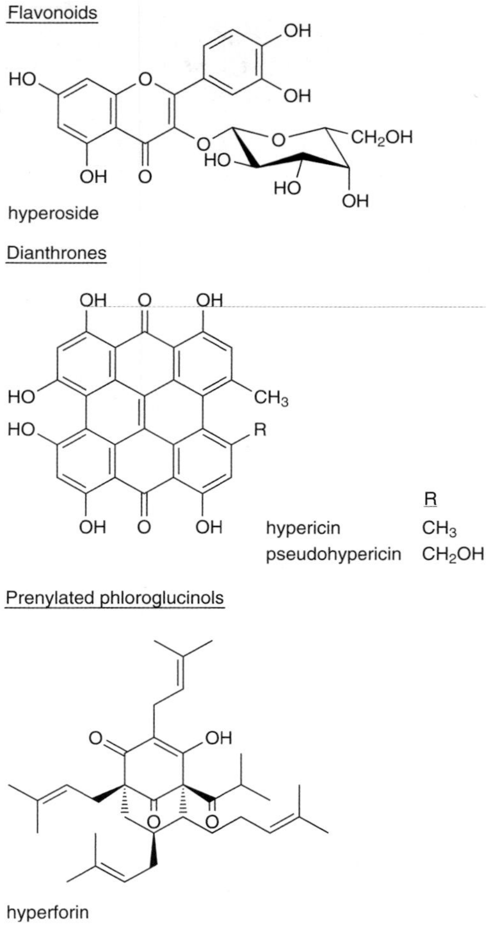

Flavonoids

hyperoside

Dianthrones

	R
hypericin	CH_3
pseudohypericin	CH_2OH

Prenylated phloroglucinols

hyperforin

Figure 1 Selected constituents of St John's wort.

Food Use

St John's wort is listed by the Council of Europe as a natural source of food flavouring (herb: category 5).[G17]

Herbal Use

St John's wort is stated to possess sedative and astringent properties. It has been used for excitability, neuralgia, fibrositis, sciatica, wounds, menopausal neurosis, anxiety and depression and as a nerve tonic.[G3, G7, G32] St John's wort also has a long history of traditional use in topical preparations for wound healing.[G1, G7] St John's wort is used extensively in homeopathic preparations as well as in herbal products. Modern interest is focused on its use as an antidepressant.

Dosage

Dosages for oral administration (adults) recommended in standard herbal reference texts[G6, G7] are the same for several traditional uses; examples are given below.

Dried herb 2–4 g as an infusion three times daily.[G7]

Liquid extract 2–4 mL (1 : 1 in 25% alcohol) three times daily.[G7]

Tincture 2–4 mL (1 : 10 in 45% alcohol) three times daily.[G7]

Doses of St John's wort extracts used in clinical trials involving patients with mild to moderate depression generally range from 240–1800 mg daily (equivalent to varying concentrations of hypericin and hyperforin, depending on the extract), typically for four to six weeks.[24]

Pharmacological Actions

The major active constituents are considered to be hyperforin (a prenylated phloroglucinol) and hypericin (a naphthodianthrone), although other biologically active constituents, e.g. flavonoids and tannins, are also present.[25] Several pharmacological activities, including antidepressant, anticancer, antiviral and antibacterial effects, have been documented for extracts of St John's wort and/or its constituents following preclinical studies. Clinical studies mainly have described antidepressant effects for St John's wort preparations.

In vitro and animal studies

Pharmacokinetics *In vivo* (rats), the bioavailability of hypericin following oral administration was increased by co-administration of procyanidin B2, isolated from *H. perforatum*, or hyperoside.[26]

Antidepressant activity The precise mechanism of action for the antidepressant effect of St John's wort is unclear. Initially, attention was focused on hypericin as the constituent of St John's wort believed to be responsible for the herb's antidepressant effects. Inhibition of monoamine oxidase (MAO) type A and B in

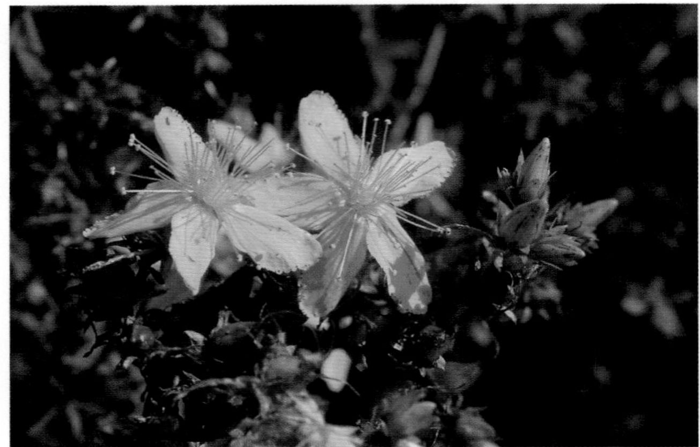

Figure 2 St John's wort (*Hypericum perforatum*).

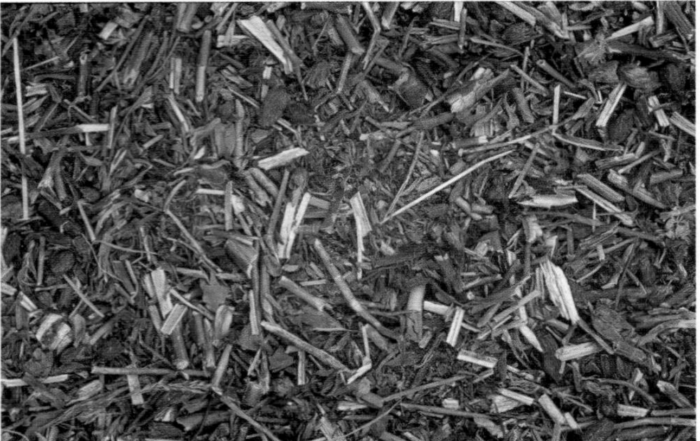

Figure 3 St John's wort – dried drug substance (herb).

rat brain mitochondria *in vitro* was described for hypericin.[27] However, other studies have demonstrated only weak or no MAO inhibition.[28–30]

In vitro receptor binding and enzyme inhibition assays carried out using hypericum extract demonstrated significant receptor affinity for adenosine, $GABA_A$, $GABA_B$, benzodiazepine and MAO types A and B, although, with the exception of $GABA_A$ and $GABA_B$, the concentrations of hypericum required were unlikely to be attained after oral administration in humans.[31] Other biochemical studies have reported that the hypericum extract LI 160 is only a weak inhibitor of MAO-A and MAO-B activity, but that it inhibits the synaptosomal uptake of serotonin (5-hydroxytryptamine or 5-HT), dopamine and noradrenaline (norepinephrine) with approximately equal affinity and also leads to a downregulation of β-receptors and an upregulation of 5-HT_2 receptors in the rat frontal cortex.[32] The effects of fluoxetine and hypericin- and flavonoid-standardised hypericum extracts (LI 160, 0.3% hypericin and 6% flavonoids and Ph-50, 0.3% hypericin and 50% flavonoids) on the concentrations of neurotransmitters in brain regions were studied in rats.[33] All three preparations induced a significant increase in 5-HT concentrations in the rat cortex, both LI 160 and Ph-50 caused increases in noradrenaline (norepinephrine) and dopamine in the rat diencephalon and Ph-50 also induced an increase in the noradrenaline (norepinephrine) content in the brainstem, areas that are implicated in depression.[33]

Other *in vitro* experiments using peripheral blood mononuclear cells have shown that an alcoholic extract of *H. perforatum* containing 0.25 mg/mL hypericin downregulated mitogen-mediated tryptophan degradation in a concentration-dependent manner.[34] Tryptophan is a precursor for biosynthesis of 5-HT.

Hyperforin has now emerged as being one of the major active constituents of importance in antidepressant activity.[35] Hyperforin has been shown to be an uptake inhibitor of 5-HT, dopamine, noradrenaline (norepinephrine), GABA and L-glutamate in synaptosomal preparations[36] and to inhibit 5-HT uptake in rat peritoneal cells in a dose-dependent manner.[37] Studies have also described discrepancies between observed and theoretical IC_{50} values, indicating that hyperforin is not the only component of hypericum extract that is responsible for the observed effects.[37,38] Adhyperforin, another phloroglucinol constituent of *H. perforatum*, also inhibits the uptake of dopamine, serotonin and norepinephrine *in vitro*, and its possible involvement in the antidepressant activity of St John's wort requires further investigation.[39]

In vitro screening of the activities of hypericin, pseudohypericin, hyperforin and several flavonoid constituents of *H. perforatum* using 42 biogenic amine receptors and transporters (available as part of the National Institute of Mental Health Psychoactive Drug Screening Program of the USA) showed that compounds significantly inhibited ligand binding at the following receptors in particular: amentoflavone – serotonin (5-HT_{1D}, 5-HT_{2C}), dopamine-D_3, opiate (delta), benzodiazepine; hypericin and pseudohypericin – dopamine-D_3, dopamine-D_4, β-adrenergic; hyperforin – dopamine-D_1, dopamine-D_5.[40] Hyperforin was less active than the other constituents tested on all receptors screened. Screening revealed some interactions at G-protein coupled receptors that were previously unreported (e.g. hypericin and β-adrenergic activity).

The effects of hyperforin on interleukin-6 (IL-6) release in different experimental models have been explored as a possible alternative mechanism for antidepressant effects, since St John's wort has been shown to inhibit substance-P mediated effects (substance P has been implicated in the aetiology of depression).[41] Hyperforin inhibited both substance-P- and lipopolysaccharide-induced IL-6 release in human astrocytoma cells (IC_{50} = 1.6 and 1.9 μmol/L, respectively), although concentrations required to achieve this were around one order of magnitude higher than those found in the plasma of patients treated with *H. perforatum* extracts.[42]

Other findings indicate that flavonoids, as well as hyperforin and hypericin, are at least some of the constituents of *H. perforatum* responsible for its antidepressant activity.[43,44]

In vivo (mice and rats) experiments which assessed the effects of a hydroalcoholic extract of *H. perforatum* (containing hypericin 0.15% and hyperforin 3.2%) and the same extract with hypericin and hyperforin removed in turn, showed that all extracts, including the extract devoid of both hypericin and hyperforin (but containing 12% flavonoids), retained activity in behavioural models.[43]

It has been reported that the mode of action of hyperforin in serotonin uptake inhibition seems to be associated with the elevation of free intracellular sodium ion concentrations[45] and that this may be secondary to activation of the Na^+/H^+ exchange as a result of a decrease in intracellular pH.[46] Further *in vitro* experiments using two cell systems (human platelets and rat phaeochromocytoma cells) have shown that hyperforin increases both intracellular sodium ion and calcium ion concentrations, and that this is mediated through activation by hyperforin of non-selective cation channels.[47]

Hyperforin was shown to inhibit 5-HT reuptake in washed platelets but not in fresh platelet-rich plasma, suggesting that plasma-protein binding could be a limiting factor for 5-HT uptake inhibition *in vivo*.[48]

A commercial extract of St John's wort has exhibited psychotropic and antidepressant activities in mice.[49] Pure hyperforin and hypericum extracts also demonstrated antidepressant activity in a despair behaviour test in rats.[37]

In other experimental models of depression, including acute and chronic forms of escape deficit induced by stressors, hypericum extract was shown to protect rats from the consequences of unavoidable stress.[50] In studies using the rat forced swimming test, an experimental model of depression, hypericum extracts induced a significant reduction in immobility.[51] Flavonoid fractions and flavonoids isolated from these fractions have also been reported to have antidepressant activity in the forced swimming test in rats.[52]

Cytotoxic and anticancer activities The findings of a substantial body of preclinical research have documented anticancer activites for *H. perforatum* preparations and their constituents. A methanolic extract of *H. perforatum* (containing hypericin 0.3% and hyperforin 3.8%) administered intraperitoneally (15 mg/kg body weight) ten days before implantation of PC-3 human Caucasian prostate adenocarcinoma cells in nude mice significantly reduced tumour growth and the number of regional lymph node metastases ($p < 0.01$ for both).[53] The same extract at a concentration of 1.41 mg/mL also significantly inhibited the proliferation of PC-3 cells *in vitro* (IC_{50} = 0.42 mg/mL). Ethanolic extracts of *H. perforatum* from fresh and dried plant material (drug to extract ratio 1.3-1.5 : 1) inhibited the proliferation of human malignant cells (e.g. leukamia cell lines K562 and U937) in a concentration-dependent manner.[54] The extracts also induced apoptosis of glioblastoma LN229 cells. The observed effects were potentiated by light activation. In a similar series of experiments using extracts of *H. perforatum* containing 0.3% hypericins but differing concentrations of hyperforin (0.21%, 2.21% or 3.25% w/w) and flavonoids (5.3% or 10% w/w), antiproliferative activity of the different extracts varied (GI_{50} values: 248.3 to 621.3 μg/mL and 378.2 to 911.7 μg/mL for K562 and U937 cell lines, respectively), indicating that the flavonoid constituents, as well as hypericin and hyperforin, contribute to the observed effects.[55] The possibility that constituents other than hypericin have cytotoxic and/or antiproliferative activity is supported by further *in vitro* work which showed that a methanolic extract of *H. perforatum* flowering parts inhibited growth of K562 cells and induced apoptosis to a greater extent than did hypericin alone.[56] In mice injected with murine and human cancer cell lines, seven days' pretreatment with hyperforin (as the stable dicyclohexylammonium salt) intraperitoneally reduced several markers of cancer infiltration and metastasis.[57] In rats given subcutaneous injections of MT-450 rat mammary carcinoma cells, treatment with hyperforin (100 μL of 2 mmol/L solution subcutaneously at the tumour site once daily) for two weeks starting 15 days after tumour injection inhibited tumour growth to a similar extent as did paclitaxel given according to the same dosage regimen.[58] There is evidence that the mechanism by which hyperforin induces apoptosis involves the activation of caspases (inactive proenzymes).[58, 59]

Numerous preclinical studies have established that hypericin is a photocytotoxic agent. Hypericin photosensitisation has been documented for various cancer cell lines *in vitro*[60–64] and in several *in vivo* experimental models of cancer.[61, 65] The photocytotoxic effects of hypericin towards human leukaemic HL-60 cells can be potientiated *in vitro* by co-incubation with acetazolamide[66] and quercetin.[67] Phototoxicity and induction of apoptosis also occur with pseudohypericin *in vitro*.[68] Hypericin photo-induced apoptosis may involve the tumour necrosis factor (TNF)-related apoptosis-inducing ligand,[69] activation of caspases, such as caspase-8,[69, 70] and inhibition of proteasome function (which is involved in caspase activation).[71]

Further *in vitro* studies have added a layer of complexity to the above findings. Hypericin can induce apoptosis or necrosis, depending on the intracellular hypericin concentration and/or the light-activating dose.[72] Furthermore, exposure of U937 cells to hypericin and sub-lethal doses of light irradiation induced subsequent photoresistance with light doses which normally induced apoptosis.[73, 74]

In an *in vitro* system involving the human cytochrome P450 enzyme CYP1A1, three commercially available *H. perforatum* extracts as well as several constituents of *H. perforatum* extracts (with the exception of rutin) inhibited the CYP1A1-catalysed epoxidation of (±)-*trans*-7,8-dihydro-7,8-dihydroxy-benzo(a)pyrene, the reaction which leads to formation of the carcinogenic product diolepoxide 2.[75]

In vitro cytotoxicity against human colon carcinoma cells (CO 115) has been described for hyperforin-related constituents isolated from *Hypericum calycinum* and *Hypericum revolutum*.[76]

Antimicrobial activity Extracts of *H. perforatum* aerial parts have antibacterial activity against Gram-positive bacteria, particularly *Bacillus subtilis* and *B. cereus*, but not Gram-negative bacteria and yeasts, according to the findings of a series of *in vitro* assays.[77]

A leaf extract of *H. perforatum* has been documented as enhancing the immunity of mice towards *Staphylococcus aureus* and *Bordetella pertussis*.[78] Hyperforin has antibacterial activity against *S. aureus*,[9] multi-drug resistant *S. aureus* and Gram-positive bacteria, including *Streptococcus pyogenes* and *Corynebacterium diphtheriae*.[79] However, the antibacterial effects of hyperforin are only observed at high concentrations.[80, 81] Other experiments have shown that *S. aureus* is able to acquire resistance to hyperforin, but that this does not occur with hyperforin concentrations similar to those found in patients treated with *H. perforatum* extracts for depression.[82] Hyperforin did not exhibit any growth inhibitory effect against Gram-negative bacteria, such as *Enterococcus faecalis*, *Escherichia coli* and *Pseudomonas aeruginosa* or against *Candida albicans*.[79] Other antibacterial constituents (imanine and novoimanine) have been isolated from St John's wort.[83, 84]

Several other species of *Hypericum* have been shown to have antimicrobial activity.[85, 86] In disc-diffusion assays, 33 of 34 chloroform extracts of *Hypericum* species (not including *H. perforatum*) showed substantial activity against a clinical isolate of methicillin-resistant *Staphylococcus aureus*.[86]

Antiviral activity Flavonoid and catechin-containing fractions have exhibited antiviral activity, inhibiting the influenza virus by 83–100%.[87] Hypericin and pseudohypericin have been reported to inhibit several encapsulated viruses *in vitro*, including herpes simplex types 1 and 2,[88, 89] varicella-zoster virus[90] and human immunodeficiency virus type 1 (HIV-1).[91–94] Hypericin has also been reported to inactivate murine cytomegalovirus (MCMV) and Sindbis virus.[94] The antiviral activity of hypericin appears to involve a photoactivation process.[94, G1] An extract of a St John's wort product (5–50 μL/mL; no further details provided) and pure hypericin (5–20 μmol/L) inhibited UV-induced HIV gene expression in HeLa cells in a concentration-dependent manner, whereas hypericin without UV-induced HIV gene activation had no effect on HIV gene expression.[95]

Other effects *In vitro* studies using a hamster vas deferens smooth muscle cell line demonstrated that hyperforin induces the release of calcium ions from mitochondrial or other sources followed by activation of cellular metabolism.[96] It is not known whether this activity contributes to the antidepressant effects of hyperforin.

Oral administration of a single dose of St John's wort (100, 200, 400, 600 or 800 mg/kg) to two strains of alcohol-preferring rats significantly reduced alcohol intake in both strains.[97] In another study in experimental alcoholism, acute intraperitoneal administration of St John's wort (10–40 mg/kg), fluoxetine (1–10 mg/kg) and imipramine (3–30 mg/kg) reduced alcohol intake in a dose-dependent manner in a 12-hour, limited access, two-bottle choice (ethanol/water) procedure.[51] In alcohol-preferring mice, the dose (5 mg/kg administered orally by gavage) of a hyperforin-rich carbon-dioxide extract of *H. perforatum* required to reduce the intake of 10% ethanol to a statistically significant extent was 125-fold lower than that required with a crude methanolic extract (625 mg/kg) with negligible hyperforin content administered by the same route.[98] In mice, oral administration of a *Hypericum perforatum* extract (Ph-50) attenuated nicotine withdrawal symptoms.[99] Depression, alcoholism and smoking are thought to have some neurochemical similarities, such as low brain serotonin concentrations.[100, 101]

An extract of St John's wort was found to suppress inflammation and leukocyte infiltration induced by carrageenan and prostaglandin E_1 (PGE_1) in mice.[102] *In vitro*, hypericin has been shown to inhibit tumour necrosis factor-induced activation of the transcription factor NF-κB,[103] specific growth factor-regulated protein kinases[104–106] and the release of arachidonic acid and leukotriene B_4.[107] In a rabbit model of proliferative vitreoretinopathy (PVR), intravitreal injection of hypericin 0.1 mL (10 or 100 μmol/L, but not 1 μmol/L) inhibited the progression of PVR when compared with severity in control eyes five days after hypericin administration.[108] It was suggested that, as protein kinase C is important in the cellular reactions occurring in PVR, modulation of protein kinase C by hypericin may be a factor in this system. Hypericin and pseudohypericin have been reported to inhibit 12-lipoxygenase activity; the products of lipoxygenase-catalysed reactions, include leukotrienes.[109] Hyperforin has also been shown to inhibit the activity of enzymes involved in inflammatory pathways: *in vitro*, hyperforin inhibited 5-lipoxygenase and cyclooxygenase 1, but not cyclooxygenase 2.[110]

Antioxidant properties have been reported for *H. perforatum* following *in vitro* experiments. St John's wort products (Nature's Plus and Movana, respectively) obtained in the USA and labelled as being hypericin- (0.3–0.5%) and hyperforin-standardised (minimum 3%) attenuated superoxide production in an inverse concentration-dependent manner in a cell-free system and in an experimental model using human vascular tissue.[111] Hyperforin isolated from *H. perforatum* reduced radical formation by polymorphonuclear cells from healthy human donors after stimulation with *N*-formyl-methionyl-leucyl-phenylalanine (IC_{50} = 1.8 μmol/L).[112] However, in other systems, hyperforin did not exhibit any free-radical scavenging activity against 2,2-diphenyl-1-picrylhydrazyl and was inactive in an enzymatic assay based on oxygen radical production by horseradish peroxidase in the presence of hydrogen peroxide.

Imanine was reported to reduce blood pressure and increase the frequency and depth of breathing following intravenous administration (50 mg/kg) to rabbits.[83] A study of the vasoconstrictor action of water-soluble imanine and imanine on the isolated rabbit ear indicated that their hypotensive action was not due to a direct effect on the vasculature.[83] When perfused through the isolated frog heart, both water-soluble imanine and imanine were found to cause cardiac systolic arrest at a dilution of 1×10^{-5}.[83] Proanthocyanidin-containing fractions isolated from St John's wort have been reported to inhibit contractions of the isolated guinea-pig heart induced by histamine, $PGF_{2\alpha}$ and potassium chloride.[113]

A tonus-raising effect on isolated guinea-pig and rabbit uteri has been documented for a crude aqueous extract.[114] Of the group of plants investigated, St John's wort was reported to exhibit the weakest uterotonic activity.

A dried methanol extract of St John's wort (no further details provided) protected human neuroblastoma cells against hydrogen peroxide induced apoptosis *in vitro*.[115]

Analgesic activity in mice has been reported for a total flavonoid fraction of *H. perforatum*;[116] the active principle was stated to be of the quercetin type.

Tannins isolated from St John's wort are stated to have mild astringent activity.[117] The anthraquinone derivatives documented for St John's wort do not possess any purgative action.[G62]

Clinical studies

Clinical trials with extracts of St John's wort have focused mainly on its effects in patients with depression, although there have been several studies exploring its use in other conditions, including seasonal affective disorder, chronic fatigue and premenstrual syndrome.[118]

Pharmacodynamics Initially, hypericin was thought to be responsible for the antidepressant activity of St John's wort, although, more recently, experimental[36, 37] and clinical evidence[119] has emerged to indicate that hyperforin is one of the major constituents required for antidepressant activity.

The precise mechanism of action of St John's wort's antidepressant effect remains unclear (*see* Pharmacological Actions, *In vitro* and animal studies).

In a randomised, double-blind, placebo-controlled, crossover study involving 16 healthy volunteers who received St John's wort extract (Neuroplant) 300 mg three times daily for seven days, St John's wort extract did not influence plasma norepinephrine (noradrenaline) concentrations, but significantly increased plasma dihydroxyphenylacetic acid concentrations (the main metabolite of dopamine), compared with placebo (p = 0.013).[120]

Studies in humans have reported conflicting results with respect to the effects of St John's wort extracts on endocrinological parameters. A double-blind, placebo-controlled, crossover study in 12 healthy male volunteers investigated the effects of a single dose of St John's wort extract (LI 160) (2700 mg, 9 × 300-mg tablets standardised to 0.3% hypericin) on plasma concentrations of growth hormone, prolactin and cortisol.[121] A significant increase in plasma growth hormone concentration and a significant decrease in plasma prolactin concentration were observed following St John's wort administration relative to placebo administration. Plasma cortisol concentrations were unchanged. These findings suggest that this dose of St John's wort extract may increase aspects of brain dopamine function in humans, although further studies are required to confirm this, assess dose–response relationships and determine whether there is evidence for effects on dopaminergic systems in patients with depression treated with St John's wort.[121] Another study, which used a randomised, three-way, crossover design, investigated the effects of a single dose of St John's wort extract (LI 160S) (600 or 300 mg) or placebo on hormone concentrations in 12 healthy male volunteers.[122] Compared with placebo, St John's wort extract (600 mg) increased cortisol secretion between 30 and 90 minutes after dosing, indicating an influence of St John's wort on certain CNS neurotransmitters. There was no difference between the three groups with regard to adrenocorticotrophic hormone (ACTH), growth hormone and prolactin secretion.[122]

By contrast, in a randomised, single-blind, placebo-controlled, crossover study involving 12 healthy male volunteers, mean serum ACTH concentrations, but not cortisol, growth hormone and prolactin concentrations, were significantly increased following oral administration of a St John's wort extract (WS-5570) at doses of 600, 900 and 1200 mg/day on four different days ($p < 0.05$ versus placebo). However, there were no significant differences in ACTH concentrations between groups when a statistical adjustment (Bonferroni correction) was made for post-hoc tests.[123] Differences in the findings of this study, compared with previous work, may be due to differences between doses, products tested and their bioavailabilities.[123]

Therapeutic effects Depression There are now over forty clinical trials of *H. perforatum* preparations involving patients with different types of depression, and many of these trials have been included in systematic reviews.

A Cochrane systematic review included 37 randomised, double-blind, controlled clinical trials of monopreparations of *H. perforatum* involving a total of 4925 patients with depressive disorders.[24] Of these, 26 trials were placebo-controlled, 14 compared *H. perforatum* preparations with standard antidepressants (imipramine 50 to 150 mg daily, four trials; fluoxetine 20 to 40 mg daily, four trials; sertraline 75 to 150 mg daily, three trials; amitriptyline 30 or 75 mg daily, two trials; maprotiline 75 mg daily, one trial) and three of these studies[124–126] also included a placebo control group. Trials involved a variety of *H. perforatum* preparations administered at doses of 240 to 1800 mg extract daily. The treatment period was typically four to six weeks (29 trials) although administration periods ranged from four to 12 weeks overall. The most frequently investigated product was LI-160 (Lichtwer Pharma, Germany). Overall, 24 trials involved only patients with major depression. In most trials ($n = 35$), the Hamilton Rating Scale for Depression (HAMD) was the instrument used to assess outcomes, and the methodological quality of the majority of the included studies was considered to be 'reasonable to good'.[24]

Of the 26 trials (involving 3320 participants) comparing *H. perforatum* preparations with placebo, 23 provided data which were eligible for meta-analysis. For these studies, the results indicated that *H. perforatum* preparations were more effective than placebo (response rate ratio (RRR), 95% confidence interval (CI): 1.55, 1.42–1.70), although when the analysis was limited to larger (i.e. more precise) trials in patients with major depression only, the results showed a small benefit for *H. perforatum* over placebo (RRR, 95% CI: 1.15, 1.02–1.129).[24] Similarly, meta-analysis of data from the 23 placebo-controlled trials which used HAMD scores to assess outcomes indicated that *H. perforatum* preparations were more effective than placebo (weighted mean difference (WMD), 95% CI: −3.25, −3.74 to −2.77), but when the analysis was restricted to the 12 such trials involving only patients with major depression, the effect was less marked (WMD, 95% CI: −2.48, −3.06 to −1.89).

Meta-analysis of data from the 14 trials (involving 2283 participants) comparing *H. perforatum* with standard antidepressant agents indicated that *H. perforatum* preparations had similar effects to those of standard antidepressants (RRR, 95% CI: 1.01, 0.93 to 1.10 and WMD, 95% CI: −0.06, −0.64 to 0.51 for trials providing response rate data (13 trials) and HAMD scores (11 trials), respectively).[24] Results were similar for sub-analysis of the trials comparing *H. perforatum* preparations with older antidepressants and comparisons with newer antidepressants (selective serotonin reuptake inhibitors).

The conclusions drawn from this work were that the evidence is inconsistent and complex. *H. perforatum* preparations and standard antidepressant agents appear to show similar effects, whereas *H. perforatum* preparations have only small benefits over placebo in patients with major depression; in older studies in patients with mild-to-moderate depression, *H. perforatum* preparations appear to be of more benefit than placebo.[24] An important point is that there is heterogeneity not only among the trials and their results, but also among the different manufacturers' products tested. Products are not necessarily equally effective, and the results of the analyses above should not be extrapolated to other *H. perforatum* preparations, which may differ considerably in their pharmaceutical quality (*see* Quality of plant material and commercial products).

One of the trials included in the systematic review was a randomised, double-blind, placebo-controlled, multicentre study comparing an extract of *H. perforatum* (LI-160, standardised for hypericin 0.12–0.28%) 900 mg daily with the SSRI sertraline (which is authorised for the treatment of depression) at a dose of 50 mg daily in 340 patients with major depressive disorder. The trial was funded by the National Center for Complementary and Alternative Medicine and the National Institute of Mental Health, USA, and was designed to assess whether or not *H. perforatum* extract was superior to placebo after 8 weeks' treatment.[126] However, at the end of the study, there were no statistically significant differences in the two primary outcome measures (changes in HAMD scores and response rate) not only between *H. perforatum* extract and placebo, but also between sertraline and placebo. Thus, this trial was criticised for lacking the sensitivity at least to detect the effectiveness of a treatment known to be effective (i.e. sertraline).

A further issue which arose subsequently relates to adherence to treatment among participants randomised to the *H. perforatum* group. Analysis of blood samples available for 97 of the 113 *H. perforatum* recipients revealed that 80 (82%) had detectable concentrations of hyperforin in at least one sample, whereas 17 (17%) had no detectable hyperforin in any of their samples.[127] The sensitivity threshold of the assay was hyperforin 10 ng/mL. Furthermore, of 104 of the 116 participants randomised to placebo for whom blood samples were available, 18 (17%) had detectable concentrations of hyperforin in at least one sample. By contrast, sertraline and/or *N*-desmethylsertraline were detected in at least one sample for all sertraline recipients for whom blood samples were available (91 of 111). Reanalysis of the efficacy data using only data from participants with plasma hyperforin concentrations consistent with their treatment allocation did not change the initial findings.[127]

A randomised, double-blind, multicentre trial comparing the effects of a hydroalcoholic extract of *H. perforatum* herb (WS-5570, drug to extract ratio 3–7 : 1, standardised for hyperforin 3–6% and hypericin 0.12–0.28%; Schwabe Pharmaceuticals) with those of paroxetine in the acute treatment of moderate to severe depression has been published since the revised Cochrane review was completed. In the study, after a placebo run-in phase, 251 participants with acute major depression received *H. perforatum* extract 300 mg three times daily (increased to 1800 mg daily in non-responders), or paroxetine 20 mg daily (40 mg daily for non-responders), for six weeks.[128] At the end of the study, the *H. perforatum* extract was reported to be at least as effective as paroxetine in reducing symptoms of moderate to severe depression (mean (standard deviation) reduction in HAMD scores from baseline values: 14.4 (8.8) and 11.4 (8.6) for *H. perforatum* and paroxetine, respectively).

The review described above[24] was an update of a previous Cochrane systematic review and meta-analysis of 27 randomised controlled trials of *H. perforatum* preparations in depressive disorders.[129] The updated review had stricter and tighter inclusion and exclusion criteria for trials – only trials which explicitly stated that the method of treatment allocation was random and which used a double-blind design were included, and trials investigating *H. perforatum* for prevention of depression, those using combination preparations containing *H. perforatum*, comparing *H. perforatum* with drugs not explicitly recommended as antidepressant agents, measuring only physiological parameters and those with a treatment period of less than four weeks were excluded.[24] Thus, the previous Cochrane review included seven trials which were excluded from the updated review.

The results of the earlier meta-analysis showed that *H. perforatum* preparations were significantly superior to placebo in the short-term treatment of mild to moderately severe depressive disorders (rate ratio 2.47 and 95% confidence interval (95% CI) 1.69–3.61). and as effective as conventional antidepressant agents (single preparations, rate ratio 1.01 and 95% CI 0.87–1.16), although for several reasons – for example, the use of low doses of conventional antidepressants and the trials involving small numbers of patients – this evidence was considered inadequate for establishing whether *H. perforatum* preparations were as effective as conventional antidepressant drugs.[129] Further studies comparing St John's wort preparations with standard antidepressant agents in well-defined patient groups and over longer periods were considered necessary.[129]

Another earlier meta-analysis employed tighter inclusion criteria for trials in an effort to increase the validity of the analysis.[130] It included only randomised, blinded, controlled trials of St John's wort as a single preparation, which involved patients with depressive disorders as defined by the standard criteria ICD-10 (International Statistical Classification of Diseases and Related Health Problems), DSM-IIIR (Diagnostic and Statistical Manual) or DSM-IV and which used the Hamilton Depression (HAMD) Scale for measuring clinical outcomes. Six such trials involving 651 patients with mainly mild to moderately severe depressive disorders were included; two trials were placebo controlled and four compared St John's wort with standard antidepressants. The studies lasted for 4–6 weeks and the doses of St John's wort extract ranged from 200 to 900 mg daily; the range for total hypericin administered was 0.75–2.7 mg daily.

This meta-analysis showed that the response rate for St John's wort was significantly greater than that for placebo (73.2% versus 37.9%, respectively, relative risk 1.48 and 95% CI 1.03–1.92) and similar to that observed with tricyclic antidepressants (64% versus 6.4% for St John's wort and tricyclic antidepressants, respectively, relative risk 1.11 and 95% CI 0.92–1.29).[130] Despite the stringent inclusion criteria for trials in this meta-analysis, it was concluded that further studies are required in order to address methodological problems before it can be concluded that St John's wort is an effective antidepressant.[130]

A systematic review of large-scale observational studies of *H. perforatum* extracts in patients with depressive disorders is also available. The review included 16 non-randomised studies (involving a total of 34 804 patients) each involving at least 100 participants with depressive disorders who were treated with *H. perforatum* preparations for at least four weeks.[131] Fifteen of the studies reported physician-assessed response rates, and these ranged from 65% to 100% for short-term studies (four to around six weeks' treatment; 13 studies) and were 60% and 69% for the two long-term studies (52 weeks' treatment). Patient-assessed response rates ranged from 63% to 98% (ten studies). These results suggest that the *H. perforatum* extracts assessed are effective for mild and moderately severe depressive disorders, although this conclusion cannot be definitive since the studies did not include random allocation to treatment and many had other methodological limitations.[131] Furthermore, the studies included in the review assessed the effects of 12 different *H. perforatum* products, with some differences in how they were standardised, administered at doses ranging from 360 to 1200 mg extract daily. Thus, the results cannot be extrapolated directly to other *H. perforatum* preparations with a different phytochemical profile.

One of the studies included in the review assessed the effects of an *H. perforatum* preparation in children aged under 12 years with symptoms of depression and psychovegetative disturbances. This study reported the highest physician- and patients-assessed response rates (100% and 98%, respectively).[132] Other open, uncontrolled studies[133] have explored the effects of *H. perforatum* preparations in children and adolescents, although the efficacy of such preparations in these patient groups requires testing in randomised controlled trials.

In a dose-ranging trial involving 348 patients with mild to moderate depression according to ICD-10 criteria, patients were randomised to receive St John's wort extract three times daily equivalent to either 1 mg (n = 119), 0.33 mg (n = 115) or 0.17 mg (n = 114) hypericin for six weeks.[134] At the end of the treatment period, there was a significant reduction in HAMD scores compared with baseline values. The response rates (according to recognised criteria) were 68%, 65% and 62% for 1, 0.33 and 0.17 mg hypericin, respectively; the differences between groups were not statistically significant. Thus, the study showed that there was no dose-dependent effect of hypericin in St John's wort extracts.

Smoking cessation A preliminary, uncontrolled study has assessed the effects of a methanol (80%) extract of *H. perforatum* herb (LI-160, standardised for hypericin 900 µg and a minimum of 2% hyperforin; drug to extract ratio 3–6 : 1) as an aid to motivational/behavioural support in adult smokers who wish to stop smoking. The rationale for investigating *H.*

perforatum in this indication is that there is an association between smoking and depression: nicotine may act as an antidepressant in some smokers, and depression can be precipitated by nicotine withdrawal, i.e. smoking cessation.(101) In the study, point prevalence and continuous abstinence rates were both 18% at 3 months, and 0% at 12 months (intention-to-treat analysis); these rates compare poorly with response rates in placebo groups in controlled clinical studies of other smoking cessation interventions.(135)

Seasonal affective disorder The effects of St John's wort extracts have been investigated in studies involving subjects with seasonal affective disorder (SAD),(136, 137) although as yet there have not been any trials that have included a placebo control group. Twenty individuals with SAD were randomised to receive St John's wort (LI 160) (300 mg) three times daily (equivalent to 0.9 mg hypericin) with or without bright light therapy.(136) After four weeks, there were significant reductions in HAMD scores in both groups compared with baseline values and there were no statistically significant differences between groups. Another study evaluated data from individuals with mild to moderate SAD who had used St John's wort (300 mg) three times daily (equivalent to 0.9 mg hypericin) with (n = 133) or without light therapy (n = 168) for eight weeks.(137) The study was not randomised and involved data collection by postal questionnaires. Data from 301 returned questionnaires were suitable for analysis. Significant reductions in the mean SAD scores were observed in both groups compared with baseline values; the differences in the SAD scores between groups were statistically non-significant.

Antiviral activity Antiviral activity has been reported for hypericin against human immunodeficiency virus (HIV).(138, 139) Several uncontrolled studies in HIV-positive patients who received St John's wort extract have reported immunologic and clinical benefits, including increases in CD4 cell counts in some patients.(140, 141) In a phase I, dose-escalating study, 30 HIV-positive patients with CD4 cell counts <350 cells/mm^3 received intravenous synthetic hypericin twice weekly (0.25 or 0.5 mg/kg body weight), three times weekly (0.25 mg/kg) or oral hypericin daily (0.5 mg/kg).(142) Sixteen patients discontinued treatment early because of toxic effects, and phototoxicity in several other patients prevented completion of dose escalation. Antiretroviral activity as assessed by significant changes in HIV p24 antigen level, HIV titre, HIV RNA copies and CD4 cell counts was not observed.

In contrast, in a phase-I dose-escalation study involving 19 patients with hepatitis C virus (HCV) infection who received hypericin administered orally at doses of 0.05 and 0.10 mg/kg daily for eight weeks, there was no evidence of antiviral activity as determined by median changes in HCV RNA concentrations in plasma.(143)

Other studies The potential for the use of St John's wort in 20 individuals presenting with fatigue(144) and in 19 women with self-reported premenstrual syndrome(145) has also been explored in uncontrolled pilot studies. Significant improvements in perceived fatigue and in symptoms of depression and anxiety were seen after six weeks' treatment with St John's wort (equivalent to 0.9 mg hypericin daily) compared with baseline values(144) and in overall premenstrual syndrome scores after treatment with St John's wort (equivalent to 0.9 mg hypericin daily) for two menstrual cycles.(145) Thus, there is scope for conducting randomised controlled trials of St John's wort in these conditions.(144, 145)

A randomised, double-blind, placebo-controlled trial assessed the effects of an 80% methanol extract of St John's wort (LI-160; containing 300 mg extract, drug to extract ratio 4–7 : 1) in 175 patients with somatoform disorders (usually characterised by chronic multiple physical symptoms not explained by underlying organic pathology). Participants received St John's wort extract 300 mg twice daily (n = 87), or placebo (n = 88), for six weeks. At the end of the study, according to an intention-to-treat analysis, St John's wort recipients, compared with placebo recipients, showed statistically significant improvements on the six individual variables comprising the primary efficacy analysis and in the combined score ($p < 0.0001$ for all comparisons).(146)

Another randomised, double-blind, parallel-group trial investigated the effects of LI-160 300 mg extract twice daily (increased in increments to a maximum of 1800 mg extract daily at the physician's discretion), or placebo, for 12 weeks in 41 individuals with social phobia (social anxiety disorder). At the end of the study, there was no statistically significant difference between the two groups in Liebowitz Social Anxiety Scale scores, the primary outcome measure ($p = 0.79$).(147)

In a randomised, double-blind, placebo-controlled trial, 179 women with menopause-related psychovegetative symptoms received a combination preparation of St John's wort and black cohosh (*Cimicifuga racemosa*) or placebo for six weeks.(148) The results indicated that the combination product had a significantly greater effect on the symptoms than did placebo.

A randomised, double-blind, phase I study involving 55 healthy volunteers who received St John's wort (900 mg) daily (containing 0.5% hyperforin), St John's wort (900 mg) daily (containing 5.0% hyperforin) or placebo for eight days investigated the effects on quantitative electroencephalogram as an indicator of drug-induced pharmacological action.(149) Reproducible central pharmacodynamic effects were apparent in both groups of St John's wort recipients compared with placebo recipients. The effects were greater in subjects who received extract containing 5.0% hyperforin than in those who received extract containing 0.5% hyperforin.

Placebo-controlled, crossover studies investigating the effects of St John's wort (0.9 and 1.8 mg) on the sleep polysomnogram of healthy subjects reported that both doses of St John's wort significantly increased rapid eye movement (REM) sleep latency compared with placebo, but had no effect on REM sleep duration or other parameters of sleep architecture.(150)

In a randomised, double-blind, placebo-controlled trial involving 23 overweight but otherwise healthy adults, subjects who received treatment with St John's wort (900 mg) daily, *Citrus aurantium* extract (975 mg) daily and caffeine (528 mg) daily lost significantly more body weight than did subjects in the placebo and no-treatment control groups.(151)

A placebo-controlled, crossover study in 19 healthy volunteers who received St John's wort for 15 days either alone or in combination with ethanol (to achieve a blood alcohol concentration of 0.05%) reported that there were no differences between the two groups in sense of well-being or adverse events.(152)

A randomised, double-blind, placebo-controlled, six-week trial involving 72 long-distance runners and triathletes reported significant improvements in endurance capacity in subjects who received vitamin E with St John's wort compared with subjects who received vitamin E alone or placebo.(153)

In a randomised, double-blind trial involving 21 patients with symmetrical mild to moderate atopic dermatitis, participants used a topical preparation of *H. perforatum* (cream containing 5% of a carbon-dioxide extract; drug to extract ratio 20–25 : 1, containing total 9.9% hyperforins) with a final hyperforin content of 1.5%, or placebo, twice daily for four weeks.[154] Treatment was randomly allocated to be applied to the left or right side of the body. At the end of the study, the *H. perforatum* preparation was found to be superior to placebo with respect to the primary outcome measure (clinical intensity of skin lesions; $p < 0.022$ for *H. perforatum* versus placebo).

In a randomised, double-blind, crossover trial involving 54 diabetic and non-diabetic patients with polyneuropathy, the analgesic effects of an *H. perforatum* preparation (Calmigen, Sanopharm; each tablet containing hypericin 900 μg, no further details of preparation provided) one tablet three times daily were compared with those of placebo.[155] The rationale for investigating the effects of *H. perforatum* on pain was centred around evidence that the antidepressant effect of *H. perforatum* preparations is due to effects on monoaminergic systems, and that effects on such systems may be the mechanism of action of agents such as tricyclic antidepressants currently used in painful polyneuropathy. In the study, patients' daily ratings of pain using numeric rating scales were used as the primary outcome measure. At the end of the treatment period, there were no statistically significant differences in total pain score between the *H. perforatum* and placebo groups (14 and 15, respectively; $p = 0.05$), in individual pain rating scales ($p = 0.09$ to 0.33), or in participants' evaluations of pain relief ($p = 0.07$).[155]

In a double-blind, controlled, crossover study, 12 healthy volunteers aged 18 to 54 years received tablets containing an extract of *H. perforatum* (Hyperiforte, each tablet contained 300 mg extract standardised for hyperforin 3–5% and hypericin 0.3%). Participants received placebo, and three and six tablets of the extract as a single dose in a random order and undertook a battery of memory tests before and after each administration. The results indicated that the *H. perforatum* extract did not have nootropic effects,[156] although as a sample size calculation does not appear to have been carried out, it is possible that the study did not have adequate statistical power to detect any differences.

A preliminary study found that a mixture of oils extracted from *H. perforatum* and *Calendula arvensis* reduced the surface area of wounds in women who had undergone Caesarean section during childbirth, when compared with control (wheatgerm oil).[157] However, the study did not involve random allocation to treatment and was not blinded, so the findings cannot be attributed definitively to the intervention.

The use of intravesical instillation of hypericin as a photosensitiser in human bladders together with blue light irradiation and fluorescence detection has been described as a diagnostic tool for the detection of bladder carcinoma. The technique had 98.5% specificity in detecting carcinoma *in situ* and dysplasia, and had a sensitivity of 93%.[158, 159]

Pharmacokinetics Detailed pharmacokinetic studies have been carried out with the hypericin-standardised St John's wort extract LI 160 and with certain other *H. perforatum* extracts.[1, G1] Administration of single oral doses of LI 160 (300, 900 and 1800 mg) to healthy male volunteers resulted in peak plasma hypericin concentrations of 1.5, 7.5 and 14.2 ng/mL for the three doses, respectively. Peak plasma concentrations were seen with hypericin after 2.0–2.6 hours and with pseudohypericin after 0.4–0.6 hours. The elimination half-life of hypericin was between 24.8 and 26.5 hours. Repeated doses of LI 160 (300 mg) three times daily resulted in steady-state concentrations after four days.[160] Oral administration of the St John's wort extract WS 5572 (300 mg, equivalent to 14.8 mg hyperforin) resulted in peak plasma concentrations of 150 ng/mL being reached 3.5 hours after administration.[161] The elimination half-life was 9 hours. Following repeated doses of 300 mg three times daily, the estimated steady-state plasma hyperforin concentrations were 100 ng/mL.

In open trials involving 18 healthy male volunteers, following oral administration of a single tablet of a dry extract of *H. perforatum* (STW-3, containing 612 mg extract equivalent to hypericin 600 μg, pseudohypericin 1200 μg, hyperforin 13.5 mg, flavonoids 73.2 mg; drug to extract ratio 5–8 : 1), pharmacokinetic parameters for hypericin, pseudohypericin and hyperforin, respectively, were: maximum plasma concentration, 3.14, 8.5 and 83.5 ng/mL; time to maximum concentration, 8.1, 3.0 and 4.4 hours; elimination half-life, 23.8, 25.4 and 19.6 hours.[162] The flavonoid compounds quercetin and isorhamnetin showed two peaks of maximum plasma concentration, separated by about four hours (quercetin: 47.7 ng/mL by 1.2 hours and 43.8 ng/mL by 5.5 hours; isorhamnetin: 7.6 ng/mL by 1.5 hours and 9.0 ng/mL by 6.4 hours). The elimination half-life for these constituents was 4.2 and 4.5 hours for quercetin and isorhamnetin, respectively. Pharmacokinetic parameters following multiple dosing (STW-3 once daily for 14 days) were similar.[162]

In an open, randomised, two-way, crossover study involving 12 healthy volunteers, the bioavailability of hyperforin after a single oral administration of a softgel capsule containing *H. perforatum* dry extract 300 mg (containing 0.3% hypericin and 5% hyperforin) was found to be superior to that following a single oral administration of a hard gelatin capsule containing the same extract.[163] The mean (standard deviation) peak plasma hyperforin concentrations were 168.4 (57.8) and 84.3 (33.5) ng/mL following administration of the softgel and hard gelatin capsules, respectively, although a p value was not reported. Hypericin, however, was not detectable in almost half of the participants for each dosage form. In nine male patients with superficial transition cell carcinoma of the bladder, intravesical instillation to the bladder of 40 mL of a 8 μmol/L hypericin solution for 2 to 3 hours followed by photodynamic diagnosis of bladder tumours, plasma concentrations of hypericin in samples taken one hour after the end of the instillation were below the detection limit (<6 nmol/L).[164]

A method for the simultaneous determination of hypericin and hyperforin in human plasma using liquid chromatography and tandem mass spectrometry (LC–MS–MS) has been developed and validated.[165] Using the method, the limits of quantification for hypericin and hyperforin were 0.05 ng/mL and 0.035 ng/mL, respectively. These low limits may allow detection of ingestion of hypericin and hyperforin for up to several days after discontinuation of treatment.

Side-effects, Toxicity

Clinical data

Data relating to the frequency and type of adverse effects associated with treatment with St John's wort extracts are available from randomised controlled trials, systematic reviews and meta-analyses of such trials, and from post-marketing surveillance and other observational studies. Collectively, the data indicate that certain St John's wort extracts are well-tolerated when taken at recommended doses for shorter periods of time (around eight weeks).[131, 166] Data from the small number of longer-term (one year) studies support the tolerability of certain St John's wort extracts, although further investigation of long-term use is warranted. Adverse events/effects reported are generally mild and most commonly gastrointestinal symptoms. These observations, however, are based on data collected in the settings of formal randomised or observational studies, usually where *H. perforatum* has been prescribed under the supervision of a physician, not taken as self-treatment.

A small number of studies has explored the effects of self-treatment with St John's wort products. In a cross-sectional study involving 452 members of a depression self-help group (response rate = 17%), 63 of the 452 respondents (28%) reported adverse effects, including psychological symptoms, allergic reactions and visual disturbances, that they believed to be related to use of St John's wort.[167] The safety of St John's wort products taken as self-treatment without supervision by a healthcare professional requires further study.

A Cochrane systematic review included 37 randomised, double-blind, controlled clinical trials of monopreparations of *H. perforatum* and involving a total of 4925 patients with depressive disorders (*see* Therapeutic effects, Depression).[24] Of the 26 placebo-controlled trials included in the review, data for analysis of the number of participants withdrawing for any reason were available from 19 trials, for withdrawing due to adverse effects from nine trials and for numbers of patients reporting adverse effects from 16 trials. Compared with placebo recipients, slightly fewer *H. perforatum* recipients withdrew from trials for any reason (odds ratio, 95% CI: 0.82, 0.64–1.06), withdrew due to adverse effects (odds ratio, 95% CI: 0.61, 0.28–1.31), and reported adverse effects (odds ratio, 95% CI: 0.79, 0.61–1.03). Compared with SSRIs, *H. perforatum* extracts were associated with a slightly lower probability of withdrawing from the study due to adverse effects (odds ratio, 95% CI: 0.60, 0.31–1.15; data from six trials) and reporting of adverse effects (odds ratio, 95% CI: 0.75, 0.52–1.08; data from five trials), whereas overall withdrawal rates were similar (odds ratio, 95% CI: 0.95, 0.65–1.40; data from six trials).[24] Compared with older antidepressant agents, *H. perforatum* extracts were associated with a lower probability of withdrawing for any reason (odds ratio, 95% CI: 0.65, 0.46–0.92; data from seven trials), withdrawing due to adverse effects (odds ratio, 95% CI: 0.25, 0.14–0.45; data from six trials) and of reporting adverse effects (odds ratio, 95% CI: 0.39, 0.31–0.50; data from seven trials). It is important to consider that there is qualitative and quantitative variation in the composition of different manufacturers' products and the results of the analyses above should not be extrapolated to other *H. perforatum* preparations.

The review described above[24] was an update, with tighter inclusion and exclusion criteria, of a previous Cochrane systematic review of 27 randomised controlled trials of *H. perforatum* preparations in depressive disorders.[129] The previous review reported that, in the trials comparing St John's wort with standard antidepressants, the proportions of patients reporting side-effects were 26.3% and 44.7%, respectively (rate ratio 0.57 and 95% CI 0.4–0.69).[129] Another meta-analysis which employed tight inclusion criteria reported that tricyclic antidepressants were associated with a higher proportion of side-effects than were St John's wort preparations (47% versus 26.4%, respectively, relative risk 1.72 and 95% CI 1.30–2.14).[130]

A randomised, double-blind, multicentre trial comparing the effects of a hydroalcoholic extract of *H. perforatum* herb (WS-5570, drug to extract ratio 3–7 : 1, standardised for hyperforin 3–6% and hypericin 0.12–0.28%; Schwabe Pharmaceuticals) with those of paroxetine in the acute treatment of moderate to severe depression has been published since the revised Cochrane review[24] was completed. In the study, 251 participants with acute major depression received *H. perforatum* extract 300 mg three times daily (increased to 1800 mg daily in non-responders), or paroxetine 20 mg daily (40 mg daily for non-responders), for six weeks.[128] During the study, 55% of *H. perforatum* recipients reported a total of 172 adverse events and 76% of paroxetine recipients reported a total of 269 adverse events, representing incidences of 0.035 and 0.060 adverse events per day of exposure for *H. perforatum* and paroxetine, respectively. Gastrointestinal adverse events were the most common adverse events reported for both groups. Data were not provided on numbers and types of adverse events considered to be related to treatment.

A systematic review of large-scale observational studies of *H. perforatum* extracts in patients with depressive disorders also provides data on adverse events. The review included 16 non-randomised studies (involving a total of 34 804 patients) each involving at least 100 participants with depressive disorders who were treated with *H. perforatum* preparations for at least four weeks (*see* Therapeutic effects, Depression).[131] Overall, 13 studies reported data on proportions of participants withdrawing due to adverse events; these ranged from 0% to 2.8% in short-term studies and from 3.4% to 5.7% in longer-term (one year) studies. Twelve studies reported data on proportions of participants with adverse events (range 0–49.3%) and 12 (not the same 12 studies) reported data on proportions of participants with side-effects (range 0–5.9%). These data, however, should be interpreted cautiously as most of the studies did not describe adequately how these data were collected, clear definitions for the terms adverse events and adverse effects were not always provided, and as no serious adverse events were reported among the 30 000 patients, this raises questions about the methods used to collect data.[131] The most frequently reported adverse events or side-effects were gastrointestinal symptoms, followed by increased sensitivity to light and other skin reactions.

Photosensitivity Sensitivity to sunlight following the ingestion of hypericum or hypericin, the photosensitising agent in *H. perforatum*,[168, G33] is known as hypericism.

Several studies have explored the photosensitising potential of hypericin-containing *H. perforatum* extract following oral administration. In a double-blind, crossover, single-dose study involving 13 healthy volunteers who received placebo or St John's wort extract (LI 160) (900, 1800 and 3600 mg containing 0, 2.81, 5.62 and 11.25 mg total hypericin, respectively), no evidence of photosensitivity was observed with or without St John's wort following skin irradiation with both UV-A and UV-B light 4 hours after dosing.[169] In a multiple-dose study in which 50 volunteers received St John's wort (LI 160) (600 mg) three times daily (equivalent to 5.6 mg total hypericin daily) for 15 days, a moderate increase in UV-A sensitivity was observed.[169] However, the doses used were higher than those recommended therapeutically. In another single-dose study, administration of St John's wort (LI 160) (1800 mg, equivalent to 5.4 mg total hypericin) to 12 healthy volunteers resulted in a mean serum total hypericin concentration of 43 ng/mL and a mean skin blister fluid concentration of 5.3 ng/

mL.[170] After administration of St John's wort (300 mg) three times daily for seven days in order to achieve steady-state concentrations, the mean serum total hypericin concentration was 12.5 ng/mL and the mean skin blister fluid concentration was 2.8 ng/mL; these concentrations are below those estimated to be phototoxic.[170] Further randomised, controlled, single- (six or 12 tablets of LI-160, equivalent to 5.4 and 10.8 mg hypericins, respectively; n = 48) and multiple-dose studies (three tablets of LI-160 daily, equivalent to 2.7 mg hypericins daily, for seven days; n = 24) found no statistically significant differences in minimum erythema threshold doses (of light irradiation), erythema index and pigmentation index between treated and untreated skin areas ($p > 0.05$ for each).[171, 172]

Collectively, the evidence indicates that the threshold for phototoxicity of hypericin is between 100 and 1000 ng/mL.[171] Since serum and skin concentrations of hypericin after oral administration of recommended doses are below 100 ng/mL, photosensitivity seems unlikely. However, caution is advised as it is possible that there may be unusual absorption of hypericin in some individuals and, particularly in fair-skinned individuals and after extended periods of solar irradiation, there may be increased susceptibility to the photosensitising properties of hypericin.[171]

A study reported that HIV-positive patients treated with oral hypericin (0.05 mg/kg) for 28 days developed mild symptoms of photosensitivity on exposure to sunlight and that two patients developed intolerable symptoms of photosensitivity when the dose was increased to 0.16 mg/kg.[173] In a dose-escalating study involving 30 HIV-infected patients treated with oral (0.5 mg/kg daily) or intravenous hypericin (starting dosage 0.25 mg/kg twice or three times weekly), 16 patients discontinued treatment before completing eight weeks of therapy because of moderate or severe phototoxicity; severe cutaneous phototoxicity was observed in 11 out of 23 evaluable patients.[142] Other serious clinical or laboratory adverse events were infrequent: elevation of alkaline phosphatase and hepatic aminotransferase concentrations to more than five times normal values was noted in two and three patients, respectively.

The effects of topical application of *H. perforatum* extract on skin sensitivity have also been investigated. In a randomised controlled trial, 16 healthy volunteers with no history of skin disease or photosensitivity were treated with *H. perforatum* oil (containing hypericin 110 μg/mL) or *H. perforatum* ointment (containing an alcoholic *H. perforatum* extract with a final hypericin concentration of 30 μg/mL). The oil or ointment was applied to a two centimetre test area on one forearm of participants for 24 hours. Controls were an untreated test area of the same forearm, and the untreated other forearm. After removal of the oil or ointment, both forearms of participants received increasing doses of solar simulated irradiation (24, 48, 96 and 144 J/cm^2). No phototoxic reactions were observed in any of the participants, and there was no change in the minimal erythema dose in either the oil or the ointment group,[174] although data to support the latter statement were not shown. There was a significant increase in the erythema index following treatment with *H. perforatum* oil (which contained the higher concentration of hypericin) but not after *H. perforatum* ointment ($p < 0.01$ and $p > 0.05$, respectively, compared with values for untreated skin), although this may not be clinically relevant since the minimal erythema dose did not change. The phototoxic potential of topical application of the *H. perforatum* preparations tested appears to be low, although caution is necessary, particularly as hypericin may penetrate more highly through broken or lesional skin, and there may be increased susceptibility to the photosensitising properties of hypericin in fair-skinned individuals and after extended periods of solar irradiation.[174]

A case report describes a 45-year-old woman who developed blisters on two occasions at the treatment site following laser therapy to her legs for multiple solar keratoses.[175] It was stated that the patient revealed that she was taking St John's wort, although a sample of the product was not obtained and, therefore, no analysis was undertaken. The blisters resolved and, after stopping treatment with St John's wort, the patient underwent a further session of laser treatment without experiencing adverse effects.

Delayed hypersensitivity or photodermatitis has been documented for St John's wort following the ingestion of a herbal tea made from the leaves.[176]

Psychiatric effects Cases of mania[177, 178] and hypomania[179, 180] have been reported in individuals taking St John's wort preparations. Two cases of mania were reported in patients with bipolar depression who began self-treatment with standardised St John's wort extract (900 mg) daily[178] and one in a patient experiencing a moderate depressive episode who was taking both sertraline and St John's wort (dosage not known).[177] A case of hypomania was reported in a woman with panic disorder and unipolar major depression who had discontinued sertraline treatment one week before starting St John's wort tincture.[179] Two cases of hypomania were reported in individuals with no history of bipolar disorder.[180] A man who had received electroconvulsive therapy and who had previously taken various antidepressant drugs, including venlafaxine, fluvoxamine, moclobemide and nortriptyline, experienced a hypomanic episode six weeks after starting St John's wort (dosage not stated). A man with symptoms of post-traumatic stress disorder was diagnosed with an acute manic episode after three months of self-treatment with St John's wort (dosage not stated).[180]

The cases described above, along with five other cases of mania, one of hypomania, two of schizophrenia, two of delirium and one of acute anxiety, were included in a review of psychotic events associated with administration of St John's wort products. Across the 17 cases, the onset of symptoms ranged from two days to six months after initiation of St John's wort treatment.[181] The dosage of St John's wort taken was stated in only six of these cases; this was within recommended dosages except in one case where an excessively high dose was reported to have been taken (18 g; no further details provided). All these reports stated that the symptoms had resolved after stopping treatment with St John's wort, although in one case the patient improved but initially remained agitated despite cessation of St John's wort.[180] None of the cases involved rechallenge with St John's wort. Typically, these cases have involved self-treatment with St John's wort products, rely on self-report of St John's wort use, have not obtained blood samples for analysis of constituents of *H. perforatum* and/or their metabolites and have not obtained samples of the product for analysis. Also, in most cases, there were other pharmacological factors and/or underlying illnesses that could have been responsible for or contributed to the observed events.

Other effects A case of subacute toxic neuropathy possibly related to the use of St John's wort and subsequent exposure to sunlight has been reported.[182] A woman developed stinging pains in areas exposed to the sun (face and hands) four weeks after starting treatment with St John's wort (500 mg/day, extract and hypericin content not stated); the report did not state whether the woman was using any other products. Her symptoms improved three weeks after stopping St John's wort and disappeared over the next two months.

There have been reports of sensory nerve hypersensitivity occurring in individuals who have taken St John's wort preparations (tablets or tinctures).[183]

There is an isolated report of confusion, disorientation and hypertensive crisis (blood pressure 210/140 mmHg) in a 41-year-old man seven days after he began taking a St John's wort product for work-related stress. It was reported that the man had consumed aged cheese and red wine before onset of the delirium, which is suggestive of hypertension associated with the use of a monoamine oxidase inhibitor.[184] However, although previous *in vitro* experiments have indicated that *H. perforatum* extracts had monoamine oxidase inhibitory activity, this has not been confirmed in subsequent *in vitro* studies (*see* Pharmcological Actions, *In vitro* and animal studies), and consensus is that St John's wort is not a monoamine oxidase inhibitor.[118] In addition, no analysis of blood samples or of the St John's product appears to have been undertaken, thus alternative explanations for the event cannot be ruled out.

St John's wort extract (BNO-1385, containing 255–285 mg extract equivalent to hypericin 900 μg) 255 to 285 mg three times daily taken for 14 days had no significant effect on heart rate variability, cognitive performance and parameters of autonomic function (vasoconstrictory response of cutaneous blood flow and skin conductance response following a single deep inspiration) according to the results of a randomised, double-blind, placebo-controlled, three-arm, crossover trial involving 12 healthy male volunteers. (Decrease in heart rate variability is an effect observed with chronic administration of tricyclic antidepressant agents, although the implications of this for morbidity and mortality in patients with depression are not yet understood.)[185, 186] In contrast, amitriptyline 25 mg daily significantly decreased heart rate variability and significantly influenced the parameters of autonomic function. The effects of another St John's wort herb extract (Hyperiforte, 300 mg extract containing hypericin 990 μg, pseudohypericin 526 μg and hyperforin 9–15 μg) 900 mg or 1800 mg as a single dose on cognitive and psychomotor performance were compared with those of amitriptyline 25 mg in a randomised, placebo-controlled, crossover study involving 13 healthy volunteers. Recipients of *H. perforatum* extract, compared with placebo, experienced a dose-dependent impairment in one of the eight tests (digit symbol substitution test), whereas amitriptyline recipients showed statistically significant impairments in performance in seven of the eight tests.[187]

In a case–control study, 37 patients with raised serum thyroid-stimulating hormone (TSH) concentrations (7–20 μU/mL) matched for age and sex to 37 individuals with normal TSH concentrations (1–3 μU/mL) selected from the same set of patient records, were interviewed regarding their exposure to St John's wort products and other prescription and non-prescription medicines. Four participants with raised TSH concentrations and two with normal TSH concentrations reported that they had taken St John's wort products within six months of the TSH test (odds ratio, 95% CI for raised TSH concentrations associated with self-reported exposure to St John's wort during the specified time period: 2.12, 0.36 to 12.36; $p > 0.05$).[188] The small sample size may mean that the study lacked the statistical power to detect an association between St John's wort exposure and raised TSH concentrations. Other methodological issues include the possibility of confounding by indication, since individuals with hypothyroidism may experience symptoms of depression and, therefore, be more likely to take St John's wort.[188] Further research to assess the possibility of effects of *H. perforatum* on thyroid function may be warranted.

There are two isolated reports of sexual dysfunction, including decreased libido and erectile dysfunction, associated with use of St John's wort products. In one man, previous symptoms of sexual dysfunction, possibly related to use of a conventional antidepressant agent which had resolved on stopping treatment, reappeared one week after initiation of treatment with St John's wort.[189] Another report describes a man who experienced decreased libido whilst taking St John's wort for nine months.[190]

Preclinical data

The consumption of large quantities of St John's wort by grazing animals has been associated with the development of photosensitivity.[191, G22, G51] Mice given 0.2–0.5 mg of the herb were found to develop severe photodynamic effects.[G22] Studies using cell cultures of human keratinocytes incubated with hypericin or St John's wort extract and exposed to UV-A resulted in a reduction in the LC_{50} (lethal concentration) with hypericin, but only a mild reduction with hypericum.[192] From these findings it has been estimated that at least 30 times the therapeutic dose would be necessary to produce phototoxic effects in humans.[192]

It has been shown in *in vitro* experiments using a human keratinocyte cell line and quercitrin-free and quercitrin-containing extracts of *H. perforatum* that quercitrin reduces the phototoxicity of *H. perforatum* extracts.[193]

Experimental evidence has suggested that a solution of hypericin can react with visible and UV light to produce free radical species and that this may lead to damage of proteins in the lens of the eye.[194] Up to October 2005, there were no spontaneous reports of cataract formation in individuals who have taken St John's wort.[195]

A hydromethanolic extract of St John's wort flowering tops (containing 0.3% hypericin) at concentrations of 1–300 μg/mL reduced experimentally induced contractions in rat vas deferens smooth muscle in a concentration-dependent manner.[196] The St John's wort extract and hyperforin also produced a concentration-dependent inhibition of phenylephrine-induced contractions in human vas deferens *in vitro*; mean (standard error of mean) IC_{50} values for the extract and hyperforin were 13.9 (2.0) and 0.45 (0.04) μg/mL, respectively.

A number of experimental studies has investigated the genotoxic potential and mutagenic activity of St John's wort extracts *in vitro* and *in vivo*. *In vivo* studies and most *in vitro* studies provided negative results, indicating a lack of mutagenic potential with defined St John's wort extracts.[G52] Mutagenic activity observed in an *in vitro* Ames test was attributed to the presence of quercetin, although other studies have found no mutagenic potential with a St John's wort extract and it has been stated that there is no valid evidence for the carcinogenicity of quercetin in humans.[G21, G52]

Dietary administration of St John's wort to rats was found to have no effect on various hepatic drug-metabolising enzymes (e.g. aminopyrine, *N*-demethylase, glutathione *S*-transferase and epoxide hydrolase) or on copper concentrations in the liver (*see* Contra-indications, Warnings, Drug interactions). No major effects were observed on hepatic iron or zinc concentrations and no significant tissue lesions were found in four rats fed St John's wort in their daily diet for 119 days (10% for first 12 days and 5% thereafter because of unpalatability).[197]

Cytotoxic constituents related to hyperforin have been isolated from two related *Hypericum* species (*see* Pharmacological Actions, *In vitro* and animal studies).

Contra-indications, Warnings

Individuals with sensitivity towards St John's wort may experience allergic reactions. The use of St John's wort is not advised in known cases of photosensitivity and, in view of the potential of hypericin as a photosensitising agent, therapeutic UV treatment should be avoided whilst using St John's wort.[G1]

It has previously been suggested that excessive doses of St John's wort may potentiate monoamine oxidase inhibitor therapy.[198] However, as monoamine oxidase inhibitory activity has not been reported *in vivo* with St John's wort, this warning is no longer considered necessary. In addition, avoidance of foodstuffs, such as those containing tyramine (e.g. cheese, wine, meat and yeast extracts) and medicines containing sympathomimetic agents (e.g. cough/cold remedies), which interact with MAOIs, is not considered necessary.

Drug interactions There are important pharmacokinetic interactions and potential for important pharmacodynamic interactions between St John's wort preparations and certain other medicines.[118, 199, 200]

Evidence for pharmacokinetic interactions between St John's wort preparations and certain other medicines, leading to a loss of or reduction in the therapeutic effect of those medicines, includes spontaneous reports[199] and published case reports.[200, G79] Drugs that may be affected include certain anticonvulsants, ciclosporin, digoxin, indinavir (and other HIV protease inhibitors, and HIV non-nucleoside reverse transcriptase inhibitors), oral contraceptives, theophylline and warfarin. A report involving four cases describes reduced plasma methadone trough concentrations in addicts who received St John's wort extract 900 mg daily before methadone maintenance treatment.[201]

There have also been reports of increased serotonergic effects (i.e. pharmacodynamic interactions) in patients taking St John's wort products concurrently with selective serotonin reuptake inhibitors (e.g. sertraline, paroxetine).[202, 203] There are isolated reports of hypotension during general anaesthesia[204] and delayed emergence following general anaesthesia.[205] In both cases, patients had been taking St John's wort before receiving several anaesthetic agents, including fentanyl and propofol. It has been suggested that treatment with St John's wort preparations should be stopped at least five days before undergoing elective surgery.[206]

In the year 2000, the UK Committee on Safety of Medicines (CSM) issued advice to pharmacists, doctors, other healthcare professionals and patients on the use of St John's wort products with certain other medicines.[207, 208] The CSM's advice for healthcare professionals regarding patients taking St John's wort and other medicines concurrently can be summarised as follows.

Warfarin, ciclosporin, digoxin, theophylline and anticonvulsants (carbamazepine, phenobarbital and phenytoin) There is a risk of reduced therapeutic effect, e.g. risk of transplant rejection, seizures and loss of asthma control. Advice is to check plasma drug concentrations (with warfarin, the patient's International Normalised Ratio should be checked) and to stop St John's wort therapy. In addition, dose adjustment may be necessary.

HIV protease inhibitors (indinavir, nelfinavir, ritonavir and saquinavir) and HIV non-nucleoside reverse transcriptase inhibitors (efavirenz and nevirapine) There is a risk of reduced blood concentrations with possible loss of HIV suppression. Advice is to measure HIV RNA viral load and to stop St John's wort.

Oral contraceptives There is a risk of reduced blood concentrations, breakthrough bleeding and unintended pregnancy. Advice is to stop St John's wort.

Triptans (sumatriptan, naratriptan, rizatriptan and zolmitriptan) and selective serotonin reuptake inhibitors (citalopram, fluoxetine, fluvoxamine, paroxetine and sertraline) There is a risk of increased serotonergic effects with the possibility of an increased risk of adverse reactions. Advice is to stop St John's wort.

Patients already taking any of the above drugs should be advised not to start taking St John's wort and users of other medicines should be advised to seek professional advice before using St John's wort. Topical medicines and non-psychotropic medicines that are excreted renally are not likely to interact with St John's wort. In addition, topical or homeopathic preparations of St John's wort are not likely to interact with prescribed medicines.

There is further evidence from prospective pharmacokinetic studies involving patients who have received St John's wort preparations and other medicines concurrently that there are interactions which result in altered pharmacokinetics, including reduced plasma concentrations, of amitriptyline,[209] ciclosporin,[210, 211] tacrolimus,[212] and irinotecan.[213] These studies have typically been open-label studies (although two involved a randomised, crossover design) involving small numbers of patients undergoing treatment with the respective conventional medicines and who were also treated with single and/or multiple doses (600 to 900 mg extract daily for around two weeks) of St John's wort preparations. In one randomised, crossover study, 10 patients who had undergone renal transplants were treated concurrently with ciclosporin and St John's wort extract with a low or high hyperforin content. Patients experienced altered ciclosporin pharmacokinetics and required ciclosporin dose increases only whilst taking the extract with the high content of hyperforin.[211]

Studies with different designs (and varying methodological quality)[214] and involving healthy volunteers have provided supporting evidence of pharmacokinetic interactions between St John's wort preparations and digoxin,[215] imatinib,[216, 217] oral contraceptives,[218, 219] phenprocoumon,[220] quazepam,[221] simvastatin,[222] tacrolimus,[223] verapamil[224] and warfarin.[225] These and other studies provide evidence indicating that St John's wort preparations induce the cytochrome P450 (CYP) drug-metabolising enzyme CYP3A4,[220, 226–229] as well as affecting P-glycoprotein (a transport protein).[200, 230] As with other medicines, whether or not clinically important drug interactions occur with St John's wort preparations depends on several factors, including the dosage regimen, route of administration and pharmaceutical quality of St John's wort preparations and co-administered medicines. As CYP3A4 is involved in the metabolism of at least half of all medicinal agents, and as P-glycoprotein is involved in the transport of many drugs, it is possible that St John's wort preparations interact with other medicines in addition to those listed above.[231]

S

There is also evidence from studies involving healthy volunteers, albeit less extensive, that St John's wort preparations induce CYP2C19.[232] Effects on certain other CYP drug metabolising enzymes are less clear: one study reported no effect on CYP2C9 activity,[229] whereas another study found that a St John's wort extract did induce CYP2C9 as determined by effects on the pharmacokinetics of *S*-warfarin;[225] conflicting results have also been reported for CYP1A2 with respect to induction[225] or a lack of induction[229] by St John's wort preparations.

In contrast, similar studies have reported a lack of pharmacokinetic interaction between St John's wort preparations and carbamazepine,[233] pravastatin,[222] and theophylline,[234] and several others have reported a lack of significant effects on CYP isoenzymes,[235–237] although the numbers of volunteers may have been too small and the duration of St John's wort administration too short to exclude definitively an inductive effect.[236, 237] There is evidence from several studies involving healthy volunteers that St John's wort preparations do not influence CYP2D6 activity to an extent likely to be clinically relevant.[200, 228, 229, 238]

Randomised, placebo-controlled studies involving healthy volunteers who received an ethanol extract of St John's wort with a low hyperforin content (Esbericum capsules containing 60 mg extract, drug to extract ratio 3.5–6.0 : 1, equivalent to 0.25 mg total hypericins and 0.88 mg hyperforin) 240 mg extract daily found no statistically significant effects on the pharmacokinetics of drugs used as substrates for CYP3A4, CYP1A2 and CYP2C9. It is not clear whether the lack of effect is due to the preparation having a low hyperforin content, or to the low dose of extract used in the studies.[239] The suggestion that the occurrence of CYP enzyme induction, or the extent of induction, may vary depending on the particular St John's wort preparation is a valid one, since the profile of constituents, including those influencing CYP enzyme activity, varies qualitatively and quantitatively between products (*see* Quality of plant material and commercial products).

A further randomised, double-blind, placebo-controlled study involving healthy volunteers ($n = 33$) explored the effects of the CYP enzyme inhibitor cimetidine and the CYP enzyme inducer carbamazepine on the pharmacokinetics of certain constituents of St John's wort extracts. Participants received St John's wort extract (LI-160) 300 mg three times daily for 11 days, followed by a further seven days' administration together with cimetidine 1000 mg daily in divided doses, carbamazepine 400 mg each night, or placebo. No statistically significant differences in the plasma concentration versus time curves from hours 0 to 24 ($AUC_{0–24}$) were observed between groups; statistically significant intragroup differences in the $AUC_{0–24}$ were observed for hypericin during cimetidine administration and for pseudohypericin during carbamazepine administration, although these effects are unlikely to be of clinical relevance.[240]

A number of *in vitro* and animal studies have also explored the effects of St John's wort preparations on CYP drug metabolising enzymes. *In vitro* studies have reported induction of the CYP enzymes CYP3A4 and CYP1A2 by St John's wort extracts,[200, 231] and of CYP2C9 by hyperforin.[241, 242] Results from *in vivo* (mice) experiments indicate that hyperforin is important for induction of CYP3A in the liver.[243] *In vitro* experiments have shown that hyperforin induction of CYP2C9 is mediated by the pregnane X nuclear receptor.[242] Induction of P-glycoprotein by St John's wort extract[244] and hyperforin[245] has been reported following *in vitro* experiments using LS180 intestinal carcinoma cells, whereas there are conflicting results on the induction of P-glycoprotein by hypericin.[244, 245]

A number of *in vitro* experiments have described inhibition of the CYP enzymes CYP3A4 and CYP2C19 by St John's wort extracts,[246, 247] and inhibition of P-glycoprotein by hypericin and hyperforin.[248] A series of *in vitro* experiments explored the effects of hypericin on human DNA topoisomerase II activity. Hypericin appeared to interact with DNA in a manner which precluded topoisomerase II DNA binding activity and antagonised the formation of topoisomerase II-covalent cleavage complexes mediated by the topoisomerase II poisons etoposide and amsacrine. The effects of hypericin and St John's wort extracts on topoisomerase II cancer chemotherapy require further investigation.[249]

Certain groups of users may have little knowledge of safety aspects, such as drug interactions, related to use of St John's wort products, and may be particularly vulnerable to certain adverse effects.[250–253]

Pregnancy and lactation Information on the use of *H. perforatum* preparations during pregnancy and breastfeeding is summarised below. In view of the lack of toxicity data, St John's wort preparations should not be used during pregnancy and lactation.

Clinical data In a prospective, cohort study, 33 breastfeeding women who had made enquiries about the safety of St John's wort during breastfeeding to a teratogen/toxicology advice service (and who took St John's wort products) were compared with 33 age- and parity-matched controls and 101 disease-matched controls (who had enquired about the safety of St John's wort products but who did not take any). Three of the women in the first group had initiated St John's wort treatment during pregnancy (stage not stated), and the mean (standard deviation) of infant exposure to St John's wort through breastfeeding was 2.1 (3.5) months.[254] There were no statistically significant differences in maternal or infant demographics, and in women's reasons for enquiring about use of St John's wort, although significantly more women who took St John's wort were using conventional antidepressants, compared with women who inquired about St John's wort but who did not use it (42.4% versus 17.8%; $p < 0.01$). No maternal adverse events were reported in any of the women and there were no statistically significant differences in the proportions of women reporting decreased milk volume (12.1%, 6.9% and 6.1% for St John's wort consumers, disease-matched controls, and age-/parity-matched controls, respectively; $p = 0.58$).[254] Five infants born to St John's wort consumers experienced colic, drowsiness or lethargy, compared with one report in each of the other two groups, although two of the former five infants were also exposed to conventional antidepressant agents during breastfeeding.

The study described above provides only limited information on the safety of St John's wort products during breastfeeding (and, to a even lesser extent, pregnancy) as it involved only small numbers of women so had the statistical power to detect only very common, acute adverse events. In addition, a report of the study did not provide any details of the St John's wort products consumed by the participants. It is likely that several, perhaps many, different St John's wort products were involved, all of which are likely to differ in their pharmaceutical quality and, therefore, in their potential effects on the infant.

There is a report of a 38-year-old woman who started taking St John's wort (900 mg/day) at her 24th week of pregnancy, taking the last dose 24 hours before delivery.[255] The pregnancy was unremarkable except for late onset of thrombocytopenia. Another report described a 43-year-old woman who discontinued fluoxetine and methylphenidate upon becoming pregnant and started taking St John's wort (900 mg/day). The report does not state the outcome of the pregnancy,[255] although it is assumed that had adverse events occurred, they would have been stated.

Another case report describes a 33-year-old woman who presented with post-natal depression at a German psychiatric service and who had been taking an extract of *H. perforatum* (Jarsin) 300 mg three times daily from five months post-partum. Analysis of breast milk samples indicated that hyperforin is excreted into breast milk at concentrations below the lower limit of quantification (0.50 ng/mL).[256] No adverse effects were observed in the infant or the mother, however, further investigation of the pharmacokinetics of constituents of *H. perforatum* extract in breast milk and in mothers' and infants' plasma is required.

Preclinical data In a randomised experiment, 40 adult female mice were given food bars containing 'hypericum herb' (no further details of plant material provided) at a dose of 180 mg/kg body weight daily, or placebo, for two weeks before conception and throughout the gestation period. At the end of the study, there were no statistically significant differences between the 'hypericum' and placebo groups in duration of gestation, number of live pups per litter, body length and head circumference measurements, dam–pup interactions, physical maturation milestones and reproductive capabilities of offspring.[257] The only exceptions to this were that male offspring in the hypericum-exposed group weighed significantly less than those in the placebo group at birth ($p < 0.02$), but this difference was not statistically significant by day three after birth, and male offspring in the hypericum-exposed group experienced a temporary delay in appearance of the upper incisors. Since multiple statistical tests were carried out, this number of statistically significant results at a level of $p < 0.05$ is likely. In similar experiments, 18 adult female rats were given a methanol extract of St John's wort (containing 0.3% total hypericins) 100 or 1000 mg/kg, or placebo, by gavage for two weeks before mating, throughout the gestation period and/or for three weeks during breastfeeding. Histological alterations in the livers and kidneys of rat pups exposed to St John's wort extract throughout gestation and/or during breastfeeding; lesions were more severe in the offspring of rats treated with the higher dose and in offspring exposed to St John's wort extract during both the gestation period and breastfeeding.[258] Slight *in vitro* uterotonic activity has been reported for St John's wort (*see* Pharmacological Actions, *In vitro* and animal studies).

S

Preparations

Proprietary single-ingredient preparations

Argentina: Amenicil; Hipax; Hiperinat. *Australia:* Bioglan Stress-Relax; Hyperiforte. *Austria:* Esbericum; Helarium; Hyperiforce; Jarsin; Johanicum; Johni; Kira; Lunare; Perikan; Psychotonin; Remotiv; Solaguttae. *Belgium:* Hyperiplant; Milperinol; Perika. *Brazil:* Adprex; Emotival; Equilibra; Fiotan; Hiperex; Hipericin; Hiperico; Hiperifarma; Hiperil; Hipersac; Hyperico; Hyperigreen; Iperisan; Jarsin; Motiven; Prazen; Triativ. *Canada:* Kira; Movana. *Chile:* Anxium; Edual. *Czech Republic:* Deprim; Lubovnik; Nat Trezalky; Trezalka v Nalevovych Sacchich; Trezalkova Nat; Trezalkovy Caj; Turineurin. *France:* Dermum; Procalmil. *Germany:* Aristo; Aristoforat; Cesradyston; Digitalysat Scilla-Digitaloid; dystolux; Esbericum; Felis; Helarium; Hewepsychon uno; Hyperforat; Hypericaps; Hyperimerck; Hyperpur; Jarsin; Jo-Sabona; Kira; Laif; Libertin; Lomahypericum; Nervei; Neuroplant; Neurosporal; Neurovegetalin; Psychotonin; Sedovegan; Syxal; Texx; Tonizin; Turineurin. *Hungary:* Helarium; Remotiv. *Italy:* Nervaxon; Proserem; Quiens; Remotive. *Mexico:* Hiperikan; Procalm; Remotiv. *Russia:* Deprim (Деприм); Helarium (Гелариум); Negrustin (Негрустин); Novo-Passit (Ново-Пассит). *Spain:* Animic; Arkocapsulas Hiperico; Hiperico; Hyneurin; Quetzal; Vitalium. *Switzerland:* Hyperiforce; HyperiMed; Hyperiplant; Hyperval; Jarsin; Lucilium; Re-Balance; Remotiv; Solevita; Yakona. *UK:* Kira. *Venezuela:* Kira.

Proprietary multi-ingredient preparations

Australia: Bioglan 3B Beer Belly Buster; Cimicifuga Compound; Feminine Herbal Complex; Infant Tonic; Irontona; Joint & Muscle Relief Cream; Nappy Rash Relief Cream; Nevaton; Skin Healing Cream; Vitatona. *Austria:* Eryval; Magentee St Severin; Nerventee St Severin; Remifemin plus; Species nervinae; Wechseltee St Severin. *Canada:* Bronco Asmol; Sirop Cocillana Codeine. *Czech Republic:* Alvisan Neo; Cajova Smes pri Redukcni Diete; Cicaderma; Eugastrin; Fytokliman Planta; Naturident; Novo-Passit; Species Nervinae Planta; Stomaran; Zaludecni Cajova Smes. *Germany:* anabolloges; Gastritol; Gutnacht; Hyperesa; Me-Sabona plus; Miroton; Neurapas; Remifemin plus; Sedariston Konzentrat; Sedariston plus. *Hong Kong:* Coci-Fedra; Cocillana Christo; Cocillana Compound; Cocillana Compound; Cocillana Compound; Mefedra-N; Mist Expect Stim. *Italy:* Hiperogyn; Mithen. *Mexico:* Nordimenty. *Portugal:* Cicaderma. *Russia:* Prostanorm (Простанорм). *South Africa:* Cocillana Co; Contra-Coff; Linctus Tussi Infans. *Spain:* Natusor Gastrolen; Natusor Somnisedan. *Switzerland:* Gel a la consoude; Huile de millepertuis A. Vogel (huile de St. Jean); Hyperiforce comp; The a l'avoine sauvage de Vollmer. *UK:* Allens Chesty Cough; Balm of Gilead; Buttercup Syrup; Chest Mixture; Covonia Mentholated; Galloway's Cough Syrup; Honey & Molasses; Modern Herbals Cough Mixture; Potters Children's Cough Pastilles; Potters Gees Linctus; Sanderson's Throat Specific; Sanderson's Throat Specific; St Johnswort Compound. *Venezuela:* Biomicovo.

References

1 Bombardelli E, Morazzoni P. *Hypericum perforatum*. *Fitoterapia* 1995; 66: 43–68.
2 Hölzl J, Petersen M. Chemical constituents of *Hypericum spp.* In Ernst E (ed), *Hypericum. The genus* Hypericum. London, New York: Taylor and Francis, 2003.
3 Vanhaelen M, Vanhaelen-Fastre R. Quantitative determination of biologically active constituents in medicinal plant crude extracts by thin-layer chromatography-densitometry. *J Chromatogr* 1983; 281: 263–271.
4 Berghöfer R, Hölzl J. Biflavonoids in *Hypericum perforatum*; part 1. Isolation of 13,II8-biapigenin. *Planta Med* 1987; 53: 216–217.

5 Berghöfer R, Hölzl J. Isolation of I3′,II8-biapigenin (amentoflavone) from *Hypericum perforatum. Planta Med* 1989; 55: 91.
6 Ollivier B *et al.* Separation et identification des acides phenols par chromatographie liquide haute performance et spectroscopie ultraviolette. Application à la pariétaire (*Parietaria officinalis* L.) et au millepertuis (*Hypericum perforatum* L.). *J Pharm Belg* 1985; 40: 173–177.
7 Hoelzl J, Ostrowski E. St John's wort (*Hypericum perforatum* L.). HPLC analysis of the main components and their variability in a population. *Dtsch Apoth Ztg* 1987; 127: 1227–1230.
8 Dorossiev I. Determination of flavonoids in *Hypericum perforatum. Pharmazie* 1985; 40: 585–586.
9 Brondz I *et al.* The relative stereochemistry of hyperforin – an antibiotic from *Hypericum perforatum* L. *Tetrahedron Lett* 1982; 23: 1299–1300.
10 Ayuga C, Rebuelta M. A comparative study of phenolic acids of *Hypericum caprifolium* Boiss and *Hypericum perforatum* L. *An Real Acad Farm* 1986; 52: 723–728.
11 Brondz I *et al.* *n*-Alkanes of *Hypericum perforatum*: a revision. *Phytochemistry* 1983; 22: 295–296.
12 Mathis C, Ourisson G. Étude chimio-taxonomique du genre *Hypericum* – II. Identification de constituants de diverses huiles essentielles d'*Hypericum. Phytochemistry* 1964; 3: 115–131.
13 Mathis C, Ourisson G. Étude chimio-taxonomique du genre *Hypericum* – IV. Repartition des sesquiterpenes, des alcools monoterpeniques et des aldehydes satures dans les huiles essentielles d'*Hypericum. Phytochemistry* 1964; 3: 377–378.
14 Mathis C, Ourisson G. Étude chimio-taxonomique du genre *Hypericum* – V. Identification de quelques constituants non volatils d'*Hypericum perforatum* L. *Phytochemistry* 1964; 3: 379.
15 ConsumerLab. Product Review: St John's wort. (accessed 28 August 2003).
16 De Los Reyes GC, Koda RT. Determining hyperforin and hypericin content in eight brands of St John's wort. *Am J Health-Syst Pharm* 2002; 59: 545–547.
17 Draves AH, Walker SE. Analysis of the hypericin and pseudohypericin content of commercially available St John's wort preparations. *Can J Clin Pharmacol* 2003; 10(3): 114–118.
18 Orth HCJ *et al.* Isolation, purity analysis and stability of hyperforin as a standard material from *Hypericum perforatum* L. *J Pharm Pharmacol* 1999; 51: 193–200.
19 Vaja V *et al.* Further degradation product of hyperforin from *Hypericum perforatum* (St. John's wort). *Fitoterapia* 2003; 74: 439–444.
20 Verotta L *et al.* Furohyperforin, a prenylated phloroglucinol from St John's wort (*Hypericum perforatum*). *J Nat Prod* 1999; 62: 770–772.
21 Verotta L *et al.* Hyperforin analogues from St John's wort (*Hypericum perforatum*). *J Nat Prod* 2000; 63: 412–415.
22 Tolonen A *et al.* Fast high-performance liquid chromatographic analysis of naphthodianthrones and phloroglucinols from *Hypericum perforatum* extracts. *Phytochemical Anal* 2003; 14: 306–309.
23 Westerhoff K *et al.* Biorelevant dissolution testing of St John's wort products. *J Pharm Pharmacol* 2002; 54: 1615–1621.
24 Linde K *et al.* St John's wort for depression. The Cochrane Database of Systematic Reviews, 2005, Issue 3. Art. No. :CD000448.pub2.
25 Nahrstedt A, Butterweck V. Biologically active and other chemical constituents of the herb of *Hypericum perforatum* L. *Pharmacopsychiatry* 1997; 30 (Suppl. Suppl.): 129–134.
26 Butterweck V *et al.* Plasma levels of hypericin in presence of procyanidin B2 and hyperoside: a pharmacokinetic study in rats. *Planta Med* 2003; 6: 189–192.
27 Suzuki O *et al.* Inhibition of monoamine oxidase by hypericin. *Planta Med* 1984; 50: 272–274.
28 Bladt S, Wagner H. Inhibition of MAO by fractions and constituents of *Hypericum* extract. *J Geriat Psychiatr Neurol* 1994; 7: S57–59.
29 Demisch L *et al.* Identification of MAO-type-A inhibitors in *Hypericum perforatum* L. (Hyperforat). *Pharmacopsychiatry* 1989; 22: 194.
30 Thiede HM, Walper A. Inhibition of MAO and COMT by *Hypericum* extracts and hypericin. *J Geriat Psychiatr Neurol* 1994; 7: S54–56.
31 Cott JM. *In vitro* receptor binding and enzyme inhibition by *Hypericum perforatum* extract. *Pharmacopsychiatry* 1997; 30 (Suppl. Suppl.): 108–112.
32 Müller WE *et al.* Effects of hypericum extract (LI 160) in biochemical models of antidepressant activity. *Pharmacopsychiatry* 1997; 30 (Suppl. Suppl.): 102–107.
33 Calapai G *et al.* Effects of *Hypericum perforatum* on levels of 5-hydroxytryptamine, noradrenaline and dopamine in the cortex, diencephalon and brainstem of the rat. *J Pharm Pharmacol* 1999; 51: 723–728.
34 Winkler C *et al.* St John's wort (*Hypericum perforatum*) counteracts cytokine-induced tryptophan catabolism *in vitro. Biol Chem* 2004; 385: 1197–1202.
35 Zanoli P. Role of hyperforin in the pharmacological activities of St John's wort. *CNS Drug Rev* 2004; 10: 203–218.
36 Chatterjee SS *et al.* Hyperforin as a possible antidepressant component of hypericum extracts. *Life Sci* 1998; 63: 499–510.
37 Chatterjee SS *et al.* Antidepressant activity of *Hypericum perforatum* and hyperforin: the neglected possibility. *Pharmacopsychiatry* 1998; 31 (Suppl. Suppl.): 7–15.
38 Gobbi M *et al.* *Hypericum perforatum* L. extract does not inhibit 5-HT transporter in rat brain cortex. *Naunyn-Schmiedebergs Arch Pharmacol* 1999; 360: 262–269.
39 Jensen AG *et al.* Adhyperforin as a contributor to the effect of *Hypericum perforatum* L. in biochemical models of antidepressant activity. *Life Sci* 2001; 68: 1593–1605.
40 Butterweck V *et al.* *In vitro* receptor screening of pure constituents of St John's wort reveals novel interactions with a number of GPCRs. *Psychopharmacology* 2002; 162: 193–202.
41 Fiebich BL *et al.* Inhibition of substance P-induced cytokine synthesis by St John's wort extracts. *Pharmacopsychiatry* 2001; 34 (Suppl. Suppl. 1): S26–S28.
42 Gobbi M *et al.* *In vitro* effects of the dicyclohexylammonium salt of hyperforin on interleukin-6 release in different experimental models. *Planta Med* 2004; 70: 680–682.
43 Butterweck V *et al.* Step by step removal of hyperforin and hypericin: activity profile of different *Hypericum* preparations in behavioral models. *Life Sci* 2003; 73: 627–639.
44 Butterweck V. Mechanism of action of St John's wort in depression: what is known?. *CNS Drugs* 2003; 17: 539–562.
45 Singer A *et al.* Hyperforin, a major antidepressant constituent of St. John's wort, inhibits serotonin uptake by elevating free intracellular Na^+. *J Pharmacol Exp Ther* 1999; 290: 1363–1368.
46 Singer A *et al.* Hyperforin alters free intracellular H^+ and Na^+ concentration in human platelets (abstract). Paper presented at the Biocenter Symposium on Drug Therapy. Pharmacology of St. John's Wort (*Hypericum perforatum* L.) and its Constituents., February 2000, Frankfurt, Germany.
47 Treiber K *et al.* Hyperforin activates nonselective cation channels (NSCCs). *Br J Pharmacol* 2005; 145: 75–83.
48 Uebelhack R, Franke L. *In vitro* effects of hypericum extract and hyperforin on 5HT uptake and efflux in human blood platelets (abstract). Paper presented at the Biocenter Symposium on Drug Therapy. Pharmacology of St. John's Wort (*Hypericum perforatum* L.) and its Constituents, February 2000, Frankfurt, Germany.
49 Okpanyi SN, Weischer ML. Animal experiments on the psychotropic action of a *Hypericum* extract. *Arzneimittelforschung* 1987; 37: 10–13.
50 Gambarana C *et al.* Efficacy of an *Hypericum perforatum* (St John's wort) extract in preventing and reverting a condition of escape deficit in rats. *Neuropsychopharmacology* 1999; 21: 247–257.
51 De Vry J *et al.* Comparison of hypericum extracts with imipramine and fluoxetine in animal models of depression and alcoholism. *Eur Neuropsychopharmacol* 1999; 9: 461–468.
52 Butterweck V *et al.* Flavonoids from *Hypericum perforatum* show antidepressant activity in the forced swimming test. *Planta Med* 2000; 66: 3–6.
53 Martarelli D *et al.* *Hypericum perforatum* methanolic extract inhibits growth of human prostatic carcinoma cell line orthotopically implanted in nude mice. *Cancer Lett* 2004; 210: 27–33.
54 Hostanska K *et al.* Aqueous ethanolic extract of St John's wort (*Hypericum perforatum* L.) induces growth inhibition and apoptosis in human malignant cells *in vitro. Pharmazie* 2002; 57: 323–331.

55 Hostanska K *et al.* Comparison of the growth-inhibitory effect of *Hypericum perforatum* L. extracts, differing in the concentration of phloroglucinols and flavonoids, on leukaemia cells. *J Pharm Pharmacol* 2003; 55: 973–980.
56 Roscetti G *et al.* Cytotoxic activity of *Hypericum perforatum* L. on K562 erythroleukemic cells: differential effects between methanolic extract and hypericin. *Phytotherapy Res* 2004; 18: 66–72.
57 Donà M *et al.* Hyperforin inhibits cancer invasion and metastasis. *Cancer Res* 2004; 64: 6225–6232.
58 Schempp CM *et al.* Inhibition of tumour cell growth by hyperforin, a novel anticancer drug from St John's wort that acts by induction of apoptosis. *Oncogene* 2002; 21: 1242–1250.
59 Hostanska K *et al.* Hyperforin a constituent of St John's wort (*Hypericum perforatum* L.) extract induces apoptosis by triggering activation of caspases and with hypericin synergistically exerts cytotoxicity towards human malignant cell lines. *Eur J Pharm Biopharmaceut* 2003; 56: 121–132.
60 Colasanti A *et al.* Hypericin photosensitization of tumor and metastatic cell lines of human prostate. *J Photochem Photobiol B Biology* 2000; 54: 103–107.
61 Liu CD *et al.* Hypericin and photodynamic therapy decreases human pancreatic cancer *in vitro* and *in vivo*. *J Surg Res* 2000; 93: 137–143.
62 Delaey E *et al.* Photocytotoxicity of hypericin in normoxic and hypoxic conditions. *J Photochem Photobiol B Biology* 2000; 56: 19–24.
63 Höpfner M *et al.* Hypericin activated by an incoherent light source has photodynamic effects on esophageal cancer cells. *Int J Colorectal Dis* 2003; 18: 239–247.
64 Kamuhabwa AR *et al.* Photodynamic activity of hypericin in human urinary bladder carcinoma cells. *Anticancer Res* 2000; 20: 2579–2584.
65 Čarvarga I *et al.* Photodynamic therapy of murine fibrosarcoma with topical and systemic administration of hypericin. *Phytomedicine* 2001; 8: 325–330.
66 Solár P *et al.* Effect of azetazolamide on hypericin photocytotoxicity. *Planta Med* 2002; 68: 658–660.
67 Miroššay A *et al.* The effect of quercetin on light-induced cytotoxicity of hypericin. *Physiol Res* 2001; 50: 635–637.
68 Schempp CM *et al.* Phototoxic and apoptosis-inducing capacity of pseudohypericin. *Planta Med* 2002; 68: 171–173.
69 Schempp CM *et al.* Hypericin photo-induced apoptosis involves the tumor necrosis factor apoptosis-inducing ligand (TRAIL) and activation of caspase-8. *FEBS Lett* 2001; 493: 26–30.
70 Ali SM *et al.* Hypericin and hypocrellin induced apoptosis in human mucosal carcinoma cells. *J Photochem Photobiol B Biology* 2001; 65: 59–73.
71 Pajonk F *et al.* Hypericin – an inhibitor of proteasome function. *Cancer Chemother Pharmacol* 2005; 55: 439–446.
72 Kamuhabwa AR *et al.* Cellular photodestruction induced by hypericin in AY-27 rat bladder carcinoma cells. *Photochem Photobiol* 2001; 74: 126–132.
73 Paba V *et al.* Photo-activation of hypericin with low doses of light promotes apparent photo-resistance in human histiocytic lymphoma U937 cells. *J Photochem Photobiol B Biology* 2001; 60: 87–96.
74 Varriale L *et al.* Molecular aspects of photodynamic therapy: low energy pre-sensitization of hypericin-loaded human endometrial carcinoma cells enhances photo-tolerance, alters gene expression and affects the cell cycle. *FEBS Lett* 2002; 512: 287–290.
75 Schwarz D *et al.* St John's wort extracts and some of their constituents potently inhibit ultimate carcinogen formation from benzo(a)pyrene-7,8-didhyrodiol by human CYP1A1. *Cancer Res* 2003; 63: 8062–8068.
76 Decosterd LA *et al.* Isolation of new cytotoxic constituents from *Hypericum revolutum* and *Hypericum calycinum* by liquid–liquid chromatography. *Planta Med* 1988; 54: 560.
77 Avato P *et al.* Extracts from St John's wort and their antimicrobial activity. *Phytotherapy Res* 2004; 18: 230–232.
78 Zakharova NS *et al.* Action of plant extracts on the natural immunity indices of animals. *Zh Mikrobiol Epidemiol Immunobiol* 1986; 4: 71–75.
79 Schempp C *et al.* Antibacterial activity of hyperforin from St John's wort, against multiresistant *Staphylococcus aureus* and Gram-positive bacteria. *Lancet* 1999; 353: 2129.
80 Voss A, Verweij PE. Antibacterial activity of hyperforin from St John's wort. *Lancet* 1999; 354: 777.
81 Fiebich B *et al.* Antibacterial activity of hyperforin from St John's wort. *Lancet* 1999; 354: 777.
82 Hübner AT *et al.* Treatment with *Hypericum perforatum* L. does not trigger decreased resistance in Staphylococcus aureus against antibiotics and hyperforin. *Phytomedicine* 2003; 10: 206–208.
83 Negrash AK *et al.* Comparative study of chemotherapeutic and pharmacological properties of antimicrobial preparations from common St John's wort. *Fitontsidy Mater Soveshch* 1969; 198–200.
84 Sakar MK *et al.* Antimicrobial activities of some *Hypericum* species growing in Turkey. *Fitoterapia* 1988; 59: 49–52.
85 Dall'Agnol R *et al.* Antimicrobial activity of some *Hypericum* species. *Phytomedicine* 2003; 10: 511–516.
86 Gibbons S *et al.* The genus *Hypericum* – a valuable resource of anti-Staphylococcal leads. *Fitoterapia* 2002; 73: 300–304.
87 Mishenkova EL *et al.* Antiviral properties of St John's wort and preparations produced from it. *Tr S'ezda Mikrobiol Ukr* 1975; 222–223.
88 Weber ND *et al.* The antiviral agent hypericin has *in vitro* activity against HSV-1 through non-specific association with viral and cellular membranes. *Antiviral Chem Chemother* 1994; 5: 83–90.
89 Wood S *et al.* Antiviral activity of naturally occurring anthraquinones and anthraquinone derivatives. *Planta Med* 1990; 56: 651–652.
90 Jia YR *et al.* *In vitro* study on the effects of hypericin and lysine hydrochloride against herpes virus. *Chin J Clin Rehab* 2004; 8(5): 966–967.
91 Lavie G *et al.* Studies of the mechanisms of the antiretroviral agents hypericin and pseudohypericin. *Proc Natl Acad Sci USA* 1989; 86: 5963–5967.
92 Lopez-Bazzocchi I *et al.* Antiviral activity of the photoactive plant pigment hypericin. *Photochem Photobiol* 1991; 54: 95–98.
93 Meruelo D *et al.* Therapeutic agents with dramatic antiretroviral activity and little toxicity at effective doses: aromatic polycyclic diones hypericin and pseudohypericin. *Proc Natl Acad Sci USA* 1988; 85: 5230–5234.
94 Hudson JB *et al.* Antiviral activities of hypericin. *Antiviral Res* 1991; 15: 101–112.
95 Taher MM *et al.* Mood-enhancing antidepressant St John's wort inhibits the activation of human immunodeficiency virus gene expression by ultraviolet light. *Life* 2002; 54: 357–364.
96 Koch E, Chatterjee SS. Hyperforin stimulates intracellular calcium mobilisation and enhances extracellular acidification in DDT1-MF2 smooth muscle cells (abstract). Paper presented at the Biocenter Symposium on Drug Therapy. Pharmacology of St. John's Wort (*Hypericum perforatum* L.) and its Constituents. February 2000, Frankfurt, Germany.
97 Rezvani AH *et al.* Attenuation of alcohol intake by extract of *Hypericum perforatum* (St John's wort) in two different strains of alcohol-preferring rats. *Alcohol Alcoholism* 1999; 34: 699–705.
98 Wright CW *et al.* Correlation of hyperforin content of *Hypericum perforatum* (St John's wort) extracts with their effects on alcohol drinking in C57BL/6J mice: a preliminary study. *J Psychopharmacol* 2003; 17: 403–408.
99 Catania MA *et al.* *Hypericum perforatum* attenuates nicotine withdrawal signs in mice. *Psychopharmacology* 2003; 169(2): 186–189.
100 Ballenger JC *et al.* Alcohol and central serotonin metabolism in man. *Arch Gen Psych Scand* 1979; 57: 224–227. Cited by Rezvani AH *et al.* *Alcohol Alcoholism* 1999; 34: 699–705.
101 Hughes JR *et al.* Antidepressants for smoking cessation. The Cochrane Database of Systematic Reviews, 2004, Issue 4. Art. No.: CD000031.
102 Shipochliev T *et al.* Anti-inflammatory action of a group of plant extracts. *Vet Med Nauki* 1981; 18: 87–94.
103 Bork PS *et al.* Hypericin as a non-oxidant inhibitor of NF-κB. *Planta Med* 1999; 65: 297–300.
104 Takahashi I *et al.* Hypericin and pseudohypericin specifically inhibit protein kinase C: possible relation to their antiretroviral activity. *Biochem Biophys Res Commun* 1989; 165: 1207–1212.
105 Agostinis P *et al.* Photosensitized inhibition of growth factor regulated protein kinases by hypericin. *Biochemical Pharmacol* 1995; 49: 1615–1622.
106 De Witte P *et al.* Inhibition of epidermal growth factor receptor tyrosine kinase activity by hypericin. *Biochemical Pharmacol* 1993; 46: 1929–1936.

107 Panossian AG *et al*. Immunosuppressive effects of hypericin on stimulated human leucocytes: inhibition of the arachidonic acid release, leukotriene B_4 and interleukin-1 production and activation of nitric oxide formation. *Phytomedicine* 1996; 3: 19–28.
108 Tahara Y *et al*. The antidepressant hypericin inhibits progression of experimental proliferative vitreoretinopathy. *Curr Eye Res* 1999; 19: 323–329.
109 Bezáková L *et al*. Effect of dianthrones and their precursors from *Hypericum perforatum* L. on lipoxygenase activity. *Pharmazie* 1999; 54: 711.
110 Albert D *et al*. Hyperforin is a dual inhibitor of cyclooxygenase-1 and 5-lipoxygenase. *Biochemical Pharmacol* 2002; 64: 1767–1775.
111 Hunt EJ *et al*. Effect of St John's wort on free radical production. *Life Sci* 2001; 69: 181–190.
112 Heilmann J *et al*. Studies on the antioxidative activity of phloroglucinol derivatives isolated from *Hypericum* species. *Planta Med* 2003; 69: 202–206.
113 Melzer R *et al*. Proanthocyanidins from *Hypericum perforatum*: effects on isolated pig coronary arteries. *Planta Med* 1988; 54: 572–573.
114 Shiplochliev T. Extracts from a group of medicinal plants enhancing the uterine tonus. *Vet Med Nauki* 1981; 18: 94–98.
115 Jang M-H *et al*. Protective effect of *Hypericum perforatum* Linn (St John's wort) against hydrogen peroxide-induced apoptosis on human neuroblastoma cells. *Neuroscience Lett* 2002; 329: 177–180.
116 Vasilchenko EA *et al*. Analgesic action of flavonoids of *Rhododendron luteum* Sweet, *Hypericum perforatum* L., *Lespedeza bicolor* Turcz. and *L. hedysaroides* (Pall.) Kitag. *Rastit Resur* 1986; 22: 12–21.
117 Grujic-Vasic J *et al*. The examining of isolated tannins and their astringent effect. *Planta Med* 1986; 52 (Suppl. Suppl.): 67–68.
118 Barnes J *et al*. St John's wort (*Hypericum perforatum* L.): a review of its chemistry, pharmacology and clinical properties. *J Pharm Pharmacol* 2001; 53: 583–600.
119 Laakman G *et al*. St John's wort in mild to moderate depression: the relevance of hyperforin for the clinical efficacy. *Pharmacopsychiatry* 1998; 31 (Suppl. Suppl.): 54–59.
120 Schroeder C *et al*. Influence of St John's wort on catecholamine turnover and cardiovascular regulation in humans. *Clin Pharmacol Ther* 2004; 76: 480–489.
121 Franklin M *et al*. Neuroendocrine evidence for dopaminergic actions of hypericum extract (LI 160) in healthy volunteers. *Biol Psychiatr* 1999; 46: 581–584.
122 Laakman G *et al*. Effects of hypericum extract on adenohypophysial hormone secretion and catechol amine metabolism (abstract). Paper presented at the Biocenter Symposium on Drug Therapy. Pharmacology of St. John's Wort (*Hypericum perforatum* L.) and its Constituents. February 2000, Frankfurt, Germany.
123 Schüle C *et al*. Endocrinological effects of high-dose *Hypericum perforatum* extract WS 5570 in healthy subjects. *Neuropsychobiology* 2004; 49: 58–63.
124 Anon. Johanniskraut VS. SSRI – neue Erkentnnisse zur Wirksamkeit und Verträglichkeit. *Nervenheilkunde* 2000; 19: 92–93.
125 Philipp M *et al*. Hypericum extract versus imipramine or placebo in patients with moderate depression: randomized multicentre study of treatment for 8 weeks. *BMJ* 1999; 319: 1534–1539.
126 Hypericum Depression Trial Study Group. Effect of *Hypericum perforatum* (St John's wort) in major depressive disorder. A randomized controlled trial. *JAMA* 2002; 287: 1807–1814.
127 Vitiello B *et al*. Hyperforin plasma level as a marker of treatment adherence in the National Institutes of Health Hypericum depression trial. *J Clin Psychopharmacol* 2005; 25(3): 243–249.
128 Szegedi A *et al*. Acute treatment of moderate to severe depression with hypericum extract WS 5570 (St John's wort): randomised controlled double blind non-inferiority trial versus paroxetine. *BMJ* 2005; 330: 503.
129 Linde K *et al*. St John's wort for depression – an overview and meta-analysis of randomised clinical trials. *BMJ* 1996; 313: 253–258.
130 Kim HL *et al*. St John's wort for depression. A meta-analysis of well-defined clinical trials. *J Nerv Ment Dis* 1999; 187: 532–539.
131 Linde K, Knüppel L. Large-scale observational studies of hypericum extracts in patients with depressive disorders – a systematic review. *Phytomedicine* 2005; 12: 148–157.15693723
132 Hübner WD, Kirste T. Experience with St John's wort (*Hypericum perforatum*) in children under 12 years with symptoms of depression and psychovegetative disturbances. *Phytotherapy Res* 2001; 15: 367–370.
133 Findling RL *et al*. An open-label pilot study of St John's wort in juvenile depression. *J Am Acad Child Adolesc Psychiatry* 2003; 42: 908–914.
134 Lenoir S *et al*. No dose-dependent effect of hypericin in hypericum extracts for depression. *Phytomedicine* 1999; 6: 141–146.
135 Barnes J *et al*. A pilot, randomised, open, uncontrolled clinical study of two dosages of St John's wort (*Hypericum perforatum* L.) herb extract as an aid to motivational/behavioural support in smoking cessation. *Planta Med* 2006; 72(4): 378–382.
136 Kasper S. Treatment of seasonal affective disorder (SAD) with hypericum extract. *Pharmacopsychiatry* 1997; 30 (Suppl. Suppl.): 89–93.
137 Wheatley D. Hypericum in seasonal affective disorder (SAD). *Curr Med Res Opin* 1999; 15: 33–37.
138 Hypericin – a plant extract with anti-HIV activity. *Scrip* 1989; 1415: 29.
139 Anon. Hypericin HIV trial in Thailand. *Scrip* 1995; 2019: 25.
140 Cooper WC, James J. An observational study of the safety and efficacy of hypericin in HIV-positive subjects (abstract). *Int Conf AIDS* 1990; 6: 369.
141 Steinbeck-Klose A, Wernet P. Successful long-term treatment over 40 months of HIV-patients with intravenous hypericin (abstract). *Int Conf AIDS* 1993; 9: 470.
142 Gulick RM *et al*. Phase I studies of hypericin, the active compound in St John's wort, as an antiretroviral agent in HIV-infected adults. *Ann Intern Med* 1999; 130: 510–514.
143 Jacobson JM *et al*. Pharmacokinetics, safety and antiviral effects of hypericin, a derivative of St John's wort plant, in patients with chronic hepatitis C virus infection. *Antimicrob Agents Chemother* 2001; 45: 517–524.
144 Stevinson C *et al*. Hypericum for fatigue – a pilot study. *Phytomedicine* 1998; 5: 443–447.
145 Stevinson C, Ernst E. A pilot study of *Hypericum perforatum* for the treatment of premenstrual syndrome. *Br J Obstet Gynaecol* 2000; 107: 870–876.
146 Müller T *et al*. Treatment of somatoform disorders with St John's wort: a randomized, double-blind and placebo-controlled trial. *Psychosomatic Med* 2004; 66: 538–547.
147 Kobak KA *et al*. St John's wort versus placebo in social phobia. Results from a placebo-controlled pilot study. *J Clin Psychopharmacol* 2005; 25(1): 51–58.
148 Boblitz N *et al*. Benefit of a fixed drug combination containing St John's wort and black cohosh for climacteric patients – results of a randomised clinical trial (abstract). *FACT* 2000; 5: 85.
149 Schellenberg R *et al*. Pharmacodynamic effects of two different hypericum extracts in healthy volunteers measured by quantitative EEG. *Pharmacopsychiatry* 1998; 31 (Suppl. Suppl.): 44–53.
150 Sharpley AL *et al*. Antidepressant-like effect of *Hypericum perforatum* (St John's wort) on the sleep polysomnogram. *Psychopharmacology* 1998; 139: 286–287.
151 Colker CM *et al*. Effects of *Citrus aurantium* extract, caffeine, and St John's wort on body fat loss, lipid levels, and mood states in overweight healthy adults. *Curr Ther Res* 1999; 60: 145–153.
152 Friede M *et al*. Alltagssicherheit eines pflanzlichen Antidepressivums aus Johanniskraut. *Fortschritte Med* 1998; 116: 131–135.
153 Hottenrot K *et al*. The influence of vitamin E and extract from hypericum on the endurance capacity of competitors. A placebo-controlled double-blind study with long-distance runners and triathletes. *Dtsche Zeitschrift Sportmed* 1997; 48: 22–27.
154 Schempp CM *et al*. Topical treatment of atopic dermatitis with St John's wort cream – a randomized, placebo controlled, double blind half-side comparison. *Phytomedicine* 2003; 10 (Suppl. Suppl. IV): 31–37.
155 Sindrup SH *et al*. St John's wort has no effect on pain in polyneuropathy. *Pain* 2000; 91: 361–365.
156 Ellis KA *et al*. An investigation into the acute nootropic effects of *Hypericum perforatum* L. (St John's wort) in healthy human volunteers. *Behav Pharmacol* 2001; 12: 173–182.

157 Lavagna SM *et al*. Efficacy of *Hypericum* and *Calendula* oils in the epithelial reconstruction of surgical wounds in childbirth with caesarean section. *Il Farmaco* 2001; 56: 451–453.
158 D'Hallewin MA *et al*. Fluorescence detection of flat bladder carcinoma in situ after intravesical instillation of hypericin. *J Urol* 2000; 164: 349–351.
159 D'Hallewin MA *et al*. Hypericin-based fluorescence diagnosis of bladder carcinoma. *BJU Int* 2002; 89: 760–763.
160 Staffeldt B *et al*. Pharmacokinetics of hypericin and pseudohypericin after oral intake of the *Hypericum perforatum* extract LI 160 in healthy volunteers. *J Geriat Psychiatr Neurol* 1994; 7: S47–53.
161 Biber A *et al*. Oral bioavailability of hyperforin from hypericum extracts in rats and human volunteers. *Pharmacopsychiatry* 1998; 31 (Suppl. Suppl.1): 36–43.
162 Schulz HU *et al*. Investigation of the bioavailability of hypericin, pseudohypericin, hyperforin and the flavonoids quercetin and isorhamnetin following single and multiple oral dosing of a hypericum extract containing tablet. *Arzneim Forsch* 2005; 55(1): 15–22.
163 Agrosi M *et al*. Oral bioavailability of active principles from herbal products in humans. A study on *Hypericum perforatum* extracts using the soft gelatin capsule technology. *Phytomedicine* 2000; 7(6): 455–462.
164 Kamuhabwa AR *et al*. Determination of hypericin in human plasma by high-performance liquid chromatography after intravesical administration in patients with transitional cell carcinoma of the bladder. *Eur J Pharmaceut Biopharmaceut* 2005; 59: 469–474.
165 Riedel KD *et al*. Simultaneous determination of hypericin and hyperforin in human plasma with liquid chromatography-tandem mass spectrometry. *J Chromatog B* 2004; 813: 27–33.
166 Ernst E *et al*. Adverse effects profile of the herbal antidepressant St John's wort (*Hypericum perforatum* L.). *Eur J Clin Pharmacol* 1998; 54: 589–594.
167 Dyson R *et al*. The reported use and effectiveness of *Hypericum* (St John's wort) on affective symptoms in a depression self-help group. *Primary Care Psych* 2002; 8: 99–102.
168 Durán N, Song P-S. Hypericin and its photodynamic action. *Photochem Photobiol* 1986; 43: 677–680.
169 Brockmöller J *et al*. Hypericin and pseudohypericin: pharmacokinetics and effects on photosensitivity in humans. *Pharmacopsychiatry* 1997; 30 (Suppl. Suppl.): 94–101.
170 Schempp C *et al*. Hypericin levels in human serum and interstitial skin blister fluid after oral single-dose and steady-state administration of *Hypericum perforatum* extract (St John's wort). *Skin Pharmacol Appl Skin Physiol* 1999; 12: 299–304.
171 Schempp CM *et al*. Effect of oral administration of *Hypericum perforatum* extract (St. John's wort) on skin erythema and pigmentation induced by UVB, UVA, visible light and solar simulated radiation. *Phytother Res* 2003; 17: 141–146.
172 Schempp CM *et al*. Single-dose and steady-state administration of *Hypericum perforatum* extract (St John's wort) does not influence skin sensitivity to UV radiation, visible light, and solar-simulated radiation. *Arch Dermatol* 2001; 337: 512.
173 Pitisuttithum P *et al*. *Int Conf AIDS 1996; 11: 285*. Cited by G50
174 Schempp CM *et al*. Effect of topical application of *Hypericum perforatum* extract (St John's wort) on skin sensitivity to solar simulated radiation. *Photodermatol Photoimmunol Photomed* 2000; 16: 125–128.
175 Cotterill JA *et al*. Severe phototoxic reaction to laser treatment in a patient taking St John's wort. *J Cosmetic Laser Ther* 2001; 3: 159–160.
176 Benner MH, Lee HJ. *Med Lett* 1979; 21: 29–30.
177 Barbenel DM *et al*. Mania in a patient receiving testosterone replacement post-orchidectomy taking St John's wort and sertraline. *J Psychopharmacol* 2000; 14: 84–86.
178 Nierenberg AA *et al*. Mania associated with St John's wort. *Biol Psychiatr* 1999; 46: 1707–1708.
179 Schneck C. St John's wort and hypomania. *J Clin Psychiatr* 1998; 59: 689.
180 O'Breasil AM, Argouarch S. Hypomania and St John's wort. *Can J Psychiatr* 1998; 43: 746–747.
181 Stevinson C, Ernst E. Can St John's wort trigger psychoses? *Int J Clin Pharmacol Ther* 2004; 42(9): 473–480.
182 Bove GM. Acute neuropathy after exposure to sun in a patient treated with St John's wort. *Lancet* 1998; 352: 1121–1122.
183 Baillie N. Hypericum – four hypersensitivity reactions. *Modern Phytother* 1997; 3: 24–26.
184 Patel S *et al*. Hypertensive crisis associated with St John's wort. *Am J Med* 2002; 112: 507–508.
185 Siepmann M *et al*. The effects of St John's wort extract on heart rate variability, cognitive function and quantitative EEG: a comparison with amitriptyline and placebo in healthy men. *Br J Clin Pharmacol* 2002; 54: 277–282.
186 Siepmann M *et al*. The effects of St John's wort extract and amitriptyline on autonomic responses of blood vessels and sweat glands in healthy volunteers. *J Clin Psychopharmacol* 2004; 24(1): 79–82.
187 Timoshanko A *et al*. A preliminary investigation on the acute pharmacodynamic effects of hypericin on cognitive and psychomotor performance. *Behav Pharmacol* 2001; 12: 635–640.
188 Ferko N, Levine MAH. Evaluation of the association between St John's wort and elevated thyroid-stimulating hormone. *Pharmacotherapy* 2001; 21(12): 1574–1578.
189 Assalian P. Sildenafil for St John-wort induced sexual dysfunction. *J Sex Marital Ther* 2000; 26: 357–358.
190 Bhopal JS. St John's wort-induced sexual dysfunction. *Can J Psychiatry* 2001; 46: 456–457.
191 Giese AC. Hypericism. *Photochem Photobiol* 1980; 5: 229–255.
192 Siegers C *et al*. Zur Frage der Phototoxizität von Hypericum. *Nervenheilkunde* 1993; 12: 320–322.
193 Wilhelm K-P *et al*. Role of flavonoids in controlling the phototoxicity of *Hypericum perforatum* extracts. *Phytomedicine* 2001; 8(4): 306–309.
194 Johnston N. Sun trap. *New Sci* 1999; 24 July: 24.
195 Uppsala Monitoring Centre. Vigibase, WHO Adverse Reactions database (accessed 24 October, 2005).
196 Capasso R *et al*. Effects of the antidepressant St John's wort (*Hypericum perforatum*) on rat and human vas deferens contractility. *J Urol* 2005; 173: 2194–2197.
197 Garrett BJ *et al*. Consumption of poisonous plants (*Senecio jacobaea*, *Symphytum officinale*, *Pteridium aquilinum*, *Hypericum perforatum*) by rats: chronic toxicity, mineral metabolism, and hepatic drug-metabolizing enzymes. *Toxicol Lett* 1982; 10: 183–188.
198 Newall CA *et al*. *Herbal Medicines. A Guide for Health-care Professionals*, 1st edn. London: The Pharmaceutical Press, 1996.
199 Henderson L *et al*. St John's wort (*Hypericum perforatum*): drug interactions and clinical outcomes. *Br J Clin Pharmacol* 2002; 54: 349–356.
200 Mannel M. Drug interactions with St John's wort. *Drug Saf* 2004; 27 (11): 773–797.
201 Eich-Hochli D *et al*. Methadone maintenance treatment and St John's wort – a case report. *Pharmacopsychiatry* 2003; 36: 35–37.
202 Gordon JB. SSRIs and St John's wort: possible toxicity? *Am Family Phys* 1998; 57: 950–953.
203 Lantz MS *et al*. St John's wort and antidepressant drug interactions in the elderly. *J Geriat Psychiatr Neurol* 1999; 12: 7–10.
204 Irefin S, Sprung J. A possible case of cardiovascular collapse during anaesthesia: long-term use of St John's wort. *J Clin Anaesthesiol* 2000; 12: 498–499.
205 Crowe S, McKeating K. Delayed emergence and St John's wort. *Anaesthesiology* 2002; 96: 1025–1027.
206 Ang-Lee MK *et al*. Herbal medicines and peri-operative care. *JAMA* 2001; 286: 208–216.
207 Breckenridge A. Herbal Safety News: Important interactions between St John's wort (*Hypericum perforatum*) preparations and prescribed medicines. http://www.mhra.gov.uk
208 Anon. CSM advice on St John's wort. *Pharm J* 2000; 264: 358.
209 Johne A *et al*. Decreased plasma levels of amitriptyline and its metabolites on comedication with an extract from St John's wort (*Hypericum perforatum*). *J Clin Psychopharmacol* 2002; 22(1): 46–54.
210 Bauer S *et al*. Alterations in cyclosporin A pharmacokinetics and metabolism during treatment with St John's wort in renal transplant patients. *Br J Clin Pharmacol* 2003; 55: 203–211.
211 Mai I *et al*. Hyperforin content determines the magnitude of the St John's wort–cyclosporin drug interaction. *Clin Pharmacol Ther* 2004; 76: 330–340.

212 Mai I *et al.* Impact of St John's wort treatment on the pharmacokinetics of tacrolimus and mycophenolic acid in renal transplant patients. *Nephrol Dial Transplant* 2003; 18: 819–822.
213 Mathijssen RHJ *et al.* Effects of St John's wort on irinotecan metabolism. *J Nat Cancer Inst* 2002; 94(16): 1247–1249.
214 Mills E *et al.* Interaction of St John's wort with conventional drugs: systematic review of clinical trials. *BMJ* 2004; 329: 27–30.
215 Johne A *et al.* Pharmacokinetic interaction of digoxin with an herbal extract from St John's wort (*Hypericum perforatum*). *Clin Pharmacol Ther* 1999; 66: 338–345.
216 Smith P *et al.* The influence of St John's wort on the pharmacokinetics and protein binding of imatinib mesylate. *Pharmacotherapy* 2004; 24 (11): 1508–1514.
217 Frye RF *et al.* Effect of St John's wort on imatinib mesylate pharmacokinetics. *Clin Pharmacol Ther* 2004; 76: 323–329.
218 Pfrunder A *et al.* Interaction of St John's wort with low-dose oral contraceptive therapy: a randomized controlled trial. *Br J Clin Pharmacol* 2003; 56: 683–690.
219 Hall SD *et al.* The interaction between St John's wort and an oral contraceptive. *Clin Pharmacol Ther* 2003; 74: 525–535.
220 Maurer A *et al.* Interaction of St John's wort extract with phenprocoumon (abstract). *Eur J Clin Pharmacol* 1999; 55: A22.
221 Kawaguchi A *et al.* Drug interaction between St John's wort and quazepam. *Br J Clin Pharmacol* 2004; 58: 403–410.
222 Sugimoto K-I *et al.* Different effects of St John's wort on the pharmacokinetics of simvastatin and pravastatin. *Clin Pharmacol Ther* 2001; 70: 518–524.
223 Hebert MF *et al.* Effects of St John's wort (*Hypericum perforatum*) on tacrolimus pharmacokinetics in healthy volunteers. *J Clin Pharmacol* 2004; 44: 89–94.
224 Tannergren C *et al.* St John's wort decreases the bioavailability of R- and S-verapamil through induction of the first-pass metabolism. *Clin Pharmacol Ther* 2004; 75: 298–309.
225 Jiang X *et al.* Effect of St John's wort and ginseng on the pharmacokinetics and pharmacodynamics of warfarin in healthy subjects. *Br J Clin Pharmacol* 2004; 57: 592–599.
226 Kerb R *et al.* Urinary 6-beta-hydroxycortisol excretion rate is affected by treatment with hypericum extract. *Eur J Clin Pharmacol* 1992; 52: 607.
227 Roby CA *et al.* St John's wort impact on CYP3A4 activity. Poster no. 129 presented at the 39th Annual Meeting of the New Clinical Drug Evaluation Unit Program, June 1999, Florida.
228 Markowitz JS *et al.* Effect of St John's wort on drug metabolism by induction of cytochrome P450 3A4 enzyme. *JAMA* 2003; 290: 1500–1504.
229 Wang Z *et al.* The effects of St John's wort (*Hypericum perforatum*) on human cytochrome P450 activity. *Clin Pharmacol Ther* 2001; 70: 317–326.
230 Hennessy M *et al.* St John's wort increases expression of P-glycoprotein: implications for drug interactions. *Br J Clin Pharmacol* 2002; 53: 75–82.
231 Zhou S *et al.* Pharmacokinetic interactions of drugs with St John's wort. *J Pscychopharmacol* 2004; 18: 262–276.
232 Wang L-S *et al.* St John's wort induces both cytochrome P450 3A4-catalyzed sulfoxidation and 2C19-dependent hydroxylation of omeprazole. *Clin Pharmacol Ther* 2004; 75: 191–197.
233 Burstein AH *et al.* Lack of effect of St John's wort on carbamazepine pharmacokinetics in healthy volunteers. *Clin Pharmacol Ther* 2000; 68: 605–612.
234 Morimoto T *et al.* Effect of St John's wort on the pharmacokinetics of theophylline in healthy volunteers. *J Clin Pharmacol* 2004; 44: 95–101.
235 Ereshefsky B *et al.* Determination of St John's wort differential metabolism at CYP2D6 and CYP3A4, using dextromethorphan probe methodology. Poster no. 130 presented at the 39th Annual Meeting of the New Clinical Drug Evaluation Unit Program, June 1999, Florida.
236 Gewertz N *et al.* Determination of the differential effects of St John's wort on the CYP1A2 and NAT2 metabolic pathways using caffeine probe methodology. Poster no. 131 presented at the 39th Annual Meeting of the New Clinical Drug Evaluation Unit Program, June 1999, Florida.
237 Markowitz JS *et al.* Effect of St John's wort (*Hypericum perforatum*) on cytochrome P450 2D6 and 3A4 activity in healthy volunteers. *Life Sci* 2000; 66(9): 133–139.
238 Wenk M *et al.* Effect of St John's wort on the activities of CYP1A2, CYP3A4,CYP2D6, N-acetyltransferase 2, and xanthine oxidase in healthy males and females. *Br J Clin Pharmacol* 2004; 57: 495–499.
239 Arold G *et al.* No relevant interaction with alprazolam, caffeine, tolbutamide, and digoxin by treatment with a low-hyperforin St John's wort extract. *Planta Med* 2005; 71: 331–337.
240 Johne A *et al.* Impact of cytochrome P-450 inhibition by cimetidine and induction by carbamazepine on the kinetics of hypericin and pseudohypericin in healthy volunteers. *Eur J Clin Pharmacol* 2004; 60: 617–622.
241 Komoroski BJ *et al.* Induction and inhibition of cytochromes P450 by the St John's wort constituent hyperforin in human hepatocyte cultures. *Drug Metab Disposition* 2004; 32: 512–518.
242 Chen Y *et al.* Induction of human CYP2C9 by rifampicin, hyperforin, and phenobarbital is mediated by the pregnane X receptor. *J Pharmacol Exp Ther* 2004; 308: 495–501.
243 Cantoni L *et al.* Hyperforin contributes to the hepatic CYP3A-inducing effect of *Hypericum perforatum* extract in the mouse. *Toxicol Sci* 2003; 75: 25–30.
244 Perloff MD *et al.* Saint John's wort: an *in vitro* analysis of P-glycoprotein induction due to extended exposure. *Br J Pharmacol* 2001; 134: 1601–1608.
245 Tian R *et al.* Functional induction and de-induction of P-glycoprotein by St John's wort and its ingredients in a human colon adenocarcinoma cell line. *Drug Metab Disposition* 2005; 33: 547–554.
246 Budzinski JW *et al.* An *in vitro* evaluation of human cytochrome P450 3A4 inhibition by selected commercial herbal extracts and tinctures. *Phytomedicine* 2000; 7: 273–282.
247 Strandell J *et al.* An approach to the *in vitro* evaluation of potential for cytochrome P450 enzyme inhibition from herbals and other natural remedies. *Phytomedicine* 2004; 11: 98–104.
248 Wang E *et al.* Quantitative characterization of direct P-glycoprotein inhibition by St John's wort constituents hypericin and hyperforin. *J Pharm Pharmacol* 2004; 56: 123–128.
249 Peebles KA *et al.* Catalytic inhibition of human DNA topoisomerase IIα by hypericin, a naphthodianthrone from St John's wort (*Hypericum perforatum*). *Biochemical Pharmacol* 2001; 62: 1059–1070.
250 Martin-Facklam M *et al.* Undeclared exposure to St John's wort in hospitalised patients. *Br J Clin Pharmacol* 2004; 58: 437–441.
251 Redvers A *et al.* How many patients self-medicate with St John's wort? *Psychiatric Bull* 2001; 25: 254–256.
252 Beckman SE *et al.* Consumer use of St John's wort: a survey on effectiveness, safety and tolerability. *Pharmacotherapy* 2000; 20: 568–574.
253 Hindmarch M, Oakeshott P. Interactions of the oral contraceptive pill with antibiotics and St John's wort: knowledge of female college students. *Family Prac* 2002; 19(6): 708.
254 Lee A *et al.* The safety of St John's wort (*Hypericum perforatum*) during breastfeeding. *J Clin Psychiatry* 2003; 64: 966–968.
255 Grush LR *et al.* St John's wort during pregnancy. *JAMA* 1998; 280(18): 1566.
256 Klier CM *et al.* St John's wort (*Hypericum perforatum*) – is it safe during breastfeeding? *Pharmacopsychiatry* 2002; 35: 29–30.
257 Rayburn WF *et al.* Effect of prenatally administered hypericum (St John's wort) on growth and physical maturation of mouse offspring. *Am J Obstet Gynecol* 2001; 184: 191–195.
258 Gregoretti B *et al.* Toxicity of *Hypericum perforatum* (St John's wort) administered during pregnancy and lactation in rats. *Toxicol Applied Pharmacol* 2004; 200: 201–205.

Stone Root

Summary and Pharmaceutical Comment

Information available on the chemistry of stone root is limited and no documented scientific evidence was located to justify the herbal uses. In view of the lack of data on pharmacological effects, efficacy and safety, the appropriateness of medicinal use of stone root should be considered. Excessive use, at least, should be avoided. Stone root should not be used during pregnancy and lactation. The potential for stone root preparations to interact with other medicines should be considered.

Species (Family)

Collinsonia canadensis L. (Labiatae/Lamiaceae)

Synonym(s)

Collinsonia punctata Ell., *C. canadensis* var. *punctata* (Ell.) Gray, Heal-All, Knob Root

Part(s) Used

Rhizome, root

Pharmacopoeial and Other Monographs

BHP 1983[G7]
Martindale 35th edition[G85]

Legal Category (Licensed Products)

GSL[G37]

Constituents

Terpenoids Pentacyclic triterpene caulophyllogenin,[1] saponin glycosides.

Other constituents An unidentified alkaloid, mucilage, resin, tannins, essential oil.

Other parts of the plant Leaves and stems contain flavonoids 2,5-dihydroxy-6,7-dimethoxyflavanone, baicalein-6,7-dimethyl ether, norwogenin-7,8-dimethyl ether and tetrochrysin (5-hydroxy-7-methoxyflavone).[2]

Food Use

Stone root is not used in foods.

Herbal Use

Stone root is stated to possess antilithic, litholytic, mild diaphoretic and diuretic properties. Traditionally, it has been used for renal calculus, lithuria, and specifically for urinary calculus.[G7, G64]

Flavonoids (in leaves and stems)

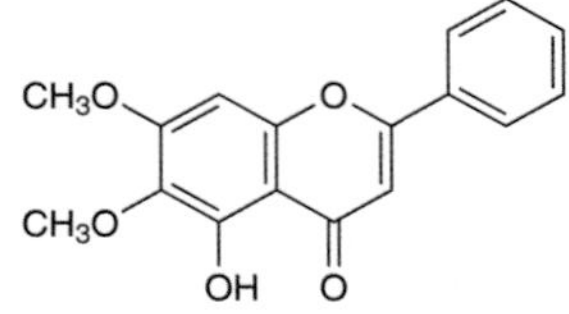

baicalein-6,7-dimethyl ether

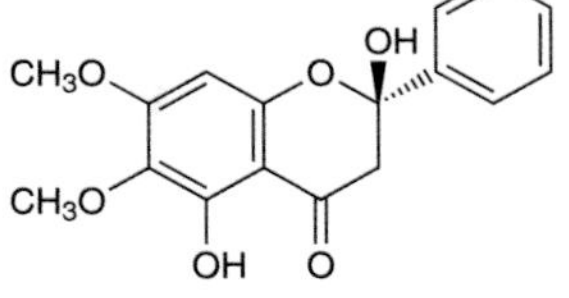

2,5-dihydroxy-6,7-dimethoxyflavanone

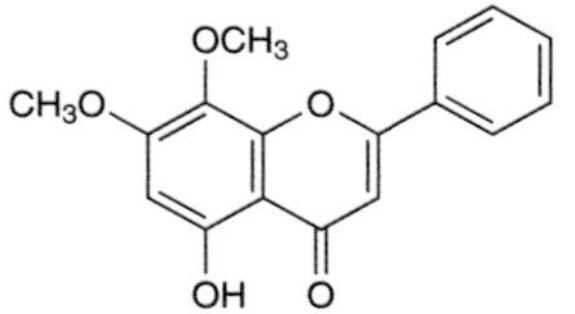

norwogenin-7,8-dimethyl ether

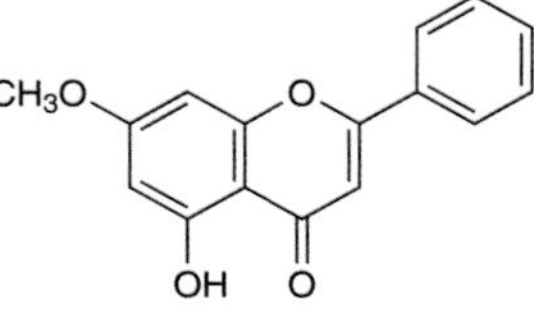

tetrochrysin
(5-hydroxy-7-methoxyflavone)

Triterpenes

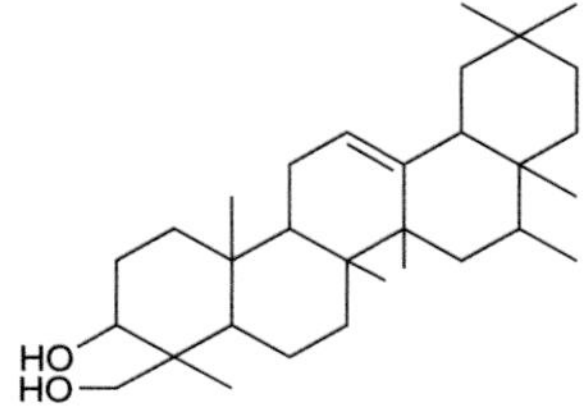

caulophyllogenin

Figure 1 Selected constituents of stone root.

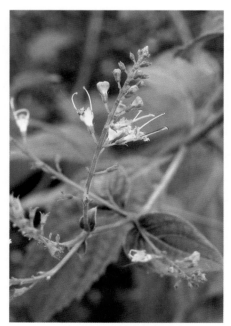

Figure 2 Stone root (*Collinsonia canadensis*).

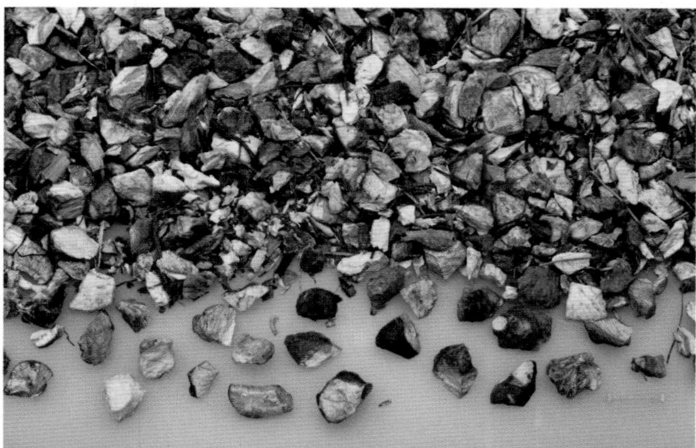

Figure 3 Stone root – dried drug substance (rhizome).

Dosage

Dosages for oral administration (adults) for traditional uses recommended in standard herbal and older pharmaceutical reference texts are given below.

Dried root 1–4 g as a decoction three times daily.(G7)

Liquid extract 1–4 mL (1 : 1 in 25% alcohol) three times daily.(G7)

Tincture 2–8 mL (1 : 5 in 40% alcohol) three times daily.(G7)

Tincture of Collinsonia 2–8 mL.(G10)

Pharmacological Actions

None documented.

Side-effects, Toxicity

None documented. However, there is a lack of clinical and preclinical safety and toxicity data for stone root and further investigation of these aspects is required.

Contra-indications, Warnings

None documented.

Drug interactions None documented. In view of the lack of information on the constituents of stone root and their pharmacological activities, the potential for stone root preparations to interact with other medicines administered concurrently should be considered.

Pregnancy and lactation The safety of stone root has not been established. In view of the lack of phytochemical, pharmacological and toxicological information, the use of stone root during pregnancy and lactation should be avoided.

Preparations

Proprietary multi-ingredient preparations

UK: Piletabs.

References

1 Buckingham J, ed. Dictionary of Natural Products on CD-ROM. Boca Raton: CRC Press, 2005.

2 Stevens JF *et al*. A novel 2-hydroxyflavanone from *Collinsonia canadensis*. *J Nat Prod* 1999; 62: 392–394.

S

Tansy

Summary and Pharmaceutical Comment

Pharmacological activities documented for tansy have been associated with the sterol and triterpene constituents. There is a lack of robust clinical research assessing the efficacy and safety of tansy. Tansy yields an extremely toxic volatile oil, which should not be used internally or externally.(G58) In view of this, the use of tansy as a herbal medicine is not justified even though documented studies have supported the traditional uses of the herb as a choleretic and anthelmintic agent. Tansy is contra-indicated in pregnancy and lactation.

Species (Family)

Tanacetum vulgare L. (Asteraceae/Compositae)

Synonym(s)

Chrysanthemum audiberti (DC.) P. Fourn., *C. tanacetum* Karsch non Vis., *C. vulgare* (L.) Bernh. non (Lam.) Gaterau, *Pyrethrum vulgare* (L.) Boiss. *Tanacetum audibertii* (Req.) DC., Tanacetum

Part(s) Used

Herb

Pharmacopoeial and Other Monographs

BHP 1983(G7)
Martindale 35th edition(G85)

Legal Category (Licensed Products)

Tansy is not included in the GSL.(G37)

Constituents

Steroids β-Sitosterol (major), campesterol, cholesterol, stigmasterol and taraxasterol.(1)

Terpenoids α-Amyrin (major), β-amyrin, sesquiterpene lactones including arbusculin-A, tanacetin, germacrene D, crispolide;(2, 3) tanacetols A and B.(4, 5)

Volatile oils 0.12–0.18%. Major components as β-thujone (up to 95%) and camphor, others include α-pinene, borneol, 1,8-cineole, umbellone and sabinene. At least ten different chemotypes have been identified in which camphor was the most frequently occurring main component and thujone second.(4)

Other constituents Gum, mucilage, resin and tannins.

Food Use

Tansy is listed by the Council of Europe as a natural source of food flavouring (category N3). This category indicates that tansy can be added to foodstuffs in the traditionally accepted manner, although there is insufficient information for an adequate assessment of potential toxicity. In addition, the Council of Europe recommends that the concentration of thujones present in food products is restricted to 0.5 mg/kg.(G16) Tansy oil is

Monoterpenes

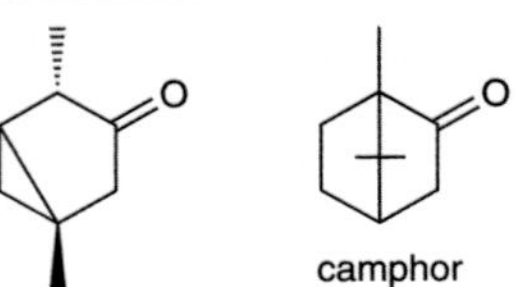

Sesquiterpene lactones

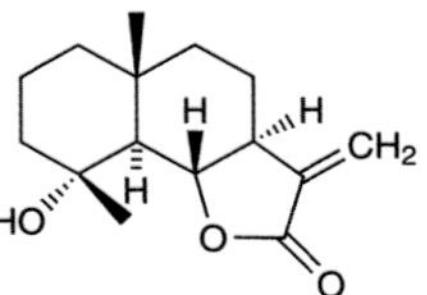

Triterpenes

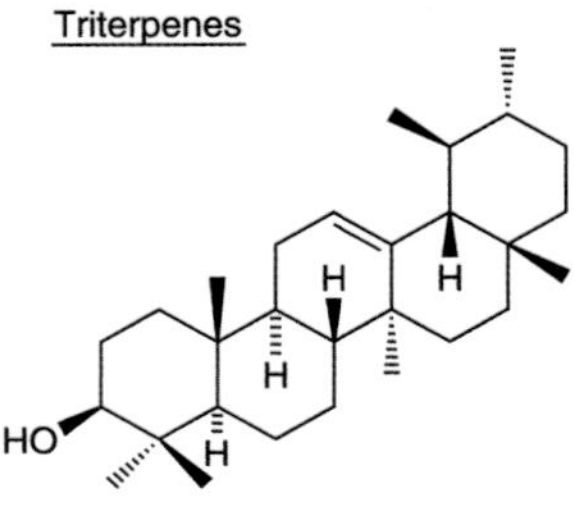

Figure 1 Selected constituents of tansy.

prohibited from use as a food flavouring by the Food Additives and Contaminants Committee (FACC) in view of the thujone content.(G44)

Herbal Use

Tansy is stated to possess anthelmintic, carminative and antispasmodic properties and to act as a stimulant to abdominal viscera. Traditionally, it has been used for nematode infestation, topically for scabies (as a decoction) and pruritus ani (as an ointment), and specifically for roundworm or threadworm infestation in children.(G7)

Dosage

Dosages for oral administration (adults) for traditional uses recommended in standard herbal reference texts are given below.

Dried herb 1–2 g as an infusion three times daily.(G7)

Liquid extract 1–2 mL (1:1 in 25% alcohol) three times daily.(G7)

Pharmacological Actions

In vitro and animal studies

In vitro antispasmodic activity on rabbit intestine, and *in vivo* choleretic activity in the dog have been documented for tansy

T

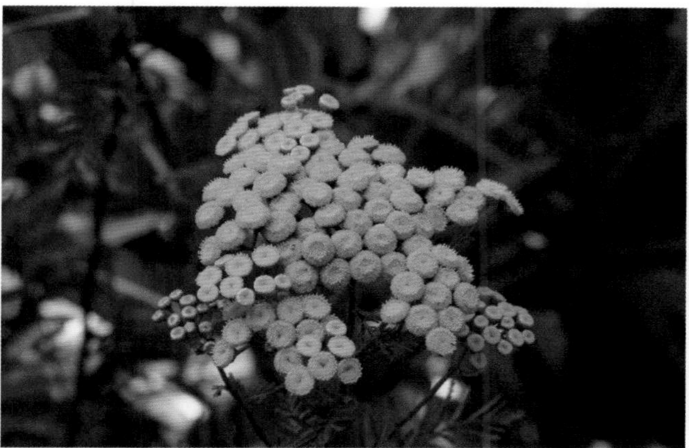

Figure 2 Tansy (*Tanacetum vulgare*).

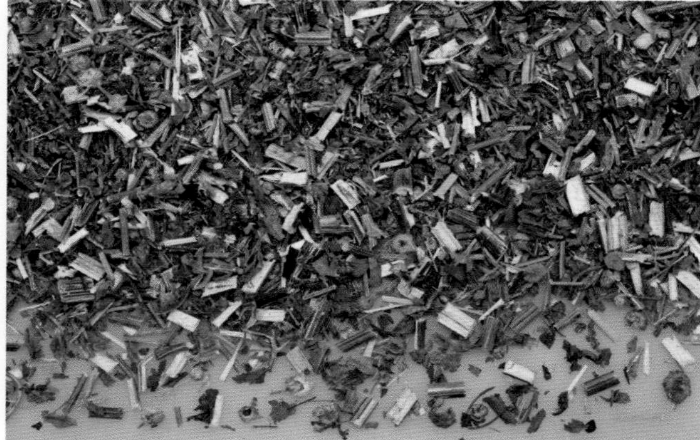

Figure 3 Tansy – dried drug substance (herb).

extracts.[6] It was suggested that the choleretic action might be attributable to caffeic acid, a known bile stimulant that is present in tansy.[6] Anthelmintic activity in dogs has been described for tansy oil, an ether extract of the oil, and for β-thujone.[6] Daily intragastric doses of a tansy extract given to rabbits have been found to reduce serum lipid concentrations and inhibit further development of hypercholesterolaemia.[6] In addition, it was noted that recovery of blood sugar concentrations was inhibited in animals given twice daily doses. *In vitro* antifungal activity in 15 pathogenic and non-pathogenic fungi has been reported.[6]

Clinical studies

There is a lack of clinical research assessing the effects of tansy and rigorous randomised clinical trials are required.

Aqueous infusions and alcoholic extracts have been reported to be clinically effective bile stimulants in patients with liver and gall bladder disorders.[6] The treatment alleviated pain and increased appetite and digestion.

Side-effects, Toxicity

Clinical data

Tansy oil contains the toxic ketone β-thujone.[G58] Symptoms of tansy oil poisoning are attributable to the thujone content and include rapid and weak pulse, severe gastritis, violent spasms and convulsions.[G22] Documented fatalities have mainly been associated with ingestion of the oil, although fatal cases of poisoning have occurred with infusions and powders.[6,7] The ratio of toxic to therapeutic dose has been reported as 2.5 : 1 and it was noted that all tansy preparations should be administered with castor oil.[6] Tansy yields potentially allergenic sesquiterpene lactones which have been implicated in the aetiology of contact dermatitis. Instances of contact dermatitis to tansy have been documented.[6, G51]

Preclinical data

An oral LD_{50} value for tansy oil is stated as 1.15 g/kg body weight.[7]

In vitro and *in vivo* antitumour activity has been documented for tansy.[6]

Contra-indications, Warnings

Tansy oil is toxic and should not be used internally or externally.[G58] Fatalities have been reported following ingestion of infusions and extracts. Tansy contains allergenic sesquiterpene lactones and may cause an allergic reaction.

Drug interactions None documented. However, the potential for preparations of tansy to interact with other medicines administered concurrently, particularly those with similar or opposing effects, should be considered. There is limited evidence from preclinical studies that tansy has hypoglycaemic activity.

Pregnancy and lactation Tansy is contra-indicated in pregnancy and lactation. Tansy is reputed to affect the menstrual cycle and utero-activity has been documented in animal studies. The volatile oil contains β-thujone, a known hepatotoxin.

Preparations

Proprietary multi-ingredient preparations

Australia: Calmo.

References

1 Chandler RF *et al.* Herbal remedies of the Maritime Indians: Sterols and triterpenes of *Tanacetum vulgare* L. (Tansy). *Lipids* 1982; 17: 102–106.

2 Chandra A *et al.* Germacranolides and an alkyl glucoside from *Tanacetum vulgare*. *Phytochemistry* 1987; 26: 1463–1465.

3 Appendino G. Crispolide, an unusual hydroperoxysesquiterpene lactone from *Tanacetum vulgare*. *Phytochemistry* 1982; 21: 1099–1102.

4 Holopainen M *et al.* A study on tansy chemotypes. *Planta Med* 1987; 53: 284–287.

5 Appendino G *et al.* Tanacetols A and B, non-volatile sesquiterpene alcohols, from *Tanacetum vulgare*. *Phytochemistry* 1983; 22: 509–512.

6 Opdyke DLJ. Tansy oil. *Food Cosmet Toxicol* 1976; 14: 869–871.

7 Hardin JW, Arena JM, eds. *Human Poisoning from Native and Cultivated Plants*, 2nd edn. North Carolina: Duke University, 1974: 150–153.

Thyme

Summary and Pharmaceutical Comment

Thyme is commonly used as a culinary herb and is characterised by its volatile oil. Documented pharmacological actions support some of the traditional medicinal uses, which have been principally attributed to the volatile oil and flavonoid constituents. However, robust clinical research assessing the efficacy and safety of thyme is limited. The oil is toxic and should not be ingested and only applied externally if diluted in a suitable carrier oil. It has been suggested that standardised thyme extracts based on the phenolic volatile components may not be appropriate because antispasmodic actions previously attributed to these compounds may be attributable to other constituents. Thyme should not be ingested during pregnancy and lactation in quantities greater than those found in foods.

Species (Family)

**Thymus vulgaris* L.
†*Thymus zygis* L. (Labiatae/Lamiaceae)

Synonym(s)

Common Thyme, French Thyme, Garden Thyme, Rubbed Thyme
**Thymus ilerdensis* Gonz. Frag. ex Costa., *T. webbianus* Rouy, *T. valentinus* Rouy., *T. aestivus* Reut. ex Willk., *T. welwitschii* Boiss. subsp *ilerdensis* (Gonz. Frag. ex Costa) Nyman
†*T. sabulicola* Coss., *T. sylvestris* Hoffman & Link

Part(s) Used

Flowering top, leaf

Pharmacopoeial and Other Monographs

BHP 1996[(G9)]
BP 2007[(G86)]
Complete German Commission E[(G3)]
ESCOP 2003[(G76)]
Martindale 35th edition[(G85)]
Ph Eur 2007[(G81)]
WHO volume 1 1999[(G63)]

Legal Category (Licensed Products)

GSL[(G37)]

Constituents

The following is compiled from several sources, including General References G2, G22, G52 and G58.

Volatile oils 0.8–2.6%. Pharmacopoeial standard, not less than 1.2%.[(G81, G86)] Phenols as major components (20–80%) primarily thymol and carvacrol; others include *p*-cymene and γ-terpinene (monoterpenes), linalool, α-terpineol, and thujan-4-ol (alcohols); biphenyl compounds of monoterpene origin.[(G52)] A detailed analysis of the volatile oil components is given elsewhere.[(G22)]

Flavonoids Cirsilineol, 8-methoxycirsilineol, thymonin and eriodictyol.

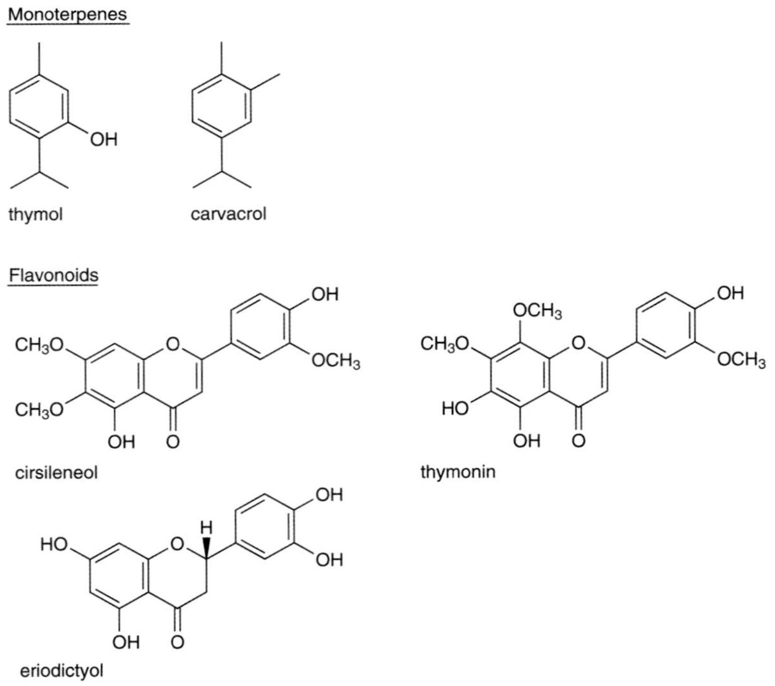

Monoterpenes

OH

thymol

carvacrol

Flavonoids

OH
CH_3O
OCH_3
CH_3O
OH O
cirsileneol

OH
OCH_3
CH_3O
OCH_3
HO
OH O
thymonin

OH
HO
H
OH
OH O
eriodictyol

Figure 1 Selected constituents of thyme.

T

Other constituents Caffeic acid, oleanolic acid, ursolic acid, rosmarinic acid, resins, saponins and tannins.

Food Use

Thyme is commonly used as a culinary herb, and thyme oil is used in food flavouring. Previously, thyme has been listed as GRAS (Generally Recognised As Safe).[G65]

Herbal Use

Thyme is stated to possess carminative, antispasmodic, antitussive, expectorant, secretomotor, bactericidal, anthelmintic and astringent properties. Traditionally, it has been used for dyspepsia, chronic gastritis, asthma, diarrhoea in children, enuresis in children, laryngitis, tonsillitis (as a gargle), and specifically for pertussis and bronchitis.[G2, G4, G7, G32, G43, G50, G52, G64] The German Commission E approved internal use for treating symptoms of bronchitis, whooping cough and catarrh of the upper respiratory tract.[G3] Thyme is used in various combinations with anise oil, eucalyptus oil, fennel oil, fennel fruit, Iceland moss, lime flower, liquorice root, marshmallow root, primrose root and star anise fruit for catarrh and diseases of the upper respiratory tract.[G3]

Dosage

Dosages for oral administration (adults) for traditional uses recommended in older and contemporary standard herbal and pharmaceutical reference texts are given below.

Dried herb 1–4 g as an infusion three times daily;[G7] 1–2 g.[G3, G52]

Liquid Extract of Thyme (BPC 1949) 0.6–4.0 mL.

Elixir of Thyme (BPC 1949) 4–8 mL.

Tincture 2–6 mL (1 : 5 in 45% alcohol) three times daily,[G7] four drops.[G3, G52]

Pharmacological Actions

In vitro and animal studies

Antitussive, expectorant and antispasmodic actions are considered to be the major pharmacological properties of thyme,[1] and have been associated with the volatile oils (e.g. thymol, carvacrol) and flavonoid constituents. Thyme oil has produced hypotensive and respiratory stimulant effects in rabbits following oral or intramuscular administration, and in cats following intravenous injection;[G41] an increase in rhythmic heart contraction was also observed in rabbits.[G41]

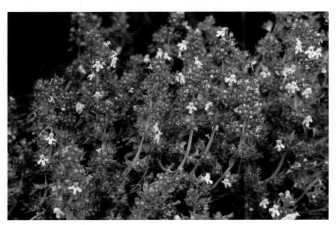

Figure 2 Thyme (*Thymus vulgaris*).

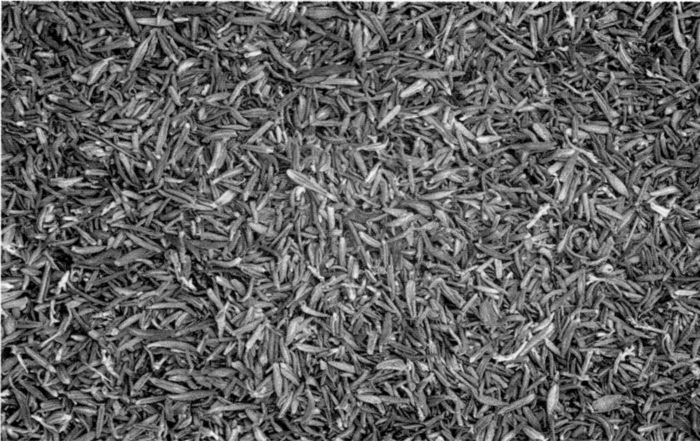

Figure 3 Thyme – dried drug substance (leaf).

In vitro antispasmodic activity of thyme and related *Thymus* species has been associated with the phenolic components of the volatile oil[2] and with the flavonoid constituents; their mode of action is thought to involve calcium-channel blockage.[1, 3, 4] The flavonoids thymonin, circilineol and 8-methoxycircilineol have potent spasmolytic activity in guineapig trachea preparations *in vitro*.[G52]

Analgesic and antipyretic properties in mice have been reported for a thyme extract.[5]

Thymol possesses anthelmintic (especially hookworms), antibacterial and antifungal properties.[G41] Thymol and thyme oil have antibacterial activity against certain organisms and thymol, carvacrol and thyme oil have antifungal activity against a range of organisms.[G50]

Thyme oil inhibits prostaglandin synthesis; rosmarinic acid has anti-inflammatory activity, inhibiting complement in rats and some of the functions of polymorphonucleocytes.[G52] Rosmarinic acid reduced oedema produced by cobra venom factor in rats, and inhibited passive cutaneous anaphylaxis and impairment of *in vivo* activation of mouse macrophages by heat killed *Corynebacterium parvum*.[G52] Activity may relate to complement inactivation.[G50]

Clinical studies

Generally, well-designed clinical studies assessing the effects of thyme are lacking. A randomised, double-blind, controlled trial involving 60 patients with productive cough compared syrup of thyme and bromhexine over a five-day period. Both groups were similar in self-reported symptom relief.[G50]

Side-effects, Toxicity

Clinical data

There is a lack of clinical safety and toxicity data for thyme and further investigation of these aspects is required.

Thyme oil is a dermal and mucous membrane irritant.[G58] Toxic symptoms documented for thymol include nausea, vomiting, gastric pain, headache, dizziness, convulsions, coma, and cardiac and respiratory arrest.[G22] Thymol is present in some toothpaste preparations, and has been reported to cause cheilitis and glossitis. Hyperaemia and severe inflammation have been described for thyme oil used in bath preparations.(G51)

Preclinical data

A concentrated extract of thyme decreased locomotor activity and caused a slight slowing down of respiration in mice following oral administration of doses of 0.5–3.0 g/kg, equivalent to 4.3–26.0 g dried plant material.(G52) In rats, oral LD_{50} values stated for thyme oil include 2.84 g/kg(G52) and 4.7 g/kg in rats, and >5 g/kg following dermal administration.(6) In mice, oral administration of a concentrated ethanol extract of herb in subacute toxicity tests resulted in increased weights of liver and testes. Also in mice, a dose of 0.9 g daily for three months resulted in mortality rates of 30% and 10% in males and females, respectively. Thyme oil had no mutagenic or DNA-damaging activity in either the Ames test or *Bacillus subtilis* rec-assay.(G52)

Contra-indications, Warnings

Thyme oil is toxic and should be used with considerable caution. It should not be taken internally and only applied externally if diluted in a suitable carrier oil.

Drug interactions None documented. However, the potential for preparations of thyme to interact with other medicines administered concurrently, particularly those with similar or opposing effects, should be considered.

Pregnancy and lactation There are no known problems with the use of thyme during pregnancy and lactation, provided that doses do not greatly exceed the amounts used in foods. Traditionally, thyme is reputed to affect the menstrual cycle and, therefore, large amounts should not be ingested.

Preparations

Proprietary single-ingredient preparations

Austria: Scottopect. *Czech Republic:* Bronchicum Husten-Pastillen. *Germany:* Anastil; Aspecton; Biotuss; Bronchicum Pastillen; Bronchipret; Gelobronchial; Hustagil Thymian-Hustensaft; Hustagil Thymiantropfen; Husties; Isephca S; Makatussin Saft; Melrosum Hustensirup; Mirfusot; Nimopect; Pertussin; Sanopinwern; Soledum Hustensaft; Soledum Hustentropfen; Tetesept Erkaltungs; Thymipin N; Thymiverlan; Tussamag Hustensaft N; Tussamag Hustentropfen N; Tussiflorin Thymian. *Israel:* Thymi Syrup. *Russia:* Bronchicum Husten (Бронхикум Пастилки от Кашля); Tussamag (Туссамаг). *Switzerland:* Thymusin N.

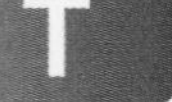

Proprietary multi-ingredient preparations

Argentina: Expectosan Hierbas y Miel. *Australia:* Broncafect; Cough Relief; Euphorbia Complex. *Austria:* Bronchipret; Bronchithym; Bronchostop; Brust- und Hustentee St Severin; Codelum; Eicebaer; Expectal-Tropfen; Krauter Hustensaft; Luuf-Hustentee; Paracodin; Pilka Forte; Pilka; Pneumopan; Pneumopect; Scottopect; Thymoval; Tussamag; Tussimont. *Belgium:* Colimax. *Canada:* Herbal Throat; Original Herb Cough Drops; Swiss Herb Cough Drops. *Chile:* Phyto Corrective Gel; Rhus Opodeldoc. *Czech Republic:* Biotussil; Bronchialtee N; Bronchicum Elixir; Bronchicum Hustensirup; Bronchicum Sekret-Loser; Bronchicum Tropfen; Erkaltungstee; Nontusyl; Perospir; Pleumolysin; Pulmoran; Stomatosan; Thymomel; Urcyston Planta. *Finland:* Katapekt. *France:* Depuratum; Saugella; Tussidoron. *Germany:* Bronchicum Elixir S; Bronchicum; Bronchipret; Bronchipret; Brust- und Hustentee; Cefadrin; Cito-Guakalin; Drosithym-N; Em-medical; Ephepect-Pastillen N; Equisil N; Expectysat N; Harzer Hustenloser; Kinder Em-eukal Hustensaft; Lomal; Makatussin Tropfen; Melissengeist; Muc-Sabona; Phytobronchin; Pulmotin; Sinuforton; Sinuforton; TUSSinfant N. *Israel:* Pilka. *Italy:* Broncosedina; Immumil; Piodermina; Saugella Attiva; Saugella Fitothym; Saugella Poligyn 7; Tussol. *Netherlands:* Balsoclase Compositum; Bronchicum. *Russia:* Bronchicum (Бронхикум); Bronchicum Husten (Бронхикум Сироп от Кашля); Maraslavin (Мараславин); Stoptussin-Fito (Стоптуссин-фито). *South Africa:* Cough Elixir. *Spain:* Natusor Asmaten; Natusor Farinol; Natusor Gripotul; Natusor Infenol; Natusor Renal; Natusor Sinulan; Pilka; Wobenzimal; Wobenzimal. *Switzerland:* DemoPectol; DemoPectol; Makaphyt Gouttes antitussives; Makaphyt Sirop; Nican; Pectoral N; Strath Gouttes contre la toux; Tisane pectorale et antitussive; Tisane pectorale pour les enfants. *Thailand:* Solvopret; Solvopret TP. *UK:* Herb and Honey Cough Elixir. *Venezuela:* Codebromil; Mixagel.

References

1 Van Den Broucke CO. The therapeutic value of *Thymus* species. *Fitoterapia* 1983; 4: 171–174.
2 Van Den Broucke CO, Lernli JA. Pharmacological and chemical investigation of thyme liquid extracts. *Planta Med* 1981; 41: 129–135.
3 Cruz T *et al*. The spasmolytic activity of the essential oil of *Thymus baeticus* Boiss in rats. *Phytother Res* 1989; 3: 106–108.
4 Blázquez MA *et al*. Effects of *Thymus* species extracts on rat duodenum isolated smooth muscle contraction. *Phytother Res* 1989; 3: 41–42.
5 Mohsin A *et al*. Analgesic, antipyretic activity and phytochemical screening of some plants used in traditional Arab system of medicine. *Fitoterapia* 1989; 60: 174.
6 Opdyke DLJ. Thyme oil, red. *Food Cosmet Toxicol* 1974; 12: 1003–1004.

Uva-Ursi

Summary and Pharmaceutical Comment

The chemistry of uva-ursi is well documented with hydroquinone derivatives, especially arbutin, identified as the major active constituents. Documented pharmacological actions justify the herbal use of uva-ursi as a urinary antiseptic. However, clinical information is lacking and further studies are required to determine the true usefulness of uva-ursi in the treatment of urinary tract infections. Although hydroquinone has been reported to be toxic in large amounts, concentrations provided by the ingestion of therapeutic doses of uva-ursi are not thought to represent a risk to human health. Excessive use of uva-ursi and use during pregnancy and lactation should be avoided.

Species (Family)

Arctostaphylos uva-ursi (L.) Spreng. (Ericaceae)

Synonym(s)

Bearberry

Part(s) Used

Leaf

Pharmacopoeial and Other Monographs

BHC 1992[(G6)]
BHP 1996[(G9)]
BP 2007[(G84)]
Complete German Commission E[(G3)]
ESCOP 2003[(G76)]
Martindale 35th edition[(G85)]
Ph Eur 2007[(G81)]

Legal Category (Licensed Products)

GSL[(G37)]

Constituents

The following is compiled from several sources, including General References G2 and G6.

Flavonoids Flavonols (e.g. myricetin, quercetin) and their glycosides including hyperin, isoquercitrin, myricitrin and quercitrin.

Iridoids Asperuloside (disputed), monotropein.[(1)]

Quinones Total content at least 6%, mainly arbutin (5–15%) and methyl-arbutin (glycosides), with lesser amounts of piceoside[(2)] (a glycoside), free hydroquinone and free *p*-methoxyphenol.[(3)]

Tannins 6–7% (range 6–40%). Hydrolysable-type (e.g. corilagin pyranoside); ellagic and gallic acids (usually associated with hydrolysable tannins).

Quinones

	R
arbutin	H
methylarbutin	CH_3
piceoside	$COCH_3$

Figure 1 Selected constituents of uva-ursi.

Terpenoids α-Amyrin, α-amyrin acetate, β-amyrin, lupeol, uvaol, ursolic acid, and a mixture of mono- and di-ketonic α-amyrin derivatives.[(4, 5)]

Other constituents Acids (malic, quinic), allantoin, resin (e.g. ursone), volatile oil (trace) and wax.

Other plant parts The root is reported to contain unedoside (iridoid glucoside).[(6)]

Food Use

Uva-ursi is not used in foods.

Herbal Use

Uva-ursi is stated to possess diuretic, urinary antiseptic, and astringent properties. Traditionally, it has been used for cystitis, urethritis, dysuria, pyelitis, lithuria, and specifically for acute catarrhal cystitis with dysuria and highly acidic urine.[(G2, G6, G7, G8, G64)]

Dosage

Dosages for oral administration (adults) for traditional uses recommended in older and contemporary standard herbal and pharmaceutical reference texts are given below.

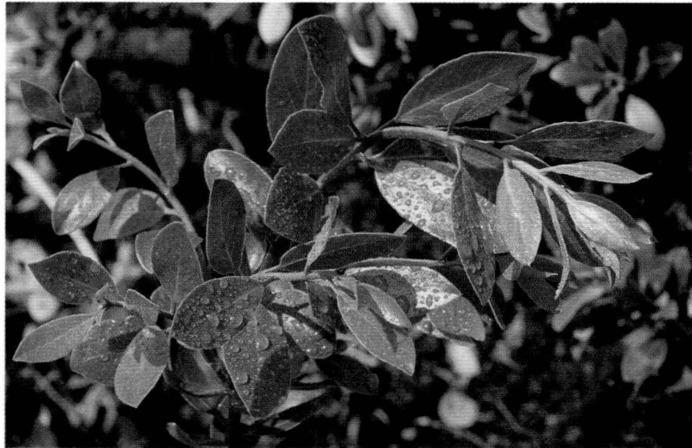

Figure 2 Uva-ursi (*Arctostaphylos uva-ursi*).

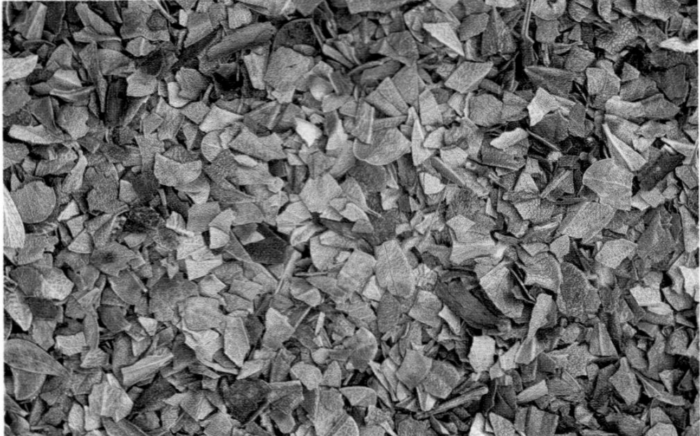

Figure 3 Uva-ursi – dried drug substance (leaf).

Dried leaves 1.5–4.0 g as an infusion three times daily.[G6, G7]

Liquid extract 1.5–4.0 mL (1 : 1 in 25% alcohol) three times daily.[G6, G7]

Concentrated Infusion of Bearberry (BPC 1934) 2–4 mL.

Fresh Infusion of Bearberry (BPC 1934) 15–30 mL.

Pharmacological Actions

In vitro and animal studies

Uva-ursi has exhibited antimicrobial activity towards a variety of organisms including *Staphylococcus aureus*, *Bacillus subtilis*, *Escherichia coli*, *Mycobacterium smegmatis*, *Shigella sonnei* and *Shigella flexneri*.[7] The antimicrobial activity of arbutin towards bacteria implicated in producing urinary tract infections, has been found to be directly dependent on the β-glucosidase activity of the infective organism.[8] Highest enzymatic activity was shown by *Enterobacter*, *Klebsiella* and *Streptococcus* genera, and lowest by *Escherichia coli*.[8] The minimum inhibitory concentration for arbutin is reported to be 0.4–0.8% depending on the micro-organism.[8] Aqueous and methanolic extracts have demonstrated molluscicidal activity against *Biomphalaria glabrata*, at a concentration of 50 ppm.[9] The activity was attributed to the tannin constituents (condensed and hydrolysable).

Anti-inflammatory activity (rat paw oedema tests) has been documented for uva-ursi against a variety of chemical inducers such as carrageenan, histamine and prostaglandins.[10]

Uva-ursi failed to exhibit any *in vitro* uterotonic action when tested on rabbit and guinea-pig uteri.[11]

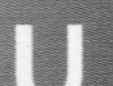

Hydroquinone has been reported to show a concentration-dependent cytotoxic activity on cultured rat hepatoma cells (HTC line); arbutin was not found to inhibit growth of the HTC cells.[12] It was stated that hydroquinone appeared to have greater cytotoxic activity towards rat hepatoma cells than agents like azauridin or colchicine, but less than valtrate from valerian (*Valeriana officinalis*). The cytoxicity of hydroquinone has also been tested on L1210, CA-755 and S-180 tumour systems.[12]

Clinical studies

Clinical research assessing the effects of uva-ursi is limited and rigorous randomised clinical trials are required.

A herbal preparation, whose ingredients included uva-ursi, hops and peppermint, has been used to treat patients suffering from compulsive strangury, enuresis and painful micturition.[13] Of 915 patients treated for six weeks, success was reported in about 70%. The design of this study, however, does not allow the observed effects to be attributed to uva-ursi.

The antiseptic and diuretic properties claimed for uva-ursi can be attributed to the hydroquinone derivatives, especially arbutin. The latter is absorbed from the gastrointestinal tract virtually unchanged and during renal excretion is hydrolysed to yield the active principle, hydroquinone, which exerts an antiseptic and astringent action on the urinary mucous membranes.[14, 15] The crude extract is reported to be more effective than isolated arbutin as an astringent and antiseptic.[G48] This may be due to the other hydroquinone derivatives, in addition to arbutin, that are present in the crude extract and which will also yield hydroquinone. Furthermore, it has been stated that the presence of gallic acid in the crude extract may prevent β-glucosidase cleavage of arbutin in the gastrointestinal tract before absorption, thereby increasing the amount of hydroquinone released during renal excretion.[G48]

Side-effects, Toxicity

Clinical data

There is a lack of clinical safety and toxicity data for uva-ursi and further investigation of these aspects is required.

Hydroquinone is reported to be toxic if ingested in large quantities: 1 g (equivalent to 6–20 g plant material) has caused tinnitus, nausea and vomiting, sense of suffocation, shortness of breath, cyanosis, convulsions, delirium and collapse.[G48] A dose of 5 g (equivalent to 30–100 g of plant material) has proved fatal.[G48] In view of the high tannin content, prolonged use of uva-ursi may cause chronic liver impairment.[G41]

Preclinical data

Cytotoxic activity has been documented for hydroquinone (*see* Pharmacological Actions, *In vitro* and animal studies).

Uva-ursi herb can sometimes be adulterated with box leaves (*Buxus sempervirens*), which contain toxic steroidal alkaloids. However, no cases of poisoning as a result of such adulteration have been reported.[G33]

Contra-indications, Warnings

Uva-ursi requires an alkaline urine for it to be effective as a urinary antiseptic; an alkaline reaction is needed to yield hydroquinone from the inactive esters such as arbutin.[14] Patients have been advised to avoid eating highly acidic foods, such as acidic fruits and their juices.[14] The presence of hydroquinone may impart a greenish-brown colour to the urine, which darkens following exposure to air due to oxidation of hydroquinone.

Excessive use of uva-ursi should be avoided in view of the high tannin content and potential toxicity of hydroquinone.

Prolonged use of uva-ursi to treat a urinary tract infection is not advisable. Patients in whom symptoms persist for longer than 48 hours should consult their doctor.

Drug interactions None documented. However, the potential for preparations of uva-ursi to interact with other medicines administered concurrently, particularly those with similar or opposing effects, should be considered.

Pregnancy and lactation Large doses of uva-ursi are reported to be oxytocic,[G22] although *in vitro* studies have reported a lack of utero-activity. In view of the potential toxicity of hydroquinone, the use of uva-ursi during pregnancy and lactation should be avoided.

Preparations

Proprietary single-ingredient preparations

Czech Republic: List Medvedice Lecive; Medvedice. *Germany:* Cystinol Akut; Uvalysat. *Mexico:* Uvavid.

Proprietary multi-ingredient preparations

Argentina: Ajolip; KLB6 Fruit Diet. *Australia:* Althaea Complex; Bioglan Cranbiotic Super; Cranberry Complex; Cranberry Complex; De Witts New Pills; Extralife Fluid-Care; Extralife PMS-Care; Extralife Uri-Care; Fluid Loss; Herbal Diuretic Formula; Medinat PMT-Eze; Profluid; Protemp; Urinase; Uva-Ursi Complex; Uva-Ursi Plus. *Austria:* Uropurat. *Brazil:* Composto Anticelulitico; Emagrevit; Lisian; Pilulas De Witt's. *Canada:* Herbal Diuretic. *Czech Republic:* Blasen- und Nierentee; Species Urologicae Planta; Urcyston Planta; Urologicka Cajova Smes. *France:* Mediflor Tisane Antirhumatismale No 2; Mediflor Tisane No 4 Diuretique; Uromil; Urophytum. *Germany:* Arctuvan; Cystinol; Harntee STADA. *Israel:* Jungborn. *Mexico:* Noxivid. *New Zealand:* De Witts Pills. *Portugal:* Asic; Rilastil Dermo Solar. *Russia:* Herbion Urological Drops (Гербион Урологические Капли). *Spain:* Genurat; Urisor. *Switzerland:* Demonatur Dragees pour les reins et la vessie; Dragees S pour les reins et la vessie; Strath Gouttes pour les reins et la vessie; Tisane pour les reins et la vessie; Urinex. *UK:* Antitis; Aqua Ban Herbal; Backache Relief; Backache; Backache; Buchu Backache Compound Tablets; Cascade; De Witt's K & B Pills; Diuretabs; Fenneherb Cystaid; Fenneherb Prementaid; HealthAid Boldo-Plus; HRI Water Balance; Kas-Bah; Modern Herbals Water Retention; Napiers Uva Ursi Tea; Prementaid; Sciargo; Sciatica Tablets; Tabritis; Tabritis Tablets; Uvacin; Watershed. *USA:* CitriMax Plus.

References

1 Jahodár L *et al.* Investigation of iridoid substances in *Arctostaphylos uva-ursi. Pharmazie* 1978; 33: 536–537.
2 Karikas GA *et al.* Isolation of piceoside from *Arctostaphylos uva-ursi. Planta Med* 1987; 53: 307–308.
3 Jahodár L, Leifertová I. The evaluation of *p*-methoxyphenol in the leaves of *Arctostaphylos uva-ursi. Pharmazie* 1979; 34: 188–189.
4 Droliac A. Triterpenes of *Arctostaphylos uva-ursi* Spreng. *Plant Méd Phytothér* 1980; 14: 155–158.
5 Malterud KE. The non-polar components of *Arctostaphylos uva-ursi* leaves. *Medd Nor Farm Selsk* 1980; 42: 15–20.
6 Jahodár L *et al.* Unedoside in *Arctostaphylos uva-ursi* roots. *Pharmazie* 1981; 36: 294–296.
7 Moskalenko SA. Preliminary screening of far-Eastern ethnomedicinal plants for antibacterial activity. *J Ethnopharmacol* 1986; 15: 231–259.
8 Jahodár L *et al.* Antimicrobial action of arbutin and the extract from the leaves of *Arctostaphylos uva-ursi in vitro. Ceskoslov Farm* 1985; 34: 174–178.
9 Schaufelberger D, Hostettmann K. On the molluscicidal activity of tannin containing plants. *Planta Med* 1983; 48: 105–107.
10 Shipochliev T, Fournadjiev G. Spectrum of the antiinflammatory effect of *Arctostaphylos uva ursi* and *Achillea millefolium*, L. *Probl Vutr Med* 1984; 12: 99–107.
11 Shipochliev T. Extracts from a group of medicinal plants enhancing the uterine tonus. *Vet Med Nauki* 1981; 18: 94–98.
12 Assaf MH *et al.* Preliminary study of the phenolic glycosides from *Origanum majorana*; quantitative estimation of arbutin; cytotoxic activity of hydroquinone. *Planta Med* 1987; 53: 343–345.
13 Lenau H *et al.* Wirksamkeit und Verträglichkeit von Cysto Fink bei Patienten mit Reizblase und/oder Harninkontinenz. *Therapiewoche* 1984; 34: 6054–6059.
14 Frohne D. Untersuchungen zur Frage der Harndesinfizierenden Wirkungen von Bärentraubenblatt-Extrakten. *Planta Med* 1970; 18: 23–25.
15 Natural drugs with glycosides. In: Stahl E, ed. *Drug Analysis in Chromatography and Microscopy.* Ann Arbor: Ann Arbor Scientific Publishers, 1973: 97.

Valerian

Summary and Pharmaceutical Comment

The traditional use of valerian as a mild sedative and hypnotic is supported by evidence from preclinical and some clinical studies. Clinical trials, however, have been heterogeneous in their design, outcomes, and products assessed, such that the evidence for the hypnotic and sedative effects of valerian root is inconclusive when considered collectively or for individual preparations. The chemistry of valerian root is well-documented. The sedative activity of valerian has been attributed to both the volatile oil and iridoid valepotriate fractions, but it is still unclear whether other constituents in valerian represent the active components. The valepotriate compounds are highly unstable and, therefore, are unlikely to be present in significant concentrations in finished products and probably degrade when taken orally. In view of this, the clinical significance of both the sedative and cytotoxic/mutagenic activities of valepotriates documented *in vitro* is unclear.

There are only limited data on safety aspects of valerian preparations from clinical trials. Randomised, placebo-controlled trials involving healthy volunteers or patients with diagnosed insomnia indicate that adverse events with valerian are mild and transient. Post-marketing surveillance-type studies are required to establish the safety of valerian preparations, particularly with long-term use. Some studies suggest that valerian may have a more favourable tolerability profile than certain benzodiazepines, particularly in view of its apparent lack of 'hangover' effects, although this requires further investigation.

Intake of valerian preparations immediately (up to two hours) before driving or operating machinery is not recommended. Excessive consumption of alcohol whilst receiving treatment with valerian root preparations should be avoided. Patients should seek medical advice if symptoms worsen beyond two weeks' continuous treatment with valerian. Patients with known sensitivity to valerian should not use valerian root preparations. The potential for preparations of valerian to interfere with other medicines administered concurrently, particularly those with similar (such as barbiturates and other sedatives) or opposing effects, should be considered.

There are isolated reports of adverse effects, mainly hepatotoxic reactions, associated with the use of single-ingredient and combination valerian-containing products. However, causal relationships for these reports could not be established as other factors could have been responsible for the observed effects.

Species (Family)

Valeriana officinalis L. (Valerianaceae)

Synonym(s)

All-Heal, Belgian Valerian, Common Valerian, Fragrant Valerian, Garden Valerian

Part(s) Used

Rhizome, root

Pharmacopoeial and Other Monographs

American Herbal Pharmacopoeia[1, G1]
BHC 1992[G6]
BHP 1996[G9]
BHMA 2003[G66]
BP 2007[G84]
Complete German Commission E[G3]
EMEA HMPC Community Herbal Monograph[G80]
ESCOP 2003[G76]
Martindale 35th edition[G85]
Ph Eur 2007[G81]
USP29/NF24[G86]
WHO volume 1 1999[G63]

Legal Category (Licensed Products)

GSL[G37]

Constituents

See also References 1–5.

Alkaloids Pyridine type. Actinidine, chatinine, skyanthine, valerianine and valerine.

Iridoids (valepotriates) Valtrates (e.g. valtrate, valtrate isovaleroxyhydrin, acevaltrate, valechlorine), didrovaltrates (e.g. didrovaltrate, homodidrovaltrate, deoxydidrovaltrate, homodeoxydidrovaltrate, isovaleroxyhydroxydidrovaltrate) and isovaltrates (e.g. isovaltrate, 7-epideacetylisovaltrate). Valtrate and didrovaltrate are documented as the major components. Valerosidate (iridoid glucoside).[6] The valepotriates are unstable and decompose on storage or processing; the main degradation products are baldrinal and homobaldrinal. The baldrinals may react further and are unlikely to be present in finished products.

Steroids β-sitosterol, clionasterol 3-β-*O*-glucoside and a mixture of 6′-*O*-acyl-β-D-glucosyl clionasterols where the acyl moieties are hexadecanoyl (major), 8*E*,11*E*-octadecadienoyl and 14-methylpentadecanoyl.[7]

Volatile oils 0.5–2%. Numerous identified components include monoterpenes (e.g. α- and β-pinene, camphene, borneol, eugenol, isoeugenol) present mainly as esters, sesquiterpenes (e.g. β-bisabolene, caryophyllene, valeranone, ledol, pacifigorgiol, patchouli alcohol, valerianol, valerenol and a series of valerenyl esters, valerenal, valerenic acid with acetoxy and hydroxy derivatives).[8–11]

Other constituents Amino acids (e.g. arginine, γ-aminobutyric acid (GABA), glutamine, tyrosine),[1, 12] caffeic and chlorogenic acids (polyphenolic), methyl 2-pyrrolketone, choline, tannins (type unspecified), gum and resin.

Monoterpenes

$OCOCH_3$

bornyl acetate

Iridoids

CH_2OR^3, R^2O, H, OR^1

	R^1	R^2	R^3
valtrate	isovaleryl	isovaleryl	acetyl
isovaltrate	isovaleryl	acetyl	isovaleryl
acevaltrate	isovaleryl	β-acetoxyvaleryl	acetyl

CH_2OR^3, R^4, R^2O, H, OR^1

	R^1	R^2	R^3	R^4
didrovaltrate	isovaleryl	acetyl	isovaleryl	H
isovaleryloxy-hydroxydidro-valtrate	isovaleryl	acetyl	2-(isovaleryl -oxy)-isovaleryl	OH

(isovaleryl = $(CH_3)_2$ CH = CH_2CO–)

CH_2OCOCH_3, CHO

baldrinal

Sesquiterpenes

R^2, H, R^1

	R^1	R^2
valerenal	CHO	H
valerenic acid	COOH	H
acetoxyvalerenic acid	COOH	$OCOCH_3$

Figure 1 Selected constituents of valerian.

Quality of plant material and commercial products

According to the British and European Pharmacopoeias, valerian consists of the dried underground parts of *V. officinalis* L., including the rhizome surrounded by the roots and stolons.(G81, G84) It contains not less than 5 mL/kg of essential oil for the whole drug and not less than 3 mL/kg for the cut drug, both calculated with reference to the dried drug, and not less than 0.17% of sesquiterpenic acids expressed as valerenic acid, calculated with reference to the dried drug.(G81) As with other plants, there can be variation in the content of active compounds (e.g. valerenic acid derivatives and valepotriates) found in valerian rhizomes and roots.(13) Detailed descriptions of *V. officinalis* root for use in botanical, microscopic and macroscopic identification have been published, along with qualitative and quantitative methods for the assessment of *V. officinalis* root raw material.(1, G1)

Food Use

Valerian is not generally used as a food. Valerian is listed by the Council of Europe as a natural source of food flavouring (root: category 5) (*see* Appendix 3, Table 1).(G17) Previously, valerian has been listed as GRAS (Generally Recognised As Safe).

Herbal Use

Valerian is stated to possess sedative, mild anodyne, hypnotic, antispasmodic, carminative and hypotensive properties. Traditionally, it has been used for hysterical states, excitability, insomnia, hypochondriasis, migraine, cramp, intestinal colic, rheumatic pains, dysmenorrhoea, and specifically for conditions presenting nervous excitability.(G2, G6, G7, G8, G32, G64) Modern interest in valerian is focused on its use as a sedative and hypnotic.

A Community Herbal Monograph adopted by the European Medicines Agency's Committee on Herbal Medicinal Products states the following therapeutic indications for valerian root:

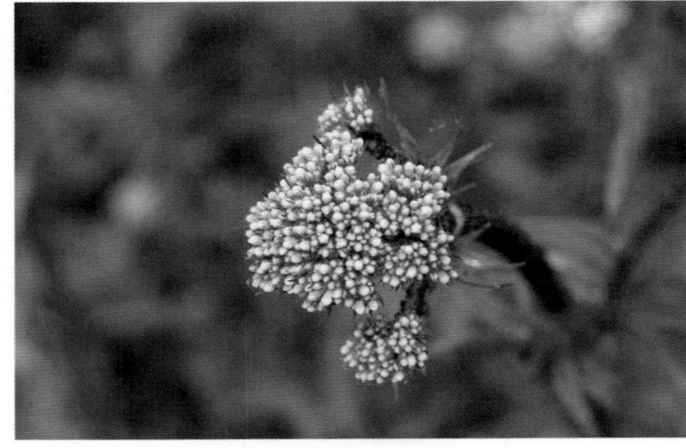

Figure 2 Valerian (*Valeriana officinalis*).

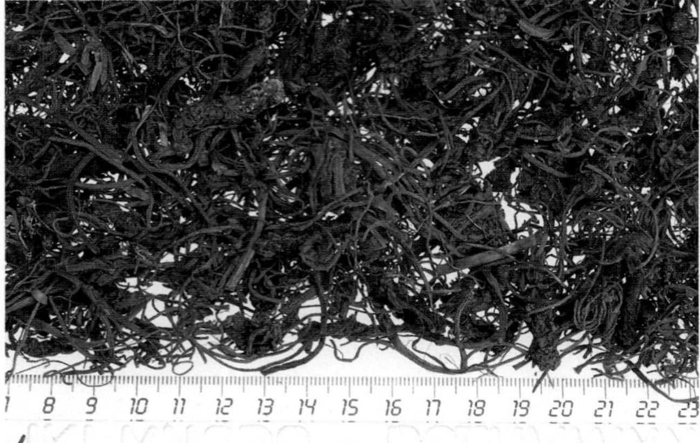

Figure 3 Valerian – dried drug substance (rhizome).

traditional use, for support of mental relaxation and to aid natural sleep; well-established use, for the relief of mild nervous tension and difficulty in falling asleep.[G80]

Dosage

Dosages for oral administration (adults) for traditional uses recommended in standard herbal reference texts are given below.

Dried rhizome/root 1–3 g as an infusion or decoction up to three times daily.[G6]

Tincture 3–5 mL (1 : 5; 70% ethanol) up to three times daily;[G6, G50] 1–3 mL, once to several times daily.[G3]

Extracts Amount equivalent to 2–3 g drug, once to several times daily;[G3] 2–6 mL of 1 : 2 liquid extract daily.[G50]

Doses given in older texts vary. For example: Valerian Liquid Extract (BPC 1963) 0.3–1.0 mL; Simple Tincture of Valerian (BPC 1949) 4–8 mL; Concentrated Valerian Infusion (BPC 1963) 2–4 mL.

Clinical trials investigating the effects of valerian root extracts on sleep parameters have used varying dosages, for example, valerian extract 400 mg/day (drug to extract ratio of 3 : 1)[14] and 1215 mg/day (drug to extract ratio of 5 to 6 : 1).[15]

Pharmacological Actions

Sedative and hypnotic properties have been described for certain valerian rhizome/root preparations following preclinical and clinical studies. However, the available scientific evidence is strong; also it remains unclear precisely which of the constituents of valerian are responsible for the observed sedative and hypnotic properties.[5] Attention had focused on the volatile oil, and then the valepotriates and their degradation products, as the constituents responsible. However, it appeared that the effects of the volatile oil could not account for the whole action of the drug, and the valepotriates, which degrade rapidly, are unlikely to be present in finished products in significant concentrations. Current thinking is that the overall effect of valerian is due to several different groups of constituents and their varying mechanisms of action. Therefore, the activity of different valerian preparations will depend on their content and concentrations of several types of constituent.[4] One mechanism of action is likely to involve increased concentrations of the inhibitory transmitter GABA in the brain. Increased concentrations of GABA are associated with a decrease in CNS activity and this action may, therefore, be involved in the reported sedative activity.

In vitro and animal studies

Sedative properties have been documented for valerian and have been attributed to both the volatile oil and valepotriate fractions.[16, 17] Screening of the volatile oil components for sedative activity concluded valerenal and valerenic acid to be the most active compounds, causing ataxia in mice at a dose of 50 mg/kg by intraperitoneal injection.[16] Further studies in mice described valerenic acid as a general CNS depressant similar to pentobarbitone, requiring high doses (100 mg/kg by intraperitoneal injection) for activity.[18] A dose of 400 mg/kg resulted in muscle spasms, convulsions and death.[18] Valerenic acid was also reported to prolong pentobarbitone-induced sleep in mice, resulting in a hangover effect. Biochemical studies have documented that valerenic acid inhibits the enzyme system responsible for the central catabolism of GABA.[19] An aqueous extract of roots and rhizomes of *V. officinalis* (standardised to 55 mg valerenic acids per 100 g extract) inhibited the uptake and stimulated the release of radiolabelled GABA in isolated synaptosomes from rat brain cortex.[20, 21] Further work suggested that this aqueous extract of valerian induces the release of GABA by reversal of the GABA carrier, and that the mechanism is Na^+ dependent and Ca^{2+} independent.[21] The extract contained a high concentration of GABA (about 5 mmol/L) which was shown to be sufficient to induce the release of radiolabelled GABA by this type of mechanism.[22] Aqueous and hydroalcoholic (ethanol) extracts of valerian root displaced radiolabelled muscimol binding to synaptic membranes (a measure of the influence of drugs on $GABA_A$ receptors). However, valerenic acid (0.1 mmol/L) did not displace radiolabelled muscimol in this model.[23] Other *in vitro* studies using rat brain tissue have shown that hydroalcoholic and aqueous total extracts of *V. officinalis* root, and an aqueous fraction derived from the hydroalcoholic extract, show affinity for $GABA_A$ receptors, although far lower than that of the neurotransmitter itself.[24] However, a lipophilic fraction of the hydroalcoholic extract, hydroxyvalerenic acid and dihydrovaltrate did not show any affinity for the $GABA_A$ receptor in this model.

The effects of valerian extracts on benzodiazepine binding to rat cortical membranes have also been explored. Very low concentrations of ethanolic extract of *V. officinalis* had no effect on radiolabelled flunitrazepam binding in this model, although concentrations of 10^{-10} to 10^{-8} mg/mL increased radiolabelled flunitrazepam binding with an EC_{50} of 4.13×10^{-10} mg/mL.[25] However, flunitrazepam binding was inhibited at higher concentrations (0.5–7.0 mg/mL) of valerian extract (IC_{50} 4.82×10^{-1} mg/mL). In other investigations, valerian extract potentiated radiolabelled GABA release from rat hippocampal slices, and inhibited synaptosomal GABA uptake, confirming the effects of valerian extract on $GABA_A$ receptors.[25]

Radiolabelled ligand binding studies have also shown that constituents of dichloromethane and petroleum ether extracts of valerian have strong binding affinities for $5\text{-}HT_{5a}$ receptors but only weak binding affinities for $5\text{-}HT_{5b}$ receptors.[26] At concentrations of 50 μg/mL, the petroleum ether and dichloromethane extracts inhibited binding of radiolabelled lysergic acid diethylamide to $5\text{-}HT_{5a}$ receptors by 86% and 51%, respectively. Generation of an IC_{50} curve for the petroleum ether extract produced a biphasic curve. Valerenic acid, a constituent of both extracts, had an IC_{50} of 17.2 μmol/L. In other radiolabelled ligand binding experiments, a 45% methanol extract of valerian root (drug to extract ratio 4–6 : 1; containing valerenic acids 0.388%, and no valepotriates) had an IC_{50} value of 450 µg/mL at melatonin-1 (ML) receptors obtained from chicken brain, whereas a 45% methanol extract of hops' cones (containing flavonoids 0.479%, calculated as rutin) had an IC_{50} value of 71 µg/mL at these receptors. A preparation (ZE-91019) containing both extracts had an IC_{50} value of 97 µg/mL, suggesting a synergistic action between the two extracts at ML1 receptors.[27]

CNS-depressant activities in mice following intraperitoneal injection have been documented for the valepotriates and for their degradation products, although activity was found to be greatly reduced following oral administration.[28] A study explored the effects of a mixture of valepotriates on the behaviour of diazepam-withdrawn male Wistar rats in the elevated plus-maze test (a measure of the anxiolytic or anxiogenic properties of drugs).[29] Rats were given diazepam (up to 5 mg/kg for 28 days) then vehicle only for three days to induce a withdrawal syndrome. Rats given diazepam or a mixture of valepotriates (stated to contain dihydrovaltrate 80%, valtrate 15% and acevaltrate 5%) administered intraperitoneally (12 mg/kg) spent a significantly greater proportion of time in the 'open' arms of the maze than did those in the control group.

Another specific valepotriate fraction, Vpt_2, has been documented to exhibit tranquillising, central myorelaxant, anticonvulsant, coronary-artery dilating and anti-arrhythmic actions in mice, rabbits, and cats.[30,31] The fraction was reported to prevent arrhythmias induced by Pituitrin vasopressin and barium chloride, and to exhibit moderate positive inotropic and negative chronotropic effects.

Antispasmodic activity on intact and isolated guinea-pig ileum has been documented for isovaltrate, valtrate and valeranone.[32] This activity was attributed to a direct action on the smooth muscle receptors rather than ganglion receptors. Valerian oil has been reported to exhibit antispasmodic activity on isolated guinea-pig uterine muscle,[33] but proved inactive when tested *in vivo*.[34]

In-vitro inactivation of complement activation has been reported for the valepotriates.[35]

In-vitro cytotoxicity (inhibition of DNA and protein synthesis, and potent alkylating activity) has been documented for the valepotriates, with valtrate stated to be the most toxic compound.[36] Valepotriates (valtrate and didrovaltrate) isolated from the related species *Valeriana wallichii*, and baldrinal (a degradation product of valtrate) have been tested for their cytotoxic activity *in vitro* using cultured rat hepatoma cells. Valtrate was the most active compound in this system, leading to a 100% mortality of hepatoma cells after 24 hours' incubation at a concentration of 33 µg/mL.[37] More detailed studies using the same system showed that didrovaltrate demonstrated cytotoxic activity when incubated at concentrations higher than 8 µg/mL of culture (1.5×10^{-5} mol/L) and led to 100% cellular mortality with 24 hours of incubation at a concentration of 66 µg/mL. The cytotoxic effect of didrovaltrate was irreversible within two hours of incubation with hepatoma cells. In mice, administration of intraperitoneal didrovaltrate led to a regression of Krebs II ascitic tumours, compared with control.[37] A subsequent *in vivo* study, in which valtrate was administered to mice (by intraperitoneal injection and by mouth), did not report any toxic effects on haematopoietic precursor cells when compared with control groups.[38] The valepotriates are known to be unstable compounds in both acidic and alkaline media and it has been suggested that their *in vivo* toxicity is limited due to poor absorption and/or distribution.[2] Baldrinal and homobaldrinal, decomposition products of valtrate and isovaltrate respectively, have exhibited direct mutagenic activity against various *Salmonella* strains *in vitro*.[39]

Clinical studies

Pharmacokinetics There are only limited data on the pharmacokinetics of valerian preparations and their constituent compounds. The pharmacokinetics of valerenic acid were explored in a single-dose study involving six healthy adults who received a 70% ethanol extract of valerian root (LI-156, Sedonium, Lichtwer Pharma; drug to extract ratio 5 : 1) 600 mg in the morning. For five participants, maximum serum concentrations of valerenic acid occurred between one and two hours after valerian administration and ranged from 0.9 to 2.3 ng/mL; valerenic acid concentrations were measurable for at least five hours after valerian administration.[40] For one subject, maximum concentrations occurred at both one and five hours after valerian administration. The mean (standard deviation (SD)) elimination half-life ($t_{1/2}$) for valerenic acid was 1.1 (0.6) hours and the mean (SD) area under the plasma concentration time curve was 4.80 (2.96) µg/mL/hour. Further investigation of the pharmacokinetics of valerian is required, including those of different manufacturers' preparations and their constituents.

Sleep disorders, hypnotic activity Numerous studies have explored the effects of valerian preparations on subjective (e.g. participants' self-assessment of sleep quality) and/or objective (e.g. sleep structure, such as duration of rapid eye movement (REM) sleep or slow-wave sleep) sleep parameters. Collectively, the findings of these studies are difficult to interpret, as different studies have assessed different valerian preparations and different dosages, and some have involved healthy volunteers whereas others have involved patients with diagnosed sleep disorders. In addition, other studies have used different subjective and/or objective outcome measures, and some have been conducted in sleep laboratories, whereas others have assessed participants receiving valerian whilst sleeping at home. Overall, several, but not all, studies have documented a hypnotic effect for valerian preparations with regard to subjective measures of sleep quality, and some have documented effects on objective measures of sleep structure. There is a view that investigating subjective measures of sleep quality may be the most appropriate or relevant form of assessment.[41] Several trials, including the most recent studies, particularly those involving individuals with sleep disorders rather than healthy volunteers, are summarised below.

A randomised, double-blind, placebo-controlled, crossover study involving 16 patients with previously established psychophysiological insomnia according to International Classification of Sleep Disorders (ICSD) criteria and confirmed by polysomnography assessed the effects of single-dose and longer-term administration of valerian root extract on objective parameters of sleep structure and subjective parameters of sleep quality.[42] Participants received a 70% ethanol extract of valerian root (LI-156; drug to extract ratio 5 : 1) 600 mg, or placebo, one hour before bedtime for 14 days, followed by a wash-out period of 13 days before crossing over to the other arm of the study. There were no statistically significant effects on objective and subjective parameters of sleep following single-dose valerian administration. Similarly, after long-term treatment, there were no statistically significant differences between groups in sleep efficiency (ratio of time spent asleep to time spent in bed). There was a statistically significant difference with valerian on parameters of slow-wave sleep, compared with baseline values, which did not occur with placebo. However, it is not clear if this difference was significantly different for valerian, compared with placebo, as no *p*-value was given.

The effects of repeated doses of the same valerian root extract (LI-156) were assessed in a randomised, double-blind, placebo-controlled, parallel-group trial involving 121 patients with insomnia not due to organic causes.[43] Participants received valerian extract 600 mg, or placebo, one hour before bedtime for 28 days. At the end of the study, clinical global impression scores were significantly higher for the valerian group than for the placebo group.

A crossover study assessing the same valerian root extract (LI-156) involved 16 individuals aged 50 to 64 years with mild sleep complaints (e.g. difficulty initiating or maintaining sleep, early morning awakenings) who received a single 300 mg or 600 mg dose of the extract, or placebo, at 10 pm on one occasion, with a 6-day wash-out period before crossing over to each of the other arms of the study.[44] Participants underwent a battery of tests designed to assess objective and subjective measures of sleep at 7.05 am on the morning after each treatment intervention. There were no statistically significant differences between the three groups for any of the outcome variables measured ($p > 0.05$).

In a randomised, double-blind, pilot study, 14 older women who were poor sleepers received valerian aqueous extract (Valdispert forte; drug to extract ratio 5–6 : 1), or placebo ($n = 6$), for eight consecutive days.[15] Valerian 405 mg was administered one hour before sleep for one night in the laboratory, then taken three times daily for the following seven days. Valerian recipients showed an increase in slow-wave sleep, compared with baseline values. However, valerian had no effect on sleep onset time, rapid eye movement (REM) sleep or on self-rated sleep quality, when compared with placebo. In another randomised, double-blind, placebo-controlled study involving older participants, 78 hospitalised patients with various chronic conditions in addition to difficulty sleeping received an aqueous valerian root extract (Baldrian Dispert) 270 mg daily, or placebo, for 14 days.[45] At the end of the study, sleep latency and sleep duration were significantly improved in the valerian group, compared with the placebo group ($p < 0.001$ for both).

A randomised, double-blind, placebo-controlled study involving 128 volunteers explored the effects of an aqueous extract of valerian root (400 mg) and a proprietary preparation of valerian and hops (Hova) on subjective measures of sleep quality. Each participant took each of the three preparations at night for three non-consecutive nights.[14] On the basis of participants' self-assessment, valerian significantly reduced sleep latency (time to onset of sleep) and improved sleep quality, compared with placebo ($p < 0.05$). Subgroup analysis suggested that the effects of valerian were most marked among participants who described themselves as 'poor' or 'irregular' sleepers.[14] It was reported that the valerian–hops preparation did not significantly affect sleep latency or sleep quality, compared with placebo, only that the valerian–hops preparation administration was associated with an increase in the number of reports of 'feeling more sleepy than usual the next morning' (i.e. a 'hangover' effect). The authors were unable to explain this discrepancy in the results for the two preparations.

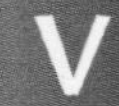

In a subsequent study, eight individuals with mild insomnia each received aqueous valerian root extract 450 mg, 900 mg or placebo, in a random-order experimental design over almost three weeks.[46] The time to the first period of five consecutive minutes without movement, measured using wrist-worn activity meters, was used as an objective measure of sleep latency. For this parameter, valerian 450 mg significantly reduced the mean sleep latency, compared with placebo, although there was no further reduction in sleep latency with valerian 900 mg. Subjective assessments indicated that participants were more likely to experience a 'hangover' effect with valerian 900 mg.[46]

The effects of a valerian root/rhizome extract (tablets containing 225 mg extract equivalent to 1000 mg crude drug, standardised for total valerenic acids 2.94 mg, valerenal 0.46 mg and valtrates 1.23 mg; Mediherb, Australia) two tablets at night half an hour before going to bed on self-assessed sleep parameters were assessed in a series of randomised, double-blind, placebo-controlled, '*n*-of-1' crossover trials involving 24 patients with chronic insomnia diagnosed by a general practitioner. The trials were conducted in a general practice setting and involved three pairs of one-week treatments with valerian extract and placebo (i. e. each *n*-of-1 trial lasted for six weeks).[47] Statistical analyses found that participants did not show any response to valerian for any of the outcome measures either individually or when individual results were pooled. *N*-of-1 trials have recognised limitations, including some which can increase the possibility of false negative results, although these were taken into consideration during the analysis of these data. Investigation of dosage regimens involving higher doses of this extract administered for longer periods may be warranted.[47]

In a randomised, double-blind, placebo-controlled trial conducted entirely over the Internet, 391 adults who scored at least 40 points on the State-Trait Anxiety Inventory (STAI) scale and who reported having sleeping problems on at least two occasions received two capsules containing valerian extract (each containing valerenic acids 3.2 mg; no further details of preparation provided) one hour before bedtime, capsules containing kava extract (each containing total kavalactones 100 mg) one three times daily, or placebo, for 28 days.[48] At the end of the study, there were no statistically significant differences between valerian and placebo with respect to the primary outcome measure changes from baseline in Insomnia Severity Index scores. The study also assessed effects on anxiety (*see* Anxiety, depression and other conditions).

The effects of preparations of valerian root extract have been compared with those of certain benzodiazepines. In a randomised, double-blind trial, 75 individuals with non-organic and non-psychiatric insomnia received valerian root extract (drug to extract ratio 5 : 1) 600 mg or oxazepam 10 mg; both treatments were taken 30 minutes before going to bed for 28 days.[49] At the end of the treatment period, sleep quality had improved significantly ($p < 0.001$) in both groups, compared with baseline values, and there was no statistically significant difference between the two groups ($p = 0.70$). The effects of a combination valerian preparation were compared with those of bromazepam in a three-week, randomised, double-blind trial involving patients with 'environmental' sleep disorders (temporary dyscoimesis and dysphylaxia) according to Diagnostic and Statistical Manual (DSM)-IV criteria.[50] The combination preparation, containing valerian 200 mg and hops extract 45.5 mg, was reported to be equivalent to bromazepam 3 mg with regard to sleep quality. These findings require confirmation in rigorous studies designed specifically to test for equivalence.

Several of the studies summarised above[14, 15, 43, 45, 46] were included in a systematic review of nine randomised, double-blind, placebo-controlled trials of monopreparations of valerian.[51] All trials included in the review had different designs and assessed the effects of different valerian preparations administered according to different dosage regimens, so the validity of considering their results collectively is questionnable. The review concluded that the evidence for valerian as a treatment for insomnia is inconclusive and that there is a need for further rigorous trials.

Several other studies have assessed the effects of valerian extract in combination with other herb extracts, such as hops (*Humulus lupulus*) and/or melissa (*Melissa officinalis*), on measures of sleep.[52–56]

In a randomised, double-blind, placebo-controlled, parallel-group trial, 184 adults with mild insomnia received two tablets of a valerian–hops preparation (each tablet containing 187 mg of a 45% methanol extract of valerian, drug to extract ratio 5–8 : 1, and 42 mg of a 45% methanol extract of hops, drug to extract ratio 7–10 : 1; $n = 59$), or placebo ($n = 65$), each night for 28 days; a third study arm received diphenhydramine 50 mg each night for 14 days followed by placebo for 14 days ($n = 60$).[52] At the end of the study, there was no statistically significant difference in sleep latency between the valerian–hops group and the placebo group ($p = 0.08$). There were no statistically significant differences between groups with respect to the sleep continuity variables, as measured by polysomnography, nor in the duration of sleep stages 3 and 4, and REM sleep. The physical component, but not the mental component, of the quality-of-life measure used was significantly improved in the valerian–hops group, compared with the placebo group after 28 days ($p = 0.028$).

A randomised, double-blind trial involving healthy volunteers who received Songha Night (*V. officinalis* root extract 120 mg and *M. officinalis* leaf extract 80 mg) three tablets daily taken as one dose 30 minutes before bedtime for 30 days ($n = 66$), or placebo ($n = 32$), found that the proportion of participants reporting an improvement in sleep quality was significantly greater for the treatment group, compared with the placebo group (33.3% versus 9.4%, respectively; $p = 0.04$).[54] However, analysis of visual analogue scale scores revealed only a slight, but statistically non-significant, improvement in sleep quality in both groups over the treatment period. Another double-blind, placebo-controlled trial involving patients with insomnia who received Euvegal forte tablets (containing valerian extract 160 mg and lemon balm extract 80 mg) two daily for two weeks reported significant improvements in sleep quality in recipients of the herbal preparation, compared with placebo recipients.[55] A placebo-controlled study involving 'poor sleepers' who received Euvegal forte reported significant improvements in sleep efficiency and in sleep stages 3 and 4 in the treatment group, compared with placebo recipients.[56]

In a single-blind, placebo-controlled, crossover study involving 12 healthy volunteers, two different single doses of a combination preparation (ZE-91019) containing extracts of valerian and hops (valerian 500 mg, hops 120 mg; valerian 1500 mg, hops 360 mg) were assessed for their effects on EEG recordings.[57] Some slight effects on the quantitative EEG were documented following administration of the higher dose valerian–hops combination, suggesting effects on the central nervous system. The same preparation (two or six tablets as a single dose; $n = 16$), in addition to caffeine 200 mg, was administered to healthy volunteers in a controlled (caffeine 200 mg plus placebo; $n = 16$) study which aimed to determine the pharmacodynamics of co-administration of the two preparations by measuring EEG responses.[58] EEG recordings at one hour after administration indicated that the lower dose of the valerian–hops preparation reduced caffeine-induced arousal and the higher dose inhibited the caffeine-induced arousal. It was stated that this indicates that the valerian–hops combination preparation acts via a central adenosine mechanism,[58] although which constituents are responsible for this effect is not known.

The effects of a related species, *V. edulis*, on sleep parameters were assessed in a preliminary randomised, double-blind, placebo-controlled, crossover trial involving five male children (7 to 14 years) with intellectual deficits (intelligence quotient < 70).[59] Participants received tablets containing *V. edulis* dried crushed root 500 mg (containing 5.52 mg valtrate/isovaltrate, didrovaltrate and acevaltrate were absent; Mediherb, Australia), or placebo (which contained 25 mg dried *V. edulis* root to achieve blinding for odour), at a dose of 20 mg/kg body weight administered each night at least one hour before bedtime for two weeks following a two-week run-in period. Participants underwent a one-week wash-out period before crossing over to the other arm of the study. Time awake, total sleep time and sleep quality all improved in the valerian group, compared with baseline values ($p < 0.05$ for each), whereas only sleep quality improved in the placebo group, compared with baseline values ($p = 0.04$).[59] However, as no statistical analyses appear to have been conducted to examine any differences between the valerian and placebo groups, these findings raise the hypothesis that dried *V. edulis* root has effects on certain sleep parameters and this requires testing in well-designed clinical trials involving adequate numbers of participants. In a randomised, double-blind, placebo-controlled trial, a preparation of constituents (Valmane, comprising didrovaltrate 80%, valtrate 15% and acevaltrate 5%; Whitehall Pharmaceuticals) obtained from the root of *V. wallichii*, another related species, was assessed for its effects on sleep parameters in 19 individuals who had undergone withdrawal from benzodiazepines.[60] Participants received the valerian preparation at a dose of 100 mg, or placebo, three times daily starting two days after completing benzodiazepine withdrawal and continuing for 15 days. At the end of the study, wake time after sleep onset was significantly reduced in the valerian group compared with the placebo group, whereas sleep latency was significantly improved in the placebo group, compared with the valerian group ($p < 0.05$ for both). The study has methodological limitations, including the small sample size, and these apparently conflicting findings require further investigation in well-designed clinical trials involving adequate numbers of participants.

Anxiety, depression and other conditions The effects of a preparation containing a mixture of valepotriate compounds (stated to contain dihydrovaltrate 80%, valtrate 15%, acevaltrate 5%) were assessed in a randomised, double-blind, placebo-controlled, parallel-group trial involving 36 patients with generalised anxiety disorder diagnosed according to DSM-III-R (Diagnostic and Statistical Manual of Mental Disorders) criteria.[61] Participants received capsules containing the valepotriate mixture 50 mg, diazepam 2.5 mg, or placebo, for four weeks according to a flexible dosing regimen (one to three capsules of the active treatments) depending on the participants' response. At the end of the study, there were no statistically significant differences between the three groups for the primary outcome variable mean total Hamilton Anxiety scale scores ($p > 0.05$) and for State-Trait Anxiety Inventory (STAI) scores. As a sample size calculation was not carried out, and as the study involved only a small sample, it is possible that the trial did not have sufficient statistical power to detect differences (if they exist) between the three groups.

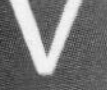

In another randomised, double-blind, placebo-controlled trial, conducted entirely over the Internet, 391 adults who scored at least 40 points on the STAI scale and who reported having sleeping problems on at least two occasions received two capsules containing valerian extract (each containing valerenic acids 3.2 mg; no further details of preparation provided) one hour before bedtime, capsules containing kava extract (each containing total kavalactones 100 mg) one three times daily, or placebo, for 28 days.[48] At the end of the study, there were no statistically significant differences between valerian and placebo with respect to the primary outcome measure changes from baseline in STAI anxiety scores. The study also assessed effects on insomnia (*see* Sleep disorders, hypnotic activity).

The effects of valerian have also been assessed on mental stress in laboratory-based studies involving healthy volunteers. In a randomised controlled trial, 36 participants received valerian root extract (LI-156) 1200 mg ($n = 18$) or kava root extract (LI-150) 120 mg daily for seven days; a third group of participants acted as a no-treatment control group.[62] Participants' heart rate and blood pressure measurements were taken before, during and after a mental stress test at baseline and seven days later following treatment. The results suggested that increases in systolic blood pressure in response to mental stress were lower in the valerian group, compared with those in the control group. These results, however, can only be considered preliminary as the control group did not receive placebo. Further investigation using a randomised, double-blind, placebo-controlled trial design is required.[62]

The effects of another valerian extract at a dose of 100 mg (no further details of preparation given), with or without propranolol 20 mg, on activation and performance under experimental social stress conditions were assessed in a randomised, double-blind, placebo-controlled study involving 48 healthy volunteers.[63] Valerian was reported to have no statistically significant effect on physiological activation and to lead to less intensive subjective feelings of somatic arousal, compared with control.

Several studies have assessed the effects of combinations of valerian and other herbal ingredients in patients with anxiety or depression. In a randomised, double-blind study involving 100 patients with anxiety, a combination of valerian and St John's wort was significantly more effective than diazepam according to a physician's rating scale and a patient's self-rating scale.[64] In a randomised, double-blind trial involving 162 patients with dysthymic disorders, the effects of a valerian and St John's wort combination preparation (Sedariston) were compared with those of amitriptyline 75–150 mg.[65] Another randomised, double-blind trial, involving 100 patients with mild-to-moderate depression compared Sedariston with desipramine 100–150 mg.[66] Pooling the results of these two studies indicated there were 88 (68%) treatment responders in the Sedariston group and 66 (50%) in the group that received standard antidepressants.[67] This difference was not statistically significant. As valerian root is not known for antidepressant effects, it is likely that any antidepressant activity observed in the studies described above is attributable to St John's wort.

Several studies have assessed the effects of valerian, or herbal combination products containing valerian, on performance the morning after treatment (*see* Side-effects, Toxicity).

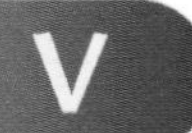

Side-effects, Toxicity

Clinical data

There are only limited clinical data on safety aspects of valerian preparations from clinical trials. Clinical trials have the statistical power to detect only common, acute adverse effects and post-marketing surveillance-type studies are required to establish the safety of valerian preparations, particularly with long-term use.

Few controlled clinical trials of valerian preparations have provided detailed information on safety. Where adverse event data were provided, randomised, placebo-controlled trials involving healthy volunteers or patients with diagnosed insomnia reported that adverse events with valerian were mild and transient, and that the types and frequency of adverse events reported for valerian were similar to those for placebo.[44, 47, 51, 68] One study involving small numbers of patients reported a lower frequency of adverse events with valerian than with placebo; the authors did not suggest an explanation for this.[42] Studies comparing valerian preparations with benzodiazepines have reported that valerian root extract (LI-156) 600 mg daily for 14 days[68] or 28 days[49] had a more favourable adverse effect profile than flunitrazepam 1 mg daily for 14 days[68] and oxazepam 10 mg daily for 28 days,[49] respectively.

There is an isolated report of cardiac complications and delirium associated with valerian root extract withdrawal in a 58-year-old man with a history of coronary artery disease, hypertension and congestive heart failure.[69] The man had been taking valerian root extract (530 mg to 2 g, five times daily), multiple other medications and had undergone surgery, therefore a causal link with valerian could not be made. There have been isolated reports of hepatotoxic reactions following the use of combination products containing valerian, although these products contained other herbal ingredients which could also be implicated.[70, G18, G21] Several other reports document hepatotoxic reactions with single-ingredient valerian products, although it is possible that these were idiosyncratic reactions.[71] There is a lack of data on the safety of the long-term use of valerian.

Cases of individuals who had taken overdoses of valerian or valerian-containing products have been documented. One case involved an 18-year-old female who ingested 40–50 capsules of powdered valerian root 470 mg, approximately 20 times therapeutic doses.[72] The patient presented three hours after ingestion with fatigue, crampy abdominal pain, chest tightness, tremor and lightheadedness. Liver function test values were normal; a urine screen tested positive for tetrahydrocannabinol. The patient was treated with activated charcoal, and symptoms resolved within 24 hours. Several cases ($n = 47$) have been documented of overdose with a combination valerian-containing product ('Sleep-Qik'; valerian dry extract 75 mg, hyoscine hydrobromide 0.25 mg, cyproheptadine hydrochloride 2 mg).[73, 74] Individuals had ingested tablets equivalent to 0.5–12 g valerian extract. Liver function tests were carried out for most patients and yielded results within normal ranges.

Effects on cognitive and psychomotor performance

Studies assessing the effects of valerian preparations on measures of performance report conflicting results: some suggest that there is slight impairment for a few hours following ingestion of single doses of valerian, whereas other studies report no effects on performance following administration. As these studies have assessed the effects of different preparations of valerian, the conflicting results may simply relate to differences in the chemical composition of the products tested. Further research is needed to establish whether or not specific valerian preparations impair performance following ingestion. In contrast, the few studies investigating the potential for impaired performance the morning following treatment (i.e. 'hangover' effects) with valerian preparations have found that such impairment does not occur, at least with the preparations and dosages tested. Several of the studies examining these aspects are summarised below.

In a randomised, double-blind, placebo-controlled, crossover study, nine healthy participants each received a 70% ethanol extract of valerian root (containing valerenic acid 0.25%; drug to extract ratio 4 : 1) 500 mg, 1000 mg, and triazolam 0.25 mg, as a single dose with a one-week wash-out period between treatments. There were no statistically significant differences in the outcomes of cognitive and psychomotor tests performed before and two, four and eight hours after each treatment dose between the valerian and placebo groups.[75] A similar finding was obtained in a randomised, double-blind, placebo-controlled, crossover study involving ten healthy participants who underwent assessments of mood and psychomotor performance before and after receiving a valerian root extract (LI-156) at doses of 600, 1200 and 1800 mg, and diazepam 10 mg, with a one-week wash-out period between treatments. Compared with placebo, valerian had no statistically significant effects on mood or on cognitive and psychomotor performance.[76]

The two studies described above involved younger (aged less than 30 years) participants. Another randomised, double-blind, placebo-controlled, crossover study involved 14 healthy older participants (mean age 71.6 years, range 65–89 years) who received valerian 400 mg and 800 mg (Jamieson, Canada; subsequently reported to contain valerenic acid, 1-acetoxyvalerenic acid and 1-hydroxyvalerenic acid 0.63%), temazepam 15 mg and 30 mg, and diphenhydramine 50 mg and 75 mg, with a three-day wash-out period between treatments. No statistically significant differences on measures of psychomotor performance or sedation were found for valerian, compared with placebo.[77]

In a randomised, double-blind trial involving 102 healthy volunteers, the effects of single-dose valerian extract (LI-156) 600 mg on reaction time, alertness and concentration were compared with those of flunitrazepam 1 mg and placebo.[68] The treatment was administered in the evening and psychometric tests were carried out the next morning. After a one-week wash-out period, 91 volunteers continued with the second phase of the study, which comprised 14 days' administration of valerian extract 600 mg or placebo. Single-dose valerian extract administration did not impair reaction time, concentration or coordination. A 'hangover' effect was reported by 59% of flunitrazepam recipients, compared with 32% and 30% of placebo and valerian recipients, respectively ($p < 0.05$ for flunitrazepam versus valerian). At the end of the 14-day study, there was no statistically significant difference ($p = 0.45$) between valerian extract and placebo on mean reaction time (a measure of performance).

A randomised, double-blind, placebo-controlled study involving 80 volunteers compared the 'hangover' effects of tablets containing valerian and hops, a syrup containing valerian only, and flunitrazepam 1 mg, all given as a single dose.[78] Performance the morning after treatment, measured both objectively and subjectively, was impaired only in the flunitrazepam group.[78] Side effects occurred more frequently in the flunitrazepam group (50%), compared with the valerian and placebo groups (10%). In a further placebo-controlled study involving 36 volunteers who received valerian–hops tablets, valerian syrup, or placebo, and who underwent a battery of cognitive psychomotor tests 1–2 hours after drug administration, there was a slight, but statistically significant, impairment in vigilance with valerian syrup and impairment in the processing of complex information with valerian–hops tablets, compared with placebo.[78]

Preclinical data

Toxicological studies documented in the older literature have reported an LD_{50} of 3.3 mg/kg for an ethanolic extract of valerian administered intraperitoneally in rats, and that daily doses of 400–600 mg/kg, administered intraperitoneally for 45 days, did not lead to any changes in weight, blood or urine measurements, compared with controls.[1] Literature cited in a review of the safety of valerian describes LD_{50} values of 64 mg/kg for valtrate, 125 mg/kg for didrovaltrate and 150 mg/kg for acevaltrate in mice after intraperitoneal injection.[G21] Another study in mice reported that valerenic acid 150 mg/kg, given by intraperitoneal injection, caused muscle spasms and that 400 mg/kg caused heavy convulsions.[18] The latter dose was lethal to six of seven mice.

In vitro cytotoxicity and mutagenicity have been documented for the valepotriates. The clinical significance of this is unclear, since the valepotriates are known to be highly unstable and, therefore, probably degrade when taken orally. Only traces of valepotriates or their degradation products (in part, baldrinals) are likely to be found in finished products.[G80]

In toxicological studies in rats, there were no changes in bile value and liver enzyme activity in animals treated with a valerian preparation (Indena, Italy; no further details provided) as a single dose (0.31 to 18.6 g/kg) or 3.1 g/kg for 28 days. *In vitro*, incubation of human hepatoma cells with the same valerian preparation at a concentration of 20 mg/mL led to increased cell death, compared with values for control.[79] No such effect was seen for the valerian preparation at a concentration of 2 mg/mL, when compared with control.

A study in rats involved the administration of valepotriates (6, 12 and 24 mg/kg administered orally) during pregnancy up to the 19th day when animals were sacrificed.[80] There were no differences between valepotriate-treated rats and control rats as determined by fetotoxicity and external examination studies, although the two highest doses of valepotriates were associated with an increase in retarded ossification evident on internal examination.

Contra-indications, Warnings

Intake of valerian preparations immediately (up to two hours) before driving or operating machinery is not recommended.[G80] The effect of valerian preparations may be enhanced by consumption of alcohol, so excessive consumption of alcohol whilst receiving treatment with valerian root preparations should be avoided.[G80] Patients should seek medical advice if symptoms worsen beyond two weeks' continuous treatment with valerian.[G80] Patients with known sensitivity to valerian should not use valerian root preparations.[G80]

Drug interactions Only limited data on the potential for pharmacodynamic and pharmacokinetic interactions with other medicines administered concurrently are available for valerian root preparations. In view of the documented pharmacological actions of valerian the potential for preparations of valerian to interfere with other medicines administered concurrently, particularly those with similar or opposing effects, should be considered. In particular, co-medication with barbiturates and other sedatives is not recommended because of the potential for excessive sedation.[G80]

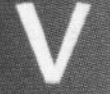

In an open-label, fixed-treatment, crossover study, 12 healthy volunteers received two tablets containing 500 mg of a 70% ethanol extract of valerian root (containing total valerenic acids 5.51 mg per tablet) each night for two weeks.[81] The probe drugs dextromethorphan 30 mg and alprazolam 2 mg were administered before and after valerian exposure to assess the effects of valerian on CYP2D6 and CYP3A4 activity, respectively. There were no statistically significant differences in dextromethorphan pharmacokinetics after valerian exposure, compared with baseline values.

The maximum plasma concentration of alprazolam was significantly increased following valerian exposure, compared with baseline values ($p < 0.05$) although there were no statistically significant differences in other pharmacokinetic parameters measured. Another study involved healthy volunteers who received valerian root extract (subsequently found to contain quantities of valerenic acid only at the limits of detection (10 ng/mL)) 125 mg three times daily for 28 days.[82] No statistically significant changes in phenotypic ratios for CYP1A2, CYP2D6, CYP2E1 and CYP3A4/5 were observed for valerian, although the valerian product tested may not be representative of other valerian preparations and their effects on CYP enzymes.[82] In *in-vitro* experiments, aqueous, ethanol and acetonitrile extracts of commercial monopreparations and combination preparations of valerian root inhibited cytochrome P450 3A4 activity and P-glycoprotein transport, as determined by an ATPase assay.[83]

Pregnancy and lactation The safety of valerian during pregnancy and lactation has not been established and, therefore, its use should be avoided.[G80]

Preparations

Proprietary single-ingredient preparations

Argentina: Nervisatis. *Australia:* Herbal Sleep Formula. *Belgium:* Dormiplant; Relaxine; Valerial. *Brazil:* Noctaval; Recalm; Sonoripan; Valeriane; Valerimed; Valerin; Valerix; Valezen; Valmane. *Canada:* Nytol Natural Source; Sleep-Eze V Natural; Unisom Natural Source. *Chile:* Sominex. *Czech Republic:* Koren Kozliku Lekarskeho; Valdispert. *Finland:* Valrian. *Germany:* Baldorm; Baldriparan Stark; Baldrivit; Baldurat; Cefaluna; Dolestan; Euvegal Balance; Luvased mono; Recvalysat; Sedonium; Sporal mono; Valdispert. *Israel:* Relaxine; Valeton. *Italy:* Ticalma. *Mexico:* Neolaikan. *Netherlands:* Dormiplant; Valdispert. *Portugal:* Valdispert. *Russia:* Novo-Passit (Ново-Пассит). *South Africa:* Calmettes. *Spain:* Ansiokey; Coenrelax; Valdispert; Valeriana Orto; Valsedan. *Sweden:* Baldrian-Dispert; Neurol; Valerecen. *Switzerland:* Baldriparan pour la nuit; Natu-Seda; ReDormin; Sedasol eco natura; Sedonium; Valdispert. *UK:* Phytorelax; Sedonium. *Venezuela:* Floral Pas.

Proprietary multi-ingredient preparations

Argentina: Armonil; Dioxicolagol; Nervocalm; SDN 200; Sedante Dia; Serenil; Sigmasedan; Valeriana Oligoplex. *Australia:* Calmo; Coleus Complex; Dan Shen Compound; Executive B; Extralife Sleep-Care; Goodnight Formula; Humulus Compound; Lifesystem Herbal Plus Formula 2 Valerian; Macro Anti-Stress; Multi-Vitamin Day & Night; Natural Deep Sleep; Pacifenity; Passiflora Complex; Passionflower Plus; Prosed-X; Relaxaplex; Valerian Plus Herbal Plus Formula 12; Valerian. *Austria:* Baldracin; Baldrian AMA; Eryval; Euvekan; Hova; Nervenruh; Nerventee St Severin; Sedadom; Sedogelat; Songha; Species nervinae; Thymoval; Valin Baldrian; Wechseltee St Severin. *Belgium:* Natudor; Seneuval; Songha. *Brazil:* Passicalm; Sominex; Sonhare. *Canada:* Herbal Nerve; Herbal Relax; Herbal Sleep Aid; Herbal Sleep Well. *Chile:* Armonyl; Recalm; Valupass. *Czech Republic:* Baldracin; Bio-Strath; Contraspan; Dr Theiss Rheuma Creme; Dr Theiss Schwedenbitter; Euvekan; Hertz- und Kreislauftee; Nervova Cajova Smes; Novo-Passit; Persen; Sanason; Schlaf-Nerventee N; Songha Night; Species Nervinae Planta; Valofyt Neo; Visinal. *France:* Biocarde; Euphytose; Mediflor Tisane Calmante Troubles du Sommeil No 14; Mediflor Tisane Circulation du Sang No 12; Neuroflorine; Passinevryl; Spasmine; Sympaneurol; Tranquital. *Germany:* Ardeysedon; Avedorm duo; Baldrian-Dispert Nacht; Baldriparan N Stark; Biosedon; Boxocalm; Cefasedativ; Dormarist; Dormeasan; Dormo-Sern; Dormoverlan; Dr. Scheffler Bergischer Krautertee Nerven- und Beruhigungstee; Dreierlei; Euvegal Entspannungs- und Einschlaftropfen; Gutnacht; Gutnacht; Heumann Beruhigungstee Teneral; Hingfong-Essenz Hofmanns; Hyperesa; Klosterfrau Beruhigungs Forte; Kytta-Sedativum; Leukona-Beruhigungsbad; Luvased; Moradorm S; Mutellon; Nervendragees; Nervenkapseln; Nervoregin forte; Neurapas; Nitrangin compositum; Oxacant-sedativ; Pascosedon; Phytonoctu; Plantival novo; Pronervon Phyto; Schlaf- und Nerventee; Schwedentrunk Elixier; Sedacur; Sedariston Konzentrat; Sedariston plus; Sedaselect D; Selon; Sensinerv forte; Tornix; Valdispert comp; Valeriana comp novum; Valeriana mild; Valverde Baldrian Hopfen bei Einschlafstorungen und zur Beruhigung; Vivinox Day. *Hungary:* Euvekan; Hova. *India:* Well-Beeing. *Israel:* Calmanervin; Calmanervin; Nerven-Dragees; Passiflora Compound; Passiflora; Songha Night. *Italy:* Anevrasi; Biocalm; Dormiplant; Fitosonno; Florelax; Glicero-Valerovit; Noctis; Parvisedil; Reve; Sedatol; Sedopuer F. *Mexico:* Nervinetas; Plantival. *Portugal:* Neurocardol; Songha; Valesono. *Russia:* Doppelherz Vitalotonik (Доппельгерц Виталотоник); Herbion Drops for the Heart (Гербион Сердечные Капли); Persen (Персен); Sanason (Санасон). *South Africa:* Avena Sativa Comp; Biral; Entressdruppels HM; Helmontskruie; Krampdruppels; Restin; Stuidruppels; Wonderkroonessens. *Spain:* Natusor Somnisedan; Nervikan; Relana; Sedasor; Sedonat; Valdispert Complex. *Switzerland:* Baldriparan; Dormeasan; Dormiplant; Dragees pour la detente nerveuse; Dragees pour le coeur et les nerfs; Dragees pour le sommeil; Dragees sedatives Dr Welti; Hova; Nervinetten; ReDormin; Relaxane; Relaxo; Songha Night; Soporin; Strath Gouttes pour le nerfs et contre l'insomnie; Tisane calmante pour les enfants; Tisane pour le sommeil et les nerfs; Valverde Coeur; Valverde Detente dragees; Valverde Sommeil; Valviska; Zeller Sommeil. *UK:* Avena Sativa Comp; Bio-Strath Valerian Formula; Boots Alternatives Sleep Well; Boots Sleepeaze Herbal Tablets; Calmanite Tablets; Constipation Tablets; Daily Tension & Strain Relief; Digestive; Fenneherb Newrelax; Fenneherb Prementaid; Gerard House Serenity; Gerard House Somnus; Golden Seal Indigestion Tablets; Herbal Indigestion Naturtabs; Herbal Pain Relief; HRI Calm Life; HRI Golden Seal Digestive; HRI Night; Indigestion and Flatulence; Kalms Sleep; Kalms; Laxative Tablets; Menopause Relief; Modern Herbals Stress; Napiers Digestion Tablets; Napiers Sleep Tablets; Napiers Tension Tablets; Natrasleep; Natural Herb Tablets; Nerfood Tablets; Nervous Dyspepsia Tablets; Newrelax; Nighttime Herb; Nodoff; Period Pain Relief; PMT Formula; Prementaid; Quiet Days; Quiet Life; Quiet Nite; Quiet Tyme; Relax B+; Roberts Alchemilla Compound Tablets; Scullcap & Gentian Tablets; Sominex Herbal; Stressless; SuNerven; Sure-Lax (Herbal); Unwind Herbal Nytol; Valerina Day Time; Valerina Day-Time; Valerina Night-Time; Valerina Night-Time; Vegetable Cough Remover; Wellwoman; Wind & Dyspepsia Relief. *USA:* Calming Aid; Stress Complex; StressEez. *Venezuela:* Cratex; Equaliv; Eufytose; Lupassin; Nervinetas; Pasidor; Pasifluidina; Rendetil.

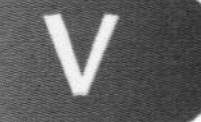

References

1 Upton R, ed. *American Herbal Pharmacopoeia and Therapeutic Compendium. Valerian root. Valeriana officinalis. Analytical, Quality Control, and Therapeutic Monograph.* Santa Cruz: American Herbal Pharmacopoeia, 1999.

2 Houghton PJ. The biological activity of valerian and related plants. *J Ethnopharmacol* 1988; 22: 121–142.

3 Morazzoni P, Bombardelli E. *Valeriana officinalis*: traditional use and recent evaluation of activity. *Fitoterapia* 1995; 66: 99–112.

4 Houghton PJ. The scientific basis for the reputed activity of valerian. *J Pharm Pharmacol* 1999; 51: 505–512.

5 Houghton PJ, ed. *Valerian. The genus Valeriana.* Amsterdam: Harwood Academic Publishers, 1997.

6 Inouye H *et al.* [The absolute configuration of valerosidate and of didovaltrate]. *Tetrahedron Lett* 1974; 30: 2317–2325 [German].

7 Pullela SV *et al.* New acylated clionasterol glycosides from *Valeriana officinalis. Planta Med* 2005; 71(10): 960–961.

8 Bos R *et al.* Isolation and identification of valerenane sesquiterpenoids from *Valeriana officinalis. Phytochemistry* 1986; 25: 133–135.

9 Bos R *et al.* Isolation of the sesquiterpene alcohol (−)-pacifigorgiol from *Valeriana officinalis. Phytochemistry* 1986; 25: 1234–1235.

10 Stoll A *et al.* New investigations on Valerian. *Schweiz Apotheker-Zeitung* 1957; 95: 115–120.

11 Hendricks H *et al.* Eugenyl isovalerate and isoeugenyl isovalerate in the essential oil of Valerian root. *Phytochemistry* 1977; 16: 1853–1854.

12 Lapke C *et al.* Free amino acids in commercial preparations of *Valeriana officinalis* L. *Pharm Pharmacol Lett* 1997; 4: 172–174.

13 Gao XQ, Björk L. Valerenic acid derivatives and valepotriates among individuals, varieties and species of *Valeriana. Fitoterapia* 2000; 71: 19–24.

14 Leathwood PD *et al.* Aqueous extract of valerian root improves sleep quality in man. *Pharmacol Biochem Behav* 1982; 17: 65–71.

15 Schulz H *et al.* The effect of valerian extract on sleep polygraphy in poor sleepers: a pilot study. *Pharmacopsychiatry* 1994; 27: 147–151.

16 Hendricks H *et al.* Pharmacological screening of valerenal and some other components of essential oil of *Valeriana officinalis. Planta Med* 1981; 42: 62–68.

17 Wagner H *et al.* Comparative studies on the sedative action of *Valeriana* extracts, valepotriates and their degradation products. *Planta Med* 1980; 39: 358–365.

18 Hendriks H *et al.* Central nervous depressant activity of valerenic acid in the mouse. *Planta Med* 1985; 51: 28–31.

19 Riedel E *et al.* Inhibition of γ-aminobutyric acid catabolism by valerenic acid derivatives. *Planta Med* 1982; 48: 219–220.

20 Santos MS *et al.* The amount of GABA present in aqueous extracts of valerian is sufficient to account for [^{3}H]GABA release in synaptosomes. *Planta Med* 1994; 60: 475–476.

21 Santos MS *et al.* Synaptosomal GABA release as influenced by valerian root extract – involvement of the GABA carrier. *Arch Int Pharmacodyn* 1994; 327: 220–231.

22 Santos MS *et al.* An aqueous extract of valerian influences the transport of GABA in synaptosomes. *Planta Med* 1994; 60: 278–279.

23 Cavadas C *et al. In vitro* study on the interaction of *Valeriana officinalis* L. extracts and their amino acids on $GABA_A$ receptor in rat brain. *Arzneimittelforschung/Drug Res* 1995; 45: 753–755.

24 Mennini T *et al. In vitro* study on the interaction of extracts and pure compounds from *Valeriana officinalis* roots with GABA, benzodiazepine and barbiturate receptors in the brain. *Fitoterapia* 1993; 64: 291–300.

25 Ortiz JG *et al.* Effects of *Valeriana officinalis* extracts on [^{3}H] flunitrazepam binding, synaptosomal [^{3}H]GABA uptake, and hippocampal [^{3}H]GABA release. *Neurochem Res* 1999; 24: 1373–1378.

26 Dietz BM *et al.* Valerian extract and valerenic acid are partial agonists of the 5-HT_{5a} receptor in vitro. *Brain Res Mol Brain Res* 2005; 138(2): 191–197.

27 Abourashed EA *et al. In vitro* binding experiments with a valerian, hops and their fixed combination extract (Ze91019) to selected central nervous system receptors. *Phytomedicine* 2004; 11: 633–638.

28 Veith J *et al.* The influence of some degradation products of valepotriates on the motor activity of light-dark synchronized mice. *Planta Med* 1986; 52: 179–183.

29 Andreatini R, Leite JR. Effect of valepotriates on the behavior of rats in the elevated plus-maze during diazepam withdrawal. *Eur J Pharmacol* 1994; 260: 233–235.

30 Petkov V. Plants with hypotensive, antiatheromatous and coronarodilating action. *Am J Chin Med* 1979; 7: 197–236.

31 Petkov V, Manolav P. To the pharmacology of iridoids. Paper presented at the 2nd Congress of the Bulgarian Society for Physiological Sciences, Sofia, October 31–November 3, 1974.

32 Hazelhoff B *et al.* Antispasmodic effects of *Valeriana* compounds: an *in vivo* and *in vitro* study on the guinea-pig ileum. *Arch Int Pharmacodyn* 1982; 257: 274–287.

33 Pilcher JD *et al.* The action of so-called female remedies on the excised uterus of the guinea-pig. *Arch Intern Med* 1916; 18: 557–583.

34 Pilcher JD, Mauer RT. The action of female remedies on the intact uteri of animals. *Surg Gynecol Obstet* 1918; 97–99.

35 Van Meer JH. Plantaardige stoffen met een effect op het complementsysteem. *Pharm Weekbl* 1984; 119: 836–942.

36 Bounthanh C *et al.* The action of valepotriates on the synthesis of DNA and proteins of cultured hepatoma cells. *Planta Med* 1983; 49: 138–142.

37 Bounthanh C *et al.* Valepotriates, a new class of cytotoxic and antitumour agents. *Planta Med* 1981; 41: 21–28.

38 Braun R *et al.* Influence of valtrate/isovaltrate on the hematopoiesis and metabolic liver activity in mice *in vivo. Planta Med* 1984; 50: 1–4.

39 Hude W *et al.* Bacterial mutagenicity of the tranquillizing constituents of Valerianaceae roots. *Mutat Res* 1986; 169: 23–27.

40 Anderson GD *et al.* Pharmacokinetics of valerenic acid after administration of valerian in healthy subjects. *Phytotherapy Research* 2005; 19(9): 801–803.

41 Leathwood PD, Chauffard F. Quantifying the effects of mild sedatives. *J Psychiatr Res* 1983; 17: 115–122.

42 Donath F *et al.* Critical evaluation of the effect of valerian extract on sleep structure and sleep quality. *Pharmacopsychiatry* 2000; 33: 47–53.

43 Vorbach EU *et al.* Therapie von Insomnien. Wirksamkeit und Verträglichkeit eines Baldrianpräparats. *Psychopharmakotherapie* 1996; 3: 109–115.

44 Diaper A, Hindmarch I. A double-blind, placebo-controlled investigation of the effects of two doses of a valerian preparation on the sleep, cognitive and psychomotor function of sleep-disturbed older adults. *Phytother Res* 2004; 18: 831–836.

45 Kamm-Kohl AV *et al.* Moderne Baldriantherapie gegen nervöse Störungen im Senium. *Med Welt* 1984; 35: 1450–1454.

46 Leathwood PD, Chauffard F. Aqueous extract of valerian reduces latency to fall asleep in man. *Planta Med* 1985; 51: 144–148.

47 Coxeter PD *et al.* Valerian does not appear to reduce symptoms for patients with chronic insomnia in general practice using a series of randomised *n*-of-1 trials. *Complement Ther Med* 2003; 11(4): 215–222.

48 Jacobs BP *et al.* An internet-based randomized, placebo-controlled trial of kava and valerian for anxiety and insomnia. *Medicine* 2005; 84 (4): 197–207.

49 Dorn M. [Baldrian versus oxazepam: efficacy and tolerability in non-organic and non-psychiatric insomniacs. A randomised, double-blind, clinical, comparative study]. *Forsch Komplement Klass Naturheilkd* 2000; 7: 79–84.

50 Schmitz M, Jäckel M. [Comparative study investigating the quality of life in patients with environmental sleep disorders (temporary dyscoimesis and dysphylaxia) under therapy with a hop-valerian preparation and a benzodiazepine preparation.] *Wiener Med Wochenschrift* 1998; 148: 291–298 [German].

51 Stevinson C, Ernst E. Valerian for insomnia: a systematic review of randomized clinical trials. *Sleep Med* 2000; 1: 91–99.

52 Morin CM *et al.* Valerian-hops combination and diphenhydramine for treating insomnia: a randomised placebo-controlled clinical trial. *Sleep* 2005; 28(11): 1465–1471.

53 Muller-Limmroth W, Ehrenstein W. Untersuchungen über die Wirkung von Seda-Kneipp auf den Schlaf schlafgëstorter Menschen. *Med Klin* 1977; 72: 1119–1125.

54 Cerny A, Schmid K. Tolerability and efficacy of valerian/lemon balm in healthy volunteers (a double-blind, placebo-controlled, multicentre study). *Fitoterapia* 1999; 70: 221–228.

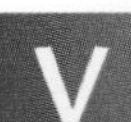

55 Dressing H *et al*. Verbesserung der Schlafqualität mit einem hochdosierten Baldrian-Melisse-Präparat. Eine plazebokontrollierte Doppelblindstudie. *Psychopharmakotherapie* 1996; 3: 123–130.
56 Dressing H *et al*. Baldrian-Melisse-Kombinationen versus Benzodiazepin. Bei Schlafstörungen gleichwertig? *Therapiewoche* 1992; 42: 726–736.
57 Vonderheid-Guth B *et al*. Pharmacodynamic effects of valerian and hops extract combination (ZE-91019) on the quantitative-topographical EEG in healthy volunteers. *Eur J Med Res* 2000; 5: 139–144.
58 Schellenberg R *et al*. The fixed combination of valerian and hops (Ze91019) acts via a central adenosine mechanism. *Planta Med* 2004; 70(7): 594–597.
59 Francis AJP, Dempster RJW. Effect of valerian, *Valeriana edulis*, on sleep difficulties in children with intellectual deficits: randomised trial. *Phytomedicine* 2002; 9: 273–279.
60 Poyares DR *et al*. Can valerian improve the sleep of insomniacs after benzodiazepine withdrawal? *Prog Neuropsychopharmacol Biol Psych* 2002; 26: 539–545.
61 Andreatini R *et al*. Effect of valepotriates (valerian extract) in generalized anxiety disorder: a randomized placebo-controlled pilot study. *Phytotherapy Res* 2002; 16: 650–654.
62 Cropley M *et al*. Effect of kava and valerian on human physiological and psychological responses to mental stress assessed under laboratory conditions. *Phytotherapy Res* 2002; 16: 23–27.
63 Kohnen R, Oswald W-D. The effects of valerian, propranolol, and their combination on activation, performance, and mood of healthy volunteers under social stress conditions. *Pharmacopsychiatry* 1988; 21: 447–448.
64 Panijel M. Die behandlung mittelschwerer angstzustände. *Therapiewoche* 1985; 41: 4659–4668.
65 Kneibel R, Burchard JM. Zur Therapie depressiver Verstimmungen in der Praxis. *Z Allgemeinmed* 1988; 64: 689–696.
66 Steger W. Depressive Verstimmungen. *Z Allgemeinmed* 1985; 61: 914–918.
67 Linde K *et al*. St John's wort for depression – an overview and meta-analysis of randomised clinical trials. *BMJ* 1996; 313: 253–258.
68 Kuhlmann J *et al*. The influence of valerian treatment on 'reaction time, alertness and concentration' in volunteers. *Pharmacopsychiatry* 1999; 32: 235–241.
69 Garges HP *et al*. Cardiac complications and delirium associated with valerian root withdrawal. *JAMA* 1998; 280: 1566–1567.
70 MacGregor FB *et al*. Hepatotoxicity of herbal medicines. *BMJ* 1989; 299: 1156–1157.
71 Shaw D *et al*. Traditional remedies and food supplements. A five-year toxicological study (1991–1995). *Drug Safety* 1997; 17: 342–356.
72 Willey LB *et al*. Valerian overdose: a case report. *Vet Human Toxicol* 1995; 37: 364–365.
73 Chan TYK *et al*. Poisoning due to an over-the-counter hypnotic, Sleep-Qik (hyoscine, cyproheptadine, valerian). *Postgrad Med J* 1995; 71: 227–228.
74 Chan TYK. An assessment of the delayed effects associated with valerian overdose. *Int J Clin Pharmacol Ther* 1998; 36: 569.
75 Hallam KT *et al*. Comparative cognitive and psychomotor effects of single doses of *Valeriana officinalis* and triazolam in healthy volunteers. *Hum Psychopharmacol Clin Exp* 2003; 18: 619–625.
76 Gutierrez S *et al*. Assessing subjective and psychomotor effects of the herbal medication valerian in healthy volunteers. *Pharmacol Biochem Behav* 2004; 78: 57–64.
77 Glass JR *et al*. Acute pharmacological effects of temazepam, diphenhydramine, and valerian in healthy elderly subjects. *J Clin Psychopharmacol* 2003; 23: 260–268.
78 Gerhard U *et al*. [Effects of two plant-based sleep remedies on vigilance]. *Schweiz Runsch Med Prax* 1996; 85: 473–481 [German].
79 Vo LT *et al*. Investigation of the effects of peppermint oil and valerian on rat liver and cultured human liver cells. *Clin Exp Pharmacol Physiol* 2003; 30: 799–804.
80 Tufik S *et al*. Effects of a prolonged administration of valepotriates in rats on the mothers and their offspring. *J Ethnopharmacol* 1994; 41: 39–44.
81 Donovan JL *et al*. Multiple night-time doses of valerian (*Valeriana officinalis*) had minimal effects on CYP3A4 activity and no effect on CYP2D6 activity in healthy volunteers. *Drug Metab Disp* 2004; 32 (12): 1333–1336.
82 Gurley BJ *et al*. In vivo effects of goldenseal, kava kava, black cohosh, and valerian on human cytochrome P450 1A2, 2D6, 2E1, and 3A4/5 phenotypes. *Clin Pharmacol Ther* 2005; 77: 415–426.
83 Lefebvre T *et al*. In vitro activity of commercial valerian extracts against human cytochrome P450 3A4. *J Pharm Pharmaceut Sci* 2004; 7 (2): 265–273.

Vervain

Summary and Pharmaceutical Comment

Limited chemical, pharmacological and toxicity data are available for vervain. Documented scientific information does not justifiy the herbal uses. In view of the lack of data on pharmacological effects, efficacy and safety, the appropriateness of medicinal use of vervain should be considered. Excessive use, at least, should be avoided. Vervain should not be used during pregnancy and breastfeeding. The potential for vervain preparations to interact with other medicines should be considered.

Species (Family)

Verbena officinalis L. (Verbenaceae)

Synonym(s)

Verbena

Part(s) Used

Herb

Pharmacopoeial and Other Monographs

BHP 1996[G9]
Martindale 35th edition[G85]

Legal Category (Licensed Products)

GSL[G37]

Constituents

The following is compiled from several sources, including General Reference G2.

Glycosides Iridoid glycosides: hastatoside, verbenalin (verbanaloside), verbenin (aucubin). Phenylpropanoid glycosides: acteoside (verbascoside) and eukovoside.[1, 2]

Volatile oils Monoterpene components include citral, geraniol, limonene and verbenone.

Other constituents Adenosibe, alkaloid (unspecified), bitters, carbohydrates (stachyose, mucilage), β-carotene, invertin (sucrose hydrolytic enzymes), saponin and tannic acid.

Food Use

Vervain is listed by the Council of Europe as a natural source of food flavouring (category N2). This category indicates that vervain can be added to foodstuffs in small quantities, with a possible limitation of an active principle (as yet unspecified) in the final product.[G16] Previously, vervain was listed by the United States of America Food and Drugs Administration (FDA) as a Herb of Undefined Safety.[G22]

Iridoids

hastoside

verbenalin (cornin, verbenaloside)

Phenylpropanoids

verbascoside

Figure 1 Selected constituents of vervain.

Herbal Use

Vervain is stated to possess sedative, thymoleptic, antispasmodic, mild diaphoretic and, reputedly, galactogogue properties. Traditionally, it has been used for depression, melancholia, hysteria, generalised seizures, cholecystalgia, jaundice, early stages of fever, and specifically for depression and debility of convalescence after fevers, especially influenza.[G2, G7, G64]

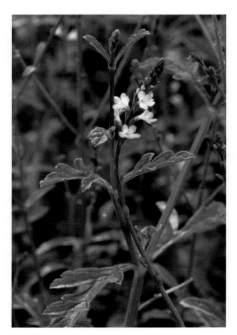

Figure 2 Vervain (*Verbena officinalis*).

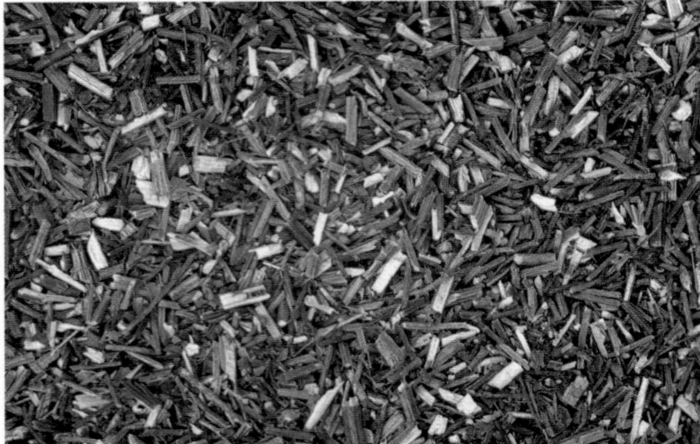

Figure 3 Vervain – dried drug substance (herb).

Dosage

Dosages for oral administration (adults) for traditional uses recommended in standard herbal reference texts are given below.

Dried herb 2–4 g as an infusion three times daily.[G7]

Liquid extract 2–4 mL (1 : 1 in 25% alcohol) three times daily.[G7]

Tincture 5–10 mL (1 : 1 in 40% alcohol) three times daily.[G7]

Pharmacological Actions

In vitro and animal studies

Chloroform, methanol and petroleum ether extracts of the aerial parts of vervain have anti-inflammatory activity *in vivo* as determined using the carrageenan-induced paw oedema model.[3] The chloroform extract was found to exhibit the greatest activity. Vervain is stated to have several properties, including galactogogue activity and luteinising activity,[4] although the scientific basis for these statements is not clear.

Verbenalin has been reported to exhibit uterine stimulant activity.[G30] A slight laxative action in mice has been documented for iridoid glycosides.[5]

A total aqueous extract of the aerial parts of the related species *Vervain hastata* was found to have sedative properties in experiments involving male rats.[6]

Clinical studies

There is a lack of clinical research assessing the effects of vervain and rigorous randomised clinical trials are required.

Side-effects, Toxicity

Clinical data

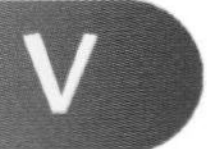

There is a lack of clinical safety and toxicity data for vervain and further investigation of these aspects is required.

Preclinical data

It is stated that, in frogs, small doses of verbenalin stimulate the uterus and that high doses paralyse the CNS, following stupor and convulsions,[G22] although the scientific basis for these statements is not known.

Contra-indications, Warnings

None documented.

Drug interactions None documented. In view of the lack of information on the constituents of vervain and their pharmacological activities, the potential for preparations of vervain to interact with other medicines taken concurrently should be considered.

Pregnancy and lactation Vervain is reputed to act as an abortifacient and oxytocic agent[G30] with *in vivo* utero-activity documented (*see In vitro* and animal studies). In view of this, vervain should not be taken during pregnancy.

Vervain is stated to act as a galactogogue,[3] although the scientific basis for this statement is not known. In view of the lack of information on the safety of vervain during breastfeeding, use should be avoided during this period.

Preparations

Proprietary multi-ingredient preparations

Australia: Avena Complex; Calmo; Nevaton. *Austria:* Sinupret. *Czech Republic:* Sinupret; Stomatosan. *France:* Calmophytum; Vigilia. *Germany:* Sinupret. *Hong Kong:* Sinupret. *Hungary:* Sinupret. *Italy:* Neoderma 47. *Russia:* Sinupret (Синупрет). *Singapore:* Sinupret. *Switzerland:* Sinupret; Tisane pour nourissons et enfants. *Thailand:* Sinupret. *UK:* Athera; Fenneherb Prementaid; HRI Night; Kalms Sleep; Modern Herbals Menopause; Modern Herbals Stress; Napiers Sleep Tablets; Newrelax; Period Pain Relief; Prementaid; Roberts Alchemilla Compound Tablets; Scullcap & Gentian Tablets; Stressless; SuNerven.

References

1 Lahloub MF *et al*. Phenylpropanoid and iridoid glycosides from the Egyptian *Verbena officinalis*. *Planta Med* 1986; 52: 47.
2 Andary C *et al*. Structures of verbascoside and orobanchoside, caffeic acid sugar esters from *Orobanche rapum-genistae*. *Phytochemistry* 1982; 21: 1123–1127.
3 Deepak M, Handa SS. Antiinflammatory activity and chemical composition of extracts of *Verbena officinalis*. *Phytotherapy Res* 2000; 14(6): 463–465.
4 Oliver-Bever BEP. *Medicinal Plants in Tropical West Africa*. Cambridge: Cambridge University Press, 1986.
5 Inouye H *et al*. Purgative activities of iridoid glycosides. *Planta Med* 1974; 25: 285–288.
6 Akanmu HA *et al*.. Hypnotic effects of total aqueous extracts of *Vervain hastata*. *Psychiatry Clin Neurosci* 2002; 56(3): 309–310.

Wild Carrot

Summary and Pharmaceutical Comment

Phytochemical studies documented for wild carrot concentrate on the composition of the volatile oil obtained from both the fresh and dried fruits (seeds). The composition of the oil varies between different cultivars. Preclinical studies have documented a variety of pharmacological actions including CNS-depressant, spasmodic and antispasmodic, hypotensive and cardiac-depressant activities. However, there is a lack of robust clinical research assessing the efficacy and safety of wild carrot. The principal traditional use of wild carrot is as a diuretic. This activity has not been documented in animal studies, but the seed oil of wild carrot does contain terpinen-4-ol, the diuretic principle documented for juniper. Toxicity data only refer to the oil and indicate low toxicity. In view of the limited information on safety, excessive use of wild carrot and use during pregnancy and lactation should be avoided.

Species (Family)

Daucus carota L. subsp. *carota* (Apiaceae/Umbelliferae)

Synonym(s)

Daucus, *Daucus carota* L. subsp. *maximus* auct. lusit. non (Desf.) Ball, *D. communis* Rouy & E.G. Camus proles communis, Queen Anne's Lace

Part(s) Used

Herb

Pharmacopoeial and Other Monographs

BHC 1992[G6]
BHP 1996[G9]
Martindale 35th edition[G85]

Legal Category (Licensed Products)

GSL[G37]

Constituents

The following is compiled from several sources, including General Reference G6.

Documented constituents refer to the fruit or seeds obtained from the dried fruit unless otherwise stated.

Flavonoids Flavones (e.g. apigenin, chrysin, luteolin), flavonols (e.g. kaempferol, quercetin) and various glycosides.[1]

Furanocoumarin 8-Methoxypsoralen and 5-methoxypsoralen (0.01–0.02 μg/g fresh weight) in fresh plant. Concentrations increased in the diseased plant.[2]

Volatile oils 0.66–1.65%.[3] Many components identified; relative composition varies between different cultivars.[3] Various components include α-pinene, β-pinene, geraniol, geranyl acetate, limonene, α-terpinen, *p*-terpinen, α-terpineol, terpinen-4-ol, *p*-decanolactone (monoterpenes); β-bisabolene, β-elemene, caryophyllene, caryophyllene oxide, carotol, daucol (sesquiterpenes); asarone (phenylpropanoid derivative).[3]

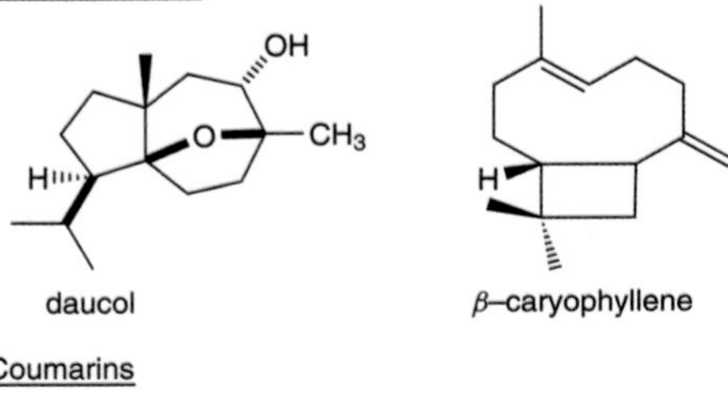

Figure 1 Selected constituents of wild carrot.

Other constituents Choline,[4] daucine (alkaloid), a tertiary base (uncharacterised),[5] fatty acids (butyric, palmitic), coumarin, xylitol (polyol).

Food Use

Wild carrot should not be confused with the common cultivated carrot, *D. carota* L. subsp. *sativus* (Hoffm.) Arcang., which has the familiar fleshy orange-red edible root. Wild carrot has an inedible tough whitish root.[G41] Wild carrot is listed by the Council of Europe as a natural source of food flavouring (categories N1, N3). Category N1 indicates that for the roots there are no restrictions on use, whereas category N3 indicates that there is insufficient information available for an adequate assessment of potential toxicity.[G16]

Herbal Use

Wild carrot is stated to possess diuretic, antilithic, and carminative properties. Traditionally, it has been used for urinary calculus, lithuria, cystitis, gout, and specifically for urinary gravel or calculus.[G6, G7, G8, G64]

Dosage

Dosages for oral administration (adults) for traditional uses recommended in standard herbal reference texts are given below.

Dried herb 2–4 g as an infusion three times daily.[G6, G7]

Liquid extract 2–4 mL (1 : 1 in 25% alcohol) three times daily.[G6, G7]

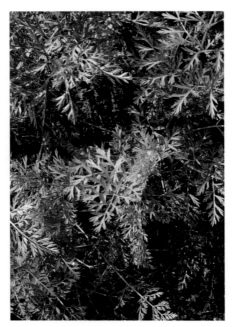

Figure 2 Wild carrot (*Daucus carota*).

Pharmacological Actions

In vitro and animal studies

Significant antifertility activity (60%) in rats has been reported for wild carrot.(6) In contrast, insignificant antifertility activity was observed in pregnant rats fed oral doses of up to 4.5 g/kg body weight from day 1 to day 10 of pregnancy.(7) Aqueous, alcoholic and petrol extracts were reported to exhibit 20%, 40% and 10% activities respectively. Weak oestrogenic activity(6, 8, 9) and inhibition of implantation(6, 9) have been documented for seed extracts.(8) Oestrogenic activity, demonstrated by the inhibition of ovarian hypertrophy in hemicastrated rats, has been attributed to the known constituent coumarin (a weak phytooestrogen).(10)

Central effects similar to those of barbiturates have been documented for the seed oil obtained from *D. carota* L. var. *sativa* DC.(11) The oil was reported to elicit CNS hypnotic effects in the rat, hypotension in the dog(4) leading to respiratory depression at higher doses, anticonvulsant activity in the frog, *in vitro* smooth muscle relaxant activity reducing acetylcholine-induced contractions (ileum/uterus, rabbit/rat), antagonism of acetylcholine in isolated frog skeletal muscle, direct depressant effect on cardiac muscle in the dog.(4, 11) *In vitro* cardiotonic activity(4) and vasodilation of coronary vessels of the isolated cat heart have been reported.(12) Papaverine-like antispasmodic activity has been documented for a tertiary base isolated from wild carrot seeds.(5) Activity of approximately one-tenth that of papaverine was noted in a number of isolated preparations: ileum, uterus, blood vessels and trachea.(5) Cholinergic-type actions have also been reported for wild carrot with *in vitro* spasmodic actions noted in both smooth and skeletal muscle.(4) This cholinergic activity has been attributed to choline.(13) The identity of a second quaternary base isolated was not established.

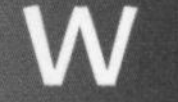

Terpinen-4-ol is a documented component of the seed oil. This constituent is considered to be the diuretic principle in juniper (*see* Juniper).

Increased resistance to carbon tetrachloride-induced hepatotoxicity has been reported in rats fed wild carrot.(14)

Limited antifungal activity has been documented, with activity exhibited against only one (*Botrytis cinerea*) out of nine fungi tested.(15)

Agglutination of *Streptococcus mutans* cells has been described for wild carrot. The agglutinin, found to be heat and trypsin stable but sensitive to dextranose, was thought to be a dextran.(16)

Clinical studies

There is a lack of clinical research assessing the effects of wild carrot and rigorous randomised controlled clinical trials are required.

Side-effects, Toxicity

Clinical data

There is a lack of clinical safety and toxicity data for wild carrot and further investigation of these aspects is required.

The oil is reported to be generally non-irritating and non-sensitising.(12) However, hypersensitivity reactions, occupational dermatitis and positive patch tests have been reported for wild carrot.(2, G51) Wild carrot is reported to have a slight photosensitising effect.(2) Furanocoumarins are known photosensitisers.

Preclinical data

The oil is reported to be of low toxicity. Acute LD_{50} values in mice (oral) and guinea-pigs (dermal) are reported to exceed 5 g/kg.(17)

Contra-indications, Warnings

Fruit extracts may cause sensitivity reactions similar to those seen with celery.(2)

Drug interactions None documented. However, the potential for preparations of wild carrot to interact with other medicines administered concurrently, particularly those with similar or opposing effects, should be considered. There is limited evidence from preclinical studies that wild carrot seed extracts have oestrogenic activity.

Pregnancy and lactation The safety of wild carrot has not been established. In view of this, the use of wild carrot during pregnancy and lactation should be avoided.

Preparations

Proprietary multi-ingredient preparations

Argentina: Hepatalgina; Hepatalgina; Metiogen; Palatrobil. *Chile:* Natur-Zin; Natursel-C. *Italy:* Evamilk. *Malaysia:* Eyebright Plus. *UK:* Sciargo; Watershed.

References

1 El-Moghazi AM *et al*. Flavonoids of *Daucus carota*. *Planta Med* 1980; 40: 382–385.

2 Ceska O *et al*. Furocoumarins in the cultivated carrot, *Daucus carota*. *Phytochemistry* 1986; 25: 81–83.

3 Benecke R *et al*. Vergleichende Untersuchungen über den Gehalt an ätherischem Öl und dessen Zusammensetzung in den Früchten verschiedener Sorten von *Daucus carota* L. ssp. sativus (Hoffm.) Arcang. *Pharmazie* 1987; 42: 256–259.

4 Gambhir SS *et al*. Studies on *Daucus carota*, Linn. Part I. Pharmacological studies with the water-soluble fraction of the alcoholic extract of the seeds: a preliminary report. *Indian J Med Res* 1966; 54: 178–187.

5 Gambhir SS *et al*. Antispasmodic activity of the tertiary base of *Daucus carota*, Linn. seeds. *Indian J Physiol Pharmacol* 1979; 23: 225–228.
6 Prakash AO. Biological evaluation of some medicinal plant extracts for contraceptive efficacy. *Contracept Deliv Syst* 1984; 5: 9.
7 Lal R *et al*. Antifertility effect of *Daucus carota* seeds in female albino rats. *Fitoterapia* 1986; 57: 243–246.
8 Kant A *et al*. The estrogenic efficacy of carrot (*Daucus carota*) seeds. *J Adv Zool* 1986; 7: 36–41.
9 Sharma MM *et al*. Estrogenic and pregnancy interceptory effects of carrot *Daucus carota* seeds. *Indian J Exp Biol* 1976; 14: 506–508.
10 Kaliwal BB, Rao MA. Inhibition of ovarian compensatory hypertrophy by carrot seed (*Daucus carota*) extract or estradiol-17β in hemicastrated albino rats. *Indian J Exp Biol* 1981; 19: 1058–1060.
11 Bhargava AK *et al*. Pharmacological investigation of the essential oil of *Daucus carota* Linn. var. sativa DC. *Indian J Pharm* 1967; 29: 127–129.
12 Carrot seed oil. *Food Cosmet Toxicol* 1976; 14: 705–706.
13 Gambhir SS *et al*. Studies on *Daucus carota*, Linn. Part II. Cholingergic activity of the quaternary base isolated from water-soluble fraction of alcoholic extracts of seeds. *Indian J Med Res* 1966; 54: 1053–1056.
14 Handa SS. Natural products and plants as liver protecting drugs. *Fitoterapia* 1986; 57: 307–351.
15 Guérin J-C, Réveillère H-P. Antifungal activity of plant extracts used in therapy. II Study of 40 plant extracts against 9 fungi species. *Ann Pharm Fr* 1985; 43: 77–81.
16 Ramstorp M *et al*. Isolation and partial characterization of a substance from carrots, *Daucus carota*, with ability to agglutinate cells of *Streptococcus mutans*. *Caries Res* 1982; 16: 423–427.
17 Opdyke DLJ. Carrot seed oil. *Food Cosmet Toxicol* 1974; 14: 705.

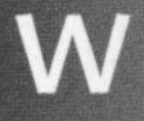

Wild Lettuce

Summary and Pharmaceutical Comment

The chemistry of wild lettuce is well documented, although it is not clear which constituents represent the active components. Early reports of hyoscyamine as a constituent have not been substantiated by subsequent study. No published information was found to support the traditional herbal uses of wild lettuce, although a sedative action in toads has been reported for a related species *L. sativa*. In view of the potential allergenicity of wild lettuce and the lack of toxicity data, excessive use and use during pregnancy and lactation should be avoided.

Related *Lactuca* species include *Lactuca sativa* (Garden Lettuce), *Lactuca serriola* L. (Prickly Lettuce), *L. quescina* L. subsp. *quercina* and *Lactuca canadensis* (Wild Lettuce of America).

Species (Family)

Lactuca virosa L. (Asteraceae/Compositae)

Synonym(s)

Bitter Lettuce, Great Lettuce, Lettuce Opium

Part(s) Used

Leaf, latex

Pharmacopoeial and Other Monographs

BHC 1992[G6]
BHP 1996[G9]
Martindale 35th edition[G85]

Legal Category (Licensed Products)

GSL[G37]

Constituents

The following is compiled from several sources, including General Reference G6.

All parts of the plant contain a milky, white latex (sap) which, when collected and dried, forms the drug known as lactucarium.[G33]

Acids Citric, malic and oxalic (up to 1%) acids; cichoric acid (phenolic).[1]

Alkaloids Hyoscyamine, later disputed.[2, G33] *N*-methyl-β-phenethylamine, also disputed.[2]

Coumarins Aesculin, cichoriin.[1]

Flavonoids Flavones (e.g. apigenin, luteolin), flavonols (e.g. quercetin) and their glycosides.[1]

Terpenoids Bitter principles including the sesquiterpene lactones lactucin and lactupicrin (lactucopicrin); β-amyrin, germanicol, and lactucone (lactucerin). Lactucone is a mixture of α- and β-lactucerol acetates, β-lactucerol being identical to taraxasterol.

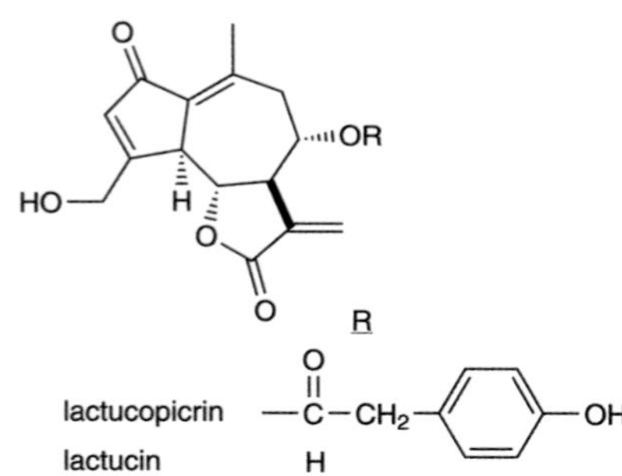

Figure 1 Selected constituents of wild lettuce.

Other constituents Mannitol, proteins, resins and sugars.

Food Use

Wild lettuce is not used in foods, although the related species *L. sativa* is commonly used as a salad ingredient.

Herbal Use

Wild lettuce is stated to possess mild sedative, anodyne and hypnotic properties. Traditionally, it has been used for insomnia, restlessness and excitability in children, pertussis, irritable cough, priapism, dysmenorrhoea, nymphomania, muscular or articular pains, and specifically for irritable cough and insomnia.[G6, G7, G8, G42, G64]

Dosage

Dosages for oral administration (adults) for traditional uses recommended in older and contemporary standard herbal and pharmaceutical reference texts are given below.

Dried leaves 0.5–3.0 g as an infusion three times daily.[G6]

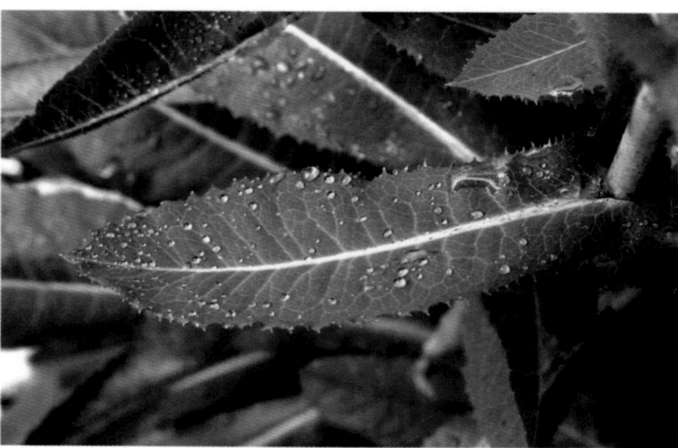

Figure 2 Wild lettuce (*Lactuca virosa*).

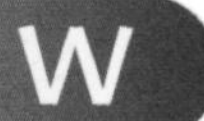

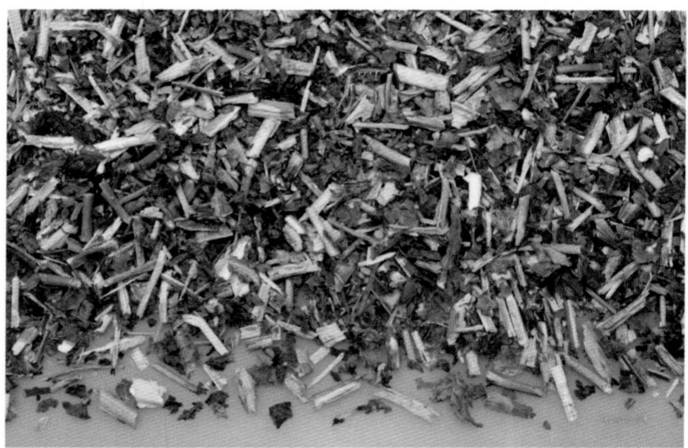

Figure 3 Wild lettuce – dried drug substance (herb).

Liquid extract 0.5–3.0 mL (1 : 1 in 25% alcohol) three times daily.(G6)

Lactucarium (dried latex extract) (BPC 1934) 0.3–1.0 g three times daily.

Soft extract (BPC 1934) 0.3–1.0 g three times daily.

Pharmacological Actions

In vitro and animal studies

Lactucarium has been noted to induce mydriasis.(G6) This effect may be attributable to hyoscyamine, although the dried sap is reportedly devoid of this alkaloid.

An alcoholic extract of a related species, *L. sativa*, has exhibited a sedative effect in toads, causing a reduction in motor activity and behaviour.(3) Higher doses resulted in flaccid paralysis. In addition, an antispasmodic action on isolated smooth and striated muscle, and *in vitro* negative chronotropic and inotropic effects on normal and stressed (tachycardic) hearts were observed. The antispasmodic action was noted to be antagonised by calcium.

Lactucin, lactupicrin and hyoscyamine have all been proposed as the sedative components in wild lettuce. However in the above study,(3) the active component was uncharacterised and acted mainly peripherally, not readily crossing the blood–brain barrier. The suggested mode of action was via interference with basic excitatory processes common to neural and muscular functions, and not via a neuromuscular block.

Low amounts (nanograms) of morphine have been detected in *Lactuca* species, although the concentrations involved are considered too low to exert any obvious pharmacological effect.(G60)

Clinical studies

There is a lack of clinical research assessing the effects of wild lettuce and rigorous randomised controlled clinical trials are required.

Side-effects, Toxicity

Clinical data

No side-effects documented for *L. virosa*. However, there is a lack of clinical safety and toxicity data for wild lettuce and further investigation of these aspects is required. Wild lettuce contains sesquiterpene lactones which are potentially allergenic.(G19) Occupational dermatitis has been documented for *L. sativa* together with an urticarial eruption after ingestion of the leaves.(4–6, G51) The milky sap of *L. sativa* is reported to be irritant.(G51)

Preclinical data

Consumption of large amounts of *L. scariola* has caused poisoning in cattle, which developed pulmonary emphysema, severe dyspnoea, and weakness.(7) Only the immature plants were reported to be toxic.

L. sativa has been reported to produce only negative responses when tested for mutagenicity using the Ames test (*Salmonella typhimurium* TA98, TA100).(8)

Contra-indications, Warnings

Overdosage may produce poisoning(G42) involving stupor, depressed respiration, coma and even death. Wild lettuce may cause an allergic reaction in sensitive individuals, in particular those with an existing sensitivity to other members of the Asteraceae/Compositae family.

Drug interactions None documented. However, the potential for preparations of wild lettuce to interact with other medicines administered concurrently, particularly those with similar or opposing effects, should be considered.

Pregnancy and lactation The safety of wild lettuce has not been established. In view of the lack of toxicity data and the possibility of allergic reactions, use of wild lettuce during pregnancy and lactation should be avoided.

Preparations

Proprietary multi-ingredient preparations

Canada: Sirop Cocillana Codeine. *Russia:* Speman Forte (Спеман Форте). *South Africa:* Choats Extract of Lettuce Cough Mixture. *UK:* Anased; Antibron; Calmanite Tablets; Gerard House Somnus; HRI Night; Kalms Sleep; Napiers Sleep Tablets; Nytol Herbal; Quiet Life; Quiet Nite; Slumber; Unwind Herbal Nytol. *Venezuela:* Cerylana.

References

1. Rees S, Harborne JB. Flavonoids and other phenolics of *Cichorium* and related members of the Lactuceae (Compositae). *Bot J Linn Soc* 1984; 89: 313–319.
2. Huang Z-J *et al.* Studies on herbal remedies I: Analysis of herbal smoking preparations alleged to contain lettuce (*Lactuca sativa* L.) and other natural products. *J Pharm Sci* 1982; 71: 270–271.
3. Gonzálex-Lima F *et al.* Depressant pharmacological effects of a component isolated from lettuce, *Lactuca sativa*. *Int J Crude Drug Res* 1986; 24: 154–166.
4. Krook G. Occupational dermatitis from *Lactuca sativa* (lettuce) and *Cichorium* (endive). *Contact Dermatitis* 1977; 3: 27–36.
5. Rinkel HJ, Balyeat RM. Occupational dermatitis due to lettuce. *JAMA* 1932; 98: 137–138.
6. Zeller W *et al.* The sensitizing capacity of Compositae plants 6. Guinea pig sensitization experiments with ornamental plants and weeds using different methods. *Arch Dermatol Res* 1985; 277: 28–35.
7. Anon. *Poisindex* CD-ROM 1995; 85. Denver: Micromedex.
8. White RD *et al.* An evaluation of acetone extracts from six plants in the Ames mutagenicity test. *Toxicol Lett* 1983; 15: 26–31.

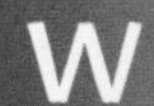

Willow

Summary and Pharmaceutical Comment

Willow is rich in phenolic constituents, such as flavonoids, tannins and salicylates. Pharmacological actions normally associated with salicylates are also applicable to willow and supports most of the herbal uses. Robust clinical research assessing the efficacy and safety of willow is limited. In view of the lack of toxicity data on willow, the usual precautions taken with other salicylate-containing drugs are applicable. Products containing willow should preferably be standardised on their salicin content, in view of the considerable variation in salicylate concentrations between different *Salix* species. The use of willow during pregnancy and lactation should be avoided.

Species (Family)

Several *Salix* species are used including *S. alba* L., *S. fragilis* L., *S. pentandra* L., *S. purpurea* L. (Salicaceae)

Synonym(s)

Salix

Part(s) Used

Bark

Pharmacopoeial and Other Monographs

American Herbal Pharmacopoeia(G1)
BHC 1992(G6)
BHP 1996(G9)
BP 2007(G84)
Complete German Commission E(G3)
ESCOP 2003(G76)
Martindale 35th edition(G85)
Ph Eur 2007(G81)

Legal Category (Licensed Products)

GSL(G37)

Constituents

The following is compiled from several sources, including General References G1, G2, G6 and G52.

Glycosides (phenolic) Various phenolic glycosides including salicin, salicortin, tremulacin, salireposide, picein and triandrin.(1) Acetylated salicin, salicortin, salireposide, and esters of salicylic acid and salicyl alcohol may also occur.

Salicylates (calculated as salicin) Vary between species, e.g. 0.5% in *S. alba*, 1–10% in *S. fragilis*, 3–9% in *S. purpurea*.(2)

Flavonoids Flavanones, eriodictoyl-7-glucoside; naringenin-5-glucoside; chalcone; isosalipurposide; catechin.(2, G52)

Tannins Condensed.

Other constituents Catechins.

There is reported to be no difference between the phenolic glycoside pattern of the bark and leaf. The latter is also reported to contain flavonoids, catechins and condensed tannins.(2, 3)

Food Use

Willow is not used in foods.

Herbal Use

Willow is stated to possess anti-inflammatory, antirheumatic, antipyretic, antihidrotic, analgesic, antiseptic and astringent properties. Traditionally it has been used for muscular and arthrodial rheumatism with inflammation and pain, influenza, respiratory catarrh, gouty arthritis, ankylosing spondylitis, and specifically for rheumatoid arthritis and other systemic connective tissue disorders characterised by inflammatory changes. The German Commission E approved internal use for diseases accompanied by fever, rheumatic ailments and headaches.(G3)

Dosage

Dosages for oral administration (adults) for traditional uses recommended in standard herbal reference texts are given below.

Dry bark 1–3 g as a decoction three times daily(G6, G7) corresponding to 60–120 mg total salicin daily.(G3)

Liquid extract 1–3 mL (1 : 1 in 25% alcohol) three times daily.(G6, G7)

Pharmacological Actions

In vitro and animal studies

Pharmacological actions documented for salicylates include anti-inflammatory, antipyretic, hyperglycaemic/hypoglycaemic and

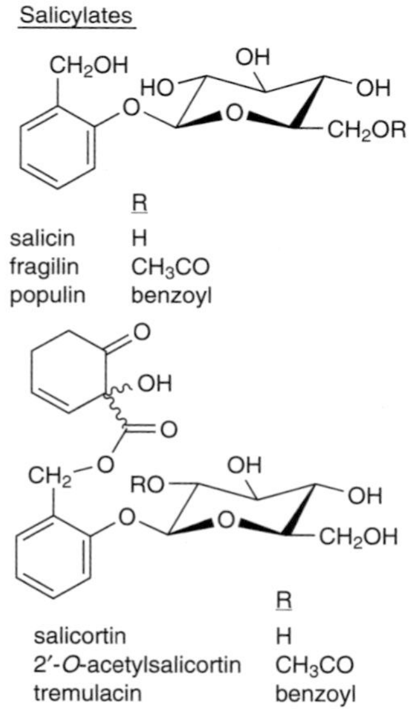

Salicylates

	R
salicin	H
fragilin	CH_3CO
populin	benzoyl

	R
salicortin	H
2′-*O*-acetylsalicortin	CH_3CO
tremulacin	benzoyl

Figure 1 Selected constituents of willow.

W

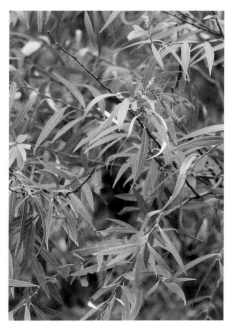

Figure 2 Willow (*Salix* spp.).

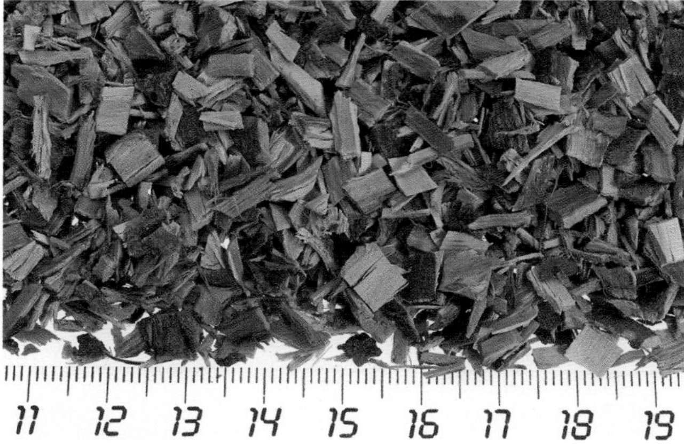

Figure 3 Willow – dried drug substance (bark).

uricosuric/antiuricosuric activities, and increased blood-clotting time and plasma albumin binding.[G46] Anti-inflammatory activity for salicin and tremulacin (isolated from *Populus* spp.) has been assessed in the hen's egg choriollantoic test.[4, G52] The results indicate that the activity may be due to the metabolites of these compounds.[4] Salicin is probably the most active anti-inflammatory compound in willow; it is metabolised to salicylic acid.[5] The enzymatic degradation of salicin, salicortin and tremulacin by β-glucosidase and by esterase has been investigated.[6]

Tannins are known to have astringent properties.

Clinical studies

Robust clinical research assessing the effects of willow is limited and rigorous randomised controlled clinical trials are required.

Willow bark extract (equivalent to 240 mg salicin/day) was compared with placebo in a two-week, randomised, double-blind trial involving 78 patients with osteoarthritis.[7] A difference in pain dimension in the treated group, compared with placebo, just reached statistical significance ($p = 0.047$).

The pharmacological actions of salicylates in humans are well documented, and are applicable to willow. Salicin is a prodrug which is metabolised to saligenin in the gastrointestinal tract and to salicylic acid after absorption.[2]

Side-effects, Toxicity

Clinical data

Clinical safety and toxicity data for willow are limited and further investigation of these aspects is required. Minor adverse effects including stomachache, nausea, dizziness, sweating and rash have been reported for willow.[G52]

Side-effects and signs of toxicity normally associated with salicylates, such as gastric and renal irritation, hypersensitivity, blood in the stools, tinnitus, nausea and vomiting, may occur. Salicin is documented to cause skin rashes.[G44]

Contra-indications, Warnings

Precautions associated with salicylate therapy are also applicable to willow. Therefore individuals with known hypersensitivity to aspirin, asthma, active peptic ulceration, diabetes, gout, haemophilia, hypoprothrombinaemia, kidney or liver disease should be aware of the possible risks associated with the ingestion of willow.[8, G46]

Drug interactions Drug interactions listed for salicylates are also applicable to willow and include oral anticoagulants, methotrexate, metoclopramide, phenytoin, probenecid, spironolactone and valproate. Concurrent administration of willow with other salicylate-containing products, such as aspirin, should be avoided. Irritant effects of salicylates on the gastrointestinal tract may be enhanced by alcohol, and barbiturates and oral sedatives have been documented to enhance salicylate toxicity as well as masking the symptoms of overdosage.[G46]

Pregnancy and lactation The safety of willow during pregnancy and lactation has not been established. Conflicting reports have been documented concerning the safety of aspirin taken during pregnancy. Salicylates excreted in breast milk have been reported to cause macular rashes in breastfed babies.[G46] In view of this information, the use of willow during pregnancy and lactation should be avoided.

Preparations

Proprietary single-ingredient preparations

Brazil: Zortrix. *Germany:* Assalix; Assplant; Rheumakaps; Rheumatab Salicis. *Switzerland:* Assalix.

Proprietary multi-ingredient preparations

Australia: Arthritic Pain Herbal Formula 1; Bioglan Arthri Plus; Extralife Migrai-Care; Extralife PMS-Care; Guaiacum Complex; Lifesystem Herbal Formula 1 Arthritic Aid; Prost-1. *Austria:* Digestodoron. *Brazil:* Calman; Calmiplan; Floriny; Pasalix; Passi Catha; Passiflorine. *Czech Republic:* Antirevmaticky Caj; Erkaltungstee; Valofyt Neo. *France:* Arkophytum; Mediflor Tisane Circulation du Sang No 12. *Germany:* Digestodoron; Dr Wiemanns Rheumatonikum. *Italy:* Biothymus DS; Biothymus DS; Bodyguard; Donalg; Influ-Zinc; Nevril; Passiflorine. *Malaysia:* Celery Plus. *Mexico:* Ifupasil. *Portugal:* Neurocardol. *South Africa:* Digestodoron. *Spain:*

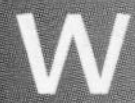

Dolosul; Jaquesor; Mesatil; Natusor Harpagosinol; Natusor Jaquesan. *Switzerland:* Dragees antirhumatismales; Strath Gouttes Rhumatisme; Tisane antirhumatismale. *UK:* Bio-Strath Willow Formula; Gerard House Reumalex; Herbal Pain Relief; Roberts Black Willow Compound Tablets; St Johnswort Compound. *Venezuela:* Passiflorum.

References

1 Meier B *et al*. Identifikation und Bestimmung von je acht Phenolglykosiden in *Salix purpurea* und *Salix daphnoides* mit moderner HPLC. *Pharm Acta Helv* 1985; 60: 269–274.
2 Meier B *et al*. Pharmaceutical aspects of the use of willows in herbal remedies. *Planta Med* 1988: 54: 559–560.
3 Karl C *et al*. Flavonoide aus *Salix alba*, die Struktur des terniflorins und eines Weiteren Acylflavonoides. *Phytochemistry* 1976; 15: 1084–1085.
4 Albrecht M *et al*. Anti-inflammatory activity of flavonol glycosides and salicin derivatives from the leaves of *Populus tremuloides*. *Planta Med* 1990; 56: 660.
5 Meier B, Liebi M. Salicinhaltige pflanzliche Arzneimittel-Überlegungen zu wirksamkeit und unbedenklichkeit. *Z Phytother* 1990; 11: 50–58.
6 Julkunen-Tiitto R, Meier B. The enzymatic decomposition of salicin and its derivatives obtained from salicaceae species. *J Nat Prod* 1992; 55: 1204–1212.
7 Schmid B *et al*. Efficacy and tolerability of a standardized willow bark extract in patients with osteoarthritis: randomized placebo-controlled, double blind clinical trial. *Phytother Res* 2001; 15: 344–350.
8 Baker S, Thomas PS. Herbal medicine precipitating massive haemolysis. *Lancet* 1987; i: 1039–1040.

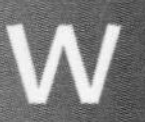

Witch Hazel

Summary and Pharmaceutical Comment

Witch hazel is characterised by its tannin constituents and astringent properties. The documented herbal uses are related to these astringent properties. There is limited evidence from clinical studies to indicate that witch hazel used topically is effective in the treatment of haemorrhoids, but its use in the treatment of eczema and dermatitis is more controversial. There are no known problems associated with the use of topical preparations of witch hazel during pregnancy and lactation.

Species (Family)

Hamamelis virginiana L. (Hamamelidaceae)

Synonym(s)

Hamamelis, Virginian Witch Hazel, Witchazel

Part(s) Used

Bark, leaf

Pharmacopoeial and Other Monographs

BHP 1996[G9]
BP 2007[G84]
Complete German Commission E[G3]
ESCOP 2003[G76]
Martindale 35th edition[G85]
Ph Eur 2007[G81]
USP29/NF24[G86]

Legal Category (Licensed Products)

GSL[G37]

Constituents

The following is compiled from several sources, including Reference 1 and General References G2 and G52.

Flavonoids (leaf) Flavonols (e.g. kaempferol, quercetin) and their glycosides including astragalin, quercitrin, afzelin and myricitrin.

Tannins, catechins Pharmacopoeial standard, not less than 3%.[G81, G84] Hamamelitannin (hydrolysable), lesser amounts of condensed tannins (bark). (+)-catechin, (+)-gallocatechin, (−)-epicatechingallate, (−)-epigallocatechingallate, proanthocyanidin oligomers of cyanidin and delphinidin type.

Volatile oils About 0.5%. Hexen-2-ol, hexenol, α- and β-ionones, eugenol, safrole and sesquiterpenes.

Other constituents Fixed oil (about 0.6%), resin (hamamelin, hamamamelitannin), wax, saponins, choline, free gallic acid and free hamamelose.

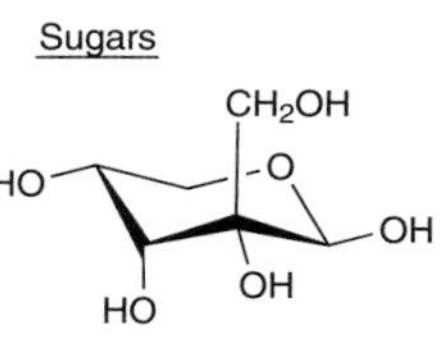

Figure 1 Selected constituents of witch hazel.

Food Use

Witch hazel is listed by the Council of Europe as a natural source of food flavouring (category N3). This category indicates that there is insufficient information available for an adequate assessment of potential toxicity.[G16]

Herbal Use

Witch hazel is stated to possess astringent, antihaemorrhagic and anti-inflammatory properties. Traditionally, it has been used for diarrhoea, mucous colitis, haemorrhoids, haematemesis, haemoptysis, and externally for external haemorrhoids, bruises and localised inflamed swellings. The German Commission E approved use for minor skin injuries, local inflammation of skin and mucous membranes, haemorrhoids and varicose veins.[G3]

Dosage

Dosages for oral (unless otherwise stated) administration (adults) for traditional uses recommended in older and contemporary standard herbal and pharmaceutical reference texts are given

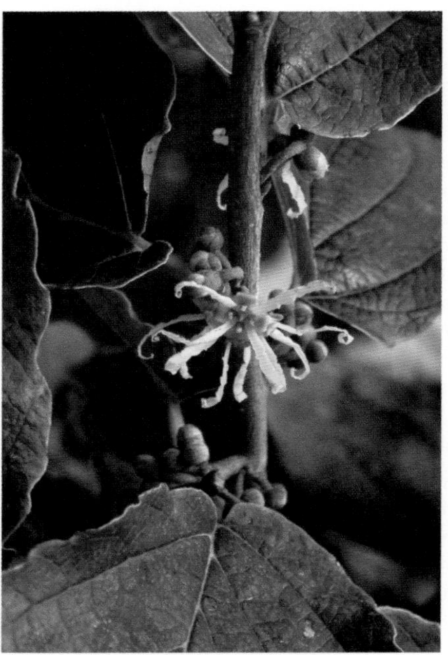

Figure 2 Witch hazel (*Hamamelis virginiana*).

W

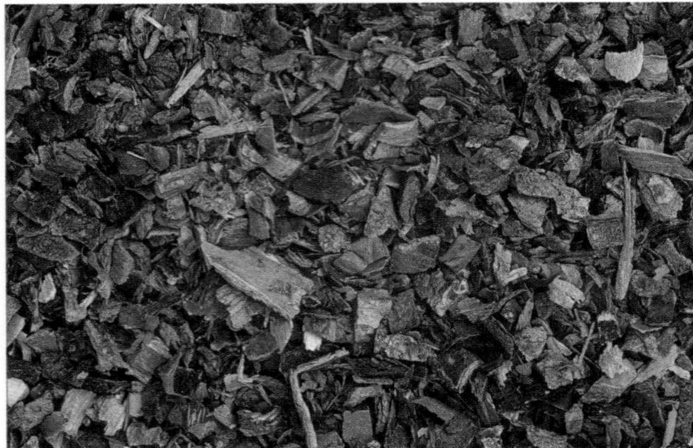

Figure 3 Witch hazel – dried drug substance (bark).

below. While doses for oral administration are given in older literature, modern use of witch hazel is by topical application.

Dried leaves 2 g as an infusion three times daily.[G6]

Hamamelis Liquid Extract (BPC 1973) 2–4 mL (1 : 1 in 45% alcohol) three times daily.[G6]

Hamamelis Water (BPC 1973) for local application, undiluted or 1 : 3 dilution for external use.[G3]

Decoction 5–10 g in 250 mL water for compresses.[G3]

Pharmacological Actions

In vitro and animal studies

Witch hazel is known to possess astringent and haemostatic properties, which have been attributed to the tannin constituents. Vasoconstriction was reduced in the hindquarters of rabbits when arteries were perfused with aqueous or ethanolic extracts of witch hazel leaf. A 70% ethanolic extract of leaf (1 : 5, 200 mg/kg, administered orally) significantly inhibited the chronic phase of carrageenan-induced rat paw oedema over a period of 19 days, compared with control ($p < 0.05$).[2] An aqueous ethanolic extract of witch hazel bark yielded a fraction rich in polymeric proanthocyanins after ultracentrifugation.[3] This fraction was significantly active against herpes simplex virus type 1 (HSV-1). It also showed radical scavenging properties, inhibited β-glucosidase and human leukocyte elastase activity, and was active in the croton oil ear oedema test in mice. In other studies, 3-O-galloyl-epicatechin-(4β,8)-catechin, a catechin oligomer and hamamelitannin isolated from witch hazel bark had IC_{50} values of 6.6, 8.8 and 1.0 μmol/L, respectively, for inhibition of 5-lipoxygenase.[4] The oligomer was active in the microsomal lyso-PAF:acetyl-CoA-acetyltransferase inhibition assay, with an IC_{50} value of 9.4 μmol/L, whereas hamamelitannin was inactive.[4]

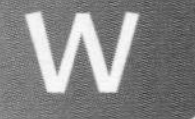

Clinical studies

Robust clinical research assessing the effects of witch hazel is limited and rigorous randomised clinical trials are required. A double-blind, controlled trial involving 90 patients with haemorrhoids compared the effects of witch hazel bark salve with those of other salves. Witch hazel was reported to be superior in relief of symptoms.[G50]

In a study involving 30 volunteers who received topical applications of a hydroglycolic extract of witch hazel leaf, skin temperature was significantly reduced, compared with baseline values. This was interpreted as a possible vasoconstrictor effect of witch hazel.[G52] The effects of an after-sun lotion containing 10% hamamelis distillate were assessed in 30 healthy volunteers using a modified UV-B erythema test for inflammation.[5] It was reported that erythema suppression ranged from 20% at seven hours to 27% at 48 hours.

In a two-week, randomised, double-blind trial, 72 patients with moderately severe eczema were treated with either a hamamelis distillate cream (5.35 g distillate with 0.64 g ketone/100 g), hydrocortisone cream 0.5%, or drug-free cream.[6] All three treatments significantly reduced itching, erythema and scaling after one week. Hydrocortisone cream was more effective than hamamelis cream.

Several clinical studies of witch hazel in the treatment of eczema have been reviewed.[G50] A double-blind, placebo-controlled trial of witch hazel salve (25% water distillate from leaf) involving 80 patients with toxic and degenerative eczema and 31 patients with endogenous eczema found that atopic dermatitis responded to the treatment to a greater extent than to placebo, but that there was no significant effect on primary irritant contact dermatitis. An uncontrolled study involving 22 patients with atopic eczema who were treated with witch hazel (4 g leaf provided 25 mL distillate/100 g salve) applied to affected arms over a three-week period reported improvements in symptoms, compared with baseline values.[G50] Uncontrolled studies provide preliminary data only and the observed effects cannot be attributed definitively to witch hazel. An uncontrolled study involving 37 patients treated with a witch hazel leaf cream twice daily for two weeks reported improvements in eczema and neurodermatitis.

Side-effects, Toxicity

The volatile oil contains safrole, a known carcinogen (*see* Sassafras), but in amounts too small to cause concern. Stomach irritation may occur in susceptible patients after oral treatment. Four of 1032 patients tested reacted to an ointment containing 25% witch hazel extract, but two of these patients were sensitive to wool fat in the ointment base.[G50]

Contra-indications, Warnings

None documented for witch hazel. In view of the tannin constituents, excessive ingestion of witch hazel is not recommended.

Pregnancy and lactation In view of the lack of information on the safety of witch hazel preparations administered orally, their use during pregnancy and lactation should be avoided. There are no known problems associated with topical use of witch hazel during pregnancy and lactation.

Preparations

Proprietary single-ingredient preparations

Australia: Optrex Original; Witch Doctor. *Austria:* Hametum. *Canada:* Optrex. *Chile:* Sperti Preparacion H Clear Gel. *France:* Optrex. *Germany:* Hamasana; Hametum; Posterine; Venoplant top. *Italy:* Acqua Virginiana; Derminiol; Optrex. *Malaysia:* Optrex. *Mexico:* Tia Puppy. *New Zealand:* Optrex. *Singapore:* Optrex. *Spain:* Derminiol; Hametol; Hemo Derminiol; Optrex. *Switzerland:* Mavena Anal-Gen; Optrex. *Thai-*

land: Optrex. *UK:* Optrex; Preparation H Clear Gel; Witch Doctor; Witch Sunsore. *USA:* A-E-R; Neutrogena Drying.

Proprietary multi-ingredient preparations

Argentina: Domuderm; Ecnagel; Esculeol P; Lavandula Oligoplex; Manzan; Venoful; VNS 45. *Australia:* Anusol; Bioglan Cirflo; Gentlees; Hemocane; Optrex; Proflo. *Austria:* Arnicet; Inotyol; Inotyol; Mirfulan; Sulgan 99; Sulgan 99; Tampositorien mit Belladonna. *Belgium:* Rectovasol. *Brazil:* Bromidrastina; Hemodotti; Hemorroidex; Malvatricin Natural Organic; Manolio; Mirorroidin; Proctosan; Supositorio Hamamelis Composto; Varizol; Varizol; Visionom. *Canada:* Onrectal; Penaten; Preparation H Cooling Gel; Tucks. *Chile:* Proctoplex. *Czech Republic:* Aviril H. *France:* Aphloine P; Climaxol; Ekseme; Evarose; Fluon; HEC; Histo-Fluine P; Jouvence de l'Abbe Soury; Jouvence de l'Abbe Soury; Jouvence de l'Abbe Soury; Keracnyl eau nettoyante; Mediflor Tisane Circulation du Sang No 12; Ophtalmine; Pastilles Monleon; Phlebosedol; Phytomelis; Veinostase. *Germany:* Aescusan; Chlorophyllin Salbe "Schuh"; Eulatin NN; Leukona-Wundsalbe; Mirfulan; Sagittaproct; Sanaderm; Trauma-cyl; Varicylum-S; Weleda Hamorrhoidalzapfchen. *Israel:* Aforinol; Derma Care; Inotyol. *Italy:* Centella Complex; Centella Complex; Centeril H; Centeril H; Decon Ovuli; Dermilia Flebozin; Dermitina; Dermoprolyn; Eulux; Ginoxil Ecoschiuma; Intim; Iridil; Lycia Luminique; Nevril; Proctopure; Sacnel; Salviette H; Steril Zeta; Varicogel; Venactive; Venoplus. *Mexico:* Almodin; Prespir; Supranettes Naturalag. *New Zealand:* Lacto Calamine; Optrex Red-Eye Relief. *Portugal:* Hemofissural. *South Africa:* Lotio Pruni Comp cum Cupro; Stibium Comp. *Singapore:* Stop-Itch Plus. *Spain:* Banoftal; Ojosbel; Roidhemo; Ruscimel; Solucion Schoum; Venofit. *Switzerland:* Collypan; Euproctol N; Haemocortin; Haemolan; HEC; Mavena Proctal-Gen; Oculosan; Optrex compresses; Tendro. *Thailand:* Opplin. *UK:* Adiantine; Eye Dew; Heemex; Lacto Calamine; Lacto Calamine; Modern Herbals Pile; Optrex Red Eyes; Swarm; Tea Tree & Witch Hazel Cream; Varicose Ointment; Vital Eyes. *USA:* Clearasil Double Clear; Preparation H Cooling Gel; Succus Cineraria Maritima; Tucks. *Venezuela:* Biomicovo; Camolyn; Supranettes.

References

1 Zeylstra H. *Hamamelis virginiana*. *Br J Phytother* 1998; 5: 23–28.

2 Duwiejua M *et al*. Anti-inflammatory activity of *Polygonum bistorta*, *Guaiacum officinale* and *Hamamelis virginiana* in rats. *J Pharm Pharmacol* 1994; 46: 286–290.

3 Erdelmeier CAJ *et al*. Antiviral and antiphlogistic activities of *Hamamelis virginiana*. *Planta Med* 1996; 62: 241–245.

4 Hartisch C *et al*. Dual inhibitory activities of tannins from *Hamamelis virginiana* and related polyphenols on 5-lipoxygenase and lyso-PAF: acetyl-CoA acetyltransferase. *Planta Med* 1997; 63: 106–110.

5 Hughes-Formella BJ *et al*. Anti-inflammatory effect of hamamelis lotion in a UVB erythema test. *Dermatology* 1998; 196: 316–322.

6 Korting HC *et al*. Comparative efficacy of hamamelis distillate and hydrocortisone cream in atopic eczema. *Eur J Clin Pharmacol* 1995; 48: 461–465.

Yarrow

Summary and Pharmaceutical Comment

The chemistry of yarrow is well-documented although there has been some disagreement over the major component in the volatile oil. Various pharmacological actions have been reported in animal studies which support many of the reputed herbal uses, although robust clinical research assessing the efficacy and safety of yarrow is limited. Yarrow is considered to be relatively non-toxic although allergic reactions in susceptible individuals have been documented. The volatile oil is contra-indicated in pregnancy and in view of the lack of safety information, use of yarrow should be avoided during lactation.[G58]

Species (Family)

Achillea millefolium L. (Asteraceae/Compositae)

Synonym(s)

Milfoil, Millefolium

Part(s) Used

Flowerhead

Pharmacopoeial and Other Monographs

BHC 1992[G6]
BHP 1996[G9]
BP 2007[G84]
Complete German Commission E[G3]
Martindale 35th edition[G85]
Ph Eur 2007[G81]

Legal Category (Licensed Products)

GSL[G37]

Constituents

The following is compiled from several sources, including General References G2 and G6.

Acids Amino acids (e.g. alanine, aspartic acid, glutamic acid, histidine, leucine, lysine, proline, valine),[1,2] fatty acids (e.g. linoleic, myristic, oleic, palmitic, stearic),[3,4] and others including ascorbic acid,[5] caffeic acid,[6] folic acid,[5] salicylic acid and succinic acid.[1]

Alkaloids/bases Betonicine and stachydrine (pyrrolidine),[1,7] trigonelline (pyridine),[1,7] betaine and choline (bases).[1,7] Uncharacterised alkaloids include achiceine, achilleine[8] (possible synonym for L-betonicine), which is stated to yield achilletine[7] on alkaline hydrolysis, and moscatine/moschatine,[7] stated to be an ill-defined glucoalkaloid.

Flavonoids Predominantly flavone glycosides apigenin- and luteolin-7-glycosides,[9] with lesser quantities of artemetin, casticin, 5-hydroxy-3,6,7,4-tetramethoxyflavone and isorhamnetin.[6] Rutin (a flavonol glycoside).[5]

Tannins Condensed and hydrolysable,[3,10] with glucose as the carbohydrate component of the latter[2]

Volatile oils Numerous identified components include borneol, bornyl acetate (trace), camphor, 1,8-cineole, eucalyptol, limonene, sabinene, terpinen-4-ol, terpineol and α-thujone (monoterpenes), caryophyllene (a sesquiterpene), achillicin, achillin, millefin and millefolide (sesquiterpene lactones), azulene and chamazulene (sesquiterpene lactone- derived) and isoartemisia ketone. The relative composition of the components varies greatly between *Achillea* species, especially the azulene content. Azulene has been reported as the major component.[11] However, true yarrow (*A. millefolium*) is thought to be hexaploid and azulene-free, whereas closely related species, such as *Achillea lanulosa* Nutt. and *Achillea collina* Becker, are tetraploid and contain up to 50% azulene in their volatile oil.[5,10,11] It is possible that the tetraploid

Monoterpenes

linalool

camphor

Sesquiterpenes

chamazulene

achillicin

leukodin

millefin

Acetylenes

$CH_3-(C{\equiv}C)_3-CH{=}CH-CH-CH-CH{=}CH_2$ pontica epoxide

$CH_3-(C{\equiv}C)_3-CH{=}CHCO.CH_3$ matricaria ester

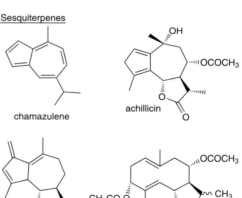

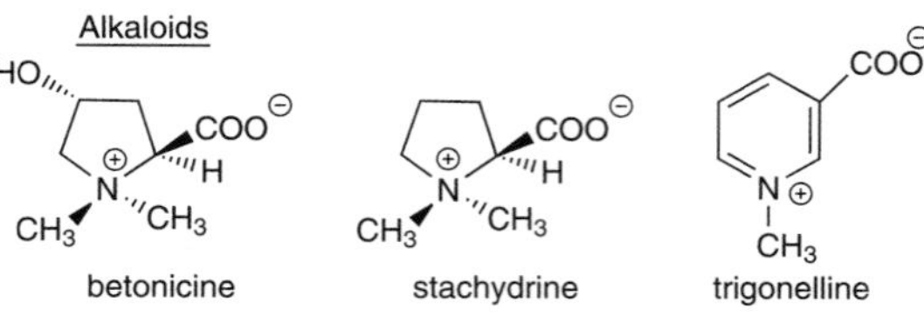

Figure 1 Selected constituents of yarrow.

species may be supplied for *A. millefolium*. The azulenes are not present in the fresh herb: they are formed as artefacts during steam distillation of the oil, from unstable precursors called proazulenes (e.g. achillin and achillicin), via equally unstable azulene–carboxylic acid intermediates.[12]

Other constituents Unknown cyanogenetic compound,[13] sugars including arabinose, galactose, dextrose, dulcitol, glucose, inositol, maltose, mannitol and sucrose.[1,2]

Food Use

Yarrow is listed by the Council of Europe as a natural source of food flavouring (herb, flowers, essential oil and other preparations: category 4, with limits on camphor, eucalyptol and thujone) (*see* Appendix 3).[G17] Previously, in the USA, yarrow was only approved for use in alcoholic beverages, and the finished product had to be thujone free.[G41]

Herbal Use

Yarrow is stated to possess diaphoretic, antipyretic, hypotensive, astringent, diuretic and urinary antiseptic properties. Traditionally, it has been used for bruises, swellings, strains, fevers, common cold, essential hypertension, amenorrhoea, dysentery, diarrhoea, and specifically for thrombotic conditions with hypertension, including cerebral and coronary thromboses.[G2, G6, G7, G8, G64]

Dosage

Dosages for oral administration (adults) for traditional uses recommended in standard herbal reference texts are given below.

Dried herb 2–4 g as an infusion three times daily.[G6, G7]

Liquid extract 2–4 mL (1 : 1 in 25% alcohol) three times daily.[G6, G7]

Tincture 2–4 mL (1 : 5 in 45% alcohol) three times daily.[G6, G7]

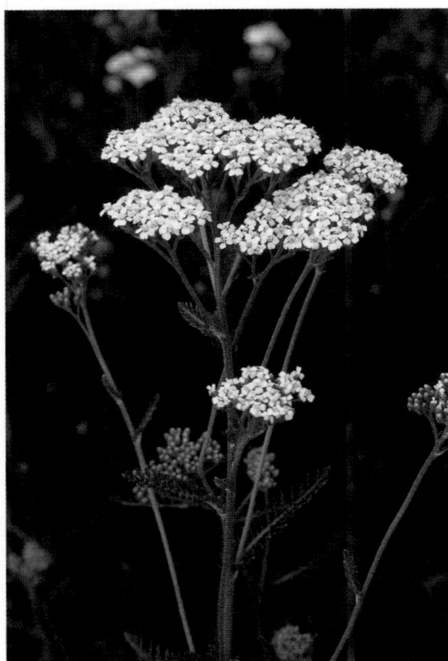

Figure 2 Yarrow (*Achillea millefolium*).

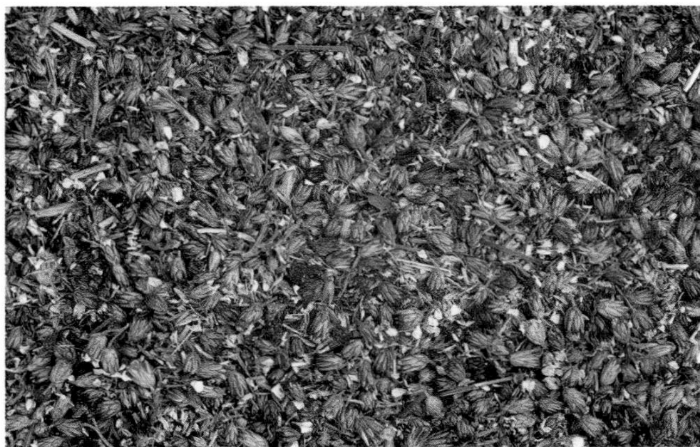

Figure 3 Yarrow – dried drug substance (flowerhead).

Pharmacological Actions

Some activities documented for yarrow are associated with the azulene constituents, although it is now thought that azulene is absent from true yarrow (*see* Constituents). It is possible that some of the documented pharmacological studies have used *Achillea* species other than *A. millefolium*.[14]

In vitro and animal studies

Anti-inflammatory activity has been documented for an aqueous extract of yarrow using mouse[15] and rat[16] paw oedema models, with inflammation induced by yeast[15] and various inflammatory substances,[16] including histamine, carrageenan and prostaglandin. In mouse studies, the active fraction was reported as a series of protein–carbohydrate complexes. Topical anti-inflammatory activity in rabbits has also been documented for the aqueous extract.[15] In general, anti-inflammatory properties are associated with azulenes (*see* Chamomile, German). Anti-inflammatory activity has been described for the azulene components documented for the volatile oil of yarrow.[5]

A diuretic effect was also noted in mice administered an aqueous extract of yarrow,[15] but only at a dose more than double that required for an anti-inflammatory effect.[15] Terpinen-4-ol, the diuretic principle in juniper, has been reported as a component of yarrow volatile oil.

CNS-depressant activity has been documented for the volatile oil: a dose of 300 mg/kg decreased the spontaneous activity of mice and lowered the body temperature of rats. In addition, 300–600 mg/kg doses inhibited pentetrazole-induced convulsions and prolonged sleep induced by a barbiturate preparation.[17]

Moderate antibacterial activity has been documented for an ethanolic extract of the herb against *Staphylococcus aureus*, *Bacillus subtilis*, *Mycobacterium smegmatis*, *Escherichia coli*, *Shigella sonnei* and *Shigella flexneri*.[18] Antimicrobial properties have been documented for the sesquiterpene lactone fraction.[5]

Achilleine 0.5 g/kg by intravenous injection has been noted to decrease the blood clotting time in rabbits by 32%.[8] The haemostatic action persisted for 45 minutes with no observable toxic effects.

Antispasmodic activity on the isolated rabbit intestine has been documented for a flavonoid-containing fraction of yarrow.[9] Antispasmodic activity is generally associated with azulene constituents (*see* Chamomile, German).

Antipyretic and hypotensive actions have been reported for the basic fraction (alkaloid/base);[G41] the sesquiterpene lactone

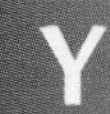

fraction is stated to possess cytotoxic activities,[5] although no further details were located. Tannins are known to possess astringent activity.

Clinical studies

There is a lack of clinical research assessing the effects of yarrow and rigorous randomised controlled clinical trials are required.

Side-effects, Toxicity

Clinical data

Allergic reactions to yarrow (e.g. dermatitis) have been documented, and positive patch tests have been produced in individuals sensitised to other plants.[5, G33, G51] An instance of yarrow tea causing a generalised eruption in a sensitised individual was reported in 1929. The allergenic properties of some sesquiterpene lactones are well documented, although none of those present in yarrow are recognised sensitisers.[G51] Yarrow has been suspected of being a photosensitiser, although extracts have been reported to lack phototoxicity and to be devoid of psoralens, compounds with known photosensitising properties.[G51]

Preclinical data

Yarrow is considered to be of low toxicity. In mice LD_{50} values have been reported of up to 3.65 g/kg (by mouth), 3.1 g/kg (by intraperitoneal injection), and greater than or equal to 1 g/kg (by subcutaneous injection).[15, 17] In rats, an LD_{50} (subcutaneous injection) has been recorded as 16.86 g/kg, with corresponding LD_0 and LD_{100} values reported as 12 and 20 g/kg, respectively.[16] By comparison, an ED_{25} for anti-inflammatory activity has been estimated as about 0.43 g/kg.[16]

The known toxic principle thujone has been documented as a minor component of yarrow volatile oil, although concentrations present are probably too low to represent a risk to human health.

A single report of animal poisoning has been documented for yarrow in which a calf died following the ingestion of a single plant.[5] No additional reports of animal toxicity were located.

Contra-indications, Warnings

Yarrow may cause an allergic reaction in sensitive individuals, especially those with an existing hypersensitivity to other members of the Asteraceae/ Compositae.[19]

Drug interactions None documented. However, the potential for preparations of yarrow to interact with other medicines administered concurrently, particularly those with similar or opposing effects, should be considered. There is limited evidence from preclinical studies that achilleine, a constituent of yarrow, has anticoagulant activity, although the clinical relevance of this, if any is not clear.

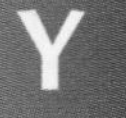

Pregnancy and lactation Yarrow should not be taken during pregnancy. It is reputed to be an abortifacient and to affect the menstrual cycle,[G30] and the volatile oil contains trace amounts (0.3%) of the abortifacient principle thujone. In view of the lack of safety information use of yarrow should be avoided during lactation.

Preparations

Proprietary single-ingredient preparations

Czech Republic: Gallentee; Nat Rebricku; Rebrickovy Caj, Rebrickova Nat. *Mexico:* Blancaler.

Proprietary multi-ingredient preparations

Australia: Flavons. *Austria:* Abfuhrtee St Severin; Amersan; Gallen- und Lebertee St Severin; Mariazeller; Menodoron. *Canada:* Original Herb Cough Drops. *Czech Republic:* Amersan; Cajova Smes pri Redukcni Diete; Cicaderma; Hemoral; Hertz- und Kreislauftee; Perospir; Projimava; Species Urologicae Planta; Stomatosan; Ungolen; Zaludecni Cajova Smes. *France:* Gonaxine; Tisane Hepatique de Hoerdt. *Germany:* Alasenn; Amara-Tropfen; Floradix Multipretten N; Gallexier; Kamillan Plus; Sedovent; Stomachysat N; Tonsilgon. *Hungary:* Hemorid; Noditran. *Italy:* Forticrin; Lozione Same Urto; Pik Gel. *Portugal:* Cicaderma; Fade Cream. *Russia:* Liv 52 (Лив 52); Liv 52 (Лив 52); Original Grosser Bittner Balsam (Оригинальный Большой Бальзам Биттнера); Tonsilgon N (Тонзилгон Н). *South Africa:* Amara; Clairo; Menodoron. *Spain:* Jaquesor; Menstrunat; Natusor Circusil; Natusor Gastrolen; Natusor Jaquesan. *Switzerland:* Gastrosan; Kernosan Heidelberger Poudre; Pommade au Baume; Tisane hepatique et biliaire; Tisane pour l'estomac. *UK:* Catarrh-eeze; Drops of Life Tablets; Rheumatic Pain Remedy; Rutin Compound Tablets; Tabritis; Tabritis Tablets; Wellwoman.

References

1 Ivanov Ch, Yankov L. Composition of *Achillea millefolium*. I. Preparation of the total extracts and composition of the part of the alcoholic extracts soluble in alcohol and water. *God Vissh Khimikotekhnol Inst Sofia* 1967; 14: 195–222.
2 Ivanov Ch, Yankov L. Composition of *Achillea millefolium*. III. Composition of the parts soluble in water and insoluble in alcohol. *God Vissh Khimikotekhnol Inst Sofia* 1967; 14: 223–241.
3 Ivanov Ch, Yankov L. Composition of *Achillea millefolium*. III. Composition of the acidic, water-insoluble part of the alcoholic extract. *God Vissh Khimikotekhnol Inst Sofia* 1967; 14: 61–72.
4 Ivanov Ch, Yankov L. Composition of *Achillea millefolium*. V. Composition and structure of the components of neutral fraction insoluble in the aqueous part of the alcoholic extract. *God Vissh Khimikotekhnol Inst Sofia* 1967; 14: 73–101.
5 Chandler RF *et al*. Ethnobotany and phytochemistry of yarrow, *Achillea millefolium*, Compositae. *Economic Bot* 1982; 36: 203–223.
6 Falk AJ *et al*. Isolation and identification of three new flavones from *Achillea millefolium* L. *J Pharm Sci* 1975; 64: 1838–1842.
7 Zirvi KA, Ikram M. Alkaloids of some of the plants of the Compositae. *Pakistan J Sci Ind Res* 1975; 18: 93–101.
8 Miller FM, Chow LM. Alkaloids of *Achillea millefolium* L. I. Isolation and characterization of Achilleine. *J Am Chem Soc* 1954; 76: 1353–1354.
9 Hoerhammer L. Flavone concentration of medical plants with regard to their spasmolytic action. *Congr Sci Farm Conf Commun 21st Pisa* 1961; 578–588.
10 Falk AJ *et al*. The constituents of the essential oil from *Achillea millefolium* L. *Lloydia* 1974; 37: 598–602.
11 Haggag MY *et al*. Thin layer and gas-chromatographic studies on the essential oil from *Achillea millefolium*. *Planta Med* 1975; 27: 361–366.
12 Sticher O. Plant mono-, di- and sesquiterpenoids with pharmacological and therapeutical activity. In: Wagner H, Wolff P, eds. *New Natural Products with Pharmacological Biological or Therapeutical Activity*. Berlin: Springer Verlag, 1977: 137–176.
13 Seigler DS. Plants of the Northeastern United States that produce cyanogenic compounds. *Economic Bot* 1976; 30: 395–407.

14 Chandler F. Vindication of maritime Indian herbal remedies. *J Ethnopharmacol* 1983; 9: 323–327.
15 Goldberg AS *et al*. Isolation of anti-inflammatory principles from *Achillea millefolium* (Compositae). *J Pharm Sci* 1969; 58: 938–941.
16 Shipochliev T, Fournadjiev G. Spectrum of the antiinflammatory effect of *Arctostaphylos uva ursi* and *Achilea millefolium*, L. *Probl Vutr Med* 1984; 12: 99–107.
17 Kudrzycka-Bieloszabska FW, Glowniak K. Pharmacodynamic properties of oleum chamomillae and oleum millefolii. *Diss Pharm Pharmacol* 1966; 18: 449–454.
18 Moskalenko SA. Preliminary screening of far-Eastern ethnomedicinal plants for antibacterial activity. *J Ethnopharmacol* 1986; 15: 231–259.
19 Mathias CGT *et al*. Plant dermatitis – patch test results (1975–78). Note on Juniperus extract. *Contact Dermatitis* 1979; 5: 336.

Yellow Dock

Summary and Pharmaceutical Comment

Limited chemical, pharmacological, and toxicity information is available for yellow dock. Documented anthraquinone constituents justify the reputed purgative action. However, there is a lack of robust clinical research assessing the efficacy and safety of yellow dock. Although the purgative effect of yellow dock is reputed to be gentle, the use of unstandardised anthraquinone-containing preparations should be avoided since their pharmacological effect is unpredictable and may cause abdominal cramp and diarrhoea. The use of yellow dock should be avoided during pregnancy and lactation.

Species (Family)

Rumex crispus L. (Polygonaceae)

Synonym(s)

Curled Dock, *Rumex odontocarpus* I. Sandór

Part(s) Used

Root

Pharmacopoeial and Other Monographs

BHP 1983[G7]
Martindale 35th edition[G85]

Legal Category (Licensed Products)

GSL[G37]

Constituents

Anthraquinones 2–4%. Chrysophanol, emodin, nepodin, physcion (aglycones).[1–3]

Tannins Catechol 5% (condensed-type).

Other plants parts The plant constituents documented include oxalic acid, oxalates, chrysophanic acid, emodin, tannin, and a complex volatile oil (more than 60 components identified).[4, G51]

Anthraquinones

	R^1	R^2
chrysophanol	H	CH_3
aloe-emodin	H	CH_2OH
emodin	OH	CH_3
physcion	OCH_3	CH_3

Figure 1 Selected constituents of yellow dock.

Food Use

Yellow dock is not used in foods.

Herbal Use

Yellow dock is stated to possess gentle purgative and cholagogue properties. Traditionally, it has been used for chronic skin disease, obstructive jaundice, constipation, and specifically for psoriasis with constipation.[G7, G64]

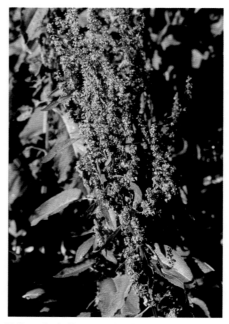

Figure 2 Yellow dock (*Rumex crispus*).

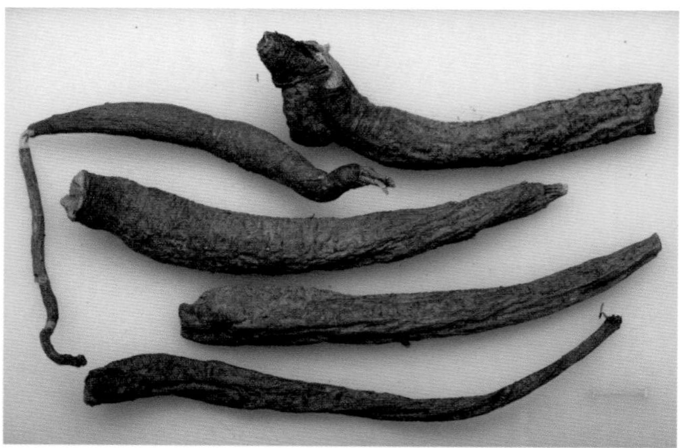

Figure 3 Yellow dock – dried drug substance (root).

Dosage

Dosages for oral administration (adults) for traditional uses recommended in standard herbal reference texts are given below.

Dried root 2–4 g as a decoction three times daily.[(G7)]

Liquid extract 2–4 mL (1 : 1 in 25% alcohol) three times daily.[(G7)]

Tincture 1–2 mL (1 : 5 in 45% alcohol) three times daily.[(G7)]

Pharmacological Actions

In vitro and animal studies

None documented for the root. Slight antibacterial activity has been reported for herb extracts, which exhibited activity towards both Gram-positive (*Staphylococcus aureus*, *Mycobacterium smegmatis*) and Gram-negative (*Escherichia coli*, *Shigella sonnei*, *Shigella flexneri*) organisms.[(4)]

Clinical studies

There is a lack of clinical research assessing the effects of yellow dock and rigorous randomised controlled clinical trials are required.

Side-effects, Toxicity

Clinical data

No side-effects documented. However, there is a lack of clinical safety and toxicity data for yellow dock and further investigation of these aspects is required.. In view of the documented anthraquinone constituents, side-effects generally associated with laxatives are also applicable to yellow dock. Overuse may cause abdominal cramps and diarrhoea, and prolonged use may lead to intestinal atrophy and hypokalaemia.

Preclinical data

Dermatitis has been reported in livestock following the ingestion of plant material in large quantities.[(G51)] Oxalic acid is known to be a toxic plant acid that forms insoluble calcium salts which cause a disturbance in calcium concentrations and hence affect the blood coagulation mechanism.[(G33)]

Contra-indications, Warnings

Warnings generally associated with stimulant laxatives are also applicable to yellow dock (*see* Senna). Therefore, yellow dock should not be taken when there is existing intestinal obstruction, and excessive use should be avoided (*see* Side-effects, Toxicity).

Drug interactions None documented. However, the potential for preparations of yellow dock to interact with other medicines administered concurrently, particularly those with similar or opposing effects, should be considered. Drug interactions listed for other stimulant laxatives are applicable to yellow dock (*see* Senna).

Pregnancy and lactation In general, unstandardised stimulant laxatives are not recommended for use during pregnancy. The use of yellow dock should therefore be avoided in favour of a standardised preparation that is recommended for the treatment of constipation during pregnancy. The use of yellow dock by breastfeeding women should also be avoided, since it has been documented that anthraquinones can be secreted into the breast milk (*see* Senna).

Preparations

Proprietary multi-ingredient preparations

Australia: Colax; Colax; Dermaco; Herbal Cleanse; Trifolium Complex. *Canada:* Herborex. *UK:* Skin Eruptions Mixture.

References

1 de Siqueira NCS *et al*. Hydroxyanthraquinones in *Rumex crispus* L. (of southern Rio Grande). *Rev Cent Cienc Biomed* 1977; 5: 69–74.
2 Midiwo JO, Rukunga GM. Distribution of anthraquinone pigments in *Rumex* species of Kenya. *Phytochemistry* 1985; 24: 1390–1391.
3 Fairbairn JW, El-Muhtadi FJ. Chemotaxonomy of anthraquinones in *Rumex*. *Phytochemistry* 1972; 11: 263–268.
4 Miyazawa M, Kameoka H. Constituents of essential oil from *Rumex crispus*. *Yakugaku Zasshi* 1983; 32: 45–47.

Yucca

Summary and Pharmaceutical Comment

Limited phytochemical information is available for yucca, steroidal saponins being the only documented constituents. There is limited evidence from clinical studies that a yucca saponin extract has beneficial effects on certain symptoms of arthritis, such as pain and stiffness, and reduces blood pressure and serum triglyceride and cholesterol concentrations. However, robust clinical research assessing the efficacy and safety of yucca is lacking. The traditional use of yucca as a foodstuff would indicate it to be of low toxicity. However there is a lack of information on the safety of medicinal use of yucca. In view of this excessive use of yucca and use during pregnancy and lactation should be avoided.

Species (Family)

Various *Yucca* species (Asparagaceae) including
**Yucca schidigera* Roezl ex Ortgies
†*Yucca brevifolia* Engelm.
Yucca glauca Nutt.

Synonym(s)

*Mohave Yucca, *Yucca mohavensis* Sarg.
†Joshua Tree, *Yucca arborescens* Trel.

Part(s) Used

Whole plant

Pharmacopoeial and Other Monographs

Martindale 35th edition[G85]

Legal Category (Licensed Products)

Yucca is not listed in the GSL.

Constituents

Terpenoids Various saponins have been isolated from different *Yucca* species, including tigogenin and chlerogenin,[1] sarsasapogenin, markogenin, higogenin, neo-tigogenin, neo-gitogenin, hecogenin, gloriogenin, and diosgenin (trace)[2] and smilagenin.

Food Use

The yucca plant has been used traditionally as a major foodstuff by Indian tribes. Previously, in the USA, both *Y. schidigera* and *Y. brevifolia* have been approved for food use.[G41]

Herbal Use

Yucca has been used for the treatment of arthritis, diabetes and stomach disorders. Concentrated plant juice has been used topically to soothe painful joints.

Dosage

None documented.

Pharmacological Actions

In vitro and animal studies

Yucca saponin extract, from *Y. schidigera*, is reported to exhibit approximately half the haemolytic activity of commercial soap bark saponin.

Antitumour activity against B16 melanoma has been documented for a polysaccharide-containing extract of *Y. glauca*.[3] The extract was found to be inactive towards L1210 or P388 leukaemias.

Clinical studies

There is a lack of clinical research assessing the effects of yucca and rigorous randomised controlled clinical trials are required.

A saponin-containing yucca extract has been reported to reduce symptoms of swelling, pain and stiffness in approximately 75 of 150 arthritic patients given the extract in a double-blind study.[4] The onset of a positive response was found to vary from days to weeks or months. A saponin-containing yucca extract has also been documented to reduce blood pressure, abnormal triglyceride, and high cholesterol concentrations in a double-blind study involving 212 arthritic and hypertensive patients.[5] Optimum results were obtained in conjunction with diet and exercise. Yucca extracts have also been reported to provide relief from headaches and to improve circulation and gastrointestinal function.[4,5]

Side-effects, Toxicity

There is a lack of clinical and preclinical safety and toxicity data for yucca and further investigation of these aspects is required.

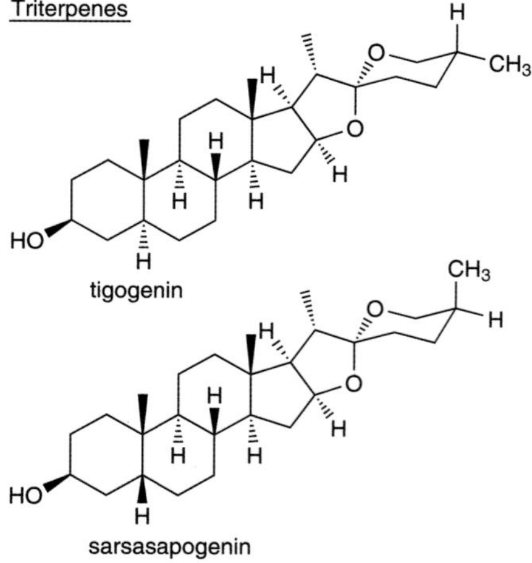

Figure 1 Selected constituents of yucca.

A saponin-containing yucca extract was given to more than 700 arthritic patients with no signs of toxicity documented.[4] The yucca saponins are regarded to be a safe food supplement since they are not thought to be absorbed from the gastrointestinal tract, thereby reducing the dangers of systemic haemolytic activity.[4]

Contra-indications, Warnings

Drug interactions None documented. However, the potential for preparations of yucca to interact with other medicines administered concurrently, particularly those with similar or opposing effects, should be considered.

Pregnancy and lactation In view of the lack of information on the constituents, pharmacology and toxicology of yucca, its use during pregnancy and lactation should be avoided.

Preparations

Proprietary multi-ingredient preparations

Australia: Prost-1. *Brazil:* Bronquiogem.

References

1 Dewidar AM, El-Munajjed D. The steroid sapogenin constituents of *Agave americana*, *A. variegata* and *Yucca gloriosa*. *Planta Med* 1970; 19: 87–91.
2 Stohs SJ *et al*. Steroidal sapogenins of *Yucca glauca* seeds. *Lloydia* 1973; 36: 443.
3 Ali MS *et al*. Isolation of antitumor polysaccharide fractions from *Yucca glauca* Nutt. (Liliaceae). *Growth* 1978; 42: 213–223.
4 Bingham R *et al*. Yucca plant saponin in the management of arthritis. *J Appl Nutr* 1975; 27: 45–51.
5 Bingham R *et al*. Yucca plant saponin in the treatment of hypertension and hypercholesterolemia. *J Appl Nutr* 1978; 30: 127–136.

Y

Appendix 1
Potential Drug–Herb Interactions

Until the emergence of reports of important interactions between St John's wort (*Hypericum perforatum* L.) and certain conventional drugs (*see* St John's Wort), very few interactions involving herbal products had been reported in the medical literature. Furthermore, there has been very little experimental and clinical research in this area.

The following list of *potential* drug–herb interactions has been compiled on the basis of known herbal constituents and their reported pharmacological actions. It should be emphasised that many drug interactions are harmless and many of those that are potentially harmful occur only in a small proportion of patients and may then vary in severity from patient to patient. Healthcare professionals should be alert to undeclared use of herbal medicines as a possible cause of unexplained toxicity or lack of effect of conventional medicines.

Suspected drug–herb interactions involving licensed or unlicensed herbal products should be reported to the regulatory authorities, as for any other suspected adverse reaction to herbal or 'conventional' medicines.

Table 1 Potential drug–herb interactions

Drug/therapeutic category affected	Herbal ingredients interacting	Possible effects
Gastrointestinal system		
Antacids, ulcer-healing drugs	Herbal ingredients irritant to gastrointestinal tract. *See* Appendix 2, Table 12	Exacerbation of symptoms. Risk of systemic side-effects
Antidiarrhoeal drugs	Herbal ingredients with laxative activity. *See* Appendix 2, Table 1	Antagonism
Laxatives	Herbal ingredients with laxative activity. *See* Appendix 2, Table 1	Potentiation; increased risk of side-effects
Cardiovascular system		
Cardiac glycosides	Cardioactive herbal ingredients. *See* Appendix 2, Table 2	Potentiation; increased risk of side-effects
	Herbal ingredients containing hydroxyanthracene laxatives. *See* Appendix 2, Table 1	Potentiation; increased risk of side-effects
	St John's wort	Risk of reduced therapeutic effect of digoxin
Diuretics	Herbal ingredients containing hydroxyanthracene laxatives. *See* Appendix 2, Table 1	Potentiation; increased risk of hypokalaemia
	Herbal ingredients with diuretic activity. *See* Appendix 2, Table 3	Potentiation; increased risk of hypokalaemia
	Herbal ingredients with hypotensive activity. *See* Appendix 2, Table 4	Difficulty in controlling diuresis; hypotension
Anti-arrhythmic activity	Herbal ingredients containing hydroxyanthracene laxatives. *See* Appendix 2, Table 1	Interference with existing therapy; increased risk of hypokalaemia
	Cardioactive herbal ingredients. *See* Appendix 2, Table 2	Interference/antagonism with existing therapy
	Herbal ingredients with diuretic activity. *See* Appendix 2, Table 3	Antagonism if hypokalaemia occurs
Beta-adrenoceptor blocking drugs	Cardioactive herbal ingredients. *See* Appendix 2, Table 2	Potential antagonism

table continues

Table 1 *continued*

Drug/therapeutic category affected	Herbal ingredients interacting	Possible effects
	Herbal ingredients with significant amine content or sympathomimetic activity. *See* Appendix 2, Table 15	Potential risk of severe hypertension
Antihypertensive therapy	Herbal ingredients with hypertensive activity. *See* Appendix 2, Table 4	Antagonism
	Herbal ingredients with mineralocorticoid activity *See* Appendix 2, Table 9	Antagonism
	Herbal ingredients with hypotensive activity. *See* Appendix 2, Table 4	Potentiation
	Herbal ingredients with significant amine content or sympathomimetic activity. *See* Appendix 2, Table 15	Antagonism
	Herbal ingredients with diuretic activity. *See* Appendix 2, Table 3	Risk of potentiation/ interference with existing therapy
Lipid-lowering drugs	Herbal ingredients with hypolipidaemic activity. *See* Appendix 2, Table 6	Additive effect
Nitrates and calcium-channel blockers	Cardioactive ingredients. *See* Appendix 2, Table 2	Interference with therapy
	Herbal ingredients with hypertensive activity. *See* Appendix 2, Table 4	Antagonism
	Herbal ingredients with anticholinergic activity	Reduced sublingual absorption of glyceryl trinitrate
Sympathomimetics	Herbal ingredients with significant sympathomimetic amine content. *See* Appendix 2, Table 15	Potentiation; increased risk of hypertension
	Herbal ingredients with hypertensive activity. *See* Appendix 2, Table 4	Increased risk of hypertension
	Herbal ingredients with hypotensive activity. *See* Appendix 2, Table 4	Antagonism
Anticoagulants	Herbal ingredients with coagulant/ anticoagulant activity. *See* Appendix 2, Table 5	Risk of antagonism or potentiation
	Herbal ingredients containing coumarins with anticoagulant activity. *See* Appendix 2, Table 16	Risk of potentiation
	Herbal ingredients with significant salicylate concentrations. *See* Appendix 2, Table 5	Risk of potentiation
	Cranberry juice	Raised INR reported in patients receiving warfarin
	Garlic	Raised INR reported in patients receiving warfarin
	Ginkgo	Antiplatelet activity; increased risk of bleeding, particularly in patients receiving warfarin and other anticoagulant or antiplatelet agents
	Horse-chestnut	Plasma protein binding
	St John's wort	Risk of reduced therapeutic effect of warfarin
Respiratory system		
	St John's wort	Risk of reduced therapeutic effect of theophylline
	Herbal ingredients that are potentially allergenic. *See* Appendix 2, Table 11	Risk of allergic reaction
Terfenadine	Cardioactive herbal ingredients. *See* Appendix 2, Table 2	May increase arrhythmogenic potential of terfenadine
	Herbal ingredients with diuretic activity. *See* Appendix 2, Table 3	Electrolyte imbalance may increase arrhythmogenic potential of terfenadine

Table 1 *continued*

Drug/therapeutic category affected	Herbal ingredients interacting	Possible effects
Allergic disorders	Herbal ingredients claimed to have sedative activity. *See* Appendix 2, Table 7	Potentiation of drowsiness associated with antihistamines
Central nervous system		
Hypnotics and anxiolytics	Herbal ingredients claimed to have sedative activity. *See* Appendix 2, Table 7	Potentiation
Antipsychotics	Herbal ingredients with diuretic activity. *See* Appendix 2, Table 3	Potentiation of lithium therapy; increased risk of toxicity; diuretics reported to reduce lithium clearance
	Herbal ingredients with anticholinergic activity	Risk of interference with therapy; anticholinergic drug reported to reduce plasma phenothiazine concentrations
	Evening primrose	Potential risk of seizures
Antidepressants	Herbal ingredients containing sympathomimetic amines. *See* Appendix 2, Table 15	Risk of hypertensive crisis with monoamine-oxidase inhibitors (MAOIs)
	Ginseng (Panax)	Suspected phenelzine interaction
	Herbal ingredients containing tryptophan	Risk of CNS excitation and confusional states with MAOIs
	White horehound	5-Hydroxytryptamine antagonism, *in vitro, in vivo*
	Herbal ingredients with sedative activity. *See* Appendix 2, Table 7	May potentiate sedative side-effects
	St John's wort	Risk of increased serotonergic effects in patients taking selective serotonin reuptake inhibitors (SSRIs)
Drugs used in nausea and vertigo	Herbal ingredients with sedative activity. *See* Appendix 2, Table 7	May potentiate sedative side-effects
	Herbal ingredients with anticholinergic activity	Antagonism
Analgesics	Herbal ingredients with diuretic activity. *See* Appendix 2, Table 3	Increased risk of toxicity with anti-inflammatory analgesics
	Herbal ingredients with corticosteroid activity. *See* Appendix 2, Table 9	Possible reduction in plasma-aspirin concentrations
	Herbal ingredients with sedative activity. *See* Appendix 2, Table 7	May potentiate sedative side-effects
	St John's wort	Risk of increased serotonergic effects, with possibility of increased risk of side-effects
Antiepileptics	Herbal ingredients with sedative activity. *See* Appendix 2, Table 7	May potentiate sedative side-effects
	Borage	May increase risk of seizure
	Evening primrose oil	May increase risk of seizure
	Sage	May increase risk of seizure
	Herbal ingredients with significant salicylate content. *See* Appendix 2, Table 5	Transient potentiation of phenytoin therapy may occur
	Herbal ingredients with significant folic acid content	Plasma phenytoin concentration may be reduced
	St John's wort	Risk of reduced therapeutic effect of anticonvulsants (carbamazepine, phenobarbitone, phenytoin)
Drugs for parkinsonism	Herbal ingredients with anticholinergic activity	Potentiation; increased risk of side-effects
	Herbal ingredients with cholinergic activity	Antagonism
Infections		
Antifungal drugs	Herbal ingredients with anticholinergic activity	Risk of reduced absorption of ketoconazole

Table 1 *continued*

Drug/therapeutic category affected	Herbal ingredients interacting	Possible effects
HIV protease inhibitorsHIV non-nucleoside reverse transcriptase inhibitors	St John's wort	Risk of reduced blood concentrations of anti-HIV drugs, with possible loss of HIV suppression
Endocrine system		
Antidiabetics	Herbal ingredients with hypo- or hyperglycaemic activity. *See* Appendix 2, Table 8	Potentiation/antagonism of activity
	Herbal ingredients with diuretic activity. *See* Appendix 2, Table 3	Antagonism
Drugs for hypo- and hyperthyroidism	Herbal ingredients with significant iodine content.	Interference with therapy
Corticosteroids	Herbal ingredients with diuretic activity. *See* Appendix 2, Table 3	Risk of increased potassium loss
	Herbal ingredients with corticosteroid activity. *See* Appendix 2 Table 9	Increased risk of side-effects, e.g. water and sodium retention
Sex hormones	Herbal ingredients with hormonal activity. *See* Appendix 2, Table 9	Possible interaction with existing therapy
Obstetrics and gynaecology		
Oral contraceptives	Herbal ingredients with hormonal activity. *See* Appendix 2, Table 9	Possible interaction with existing therapy; may reduce effectiveness of oral contraceptive
	St John's wort	Risk of reduced blood concentrations of oral contraceptives, breakthrough bleeding and unintended pregnancy
Malignant disease and immunosuppression		
Irinotecan	St John's wort	Risk of altered irinotecan pharmacokinetics
Methotrexate	Herbal ingredients with significant salicylate content. *See* Appendix 2, Table 5	Increased risk of toxicity
Drugs affecting immune response	Herbal ingredients with immunomodulatory activity. *See* Appendix 2, Table 10	Potentiation or antagonism
	St John's wort	Risk of reduced therapeutic effect of ciclosporin
Musculoskeletal and joint diseases		
Systemic lupus erythematosus	Alfalfa	Antagonism; contra-indicated
Probenecid	Herbal ingredients with significant salicylate content. *See* Appendix 2, Table 5	Risk of inhibition of probenecid
Eye		
Acetazolamide	Herbal ingredients with significant salicylate content. *See* Appendix 2, Table 5	Increased risk of toxicity
Skin	Herbal ingredients with potential allergenic activity. *See* Appendix 2, Table 11	Allergic reaction; exacerbation of existing symptoms
	Herbal ingredients with phototoxic activity. *See* Appendix 2, Table 11	Phototoxic reaction; exacerbation of existing symptoms
Anaesthetics		
General anaesthetics	Herbal ingredients with hypotensive activity. *See* Appendix 2, Table 4	Potentiation of hypotensive effect
Competitive muscle relaxants	Herbal ingredients with diuretic activity. *See* Appendix 2, Table 3	Risk of potentiation if hypokalaemia occurs
Depolarising muscle relaxants	Cardioactive herbal ingredients. *See* Appendix 2, Table 2	Risk of arrhythmias

Appendix 2 Pharmacological Activities and Constituents of Herbal Ingredients

Table 1 Laxatives

Drug	Comment
Aloes	Hydroxyanthracene constituents
Cascara	Hydroxyanthracene constituents
Frangula	Hydroxyanthracene constituents
Horehound, White	Large doses
Ispaghula	Bulk laxative
Plantain	Bulk laxative
Rhubarb	Hydroxyanthracene constituents
Senna	Hydroxyanthracene constituents
Yellow Dock	Hydroxyanthracene constituents

Table 2 Cardioactive agents

Drug	Comment
Broom	Alkaloid constituents: cardiac depressant activity
Butterbur	*S*-petasin: negative chronotropic activity *in vivo*, negative inotropic activity *ex vivo*
Calamus	Anti-arrhythmic activity
Cereus	Tyramine: cardiotonic amine
Cola	Caffeine
Coltsfoot	Cardiac calcium-channel blocking activity
Devil's Claw	Activity *in vivo*
Fenugreek	Activity *in vitro*
Figwort	Cardioactive glycoside constituents, activity *in vitro*
Fumitory	Alkaloid constituent: cardioactive
Ginger	Activity *in vivo*
Ginseng, Panax	Activity *in vivo*
Golden Seal	Berberine: cardioactive alkaloid
Hawthorn	Tyramine: cardiotonic amine; activity *in vivo*
Horehound, White	Activity *in vivo*
Lime Flower	Activity reputed with excessive ingestion
Maté	Caffeine
Mistletoe	Viscotoxin, negative inotropic effect *in vivo*
Motherwort	Cardiac glycoside constituents; activity *in vitro*
Pleurisy Root	Cardenolides, active *in vitro* and *in vivo*
Prickly Ash, Northern	Interaction with $Na^{+}K^{+}$ ATPase
Prickly Ash, Southern	Interaction with $Na^{+}K^{+}$ ATPase
Quassia	Activity *in vitro*
Rhodiola	Inotropic, anti-arrhythmic and other cardiac effects *ex vivo*, confirmation required
Shepherd's Purse	Activity *in vitro*
Squill	Cardiac glycoside constituents
Wild Carrot	Depressant activity *in vivo*

Table 3 Diuretics

Drug	Comment
Agrimony	Activity *in vivo*
Artichoke	Reputed action
Boldo	Reputed action, oil
Broom	Reputed action
Buchu	Reputed action
Burdock	Reputed action
Celery	Reputed action
Corn Silk	Reputed action
Couchgrass	Activity *in vivo*
Dandelion	Activity *in vivo*
Elder	Activity *in vivo*
Guaiacum	Reputed action
Java Tea	Activity *in vivo*
Juniper	Reputed action; terpinen-4-ol
Nettle	Activity in humans
Pokeroot	Activity *in vivo*
Shepherd's Purse	Activity *in vivo*
Squill	Activity *in vivo*
Uva-Ursi	Reputed action
Yarrow	Activity *in vivo*

Table 4 Hypotensives and hypertensives

Drug	Comment
Hypotensive	
Agrimony	Hypotensive, *in vivo*
Asafoetida	Hypotensive, *in vivo*
Avens	Hypotensive, *in vivo*
Butterbur	Hypotensive, in vivo; *S*-petasin, iso-*S*-petasin
Calamus	Hypotensive, *in vivo*
Cat's Claw	Hypotensive, *in vivo*
Corn Silk	Hypotensive, *in vivo*
Cowslip	Hypotensive, then hypertensive *in vivo*
Devil's Claw	Hypotensive, *in vivo*
Elecampane	Hypotensive, *in vivo*
Fenugreek	Hypotensive
Fucus	Hypotensive
Fumitory	Hypotensive, *in vivo*
Garlic	Hypotensive, human and *in vivo*
Ginger	Hypotensive
Ginseng, Panax	Hypotensive, human and *in vivo*
Golden Seal	Hypotensive, alkaloid effect
Hawthorn	Hypotensive, *in vivo*
Horehound, White	Vasodilator (volatile oil)
Horse-chestnut	Hypotensive, *in vivo*
Horseradish	Hypotensive, *in vivo*
Java Tea	Hypotensive, *in vivo*
Juniper	Hypotensive, *in vivo*
Mistletoe	Hypotensive, *in vivo*
Nettle	Hypotensive, *in vivo*
Parsley	Hypotensive, *in vivo*
Plantain	Hypotensive, *in vivo*
Pokeroot	Hypotensive, *in vivo*
Prickly Ash, Northern	Hypotensive, *in vivo*
Prickly Ash, Southern	Hypotensive, *in vivo*
Sage	Hypotensive
Shepherd's Purse	Hypotensive
Squill	Vasodilator, *in vivo*
St John's Wort	Hypotensive, *in vivo*
Thyme	Hypotensive, *in vivo*
Vervain	Hypotensive
Wild Carrot	Hypotensive, *in vivo*
Yarrow	Hypotensive, *in vivo*
Hypertensive	
Bayberry	Hypertensive, myricitrin mineralocorticoid side-effect
Broom	Hypertensive, alkaloid effect
Capsicum	Hypertensive, increased catecholamine secretion
Cohosh, Blue	Hypertensive, alkaloid effect
Cola	Hypertensive, caffeine
Coltsfoot	Hypertensive, pressor activity
Ephedra	Hypertensive, human and *in vivo*
Ginger	Hypertensive
Ginseng, Panax	Hypertensive, human and *in vivo*
Liquorice	Hypertensive, mineralocorticoid side-effect
Maté	Hypertensive, caffeine
Vervain	Hypertensive

Table 5 Anticoagulants and coagulants

Drug	Comment
Anticoagulants	
Bilberry	Inhibits platelet aggregation, human, *in vivo*, *in vitro*
Cat's Claw	Inhibits platelet aggregation, *in vitro*
Clove	Eugenol inhibitor of platelet activity
Feverfew	Inhibits platelet aggregation
Fucus	Anticoagulant action
Garlic	Inhibits platelet aggregation, humans *in vivo*
Ginger	Inhibition of platelet activity
Ginkgo	Inhibition of platelet activity
Ginseng, Panax	Reduction of blood coagulation
Horseradish	Peroxidase stimulates synthesis of arachidonic acid metabolites
Liquorice	Inhibition of platelet activity
Meadowsweet	Salicylate constituents
Poplar	Salicylate constituents
Willow	Salicylate constituents
Coagulants	
Golden Seal	Heparin antagonist
Mistletoe	Lectins, agglutinating activity
Yarrow	Coagulant, *in vivo*

Table 6 Hypolipidaemic and hyperlipidaemic agents

Drug	Comment
Hypocholesterolaemic	
Alfalfa	Hypocholesterolaemic, *in vivo*
Artichoke	Hypocholesterolaemic, human, *in vivo*
Bilberry	Hypocholesterolaemic, *in vivo*
Capsicum	Hypocholesterolaemic, *in vivo*
Cohosh, Black	Hypocholesterolaemic, *in vivo*
Fenugreek	Hypocholesterolaemic, human, *in vivo*
Garlic	Hypocholesterolaemic, human, *in vivo*

table continues

Table 6 *continued*

Drug	Comment
Ginger	Hypocholesterolaemic, *in vivo*
Ispaghula	Hypocholesterolaemic, human
Milk thistle	Hypocholesterolaemic, *in vivo*
Myrrh	Hypolipidaemic, human, *in vivo*
Plantain	Hypocholesterolaemic, *in vivo*
Scullcap	Hypocholesterolaemic, *in vivo*
Senega	Hypolipidaemic, *in vivo*
Tansy	Hypocholesterolaemic, *in vivo*
	Hypercholesterolaemic
Hydrocotyle	Hypercholesterolaemic, *in vivo*

Table 7 Sedatives

Drug	Comment
Calamus	Potentiates barbiturate sleeping time
Celery	*In vivo*
Centaury	Reputed action
Chamomile, German	Human
Couchgrass	*In vivo*
Elecampane	*In vivo*
Ginseng, Eleutherococcus; Ginseng, Panax	CNS depressant and stimulant
Golden Seal	*In vivo*
Hawthorn	CNS depressant; potentiates barbiturate sleeping time
Hops	*In vivo*
Hydrocotyle	*In vivo*
Jamaica Dogwood	*In vivo*
Kava	Conflicting results *in vivo*
Nettle	CNS depression, *in vivo*
Passionflower	*In vivo*
Sage	*In vivo*
Scullcap	Reputed action
Senega	CNS depressant, *in vivo*
Shepherd's Purse	Potentiates barbiturate sleeping time
Valerian	Human, *in vivo*
Wild Carrot	*In vivo*
Wild Lettuce	*In vivo*, related species

Table 8 Hypoglycaemics and hyperglycaemics

Drug	Comment
Hypoglycaemic	
Agrimony	Hypoglycaemic, *in vivo*
Alfalfa	Manganese, human
Aloes/Aloe vera	*In vivo*
Burdock	*In vivo*
Celery	*In vivo*
Corn Silk	*In vivo*
Damiana	*In vivo*
Dandelion	*In vivo*
Devil's Claw	*In vivo*
Elecampane	*In vivo*
Eucalyptus	*In vivo*
Fenugreek	Human
Garlic	Human, *in vivo*,
Ginger	*In vivo*
Ginseng, Eleutherococcus	*In vivo*
Ginseng, Panax	Human
Ispaghula	Human
Java Tea	*In vivo*
Juniper	*In vivo*
Marshmallow	Human, *in vivo*
Myrrh	*In vivo*
Nettle	*In vivo*
Sage	*In vivo*
Senega	*In vivo*
Tansy	*In vivo*
Hyperglycaemic	
Elecampane	*In vivo*
Ginseng, Panax	Human, *in vivo*
Hydrocotyl	Human
Rosemary	*In vivo*

Table 9 Hormonally active agents

Drug	Comment
Agnus Castus	Oestrogenic, in vitro; conflicting results
Alfalfa	Oestrogenic, *in vivo*
Aniseed	Oestrogenic, *in vivo*
Bayberry	Mineralocorticoid, *in vivo*
Butterbur	*S*-petasin, inhibition of testosterone release, *in vivo*, *in vitro*
Cohosh, Black	Oestrogenic, *in vivo*, *in vitro*; conflicting results
Fucus	Hyper-/hypothyroidism reported
Ginkgo	Oestrogenic, *in vitro*
Ginseng, Eleutherococcus; Ginseng, Panax	Oestrogenic, *in vivo*, *in vitro*
Horseradish	May depress thyroid activity; conflicting results

table continues

Table 9 *continued*

Drug	Comment
Liquorice	Mineralocorticoid activity, human; oestrogenic *in vivo*, *in vitro*
Motherwort	Oxytocic, *in vitro*; conflicting results
Pleurisy Root	Oestrogenic, *in vivo*; conflicting results
Red Clover	Oestrogenic *in vivo*; conflicting results
Saw Palmetto	Oestrogenic and anti-androgenic *in vivo*; human use in prostate cancer
Vervain	Inhibition of gonadotrophic activity; conflicting results
Wild Carrot	Oestrogenic, *in vivo*

Table 10 Immunomodulating agents

Drug	Comments
Alfalfa	*In vitro*
Boneset	*In vitro*
Calendula	*In vitro*
Cat's Claw	*In vitro*
Celandine, Greater	*In vitro*
Chamomile, German	*In vitro*
Drosera	*In vitro*
Echinacea	*In vitro*, *in vivo*, conflicting results in humans
Ephedra	Inhibits complement pathway, *in vitro*
Ginseng, Eleutherococcus	Human *in vivo*, *in vitro*
Mistletoe	Human, *in vivo*, *in vitro*
Saw Palmetto	*In vivo*

Table 11 Allergenic and photosensitising agents

Drug	Comment
Agnus Castus	Allergic effects reported
Angelica	Furanocoumarins, photosensitivity, contact allergy
Aniseed	Furanocoumarins, photosensitivity, contact allergy
Apricot	Contact allergy, kernels
Arnica	Contact allergy
Artichoke	Sesquiterpene lactone constituents
Asafoetida	Irritant gum, contact allergy
Boneset	Sesquiterpene lactone constituents
Calendula	Individuals sensitive to plants from the Compositae/Asteraceae families
Cassia	Allergic reactions, mainly contact dermatitis
Celery	Furanocoumarins, photosensitivity
Chamomile, German	Sesquiterpene lactone constituents
Chamomile, Roman	Sesquiterpene lactone constituents
Cinnamon	Contact allergy
Corn Silk	Allergic reactions
Cowslip	Allergic reactions
Dandelion	Sesquiterpene lactone constituents
Echinacea	Individuals sensitive to plants from the Compositae/Asteraceae families
Elecampane	Sesquiterpene lactone constituents
Feverfew	Sesquiterpene lactone constituents
Fucus	Iodine may aggravate/trigger acne
Garlic	Sulfur-containing compounds, allergic reaction
Ginger	Dermatitis in sensitive individuals
Ginkgo	Fruit pulp and seeds: severe allergic reactions
Gravel Root	Sesquiterpene lactone constituents
Guaiacum	Irritant resin
Holy Thistle	Sesquiterpene lactone constituents
Hops	Contact allergy
Hydrangea	Contact allergy
Hydrocotyle	Photosensitivity
Ispaghula	Rare cases of allergy
Juniper	Contact allergy
Kava	Cases of allergic skin reactions
Lady's Slipper	Contact allergy
Mistletoe	Injection site reactions, rare cases of anaphylactic reactions
Motherwort	Dermatitis, photosensitisation
Parsley	Furanocoumarins, photosensitivity
Pilewort	Contact allergy, protanemonin
Plantain	Contact allergy
Pleurisy Root	Contact allergy
Pulsatilla	Contact allergy, protoanemonin
Rosemary	Dermatitis, photosensitisation
St John's Wort	Photodermatitis, hypericin
Tansy	Sesquiterpene lactone constituents
Wild Carrot	Furanocoumarins, photosensitivity
Yarrow	Sesquiterpene lactone constituents

Table 12 Irritants

Drug	Comment
Alfalfa	Canavanine in seeds
Arnica	Irritant to mucous membranes
Asafoetida	Irritant gum
Blue Flag	Irritant gum and oil
Bogbean	Irritant to GI tract
Boldo	Irritant oil

table continues

Table 12 *continued*

Drug	Comment
Buchu	Irritant oil
Capsicum	Capsaicinoids, mucosal irritants
Cassia	Irritant to mucous membranes; oil
Celandine, Greater	Irritant juice
Cinnamon	Irritant to mucous membranes; oil
Cohosh, Blue	Irritant to mucous membranes; spasmogenic *in vitro*
Cowslip	Irritant saponins
Drosera	Plumbagin
Eucalyptus	Irritant oil
False Unicorn	Large doses may cause vomiting
Figwort	Purgative effect
Garlic	Raw clove
Ground Ivy	Irritant oil
Guaiacum	Avoid if inflammatory condition
Horse-chestnut	Saponin constituents, contra-indicated in existing renal disease
Horseradish	Irritant oil
Hydrangea	May cause gastro-enteritis, hydrangin
Jamaica Dogwood	Irritant to humans
Juniper	Irritant oil
Lemon Verbena	Irritant oil
Lime Flower	Irritant to kidney, oil
Mistletoe	Injection site reactions
Nettle	Tea irritant to stomach
Parsley	Irritant oil
Pennyroyal	Toxic and irritant oil
Pilewort	Irritant sap
Pleurisy Root	Gastrointestinal irritant
Pokeroot	Irritant saponins
Pulsatilla	Irritant to mucous membranes
Queen's Delight	Diterpene constituents
Sage	Irritant oil
Sarsaparilla	Saponins
Senega	Saponins
Skunk Cabbage	Inflammatory and blistering to skin
Squill	Saponins
Thyme	Irritant oil
Willow	Salicylates
Witch Hazel	Irritant to stomach

Table 13 Anti-inflammatory agents

Aloe Vera, Angelica, Arnica, Bilberry, Bloodroot, Blue Flag, Boldo, Boneset, Borage, Buchu, Butterbur, Calendula, Cassia, Cat's Claw, Celandine (Greater), Centaury, Chamomile (German), Chamomile (Roman), Cohosh (Black), Coltsfoot, Comfrey, Cowslip, Dandelion, Devil's Claw, Echinacea, Elder, Ephedra, Evening Primrose, Feverfew, Figwort, Gentian, Ginger, Ground Ivy, Horse-chestnut, Hydrocotyle, Java tea, Juniper, Liquorice, Milk Thistle, Myrrh, Nettle, Passionflower, Plantain, Pokeroot, Prickly Ash (Southern), Rosemary, Sarsaparilla, Shepherd's Purse, St John's wort, Uva-Ursi, Willow, Yarrow, Yucca

Table 14 Antispasmodics

Angelica, Aniseed, Asafoetida, Butterbur, Calendula, Capsicum, Cassia, Celandine (Greater), Celery, Chamomile (German), Cinnamon, Clove, Cohosh (Blue), Cowslip, Devil's claw, Elecampane, Euphorbia, Hops, Jamaica Dogwood, Lime Flower, Raspberry, Chamomile (Roman), Rosemary, Sage, Scullcap, Tansy, Thyme, Valerian

Table 15 Herbal ingredients containing amines or alkaloids, or with sympathomimetic action

Drug	Comment
Agnus Castus	Dopamine agonist (labdane diterpenes), *in vitro*
Alfalfa	Alkaloids
Aniseed	Anethole, sympathomimetic
Arnica	Betaines, choline
Bloodroot	Alkaloids
Bogbean	Alkaloids
Boldo	Alkaloids
Borage	Alkaloids
Broom	Alkaloids, amines
Butterbur	Alkaloids
Calamus	Amines
Capsicum	Sympathomimetic
Cat's Claw	Alkaloids
Celandine, Greater	Alkaloids
Centaury	Alkaloids
Cereus	Tyramine
Cohosh, Black	Alkaloids
Cohosh, Blue	Alkaloids
Cola	Alkaloids
Coltsfoot	Alkaloids
Comfrey	Alkaloids
Corn Silk	Amines
Ephedra	Alkaloids
Eyebright	Alkaloids
Fenugreek	Choline, trigonelline
Fumitory	Alkaloids
Gentian	Alkaloids
Ginkgo	Seed: alkaloids; leaf: MAOI activity

table continues

Table 15 *continued*

Drug	Comment
Ginseng, Panax	MAOI potentiation, suspected phenelzine interaction
Golden Seal	Alkaloids
Gravel Root	Alkaloids
Hawthorn	Tyramine
Horehound, White	Alkaloids
Hydrocotyle	Alkaloids
Ispaghula	Alkaloids
Jamaica Dogwood	Alkaloids
Kava	Alkaloids; possible dopamine antagonist effects
Liferoot	Alkaloids
Lobelia	Alkaloids
Maté	Alkaloids, amines
Mistletoe	Amines, alkaloids (possible)
Motherwort	Alkaloids
Nettle	Choline
Parsley	Myristicin, sympathomimetic
Passionflower	Alkaloids (traces or absent)
Plantain	Alkaloids
Pleurisy Root	Sympathomimetic
Pokeroot	Betalains
Prickly Ash, Northern	Alkaloids
Prickly Ash, Southern	Alkaloids
Quassia	Alkaloids
Sassafras	Alkaloids
Shepherd's Purse	Choline, tyramine
Skunk Cabbage	Alkaloids
Stone Root	Alkaloids
Valerian	Alkaloids
Vervain	Sympathomimetic
Yarrow	Betonicine, stachydrine, betaine

Table 16 Herbal ingredients containing coumarins[(a)]

Alfalfa, Angelica, Aniseed, Arnica, Asafoetida, Bogbean, Boldo, Buchu, Capsicum, Cassia, Celery, Chamomile (German), Chamomile (Roman), Dandelion, Fenugreek, Ginseng (Eleutherococcus), Horse-chestnut, Horseradish, Java tea, Liquorice, Meadowsweet, Nettle, Parsley, Prickly Ash (Northern), Quassia, Wild Carrot, Wild Lettuce

Coumarin constituents detected so far in these herbal ingredients do not possess the minimum structural requirements (a C-4 hydroxyl substituent and a C-3 non-polar carbon substituent)[(G87)] for anticoagulant activity.

Table 17 Herbal ingredients containing flavonoids

Agnus Castus, Agrimony, Angelica, Aniseed, Apricot, Arnica, Artichoke, Bayberry, Bilberry, Bogbean, Boldo, Boneset, Broom, Buchu, Burdock, Burnet, Butterbur, Calendula, Celandine (Greater), Celery, Cereus, Chamomile (German), Chamomile (Roman), Chaparral, Clivers, Cohosh (Black), Coltsfoot, Corn Silk, Couchgrass, Cowslip, Damiana, Dandelion, Devil's Claw, Drosera, Elder, Ephedra, Eucalyptus, Euphorbia, Eyebright, Fenugreek, Feverfew, Figwort, Frangula, Fumitory, Ginkgo, Gravel Root, Ground Ivy, Hawthorn, Hops, Horehound (Black), Horehound (White), Horse-chestnut, Hydrangea, Hydrocotyle, Java Tea, Juniper, Kava, Lemon Verbena, Lime Flower, Liquorice, Marshmallow, Maté, Meadowsweet, Melissa, Milk thistle, Mistletoe, Motherwort, Nettle, Parsley, Passionflower, Plantain, Pulsatilla, Raspberry, Red Clover, Rhodiola, Rhubarb, Rosemary, Sage, Sarsaparilla, Saw Palmetto, Scullcap, Senna, Shepherd's Purse, Squill, St John's Wort, Stone Root, Thyme, Uva-Ursi, Wild Carrot, Wild Lettuce, Willow, Witch Hazel, Yarrow

Table 18 Herbal ingredients containing iridoids

Agnus Castus, Bilberry, Bogbean, Centaury, Clivers, Devil's Claw, Eyebright, Figwort, Gentian, Ispaghula, Motherwort, Plantain, Scullcap, Uva-Ursi, Valerian, Vervain

Table 19 Herbal ingredients containing saponins

Alfalfa, Aloe Vera, Bogbean, Burnet, Calendula, Chaparral, Cohosh (Blue), Corn Silk, Cowslip, False Unicorn, Fenugreek, Ginseng (Eleutherococcus), Ginseng (Panax), Hawthorn, Horehound (White), Horse-chestnut, Hydrangea, Hydrocotyle, Jamaica Dogwood, Lime Flower, Milk Thistle, Mistletoe, Pokeroot, Pulsatilla, Red Clover, Sarsaparilla, Senega, Senna, Stone Root, Thyme, Vervain, Witch Hazel, Yucca

Table 20 Herbal ingredients containing tannins

Agrimony, Apricot, Arnica, Artichoke, Avens, Bayberry, Bilberry, Blue Flag, Boldo, Borage, Burnet, Butterbur, Calamus, Cascara, Cassia, Chamomile (German), Cinnamon, Clivers, Cola, Coltsfoot, Comfrey, Corn Silk, Cowslip, Damiana, Drosera, Elder, Ephedra, Eucalyptus, Eyebright, Feverfew, Frangula, Gentian, Ground Ivy, Hawthorn, Holy Thistle, Hops, Horse-chestnut, Ispaghula, Juniper, Lady's Slipper, Lime Flower, Marshmallow, Meadowsweet, Motherwort, Nettle, Pilewort, Plantain, Poplar, Prickly Ash (Northern), Prickly Ash (Southern), Queen's Delight, Raspberry, Rhubarb, Sage, Sassafras, Saw Palmetto, Scullcap, Slippery Elm, Squill, St. John's Wort, Stone Root, Tansy, Thyme, Uva-Ursi, Valerian, Vervain, Willow, Witch Hazel, Yarrow, Yellow Dock

Table 21 Herbal ingredients containing essential oils

Agnus Castus, Agrimony, Angelica, Aniseed, Arnica, Artichoke, Asafoetida, Avens, Blue Flag, Boldo, Boneset, Buchu, Burdock, Burnet, Butterbur, Calamus, Calendula, Capsicum, Cassia, Celery, Chamomile (German), Chamomile (Roman), Chaparral, Cinnamon, Clove, Coltsfoot, Couchgrass, Damiana, Elder, Elecampane, Ephedra, Eucalyptus, Eyebright, Feverfew, Garlic, Gentian, Ginger, Ginseng (Eleutherococcus), Ginseng (Panax), Golden Seal, Ground Ivy, Holy Thistle, Hops, Horehound (Black), Horseradish, Hydrocotyle, Java Tea, Juniper, Lemon Verbena, Lime Flower, Liquorice, Lobelia, Meadowsweet, Melissa, Motherwort, Myrrh, Parsley, Pennyroyal, Prickly Ash (Northern), Queen's Delight, Red Clover, Rhodiola, Rosemary, Sage, Sassafras, Saw Palmetto, Senna (trace), Skunk Cabbage, Squill, St John's Wort, Stone Root, Tansy, Thyme, Uva-Ursi, Valerian, Vervain, Wild Carrot, Witch Hazel, Yarrow

Appendix 3
Council of Europe – Categories for Natural Sources of Flavourings

Table 1 Council of Europe. categories for natural sources of flavourings (Report No. 1. Strasbourg: Council of Europe, 2000)[(a)]

Category	Natural source of flavouring
1	Plants, animals and other organisms, and parts of these or products thereof, normally consumed as food items, herbs or spices in Europe for which it is considered that there should be no restrictions on use.Flavouring preparations, which are not themselves consumed as food but which are derived from plants, animals and other organisms, and parts of these or products thereof, normally consumed as food items, herbs or spices in Europe. These preparations, on the basis of the information available, are not considered a risk to health in the quantities used.
2	Plants, animals and other organisms, and parts of these or products thereof, and preparations derived therefrom, not normally consumed as food items, herbs or spices in Europe.These source materials and preparations, on the basis of the information available, are not considered to constitute a risk to health in the quantities used.
3	Plants, animals and other organisms, and parts of these or products thereof, normally consumed as food items, herbs or spices in Europe which contain defined 'active principles' or 'other chemical components' requiring limits on use levels.Flavouring preparations, which are not themselves consumed as food but which are derived from plants, animals and other organisms, and parts of these or products thereof, normally consumed as food items, herbs or spices in Europe which contain defined 'active principles' or 'other chemical components' requiring limits on use levels. These source materials and preparations are not considered to constitute a risk to health in the quantities used provided that the limits set for the 'active principles' or 'other chemical components' are not exceeded.
4	Plants, animals and other organisms, and parts of these or products thereof, and preparations derived therefrom, not normally consumed as food items, herbs or spices in Europe which contain defined 'active principles' or 'other chemical components' requiring limits on use levels.These source materials and preparations are not considered to constitute a risk to health in the quantities used provided that the limits set for the 'active principles' or 'other chemical components' are not exceeded.
5	Plants, animals and other organisms, and parts of these or products thereof, and preparations derived therefrom, for which additional toxicological and/or chemical information is required.These could temporarily be acceptable provided that any limits set for the 'active principles' or the 'other chemical components' are not exceeded.
6	Plants, animals and other organisms, and parts of these or products thereof, and preparations derived therefrom, which are considered to be unfit for human consumption in any amount.

Reproduced with permission of Council of Europe.

Appendix 4
Preparations Directory

4

Introduction

Appendix 4 contains an alphabetical listing of selected preparations from over 35 countries. Information on products believed to be currently available was gathered from standard compendia and specific supplier literature and websites. The inclusion of a supplier or product is not intended as an endorsement of that supplier or its products; similarly, the omission of a supplier or product is not intended to reflect adversely on that supplier or product. Preparations are arranged in two sections. The first section lists preparations that have a single herbal ingredient which is included in *Herbal Medicines*. The second section lists preparations that contain multiple ingredients. Only those herbal ingredients included as monographs in *Herbal Medicines* are shown. It should be noted that these preparations may contain other ingredients, possibly not just herbal ingredients, that are not shown in this listing. Preparations are listed by proprietary name (product name), supplier, country, herbal ingredient(s). Preparations without a proprietary name that are identified by a supplier by the herbal ingredient name (e.g. angelica) are indicated with a • symbol. Contact details for the supplier are shown in Appendix 5.

Single-ingredient preparations

aar gamma N *aar pharma GmbH & Co. KG, Germany,* Artichoke (p. 67)

aar vir *aar pharma GmbH & Co. KG, Germany,* Echinacea (p. 217)

ABC *Beiersdorf GmbH, Austria,* Capsicum (p. 125)

Abfuhrtee N *Bad Heilbrunner Naturheilmittel GmbH & Co., Germany,* Senna (p. 537)

Abnobaviscum *Abnoba Heilmittel GmbH, Germany,* Milk Thistle (p. 429)

Abolibe *Sidefarma SA, Portugal,* Ginkgo (p. 299)

Acorus *Zeppenfeldt Pharma GmbH, Germany,* Couchgrass (p. 193)

Acqua Virginiana *Kelemata S.p.A., Italy,* Witch Hazel (p. 601)

Adprex *Hebron S.A. Indústria Química e Farmacêutica, Brazil,* St John's Wort (p. 549)

A-E-R *Birchwood Laboratories Inc., USA,* Witch Hazel (p. 601)

Aescorin Forte *Steigerwald Arzneimittelwerk GmbH, Germany,* Horse-chestnut (p. 363)

Aesculaforce *Aponova Pharma Handels GmbH, Austria,* Horse-chestnut (p. 363) *Bioforce AG, Switzerland,* Horse-chestnut (p. 363)

AesculaMed *Bioforce AG, Switzerland,* Horse-chestnut (p. 363)

Aescusan *Jenapharm GmbH & Co. KG, Germany,* Horse-chestnut (p. 363)

Aescuven *Cesra Arzneimittel GmbH & Co. KG, Germany,* Horse-chestnut (p. 363)

Agarol Extra *Numark Laboratories Inc., USA,* Senna (p. 537)

Agarol with Sennosides *Numark Laboratories Inc., USA,* Senna (p. 537)

Agiobulk *Altana Madaus Pty Ltd, South Africa,* Ispaghula (p. 374)

Agiocur *Madaus GmbH, Austria,* Ispaghula (p. 374) *Meda Oy, Finland,* Ispaghula (p. 374) *Madaus AG, Germany,* Ispaghula (p. 374) *Trinity Trading Co. Ltd, Hong and Salomon, Levin, & Elstein Ltd, Israel,* Ispaghula (p. 374) *Neo-Farmacêutica, Lda, Portugal,* Ispaghula (p. 374) *Oui Heng Import Co. Ltd, Thailand,* Ispaghula (p. 374)

Agiofibe *Knoll Australia, Australia,* Ispaghula (p. 374)

Agiofibra *Altana Pharma Ltda, Brazil,* Ispaghula (p. 374) *Altana Pharma S.A. de C. V., Mexico,* Ispaghula (p. 374)

Agiofibras *Laboratorios Phoenix S.A.I.C.F., Argentina,* Ispaghula (p. 374)

Agiofibre *Madaus S.r.l., Italy,* Ispaghula (p. 374)

Agiogel *Altana Madaus Pty Ltd, South Africa,* Ispaghula (p. 374)

Agiolax mite *Max Zeller Söhne AG, Pflanzliche Heilmittel, Switzerland,* Ispaghula (p. 374)

Agnofem *Madaus GmbH, Austria,* Agnus Castus (p. 36)

Agnolyt *Madaus AG, Germany,* Agnus Castus (p. 36) *Max Zeller Söhne AG, Pflanzliche Heilmittel, Switzerland,* Agnus Castus (p. 36)

Agno-Sabona *Sabona GmbH, Germany,* Agnus Castus (p. 36)

Agnucaston *Austroplant-Arzneimittel GmbH, Austria,* Agnus Castus (p. 36) *Arzneimittel Schwabe International GmbH, Czech Republic,* Agnus Castus (p. 36) *Bionorica AG, Germany,* Agnus Castus (p. 36) *ASI Budapest Kft, Hungary,* Agnus Castus (p. 36) *Zuellig Pharma Ltd, Thailand,* Agnus Castus (p. 36)

Agnucaston (Агнукастон) *Bionorica AG, Russia,* Agnus Castus (p. 36)

Agnufemil *Steigerwald Arzneimittelwerk GmbH, Germany,* Agnus Castus (p. 36)

Agnukliman *Gebro Pharma GmbH, Austria,* Cohosh, Black (p. 168)

Agnumens *Gebro Pharma GmbH, Austria,* Agnus Castus (p. 36)

• **Agnus Castus** (p. 36)
UK: Biocare Ltd; Culpeper and Napiers; Frank Roberts (Herbal Dispensaries) Ltd; Healthy Direct; Holland and Barrett; Quest Vitamins Ltd

• **Agrimony** (p. 42)
UK: Culpeper and Napiers

Ajomast *Monserrat y Eclair S.A., Argentina,* Garlic (p. 279)

Ajuta *Hermes Arzneimittel GmbH, Germany,* Devil's Claw (p. 207)

Akipic *Laboratoires Asepta, Monaco,* Aloes (p. 50), Calendula (p. 121)

Alcachofa Plus *Tecnonat S.A., Argentina,* Artichoke (p. 67)

Alcodin *Alcon Italia S.p.A., Italy,* Bilberry (p. 79)

Alepa *Duopharm GmbH, Germany,* Milk Thistle (p. 429)

• **Alfalfa** (p. 45)
UK: Culpeper and Napiers

Alho Rogoff *Crefar, Lda, Portugal,* Garlic (p. 279)

Alliocaps *Lab. Dr. Madaus & Co. SA, Argentina,* Garlic (p. 279)

Allya *Pascoe Pharmazeutische Präparate GmbH, Germany,* Devil's Claw (p. 207)

• **Aloe Vera** (p. 48)
UK: Biocare Ltd; Culpeper and Napiers; Frank Roberts (Herbal Dispensaries) Ltd; Healthy Direct; Holland and Barrett; Worldwide Health Corp. Ltd
USA: Nature's Bounty

Alrinte *Ativus Farmacêutica Ltda, Brazil,* Rosemary (p. 508)

Alz *CuraMED Pharma GmbH, Germany,* Ginkgo (p. 299)

Amenicil *Laboratorios Phoenix S.A.I.C.F., Argentina,* St John's Wort (p. 549)

Anastil *Dr. Friedrich Eberth Arzneimittel, Germany,* Thyme (p. 574)

• **Angelica** (p. 53)
UK: Culpeper and Napiers

Animic *Viñas, Spain,* St John's Wort (p. 549)

• **Aniseed** (p. 57)
UK: Culpeper and Napiers

Ansiokey *Inkeysa, Spain,* Valerian (p. 580)

Ansiopax *Hebron S.A. Indústria Química e Farmacêutica, Brazil,* Kava (p. 389)

Antares *Krewel Meuselbach GmbH, Czech Republic,* Kava (p. 389)

4

Anxium *Laboratorio Esp. Med. Knop Ltda, Chile,* St John's Wort (p. 549)

Aperisan *Dentinox Gesellschaft für Pharmazeutische Präparate Lenk & Schuppan, Germany,* Sage (p. 512)

Apihepar *Madaus GmbH, Viatris Pharma GmbH, Austria,* Milk Thistle (p. 429)

Aplause *Marjan Indústria e Comércio Ltda, Brazil,* Cohosh, Black (p. 168)

Ardey-aktiv *Ardeypharm GmbH, Germany,* Ginseng, Panax (p. 325)

Ardeycholan *Ardeypharm GmbH, Germany,* Artichoke (p. 67)

Ardeycordal mono *Ardeypharm GmbH, Germany,* Hawthorn (p. 346)

Ardeyhepan *Emonta Pharma GmbH, Austria,* Milk Thistle (p. 429) *Ardeypharm GmbH, Germany,* Milk Thistle (p. 429)

Aristo *Steiner & Co. Deutsche Arzneimittel Gesellschaft, Germany,* St John's Wort (p. 549)

Aristoforat *Steiner & Co. Deutsche Arzneimittel Gesellschaft, Germany,* St John's Wort (p. 549)

Arkocapsulas Hiperico *Arkochim España, Spain,* St John's Wort (p. 549)

Arnican *Coopération Pharmaceutique Francaise, France,* Arnica (p. 64)

Arnigel *Prisfar, SA, Portugal,* Arnica (p. 64)

Arnikaderm *Laboratorio Esp. Med. Knop Ltda, Chile,* Arnica (p. 64)

Arnikatinktur *Chemische Fabrik Dr. Hetterich GmbH & Co. KG, Germany,* Arnica (p. 64)

Arsen *Arlex de México, S.A.deC.V., Mexico,* Senna (p. 537)

Arthrodynat N *Ziethen, Germany,* Nettle (p. 452)

Arthrosenex AR *Riemser Arzneimittel AG, Germany,* Arnica (p. 64)

Arthrosetten H *Riemser Arzneimittel AG, Germany,* Devil's Claw (p. 207)

Arthrotabs *Duopharm GmbH, Germany,* Devil's Claw (p. 207)

• **Artichoke** (p. 67)
UK: Frank Roberts (Herbal Dispensaries) Ltd

Asendra *Pascoe Pharmazeutische Präparate GmbH, Germany,* Nettle (p. 452)

Aspecton *Krewel Meuselbach GmbH, Germany,* Thyme (p. 574)

Assalix *Bionorica AG, Germany,* Willow (p. 598) *Biomed AG, Switzerland,* Willow (p. 598)

Assplant *Robugen GmbH Pharmazeutische Fabrik, Germany,* Willow (p. 598)

Aubeline *Laboratoires Arkopharma, France,* Hawthorn (p. 346)

Avala *Laboratorios DHU Ibérica, S.A., Spain,* Cohosh, Black (p. 168)

Azuprostat Sabal *Sandoz Pharmaceuticals GmbH, Germany,* Saw Palmetto (p. 521)

Azuprostat Urtica *Sandoz Pharmaceuticals GmbH, Germany,* Nettle (p. 452)

Baldorm *Dr Gustav Klein, Germany,* Valerian (p. 580)

Baldrian-Dispert *Solvay Pharma AB, Sweden,* Valerian (p. 580)

Baldriparan pour la nuit *Whitehall-Robins AG, Switzerland,* Valerian (p. 580)

Baldriparan Stark *Whitehall-Much GmbH, Germany,* Valerian (p. 580)

Baldrivit *Rodisma-Med Pharma GmbH, Germany,* Valerian (p. 580)

Baldurat *G. Pohl-Boskamp GmbH & Co., Germany,* Valerian (p. 580)

Balsamo Nordin *Química Franco Mexicana Nordin S.A. de C.V., Mexico,* Arnica (p. 64)

Basticrat *Bastian-Werk GmbH, Germany,* Hawthorn (p. 346)

Bazoton *Abbott GmbH & Co. KG, Germany,* Nettle (p. 452)

Bekunis *Schülke & Mayr GmbH, Austria,* Senna (p. 537) *Dexxon, Israel,* Senna (p. 537) *Laboratorios Farmasa, S.A. de C.V., Mexico,* Senna (p. 537) *Merz Pharma (Schweiz) AG, Switzerland,* Senna (p. 537)

Bekunis Herbal Tea *Thursday Plantation laboratories Ltd, Australia,* Senna (p. 537)

Bekunis Instant *Thursday Plantation laboratories Ltd, Australia,* Senna (p. 537) *roha Arzneimittel GmbH, Germany,* Senna (p. 537)

Bekunis Plantaardig *roha Arzneimittel GmbH, Germany,* Senna (p. 537)

Bekunis Senna *roha Arzneimittel GmbH, Germany,* Senna (p. 537)

Bekunis-Krautertee N *roha Arzneimittel GmbH, Germany,* Senna (p. 537)

Beltrax Uno *Lab. Baliarda S.A., Argentina,* Saw Palmetto (p. 521)

beni-cur *Sabona GmbH, Germany,* Garlic (p. 279)

Benylin Energy Boosting *Pfizer Consumer Healthcare, Division of Pfizer Canada Inc., Canada,* Ginseng, Eleutherococcus (p. 315)

Bericard *Provita Pharma GmbH, Austria,* Hawthorn (p. 346)

• **Bilberry** (p. 79)
UK: Culpeper and Napiers; Healthy Direct; Holland and Barrett; Quest Vitamins Ltd; Worldwide Health Corp. Ltd
USA: Nature Made; Nature's Bounty; Sundown

Biloban *Cipan, Companhia Industrial Produtora de Antibioticos SA, Portugal,* Ginkgo (p. 299)

Bilobene *Ratiopharm Arzneimittel Vertriebs-GmbH, Austria,* Fumitory (p. 276) *Merckle GmbH, Germany,* Fumitory (p. 276) *ratiopharm Hungária Kft, Hungary,* Fumitory (p. 276)

Bilobil (Билобил) *KRKA d.d., Russia,* Ginkgo (p. 299)

Bilogink *Productos Maver S.A. de C.V., Mexico,* Ginkgo (p. 299)

Binko *Hexal do Brasil Ltda, Brazil,* Ginkgo (p. 299)

Bio Star *Ferrer Farma, Spain,* Ginseng, Panax (p. 325)

Bio-Dermis *Laboratorios Sidus S.A., Argentina,* Aloe Vera (p. 48)

Biofem *Biocur Arzneimittel GmbH, Germany,* Agnus Castus (p. 36)

BioGinkgo *Pharmanex Inc., USA,* Ginkgo (p. 299)

Bioglan Liver-Vite *Bioglan Ltd, Australia,* Milk Thistle (p. 429)

Bioglan Pro-Guard *Bioglan Ltd, Australia,* Saw Palmetto (p. 521)

Bioglan Stress-Relax *Bioglan Ltd, Australia,* St John's Wort (p. 549)

Biolid *Rovi, Spain,* Ispaghula (p. 374)

Biorevit Gel *Laboratorio DNR Farma SRL, Argentina,* Aloe Vera (p. 48)

Biotuss *W. Spitzner, Arzneimittelfabrik GmbH, Germany,* Thyme (p. 574)

Black-Draught *Chattem Consumer Products, USA,* Senna (p. 537)

Blancaler *Galderma Mexico S.A. de C.V., Mexico,* Yarrow (p. 604)

Blastoestimulina *Almirall Prodesfarma S.A., Spain,* Hydrocotyle (p. 371)

• **Blue Flag** (p. 87)
UK: Culpeper and Napiers

• **Boldo** (p. 91)
UK: Culpeper and Napiers; Holland and Barrett

Bomarthros *Hevert-Arzneimittel GmbH & Co. KG, Germany,* Devil's Claw (p. 207)

• **Boneset** (p. 94)
UK: Culpeper and Napiers

• **Borage** (p. 96)
UK: Culpeper and Napiers
USA: Sundown

Born *Riemser Arzneimittel AG, Germany,* Hawthorn (p. 346)

Brefus *Hebron S.A. Indústria Química e Farmacêutica, Brazil,* Liquorice (p. 411)

Bronchicum Husten (Бронхикум Пастилки от Кашля) *Sanofi-Aventis, Russia,* Thyme (p. 574)

Bronchicum Husten-Pastillen *Aventis Pharma sro, Czech Republic,* Thyme (p. 574)

Bronchicum Pastillen *Cassella-med GmbH & Co. KG, Germany,* Thyme (p. 574)

Bronchipret *Bionorica AG, Germany,* Thyme (p. 574)

Bukosan *Slovakofarma sro, Czech Republic,* Rhubarb (p. 506)

• **Burdock** (p. 102)
UK: Culpeper and Napiers; Holland and Barrett

Butt-Out *Paradise Promotions Ltd, Canada,* Marshmallow (p. 418)

Caj z Hlohu *Megafyt-R sro, Czech Republic,* Hawthorn (p. 346)

Caj z Kvetu Bezu Cerneho *Megafyt-R sro, Czech Republic,* Elder (p. 237)

Caj z Listu Senny *Megafyt-R sro, Czech Republic,* Senna (p. 537)

Caj ze Salveje *Megafyt-R sro, Czech Republic,* Sage (p. 512)

Calendolon *Weleda (UK) Ltd, UK,* Calendula (p. 121)

• **Calendula** (p. 121)
UK: Culpeper and Napiers

Calendulene *Laboratoires Théa, France,* Calendula (p. 121)

Calendumed *Dr Peithner KG nunmehr GmbH & Co., Austria,* Calendula (p. 121)

Calmettes *Solvay Pharma (Pty) Ltd, South Africa,* Valerian (p. 580)

Calmonex *Instituto Terapeutico Delta Ltda, Brazil,* Kava (p. 389)

Capistan *Pierre Fabre Medicament sro, Czech Republic,* Saw Palmetto (p. 521)

Capsamol *Wörwag Pharma GmbH & Co. KG, Germany,* Capsicum (p. 125)

Capson *Pharmatrix, Div. de Therabel Pharma S.A., Argentina,* Aloe Vera (p. 48)

Cardiocalm *Pharmastra, Usines Chimiques et Pharmaceutiques de Strasbourg, France,* Hawthorn (p. 346)

Cardiplant *Arzneimittel Schwabe International GmbH, Czech Republic,* Hawthorn (p. 346) *Schwabe Pharma AG, Switzerland,* Hawthorn (p. 346)

Carito mono *MaxMedic Pharma GmbH & Co. KG, Germany,* Java Tea (p. 381)

Carvicum *Duopharm GmbH, Germany,* Dandelion (p. 204)

• **Cascara** (p. 128)
USA: Nature's Bounty; Sundown

Castufemin *Ardeypharm GmbH, Germany,* Agnus Castus (p. 36)

• **Cat's Claw** (p. 132)
UK: Frank Roberts (Herbal Dispensaries) Ltd; Holland and Barrett; Worldwide Health Corp. Ltd

Cefacynar *Cefak KG, Germany,* Artichoke (p. 67)

Cefakliman mono *Cefak KG, Germany,* Cohosh, Black (p. 168) *Vicis Pharma Kft, Hungary,* Cohosh, Black (p. 168)

Cefalektin *Cefak KG, Germany,* Milk Thistle (p. 429)

Cefaluna *Cefak KG, Germany,* Valerian (p. 580)

Cefanorm *Cefak KG, Germany,* Agnus Castus (p. 36) *Vicis Pharma Kft, Hungary,* Agnus Castus (p. 36)

Cefasept *Cefak KG, Germany,* Echinacea (p. 217)

Cefasliymarin *Cefak KG, Germany,* Milk Thistle (p. 429)

Cefatec *Cefak KG, Germany,* Devil's Claw (p. 207)

• **Celery** (p. 146)
UK: Biocare Ltd

Celulase *Laboratorios Rider SA, Chile,* Hydrocotyle (p. 371)

Celulase Plus *Laboratorios Rider SA, Chile,* Hydrocotyle (p. 371)

Cenat *Madaus, Spain,* Ispaghula (p. 374)

Centabel *Laboratorios Silesia SA, Chile,* Hydrocotyle (p. 371)

• **Centaury** (p. 149)
UK: Culpeper and Napiers

Centellase *Aventis Pharma S.p.A., Italy,* Hydrocotyle (p. 371) *Polymedic Trading Enterprise Pte Ltd, Singapore,* Hydrocotyle (p. 371)

Centella-Vit *Fontovit Laboratórios Ltda, Brazil,* Hydrocotyle (p. 371)

Centica *Zyfas Medical Co, Singapore,* Hydrocotyle (p. 371)

Cerebokan *Austroplant-Arzneimittel GmbH, Austria,* Ginkgo (p. 299)

Ceremin *Austroplant-Arzneimittel GmbH, Austria,* Ginkgo (p. 299)

Cesradyston *Cesra Arzneimittel GmbH & Co. KG, Germany,* St John's Wort (p. 549)

Chofitol *Laboratorios Millet-Franklin S.A., Argentina,* Artichoke (p. 67)

Cholagogum *Cassella-med GmbH & Co. KG, Germany,* Artichoke (p. 67)

Cholax *Laboratorios Maver SA, Chile,* Senna (p. 537)

Chophytol *Produtos Farmacêuticos Millet Roux Ltda, Brazil,* Artichoke (p. 67) *Laboratoires Rosa-Phytopharma, France,* Artichoke (p. 67) *Laboratoire Golaz SA, Switzerland,* Artichoke (p. 67)

Chophytol (Хофитол**)** *FIC Medical, Russia,* Artichoke (p. 67)

Chronocard N *Cesra Arzneimittel GmbH & Co. KG, Germany,* Hawthorn (p. 346)

Cicloplant *Abbott Laboratories de Mexico S.A. de C.V., Mexico,* Agnus Castus (p. 36)

Cimifemine *Max Zeller Söhne AG, Pflanzliche Heilmittel, Switzerland,* Cohosh, Black (p. 168)

Cimipax *Laboratoires IPRAD, France,* Cohosh, Black (p. 168)

Cimisan *APS Pharma GmbH, Germany,* Cohosh, Black (p. 168)

• **Cinnamon** (p. 162)
UK: Healthy Direct

Cinnamon Extract *Natrol, USA,* Cinnamon (p. 162)

Ciruela Fibra *Lab. Garden House S.A., Argentina,* Senna (p. 537)

Ciruelax Comp *Ivax Pharmaceuticals Mexico S.A. de C.V., Mexico,* Senna (p. 537)

Ciruelax TE *Ivax Pharmaceuticals Mexico S.A. de C.V., Mexico,* Senna (p. 537)

Citranacea *Nutravite, Canada,* Echinacea (p. 217)

Citromel *Laboratorio Esp. Med. Knop Ltda, Chile,* Melissa (p. 425)

Clarvix *Laboratorios Beta S.A., Argentina,* Ginkgo (p. 299)

Clibium *Laboratórios Klinger do Brasil Ltda, Brazil,* Ginkgo (p. 299)

Clifemin *Herbarium Laboratório Botanico Ltda, Brazil,* Cohosh, Black (p. 168)

Climadil *Marjan Indústria e Comércio Ltda, Brazil,* Red Clover (p. 498)

Climavita *Permamed AG, Switzerland,* Cohosh, Black (p. 168)

Coenrelax *A.S.A.C. Pharma, Spain,* Valerian (p. 580)

• **Cohosh, Black** (p. 168)
UK: Culpeper and Napiers; Frank Roberts (Herbal Dispensaries) Ltd; Healthy Direct; Holland and Barrett; Medic Herb UK Ltd; Quest Vitamins Ltd
USA: Nature Made; Nature's Bounty; Sundown

Colofiber *Madaus Pharma SA, Belgium,* Ispaghula (p. 374)

Colonorm *Mundipharma GmbH, Austria,* Senna (p. 537)

Concentrin *ct-Arzneimittel GmbH, Germany,* Horse-chestnut (p. 363)

Contre-Coups de l'Abbe Perdrigeon *Laboratoires Pionneau, France,* Aloes (p. 50)

Cordapur Novo *APS Pharma GmbH, Germany,* Hawthorn (p. 346)

Coriosta Vitaltonikum N *Dr Niedermaier GmbH, Germany,* Ginseng, Panax (p. 325)

Corocrat *biomo Pharma GmbH, Germany,* Hawthorn (p. 346)

• **Couchgrass** (p. 193)
UK: Culpeper and Napiers

Craegium *Biocur Arzneimittel GmbH, Germany,* Hawthorn (p. 346)

Cran Max *Swiss Herbal Remedies Ltd, Canada,* Cranberry (p. 197)

• **Cranberry** (p. 197)
UK: Biocare Ltd; Frank Roberts (Herbal Dispensaries) Ltd; Healthy Direct; Holland and Barrett; Quest Vitamins Ltd
USA: Nature Made; Sundown; Walgreens Finest Natural

Crataegan *Austroplant-Arzneimittel GmbH, Austria,* Hawthorn (p. 346)

Crataegisan *Bioforce AG, Switzerland,* Hawthorn (p. 346)

Crataegitan *Amino AG, Switzerland,* Hawthorn (p. 346)

Crataegutt *Dr Peithner KG nunmehr GmbH & Co., Austria,* Hawthorn (p. 346) *Dr Willmar Schwabe GmbH & Co., Germany,* Hawthorn (p. 346) *ASI Budapest Kft, Hungary,* Hawthorn (p. 346)

Crataegysat F *Johannes Bürger Ysatfabrik GmbH, Germany,* Hawthorn (p. 346)

Cratae-Loges *Dr. Loges & Co. GmbH, Germany,* Hawthorn (p. 346)

Crataepas *Pascoe Pharmazeutische Präparate GmbH, Germany,* Hawthorn (p. 346)

Cratenox *Laboratorio Esp. Med. Knop Ltda, Chile,* Hawthorn (p. 346)

Cuassicum Prevent 2 en 1 *Nucleopharm SRL, Argentina,* Quassia (p. 491)

Cynacur *Biocur Arzneimittel GmbH, Germany,* Artichoke (p. 67)

Cynalip duo *Sabona GmbH, Germany,* Artichoke (p. 67)

Cynarex *Lab. Roux-Ocefa S.A., Argentina,* Artichoke (p. 67)

Cynarix *Montavit GmbH, Austria,* Artichoke (p. 67)

Cynarix N *Sabona GmbH, Germany,* Artichoke (p. 67)

Cystinol Akut *Hoyer-Madaus GmbH & Co. KG, Germany,* Uva-Ursi (p. 577)

• **Damiana** (p. 201)
UK: Culpeper and Napiers

• **Dandelion** (p. 204)
UK: Culpeper and Napiers; Holland and Barrett

Darlin *Nycomed Christiaens, Belgium,* Senna (p. 537)

Darmol *Dr A & L Schmidgall, Austria,* Senna (p. 537) *Iromedica AG, Switzerland,* Senna (p. 537)

Dekatin *Ativus Farmacêutica Ltda, Brazil,* Hawthorn (p. 346)

Demodon Neo *Vifor SA, Switzerland,* Senna (p. 537)

Demonatur Ginkgo *Vifor SA, Switzerland,* Ginkgo (p. 299)

Depiderm *Laboratoires Dermatologiques Uriage, France,* Liquorice (p. 411)

Deprim *Lek Pharma sro, Czech Republic,* St John's Wort (p. 549)

Deprim (Деприм**)** *Lek, Russia,* St John's Wort (p. 549)

Depuran *Woelm Pharma GmbH & Co., Germany,* Senna (p. 537) *Aspen Pharmacare (Pty) Ltd, South Africa,* Senna (p. 537)

Depuratif des Alpes *Laboratoires Sodia, France,* Frangula (p. 270)

Derminiol *Marvecs Services Srl, Italy,* Witch Hazel (p. 601) *Laboratorios DHU Ibérica, S.A., Spain,* Witch Hazel (p. 601)

Dermum *Laboratoires du Dermophil Indien, France,* St John's Wort (p. 549)

• **Devil's Claw** (p. 207)
UK: Culpeper and Napiers; Frank Roberts (Herbal Dispensaries) Ltd; Healthy Direct; Holland and Barrett; Medic Herb UK Ltd; Quest Vitamins Ltd

Dexol *Laboratorios SMB Farma SA, Chile,* Borage (p. 96)

Difrarel *Sigma-Tau Arzneimittel GmbH, Germany,* Bilberry (p. 79) *Tecnifar, SA, Portugal,* Bilberry (p. 79)

Digitalysat Scilla-Digitaloid *Johannes Bürger Ysatfabrik GmbH, Germany,* St John's Wort (p. 549)

Dinaton *Asta Medica Ltda, Brazil,* Ginkgo (p. 299)

Dismegyn *Gynea Laboratorios, Spain,* Agnus Castus (p. 36)

Diurevit Mono *Bional Pharma Deutschland GmbH & Co. KG, Germany,* Java Tea (p. 381)

Doc *FIT Pharma GmbH, Germany,* Arnica (p. 64)
Dolestan *Krewel Meuselbach GmbH, Germany,* Valerian (p. 580)
Dolo-Arthrodynat *Ziethen, Germany,* Devil's Claw (p. 207)
Dolo-Arthrosetten H *Riemser Arzneimittel AG, Germany,* Devil's Claw (p. 207)
Dolorub Capsico *Laboratorios Maver SA, Chile,* Capsicum (p. 125)
Doloteffin *Ardeypharm GmbH, Germany,* Devil's Claw (p. 207)
Dormiplant *VSM Belgium, Belgium,* Melissa (p. 425), Valerian (p. 580) *VSM Geneesmiddelen BV, Netherlands,* Valerian (p. 580)
Dosaflex *Shire Pharmaceuticals, USA,* Senna (p. 537)
Dr Theiss Ringelblumen Salbe *Naturwaren OHG, Czech Republic,* Calendula (p. 121)
Duiwelsdrekdruppels *Aspen Pharmacare (Pty) Ltd, South Africa,* Asafoetida (p. 72)
Duogink *Duopharm GmbH, Germany,* Ginkgo (p. 299)
durasilymarin *Merck dura GmbH, Germany,* Milk Thistle (p. 429)
dysto-lux *Dr. Loges & Co. GmbH, Germany,* St John's Wort (p. 549)

Ebamin *Ebewe Pharma (ASIA) Ltd, Hong Kong,* Ginkgo (p. 299)
Echan *Biocur Arzneimittel GmbH, Germany,* Echinacea (p. 217)
Echifit *Krewel Meuselbach GmbH, Germany,* Echinacea (p. 217)
Echiherb *Duopharm GmbH, Germany,* Echinacea (p. 217)
Echinacea *Potter's (Herbal Supplies) Ltd, UK,* Echinacea (p. 217) *Natrol, USA,* Echinacea (p. 217)
• **Echinacea** (p. 217)
UK: Biocare Ltd; Culpeper and Napiers; Frank Roberts (Herbal Dispensaries) Ltd; Healthy Direct; Quest Vitamins Ltd; Worldwide Health Corp. Ltd
USA: Nature Made; Nature's Bounty; Sundown; Walgreens Finest Natural
Echinacin *Thursday Plantation laboratories Ltd, Australia,* Echinacea (p. 217) *Madaus GmbH, Austria,* Echinacea (p. 217) *Madaus Pharma SA, Belgium,* Echinacea (p. 217) *Madaus AG, Germany,* Echinacea (p. 217) *Apivita SA, Greece,* Echinacea (p. 217) *Naturprodukt Kft, Hungary,* Echinacea (p. 217) *Madaus, Spain,* Echinacea (p. 217) *Max Zeller Söhne AG, Pflanzliche Heilmittel, Switzerland,* Echinacea (p. 217)
Echinaforce *Aponova Pharma Handels GmbH, Austria,* Echinacea (p. 217) *Bioforce GmbH, Germany,* Echinacea (p. 217) *Bioforce AG, Switzerland,* Echinacea (p. 217) *Bioforce UK Ltd, UK,* Echinacea (p. 217)
EchinaMed *Bioforce AG, Switzerland,* Echinacea (p. 217)
Echinapur *Dr Scheffler Nachf. GmbH & Co. KG, Germany,* Echinacea (p. 217)
Echinatur *Dr. E. Ritsert GmbH & Co. KG, Germany,* Echinacea (p. 217)
Edual *Laboratorios Recalcine SA, Chile,* St John's Wort (p. 549)
Ekian *Laboratorios Diviser-Aquilea S.L., Spain,* Echinacea (p. 217)
Elagen *Eladon Ltd, UK,* Ginseng, Eleutherococcus (p. 315)
Eleu *Harras Pharma Curarina Arzneimittel GmbH, Germany,* Ginseng, Eleutherococcus (p. 315)
Eleu-Kokk *Boehringer Ingelheim Pharma GmbH & Co. KG, Germany,* Ginseng, Eleutherococcus (p. 315)
Eleutheroforce *Bioforce GmbH, Germany,* Ginseng, Eleutherococcus (p. 315)
Eleutherokokk *Arko Pharma GmbH, Germany,* Ginseng, Eleutherococcus (p. 315)
Eleutherosan *Alpa sro, Czech Republic,* Ginseng, Eleutherococcus (p. 315)
Elixir frangulae compositum *G. Streuli & Co. AG, Switzerland,* Frangula (p. 270)
Emotival *Laboratórios Klinger do Brasil Ltda, Brazil,* St John's Wort (p. 549)
Emoton *Tentan AG, Switzerland,* Agnus Castus (p. 36)
Enax *Ativus Farmacêutica Ltda, Brazil,* Echinacea (p. 217)
Enelbin-Salbe *Cassella-med GmbH & Co. KG, Germany,* Arnica (p. 64)
Enziagil Magenplus *Riemser Arzneimittel AG, Germany,* Gentian (p. 290)
Episcorit *Sanum-Kehlbeck GmbH & Co. KG, Germany,* Echinacea (p. 217)
Epitaloe *Mediwhite Srl, Italy,* Aloe Vera (p. 48)
Equilibra *Darrow Laboratórios S.A., Brazil,* St John's Wort (p. 549)
Equinacea *Herbarium Laboratório Botanico Ltda, Brazil,* Echinacea (p. 217)
Equitam *Eurofarma Laboratórios Ltda, Brazil,* Ginkgo (p. 299)
Esbericard novo *Schaper & Brümmer GmbH & Co. KG, Germany,* Hawthorn (p. 346)
Esbericum *Europharm, Austria,* St John's Wort (p. 549) *Schaper & Brümmer GmbH & Co. KG, Germany,* St John's Wort (p. 549)
Esberitox mono *Schaper & Brümmer GmbH & Co. KG, Germany,* Echinacea (p. 217)
Escar T *Laboratorio Prater SA, Chile,* Hydrocotyle (p. 371)
Essaven *Cassella-med GmbH & Co. KG, Germany,* Horse-chestnut (p. 363)
Estimul *Química Franco Mexicana Nordin S.A. de C.V., Mexico,* Arnica (p. 64)
EuMunil *Madaus S.r.l., Italy,* Echinacea (p. 217)
Eurixor *Richter Pharma, Austria,* Milk Thistle (p. 429) *biosyn Arzneimittel GmbH, Germany,* Milk Thistle (p. 429)
Euromucil *Laboratorios Saval SA, Chile,* Ispaghula (p. 374)
Euvegal Balance *Dr Willmar Schwabe GmbH & Co., Germany,* Valerian (p. 580)
Evana *Arzneimittel Schwabe International GmbH, Czech Republic,* Agnus Castus (p. 36)
• **Evening Primrose** (p. 251)
UK: Frank Roberts (Herbal Dispensaries) Ltd; Healthy Direct; Worldwide Health Corp. Ltd
USA: Nature Made; Nature's Bounty; Sundown
Eviprostat-S *Pharmazeutische Fabrik Evers & Co. GmbH, Germany,* Saw Palmetto (p. 521)
Ex-Lax *Novartis Consumer Health, UK,* Senna (p. 537) *Novartis Consumer Health Inc., USA,* Senna (p. 537)
Experience *Awareness Corp., Canada,* Senna (p. 537)
Exprep *Mundipharma Oy, Finland,* Senna (p. 537)

Falquilax *Falqui Prodotti Farmaceutici S.p.A., Italy,* Senna (p. 537)
Farmakava *Laboratório Farmaervas Ltda, Brazil,* Kava (p. 389)
Faros *Lichtwer Pharma AG, Germany,* Hawthorn (p. 346) *Vifor SA, Switzerland,* Hawthorn (p. 346)
Felis *Biocur Arzneimittel GmbH, Germany,* St John's Wort (p. 549)
Femi *Sabona GmbH, Germany,* Cohosh, Black (p. 168)
Femicine *Vifor SA, Switzerland,* Cohosh, Black (p. 168)
Femicur N *Schaper & Brümmer GmbH & Co. KG, Germany,* Agnus Castus (p. 36)
Femikliman uno *Biocur Arzneimittel GmbH, Germany,* Cohosh, Black (p. 168)
Femilla N *Steigerwald Arzneimittelwerk GmbH, Germany,* Cohosh, Black (p. 168)
Feminon A *Cesra Arzneimittel GmbH & Co. KG, Germany,* Agnus Castus (p. 36)
Feminon C *Cesra Arzneimittel GmbH & Co. KG, Germany,* Cohosh, Black (p. 168)
Femiplante *Farmasierra S.A., Spain,* Agnus Castus (p. 36)
Femisana gyn *Cheplapharm Arzneimittel GmbH, Germany,* Cohosh, Black (p. 168)
Femisana mens *Cheplapharm Arzneimittel GmbH, Germany,* Agnus Castus (p. 36)
• **Fenugreek** (p. 260)
UK: Culpeper and Napiers; Holland and Barrett
Fenugrene *Laboratoires Legras, France,* Fenugreek (p. 260)
• **Feverfew** (p. 263)
UK: Culpeper and Napiers; Frank Roberts (Herbal Dispensaries) Ltd; Holland and Barrett; Medic Herb UK Ltd; Worldwide Health Corp. Ltd
USA: Sundown
Fiberall *Novartis Pharmaceuticals Corp., USA,* Ispaghula (p. 374)
Fibrasol *Laboratorios Maver SA, Chile,* Ispaghula (p. 374)
Fibrelief *Manx Pharma Ltd, UK,* Ispaghula (p. 374)
Fibrolax *Giuliani S.p.A., Italy,* Ispaghula (p. 374)
Fibromucil *Productos Farmaceuticos Collins S.A. de C.V., Mexico,* Ispaghula (p. 374)
Fiotan *Altana Pharma Ltda, Brazil,* St John's Wort (p. 549)
Fitokey Ginkgo *Inkeysa, Spain,* Ginkgo (p. 299)
Fitokey Harpagophytum *Inkeysa, Spain,* Devil's Claw (p. 207)
Flebostasin *Sankyo Pharma Italia S.p.A., Italy,* Horse-chestnut (p. 363)
Fletchers Castoria *Mentholatum Inc., USA,* Senna (p. 537)
Flexal Brennessel *Biocur Arzneimittel GmbH, Germany,* Nettle (p. 452)
flexi-loges *Dr. Loges & Co. GmbH, Germany,* Devil's Claw (p. 207)
Floral Pas *Productos Gache S.A., Venezuela,* Passionflower (p. 461), Valerian (p. 580)
Florilax *Floris, Israel,* Senna (p. 537)
Florsalmin *Slovakofarma sro, Czech Republic,* Sage (p. 512)
Flosa *Merckle GmbH, Germany,* Ispaghula (p. 374)
Flosine *Bittermedizin Arzneimittel Vertriebs-GmbH, Germany,* Ispaghula (p. 374)
Ford Fibre *Mayne Pharma P/L, Australia,* Ispaghula (p. 374)
Fuca *Melisana SA, Belgium,* Senna (p. 537)

Fuca N *Melisana AG, Switzerland,* Senna (p. 537)

Fybogel *Reckitt Benckiser Pharmaceuticals, Australia,* Ispaghula (p. 374) *Reckitt Benckiser, Ireland,* Ispaghula (p. 374) *Zuellig Pharma Pte Ltd, Singapore,* Ispaghula (p. 374) *Reckitt Benckiser Pharmaceuticals (Pty) Ltd, South Africa,* Ispaghula (p. 374) *Reckitt Benckiser (Thailand) Ltd, Thailand,* Ispaghula (p. 374) *Reckitt Benckiser plc, UK,* Ispaghula (p. 374)

Gal *Aspen Pharmacare (Pty) Ltd, South Africa,* Senna (p. 537)

Gallentee *Abtswinder Naturheilmittel GmbH, Czech Republic,* Calendula (p. 121), Dandelion (p. 204), Liquorice (p. 411), Yarrow (p. 604)

• **Garlic** (p. 279)
UK: Biocare Ltd; Frank Roberts (Herbal Dispensaries) Ltd; Healthy Direct; Worldwide Health Corp. Ltd
USA: Sundown; Walgreens Finest Natural

Garlimega *The Cantassium Company, UK,* Garlic (p. 279)

GarliPure *Natrol, USA,* Garlic (p. 279)

Garlix *Blackmores Ltd, Australia,* Garlic (p. 279)

Gastrovegetalin *Verla-Pharm, Arzneimittelfabrik, Apotheker H.J.v. Ehrlich GmbH & Co. KG, Germany,* Melissa (p. 425)

Gelobronchial *G. Pohl-Boskamp GmbH & Co., Germany,* Thyme (p. 574)

• **Gentian** (p. 290)
UK: Culpeper and Napiers

Geriaforce *Bioforce AG, Switzerland,* Ginkgo (p. 299)

Gerimax Ginseng (Геримакс Женьшень) *Sanofi-Aventis, Russia,* Ginseng, Panax (p. 325)

Gerimax Tonique *Merck Lipha Santé, France,* Ginseng, Panax (p. 325)

Gibilon *Instituto Terapeutico Delta Ltda, Brazil,* Ginkgo (p. 299)

Ginbiloba *Bunker Indústria Farmacêutica Ltda, Brazil,* Ginkgo (p. 299)

Gincare *Y.S.P. Industries (M) Sdn Bhd, Malaysia,* Ginkgo (p. 299)

Gincoben *Ipsen Portugal, SA, Portugal,* Ginkgo (p. 299)

Gincolin *Laboratório Teuto-Brasileiro Ltda, Brazil,* Ginkgo (p. 299)

Gincuran *Bioplanta Arzneimittel GmbH, Germany,* Ginkgo (p. 299)

Ginemaxim *Laboratorio Esp. Med. Knop Ltda, Chile,* Cohosh, Black (p. 168)

• **Ginger** (p. 293)
UK: Biocare Ltd; Culpeper and Napiers; Frank Roberts (Herbal Dispensaries) Ltd; Holland and Barrett; Quest Vitamins Ltd; Worldwide Health Corp. Ltd
USA: Sundown

Gingiloba *1 A Pharma GmbH, Germany,* Ginkgo (p. 299)

Gingium *Biocur Arzneimittel GmbH, Germany,* Ginkgo (p. 299) *Hexal Hungária Kft, Hungary,* Ginkgo (p. 299)

Gingivitol N *Hennig Arzneimittel GmbH & Co. KG, Germany,* Golden Seal (p. 337)

Gingobeta *betapharm Arzneimittel GmbH, Germany,* Ginkgo (p. 299)

Gingohexal *Hexal Pharma GmbH, Austria,* Ginkgo (p. 299)

Gingol *F. Joh. Kwizda, Austria,* Ginkgo (p. 299)

Gingopret *Bionorica AG, Germany,* Ginkgo (p. 299)

Gingosol *Ecosol AG, Switzerland,* Ginkgo (p. 299)

Ginkapran *Zyfas Medical Co, Singapore,* Ginkgo (p. 299)

• **Ginkgo** (p. 299)
UK: Biocare Ltd; Culpeper and Napiers; Frank Roberts (Herbal Dispensaries) Ltd; Healthy Direct; Medic Herb UK Ltd; Quest Vitamins Ltd; Worldwide Health Corp. Ltd
USA: Natrol; Nature Made; Nature's Bounty; Sundown; Walgreens Finest Natural

Ginkgold *ASI Budapest Kft, Hungary,* Ginkgo (p. 299)

Ginkoba *Química E Farmacêutica Nikkho do Brasil Ltda, Brazil,* Ginkgo (p. 299) *Fher, Divisione della Boehringer Ingelheim, Italy,* Ginkgo (p. 299)

Ginkobil *Infabra Indústria Farmacêutica Brasileira Ltda, Brazil,* Ginkgo (p. 299) *ratiopharm GmbH, Germany,* Ginkgo (p. 299)

Ginkodilat *Sandoz Pharmaceuticals GmbH, Germany,* Ginkgo (p. 299)

Ginkofarma *Laboratório Farmaervas Ltda, Brazil,* Ginkgo (p. 299)

Ginkoftal *Dávi Farmacêutica, Lda, Portugal,* Ginkgo (p. 299)

Ginkogink *Beaufour Ipsen Pharma, France,* Ginkgo (p. 299)

Ginkogreen *Greenpharma Química e Farmacêutica Ltda, Brazil,* Ginkgo (p. 299)

Ginkokan *Farmasan Arzneimittel GmbH & Co., Germany,* Ginkgo (p. 299)

Ginkolab *Multilab Ind. e Com. Prods. Farmacêuticos Ltda, Brazil,* Ginkgo (p. 299)

Ginkolin *Weston Pharmaceutical Ltd, Hong Kong,* Ginkgo (p. 299)

Ginkoplus *Fontovit Laboratórios Ltda, Brazil,* Ginkgo (p. 299)

Ginkopur *W. Spitzner, Arzneimittelfabrik GmbH, Germany,* Ginkgo (p. 299)

Ginkosen *Polymedic Trading Enterprise Pte Ltd, Singapore,* Ginkgo (p. 299)

Ginkovital *Pharmadass Ltd, UK,* Ginkgo (p. 299)

Ginsana *Boehringer Ingelheim S.A., Argentina,* Ginseng, Panax (p. 325) *Boehringer Ingelheim Austria GmbH, Austria,* Ginseng, Panax (p. 325) *Boehringer Ingelheim SA/NV, Belgium,* Ginseng, Panax (p. 325) *Boehringer Ingelheim do Brasil Quím. e Farm. Ltda, Brazil,* Ginseng, Panax (p. 325) *Boehringer Ingelheim (Canada) Ltd, Canada,* Ginseng, Panax (p. 325) *Boehringer Ingelheim sro, Czech Republic,* Ginseng, Panax (p. 325) *Boehringer Ingelheim Pharma GmbH & Co. KG, Germany,* Ginseng, Panax (p. 325) *Fher, Divisione della Boehringer Ingelheim, Italy,* Ginseng, Panax (p. 325) *Boehringer Ingelheim, Division Diethelm Malaysia Sdn Bhd, Malaysia,* Ginseng, Panax (p. 325) *Boehringer Ingelheim, Lda, Portugal,* Ginseng, Panax (p. 325) *Diethelm Singapore Pte Ltd, Singapore,* Ginseng, Panax (p. 325) *GPL Ginsana Products Lugano SA, Tochterunternehmen der Pharmaton SA, Switzerland,* Ginseng, Panax (p. 325) *Boehringer Ingelheim (Thai) Ltd, Thailand,* Ginseng, Panax (p. 325)

Ginsana (Гинсана) *Boehringer Ingelheim Pharma GmbH, Russia,* Ginseng, Panax (p. 325)

• **Ginseng, Eleutherococcus** (p. 315)
UK: Culpeper and Napiers; Frank Roberts (Herbal Dispensaries) Ltd; Healthy Direct; Quest Vitamins Ltd; Worldwide Health Corp. Ltd

• **Ginseng, Panax** (p. 325)
UK: Biocare Ltd; Healthy Direct; Holland and Barrett; Worldwide Health Corp. Ltd
USA: Nature Made; Nature's Bounty; Sundown

Ginsex *Instituto Terapeutico Delta Ltda, Brazil,* Ginseng, Panax (p. 325)

Ginsroy *Schumit 1967 Co. Ltd, Thailand,* Ginseng, Panax (p. 325)

GNC Herbal Laxative *General Nutrition Canada, Canada,* Senna (p. 537)

• **Golden Seal** (p. 337)
UK: Frank Roberts (Herbal Dispensaries) Ltd; Worldwide Health Corp. Ltd
USA: Nature Made; Nature's Bounty

Grafic Retard *Microsules y Bernabo S.A., Argentina,* Horse-chestnut (p. 363)

Grains de Vals Nouvelle formule *F. Uhlmann-Eyraud SA, Switzerland,* Senna (p. 537)

• **Gravel Root** (p. 340)
UK: Culpeper and Napiers

Gravol Natural Source *Carter Horner Inc., Canada,* Ginger (p. 293)

• **Ground Ivy** (p. 342)
UK: Culpeper and Napiers

Gyncobem *Cifarma Cientifica Farmacêutica Ltda, Brazil,* Ginkgo (p. 299)

Gyndelta *Laboratoires CCD, France,* Cranberry (p. 197)

Gynocastus *Fritz Zilly GmbH, Germany,* Agnus Castus (p. 36)

Hamasana *Robugen GmbH Pharmazeutische Fabrik, Germany,* Witch Hazel (p. 601)

Hamburg Tea *Aspen Pharmacare (Pty) Ltd, South Africa,* Senna (p. 537)

Hametol *Dr W Schwabe, Spain,* Witch Hazel (p. 601)

Hametum *Dr Peithner KG nunmehr GmbH & Co., Austria,* Witch Hazel (p. 601) *Dr Willmar Schwabe GmbH & Co., W. Spitzner, Arzneimittelfabrik GmbH, Germany,* Witch Hazel (p. 601)

Harpadol *Laboratoires Arkopharma, France,* Devil's Claw (p. 207)

Harpagocid *Laboratoires Phytomedica, France,* Devil's Claw (p. 207)

Harpagofito Orto *Normon S.A., Spain,* Devil's Claw (p. 207)

Harpagoforte Asmedic *Dyckerhoff Pharma GmbH & Co., Germany,* Devil's Claw (p. 207)

HarpagoMega *Astrid Twardy GmbH, Germany,* Devil's Claw (p. 207)

Harpagosan *Neopharma GmbH & Co. KG, Germany,* Devil's Claw (p. 207)

• **Hawthorn** (p. 346)
UK: Culpeper and Napiers; Frank Roberts (Herbal Dispensaries) Ltd; Holland and Barrett; Quest Vitamins Ltd; Worldwide Health Corp. Ltd
USA: Sundown

Hebucol *Will-Pharma SA, Belgium,* Artichoke (p. 67)

Hegrimarin *Strathmann Ag & Co Képviselete, Hungary,* Milk Thistle (p. 429)

Helarium *Austroplant-Arzneimittel GmbH, Austria,* St John's Wort (p. 549) *Bionorica AG, Germany,* St John's Wort (p. 549) *ASI Budapest Kft, Hungary,* St John's Wort (p. 549)

Helarium (Геларнум) *Bionorica AG, Russia,* St John's Wort (p. 549)

Helixor *Germania Pharmazeutika GmbH, Austria,* Milk Thistle (p. 429) *Helixor Heilmittel GmbH & Co., Germany,* Milk Thistle (p. 429)

Hemo Derminiol *Laboratorios DHU Ibérica, S.A., Spain,* Witch Hazel (p. 601)

HepaBesch S *Strathmann AG & Co., Germany,* Milk Thistle (p. 429)

4

Hepagallin N *Homöopathisches Laboratorium A. Pflüger GmbH, Germany,* Artichoke (p. 67)

Hepa-Loges *Dr. Loges & Co. GmbH, Germany,* Milk Thistle (p. 429)

Hepanephrol *Laboratoires Zambon France, France,* Artichoke (p. 67)

Hepar SL *Sertürner Arzneimittel GmbH, Germany,* Artichoke (p. 67)

Hepar-Pasc *Pascoe Pharmazeutische Präparate GmbH, Germany,* Milk Thistle (p. 429)

Hepar-POS *Croma-Pharma GmbH, Austria,* Artichoke (p. 67) *Ursapharm Arzneimittel GmbH & Co. KG, Germany,* Artichoke (p. 67)

Heparstad *Stada GmbH, Germany,* Artichoke (p. 67)

Hepa-S *Vifor SA, Switzerland,* Artichoke (p. 67)

Hepatos *Hevert-Arzneimittel GmbH & Co. KG, Germany,* Milk Thistle (p. 429)

Heplant *W. Spitzner, Arzneimittelfabrik GmbH, Germany,* Milk Thistle (p. 429)

Herbaccion Bioenergizante *Instituto Seroterapico Argentino S.A.I.C., Argentina,* Ginseng, Panax (p. 325)

Herbaccion Venotonico *Instituto Seroterapico Argentino S.A.I.C., Argentina,* Horse-chestnut (p. 363)

Herbal Eye Care Formula *Mayne Pharma P/L, Australia,* Bilberry (p. 79)

Herbal Headache Relief *Mayne Pharma P/L, Australia,* Feverfew (p. 263)

Herbal Liver Formula *Mayne Pharma P/L, Australia,* Milk Thistle (p. 429)

Herbal Premens *SwissHealth, UK,* Agnus Castus (p. 36)

Herbal Sleep Formula *Mayne Pharma P/L, Australia,* Valerian (p. 580)

Herbal Stress Relief *Mayne Pharma P/L, Australia,* Ginseng, Panax (p. 325)

Hevert-Aktivon Mono *Hevert-Arzneimittel GmbH & Co. KG, Germany,* Ginseng, Panax (p. 325)

Heverto *Hevert-Arzneimittel GmbH & Co. KG, Germany,* Senna (p. 537)

Hevertogyn *Hevert-Arzneimittel GmbH & Co. KG, Germany,* Agnus Castus (p. 36)

Hewechol Artischockendragees *Hevert-Arzneimittel GmbH & Co. KG, Germany,* Artichoke (p. 67)

Hewepsychon uno *Hevert-Arzneimittel GmbH & Co. KG, Germany,* St John's Wort (p. 549)

Heweven Phyto *Hevert-Arzneimittel GmbH & Co. KG, Germany,* Horse-chestnut (p. 363)

Hipax *Lab. Baliarda S.A., Argentina,* St John's Wort (p. 549)

Hiperex *Eurofarma Laboratórios Ltda, Brazil,* St John's Wort (p. 549)

Hipericin *Herbarium Laboratório Botanico Ltda, Brazil,* St John's Wort (p. 549)

Hiperico *Herbarium Laboratório Botanico Ltda, Brazil,* St John's Wort (p. 549) *Laboratorios Diviser-Aquilea S.L., Naytsal, Spain,* St John's Wort (p. 549)

Hiperifarma *Laboratório Farmaervas Ltda, Brazil,* St John's Wort (p. 549)

Hiperikan *Laboratorios Farmasa, S.A. de C.V., Mexico,* St John's Wort (p. 549)

Hiperil *Laboratório Teuto-Brasileiro Ltda, Brazil,* St John's Wort (p. 549)

Hiperinat *Lab. Natufarma, Argentina,* St John's Wort (p. 549)

Hipersac *Bunker Indústria Farmacêutica Ltda, Brazil,* St John's Wort (p. 549)

Hloh-List S *Leros sro, Czech Republic,* Hawthorn (p. 346)

Hoevenol *Carl Hoernecke GmbH, Germany,* Horse-chestnut (p. 363)

• **Hops** (p. 354)
UK: Culpeper and Napiers

• **Horehound, Black** (p. 358)
UK: Culpeper and Napiers

Hormolax *Laboratorios Hormona S.A. de C.V., Mexico,* Ispaghula (p. 374)

• **Horse-chestnut** (p. 363)
UK: Culpeper and Napiers; Healthy Direct; Holland and Barrett
USA: Sundown

Hox Alpha *Strathmann AG & Co., Germany,* Nettle (p. 452)

Hustagil Thymian-Hustensaft *Dentinox Gesellschaft für Pharmazeutische Präparate Lenk & Schuppan, Germany,* Thyme (p. 574)

Hustagil Thymiantropfen *Dentinox Gesellschaft für Pharmazeutische Präparate Lenk & Schuppan, Germany,* Thyme (p. 574)

Husties *Eu Rho OTC Pharma GmbH, Germany,* Thyme (p. 574)

Hydrocil Instant *Numark Laboratories Inc., USA,* Ispaghula (p. 374)

Hyneurin *Korhispana, Spain,* St John's Wort (p. 549)

Hypercircin *Riemser Arzneimittel AG, Germany,* Milk Thistle (p. 429)

Hyperforat *Dr Gustav Klein, Germany,* St John's Wort (p. 549)

Hypericaps *Duopharm GmbH, Germany,* St John's Wort (p. 549)

Hyperico *Viternat Laboratórios Ltda, Brazil,* St John's Wort (p. 549)

Hyperiforce *Bio-Garten GmbH, Austria,* St John's Wort (p. 549) *Bioforce AG, Switzerland,* St John's Wort (p. 549)

Hyperiforte *Blackmores Ltd, Australia,* St John's Wort (p. 549)

Hyperigreen *Greenpharma Química e Farmacêutica Ltda, Brazil,* St John's Wort (p. 549)

HyperiMed *Bioforce AG, Switzerland,* St John's Wort (p. 549)

Hyperimerck *Merck dura GmbH, Germany,* St John's Wort (p. 549)

Hyperiplant *VSM Belgium, Belgium,* St John's Wort (p. 549) *Schwabe Pharma AG, Switzerland,* St John's Wort (p. 549)

Hyperprost Uno *Robugen GmbH Pharmazeutische Fabrik, Germany,* Saw Palmetto (p. 521)

Hyperpur *Alpharma-Isis GmbH & Co. KG, Germany,* St John's Wort (p. 549)

Hyperval *Sidroga AG, Switzerland,* St John's Wort (p. 549)

Hyzum N *Merckle GmbH, Germany,* Arnica (p. 64)

IL HWA *allcura Naturheilmittel GmbH, Germany,* Ginseng, Panax (p. 325)

Ilja Rogoff Forte *Roche Consumer Health Deutschland GmbH, Germany,* Garlic (p. 279)

Immunal *Lek Pharma sro, Czech Republic,* Echinacea (p. 217)

Immunal (Иммунал) *Lek, Russia,* Echinacea (p. 217)

Immunorm (Иммунорм) *Ratiopharm Group, Russia,* Echinacea (p. 217)

Imunnal *Herbarium Laboratório Botanico Ltda, Brazil,* Echinacea (p. 217)

Imunocel *Laboratório Teuto-Brasileiro Ltda, Brazil,* Echinacea (p. 217)

Imunogreen *Greenpharma Química e Farmacêutica Ltda, Brazil,* Echinacea (p. 217)

Inmune Booster *Solara Farmaceutica SA de CV, Mexico,* Echinacea (p. 217)

Inspirol P *Riemser Arzneimittel AG, Germany,* Myrrh (p. 449)

Iperisan *Marjan Indústria e Comércio Ltda, Brazil,* St John's Wort (p. 549)

Iscador *Weleda GmbH & Co. KG, Austria,* Milk Thistle (p. 429) *Weleda AG-Heilmittelbetriebe, Germany,* Milk Thistle (p. 429) *Weleda AG, Switzerland,* Milk Thistle (p. 429)

Isephca S *Iso-Arzneimittel GmbH & Co. KG, Germany,* Thyme (p. 574)

Isogel *GlaxoSmithKline Pharmaceuticals (India) Ltd, India,* Ispaghula (p. 374) *GlaxoSmithKline, New Zealand,* Ispaghula (p. 374) *Chefaro UK Ltd, UK,* Ispaghula (p. 374)

Isoginkgo *Merck dura GmbH, Germany,* Ginkgo (p. 299)

Isorel *Novipharm GmbH, Austria,* Milk Thistle (p. 429)

Ispagel *LPC Medical (UK) Ltd, UK,* Ispaghula (p. 374)

Jarsin *F. Joh. Kwizda, Austria,* St John's Wort (p. 549) *Laboratórios Biosintetica Ltda, Brazil,* St John's Wort (p. 549) *Lichtwer Pharma AG, Germany,* St John's Wort (p. 549) *Vifor SA, Switzerland,* St John's Wort (p. 549)

Jinda *F. Joh. Kwizda, Austria,* Cohosh, Black (p. 168) *Riemser Arzneimittel AG, Germany,* Cohosh, Black (p. 168)

Johanicum *Apomedica GmbH, Austria,* St John's Wort (p. 549)

Johni *Interpharm GmbH, Austria,* St John's Wort (p. 549)

Jo-Sabona *Sabona GmbH, Germany,* St John's Wort (p. 549)

Jucurba *Strathmann AG & Co., Germany,* Capsicum (p. 125), Devil's Claw (p. 207)

Jungborn *Taro Pharmaceutical International, Israel,* Senna (p. 537)

• **Juniper** (p. 386)
UK: Culpeper and Napiers

Kalter *Laboratorios Phoenix S.A.I.C.F., Argentina,* Ginkgo (p. 299)

• **Kava** (p. 389)
UK: Worldwide Health Corp. Ltd
USA: Natrol

Kavakan *Ativus Farmacêutica Ltda, Brazil,* Kava (p. 389)

Kavalac *Fontovit Laboratórios Ltda, Brazil,* Kava (p. 389)

Kavasedon *Novaquimica Sigma Pharma-Nature's Plus Ltda, Brazil,* Kava (p. 389) *Horna Business Service, Czech Republic,* Kava (p. 389) *Laboratorios Cofasa S.A., Venezuela,* Kava (p. 389)

Kaveri *Lichtwer Pharma AG, Germany,* Ginkgo (p. 299)

Kiadon *Merck S.A. Industrias Químicas, Brazil,* Ginkgo (p. 299) *Merck Química Chilena Ltda, Chile,* Ginkgo (p. 299) *Merck S.A., Venezuela,* Ginkgo (p. 299)

KintaVital *Sanofi-Aventis (Schweiz) AG, Switzerland,* Ginseng, Panax (p. 325)

Kira *F. Joh. Kwizda, Austria,* St John's Wort (p. 549) *Lichtwer Pharma, Canada,* St John's Wort (p. 549) *Riemser Arzneimittel AG, Germany,* St John's Wort (p. 549) *Lichtwer Pharma UK, UK,* St John's Wort (p. 549) *Grupo Farma S.A., Venezuela,* St John's Wort (p. 549)

Kirsan *Ativus Farmacêutica Ltda, Brazil,* Ginkgo (p. 299)

Klimadynon *Austroplant-Arzneimittel GmbH, Austria,* Cohosh, Black (p. 168) *Bionorica AG, Germany,* Cohosh, Black (p. 168) *Jacobson Medical (Hong Kong) Ltd, Hong Kong,* Cohosh, Black (p. 168) *MBD Marketing (S) Pte Ltd, Singapore,* Cohosh, Black (p. 168)

Klimadynon (Климадинон) *Bionorica AG, Russia,* Cohosh, Black (p. 168)

Klosterfrau Nervenruh Dragees *Melisana AG, Switzerland,* Hops (p. 354)

Kneipp Pflanzen-Dragees Weissdorn *Kneipp-Werke, Germany,* Hawthorn (p. 346)

Kolob *Unipharm de Mexico SA de CV, Mexico,* Ginkgo (p. 299)

Konstitutin *CytoChemia AG, Germany,* Ginseng, Eleutherococcus (p. 315)

Konsyl *GlaxoSmithKline S.A., Argentina,* Ispaghula (p. 374) *Pharmateam Marketing, Israel,* Ispaghula (p. 374) *Konsyl Pharmaceuticals, USA,* Ispaghula (p. 374)

Konsyl-D *Konsyl Pharmaceuticals, USA,* Ispaghula (p. 374)

Kontryhelova Nat *Megafyt-R sro, Czech Republic,* Parsley Piert (p. 459)

Koprivovy Caj, Koprivova Nat *Megafyt-R sro, Czech Republic,* Nettle (p. 452)

Koren Kozliku Lekarskeho *Leros sro, Czech Republic,* Valerian (p. 580)

Koren Puskvorce *Leros sro, Czech Republic,* Calamus (p. 118)

Koro-Nyhadin *Robugen GmbH Pharmazeutische Fabrik, Germany,* Hawthorn (p. 346)

Korseng *Self-Care Products Ltd, UK,* Ginseng, Panax (p. 325)

Krauterlax *Dolorgiet GmbH & Co. KG, Germany,* Aloes (p. 50)

Kvet Bazy Ciernej *Slovakofarma sro, Czech Republic,* Elder (p. 237)

Kvet Lipy *Slovakofarma sro, Czech Republic,* Lime Flower (p. 409)

Kwai *F. Joh. Kwizda, Austria,* Garlic (p. 279) *Lichtwer Pharma, Canada,* Garlic (p. 279) *Lichtwer Pharma AG, Germany,* Garlic (p. 279) *Solvay Pharma S.p.A., Italy,* Garlic (p. 279) *Lichtwer Pharma UK, UK,* Garlic (p. 279) *Grupo Farma S.A., Venezuela,* Garlic (p. 279)

Kyolic *Boehringer Ingelheim (Canada) Ltd, Canada,* Garlic (p. 279) *JDH Pharmaceutical Sdn Bhd, Malaysia,* Garlic (p. 279) *Quest Vitamins Ltd, UK,* Garlic (p. 279)

Kytta Pommade *Iromedica AG, Switzerland,* Comfrey (p. 188)

Kytta-Cor *Merck KGaA, Germany,* Hawthorn (p. 346)

Kytta-Plasma f *Merck KGaA, Germany,* Comfrey (p. 188)

Kytta-Salbe f *Merck KGaA, Germany,* Comfrey (p. 188)

Laci Echinacea with Hint of Mint *Natrol, USA,* Echinacea (p. 217)

Lagenbach *Representaciones Mex-America S.A. de C.V., Mexico,* Senna (p. 537)

Lagosa *Wörwag Pharma GmbH & Co, Czech Republic,* Milk Thistle (p. 429) *Wörwag Pharma GmbH & Co. KG, Germany,* Milk Thistle (p. 429)

Laif *Steigerwald Arzneimittelwerk GmbH, Germany,* St John's Wort (p. 549)

Laitan *Altana Pharma Ltda, Brazil,* Kava (p. 389)

Lakinal *Slovakofarma sro, Czech Republic,* Melissa (p. 425)

Laxabene *Alter, Spain,* Ispaghula (p. 374)

Laxal *Gulf Pharmaceutical Industries, Julphar, United Arab Emirates,* Senna (p. 537)

Laxamucil *Orion-yhtymä Oyj, Finland,* Ispaghula (p. 374)

Laxans *Schülke & Mayr GmbH, Austria,* Ispaghula (p. 374)

Laxante Bescansa Normal *Bescansa, Spain,* Senna (p. 537)

Laxante Olan *Puerto Galiano, Spain,* Senna (p. 537)

Laxante Salud *Boots Healthcare, Spain,* Senna (p. 537)

Laxikal Forte *Teva Pharmaceuticals Ind. Ltd, Israel,* Senna (p. 537)

Laxiplant Soft *Schwabe Pharma AG, Switzerland,* Ispaghula (p. 374)

Laxiruela Ciruela Fibra *Lab. Garden House S.A., Argentina,* Senna (p. 537)

Laxolen *Laboratorios Basi, Portugal,* Cascara (p. 128)

Laxucil *Novopharm Ltd, Canada,* Ispaghula (p. 374)

Legalon *Madaus GmbH, Austria,* Milk Thistle (p. 429) *Madaus Pharma SA, Belgium,* Milk Thistle (p. 429) *Altana Pharma Ltda, Brazil,* Milk Thistle (p. 429) *Laboratoires Madaus, France,* Milk Thistle (p. 429) *Madaus AG, Germany,* Milk Thistle (p. 429) *Naturprodukt Kft, Hungary,* Milk Thistle (p. 429) *Madaus S.r.l., Italy,* Milk Thistle (p. 429) *Neo-Farmacêutica, Lda, Portugal,* Milk Thistle (p. 429) *Max Zeller Söhne AG, Pflanzliche Heilmittel, Switzerland,* Milk Thistle (p. 429)

Legapas *Pascoe Pharmazeutische Präparate GmbH, Germany,* Cascara (p. 128)

Leikan *Arzneimittel Schwabe International GmbH, Czech Republic,* Kava (p. 389)

Lektinol *Madaus AG, Germany,* Milk Thistle (p. 429)

Libeprosta *Pharma Fabre Hellas S.A., Greece,* Saw Palmetto (p. 521)

Libertin *Robugen GmbH Pharmazeutische Fabrik, Germany,* St John's Wort (p. 549)

Lipei *Steiner & Co. Deutsche Arzneimittel Gesellschaft, Germany,* Artichoke (p. 67)

Lipovy *Megafyt-R sro, Czech Republic,* Lime Flower (p. 409)

Liquidepur *Woelm Pharma GmbH & Co., Germany,* Senna (p. 537)

• **Liquorice** (p. 411)
UK: Culpeper and Napiers; Holland and Barrett; Medic Herb UK Ltd

List Medvedice Lecive *Leros sro, Czech Republic,* Uva-Ursi (p. 577)

List Salveje Lekarske *Leros sro, Czech Republic,* Sage (p. 512)

List Senny *Leros sro, Czech Republic,* Senna (p. 537)

List Vachty Trojliste *Leros sro, Czech Republic,* Bogbean (p. 89)

Litonate *Laboratorios Biotech C.A., Venezuela,* Hydrocotyle (p. 371)

Lomacard *Lomapharm, Rudolf Lohmann GmbH KG, Germany,* Hawthorn (p. 346)

Lomaherpan *Madaus GmbH, Austria,* Melissa (p. 425) *Lomapharm, Rudolf Lohmann GmbH KG, Germany,* Melissa (p. 425)

Lomahypericum *Lomapharm, Rudolf Lohmann GmbH KG, Germany,* St John's Wort (p. 549)

Losapan *Duopharm GmbH, Germany,* Artichoke (p. 67)

Lostamucil *Lab. Temis Lostaló S.A., Argentina,* Ispaghula (p. 374)

Lubovnik *Slovakofarma sro, Czech Republic,* St John's Wort (p. 549)

Lucilium *Ecosol AG, Switzerland,* St John's Wort (p. 549)

Lunare *Interpharm GmbH, Austria,* St John's Wort (p. 549)

Lunelax *Nycomed Pharma AS, Norway,* Ispaghula (p. 374) *AstraZeneca Sverige AB, Sweden,* Ispaghula (p. 374)

Lutene *Herbarium Laboratório Botanico Ltda, Brazil,* Agnus Castus (p. 36)

Luvased mono *Biocur Arzneimittel GmbH, Germany,* Valerian (p. 580)

Lymphozil *Cesra Arzneimittel GmbH & Co. KG, Germany,* Echinacea (p. 217)

Macro Garlic *Wyeth Pharmaceuticals, Division of Wyeth Australia P/L, Australia,* Garlic (p. 279)

Madecassol *Bayer Austria GmbH, Austria,* Hydrocotyle (p. 371) *Roche SA/NV, Belgium,* Hydrocotyle (p. 371) *Bayer SA, Chile,* Hydrocotyle (p. 371) *Laboratoires Roche Nicholas, France,* Hydrocotyle (p. 371) *A. Nikolakopoulos & Co. O.E, Greece,* Hydrocotyle (p. 371) *CNW (Hong Kong) Ltd, Hong Kong,* Hydrocotyle (p. 371) *Sanofi-Synthelabo de Mexico S.A. de C.V., Mexico,* Hydrocotyle (p. 371) *Confar, Lda, Portugal,* Hydrocotyle (p. 371) *Laboratorios Politecnicos Nacionales C.A., Venezuela,* Hydrocotyle (p. 371)

Makatussin Saft *Altana Pharma Deutschland GmbH, Germany,* Thyme (p. 574)

Makatussin Saft Drosera *Altana Pharma Deutschland GmbH, Germany,* Drosera (p. 215)

Makatussin Tropfen Drosera *Altana Pharma Deutschland GmbH, Germany,* Drosera (p. 215)

Mariendistel Curarina *Harras Pharma Curarina Arzneimittel GmbH, Germany,* Milk Thistle (p. 429)

• **Marshmallow** (p. 418)
UK: Culpeper and Napiers; Holland and Barrett

Matai *Engelhard Arzneimittel GmbH & Co. KG, Germany,* Devil's Claw (p. 207)

Mavena Anal-Gen *Psorimed AG, Switzerland,* Witch Hazel (p. 601)

Maxifem *Ecosol AG, Switzerland,* Cohosh, Black (p. 168)

Maximum Relief Ex-Lax *Novartis Consumer Health Inc., USA,* Senna (p. 537)

• **Meadowsweet** (p. 423)
UK: Culpeper and Napiers

Medovka Lekarska *Slovakofarma sro, Czech Republic,* Melissa (p. 425)

Medunkovy, Medunkova *Megafyt-R sro, Czech Republic,* Melissa (p. 425)

Medvedice *Leciva as, Czech Republic,* Uva-Ursi (p. 577)

• **Melissa** (p. 425)
UK: Culpeper and Napiers; Medic Herb UK Ltd

Melrosum Hustensirup *Cassella-med GmbH & Co. KG, Germany,* Thyme (p. 574)

Memfit *Boehringer Ingelheim SA/NV, Belgium,* Ginkgo (p. 299)

Memokit *Laboratorio Ximena Polanco, Chile,* Ginkgo (p. 299)

Mencirax *Ativus Farmacêutica Ltda, Brazil,* Cohosh, Black (p. 168)

Menofem *Boehringer Ingelheim S.A., Argentina,* Cohosh, Black (p. 168) *Arzneimittel Schwabe International GmbH, Czech Republic,* Cohosh, Black (p. 168)

Menoflavon *Cedar Health Ltd, UK,* Red Clover (p. 498)

Menoliv *Laboratório Teuto-Brasileiro Ltda, Brazil,* Cohosh, Black (p. 168)

Mensana *Darrow Laboratórios S.A., Brazil,* Ginkgo (p. 299)

Mensifem *Boehringer Ingelheim, Chile,* Cohosh, Black (p. 168)

Me-Sabona *Sabona GmbH, Germany,* Melissa (p. 425)

Mesickovy *Megafyt-R sro, Czech Republic,* Calendula (p. 121)

Metamucil *Procter & Gamble Interamericanos Inc., Argentina,* Ispaghula (p. 374) *Procter & Gamble Australia P/L, Australia,* Ispaghula (p. 374) *Procter & Gamble Austria GmbH, Austria,* Ispaghula (p. 374) *Procter & Gamble do Brasil S.A., Brazil,* Ispaghula (p. 374) *Procter & Gamble Inc., Canada,* Ispaghula (p. 374) *Laboratorios Recalcine SA, Chile,* Ispaghula (p. 374) *Wick Pharma Zweigniederlassung der Procter & Gamble GmbH, Germany,* Ispaghula (p. 374) *Pharmacia Asia Ltd, Hong Kong,* Ispaghula (p. 374) *Procter & Gamble de Mexico S.A. de C.V., Mexico,* Ispaghula (p. 374) *Procter & Gamble Pharmaceuticals, Netherlands,* Ispaghula (p. 374) *Procter & Gamble NPD, Inc., New Zealand,* Ispaghula (p. 374) *Procter Gamble, Spain,* Ispaghula (p. 374) *Procter & Gamble AG, Switzerland,* Ispaghula (p. 374) *Pfizer (Thailand) Ltd, Thailand,* Ispaghula (p. 374) *Procter & Gamble, USA,* Ispaghula (p. 374)

Midro *Wolfs SA, Belgium,* Senna (p. 537) *Midro Vertrieb AG, Switzerland,* Senna (p. 537)

Midro Abfuhr *Midro Lörrach GmbH, Germany,* Senna (p. 537)

Midro Tee *Midro Lörrach GmbH, Germany,* Senna (p. 537)

• **Milk Thistle** (p. 429)
UK: Biocare Ltd; Culpeper and Napiers; Frank Roberts (Herbal Dispensaries) Ltd; Healthy Direct; Holland and Barrett; Quest Vitamins Ltd; Worldwide Health Corp. Ltd
USA: Nature Made; Nature's Bounty; Sundown

Milperinol *Dolisos SA, Belgium,* St John's Wort (p. 549)

Miralis *Ativus Farmacêutica Ltda, Brazil,* Bilberry (p. 79)

Mirfusot *Merckle GmbH, Germany,* Thyme (p. 574)

Mirtilene Forte *Società Industria Farmaceutica Italiana S.p.A., Italy,* Bilberry (p. 79)

Mirtilene Forte (Миртилене Форте) *Schering-Plough Central East AG, Russia,* Bilberry (p. 79)

Mistel Curarina *Harras Pharma Curarina Arzneimittel GmbH, Germany,* Milk Thistle (p. 429)

Mistel-Krautertabletten *Salus-Haus Dr. med. Otto Greither Nachf. GmbH & Co KG, Germany,* Milk Thistle (p. 429)

Misteltropfen *Bio-Diät-Berlin GmbH, Germany,* Milk Thistle (p. 429)

Misteltropfen Hofmanns *Hofmann & Sommer GmbH & Co. KG, Germany,* Milk Thistle (p. 429)

Modern Herbals Sleep Aid *G.R. Lane Health Products Ltd, UK,* Passionflower (p. 461)

• **Motherwort** (p. 447)
UK: Culpeper and Napiers; Frank Roberts (Herbal Dispensaries) Ltd

Motional *Laboratorios Beta S.A., Argentina,* Ispaghula (p. 374)

Motiven *Fontovit Laboratórios Ltda, Brazil,* St John's Wort (p. 549)

Movana *Boehringer Ingelheim (Canada) Ltd, Canada,* St John's Wort (p. 549)

Mucilag *Química y Farmacia, S.A. de C.V., Mexico,* Ispaghula (p. 374)

Mucilar *Spirig Pharma AG, Switzerland,* Ispaghula (p. 374)

Mucilax *Douglas Pharmaceuticals Ltd, New Zealand,* Ispaghula (p. 374)

Mucilin *Polymedic Trading Enterprise Pte Ltd, Singapore,* Ispaghula (p. 374) *Berlin Pharmaceutical Industry Co. Ltd, Thailand,* Ispaghula (p. 374)

Mucillium *Pharmascience Inc., Canada,* Ispaghula (p. 374)

Mucinum *Confar, Lda, Portugal,* Cascara (p. 128)

Mucivital *Laboratoires Arkopharma, France,* Ispaghula (p. 374) *Pharma Guri, Israel,* Ispaghula (p. 374)

Mucofalk *Lab. Cevallos Salud S.R.L., Argentina,* Ispaghula (p. 374) *Dr. Falk Pharma GmbH, Germany,* Ispaghula (p. 374) *Jacobson Medical (Hong Kong) Ltd, Hong Kong,* Ispaghula (p. 374) *JDH Pharmaceutical Sdn Bhd, Malaysia,* Ispaghula (p. 374) *Tramedico BV, Netherlands,* Ispaghula (p. 374) *Dr. Falk Pharma Portugal Lda, Portugal,* Ispaghula (p. 374) *JDH Pharmaceutical Division, Singapore,* Ispaghula (p. 374)

• **Myrrh** (p. 449)
UK: Culpeper and Napiers

Myrtaven *Institut Biochimique SA, Switzerland,* Bilberry (p. 79)

Nadem *Ivax Argentina SA, Argentina,* Horse-chestnut (p. 363)

Nat Cubetu Benediktu *Leros sro, Czech Republic,* Milk Thistle (p. 429)

Nat Jmeli *Megafyt-R sro, Czech Republic,* Milk Thistle (p. 429)

Nat Rebricku *Leros sro, Czech Republic,* Yarrow (p. 604)

Nat Repiku Lekarskeho *Leros sro, Czech Republic,* Agrimony (p. 42)

Nat Salveje Lekarske *Leros sro, Czech Republic,* Sage (p. 512)

Nat Trezalky *Leros sro, Czech Republic,* St John's Wort (p. 549)

Nat Zemezluce *Leros sro, Czech Republic,* Centaury (p. 149)

Natracalm *Chefaro UK Ltd, UK,* Passionflower (p. 461)

Natucor *Rodisma-Med Pharma GmbH, Germany,* Hawthorn (p. 346)

Natu-fem *Rodisma-Med Pharma GmbH, Germany,* Cohosh, Black (p. 168)

Natu-Hepa *Rodisma-Med Pharma GmbH, Germany,* Artichoke (p. 67) *Vita Health Care AG, Switzerland,* Artichoke (p. 67)

Natulax *Lab. Natufarma, Argentina,* Cascara (p. 128)

Natu-lind *Rodisma-Med Pharma GmbH, Germany,* Nettle (p. 452)

Natu-prosta *Rodisma-Med Pharma GmbH, Germany,* Nettle (p. 452)

Naturest *G.R. Lane Health Products Ltd, UK,* Passionflower (p. 461)

Naturlax *Laboratorios Maver SA, Chile,* Senna (p. 537) *Great Eastern Healthcare Ltd, Hong Kong,* Ispaghula (p. 374)

Naturreiner *Kneipp-Werke, Germany,* Artichoke (p. 67)

Natu-Seda *Vita Health Care AG, Switzerland,* Valerian (p. 580)

Natuzilium *Laboratório Teuto-Brasileiro Ltda, Brazil,* Kava (p. 389)

Neda Fruchtewurfel *Novartis Consumer Health GmbH, Germany,* Senna (p. 537)

Negrustin (Негрустин) *Hexal AG, Russia,* St John's Wort (p. 549)

Neolaikan *Laboratorios Farmasa, S.A. de C.V., Mexico,* Valerian (p. 580)

Nephronorm med *APS Pharma GmbH, Germany,* Java Tea (p. 381)

Nervaxon *Fidia Farmaceutici S.p.A., Italy,* St John's Wort (p. 549)

Nervei *Rodisma-Med Pharma GmbH, Germany,* St John's Wort (p. 549)

Nervisatis *Lab E J Gezzi SRL, Argentina,* Valerian (p. 580)

Neurol *Abigo Medical AB, Sweden,* Valerian (p. 580)

Neuroplant *Dr Willmar Schwabe GmbH & Co., Germany,* St John's Wort (p. 549)

Neurosporal *Chemisch-Pharmazeutische Fabrik Göppingen Carl Müller, Apotheker, GmbH & Co. KG, Germany,* St John's Wort (p. 549)

Neurovegetalin *Verla-Pharm, Arzneimittelfabrik, Apotheker H.J.v. Ehrlich GmbH & Co. KG, Germany,* St John's Wort (p. 549)

Neutrogena Drying *Neutrogena Corp., USA,* Witch Hazel (p. 601)

Nimopect *Hevert-Arzneimittel GmbH & Co. KG, Germany,* Thyme (p. 574)

Noctaval *Novaquimica Sigma Pharma-Nature's Plus Ltda, Brazil,* Valerian (p. 580)

Nodoff *Potter's (Herbal Supplies) Ltd, UK,* Passionflower (p. 461)

Nokatar *Laboratorio Prater SA, Chile,* Ginkgo (p. 299)

Noricaven *Bionorica AG, Germany,* Horse-chestnut (p. 363)

Normurol *CuraMED Pharma GmbH, Germany,* Saw Palmetto (p. 521)

Novo-Mucilax *Novopharm Ltd, Canada,* Ispaghula (p. 374)

Novo-Passit (Ново-Пассит) *Ivax AC, Russia,* Elder (p. 237), Hawthorn (p. 346), Hops (p. 354), Melissa (p. 425), Passionflower (p. 461), St John's Wort (p. 549), Valerian (p. 580)

Nylax with Senna *Crookes Healthcare Ltd, UK,* Senna (p. 537)

Nytol Natural Source *GlaxoSmithKline Consumer Healthcare, Canada,* Valerian (p. 580)

Oddibil *Gerot-Pharmazeutika GmbH, Austria,* Fumitory (p. 276) *Aventis Pharma Ltda, Brazil,* Fumitory (p. 276) *Coopération Pharmaceutique Francaise, France,* Fumitory (p. 276)

Oprane *Vifor SA, Switzerland,* Agnus Castus (p. 36)

Optrex *Schering-Plough Healthcare Products Canada Inc., Canada,* Witch Hazel (p. 601) *Laboratoires Pierre Fabre, France,* Witch Hazel (p. 601) *Boots Healthcare S. p.A., Italy,* Witch Hazel (p. 601) *Boots Trading (Malaysia) Sdn Bhd, Malaysia,* Witch Hazel (p. 601) *Boots Healthcare New Zealand Ltd, New Zealand,* Witch Hazel (p. 601) *The Boots Company (Far East) Pte Ltd, Singapore,* Witch Hazel (p. 601) *Boots Healthcare, Spain,* Witch Hazel (p. 601) *Boots Healthcare (Switzerland) AG, Hermal, Switzerland,* Witch Hazel (p. 601) *Olic (Thailand) Ltd, Thai-land,* Witch Hazel (p. 601) *Crookes Healthcare Ltd, UK,* Witch Hazel (p. 601)

Optrex Original *Boots Healthcare Australia P/L, Australia,* Witch Hazel (p. 601)

Orgaplasma *Ardeypharm GmbH, Germany,* Ginseng, Panax (p. 325)

Orthangin novo *Altana Pharma Deutschland GmbH, Germany,* Hawthorn (p. 346)

Orthosiphonblatter Indischer Nierentee *FidesLine Biologische Heilmittel Heel GmbH, Germany,* Java Tea (p. 381)

Oxacant-mono *Dr Gustav Klein, Germany,* Hawthorn (p. 346)

Parche Leon Fortificante *Beiersdorf SA, Chile,* Capsicum (p. 125)

Pargo *Bio-Diät-Berlin GmbH, Germany,* Devil's Claw (p. 207)

• **Parsley Piert** (p. 459)
UK: Culpeper and Napiers; Frank Roberts (Herbal Dispensaries) Ltd

Pascomucil *Pascoe Pharmazeutische Präparate GmbH, Germany,* Ispaghula (p. 374)

Pascotox forte-Injektopas *Pascoe Pharmazeutische Präparate GmbH, Germany,* Echinacea (p. 217)

Pascotox mono *Pascoe Pharmazeutische Präparate GmbH, Germany,* Echinacea (p. 217)

Passelyt *Gebro Pharma SA, Switzerland,* Passionflower (p. 461)

Passiflora Curarina *Harras Pharma Curarina Arzneimittel GmbH, Germany,* Passionflower (p. 461)

Passiflorin *Austroplant-Arzneimittel GmbH, Austria,* Passionflower (p. 461)

Perika *VSM Belgium, Belgium,* St John's Wort (p. 549)

Perikan *Austroplant-Arzneimittel GmbH, Austria,* St John's Wort (p. 549)

Peristaltine *Novartis Santé Familiale SA, France,* Cascara (p. 128)

Permicaps *Laboratorios Bagó S.A., Argentina,* Saw Palmetto (p. 521)

Permixon *Pierre Fabre Argentina S.A., Argentina,* Saw Palmetto (p. 521) *Germania Pharmazeutika GmbH, Austria,* Saw Palmetto (p. 521) *Laboratoires Pierre Fabre, France,* Saw Palmetto (p. 521) *Medibrands, Israel,* Saw Palmetto (p. 521) *Pierre Fabre Italia S.p.A., Italy,* Saw Palmetto (p. 521) *Pierre Fabre Farma de Mexico S.A. de C.V., Mexico,* Saw Palmetto (p. 521) *Pierre Fabre Médicament Portugal, Lda, Portugal,* Saw Palmetto (p. 521) *Pierre Fabre Iberica, Spain,* Saw Palmetto (p. 521) *Robapharm SA, Switzerland,* Saw Palmetto (p. 521) *BJC Trading Co Ltd, Thailand,* Saw Palmetto (p. 521) *Laboratorio Leti S.A.V., Venezuela,* Saw Palmetto (p. 521)

Permixon (Пермиксон) *Pierre Fabre Medicament, Russia,* Saw Palmetto (p. 521)

Pertussin *medphano Arzneimittel GmbH, Germany,* Thyme (p. 574)

Petadolex *Weber & Weber GmbH & Co. KG, Germany,* Butterbur (p. 107)

Petaforce V *Bioforce GmbH, Germany,* Butterbur (p. 107)

Pharmadose teinture d'arnica *Laboratoires Gilbert, France,* Arnica (p. 64)

Phlebostasin *Altana Pharma Ltd, Switzerland,* Horse-chestnut (p. 363)

Phytocalm *Arkopharma UK Ltd, UK,* Passionflower (p. 461)

Phytocold *Arkopharma UK Ltd, UK,* Echinacea (p. 217)

Phytohepar *Steigerwald Arzneimittelwerk GmbH, Germany,* Milk Thistle (p. 429)

Phytohustil *Steigerwald Arzneimittelwerk GmbH, Germany,* Marshmallow (p. 418)

Phytorelax *Arkopharma UK Ltd, UK,* Valerian (p. 580)

• **Pilewort** (p. 472)
UK: Culpeper and Napiers; Frank Roberts (Herbal Dispensaries) Ltd

Plantaben *Altana Pharma SA, Argentina,* Ispaghula (p. 374) *Altana Pharma Ltda, Brazil,* Ispaghula (p. 374) *EciFarma SA, Chile,* Ispaghula (p. 374) *Altana Pharma S.A. de C.V., Mexico,* Ispaghula (p. 374) *Madaus, Spain,* Ispaghula (p. 374)

Planten *Whitehall Italia S.p.A., Italy,* Ispaghula (p. 374)

Plantivenol *Dr W Schwabe, Spain,* Horse-chestnut (p. 363)

Planturol *Farmasan Arzneimittel GmbH & Co., Germany,* Saw Palmetto (p. 521)

• **Pleurisy Root** (p. 477)
UK: Culpeper and Napiers

Plissamur *Ardeypharm GmbH, Germany,* Horse-chestnut (p. 363)

Plod Jalovce *Leros sro, Czech Republic,* Juniper (p. 386)

• **Pokeroot** (p. 479)
UK: Culpeper and Napiers

Pollivita *Permamed AG, Switzerland,* Butterbur (p. 107)

Posterine *Dr Kade Pharmazeutische Fabrik GmbH, Germany,* Witch Hazel (p. 601)

Prazen *Instituto Terapeutico Delta Ltda, Brazil,* St John's Wort (p. 549)

Prefemine *Max Zeller Söhne AG, Pflanzliche Heilmittel, Switzerland,* Agnus Castus (p. 36)

PreMens *Phytotec Hungária Kft, Hungary,* Agnus Castus (p. 36) *Max Zeller Söhne AG, Pflanzliche Heilmittel, Switzerland,* Agnus Castus (p. 36)

Preparation H Clear Gel *Wyeth Laboratories, UK,* Witch Hazel (p. 601)

• **Prickly Ash, Northern** (p. 484)
UK: Frank Roberts (Herbal Dispensaries) Ltd

Primadrill *Laboratoires Pierre Fabre, France,* Marshmallow (p. 418)

Probeks *Hebron S.A. Indústria Química e Farmacêutica, Brazil,* Aloe Vera (p. 48)

Procalm *Productos Maver S.A. de C.V., Mexico,* St John's Wort (p. 549)

Procalmil *Laboratoires Arkopharma, France,* St John's Wort (p. 549)

Prodiem Plain *Novartis Consumer Health Canada Inc., Canada,* Ispaghula (p. 374)

Proginkgo *Biovital Pty Ltd, Australia,* Ginkgo (p. 299)

Prol *Biovital Pty Ltd, Australia,* Milk Thistle (p. 429)

Promensil *Novogen Laboratories P/L, Australia,* Red Clover (p. 498)

Pro-Sabona Uno *Sabona GmbH, Germany,* Nettle (p. 452)

Proserem *Arkofarm S.r.l., Italy,* St John's Wort (p. 549)

Prosta *Biovital Pty Ltd, Australia,* Saw Palmetto (p. 521)

Prosta Urgenin Uno *Hoyer-Madaus GmbH & Co. KG, Germany,* Saw Palmetto (p. 521)

Prostafort *Laboratorio Esp. Med. Knop Ltda, Chile,* Saw Palmetto (p. 521)

Prostaforton *Biocur Arzneimittel GmbH, Germany,* Nettle (p. 452)

Prostagalen *Hevert-Arzneimittel GmbH & Co. KG, Germany,* Nettle (p. 452)

Prostagutt mono *Dr Willmar Schwabe GmbH & Co., Germany,* Saw Palmetto (p. 521)

Prostagutt uno *Dr Willmar Schwabe GmbH & Co., Germany,* Saw Palmetto (p. 521)

Prostaherb N *Cesra Arzneimittel GmbH & Co. KG, Germany,* Nettle (p. 452)

Prostakan *ASI Budapest Kft, Hungary,* Saw Palmetto (p. 521)

Prostakan Mono *Arzneimittel Schwabe International GmbH, Czech Republic,* Saw Palmetto (p. 521)

Prostalium *Laboratório Teuto-Brasileiro Ltda, Brazil,* Saw Palmetto (p. 521)

ProstaMed *Bioforce AG, Switzerland,* Saw Palmetto (p. 521)

Prostamed Urtica *Dr Gustav Klein, Germany,* Nettle (p. 452)

Prostamol Uno *Berlin-Chemie Menarini Group, Czech Republic,* Saw Palmetto (p. 521) *Berlin-Chemie Képviselet, Hungary,* Saw Palmetto (p. 521)

Prostamol Uno (Простамол Уно) *Berlin-Pharma ZAO Moscow, Russia,* Saw Palmetto (p. 521)

Prostaplant *Bioplanta Arzneimittel GmbH, Germany,* Saw Palmetto (p. 521)

Prostasan *Biofarma Natural CMD SA de CV, Mexico,* Saw Palmetto (p. 521) *Bioforce AG, Switzerland,* Saw Palmetto (p. 521)

Prostaserene *Therabel Pharma SA, Belgium,* Saw Palmetto (p. 521)

Prostata *Stada GmbH, Germany,* Nettle (p. 452)

Prostatal *Herbarium Laboratório Botanico Ltda, Brazil,* Saw Palmetto (p. 521)

Prosta-Truw *Truw Arzneimittel Vertriebs GmbH, Germany,* Nettle (p. 452)

Prosta-Urgenin *Madaus GmbH, Austria,* Saw Palmetto (p. 521) *Madaus Pharma SA, Belgium,* Saw Palmetto (p. 521) *Madaus AG, Germany,* Saw Palmetto (p. 521)

Prosta-Urgenine *Max Zeller Söhne AG, Pflanzliche Heilmittel, Switzerland,* Saw Palmetto (p. 521)

Prostawern *Pharma Wernigerode GmbH, Germany,* Nettle (p. 452)

Prosteren *Cornelli Consulting Sas, Italy,* Saw Palmetto (p. 521)

Prostess *TAD Pharma GmbH, Germany,* Saw Palmetto (p. 521)

Prostex *Productos Medix S.A. de C.V., Mexico,* Saw Palmetto (p. 521)

Prostiva *Aneid, Lda, Portugal,* Saw Palmetto (p. 521)

Protat *Potter's (Herbal Supplies) Ltd, UK,* Corn Silk (p. 191)

Provenen *HWS-OTC-Service GmbH, Austria,* Horse-chestnut (p. 363)

Prunasine *Nycomed Christiaens, Belgium,* Senna (p. 537)

Psychotonin *Madaus GmbH, Austria,* St John's Wort (p. 549) *Steigerwald Arzneimittelwerk GmbH, Germany,* St John's Wort (p. 549)

Psylia *Techni-Pharma, Monaco,* Ispaghula (p. 374)

• **Pulsatilla** (p. 489)
UK: Frank Roberts (Herbal Dispensaries) Ltd

Pursennid *Novartis Finland Oy, Finland,* Senna (p. 537) *Novartis Sverige AB, Sweden,* Senna (p. 537)

• **Quassia** (p. 491)
UK: Culpeper and Napiers

Quetzal *A.S.A.C. Pharma, Spain,* St John's Wort (p. 549)

Quiens *Marco Antonetto S.p.A., Italy,* St John's Wort (p. 549)

Raigin *Gelcaps Exp. de Mexico SA de CV, Mexico,* Ginseng, Panax (p. 325)

Ramend *Queisser Pharma GmbH & Co., Germany,* Senna (p. 537)

• **Raspberry** (p. 495)
UK: Holland and Barrett

Rebrickovy Caj, Rebrickova Nat *Megafyt-R sro, Czech Republic,* Yarrow (p. 604)

Recalm *Herbarium Laboratório Botanico Ltda, Brazil,* Valerian (p. 580)

Recvalysat *Johannes Bürger Ysatfabrik GmbH, Germany,* Valerian (p. 580)

• **Red Clover** (p. 498)
UK: Biocare Ltd; Holland and Barrett

Red Kooga *Peter Black Healthcare Ltd, UK,* Ginseng, Panax (p. 325)

ReDormin *Max Zeller Söhne AG, Pflanzliche Heilmittel, Switzerland,* Valerian (p. 580)

Regripax *Biofarma Natural CMD SA de CV, Mexico,* Echinacea (p. 217)

Regucol *Procter & Gamble Pharmaceuticals, Netherlands,* Ispaghula (p. 374)

Regulacor-POS *Ursapharm Arzneimittel GmbH & Co. KG, Germany,* Hawthorn (p. 346)

Regulan *Procter & Gamble Pharmaceuticals UK Ltd, UK,* Ispaghula (p. 374)

Regulatum *Laboratório Teuto-Brasileiro Ltda, Brazil,* Agnus Castus (p. 36)

Regulax *Krewel Meuselbach GmbH, Czech Republic,* Senna (p. 537)

Regulax N *Krewel Meuselbach GmbH, Germany,* Senna (p. 537)

Reguloid *Watson Pharmaceuticals Inc., USA,* Ispaghula (p. 374)

Relaxine *Laboratoires Pharmaceutiques Trenker SA, Belgium,* Valerian (p. 580) *Trima, Israel,* Valerian (p. 580)

Remifemin *Schaper & Brümmer GmbH & Co. KG, Germany,* Cohosh, Black (p. 168) *Phytotec Hungária Kft, Hungary,* Cohosh, Black (p. 168) *Bionax Singapore Pte Ltd, Singapore,* Cohosh, Black (p. 168) *Farmasierra S.A., Spain,* Cohosh, Black (p. 168) *Diethelm & Co. Ltd, Thailand,* Cohosh, Black (p. 168)

Remiprostan uno *Schaper & Brümmer GmbH & Co. KG, Germany,* Saw Palmetto (p. 521)

Remotiv *Torrex Pharma GmbH, Austria,* St John's Wort (p. 549) *Phytotec Hungária Kft, Hungary,* St John's Wort (p. 549) *Abbott Laboratories de Mexico S.A. de C.V., Mexico,* St John's Wort (p. 549) *Max Zeller Söhne AG, Pflanzliche Heilmittel, Switzerland,* St John's Wort (p. 549)

Remotive *Sigma Tau S.p.A., Italy,* St John's Wort (p. 549)

Renopen *Ativus Farmacêutica Ltda, Brazil,* Saw Palmetto (p. 521)

Repha Orphon *Repha GmbH Biologische Arzneimittel, Germany,* Java Tea (p. 381)

Repik Lekarsky *Slovakofarma sro, Czech Republic,* Agrimony (p. 42)

Repikovy Caj, Repikova Nat *Megafyt-R sro, Czech Republic,* Agrimony (p. 42)

Resistan mono *Truw Arzneimittel Vertriebs GmbH, Germany,* Echinacea (p. 217)

Resplant *W. Spitzner, Arzneimittelfabrik GmbH, Germany,* Echinacea (p. 217)

ReBalance *Max Zeller Söhne AG, Pflanzliche Heilmittel, Switzerland,* St John's Wort (p. 549)

Rheogen *Robugen GmbH Pharmazeutische Fabrik, Germany,* Aloes (p. 50)

Rheuferm Phyto *Wiedemann Pharma GmbH, Germany,* Devil's Claw (p. 207)

Rheuma-Hek *Strathmann AG & Co., Germany,* Nettle (p. 452)

Rheumakaps *Steigerwald Arzneimittelwerk GmbH, Germany,* Willow (p. 598)

Rheuma-Sern *Truw Arzneimittel Vertriebs GmbH, Germany,* Devil's Claw (p. 207)

Rheuma-Stada *Stada GmbH, Germany,* Nettle (p. 452)

Rheumatab Salicis *Schuck GmbH, Germany,* Willow (p. 598)

• **Rhodiola** (p. 500)
UK: Biocare Ltd; Frank Roberts (Herbal Dispensaries) Ltd; Quest Vitamins Ltd

Rilaprost *Laboratori Guidotti S.p.A., Italy,* Saw Palmetto (p. 521)

Rivoltan *Krewel Meuselbach GmbH, Germany,* Devil's Claw (p. 207)

Rokan *Laboratorios Andromaco SA, Chile,* Ginkgo (p. 299) *W. Spitzner, Arzneimittelfabrik GmbH, Germany,* Ginkgo (p. 299)

• **Rosemary** (p. 508)
UK: Culpeper and Napiers

Rutying *Super Mayoreo Naturista S.A. de C.V., Mexico,* Ginseng, Panax (p. 325)

Saba *Lampugnani Farmaceutici S.p.A., Italy,* Saw Palmetto (p. 521)

Sabacur uno *Biocur Arzneimittel GmbH, Germany,* Saw Palmetto (p. 521)

Sabal uno *Apogepha Arzneimittel GmbH, Germany,* Saw Palmetto (p. 521)

Sabalin *Medic Herb UK Ltd, UK,* Saw Palmetto (p. 521) *Lichtwer Pharma UK,*

Sabalvit *Bional Pharma Deutschland GmbH & Co. KG, Germany,* Saw Palmetto (p. 521)

Sabal *Duopharm GmbH, Stada GmbH, Germany,* Saw Palmetto (p. 521)

SabCaps *Vifor SA, Switzerland,* Saw Palmetto (p. 521)

Sabonal Uno *Sabona GmbH, Germany,* Saw Palmetto (p. 521)

Saforelle *Avanderm Mexico, S.A. de C.V., Mexico,* Burdock (p. 102) *Biosaúde Produtos Farmaceuticos SA, Portugal,* Burdock (p. 102)

• **Sage** (p. 512)
UK: Culpeper and Napiers; Healthy Direct; Holland and Barrett; Medic Herb UK Ltd

Salbei Curarina *Harras Pharma Curarina Arzneimittel GmbH, Germany,* Sage (p. 512)

Salus Mistel-Tropfen *Salus-Haus Dr. med. Otto Greither Nachf. GmbH & Co KG, Germany,* Milk Thistle (p. 429)

Salvejova Nat *Megafyt-R sro, Czech Republic,* Sage (p. 512)

Salvysat *Mayrhofer Pharmazeutika, Austria,* Sage (p. 512) *Johannes Bürger Ysatfabrik GmbH, Germany,* Sage (p. 512)

Sanjin Royal Jelly *Super Mayoreo Naturista S.A. de C.V., Mexico,* Ginseng, Panax (p. 325)

Sanopinwern *Pharma Wernigerode GmbH, Germany,* Thyme (p. 574)

Sanvita Immun *Sanamed GmbH, Austria,* Echinacea (p. 217)

Sapec *Riemser Arzneimittel AG, Germany,* Garlic (p. 279)

Sarai *Steiner & Co. Deutsche Arzneimittel Gesellschaft, Germany,* Agnus Castus (p. 36)

• **Sarsaparilla** (p. 515)
UK: Culpeper and Napiers; Holland and Barrett; Medic Herb UK Ltd

Saugella Dermoliquido *Rottapharm S.r.l., Italy,* Sage (p. 512)

• **Saw Palmetto** (p. 521)
UK: Biocare Ltd; Culpeper and Napiers; Frank Roberts (Herbal Dispensaries) Ltd; Healthy Direct; Holland and Barrett; Quest Vitamins Ltd; Worldwide Health Corp. Ltd
USA: Nature Made; Nature's Bounty; Sundown

Scottopect *Nycomed Austria GmbH, Austria,* Thyme (p. 574)

• **Scullcap** (p. 530)
UK: Culpeper and Napiers

Sedante Noche *La Serranita, Lab. de Esp. Medic. y Cosmet., Argentina,* Passionflower (p. 461)

Sedasol eco natura *Ecosol AG, Switzerland,* Valerian (p. 580)

Sedinfant *Sabona GmbH, Germany,* Melissa (p. 425)

Sedonium *Lichtwer Pharma AG, Germany,* Valerian (p. 580) *Vifor SA, Switzerland,* Valerian (p. 580) *Lichtwer Pharma UK, UK,* Valerian (p. 580)

Sedovegan *Dr. August Wolff Arzneimittel GmbH & Co., Germany,* St John's Wort (p. 549)

Senan *Ativus Farmacêutica Ltda, Brazil,* Senna (p. 537)

Senicor *Duopharm GmbH, Germany,* Hawthorn (p. 346)

• **Senna** (p. 537)
UK: Culpeper and Napiers; Quest Vitamins Ltd

Senna-Gen *Ivax Pharmaceuticals Inc., USA,* Senna (p. 537)

Sennalax *Aspen Pharmacare (Pty) Ltd, South Africa,* Senna (p. 537)

Sennaprep *Pharmascience Inc., Canada,* Senna (p. 537)

Sennapur *Pharmia Oy, Finland,* Senna (p. 537)

Sennatab *Pharmascience Inc., Canada,* Senna (p. 537)

Sennocol *Viatris BV, Netherlands,* Senna (p. 537)

Sennove Lusky *Leros sro, Czech Republic,* Senna (p. 537)

Sennovy List *Megafyt-R sro, Czech Republic,* Senna (p. 537)

Senokot *Purdue Pharma, Canada,* Senna (p. 537) *Viatris, France,* Senna (p. 537) *Reckitt Benckiser Hong Kong Ltd, Hong Kong,* Senna (p. 537) *mundipharma AS, Norway,* Senna (p. 537) *Zuellig Pharma Pte Ltd, Singapore,* Senna (p. 537) *Reckitt Benckiser plc, UK,* Senna (p. 537) *The Purdue Frederick Co., USA,* Senna (p. 537)

Senokotxtra *The Purdue Frederick Co., USA,* Senna (p. 537)

Sensivision au plantain *Laboratoires Chauvin Bausch & Lomb, France,* Plantain (p. 474)

Sereprostat *Robapharm España, Spain,* Saw Palmetto (p. 521)

Serpens *Lisapharma S.p.A., Italy,* Saw Palmetto (p. 521)

Seven Seas Cranberry Forte *Seven Seas Ltd, UK,* Cranberry (p. 197)

Silegon *Biogal-Teva Pharma Rt, Hungary,* Milk Thistle (p. 429)

Silibene *Merckle GmbH, Germany,* Milk Thistle (p. 429)

Silicur *Biocur Arzneimittel GmbH, Germany,* Milk Thistle (p. 429)

Silimarin *Benedetti S.p.A., Italy,* Milk Thistle (p. 429)

Silimarit *Bionorica AG, Germany,* Milk Thistle (p. 429)

Siliver *Laboratório Americano de Farmacoterapia S/A, Brazil,* Milk Thistle (p. 429)

Silmar *Hennig Arzneimittel GmbH & Co. KG, Germany,* Milk Thistle (p. 429)

Siludane *Laboratorios Dermatologicos Darier S.A. de C.V., Mexico,* Ispaghula (p. 374)

Silvaysan *Sanum-Kehlbeck GmbH & Co. KG, Germany,* Milk Thistle (p. 429)

Silyhexal *Hexal Pharma GmbH, Austria,* Milk Thistle (p. 429)

Silymarin Phytosome *Eagle Pharmaceuticals P/L, Australia,* Milk Thistle (p. 429)

Sinei *Steiner & Co. Deutsche Arzneimittel Gesellschaft, Germany,* Cohosh, Black (p. 168)

Sita *Hoyer-Madaus GmbH & Co. KG, Germany,* Saw Palmetto (p. 521)

Skin Clear *Potter's (Herbal Supplies) Ltd, UK,* Echinacea (p. 217)

Sklerovenol N *Febena Pharma GmbH, Germany,* Horse-chestnut (p. 363)

Sleep-Eze V Natural *Medtech Lab, Canada,* Valerian (p. 580)

• **Slippery Elm** (p. 545)
UK: Culpeper and Napiers

Snore Calm *British Snoring & Sleep Apnoea Association Ltd, UK,* Eyebright (p. 256)

Soflax *Cipla-Medpro (Pty) Ltd, South Africa,* Senna (p. 537)

Sogoon *Steiner & Co. Deutsche Arzneimittel Gesellschaft, Germany,* Devil's Claw (p. 207)

Solaguttae *Emonta Pharma GmbH, Austria,* St John's Wort (p. 549)

Solarcaine Aloe Vera *Balmar, New Zealand,* Aloe Vera (p. 48)

Solcosplen C *Strathmann AG & Co., Germany,* Cohosh, Black (p. 168)

Soledum Hustensaft *Cassella-med GmbH & Co. KG, Germany,* Thyme (p. 574)

Soledum Hustentropfen *Cassella-med GmbH & Co. KG, Germany,* Thyme (p. 574)

Solevita *Permamed AG, Switzerland,* St John's Wort (p. 549)

Sominex *Laboratorio Prater SA, Chile,* Valerian (p. 580)

Sonoripan *Marjan Indústria e Comércio Ltda, Brazil,* Valerian (p. 580)

Spagulax *Laboratoires Pharmafarm, France,* Ispaghula (p. 374)

Spagulax Mucilage *Laboratoires Pharmafarm, France,* Ispaghula (p. 374)

Spalda Sabal *Leo Pharma A/S, Denmark,* Saw Palmetto (p. 521)

Spartiol *Dr Gustav Klein, Germany,* Broom (p. 98)

Spasmosedine *Laboratoires DB Pharma, France,* Hawthorn (p. 346)

Sperti Preparacion H Clear Gel *Wyeth Consumer Healthcare, Chile,* Witch Hazel (p. 601)

Sporal mono *Chemisch-Pharmazeutische Fabrik Göppingen Carl Müller, Apotheker, GmbH & Co. KG, Germany,* Valerian (p. 580)

• **St John's Wort** (p. 550)
UK: Biocare Ltd; Culpeper and Napiers; Frank Roberts (Herbal Dispensaries) Ltd; Healthy Direct; Medic Herb UK Ltd; Quest Vitamins Ltd; Worldwide Health Corp. Ltd
USA: Natrol; Nature Made; Nature's Bounty; Sundown; Walgreens Finest Natural

Steicorton *Steigerwald Arzneimittelwerk GmbH, Germany,* Hawthorn (p. 346)

Steiprostat *Steigerwald Arzneimittelwerk GmbH, Germany,* Saw Palmetto (p. 521)

Stenocrat mono *Dr Willmar Schwabe GmbH & Co., Germany,* Hawthorn (p. 346)

Sthenorex *Laboratoires Pharmygiène-SCAT, France,* Fenugreek (p. 260)

Strogen *Strathmann AG & Co., Germany,* Saw Palmetto (p. 521)

Strogen Uno *Strathmann Ag & Co Képviselete, Hungary,* Saw Palmetto (p. 521)

Strongus *franconpharm Arzneimittel GmbH, Germany,* Garlic (p. 279)

Strotan *Strathmann AG & Co., Germany,* Agnus Castus (p. 36)

Styptysat *Johannes Bürger Ysatfabrik GmbH, Germany,* Senna (p. 537)

Sure-Lax *Chefaro UK Ltd, UK,* Senna (p. 537)

Sweatosan N *Novartis Consumer Health GmbH, Germany,* Sage (p. 512)

Syllact *MedPointe Healthcare Inc, USA,* Ispaghula (p. 374)

Symfona *Medichemie AG, Switzerland,* Ginkgo (p. 299)

Syxal *Syxyl GmbH & Co. KG, Germany,* St John's Wort (p. 549)

Takata *Madariaga, Spain,* Senna (p. 537)

Talso *Sanofi-Synthelabo GmbH, Germany,* Saw Palmetto (p. 521)

Tanacain *Ipsen EpE, Greece,* Ginkgo (p. 299)

Tanacet *Ashbury Biologicals Inc., Canada,* Feverfew (p. 263) *Herbal Laboratories Ltd, UK,* Feverfew (p. 263)

Tanaceto *Herbarium Laboratório Botanico Ltda, Brazil,* Feverfew (p. 263)

Tanakan *Laboratorios Phoenix S.A.I.C.F., Argentina,* Ginkgo (p. 299) *Ipsen NV, Belgium,* Ginkgo (p. 299) *Knoll SA Produtos Químicos e Farmacêuticos, Brazil,* Ginkgo (p. 299) *Beaufour Ipsen Pharma, France,* Ginkgo (p. 299) *IDS (Hong Kong) Ltd Healthcare Division, Hong Kong,* Ginkgo (p. 299) *Europharm Trade Kft, Hungary,* Ginkgo (p. 299) *Laboratorios Farmasa, S.A. de C.V., Mexico,* Ginkgo (p. 299) *Sime Darby Marketing, A Division of Sime Darby Singapore Ltd, Singapore,* Ginkgo (p. 299) *Pacific Healthcare (Thailand) Co. Ltd, Thailand,* Ginkgo (p. 299) *Laboratorio Leti S.A.V., Venezuela,* Ginkgo (p. 299)

Tanakan (Танакан) *Beaufour Ipsen International SNC, Russia,* Ginkgo (p. 299)

Tanakan *Antah Pharma Sdb Bhd, Emerging Pharma Sdn Bhd, Malaysia,* Ginkgo (p. 299)

Tanakene *Ipsen Pharma, Spain,* Ginkgo (p. 299) *F. Uhlmann-Eyraud SA, Switzerland,* Ginkgo (p. 299)

Tavonin *VSM Belgium, Belgium,* Ginkgo (p. 299) *VSM Geneesmiddelen BV, Netherlands,* Ginkgo (p. 299)

Tebofortan *Austroplant-Arzneimittel GmbH, Austria,* Ginkgo (p. 299) *ASI Budapest Kft, Hungary,* Ginkgo (p. 299)

Tebokan *Arzneimittel Schwabe International GmbH, Czech Republic,* Ginkgo (p. 299) *Vianex S.A., Greece,* Ginkgo (p. 299) *Schwabe Pharma AG, Switzerland,* Ginkgo (p. 299)

Tebonin *Austroplant-Arzneimittel GmbH, Austria,* Ginkgo (p. 299) *Altana Pharma Ltda, Brazil,* Ginkgo (p. 299) *Dr Willmar Schwabe GmbH & Co., Germany,* Ginkgo (p. 299) *ASI Budapest Kft, Hungary,* Ginkgo (p. 299) *Laboratorios Farmasa, S.A. de C.V., Mexico,* Ginkgo (p. 299)

Tegens *Sanofi-Synthelabo S.p.A., Italy,* Bilberry (p. 79)

Teltonal *Biocur Arzneimittel GmbH, Germany,* Devil's Claw (p. 207)

Tenag *Marjan Indústria e Comércio Ltda, Brazil,* Agnus Castus (p. 36)

Tenliv *Ativus Farmacêutica Ltda, Brazil,* Feverfew (p. 263)

Tensiane *Greenpharma Química e Farmacêutica Ltda, Brazil,* Cohosh, Black (p. 168)

Tesalin *Max Zeller Söhne AG, Pflanzliche Heilmittel, Switzerland,* Butterbur (p. 107)

Tetesept Erkaltungs *tetesept Pharma GmbH, Germany,* Thyme (p. 574)

Teufelskralle&xref details= *ratiopharm GmbH, Stada GmbH, Germany,* Devil's Claw (p. 207)

Texx *Krewel Meuselbach GmbH, Germany,* St John's Wort (p. 549)

Thankgod *Panacea Biotec Ltd, India,* Euphorbia (p. 249)

Thermo Burger *Johannes Bürger Ysatfabrik GmbH, Germany,* Capsicum (p. 125)

• **Thyme** (p. 574)
UK: Culpeper and Napiers

Thymi Syrup *Vitamed Ltd, Israel,* Thyme (p. 574)

Thymipin N *Novartis Consumer Health GmbH, Germany,* Thyme (p. 574)

Thymiverlan *Verla-Pharm, Arzneimittelfabrik, Apotheker H.J.v. Ehrlich GmbH & Co. KG, Germany,* Thyme (p. 574)

Thymusin N *G. Streuli & Co. AG, Switzerland,* Thyme (p. 574)

Tia Puppy *Química Franco Mexicana Nordin S.A. de C.V., Mexico,* Witch Hazel (p. 601)

Ticalma *Kelemata S.p.A., Italy,* Valerian (p. 580)

Tisana Kelemata *Kelemata S.p.A., Italy,* Senna (p. 537)

Tisane laxative H nouvelle formulation *Häseler AG, Switzerland,* Senna (p. 537)

Tisasen *ICN Czech Republic as, Czech Republic,* Senna (p. 537)

Tonizin *betapharm Arzneimittel GmbH, Germany,* St John's Wort (p. 549)

Tramisal *Beaufour Ipsen Pharma, France,* Ginkgo (p. 299)

Transilane *Laboratoires Innotech International, Sté du groupe Innothéra, France,* Ispaghula (p. 374)

Transix *Nycomed Christiaens, Belgium,* Senna (p. 537)

Traumaplant *F. Joh. Kwizda, Austria,* Comfrey (p. 188) *Horna Business Service, Czech Republic,* Comfrey (p. 188) *Harras Pharma Curarina Arzneimittel GmbH, Germany,* Comfrey (p. 188) *Laboratorios Cofasa S.A., Venezuela,* Comfrey (p. 188)

Travacalm Natural *Hamilton Pharmaceuticals P/L, Australia,* Ginger (p. 293)

Travel Sickness *The Cantassium Company, UK,* Ginger (p. 293)

Trezalka v Nalevovych Sacchich *Leros sro, Czech Republic,* St John's Wort (p. 549)

Trezalkova Nat *Megafyt-R sro, Czech Republic,* St John's Wort (p. 549)

Trezalkovy Caj *Megafyt-R sro, Czech Republic,* St John's Wort (p. 549)

Triativ *Ativus Farmacêutica Ltda, Brazil,* St John's Wort (p. 549)

Triffadiane *Laboratorios Politecnicos Nacionales C.A., Venezuela,* Hydrocotyle (p. 371)

Trinovin *Novogen Laboratories P/L, Australia,* Red Clover (p. 498)

Trio D *Laboratoires d'Evolution Dermatologique, France,* Liquorice (p. 411)

Triple Blend Echinacea *Swiss Herbal Remedies Ltd, Canada,* Echinacea (p. 217)

Turineurin *Schering sro, Czech Republic,* St John's Wort (p. 549) *Jenapharm GmbH & Co. KG, Germany,* St John's Wort (p. 549)

Tussamag Hustensaft N *ct-Arzneimittel GmbH, Germany,* Thyme (p. 574)

Tussamag Hustentropfen N *ct-Arzneimittel GmbH, Germany,* Thyme (p. 574)

Tussamag (Туссамаг) *Ratiopharm Group, Russia,* Thyme (p. 574)

Tussiflorin Thymian *Pascoe Pharmazeutische Präparate GmbH, Germany,* Thyme (p. 574)

Unisom Natural Source *Pfizer Consumer Healthcare, Division of Pfizer Canada Inc., Canada,* Valerian (p. 580)

Uricleanse *Douglas Pharmaceuticals Australia Ltd, Australia,* Cranberry (p. 197)

Urogutt *Laboratorios Farmasa, S.A. de C.V., Mexico,* Saw Palmetto (p. 521)

Uro-POS *Croma-Pharma GmbH, Austria,* Nettle (p. 452) *Ursapharm Arzneimittel GmbH & Co. KG, Germany,* Nettle (p. 452)

Urtivit *Bional Pharma Deutschland GmbH & Co. KG, Germany,* Nettle (p. 452)

utk *TAD Pharma GmbH, Germany,* Nettle (p. 452)

Uvalysat *Johannes Bürger Ysatfabrik GmbH, Germany,* Uva-Ursi (p. 577)

• **Uva-Ursi** (p. 577)
UK: Frank Roberts (Herbal Dispensaries) Ltd

Uvavid *Productos Maver S.A. de C.V., Mexico,* Uva-Ursi (p. 577)

Valdispert *Solvay Pharma sro, Czech Republic,* Valerian (p. 580) *Solvay Arzneimittel GmbH, Germany,* Valerian (p. 580) *Solvay Pharma BV, Netherlands,* Valerian (p. 580) *Solvayfarma, Lda, Portugal,* Valerian (p. 580) *Solvay Pharma, Spain,* Valerian (p. 580) *Solvay Pharma AG, Switzerland,* Valerian (p. 580)

Valerecen *Abigo Medical AB, Sweden,* Valerian (p. 580)

Valerial *Zambon SA, Belgium,* Valerian (p. 580)

• **Valerian** (p. 580)
UK: Culpeper and Napiers; Frank Roberts (Herbal Dispensaries) Ltd; Healthy Direct; Holland and Barrett; Quest Vitamins Ltd
USA: Nature Made; Nature's Bounty; Sundown

Valeriana Orto *Normon S.A., Spain,* Valerian (p. 580)

Valeriane *Química E Farmacêutica Nikkho do Brasil Ltda, Brazil,* Valerian (p. 580)

Valerimed *Cimed Indústria de Medicamentos Ltda, Brazil,* Valerian (p. 580)

Valerin *Fontovit Laboratórios Ltda, Brazil,* Valerian (p. 580)

Valerix *Ativus Farmacêutica Ltda, Brazil,* Valerian (p. 580)

Valeton *Rekah Ltd, Israel,* Valerian (p. 580)

Valezen *Laboratório Teuto-Brasileiro Ltda, Brazil,* Valerian (p. 580)

Valmane *Solvay Farma Ltda, Brazil,* Valerian (p. 580)

Valrian *Oy Leiras Finland AB, Finland,* Valerian (p. 580)

Valsedan *Cederroth, Spain,* Valerian (p. 580)

Valverde Artischocke *Novartis Consumer Health GmbH, Germany,* Artichoke (p. 67)

Valverde Boutons de fievre creme *Sidroga AG, Switzerland,* Melissa (p. 425)

Valverde Monchspfeffer bei Menstruationsbeschwerden *Novartis Consumer Health GmbH, Germany,* Agnus Castus (p. 36)

Valverde Prostate capsules *Sidroga AG, Switzerland,* Nettle (p. 452)

Varicid *Lacer, Spain,* Horse-chestnut (p. 363)

Varilise *Ativus Farmacêutica Ltda, Brazil,* Horse-chestnut (p. 363)

Varison *Grünenthal Lda, Grünenthal Lda, Portugal,* Bilberry (p. 79)

Vasactife *Ferring Portuguesa, Lda, Portugal,* Ginkgo (p. 299)

Vasodil *Altana Pharma S.A. de C.V., Mexico,* Ginkgo (p. 299)

Venafort *Laboratório Teuto-Brasileiro Ltda, Brazil,* Horse-chestnut (p. 363)

Venalot novo *Schaper & Brümmer GmbH & Co. KG, Germany,* Horse-chestnut (p. 363)

Venastat *Boehringer Ingelheim S.A., Argentina,* Horse-chestnut (p. 363) *Boehringer Ingelheim, Chile,* Horse-chestnut (p. 363) *Boehringer Ingelheim Pharma Magyarországi Kereskedelmi Képviselet, Hungary,* Horse-chestnut (p. 363) *Boehringer Ingelheim Promeco, S.A. de C.V., Mexico,* Horse-chestnut (p. 363)

Venavit N *UB Interpharm SA, Switzerland,* Horse-chestnut (p. 363)

Venen-Dragees *ct-Arzneimittel GmbH, Germany,* Horse-chestnut (p. 363)

Venen-Fluid *ct-Arzneimittel GmbH, Germany,* Horse-chestnut (p. 363)

Venen-Tabletten *Stada GmbH, Germany,* Horse-chestnut (p. 363)

Venentabs *ratiopharm GmbH, Germany,* Horse-chestnut (p. 363)

Venen-Tropfen N *Bioforce GmbH, Germany,* Horse-chestnut (p. 363)

Venitan *Lek Pharma sro, Czech Republic,* Horse-chestnut (p. 363)

Veno-biomo *biomo Pharma GmbH, Germany,* Horse-chestnut (p. 363)

Venodura *Merck dura GmbH, Germany,* Horse-chestnut (p. 363)

Venoplant *VSM Belgium, Belgium,* Horse-chestnut (p. 363) *Dr Willmar Schwabe GmbH & Co., Germany,* Horse-chestnut (p. 363)

Venoplant top *Dr Willmar Schwabe GmbH & Co., Germany,* Witch Hazel (p. 601)

Venopyronum *Abbott GmbH & Co. KG, Germany,* Horse-chestnut (p. 363)

Venosin *Fujisawa GmbH, Austria,* Horse-chestnut (p. 363)

Venostasin *Química Ariston S.A.C.I.F., Argentina,* Horse-chestnut (p. 363) *Fujisawa GmbH, Austria,* Horse-chestnut (p. 363) *Ariston Industrias Químicas e Farm. Ltda, Brazil,* Horse-chestnut (p. 363) *Fujisawa Deutschland GmbH, Germany,* Horse-chestnut (p. 363) *Altana Pharma Ltd, Switzerland,* Horse-chestnut (p. 363)

Veraskin *Laboratoires Mazal Pharmaceutique, France,* Aloe Vera (p. 48)

• **Vervain** (p. 591)
UK: Culpeper and Napiers

Vibtil *Therabel Pharma SA, Belgium,* Lime Flower (p. 409) *SERP, Monaco,* Lime Flower (p. 409)

Viru-Salvysat *Johannes Bürger Ysatfabrik GmbH, Germany,* Sage (p. 512)

Viscysat *Johannes Bürger Ysatfabrik GmbH, Germany,* Milk Thistle (p. 429)

Vi-Siblin *Pfizer ApS Danmark, Denmark,* Ispaghula (p. 374) *Pfizer Oy, Finland,* Ispaghula (p. 374) *Nycomed Pharma AS, Norway,* Ispaghula (p. 374) *Recip AB, Sweden,* Ispaghula (p. 374)

Vitacor *UB Interpharm SA, Switzerland,* Hawthorn (p. 346)

Vitalium *Farma Lepori, Spain,* St John's Wort (p. 549)

Vitenon *Ativus Farmacêutica Ltda, Brazil,* Agnus Castus (p. 36)

Vitex *Herbarium Laboratório Botanico Ltda, Brazil,* Agnus Castus (p. 36)

Volcolon *Pfizer BV, Netherlands,* Ispaghula (p. 374)

Vulcase *Teofarma, Italy,* Aloes (p. 50)

Wiedimmun *Wiedemann Pharma GmbH, Germany,* Echinacea (p. 217)

• **Wild Lettuce** (p. 596)
UK: Culpeper and Napiers

Witch Doctor *C.B. Fleet Co. (Australia) P/L, Australia,* Witch Hazel (p. 601) *E.C. De Witt & Co. Ltd, UK,* Witch Hazel (p. 601)

Witch Sunsore *E.C. De Witt & Co. Ltd, UK,* Witch Hazel (p. 601)

X-Prep *Mundipharma GmbH, Austria,* Senna (p. 537) *Purdue Pharma, Canada,* Senna (p. 537) *Mundipharma GmbH, Czech Republic,* Senna (p. 537) *Lavipharm Group, Greece,* Senna (p. 537) *Viatris S.p.A., Italy,* Senna (p. 537) *Ferring S.A. de C. V., Mexico,* Senna (p. 537) *mundipharma AS, Norway,* Senna (p. 537) *Viatris Farmacêutica SA, Portugal,* Senna (p. 537) *Mundipharma Medical Co, Switzerland,* Senna (p. 537) *The Purdue Frederick Co., USA,* Senna (p. 537)

Yakona *Tentan AG, Switzerland,* St John's Wort (p. 549)

Zihlava *Slovakofarma sro, Czech Republic,* Nettle (p. 452)

Zinaxin *Vita Healthcare Ltd, UK,* Ginger (p. 293)

Zintona *Herbalist & Doc Gesundheitsgesellschaft mbH, Germany,* Ginger (p. 293) *Chrisana GmbH, Switzerland,* Ginger (p. 293)

Zortrix *Ativus Farmacêutica Ltda, Brazil,* Willow (p. 598)

Multiple-ingredient preparations

A Saude da Mulher *EMS Ind. Farmacêutica Ltda, Brazil,* Passionflower (p. 461)

Abanta *Laboratorios Columbia de Argentina SA, Argentina,* Aloe Vera (p. 48)

Abdomilon *Cesra Arzneimittel GmbH & Co. KG, Germany,* Angelica (p. 53), Calamus (p. 118), Frangula (p. 270), Gentian (p. 290), Melissa (p. 425), Rhubarb (p. 506)

Abdomilon N *Caesaro Med GmbH, Austria,* Angelica (p. 53), Calamus (p. 118), Gentian (p. 290), Melissa (p. 425) *Cesra Arzneimittel GmbH & Co. KG, Germany,* Angelica (p. 53), Calamus (p. 118), Gentian (p. 290), Melissa (p. 425)

Abfuhr-Heilkrautertee *Abtswinder Naturheilmittel GmbH, Czech Republic,* Calendula (p. 121), Frangula (p. 270), Juniper (p. 386), Nettle (p. 452), Senna (p. 537)

Abfuhrtee St Severin *EF-EM-ES - Dr Smetana & Co., Austria,* Senna (p. 537), Yarrow (p. 604)

Absorbine Arthritis *WF Young Inc., Canada,* Capsicum (p. 125)

Acetoben *Productos Ronava C.A., Venezuela,* Senega (p. 533)

Acidosis *Potter's (Herbal Supplies) Ltd, UK,* Gentian (p. 290), Meadowsweet (p. 423), Meadowsweet (p. 423), Rhubarb (p. 506)

Acne Oral Spray *Brauer Natural Medicine P/L, Australia,* Burdock (p. 102)

Acnetrol *Lagos Laboratorios Argentina S.R.L., Argentina,* Calendula (p. 121), Rosemary (p. 508), Sage (p. 512)

Ac-Sal *Isdin Chile Ltda, Chile,* Aloe Vera (p. 48)

Actibil *Laboratoires Arkopharma, France,* Artichoke (p. 67), Fumitory (p. 276)

Actimind *Potter's Herbal Medicines, UK,* Ginkgo (p. 299), Ginseng, Panax (p. 325)

Activex 40 Plus *Adcock Ingram Pharmaceuticals Ltd, South Africa,* Ginseng, Panax (p. 325)

Acuaderm *Laboritorios Felipe Bajer S.A.I.C., Argentina,* Aloe Vera (p. 48)

Adiantine *Potter's (Herbal Supplies) Ltd, UK,* Witch Hazel (p. 601)

Adios *DDD Ltd, UK,* Boldo (p. 91), Dandelion (p. 204)

Ad-Muc *Merz Pharmaceuticals GmbH, Germany,* Myrrh (p. 449) *Weston Pharmaceutical Ltd, Hong Kong,* Myrrh (p. 449)

Adult Citrex Multivitamin + Ginseng + Omega 3 *Pharmaniaga Marketing Sdn Bhd, Malaysia,* Ginseng, Panax (p. 325)

Aescusan *Riemser Arzneimittel AG, Germany,* Horse-chestnut (p. 363), Witch Hazel (p. 601)

Aforinol *Rekah Ltd, Israel,* Witch Hazel (p. 601)

After Burn *Tender Corporation, Czech Republic,* Aloe Vera (p. 48)

Aftil *Laboratorios Elmor S.A., Venezuela,* Cinnamon (p. 162)

Agiolax *Laboratorios Phoenix S.A.I.C.F., Argentina,* Ispaghula (p. 374), Senna (p. 537) *Knoll Australia, Australia,* Ispaghula (p. 374), Senna (p. 537) *Madaus GmbH, Austria,* Ispaghula (p. 374), Senna (p. 537) *Madaus Pharma SA, Belgium,* Ispaghula (p. 374), Senna (p. 537) *Altana Pharma Ltda, Brazil,* Ispaghula (p. 374), Senna (p. 537) *Meda Oy, Finland,* Ispaghula (p. 374), Senna (p. 537) *Laboratoires Madaus, France,* Ispaghula (p. 374), Senna (p. 537) *Madaus AG, Germany,* Ispaghula (p. 374), Senna (p. 537) *Trinity Trading Co. Ltd, Hong Kong,* Ispaghula (p. 374), Senna (p. 537) *Salomon, Levin, & Elstein Ltd, Israel,* Ispaghula (p. 374), Senna (p. 537) *Madaus S.r.l., Italy,* Ispaghula (p. 374), Senna (p. 537) *Altana Pharma S.A. de C.V., Mexico,* Ispaghula (p. 374), Senna (p. 537) *Byk Nederland BV, Netherlands,* Ispaghula (p. 374), Senna (p. 537) *Meda A/S, Norway,* Ispaghula (p. 374), Senna (p. 537) *Neo-Farmacêutica, Lda, Portugal,* Ispaghula (p. 374), Senna (p. 537) *Altana Madaus Pty Ltd, South Africa,* Ispaghula (p. 374), Senna (p. 537) *Madaus, Spain,* Ispaghula (p. 374), Senna (p. 537) *Meda AB, Sweden,* Ispaghula (p. 374), Senna (p. 537) *Max Zeller Söhne AG, Pflanzliche Heilmittel, Switzerland,* Ispaghula (p. 374), Senna (p. 537) *Oui Heng Import Co. Ltd, Thailand,* Ispaghula (p. 374), Senna (p. 537) *Zuoz Pharma S.A., Venezuela,* Ispaghula (p. 374), Senna (p. 537)

Agua del Carmen *Fardi, Spain,* Angelica (p. 53), Cinnamon (p. 162), Lemon Verbena (p. 405), Lime Flower (p. 409), Melissa (p. 425)

Ajo 1000 + C *Lab. Garden House S.A., Argentina,* Garlic (p. 279)

Ajolip *Lab. Natufarma, Argentina,* Garlic (p. 279), Uva-Ursi (p. 577)

Akildia *Laboratoires Asepta, Monaco,* Hydrocotyle (p. 371)

Alasenn *Pharma Schwörer GmbH, Germany,* Dandelion (p. 204), Senna (p. 537), Yarrow (p. 604)

Albizia Complex *Mediherb P/L, Australia,* Feverfew (p. 263), Scullcap (p. 530)

Alcafelol *Luper Indústria Farmacêutica Ltda, Brazil,* Artichoke (p. 67), Boldo (p. 91)

Alcaflor *Luper Indústria Farmacêutica Ltda, Brazil,* Artichoke (p. 67), Boldo (p. 91)

Alkagin *Istituto Ganassini S.p.A. di Ricerche Biochimiche, Italy,* Calendula (p. 121), Lime Flower (p. 409) *Dermoteca, SA, Portugal,* Aloe Vera (p. 48), Calendula (p. 121), Lime Flower (p. 409)

Allens Chesty Cough *Allens & Co. (Anglesey) Ltd, UK,* St John's Wort (p. 549)

Allens Dry Tickly Cough *Allens & Co. (Anglesey) Ltd, UK,* Capsicum (p. 125)

Allens Pine & Honey *Allens & Co. (Anglesey) Ltd, UK,* Liquorice (p. 411)

Allercept *Jamieson Laboratories, Canada,* Nettle (p. 452)

AllerClear *Potter's Herbal Medicines, UK,* Echinacea (p. 217), Garlic (p. 279)

Allium Plus *Max Zeller Söhne AG, Pflanzliche Heilmittel, Switzerland,* Garlic (p. 279), Ginkgo (p. 299)

Almodin *Química Franco Mexicana Nordin S.A. de C.V., Mexico,* Horse-chestnut (p. 363), Witch Hazel (p. 601)

Aloe Grande *Gordon Laboratories, USA,* Aloe Vera (p. 48)

Aloe Vera Plus *GNLD International P/L, Australia,* Aloe Vera (p. 48)

Aloebel *Lab. Fortbenton Co. S.A., Argentina,* Aloe Vera (p. 48)

Aloelax *Laboratorio Esp. Med. Knop Ltda, Chile,* Aloes (p. 50)

Alofedina *Coll Farma, Spain,* Aloes (p. 50)

Althaea Complex *Blackmores Ltd, Australia,* Buchu (p. 100), Marshmallow (p. 418), Uva-Ursi (p. 577)

Alvear con Ginseng *Specialità Igienico Terapeutiche S.r.l., Italy,* Bilberry (p. 79), Ginseng, Panax (p. 325)

Alvisan Neo *Leros sro, Czech Republic,* Hawthorn (p. 346), Melissa (p. 425), Milk Thistle (p. 429), St John's Wort (p. 549)

Amara *Pharma-Natura (Pty) Ltd, South Africa,* Centaury (p. 149), Dandelion (p. 204), Gentian (p. 290), Juniper (p. 386), Sage (p. 512), Yarrow (p. 604)

Amara-Pascoe *Pascoe Pharmazeutische Präparate GmbH, Germany,* Cinnamon (p. 162), Gentian (p. 290)

Amara-Tropfen *Weleda AG-Heilmittelbetriebe, Germany,* Centaury (p. 149), Dandelion (p. 204), Gentian (p. 290), Juniper (p. 386), Sage (p. 512), Yarrow (p. 604)

Amaro Medicinale *Giuliani S.p.A., Italy,* Boldo (p. 91), Cascara (p. 128), Gentian (p. 290), Rhubarb (p. 506)

Amerigel *Amerx Health Care Corp., USA,* Meadowsweet (p. 423)

Amersan *Austroplant-Arzneimittel GmbH, Austria,* Agrimony (p. 42), Bilberry (p. 79), Yarrow (p. 604) *Arzneimittel Schwabe International GmbH, Czech Republic,* Agrimony (p. 42), Bilberry (p. 79), Yarrow (p. 604)

Amphodyn *Fujisawa Deutschland GmbH, Germany,* Horse-chestnut (p. 363)

anabol-loges *Dr. Loges & Co. GmbH, Germany,* St John's Wort (p. 549)

Anaemodoron *Weleda GmbH & Co. KG, Austria,* Nettle (p. 452)

Anased *Potter's (Herbal Supplies) Ltd, UK,* Hops (p. 354), Ispaghula (p. 374), Passionflower (p. 461), Pulsatilla (p. 489), Wild Lettuce (p. 596)

Anastim con RTH *Pierre Fabre Argentina S.A., Argentina,* Saw Palmetto (p. 521)

Andrographis Complex *Mediherb P/L, Australia,* Echinacea (p. 217)

Andrographis Compound *Phytomedicine P/L, Australia,* Echinacea (p. 217), Scullcap (p. 530)

Anevrasi *Donini S.r.l., Italy,* Hawthorn (p. 346), Passionflower (p. 461), Valerian (p. 580)

Angioton *GD Tecnologie Interdisciplinari Farmaceutiche S.r.l., Italy,* Bilberry (p. 79), Ginkgo (p. 299), Hydrocotyle (p. 371)

Angocin Anti-Infekt N *Repha GmbH Biologische Arzneimittel, Germany,* Horseradish (p. 367)

Antiacneicos Ac-Sal *Isdin Lda, Portugal,* Aloe Vera (p. 48)

Antibron *Potter's (Herbal Supplies) Ltd, UK,* Coltsfoot (p. 185), Euphorbia (p. 249), Marshmallow (p. 418), Pleurisy Root (p. 477), Senega (p. 533), Wild Lettuce (p. 596)

Antiestrias *Isdin Lda, Portugal,* Hydrocotyle (p. 371)

Antifect *Potter's (Herbal Supplies) Ltd, UK,* Echinacea (p. 217), Garlic (p. 279)

Antiglan *Potter's (Herbal Supplies) Ltd, UK,* Hydrangea (p. 369), Saw Palmetto (p. 521)

Antihypertonicum S *Schuck GmbH, Germany,* Hawthorn (p. 346), Milk Thistle (p. 429)

Antioxidant Forte Tablets *Mayne Pharma P/L, Australia,* Milk Thistle (p. 429)

Antirevmaticky Caj *Leros sro, Czech Republic,* Devil's Claw (p. 207), Meadowsweet (p. 423), Willow (p. 598)

Antitis *Potter's (Herbal Supplies) Ltd, UK,* Buchu (p. 100), Clivers (p. 164), Couchgrass (p. 193), Senna (p. 537), Uva-Ursi (p. 577)

Antitos *Lab. Pharma del Plata S.R.L., Argentina,* Senega (p. 533)

Antomiopic *Novartis Farmaceutica, Spain,* Bilberry (p. 79)

Anusol *Pfizer P/L, Australia,* Witch Hazel (p. 601)

Apaisance *Laboratoires Liérac, France,* Lime Flower (p. 409), Pilewort (p. 472)

Apergan *Farmaceutici G.B. Panzera S.r.l., Italy,* Ginseng, Panax (p. 325)

Aphloine P *Laboratoires DB Pharma, France,* Witch Hazel (p. 601)

Aphtagone *Trima, Israel,* Aloe Vera (p. 48)

Api Baby *Sanitalia S.n.c. di Battaglia & C., Italy,* Bilberry (p. 79)

Appetiser Mixture *Potter's (Herbal Supplies) Ltd, UK,* Gentian (p. 290)

Aptha-X *C.T.S. Chemical Industries Ltd, Israel,* Aloe Vera (p. 48)

Aqua Ban Herbal *G.R. Lane Health Products Ltd, UK,* Burdock (p. 102), Clivers (p. 164), Uva-Ursi (p. 577)

Aqualette *Medic Herb UK Ltd, UK,* Dandelion (p. 204) *Lichtwer Pharma UK,*

Aqualibra *Medice, Arzneimittel Pütter GmbH & Co. KG, Germany,* Java Tea (p. 381)

Arbum *Laboratoires Jaldes, France,* Burdock (p. 102)

Arceligasol *Lab E J Gezzi SRL, Argentina,* Artichoke (p. 67), Coltsfoot (p. 185)

Arctuvan *Fujisawa Deutschland GmbH, Germany,* Uva-Ursi (p. 577)

Ardeysedon *Ardeypharm GmbH, Germany,* Hops (p. 354), Valerian (p. 580)

Argeal *Pierre Fabre Argentina S.A., Argentina,* Saw Palmetto (p. 521) *Laboratoires Pierre Fabre, France,* Saw Palmetto (p. 521)

Arheumacare *Health Perception Ltd, UK,* Ginger (p. 293)

Aristaloe *Neo Dermos S.R.L., Argentina,* Aloe Vera (p. 48)

Arkophytum *Laboratoires Arkopharma, France,* Devil's Claw (p. 207), Willow (p. 598)

4

Armonil *Ivax Argentina SA, Argentina,* Lime Flower (p. 409), Passionflower (p. 461), Valerian (p. 580)

Armonyl *Laboratorios Maver SA, Chile,* Hawthorn (p. 346), Passionflower (p. 461), Valerian (p. 580)

Arnicadol *Laboratoires Phytomedica, France,* Arnica (p. 64)

Arnicet *Metochem-Pharma GmbH, Austria,* Arnica (p. 64), Witch Hazel (p. 601)

Arnicon *Pan Química Farmaceutica, Spain,* Arnica (p. 64)

Arnidol *Horna Business Service, Czech Republic,* Arnica (p. 64)

Arowash *Zydus Cadila Group, India,* Liquorice (p. 411)

Arterase *Laboratoires Clément-Thékan, France,* Garlic (p. 279), Horse-chestnut (p. 363)

Arterosan Plus *Doetsch Grether AG, Switzerland,* Ginkgo (p. 299), Hawthorn (p. 346), Melissa (p. 425)

Arthriforte *Blackmores Ltd, Australia,* Devil's Claw (p. 207)

Arthritic Pain Herbal Formula 1 *Mayne Pharma P/L, Australia,* Celery (p. 146), Devil's Claw (p. 207), Juniper (p. 386), Willow (p. 598)

Artin *Sanova Pharma GmbH, Austria,* Aloes (p. 50), Frangula (p. 270)

Artrex *MD Pharmaceuticals Pte Ltd, Singapore,* Ginger (p. 293)

Asa Tones *Eagle Pharmaceuticals P/L, Australia,* Drosera (p. 215), Euphorbia (p. 249), Hawthorn (p. 346), Liquorice (p. 411)

Asic *Cesam, Lda, Portugal,* Uva-Ursi (p. 577)

Asmatiron *Ibefar Inst. Brasileiro de Esp. Ftcas. Ltda, Brazil,* Marshmallow (p. 418)

Asparagus-P *Plantina Biologische Arzneimittel AG, Germany,* Parsley (p. 456)

Asthma & Catarrh Relief *Herbal Concepts Ltd, UK,* Liquorice (p. 411), Marshmallow (p. 418)

Asthmatee EF-EM-ES *EF-EM-ES - Dr Smetana & Co., Austria,* Aniseed (p. 57), Arnica (p. 64)

Astragalus Complex *Mediherb P/L, Australia,* Echinacea (p. 217), Ginseng, Eleutherococcus (p. 315)

Astrijesan *Farmo Química del Pacifico SA, Chile,* Myrrh (p. 449)

Athera *G.R. Lane Health Products Ltd, UK,* Clivers (p. 164), Parsley (p. 456), Senna (p. 537), Vervain (p. 591)

Avedorm duo *Dr. Friedrich Eberth Arzneimittel, Germany,* Hops (p. 354), Valerian (p. 580)

Avena Complex *Blackmores Ltd, Australia,* Rosemary (p. 508), Vervain (p. 591)

Avena Sativa Comp *Pharma-Natura (Pty) Ltd, South Africa,* Hops (p. 354), Passionflower (p. 461), Valerian (p. 580) *Weleda (UK) Ltd, UK,* Hops (p. 354), Passionflower (p. 461), Valerian (p. 580)

Avenoc *Boiron CZ sro, Czech Republic,* Pilewort (p. 472)

Avensyl *Laboratorios Elmor S.A., Venezuela,* Ispaghula (p. 374)

Aviril H *Leciva as, Czech Republic,* Witch Hazel (p. 601)

B-100 Complex *Natrol, USA,* Alfalfa (p. 45)

Baby Paste + Chamomile *Vitamed Ltd, Israel,* Sage (p. 512)

Babygella *Rottapharm S.r.l., Italy,* Calendula (p. 121)

Backache *Potter's (Herbal Supplies) Ltd, UK,* Buchu (p. 100), Burdock (p. 102), Clivers (p. 164), Dandelion (p. 204), Gravel Root (p. 340), Hydrangea (p. 369), Juniper (p. 386), Uva-Ursi (p. 577)

Backache Relief *Herbal Concepts Ltd, UK,* Buchu (p. 100), Parsley Piert (p. 459), Uva-Ursi (p. 577)

Bacopa Complex *Mediherb P/L, Australia,* Ginseng, Eleutherococcus (p. 315)

Bagohepat *Laboratorios Bagó S.A., Argentina,* Artichoke (p. 67)

Baldracin *Austroplant-Arzneimittel GmbH, Austria,* Hops (p. 354), Melissa (p. 425), Valerian (p. 580) *Arzneimittel Schwabe International GmbH, Czech Republic,* Hops (p. 354), Melissa (p. 425), Valerian (p. 580)

Baldrian AMA *F. Joh. Kwizda, Austria,* Hops (p. 354), Valerian (p. 580)

Baldrian-Dispert Nacht *Solvay Arzneimittel GmbH, Germany,* Hops (p. 354), Valerian (p. 580)

Baldriparan *Whitehall-Robins AG, Switzerland,* Hops (p. 354), Melissa (p. 425), Valerian (p. 580)

Baldriparan N Stark *Whitehall-Much GmbH, Germany,* Hops (p. 354), Melissa (p. 425), Valerian (p. 580)

Balm of Gilead *Potter's (Herbal Supplies) Ltd, UK,* Marshmallow (p. 418), St John's Wort (p. 549)

Balsamo Analgesico Sanitas *Upsifarma, Lda, Portugal,* Capsicum (p. 125)

Balsamo Branco *Laboratório Catarinense S.A., Brazil,* Aniseed (p. 57), Cinnamon (p. 162), Clove (p. 166), Melissa (p. 425)

Balsoclase Compositum *UCB Pharma BV, Netherlands,* Thyme (p. 574)

Banoftal *Alcon Cusi, Spain,* Calendula (p. 121), Witch Hazel (p. 601)

Bebimix *Sella A. Lab. Chim. Farm. S.r.l., Italy,* Bilberry (p. 79)

Bekunis Complex *Diafarm, Spain,* Senna (p. 537)

Bentasil Licorice with Echinacea *Carter Horner Inc., Canada,* Liquorice (p. 411)

Bentasil Licorice with Echina-cea *Carter Horner Inc., Canada,* Echinacea (p. 217)

Benylin First Defense *Pfizer Consumer Healthcare, Division of Pfizer Canada Inc., Canada,* Echinacea (p. 217)

Benzomel *Casa Granado Lab. Farmacias e Drogarias S.A., Brazil,* Passionflower (p. 461)

Berberis Complex *Blackmores Ltd, Australia,* Boldo (p. 91), Dandelion (p. 204)

Berggeist *Kur- und Stadtapotheke, Austria,* Arnica (p. 64), Nettle (p. 452)

Betaine Digestive Aid *GNLD International P/L, Australia,* Liquorice (p. 411), Rhubarb (p. 506)

Bicholate *Sabex Inc., Canada,* Cascara (p. 128)

Bilaxil *Bayer SA, Chile,* Ispaghula (p. 374), Senna (p. 537)

Bilberry Plus Eye Health *Mayne Pharma P/L, Australia,* Bilberry (p. 79), Ginkgo (p. 299)

Bilbery 40mg *Natrol, USA,* Bilberry (p. 79)

Bilidren *Lab. Lafage S.R.L., Argentina,* Artichoke (p. 67), Cascara (p. 128)

Bilifel *Neckerman Indústria Farmacêutica Ltda, Brazil,* Boldo (p. 91), Cascara (p. 128), Rhubarb (p. 506)

Bilifuge *Laboratoires Plan SA, Switzerland,* Artichoke (p. 67), Java Tea (p. 381)

Biliosan Compuesto *Lab. Hexa-Medinova S.A., Argentina,* Artichoke (p. 67), Boldo (p. 91)

Bilisan Duo *Repha GmbH Biologische Arzneimittel, Germany,* Milk Thistle (p. 429)

Biocalm *Lizofarm S.r.l., Italy,* Passionflower (p. 461), Valerian (p. 580)

Biocarde *Laboratoires Lehning, France,* Hawthorn (p. 346), Melissa (p. 425), Motherwort (p. 447), Passionflower (p. 461), Valerian (p. 580)

BioCyst *CytoChemia AG, Germany,* Java Tea (p. 381)

Bioglan 3B Beer Belly Buster *Bioglan Ltd, Australia,* St John's Wort (p. 549)

Bioglan Arthri Plus *Bioglan Ltd, Australia,* Devil's Claw (p. 207), Willow (p. 598)

Bioglan Bioage Peripheral *Bioglan Ltd, Australia,* Hawthorn (p. 346)

Bioglan Cirflo *Bioglan Ltd, Australia,* Horse-chestnut (p. 363), Pulsatilla (p. 489), Witch Hazel (p. 601)

Bioglan Cranbiotic Super *Bioglan Ltd, Australia,* Buchu (p. 100), Cranberry (p. 197), Dandelion (p. 204), Uva-Ursi (p. 577)

Bioglan Ginger-Vite Forte *Bioglan Ltd, Australia,* Ginger (p. 293)

Bioglan Ginsynergy *Bioglan Ltd, Australia,* Ginseng, Eleutherococcus (p. 315), Ginseng, Panax (p. 325)

Bioglan Joint Mobility *Bioglan Ltd, Australia,* Capsicum (p. 125)

Bioglan Mens Super Soy/Clover *Bioglan Ltd, Australia,* Damiana (p. 201), Red Clover (p. 498), Saw Palmetto (p. 521)

Bioglan Psylli-Mucil Plus *Bioglan Ltd, Australia,* Ginger (p. 293), Ispaghula (p. 374), Slippery Elm (p. 545)

Bioglan Pygno-Vite *Bioglan Ltd, Australia,* Bilberry (p. 79)

Bioglan Soy Power Plus *Bioglan Ltd, Australia,* Red Clover (p. 498)

Bioglan The Blue One *Bioglan Ltd, Australia,* Capsicum (p. 125), Damiana (p. 201)

Bioglan Vision-Eze *Bioglan Ltd, Australia,* Bilberry (p. 79), Ginkgo (p. 299)

Bioglan Zellulean with Escin *Bioglan Ltd, Australia,* Ginkgo (p. 299), Horse-chestnut (p. 363)

Biolactine *Sella A. Lab. Chim. Farm. S.r.l., Italy,* Bilberry (p. 79)

Biomicovo *Laboratorio Biotecnoquímica, Venezuela,* Arnica (p. 64), Calendula (p. 121), St John's Wort (p. 549), Witch Hazel (p. 601)

Biophase Shampoo *Ecofarm Group Srl, Italy,* Cinnamon (p. 162), Clove (p. 166)

bioplant-Kamillenfluid *Serumwerk Bernburg AG, Germany,* Calendula (p. 121)

Biosedon *Sabona GmbH, Germany,* Hops (p. 354), Passionflower (p. 461), Valerian (p. 580)

Bio-Strath *Bio-Strath AG, Czech Republic,* Passionflower (p. 461), Valerian (p. 580)

Bio-Strath Artichoke Formula *Cedar Health Ltd, UK,* Artichoke (p. 67), Holy Thistle (p. 352)

Bio-Strath Valerian Formula *Cedar Health Ltd, UK,* Passionflower (p. 461), Valerian (p. 580)

Bio-Strath Willow Formula *Cedar Health Ltd, UK,* Cowslip (p. 195), Willow (p. 598)

Biotene with Calcium *Laclede Inc., USA,* Aloe Vera (p. 48)

Biothymus DS *Biochimici PSN S.p.A., Italy,* Nettle (p. 452), Willow (p. 598)

Biothymus M Urto *Biochimici PSN S.p.A., Italy,* Saw Palmetto (p. 521)

Bioton *Sella A. Lab. Chim. Farm. S.r.l., Italy,* Ginseng, Panax (p. 325)

Biotussil *Biomedica sro, Czech Republic,* Cowslip (p. 195), Elder (p. 237), Gentian (p. 290), Liquorice (p. 411), Thyme (p. 574)

Biovital *Roche (Magyarország) Kft, Hungary,* Hawthorn (p. 346), Motherwort (p. 447)

Biovital *Roche (Magyarország) Kft, Hungary,* Motherwort (p. 447)

Biovital Aktiv *Roche Consumer Health Deutschland GmbH, Germany,* Hawthorn (p. 346), Hawthorn (p. 346), Motherwort (p. 447)

Biovital Classic *Roche Consumer Health Deutschland GmbH, Germany,* Hawthorn (p. 346), Motherwort (p. 447)

Biovital Ginseng *Bayer (Schweiz) AG, Pharma, Switzerland,* Ginseng, Panax (p. 325)

Biral *Altana Madaus Pty Ltd, South Africa,* Passionflower (p. 461), Valerian (p. 580)

Bisuisan *DM Indústria Farmacêutica Ltda, Brazil,* Rhubarb (p. 506)

Black Cohosh *Natrol, USA,* Cohosh, Black (p. 168)

Blackoids du Docteur Meur *SERP, Monaco,* Liquorice (p. 411)

Blahungstee N *Abtswinder Naturheilmittel GmbH, Czech Republic,* Aniseed (p. 57), Calendula (p. 121), Cinnamon (p. 162), Melissa (p. 425)

Blasen- und Nierentee *Abtswinder Naturheilmittel GmbH, Czech Republic,* Calendula (p. 121), Liquorice (p. 411), Uva-Ursi (p. 577)

Blastoestimulina *Almirall Prodesfarma S.A., Spain,* Hydrocotyle (p. 371)

Bodi Kleen *Geritrex Corp., USA,* Aloe Vera (p. 48)

Bodyguard *Sanitalia S.n.c. di Battaglia & C., Italy,* Devil's Claw (p. 207), Echinacea (p. 217), Willow (p. 598)

Bolcitol *Laboratoires Gabriel Lesourd, France,* Boldo (p. 91), Fumitory (p. 276), Sage (p. 512)

Boldex *Potter's (Herbal Supplies) Ltd, UK,* Boldo (p. 91), Dandelion (p. 204)

Boldina *Lab. Pharma del Plata S.R.L., Argentina,* Artichoke (p. 67), Boldo (p. 91)

Boldocynara *Bioforce AG, Switzerland,* Artichoke (p. 67), Boldo (p. 91), Dandelion (p. 204)

Boldopeptan *Laboratório Neo Química Comércio e Indústria Ltda, Brazil,* Boldo (p. 91), Cascara (p. 128), Rhubarb (p. 506)

Boljuprima *Laboratórios Prima Ltda, Brazil,* Boldo (p. 91)

Bolus Laxans *EGIS Pharmaceuticals, Hungary,* Rhubarb (p. 506), Senna (p. 537)

Bomacorin *Hevert-Arzneimittel GmbH & Co. KG, Germany,* Hawthorn (p. 346)

Bonningtons Irish Moss *GlaxoSmithKline, New Zealand,* Liquorice (p. 411)

Boots Alternatives Easy Digest *Alliance Boots plc, UK,* Artichoke (p. 67)

Boots Alternatives Laxative *Alliance Boots plc, UK,* Senna (p. 537)

Boots Alternatives Premenstrual *Alliance Boots plc, UK,* Evening Primrose (p. 251)

Boots Alternatives Sharp Mind *Alliance Boots plc, UK,* Ginkgo (p. 299)

Boots Alternatives Sleep Well *Alliance Boots plc, UK,* Hops (p. 354), Melissa (p. 425), Valerian (p. 580)

Boots Sleepeaze Herbal Tablets *Alliance Boots plc, UK,* Hops (p. 354), Melissa (p. 425), Valerian (p. 580)

Borage Oil *Natrol, USA,* Borage (p. 96)

Borsdruppels *Aspen Pharmacare (Pty) Ltd, South Africa,* Liquorice (p. 411)

Borstol Cough Remedy *Group Laboratories SA (Pty) Ltd, South Africa,* Buchu (p. 100), Senega (p. 533)

Boswellia Complex *Mediherb P/L, Australia,* Celery (p. 146), Ginger (p. 293)

Boswellia Compound *Phytomedicine P/L, Australia,* Devil's Claw (p. 207), Ginger (p. 293), Guaiacum (p. 344)

Botanica Hayfever *Pacific Pharmaceuticals Co. Ltd, New Zealand,* Melissa (p. 425)

Boxocalm *Cheplapharm Arzneimittel GmbH, Germany,* Hops (p. 354), Valerian (p. 580)

Brady's-Magentropfen *Brady C. KG, Austria,* Aniseed (p. 57), Cinnamon (p. 162), Gentian (p. 290), Myrrh (p. 449)

Bromidrastina *Ibefar Inst. Brasileiro de Esp. Ftcas. Ltda, Brazil,* Golden Seal (p. 337), Witch Hazel (p. 601)

Bromocod N *G. Streuli & Co. AG, Switzerland,* Drosera (p. 215)

Broncafect *Mediherb P/L, Australia,* Echinacea (p. 217), Ginger (p. 293), Liquorice (p. 411), Pleurisy Root (p. 477), Thyme (p. 574)

Bronchial *E-Z-EM Canada Inc., Canada,* Senega (p. 533)

Bronchialtee N *Abtswinder Naturheilmittel GmbH, Czech Republic,* Cowslip (p. 195), Liquorice (p. 411), Thyme (p. 574)

Bronchicum *Cassella-med GmbH & Co. KG, Germany,* Cowslip (p. 195), Thyme (p. 574) *Aventis Pharma, Netherlands,* Cowslip (p. 195), Thyme (p. 574)

Bronchicum Elixir *Aventis Pharma sro, Czech Republic,* Cowslip (p. 195), Thyme (p. 574)

Bronchicum Elixir S *Cassella-med GmbH & Co. KG, Germany,* Cowslip (p. 195), Thyme (p. 574)

Bronchicum Husten (Бронхикум Сироп от Кашля) *Sanofi-Aventis, Russia,* Cowslip (p. 195), Thyme (p. 574)

Bronchicum Hustensirup *Aventis Pharma sro, Czech Republic,* Cowslip (p. 195), Thyme (p. 574)

Bronchicum Pflanzlicher Hustenstiller *Aventis Pharma sro, Czech Republic,* Drosera (p. 215)

Bronchicum Sekret-Loser *Aventis Pharma sro, Czech Republic,* Cowslip (p. 195), Thyme (p. 574)

Bronchicum Tropfen *Aventis Pharma sro, Czech Republic,* Thyme (p. 574)

Bronchicum (Бронхикум) *Sanofi-Aventis, Russia,* Cowslip (p. 195), Thyme (p. 574)

Bronchipret *Austroplant-Arzneimittel GmbH, Austria,* Thyme (p. 574) *Bionorica AG, Germany,* Cowslip (p. 195), Thyme (p. 574)

Bronchithym *Austroplant-Arzneimittel GmbH, Austria,* Cowslip (p. 195), Thyme (p. 574)

Bronchostop *Metochem-Pharma GmbH, Austria,* Thyme (p. 574)

Bronchozone *DC Labs Ltd, Canada,* Liquorice (p. 411), Senega (p. 533)

Bronco Asmol *Herbes Universelles, Canada,* St John's Wort (p. 549)

Broncofenil *Zurita Laboratório Farmacêutico Ltda, Brazil,* Marshmallow (p. 418)

Broncol *Instituto Terapeutico Delta Ltda, Brazil,* Ginger (p. 293)

Broncosedina *F.A.M.A. Istituto Chimico Biologico S.r.l., Italy,* Juniper (p. 386), Thyme (p. 574)

Broncovital *Puerto Galiano, Spain,* Drosera (p. 215), Senega (p. 533)

Bronpul *Soria Natural, Spain,* Elecampane (p. 240), Liquorice (p. 411), Marshmallow (p. 418)

Bronquidex *Farmalab Industrias Químicas e Farmacêuticas Ltda, Brazil,* Marshmallow (p. 418)

Bronquiogem *Prodotti Laboratório Farmacêutico Ltda, Brazil,* Passionflower (p. 461), Yucca (p. 610)

Brontoss *Laboratório Teuto-Brasileiro Ltda, Brazil,* Marshmallow (p. 418)

Brown Mixture *British Dispensary, Thailand,* Liquorice (p. 411)

Brunavera *Euroderm Laboratorios S.R.L., Argentina,* Aloe Vera (p. 48), Calendula (p. 121)

Brust- und Hustentee *Bad Heilbrunner Naturheilmittel GmbH & Co., Germany,* Cowslip (p. 195), Thyme (p. 574)

Brust- und Hustentee St Severin *EF-EM-ES - Dr Smetana & Co., Austria,* Elecampane (p. 240), Thyme (p. 574)

Buchu Backache Compound Tablets *Frank Roberts (Herbal Dispensaries) Ltd, UK,* Buchu (p. 100), Parsley Piert (p. 459), Uva-Ursi (p. 577)

Buco Regis *Reig Jofre, Spain,* Myrrh (p. 449)

Bulgarolax *Laboratorios Chile SA, Chile,* Aloes (p. 50), Cascara (p. 128)

Bupleurum Complex *Mediherb P/L, Australia,* Milk Thistle (p. 429)

Bupleurum Compound *Phytomedicine P/L, Australia,* Milk Thistle (p. 429)

Burgerstein TopVital *Antistress AG, Gesellschaft fur Gesundheitsschutz, Switzerland,* Ginseng, Panax (p. 325)

Bushi *Laboratorios Andrómaco S.A.I.C.I., Argentina,* Calendula (p. 121)

Buttercup Syrup *Chefaro UK Ltd, UK,* Capsicum (p. 125), St John's Wort (p. 549)

Cadifen *Ca.Di.Group S.r.l., Italy,* Aniseed (p. 57), Liquorice (p. 411)

Cadimint *Ca.Di.Group S.r.l., Italy,* Aniseed (p. 57), Liquorice (p. 411)

Cajova Smes pri Nachlazeni *Megafyt-R sro, Czech Republic,* Elder (p. 237), Lime Flower (p. 409), Liquorice (p. 411)

Cajova Smes pri Redukcni Diete *Megafyt-R sro, Czech Republic,* Liquorice (p. 411), St John's Wort (p. 549), Yarrow (p. 604)

Cal Alkyline *Eagle Pharmaceuticals P/L, Australia,* Ginger (p. 293), Slippery Elm (p. 545)

Calcio 520 *Laboratorio Esp. Med. Knop Ltda, Chile,* Alfalfa (p. 45)

Calcium with Magnesium *Natrol, USA,* Cranberry (p. 197)

Calendula Concreta *Laboratório Simões Ltda, Brazil,* Calendula (p. 121)

Calendula Nappy Change Cream *Weleda (UK) Ltd, UK,* Calendula (p. 121)

Califig *Seven Seas Ltd, UK,* Senna (p. 537)

Calman *Ativus Farmacêutica Ltda, Brazil,* Hawthorn (p. 346), Passionflower (p. 461), Willow (p. 598)

Calmanervin *Meditec/Sam-On Ltd, Israel,* Passionflower (p. 461), Valerian (p. 580)

Calmanite Tablets *Frank Roberts (Herbal Dispensaries) Ltd, UK,* Hops (p. 354), Pulsatilla (p. 489), Valerian (p. 580), Wild Lettuce (p. 596)

Calmapax *Instituto Terapeutico Delta Ltda, Brazil,* Melissa (p. 425), Passionflower (p. 461)

Calmatol *Farmo Química del Pacifico SA, Chile,* Lime Flower (p. 409)

Calmazin *Ibefar Inst. Brasileiro de Esp. Ftcas. Ltda, Brazil,* Hawthorn (p. 346), Passionflower (p. 461)

Calming Aid *Sundown, USA,* Kava (p. 389), Passionflower (p. 461), Valerian (p. 580)

Calmiphase *Laboratoires Arkopharma, France,* Hydrocotyle (p. 371)

Calmiplan *Bunker Indústria Farmacêutica Ltda, Brazil,* Hawthorn (p. 346), Passionflower (p. 461), Willow (p. 598)

Calmo *Eagle Pharmaceuticals P/L, Australia,* Gentian (p. 290), Milk Thistle (p. 429), Passionflower (p. 461), Pulsatilla (p. 489), Scullcap (p. 530), Tansy (p. 572), Valerian (p. 580), Vervain (p. 591)

Calmophytum *Laboratoires Holistica International, France,* Lime Flower (p. 409), Vervain (p. 591)

Camolyn *Laboratorios L.O. Oftalmi C.A., Venezuela,* Witch Hazel (p. 601)

Canephron *Bionorica AG, Germany,* Centaury (p. 149), Rosemary (p. 508)

Canephron N (Канефрон Н) *Bionorica AG, Russia,* Centaury (p. 149), Rosemary (p. 508)

Canephron novo *Bionorica AG, Germany,* Java Tea (p. 381)

Canol *Laboratoires Jolly-Jatel, France,* Artichoke (p. 67)

Capill *Pharma Italia Laboratori Farmaceutici S.r.l., Italy,* Bilberry (p. 79), Horse-chestnut (p. 363), Hydrocotyle (p. 371)

Capill Venogel *Pharma Italia Laboratori Farmaceutici S.r.l., Italy,* Horse-chestnut (p. 363), Hydrocotyle (p. 371)

Capso *Euroderm-RDC S.p.A., Italy,* Aloe Vera (p. 48)

Capsules-vital *Biomed AG, Switzerland,* Ginkgo (p. 299)

Caramelle alle Erbe Digestive *Giuliani S.p.A., Italy,* Boldo (p. 91), Gentian (p. 290), Rhubarb (p. 506)

Caramelos Agua del Carmen *Fardi, Spain,* Melissa (p. 425)

Cardiaforce *Bioforce AG, Switzerland,* Hawthorn (p. 346), Melissa (p. 425)

Cardioace *Vitabiotics Ltd, UK,* Garlic (p. 279)

Cardiodoron *Weleda GmbH & Co. KG, Austria,* Cowslip (p. 195) *Weleda AG-Heilmittelbetriebe, Germany,* Cowslip (p. 195) *Pharma-Natura (Pty) Ltd, South Africa,* Cowslip (p. 195)

Cardio-Longoral *Artesan Pharma GmbH & Co. KG, Cassella-med GmbH & Co. KG, Germany,* Hawthorn (p. 346)

Carilax *Mag. Dr. Till Strallhofer, Austria,* Senna (p. 537)

Carmicide *Indoco Remedies Ltd, India,* Cinnamon (p. 162), Ginger (p. 293)

Carmol *Iromedica AG, Switzerland,* Melissa (p. 425)

Carmol Magen-Galle-Darm *Omegin Dr Schmidgall GmbH & Co. KG, Germany,* Artichoke (p. 67), Dandelion (p. 204)

Cascade *G.R. Lane Health Products Ltd, UK,* Burdock (p. 102), Clivers (p. 164), Uva-Ursi (p. 577)

Cascara Sagrada Bouzen *Bouzen S.A.C,.I.F.A.F., Argentina,* Cascara (p. 128)

Cascara-Salax *Ferring Arzneimittel GmbH, Austria,* Cascara (p. 128)

Castanha de India Composta *Infabra Indústria Farmacêutica Brasileira Ltda, Brazil,* Horse-chestnut (p. 363)

Catarrh Mixture *Potter's (Herbal Supplies) Ltd, UK,* Blue Flag (p. 87), Boneset (p. 94), Burdock (p. 102), Capsicum (p. 125)

Catarrh Tablets *Frank Roberts (Herbal Dispensaries) Ltd, UK,* Echinacea (p. 217), Lobelia (p. 416), Pokeroot (p. 479)

Catarrh-eeze *Chefaro UK Ltd, UK,* Elecampane (p. 240), Yarrow (p. 604)

Catiz Plus *Merck Química Argentina S.A.I.C., Argentina,* Saw Palmetto (p. 521)

Cats Claw Complex *Mediherb P/L, Australia,* Echinacea (p. 217)

Cayenne Plus *Nutravite, Canada,* Ginger (p. 293)

Cefadrin *Cefak KG, Germany,* Ephedra (p. 243), Thyme (p. 574)

Cefasabal *Cefak KG, Germany,* Horse-chestnut (p. 363), Saw Palmetto (p. 521)

Cefasedativ *Cefak KG, Germany,* Hops (p. 354), Valerian (p. 580)

Cefawell *Cefak KG, Germany,* Arnica (p. 64), Calendula (p. 121)

Celery Plus *Swiss Bio Pharma Sdn Bhd, Malaysia,* Burdock (p. 102), Celery (p. 146), Devil's Claw (p. 207), Willow (p. 598)

Celltech Gold *Laboratorios Recalcine SA, Chile,* Borage (p. 96), Ginkgo (p. 299)

Celu-Atlas *Atlas Farmaceutica, Argentina,* Hydrocotyle (p. 371)

Celulase Con Neomicina *Laboratorios Rider SA, Chile,* Hydrocotyle (p. 371)

Cemalyt *Saros Laboratorios, Spain,* Hydrocotyle (p. 371)

Centella Complex *Peter Italia sas, Italy,* Horse-chestnut (p. 363), Hydrocotyle (p. 371), Hydrocotyle (p. 371), Witch Hazel (p. 601)

Centella Queen Complex *Lab. Temis Lostaló S.A., Argentina,* Hydrocotyle (p. 371)

Centella Queen Reductora *Lab. Temis Lostaló S.A., Argentina,* Hydrocotyle (p. 371)

Centellase de Centella Queen *Lab. Temis Lostaló S.A., Argentina,* Ginkgo (p. 299), Hydrocotyle (p. 371)

Centellase Gel *Lab. Temis Lostaló S.A., Argentina,* Hydrocotyle (p. 371)

Centeril H *Errekappa Euroterapici S.p.A., Italy,* Horse-chestnut (p. 363), Hydrocotyle (p. 371), Witch Hazel (p. 601)

Cervusen *Australian Medic-Care Co. Ltd, Hong Kong,* Ginseng, Panax (p. 325)

Cerylana *Laboratorios Intra S.A., Venezuela,* Wild Lettuce (p. 596)

Chamberlains Cough Remedy Regular *Pfizer Laboratories (Pty) Ltd, South Africa,* Liquorice (p. 411)

Chap Stick *Whitehall, New Zealand,* Aloe Vera (p. 48)

Chase Coldsorex *Stella Pharmaceutical Canada Inc., Canada,* Myrrh (p. 449)

Chase Kolik GripeWater *Stella Pharmaceutical Canada Inc., Canada,* Ginger (p. 293)

Chest Mixture *Potter's (Herbal Supplies) Ltd, UK,* Marshmallow (p. 418), Pleurisy Root (p. 477), Senega (p. 533), St John's Wort (p. 549)

Chesty Cough Relief *Herbal Concepts Ltd, UK,* Coltsfoot (p. 185), Liquorice (p. 411), Senega (p. 533)

China-Eisenwein *Mayrhofer Pharmazeutika, Austria,* Centaury (p. 149), Cinnamon (p. 162), Gentian (p. 290)

Chlorophyl liquid *Coradol-Pharma GmbH, Germany,* Hawthorn (p. 346)

Chlorophyllin Salbe *Coradol-Pharma GmbH, Germany,* Witch Hazel (p. 601)

Choats Extract of Lettuce Cough Mixture *Pfizer Laboratories (Pty) Ltd, South Africa,* Wild Lettuce (p. 596)

Chofabol *Allen Laboratorios, S.A. de C.V., Mexico,* Artichoke (p. 67), Boldo (p. 91)

Chofranina *De Mayo Industrias Químicas e Farmacêuticas Ltda, Brazil,* Artichoke (p. 67), Cascara (p. 128)

Cholagol *Ivax-CR a s Közvetlen Kereskedelmi Képviselet, Hungary,* Frangula (p. 270) *Ivax-CR as, Ivax-CR as, Czech Republic,* Frangula (p. 270)

Cholagutt *Korangi S.A., Portugal,* Calamus (p. 118), Milk Thistle (p. 429)

Cholasyn II *Rolmex International Inc., Canada,* Cascara (p. 128), Senna (p. 537)

Cholhepan N *Schuck GmbH, Germany,* Aloes (p. 50), Milk Thistle (p. 429)

Chol-Kugeletten Neu *Dolorgiet GmbH & Co. KG, Germany,* Aloes (p. 50)

Cholosom SL *Hevert-Arzneimittel GmbH & Co. KG, Germany,* Dandelion (p. 204)

Cholosom-Tee *Hevert-Arzneimittel GmbH & Co. KG, Germany,* Dandelion (p. 204), Milk Thistle (p. 429)

Cicaderma *Boiron CZ sro, Czech Republic,* Calendula (p. 121), Pulsatilla (p. 489), St John's Wort (p. 549), Yarrow (p. 604) *Prisfar, SA, Portugal,* Calendula (p. 121), St John's Wort (p. 549), Yarrow (p. 604)

Cicapost *Isdin Chile Ltda, Chile,* Hydrocotyle (p. 371)

Cimicifuga Compound *Phytomedicine P/L, Australia,* Cohosh, Black (p. 168), St John's Wort (p. 549)

Cional *Nycomed Austria GmbH, Austria,* Arnica (p. 64), Sage (p. 512)

Circanetten *Eversil Produtos Farmacêuticos Indústria e Comércio Ltda, Brazil,* Senna (p. 537) *Sriprasit Dispensary R O P, Thailand,* Senna (p. 537)

Circulan *Adroka AG, Switzerland,* Hawthorn (p. 346), Passionflower (p. 461)

Ciruelax Jalea *Ivax Pharmaceuticals Mexico S.A. de C.V., Mexico,* Senna (p. 537)

Cirulaxia *Altana Pharma SA, Argentina,* Senna (p. 537)

Cito-Guakalin *Stada GmbH, Germany,* Thyme (p. 574)

Citos *Química Franco Mexicana Nordin S.A. de C.V., Mexico,* Drosera (p. 215)

CitriMax Plus *Natrol, USA,* Uva-Ursi (p. 577)

Citrimax Plus with ChromeMate *Natrol, USA,* Cascara (p. 128)

Citro-C *Laboratorio Esp. Med. Knop Ltda, Chile,* Echinacea (p. 217)

Clairo *Pharma-Natura (Pty) Ltd, South Africa,* Aniseed (p. 57), Centaury (p. 149), Clove (p. 166), Senna (p. 537), Yarrow (p. 604)

Cleansa Plus *Swiss Bio Pharma Sdn Bhd, Malaysia,* Burdock (p. 102), Nettle (p. 452), Passionflower (p. 461), Red Clover (p. 498), Sarsaparilla (p. 515)

Cleansing Herbs *Potter's (Herbal Supplies) Ltd, UK,* Elder (p. 237), Senna (p. 537)

Clearasil Double Clear *Procter & Gamble, USA,* Witch Hazel (p. 601)

Clevosan *Lab. Baliarda S.A., Argentina,* Hydrocotyle (p. 371)

Climaxol *Laboratoires Lehning, France,* Golden Seal (p. 337), Horse-chestnut (p. 363), Witch Hazel (p. 601)

Climil Complex *Wassen Italia S.r.l., Italy,* Cohosh, Black (p. 168)

Climil-80 *Wassen Italia S.r.l., Italy,* Cohosh, Black (p. 168)

Clogar *Self-Care Products Ltd, UK,* Garlic (p. 279)

Coci-Fedra *MPL, Marching Pharmaceutical Ltd, Hong Kong,* Senega (p. 533), St John's Wort (p. 549)

Cocillana Christo *Christo Pharmaceuticals Ltd, Hong Kong,* Euphorbia (p. 249), Senega (p. 533), St John's Wort (p. 549)

Cocillana Co *Adcock Ingram Pharmaceuticals Ltd, South Africa,* St John's Wort (p. 549)

Cocillana Compound *Synco (HK) Ltd, Hong Kong,* Euphorbia (p. 249), Senega (p. 533), St John's Wort (p. 549) *Universal Pharmaceutical Lab Ltd, Hong Kong,* Euphorbia (p. 249), Senega (p. 533), St John's Wort (p. 549) *Vida Laboratories Ltd, Hong Kong,* Euphorbia (p. 249), St John's Wort (p. 549)

Cocillana-Etyfin *Ellem Läkemedel AB, Sweden,* Senega (p. 533)

Codebromil *Laboratorios Vincenti C.A., Venezuela,* Drosera (p. 215), Thyme (p. 574)

Codelum *Sanova Pharma GmbH, Austria,* Thyme (p. 574)

Colachofra *EMS Ind. Farmacêutica Ltda, Brazil,* Artichoke (p. 67), Boldo (p. 91)

Coladren *Cooperativa Farmaceutica Soc. (CoFa Farmaceutici), Italy,* Boldo (p. 91), Cascara (p. 128)

Colax *Mediherb P/L, Australia,* Cascara (p. 128), Dandelion (p. 204), Yellow Dock (p. 608) *Mediherb P/L, Officina Farmaceutica Fiorentina S.r.l. Istituto Biochimico, Italy,* Artichoke (p. 67), Boldo (p. 91), Rhubarb (p. 506), Senna (p. 537)

Cold and Flu Relief *Brauer Natural Medicine P/L, Australia,* Echinacea (p. 217)

Cold Sore Lotion *DC Labs Ltd, Canada,* Myrrh (p. 449)

Coleus Complex *Mediherb P/L, Australia,* Hawthorn (p. 346), Valerian (p. 580)

Colimax *Qualiphar SA, Belgium,* Thyme (p. 574)

Colimil *Milte Italia S.p.A., Italy,* Melissa (p. 425)

Collypan *Vifor SA, Switzerland,* Eyebright (p. 256), Witch Hazel (p. 601)

Colosan plus *Vifor SA, Switzerland,* Frangula (p. 270)

Combudoron *Weleda AG-Heilmittelbetriebe, Germany,* Arnica (p. 64), Nettle (p. 452) *Pharma-Natura (Pty) Ltd, South Africa,* Arnica (p. 64), Nettle (p. 452) *Weleda AG, Switzerland,* Arnica (p. 64), Nettle (p. 452)

Comfrey Plus *Concept for Pharmacy Ltd, Israel,* Comfrey (p. 188)

Composto Anticelulitico *Infabra Indústria Farmacêutica Brasileira Ltda, Brazil,* Ginkgo (p. 299), Hydrocotyle (p. 371), Uva-Ursi (p. 577)

Composto Emagrecedor *Viternat Laboratórios Ltda, Brazil,* Artichoke (p. 67), Cascara (p. 128), Hydrocotyle (p. 371), Passionflower (p. 461)

Compound Laxative Syrup of Figs *Alliance Boots plc, UK,* Senna (p. 537)

Concentrated Milk of Magnesia-Cascara *Roxane Laboratories Inc., a Subsidiary of Boehringer Ingelheim, USA,* Cascara (p. 128)

Confetti Lassativi CM *Giuliani S.p.A., Italy,* Boldo (p. 91), Cascara (p. 128), Senna (p. 537)

Confortel *Forder Lab. Esp. Dermatologicas, Argentina,* Pilewort (p. 472)

Constipation *Nobel Pharm Enrg, Canada,* Frangula (p. 270), Senna (p. 537)

Constipation Tablets *Frank Roberts (Herbal Dispensaries) Ltd, UK,* Aloes (p. 50), Senna (p. 537), Valerian (p. 580)

Contra-Coff *Universal Pharmaceuticals (Pty) Ltd, South Africa,* St John's Wort (p. 549)

Contraspan *Ivax-CR as, Ivax-CR as, Czech Republic,* Valerian (p. 580)

Control *Les Laboratoires Bio-Santé, Canada,* Cascara (p. 128)

Controlacne *Pharmalab, Division de Stonglass SA, Argentina,* Aloe Vera (p. 48), Calendula (p. 121)

Contusin *Lacer, Spain,* Horse-chestnut (p. 363)

Convallocor-SL *Hevert-Arzneimittel GmbH & Co. KG, Germany,* Hawthorn (p. 346)

Convastabil *Dr Gustav Klein, Germany,* Hawthorn (p. 346)

Cosylan *Pfizer AS, Norway,* Cascara (p. 128)

Cough Elixir *Pharma-Natura (Pty) Ltd, South Africa,* Aniseed (p. 57), Drosera (p. 215), Marshmallow (p. 418), Pulsatilla (p. 489), Thyme (p. 574)

Cough Relief *Brauer Natural Medicine P/L, Australia,* Echinacea (p. 217), Marshmallow (p. 418), Nettle (p. 452), Thyme (p. 574)

Cough-eeze *Perrigo, UK,* Elecampane (p. 240)

Covonia Mentholated *Thornton & Ross Ltd, UK,* Liquorice (p. 411), St John's Wort (p. 549)

Cran Support *Natrol, USA,* Cat's Claw (p. 132), Corn Silk (p. 191), Cranberry (p. 197)

CranAssure *Nature Made, USA,* Cranberry (p. 197)

Cranberry *Natrol, USA,* Cranberry (p. 197)

Cranberry Complex *Mayne Pharma P/L, Australia,* Buchu (p. 100), Cranberry (p. 197), Uva-Ursi (p. 577) *Mediherb P/L, Australia,* Buchu (p. 100), Cranberry (p. 197), Uva-Ursi (p. 577)

Cran-C *Holista Health Corp, Canada,* Cranberry (p. 197)

Cratex *Corporacion de Salud C.A., Venezuela,* Hawthorn (p. 346), Passionflower (p. 461), Valerian (p. 580)

Creme Rap *Laboratoires IPRAD, France,* Arnica (p. 64), Broom (p. 98), Horse-chestnut (p. 363)

Cremor capsici comp *Pharmachemie BV, Netherlands,* Capsicum (p. 125)

Cremor Capsici compositus *ratiopharm GmbH, Germany,* Capsicum (p. 125)

Crislaxo *Químifar, Spain,* Aloes (p. 50), Aniseed (p. 57), Cascara (p. 128), Rhubarb (p. 506), Senna (p. 537)

Critichol *Aziende Chimiche Riunite Angelini Francesco S.p.A., Italy,* Boldo (p. 91), Cascara (p. 128), Rhubarb (p. 506)

Cuassicum *Nucleopharm SRL, Argentina,* Quassia (p. 491)

Culpeper After Dinner Tea *Culpeper and Napiers, UK,* Chamomile, German (p. 152)

Culpeper DeTox Tea *Culpeper and Napiers, UK,* Dandelion (p. 204), Liquorice (p. 411), Nettle (p. 452)

Cuscutine *Geymonat S.p.A., Italy,* Senna (p. 537)

Cycloven Forte N *ct-Arzneimittel GmbH, Germany,* Horse-chestnut (p. 363)

Cynarix comp *Montavit GmbH, Austria,* Artichoke (p. 67)

Cynaro Bilina *Nutridiver SL, Spain,* Aloes (p. 50), Artichoke (p. 67)

Cynarosan *Slovakofarma sro, Czech Republic,* Agrimony (p. 42), Artichoke (p. 67), Dandelion (p. 204), Rhubarb (p. 506)

Cynarzym N *Altana Pharma Deutschland GmbH, Germany,* Artichoke (p. 67), Boldo (p. 91)

Cystinol *Hoyer-Madaus GmbH & Co. KG, Germany,* Uva-Ursi (p. 577)

Daily Fatigue Relief *Herbal Concepts Ltd, UK,* Damiana (p. 201), Saw Palmetto (p. 521)

Daily Tension & Strain Relief *Herbal Concepts Ltd, UK,* Asafoetida (p. 72), Passionflower (p. 461), Valerian (p. 580)

Dam *Laboratorio Terapeutico M.R. S.r.l., Italy,* Cinnamon (p. 162), Damiana (p. 201)

DAM Antacidum *Corifel SA, Switzerland,* Liquorice (p. 411)

Damiana and Kola Tablets *Dorwest Herbs Ltd, UK,* Damiana (p. 201), Saw Palmetto (p. 521)

Damiana-Sarsaparilla Formula *Boehringer Ingelheim (Canada) Ltd, Canada,* Damiana (p. 201), Ginseng, Panax (p. 325), Liquorice (p. 411), Sarsaparilla (p. 515), Saw Palmetto (p. 521)

Dan Shen Compound *Phytomedicine P/L, Australia,* Hawthorn (p. 346), Valerian (p. 580)

Dandelion Complex *Swiss Bio Pharma Sdn Bhd, Malaysia,* Artichoke (p. 67), Burdock (p. 102), Capsicum (p. 125), Dandelion (p. 204), Ginger (p. 293)

Davilla *Rekah Ltd, Israel,* Cinnamon (p. 162), Rhubarb (p. 506)

De Witt's K & B Pills *E.C. De Witt & Co. Ltd, UK,* Buchu (p. 100), Uva-Ursi (p. 577)

De Witts New Pills *C.B. Fleet Co. (Australia) P/L, Australia,* Buchu (p. 100), Uva-Ursi (p. 577)

De Witts Pills *Regional Health Ltd, New Zealand,* Buchu (p. 100), Uva-Ursi (p. 577)

Decon Ovuli *IP Farma Sas, Italy,* Calendula (p. 121), Witch Hazel (p. 601)

Dekar 2 *Pentamedical S.r.l., Italy,* Quassia (p. 491)

Dellova *Laboratoires Clément-Thionville, France,* Java Tea (p. 381)

Demo Elixir pectoral N *Vifor SA, Switzerland,* Drosera (p. 215)

Demonatur Capsules contre les refroidissements *Vifor SA, Switzerland,* Echinacea (p. 217)

Demonatur Dragees pour les reins et la vessie *Vifor SA, Switzerland,* Echinacea (p. 217), Java Tea (p. 381), Uva-Ursi (p. 577)

Demonatur Gouttes pour le foie et la bile *Vifor SA, Switzerland,* Artichoke (p. 67), Dandelion (p. 204), Gentian (p. 290), Milk Thistle (p. 429)

DemoPectol *Vifor SA, Switzerland,* Cowslip (p. 195), Liquorice (p. 411), Thyme (p. 574)

DemoPectol *Vifor SA, Switzerland,* Thyme (p. 574)

DemoTussil *Vifor SA, Switzerland,* Drosera (p. 215), Liquorice (p. 411)

Demoven N *Vifor SA, Switzerland,* Horse-chestnut (p. 363)

4

Dentinox *Altana Pharma GmbH, Austria,* Myrrh (p. 449)

Dentosan Carie & Alito *Pfizer Italiana S.r.l., Italy,* Bloodroot (p. 84)

Depuratif Parnel *Laboratoires Phytoprevent, France,* Burdock (p. 102), Fumitory (p. 276)

Depurativo Richelet *Vitafarma, Spain,* Gentian (p. 290)

Depuratum *Laboratoires Lehning, France,* Fumitory (p. 276), Juniper (p. 386), Rosemary (p. 508), Thyme (p. 574)

Derma Care *Fischer Pharmaceuticals Ltd, Israel,* Witch Hazel (p. 601)

Dermaco *Mediherb P/L, Australia,* Burdock (p. 102), Clivers (p. 164), Sarsaparilla (p. 515), Yellow Dock (p. 608)

Dermaglos Plus *Laboratorios Andromaco SA, Chile,* Hydrocotyle (p. 371)

Dermaloe *Forder Lab. Esp. Dermatologicas, Argentina,* Aloe Vera (p. 48)

Derm'attive 10 *Sidone Indústria e Comércio Ltda., Brazil,* Hydrocotyle (p. 371)

Derm'attive Solaire *Sidone Indústria e Comércio Ltda., Brazil,* Aloe Vera (p. 48), Ginkgo (p. 299)

Dermilia Flebozin *Depofarma S.r.l., Italy,* Bilberry (p. 79), Echinacea (p. 217), Hydrocotyle (p. 371), Witch Hazel (p. 601)

Dermitina *Donini S.r.l., Italy,* Witch Hazel (p. 601)

Dermocica *Laboratoires Phytomedica, France,* Arnica (p. 64)

Dermol *Laboratório Simões Ltda, Brazil,* Arnica (p. 64)

Dermoprolyn *Infosint S.p.A., Italy,* Witch Hazel (p. 601)

Dermtex HC with Aloe *Pfeiffer Company, USA,* Aloe Vera (p. 48)

Dermvien *Hautel S.A., Argentina,* Aloe Vera (p. 48)

Desitin Creamy *Pfizer Pte Ltd, Singapore,* Aloe Vera (p. 48)

Detska Cajova Smes *Megafyt-R sro, Czech Republic,* Liquorice (p. 411), Marshmallow (p. 418)

Detsky Caj s Hermankem *Leros sro, Czech Republic,* Elder (p. 237), Hops (p. 354), Liquorice (p. 411), Marshmallow (p. 418)

Devils Claw Plus *Eagle Pharmaceuticals P/L, Australia,* Celery (p. 146), Devil's Claw (p. 207)

Diabesor *Soria Natural, Spain,* Burdock (p. 102), Sage (p. 512)

Diabetan *Leros sro, Czech Republic,* Bilberry (p. 79), Burdock (p. 102), Dandelion (p. 204), Liquorice (p. 411), Sage (p. 512)

Diabeticka Cajova Smes-Megadiabetin *Megafyt-R sro, Czech Republic,* Bilberry (p. 79), Dandelion (p. 204), Nettle (p. 452), Sage (p. 512)

Diacure *Laboratoires Lehning, France,* Bilberry (p. 79), Centaury (p. 149), Dandelion (p. 204)

Diaparene Corn Starch *Personal Care Group Inc., USA,* Aloes (p. 50)

Dicalmir *Dicofarm S.p.A., Italy,* Aniseed (p. 57), Liquorice (p. 411)

Difrarel *Laboratoires Leurquin Mediolanum, France,* Bilberry (p. 79) *Sigma-Tau Ethifarma B.V., Netherlands,* Bilberry (p. 79)

Difrarel E *Laboratoires Leurquin Mediolanum, France,* Bilberry (p. 79) *Ubepharm, Hungary,* Bilberry (p. 79)

Digelax *Balverda Srl, Italy,* Artichoke (p. 67), Boldo (p. 91), Cascara (p. 128), Rhubarb (p. 506)

Digest *Mediherb P/L, Australia,* Dandelion (p. 204), Echinacea (p. 217), Gentian (p. 290), Milk Thistle (p. 429)

Digestaid *Eagle Pharmaceuticals P/L, Australia,* Gentian (p. 290) *Healthy Direct, UK,* Gentian (p. 290)

Digestar *Brasmedica S.A. Industrias Farmacêuticas, Brazil,* Gentian (p. 290)

Digestive *Dorwest Herbs Ltd, UK,* Ginger (p. 293), Golden Seal (p. 337), Rhubarb (p. 506), Valerian (p. 580)

Digestive Aid *Blackmores Ltd, Australia,* Gentian (p. 290), Ginger (p. 293), Slippery Elm (p. 545)

Digestodoron *Weleda GmbH & Co. KG, Austria,* Willow (p. 598) *Weleda AG-Heilmittelbetriebe, Germany,* Willow (p. 598) *Pharma-Natura (Pty) Ltd, South Africa,* Willow (p. 598)

Digestovital *Puerto Galiano, Spain,* Aniseed (p. 57)

Digestron *Lopes Produtos Farmaceuticos S.A., Brazil,* Artichoke (p. 67), Holy Thistle (p. 352), Horse-chestnut (p. 363)

Dilaescol *Dr. Kolassa & Merz GmbH, Austria,* Horse-chestnut (p. 363)

Dioptec *Laboratoires Dergam, France,* Calendula (p. 121)

Diovol Forte DGL *Wallace Pharmaceuticals Ltd, India,* Liquorice (p. 411)

Dioxicolagol *Lab. Fabra S.R.L., Argentina,* Artichoke (p. 67), Boldo (p. 91), Valerian (p. 580)

Dis-Cinil Complex *A. Menarini Industrie Farmaceutiche Riunite S.r.l., Italy,* Boldo (p. 91), Cascara (p. 128), Rhubarb (p. 506)

Disogel *Concept Pharmaceuticals Ltd, India,* Liquorice (p. 411)

Diu Venostasin *Fujisawa Deutschland GmbH, Germany,* Horse-chestnut (p. 363)

Diuretabs *Potter's (Herbal Supplies) Ltd, UK,* Buchu (p. 100), Parsley Piert (p. 459), Uva-Ursi (p. 577)

Diurette *Cederroth, Spain,* Dandelion (p. 204)

Diurinat *Soria Natural, Spain,* Corn Silk (p. 191), Couchgrass (p. 193)

Doans Backache Pills *Mentholatum South Africa (Pty) Ltd, South Africa,* Buchu (p. 100)

Docrub *Aspen Pharmacare (Pty) Ltd, South Africa,* Buchu (p. 100)

Doktor Mom Herbal Cough Lozenges (Доктор Мом Растительные Пастилки От Кашля**)** *Unique Pharmaceutical Laboratories, Russia,* Ginger (p. 293), Liquorice (p. 411)

Doktor Mom (Доктор Мом**)** *Unique Pharmaceutical Laboratories, Russia,* Aloes (p. 50), Ginger (p. 293), Liquorice (p. 411)

Dolo-cyl *Pharma Liebermann GmbH, Germany,* Arnica (p. 64)

Dolodent *OBA Pharma ApS, Denmark,* Myrrh (p. 449)

Dolokey *Inkeysa, Spain,* Capsicum (p. 125)

Dolosul *Soria Natural, Spain,* Devil's Claw (p. 207), Meadowsweet (p. 423), Willow (p. 598)

Domuderm *Lab. Fortbenton Co. S.A., Argentina,* Witch Hazel (p. 601)

Donalg *Dynacren Laboratorio Farmaceutico del Dott. A. Francioni e di M. Gerosa S.r.l., Italy,* Ginger (p. 293), Sage (p. 512), Willow (p. 598)

Dong Quai Complex *Blackmores Ltd, Australia,* Agnus Castus (p. 36), Cohosh, Black (p. 168)

Doppelherz Ginseng Aktiv (Доппельгерц Женьшень Актив**)** *Queisser Pharma GmbH.& Co., Russia,* Ginseng, Panax (p. 325)

Doppelherz Melissa (Доппельгерц Мелисса**)** *Queisser Pharma GmbH.& Co., Russia,* Angelica (p. 53), Cinnamon (p. 162), Clove (p. 166), Melissa (p. 425)

Doppelherz Vitalotonik (Доппельгерц Виталотоник**)** *Queisser Pharma GmbH.& Co., Russia,* Ginseng, Panax (p. 325), Hawthorn (p. 346), Hops (p. 354), Melissa (p. 425), Valerian (p. 580)

Dormarist *Steiner & Co. Deutsche Arzneimittel Gesellschaft, Germany,* Melissa (p. 425), Valerian (p. 580)

Dormeasan *Bioforce GmbH, Germany,* Hops (p. 354), Valerian (p. 580) *Bioforce AG, Switzerland,* Hops (p. 354), Valerian (p. 580)

Dormil *Milte Italia S.p.A., Italy,* Passionflower (p. 461)

Dormiplant *Marvecs Services Srl, Italy,* Melissa (p. 425), Valerian (p. 580) *Schwabe Pharma AG, Switzerland,* Melissa (p. 425), Valerian (p. 580)

Dormo-Sern *Riemser Arzneimittel AG, Germany,* Passionflower (p. 461), Valerian (p. 580)

Dormoverlan *Verla-Pharm, Arzneimittelfabrik, Apotheker H.J.v. Ehrlich GmbH & Co. KG, Germany,* Hops (p. 354), Passionflower (p. 461), Valerian (p. 580)

Dorofen *Liptis Pharmaceuticals Inc., USA,* Ginkgo (p. 299)

Doulax *Les Laboratoires Bio-Santé, Canada,* Cascara (p. 128), Senna (p. 537)

Dr. Scheffler Bergischer Krautertee Blasen- und Nierentee *Dr Scheffler Nachf. GmbH & Co. KG, Germany,* Java Tea (p. 381)

Dr. Scheffler Bergischer Krautertee Nerven- und Beruhigungstee *Dr Scheffler Nachf. GmbH & Co. KG, Germany,* Melissa (p. 425), Passionflower (p. 461), Valerian (p. 580)

Dr Scurr's Zinopin *Healthy Direct, UK,* Ginger (p. 293)

Dr Theiss Beinwell Salbe *Naturwaren OHG, Czech Republic,* Comfrey (p. 188)

Dr Theiss Rheuma Creme *Naturwaren OHG, Czech Republic,* Aloes (p. 50), Angelica (p. 53), Cinnamon (p. 162), Cohosh, Black (p. 168), Myrrh (p. 449), Rhubarb (p. 506), Senna (p. 537), Valerian (p. 580)

Dr Theiss Schweden Krauter *Naturwaren OHG, Czech Republic,* Aloes (p. 50), Angelica (p. 53), Gentian (p. 290), Myrrh (p. 449), Rhubarb (p. 506), Senna (p. 537)

Dr Theiss Schwedenbitter *Naturwaren OHG, Czech Republic,* Aloes (p. 50), Angelica (p. 53), Calamus (p. 118), Cinnamon (p. 162), Cohosh, Black (p. 168), Gentian (p. 290), Myrrh (p. 449), Rhubarb (p. 506), Senna (p. 537), Valerian (p. 580)

Dr Wiemanns Rheumatonikum *Beethoven-Pharma Dr Wiemann GmbH, Germany,* Devil's Claw (p. 207), Willow (p. 598)

Dragees antirhumatismales *Max Zeller Söhne AG, Pflanzliche Heilmittel, Switzerland,* Passionflower (p. 461), Willow (p. 598)

Dragees aux figues avec du sene *Max Zeller Söhne AG, Pflanzliche Heilmittel, Switzerland,* Butterbur (p. 107), Senna (p. 537)

Dragees Fuca *Laboratoires Fuca, France,* Cascara (p. 128), Frangula (p. 270)

Dragees pour la detente nerveuse *Max Zeller Söhne AG, Pflanzliche Heilmittel, Switzerland,* Butterbur (p. 107), Melissa (p. 425), Passionflower (p. 461), Valerian (p. 580)

Dragees pour le sommeil *Max Zeller Söhne AG, Pflanzliche Heilmittel, Switzerland,* Hawthorn (p. 346)

Dragees pour le coeur et les nerfs *Max Zeller Söhne AG, Pflanzliche Heilmittel, Switzerland,* Hops (p. 354), Passionflower (p. 461), Valerian (p. 580)

Dragees pour le sommeil *Max Zeller Söhne AG, Pflanzliche Heilmittel, Switzerland,* Hops (p. 354), Valerian (p. 580)

Dragees S pour les reins et la vessie *Hänseler AG, Switzerland,* Uva-Ursi (p. 577)

Dragees sedatives Dr Welti *Dr Heinz Welti AG, Switzerland,* Hawthorn (p. 346), Hops (p. 354), Valerian (p. 580)

Dragees Vegetales Rex *Laboratoires Lehning, France,* Cascara (p. 128), Frangula (p. 270)

Drainactil *Laboratoires Aérocid, France,* Boldo (p. 91)

Draverex *Istituto di Medicina Omeopatica S.p.A., Italy,* Cascara (p. 128), Frangula (p. 270)

Dreierlei *Hofmann & Sommer GmbH & Co. KG, Germany,* Valerian (p. 580)

Drenocol *Lab. Lafage S.R.L., Argentina,* Boldo (p. 91)

Drops of Life Tablets *Frank Roberts (Herbal Dispensaries) Ltd, UK,* Yarrow (p. 604)

Drosana Resiston avec vitamine C *Vifor SA, Switzerland,* Echinacea (p. 217)

Drosithym-N *Johannes Bürger Ysatfabrik GmbH, Germany,* Cowslip (p. 195), Drosera (p. 215), Thyme (p. 574)

Dual-Lax Extra Strong *G.R. Lane Health Products Ltd, UK,* Cascara (p. 128), Senna (p. 537)

Dual-Lax Normal Strength *G.R. Lane Health Products Ltd, UK,* Aloes (p. 50), Cascara (p. 128), Senna (p. 537)

Ductoveran *Lab. Ducto Ind. Farm. Ltda, Brazil,* Boldo (p. 91)

Duolaxan *Pharmacia Italia S.p.A., Italy,* Ispaghula (p. 374)

Dynamisan *Novartis Argentina S.A., Argentina,* Ginseng, Panax (p. 325)

Dynexan *Nycomed Austria GmbH, Austria,* Arnica (p. 64), Sage (p. 512) *Adcock Ingram Pharmaceuticals Ltd, South Africa,* Arnica (p. 64), Sage (p. 512)

Dystolise *Laboratoires Motima, France,* Angelica (p. 53), Melissa (p. 425)

Dyzco *Mediherb P/L, Australia,* Cohosh, Black (p. 168), Cohosh, Blue (p. 180), Ginger (p. 293)

E

Echinaboost *Medic Herb UK Ltd, UK,* Echinacea (p. 217)

Echinacea *Potter's (Herbal Supplies) Ltd, UK,* Echinacea (p. 217), Fumitory (p. 276)

Echinacea 4000 *Biovital Pty Ltd, Australia,* Echinacea (p. 217)

Echinacea ACE + Zinc *Blackmores Ltd, Australia,* Echinacea (p. 217)

Echinacea Complex *Mayne Pharma P/L, Australia,* Echinacea (p. 217)

Echinacea Golden Seal *Natrol, USA,* Echinacea (p. 217)

Echinacea Goldenseal Formula *Boehringer Ingelheim (Canada) Ltd, Canada,* Echinacea (p. 217), Golden Seal (p. 337)

Echinacea Lozenge *Blackmores Ltd, Australia,* Echinacea (p. 217)

Echinacea Plus *Zuellig Pharma Sdn Bhd, Swiss Bio Pharma Sdn Bhd, Malaysia,* Echinacea (p. 217), Garlic (p. 279)

Eciclean *EciFarma SA, Chile,* Sage (p. 512)

Ecnagel *Valuge S.A., Argentina,* Witch Hazel (p. 601)

Eczema Relief *Mediherb P/L, Australia,* Calendula (p. 121), Myrrh (p. 449)

Efcamon (Эфкамон) *Nizhpharm OAO, Russia,* Capsicum (p. 125)

Efluvium Anti-caspa *Dermoteca, SA, Portugal,* Saw Palmetto (p. 521)

Efluvium Anti-seborreico *Dermoteca, SA, Portugal,* Saw Palmetto (p. 521)

Ehrlich Balsamo *Laboratorios Politecnicos Nacionales C.A., Venezuela,* Capsicum (p. 125)

Eicebaer *Merck GmbH, Austria,* Senega (p. 533), Thyme (p. 574)

Ekseme *Laboratoires Monin-Chanteaud, France,* Witch Hazel (p. 601)

Ektrofil *Farmaceutici Ecobi s.a.s., Italy,* Aloe Vera (p. 48)

Elixir Bonjean *Laboratoires Dexo, France,* Aniseed (p. 57), Melissa (p. 425)

Elixir Damiana and Saw Palmetto *Potter's (Herbal Supplies) Ltd, UK,* Corn Silk (p. 191), Damiana (p. 201), Saw Palmetto (p. 521)

Elixir de Inhame *Laboratórios Goulart S.A., Brazil,* Sarsaparilla (p. 515)

Elixir de Marinheiro *Laboratório Phos-Kola Ltda, Brazil,* Sarsaparilla (p. 515)

Elixir de Passiflora *Laboratório Sinterapico Industrial e Farmacêutico Ltda, Brazil,* Melissa (p. 425), Passionflower (p. 461)

Elixir Grez *Laboratoires Monin-Chanteaud, France,* Cinnamon (p. 162), Gentian (p. 290)

Elixir Spark *Laboratoires Phytoprevent, France,* Artichoke (p. 67), Boldo (p. 91)

Elovera *Glenmark Pharmaceuticals Ltd, India,* Aloe Vera (p. 48)

Elovera-SPF *Glenmark Pharmaceuticals Ltd, India,* Aloe Vera (p. 48)

Emagrevit *Viternat Laboratórios Ltda, Brazil,* Artichoke (p. 67), Boldo (p. 91), Cascara (p. 128), Hydrocotyle (p. 371), Passionflower (p. 461), Uva-Ursi (p. 577)

Embrocacion Gras *Químifar, Spain,* Capsicum (p. 125)

Em-medical *Dr. C. Soldan GmbH, Germany,* Aniseed (p. 57), Thyme (p. 574)

Emmenoiasi *Ferlito Farmaceutici, Divisione Palmares S.p.A., Italy,* Couchgrass (p. 193), Hops (p. 354), Hydrocotyle (p. 371), Melissa (p. 425)

Emulax *AstraZeneca Sverige AB, Sweden,* Cascara (p. 128)

Encypalmed *Trima, Israel,* Frangula (p. 270), Rhubarb (p. 506)

Energy Plus *Nutravite, Canada,* Ginseng, Panax (p. 325)

Energy Support *Sundown, USA,* Ginseng, Eleutherococcus (p. 315), Ginseng, Panax (p. 325)

Energysor *Soria Natural, Spain,* Damiana (p. 201), Ginseng, Eleutherococcus (p. 315), Ginseng, Panax (p. 325)

Entertainer's Secret *KLI Corp., USA,* Aloe Vera (p. 48)

Entressdruppels HM *Aspen Pharmacare (Pty) Ltd, South Africa,* Asafoetida (p. 72), Valerian (p. 580)

Entschlackender Abfuhrtee EF-EM-ES *EF-EM-ES - Dr Smetana & Co., Austria,* Elder (p. 237), Senna (p. 537)

Enzian Anaemodoron Drops *Pharma-Natura (Pty) Ltd, South Africa,* Gentian (p. 290), Nettle (p. 452)

Epagest *Lampugnani Farmaceutici S.p.A., Italy,* Artichoke (p. 67), Milk Thistle (p. 429)

Eparema *Altana Pharma Ltda, Brazil,* Boldo (p. 91), Cascara (p. 128), Rhubarb (p. 506) *Specialità Igienico Terapeutiche S.r.l., Italy,* Boldo (p. 91), Cascara (p. 128), Rhubarb (p. 506)

Eparema-Levul *Specialità Igienico Terapeutiche S.r.l., Italy,* Boldo (p. 91), Cascara (p. 128), Rhubarb (p. 506)

EP&C Essence *Potter's (Herbal Supplies) Ltd, UK,* Bayberry (p. 77), Elder (p. 237)

Ephepect-Pastillen N *Bolder Arzneimittel GmbH & Co. KG, Germany,* Thyme (p. 574)

Ephydrol *Laboratoires CS Dermatologie, France,* Plantain (p. 474)

Epilobin *Leros sro, Czech Republic,* Buchu (p. 100), Calendula (p. 121)

Equaliv *Meyer Productos Terapéuticos S.A., Venezuela,* Hawthorn (p. 346), Passionflower (p. 461), Valerian (p. 580)

Equisil N *Dr Gustav Klein, Germany,* Cowslip (p. 195), Thyme (p. 574)

Erkaltungstee *Abtswinder Naturheilmittel GmbH, Czech Republic,* Elder (p. 237), Liquorice (p. 411), Thyme (p. 574), Willow (p. 598)

Erpecalm *Prisfar, SA, Portugal,* Melissa (p. 425), Plantain (p. 474)

Eryange *Laboratoires Klorane, France,* Calendula (p. 121)

Eryval *Gebro Pharma GmbH, Austria,* Centaury (p. 149), St John's Wort (p. 549), Valerian (p. 580)

Esberitop *Max Zeller Söhne AG, Pflanzliche Heilmittel, Switzerland,* Echinacea (p. 217)

Esberitox *Schaper & Brümmer GmbH & Co. KG, Germany,* Echinacea (p. 217)

Esberitox N *Schaper & Brümmer GmbH & Co. KG, Germany,* Echinacea (p. 217)

Escar T-Neomicina *Laboratorio Prater SA, Chile,* Hydrocotyle (p. 371)

Escotussin *G. Streuli & Co. AG, Switzerland,* Drosera (p. 215)

Esculeol P *Química Medical Arg. S.A.C.I., Argentina,* Witch Hazel (p. 601)

Espol (Эспол) *Nizhpharm OAO, Russia,* Capsicum (p. 125)

Essens Amara of Groen Amara *Aspen Pharmacare (Pty) Ltd, South Africa,* Holy Thistle (p. 352), Quassia (p. 491)

Estomafitino *Jofadel Ind. Farmacêutica S.A., Brazil,* Gentian (p. 290), Senna (p. 537)

Estri-Atlas *Atlas Farmaceutica, Argentina,* Hydrocotyle (p. 371)

Estrocare *Pharmanex Inc., USA,* Cohosh, Black (p. 168)

Eucarbon *F Trenka Chemisch-Pharmazeutische Fabrik GmbH, Austria,* Rhubarb (p. 506), Senna (p. 537) *Tetra Pharm, Israel,* Rhubarb (p. 506), Senna (p. 537) *Giuliani S.p.A., Italy,* Rhubarb (p. 506), Senna (p. 537)

Eucarbon Herbal *F Trenka Chemisch-Pharmazeutische Fabrik GmbH, Austria,* Rhubarb (p. 506), Senna (p. 537)

Euceta avec camomille et arnica *Novartis Consumer Health Schweiz AG, Switzerland,* Arnica (p. 64)

Eufytose *Productos Roche S.A., Venezuela,* Hawthorn (p. 346), Passionflower (p. 461), Valerian (p. 580)

Eugastrin *Slovakofarma sro, Czech Republic,* Agrimony (p. 42), Calamus (p. 118), Melissa (p. 425), St John's Wort (p. 549)

Euka *Pharmonta Mag. pharm. Dr Fischer, Austria,* Aniseed (p. 57), Rosemary (p. 508)

Eulatin NN *Riemser Arzneimittel AG, Germany,* Witch Hazel (p. 601)

Eulux *Mediwhite Srl, Italy,* Eyebright (p. 256), Witch Hazel (p. 601)

Eupatol *Donini S.r.l., Italy,* Boldo (p. 91), Cascara (p. 128), Rhubarb (p. 506)

Euphorbia Complex *Blackmores Ltd, Australia,* Euphorbia (p. 249), Passionflower (p. 461), Thyme (p. 574)

Euphrasia Complex *Mediherb P/L, Australia,* Capsicum (p. 125), Echinacea (p. 217), Eyebright (p. 256), Golden Seal (p. 337)

Euphrasia Compound *Phytomedicine P/L, Australia,* Capsicum (p. 125), Eyebright (p. 256), Scullcap (p. 530)

Euphytose *Laboratoires Roche Nicholas, France,* Hawthorn (p. 346), Passionflower (p. 461), Valerian (p. 580)

Euproctol N *Sanopharm AG, Switzerland,* Witch Hazel (p. 601)

Eurocolor Post Solar *Euroderm Laboratorios S.R.L., Argentina,* Aloe Vera (p. 48), Calendula (p. 121)

Europrotec Post Solar *Euroderm Laboratorios S.R.L., Argentina,* Aloe Vera (p. 48), Calendula (p. 121)

Euvegal Entspannungs- und Einschlaftropfen *Dr Willmar Schwabe GmbH & Co., Germany,* Melissa (p. 425), Valerian (p. 580)

Euvekan *Austroplant-Arzneimittel GmbH, Austria,* Melissa (p. 425), Valerian (p. 580) *Arzneimittel Schwabe International GmbH, Czech Republic,* Melissa (p. 425), Valerian (p. 580) *ASI Budapest Kft, Hungary,* Melissa (p. 425), Valerian (p. 580)

Evacrine *Laboratoires Motima, France,* Ginger (p. 293)

Evamilk *Laboratori Gambar S.r.l., Italy,* Bilberry (p. 79), Wild Carrot (p. 593)

Evarose *Laboratoires Bailly SPEAB, France,* Arnica (p. 64), Horse-chestnut (p. 363), Witch Hazel (p. 601)

Evening Primrose Oil *Natrol, USA,* Evening Primrose (p. 251)

Eviprostat *Eversil Produtos Farmacêuticos Indústria e Comércio Ltda, Brazil,* Pulsatilla (p. 489) *Nippon Shinyaku Co. Ltd, Japan,* Pulsatilla (p. 489) *Wellchem Pharmaceuticals Pte Ltd, Singapore,* Pulsatilla (p. 489)

Eviprostat N *Pharmazeutische Fabrik Evers & Co. GmbH, Germany,* Pulsatilla (p. 489)

Exail *Laboratorios Sigma, Argentina,* Garlic (p. 279)

Excess *Neo-Farmacêutica, Lda, Portugal,* Ispaghula (p. 374)

Executive B *Mayne Pharma P/L, Mayne Pharma P/L, Australia,* Passionflower (p. 461), Valerian (p. 580)

Ex-Lax Gentle Strength *Novartis Consumer Health Canada Inc., Canada,* Senna (p. 537)

Expectal-Tropfen *Dr. Kolassa & Merz GmbH, Austria,* Thyme (p. 574)

Expectobron *Hebron S.A. Indústria Química e Farmacêutica, Brazil,* Marshmallow (p. 418)

Expectol *Laboratório Teuto-Brasileiro Ltda, Brazil,* Marshmallow (p. 418)

Expectomel *Cazi Química Farmacêutica Indústria e Comércio Ltda, Brazil,* Senega (p. 533)

Expectosan Hierbas y Miel *Laboratorios Excelentia S.A., Argentina,* Cowslip (p. 195), Thyme (p. 574)

Expectysat N *Johannes Bürger Ysatfabrik GmbH, Germany,* Cowslip (p. 195), Thyme (p. 574)

Extralife Arthri-Care *Felton, Grimwade & Bickford P/L, Australia,* Devil's Claw (p. 207), Feverfew (p. 263), Ginger (p. 293)

Extralife Extra-Brite *Felton, Grimwade & Bickford P/L, Australia,* Ginkgo (p. 299), Ginseng, Panax (p. 325)

Extralife Eye-Care *Felton, Grimwade & Bickford P/L, Australia,* Bilberry (p. 79), Ginkgo (p. 299)

Extralife Flow-Care *Felton, Grimwade & Bickford P/L, Australia,* Nettle (p. 452), Saw Palmetto (p. 521)

Extralife Fluid-Care *Felton, Grimwade & Bickford P/L, Australia,* Dandelion (p. 204), Parsley (p. 456), Uva-Ursi (p. 577)

Extralife Leg-Care *Felton, Grimwade & Bickford P/L, Australia,* Bilberry (p. 79), Ginkgo (p. 299), Horse-chestnut (p. 363), Hydrocotyle (p. 371)

Extralife Liva-Care *Felton, Grimwade & Bickford P/L, Australia,* Artichoke (p. 67), Dandelion (p. 204), Milk Thistle (p. 429)

Extralife Meno-Care *Felton, Grimwade & Bickford P/L, Australia,* Cohosh, Black (p. 168)

Extralife Migrai-Care *Felton, Grimwade & Bickford P/L, Australia,* Feverfew (p. 263), Willow (p. 598)

Extralife PMS-Care *Felton, Grimwade & Bickford P/L, Australia,* Cohosh, Black (p. 168), Uva-Ursi (p. 577), Willow (p. 598)

Extralife Sleep-Care *Felton, Grimwade & Bickford P/L, Australia,* Gentian (p. 290), Hops (p. 354), Passionflower (p. 461), Valerian (p. 580)

Extralife Uri-Care *Felton, Grimwade & Bickford P/L, Australia,* Buchu (p. 100), Cranberry (p. 197), Uva-Ursi (p. 577)

Eye Dew *Crookes Healthcare Ltd, UK,* Witch Hazel (p. 601)

Eye Health Herbal Plus Formula 4 *Mayne Pharma P/L, Australia,* Eyebright (p. 256), Ginkgo (p. 299)

Eye Support Formula *Natrol, USA,* Pulsatilla (p. 489)

Eye Support Formula Herbal Blend *Natrol, USA,* Bilberry (p. 79), Eyebright (p. 256)

Eyebright Plus *Swiss Bio Pharma Sdn Bhd, Malaysia,* Eyebright (p. 256), Wild Carrot (p. 593)

Fade Cream *Cosmofarma, Lda (Laboratórios Cosmos), Portugal,* Yarrow (p. 604)

Fadiamone *Laboratoires CS Dermatologie, France,* Hydrocotyle (p. 371)

Fagorutin Rosskastanien-Balsam N *GlaxoSmithKline Consumer Healthcare GmbH & Co. KG, Germany,* Horse-chestnut (p. 363)

Famel *Boots Healthcare (Switzerland) AG, Hermal, Switzerland,* Drosera (p. 215)

Fam-Lax *Typharm Ltd, UK,* Rhubarb (p. 506)

Fam-Lax Senna *Typharm Ltd, UK,* Rhubarb (p. 506), Senna (p. 537)

Fave di Fuca *Roche S.p.A., Italy,* Cascara (p. 128), Frangula (p. 270)

Feminine Herbal Complex *GNLD International P/L, Australia,* Agnus Castus (p. 36), Dandelion (p. 204), Ginger (p. 293), Liquorice (p. 411), Sage (p. 512), Scullcap (p. 530), St John's Wort (p. 549)

Fenneherb Cystaid *Potter's Herbal Medicines, UK,* Buchu (p. 100), Clivers (p. 164), Couchgrass (p. 193), Shepherd's Purse (p. 541), Uva-Ursi (p. 577)

Fenneherb Monthly *Potter's Herbal Medicines, UK,* Raspberry (p. 495)

Fenneherb Newrelax *Potter's Herbal Medicines, UK,* Hops (p. 354), Scullcap (p. 530), Valerian (p. 580)

Fenneherb Prementaid *Potter's Herbal Medicines, UK,* Motherwort (p. 447), Pulsatilla (p. 489), Uva-Ursi (p. 577), Valerian (p. 580), Vervain (p. 591)

Fenneherb Slim Aid *Potter's Herbal Medicines, UK,* Boldo (p. 91), Dandelion (p. 204), Fucus (p. 273)

Fenneherb Sweetdreams *Potter's Herbal Medicines, UK,* Passionflower (p. 461)

Fen-y-Tos *Química Franco Mexicana Nordin S.A. de C.V., Mexico,* Drosera (p. 215)

Ferroplex-frangula *ERA Medical ApS, Denmark,* Frangula (p. 270)

Fiberfull *Ponce & Benzo Sucesores C.A., Venezuela,* Ispaghula (p. 374)

Fibralax *Ponce & Benzo Sucesores C.A., Venezuela,* Ispaghula (p. 374), Senna (p. 537)

Fibre Dophilus *Pharmadass Ltd, UK,* Ispaghula (p. 374)

Fibre Plus *Pharmadass Ltd, UK,* Ispaghula (p. 374), Senna (p. 537)

Fibrolax Complex *Giuliani S.p.A., Italy,* Ispaghula (p. 374), Senna (p. 537)

Figatil *Laboratório Catarinense S.A., Brazil,* Artichoke (p. 67), Boldo (p. 91)

Figen *ERA Medical ApS, Amternes Laegemiddelregistreringskontor I/S, Denmark,* Senna (p. 537)

Filigel *Laboratoires Codifra, France,* Ispaghula (p. 374)

Fishogar *Self-Care Products Ltd, UK,* Garlic (p. 279)

Fitacnol *Laboratoires Arkopharma, France,* Burdock (p. 102), Nettle (p. 452)

Fitolax *Instituto de Medicamentos e Alergia IMA Ltda, Brazil,* Senna (p. 537)

Fitosonno *Pharbenia S.r.l., Societa del Gruppo Bayer, Italy,* Passionflower (p. 461), Valerian (p. 580)

Fitotos *Laboratorio Koni-Cofarm SA, Chile,* Drosera (p. 215)

Flatulence Gastulence *Greater Pharma Ltd Part, Thailand,* Asafoetida (p. 72), Capsicum (p. 125), Cascara (p. 128), Ginger (p. 293)

Flavion *Laboratorio Terapeutico M.R. S.r.l., Italy,* Horse-chestnut (p. 363)

Flavo-C *Primal Chemical Co. Ltd, Hong Kong,* Ginkgo (p. 299)

Flavons *Eagle Pharmaceuticals P/L, Australia,* Boneset (p. 94), Echinacea (p. 217), Yarrow (p. 604)

Flebior *Therasophia, France,* Bilberry (p. 79)

Flebitol *Laboratorios Phoenix S.A.I.C.F., Argentina,* Ginkgo (p. 299)

Flebolider *Amnol Chimica Biologica S.r.l., Italy,* Arnica (p. 64), Hydrocotyle (p. 371)

Flexi-muv *Zydus Cadila Group, India,* Capsicum (p. 125), Celery (p. 146)

Floradix Multipretten N *Salus-Haus Dr. med. Otto Greither Nachf. GmbH & Co KG, Germany,* Aniseed (p. 57), Yarrow (p. 604)

Florelax *Sanofi-Synthelabo S.p.A., Italy,* Angelica (p. 53), Valerian (p. 580)

Floriny *Ativus Farmacêutica Ltda, Brazil,* Hawthorn (p. 346), Passionflower (p. 461), Willow (p. 598)

Florlax *Cazi Química Farmacêutica Indústria e Comércio Ltda, Brazil,* Senna (p. 537)

Fluid Loss *Vitaplex Products, Australia,* Buchu (p. 100), Celery (p. 146), Dandelion (p. 204), Uva-Ursi (p. 577)

Fluido *Spineda, Pérez y Hnos. Y Cia SRL, Argentina,* Arnica (p. 64)

Fluon *Laboratoires Aérocid, France,* Horse-chestnut (p. 363), Witch Hazel (p. 601)

Fon Wan Ginsenergy *Giuliani S.p.A., Italy,* Ginseng, Panax (p. 325)

Fontlax *Fontovit Laboratórios Ltda, Brazil,* Senna (p. 537)

Fontolax *Fontovit Laboratórios Ltda, Brazil,* Liquorice (p. 411)

For Peripheral Circulation Herbal Plus Formula 5 *Mayne Pharma P/L, Australia,* Capsicum (p. 125), Ginkgo (p. 299), Hawthorn (p. 346)

Fortacet *Interdelta SA, Switzerland,* Arnica (p. 64)

Forticrin *Farmaceutici G.B. Panzera S.r.l., Italy,* Ginkgo (p. 299), Ginseng, Panax (p. 325), Yarrow (p. 604)

Fosfarsile Forte *Fitobucaneve S.r.l., Italy,* Ginseng, Panax (p. 325)

Four-Ton *Body Spring S.r.l., Italy,* Damiana (p. 201), Ginseng, Panax (p. 325)

Fovysat *Johannes Bürger Ysatfabrik GmbH, Germany,* Ginger (p. 293), Hawthorn (p. 346)

Fray Romano *Laboratorio Ximena Polanco, Chile,* Aloe Vera (p. 48)

Fre-bre *Self-Care Products Ltd, UK,* Parsley (p. 456)

Frugelletten *Herbert Bregenzer, Austria,* Senna (p. 537)

Frutalax *Hexal do Brasil Ltda, Brazil,* Liquorice (p. 411), Senna (p. 537)

Fruttasan *Graf Fruttasan AG, Switzerland,* Senna (p. 537)

Fybogel Mebeverine *Reckitt Benckiser, Ireland,* Ispaghula (p. 374) *Reckitt Benckiser plc, UK,* Ispaghula (p. 374)

Fytokliman Planta *Leros sro, Czech Republic,* Hawthorn (p. 346), Hops (p. 354), Melissa (p. 425), Parsley Piert (p. 459), St John's Wort (p. 549)

Galium Complex *Blackmores Ltd, Australia,* Calendula (p. 121), Clivers (p. 164), Echinacea (p. 217)

Gallemolan forte *Cesra Arzneimittel GmbH & Co. KG, Germany,* Dandelion (p. 204)

Gallen- und Lebertee St Severin *EF-EM-ES - Dr Smetana & Co., Austria,* Agrimony (p. 42), Dandelion (p. 204), Yarrow (p. 604)

Gallesyn *Mr J W Wenig GmbH, Austria,* Frangula (p. 270)

Gallexier *Salus-Haus Dr. med. Otto Greither Nachf. GmbH & Co KG, Germany,* Artichoke (p. 67), Bogbean (p. 89), Dandelion (p. 204), Gentian (p. 290), Ginger (p. 293), Holy Thistle (p. 352), Milk Thistle (p. 429), Yarrow (p. 604)

Galloway's Cough Syrup *Chefaro UK Ltd, UK,* St John's Wort (p. 549)

Gameral *Productos Gache S.A., Venezuela,* Cascara (p. 128)

Garcinol Max *Lab. Garden House S.A., Argentina,* Hydrocotyle (p. 371)

Garlic Allium Complex *GNLD International P/L, Australia,* Garlic (p. 279), Rosemary (p. 508)

Garlic and Horseradish + C Complex *Mayne Pharma P/L, Mayne Pharma P/L, Australia,* Fenugreek (p. 260), Garlic (p. 279), Horseradish (p. 367), Marshmallow (p. 418)

Garlic, Horseradish, A & C Capsules *Vitaplex Products, Australia,* Horseradish (p. 367)

GarLife *Nature Made, USA,* Garlic (p. 279)

Gartech *Eagle Pharmaceuticals P/L, Australia,* Echinacea (p. 217), Garlic (p. 279)

Gastripan *Ratiopharm Arzneimittel Vertriebs-GmbH, Austria,* Liquorice (p. 411)

Gastritol *Dr Gustav Klein, Germany,* Angelica (p. 53), Holy Thistle (p. 352), Liquorice (p. 411), St John's Wort (p. 549)

Gastrosan *Bioforce AG, Switzerland,* Angelica (p. 53), Centaury (p. 149), Dandelion (p. 204), Gentian (p. 290), Holy Thistle (p. 352), Melissa (p. 425), Yarrow (p. 604)

Gastrosecur *Duopharm GmbH, Germany,* Cinnamon (p. 162), Gentian (p. 290), Ginger (p. 293)

Gastrotuss *DMG Italia S.r.l., Italy,* Marshmallow (p. 418)

GB 100 *Laboratorios Sigma, Argentina,* Ginkgo (p. 299)

GB Tablets *Potter's (Herbal Supplies) Ltd, UK,* Burdock (p. 102)

Gel a la consoude *Phytomed AG, Switzerland,* Calendula (p. 121), Comfrey (p. 188), Echinacea (p. 217), St John's Wort (p. 549)

Gelax *Laboratorios Sidus S.A., Argentina,* Senna (p. 537)

Gelconordin *Química Franco Mexicana Nordin S.A. de C.V., Mexico,* Aloe Vera (p. 48)

Gelovis *Amnol Chimica Biologica S.r.l., Italy,* Capsicum (p. 125), Hydrocotyle (p. 371)

Gem *Iromedica AG, Switzerland,* Liquorice (p. 411)

Gengivario *Giovanni Ogna & Figli S.p.A., Italy,* Myrrh (p. 449)

Genolaxante *Craveri S.A.I.C., Argentina,* Aloes (p. 50)

Gentaplex *Liptis Pharmaceuticals Inc., USA,* Ginkgo (p. 299)

Gentlees *Delamac Pharmaceuticals P/L, Australia,* Witch Hazel (p. 601)

Genurat *Soria Natural, Spain,* Uva-Ursi (p. 577)

Gerard House Reumalex *Chefaro UK Ltd, UK,* Cohosh, Black (p. 168), Guaiacum (p. 344), Sarsaparilla (p. 515), Willow (p. 598)

Gerard House Serenity *Chefaro UK Ltd, UK,* Hops (p. 354), Passionflower (p. 461), Valerian (p. 580)

Gerard House Skin *Chefaro UK Ltd, UK,* Burdock (p. 102)

Gerard House Somnus *Chefaro UK Ltd, UK,* Hops (p. 354), Valerian (p. 580), Wild Lettuce (p. 596)

Gerard House Water Relief Tablets *Chefaro UK Ltd, UK,* Burdock (p. 102), Clivers (p. 164), Ground Ivy (p. 342)

Geri *Gisand AG, Switzerland,* Ginseng, Panax (p. 325)

Geri-Lav Free *Geritrex Corp., USA,* Aloe Vera (p. 48)

Gerimax Plus *Nycomed Austria GmbH, Austria,* Ginseng, Panax (p. 325)

Gerin *EMS Ind. Farmacêutica Ltda, Brazil,* Ginseng, Panax (p. 325)

Ginal Cent *Laboratorios Beta S.A., Argentina,* Hydrocotyle (p. 371)

Gincosan *Boehringer Ingelheim, Chile,* Ginkgo (p. 299), Ginseng, Panax (p. 325) *Boehringer Ingelheim sro, Czech Republic,* Ginkgo (p. 299), Ginseng, Panax (p. 325) *Pharmaton SA, Switzerland,* Ginkgo (p. 299), Ginseng, Panax (p. 325)

Gingisan *Teva Pharmaceuticals Ind. Ltd, Israel,* Liquorice (p. 411)

Gingo A *Eagle Pharmaceuticals P/L, Australia,* Ginkgo (p. 299), Ginseng, Eleutherococcus (p. 315), Hawthorn (p. 346), Liquorice (p. 411)

Ginkan *Lab. Baliarda S.A., Argentina,* Hydrocotyle (p. 371)

Ginkgo Biloba Plus *Eagle Pharmaceuticals P/L, Australia,* Ginkgo (p. 299), Ginseng, Eleutherococcus (p. 315), Ginseng, Panax (p. 325), Hawthorn (p. 346)

Ginkgo Complex *Blackmores Ltd, Australia,* Ginkgo (p. 299), Ginseng, Panax (p. 325), Hawthorn (p. 346)

Ginkgo Plus Herbal Plus Formula 10 *Mayne Pharma P/L, Australia,* Ginger (p. 293), Ginkgo (p. 299)

Ginkgo-PS *Usana, Singapore,* Ginkgo (p. 299)

Ginkoba *Boehringer Ingelheim (Canada) Ltd, Canada,* Ginkgo (p. 299), Ginseng, Panax (p. 325)

Ginkoba Active *Fher, Divisione della Boehringer Ingelheim, Italy,* Ginkgo (p. 299)

Ginkoftal *Tubilux Pharma S.p.A., Italy,* Ginkgo (p. 299)

Ginkor *Beaufour Ipsen Pharma, France,* Ginkgo (p. 299)

Ginkor Fort *Beaufour Ipsen International, Czech Republic,* Ginkgo (p. 299) *Beaufour Ipsen Pharma, France,* Ginkgo (p. 299) *IDS (Hong Kong) Ltd Healthcare Division, Hong Kong,* Ginkgo (p. 299) *Europharm Trade Kft, Hungary,* Ginkgo (p. 299) *Pacific Healthcare (Thailand) Co. Ltd, Thailand,* Ginkgo (p. 299)

Ginkor Fort (Гинкор Форт**)** *Beaufour Ipsen International SNC, Russia,* Ginkgo (p. 299)

Ginkor Fort *Antah Pharma Sdb Bhd, Emerging Pharma Sdn Bhd, Malaysia,* Ginkgo (p. 299)

Ginkor Gel (Гинкор Гель**)** *Beaufour Ipsen International SNC, Russia,* Ginkgo (p. 299)

Ginkoret *Tubilux Pharma S.p.A., Italy,* Ginkgo (p. 299)

Ginoxil Ecoschiuma *Euroderm-RDC S.p.A., Italy,* Aloe Vera (p. 48), Witch Hazel (p. 601)

Ginsana Ton *Fher, Divisione della Boehringer Ingelheim, Italy,* Ginseng, Panax (p. 325)

Ginseng-Complex *Coradol-Pharma GmbH, Germany,* Ginseng, Panax (p. 325), Hawthorn (p. 346)

Gin-Vita *Zyfas Medical Co, Singapore,* Ginseng, Panax (p. 325)

Glicero-Valerovit *Teofarma, Italy,* Valerian (p. 580)

Glycoplex *Vitaplex Products, Australia,* Dandelion (p. 204), Liquorice (p. 411)

Glycyrrhiza Complex *Blackmores Ltd, Australia,* Ginseng, Panax (p. 325), Liquorice (p. 411)

Golatux *Laboratorio di Chimica Medica dell' Antipiol S.n.c., Italy,* Echinacea (p. 217)

Gold Bond Medicated Triple Action Relief *Chattem Consumer Products, USA,* Aloe Vera (p. 48)

Golden Seal Indigestion Tablets *Richard Lane's, UK,* Ginger (p. 293), Golden Seal (p. 337), Myrrh (p. 449), Rhubarb (p. 506), Valerian (p. 580)

Gonaxine *Laboratoires Motima, France,* Alfalfa (p. 45), Parsley Piert (p. 459), Sage (p. 512), Yarrow (p. 604)

Goodnight Formula *Vitaplex Products, Australia,* Passionflower (p. 461), Scullcap (p. 530), Valerian (p. 580)

Goodypops *Health Imports Ltd, UK,* Echinacea (p. 217)

Gotas Digestivas *Bunker Indústria Farmacêutica Ltda, Brazil,* Boldo (p. 91), Gentian (p. 290)

Gotas Nican *Laboratórios Prima Ltda, Brazil,* Passionflower (p. 461) *Laboratorios Andromaco SA, Chile,* Drosera (p. 215)

Gothaplast Rheumamed AC *Gothaplast Verbandpflasterfabrik GmbH, Germany,* Arnica (p. 64), Capsicum (p. 125)

Gouttes contre la toux *Hänseler AG, Switzerland,* Drosera (p. 215)

Grains de Vals *Qualiphar SA, Belgium,* Aloes (p. 50), Cascara (p. 128), Frangula (p. 270) *Laboratoires Noguès, France,* Boldo (p. 91), Cascara (p. 128), Senna (p. 537)

Grani di Vals *Geymonat S.p.A., Italy,* Aloes (p. 50), Cascara (p. 128)

Granocol *Schering P/L, Australia,* Frangula (p. 270) *Schering (NZ) Ltd, New Zealand,* Frangula (p. 270)

Granu Fink Prosta *GlaxoSmithKline Consumer Healthcare GmbH & Co. KG, Germany,* Saw Palmetto (p. 521) *GlaxoSmithKline, Switzerland,* Saw Palmetto (p. 521)

Gripaleta *Productos Maver S.A. de C.V., Mexico,* Echinacea (p. 217)

Grippetee St Severin *EF-EM-ES - Dr Smetana & Co., Austria,* Elder (p. 237), Lime Flower (p. 409)

Guaiacum Complex *Mediherb P/L, Australia,* Celery (p. 146), Devil's Claw (p. 207), Feverfew (p. 263), Guaiacum (p. 344), Willow (p. 598)

Gutnacht *Salus-Haus Dr. med. Otto Greither Nachf. GmbH & Co KG, Germany,* Hops (p. 354), Melissa (p. 425), Passionflower (p. 461), St John's Wort (p. 549), Valerian (p. 580)

Gynastan *Slovakofarma sro, Czech Republic,* Parsley Piert (p. 459)

Gynosoja *Laboratoires Codifra, France,* Alfalfa (p. 45)

H

Hactos *Hubert A.C. Thomas & Co., UK,* Capsicum (p. 125)

Haemocortin *G. Streuli & Co. AG, Switzerland,* Witch Hazel (p. 601)

Haemolan *G. Streuli & Co. AG, Switzerland,* Witch Hazel (p. 601)

Hansaplast Herbal Heat Plaster *Beiersdorf UK Ltd, UK,* Arnica (p. 64), Capsicum (p. 125)

Happy'tizer *Zydus Cadila Group, India,* Fenugreek (p. 260), Ginger (p. 293)

Harntee STADA *Stada GmbH, Germany,* Java Tea (p. 381), Uva-Ursi (p. 577)

Harntee-Steiner *Steiner & Co. Deutsche Arzneimittel Gesellschaft, Germany,* Java Tea (p. 381)

Harzer Hustenloser *Pharma Wernigerode GmbH, Germany,* Cowslip (p. 195), Thyme (p. 574)

Hawaiian Tropic Cool Aloe with I.C.E. *Tanning Research Labs Inc., USA,* Aloe Vera (p. 48)

Hay Fever & Sinus Relief *Herbal Concepts Ltd, UK,* Echinacea (p. 217), Elder (p. 237), Garlic (p. 279)

Hayfever & Sinus Relief *Herbal Concepts Ltd, UK,* Echinacea (p. 217), Elder (p. 237), Garlic (p. 279)

HDG *Laboratorios Sigma, Argentina,* Artichoke (p. 67)

HealthAid Boldo-Plus *Pharmadass Ltd, UK,* Boldo (p. 91), Clivers (p. 164), Dandelion (p. 204), Uva-Ursi (p. 577)

Healthy Eyes *Sundown, USA,* Bilberry (p. 79), Ginkgo (p. 299)

Heart Health *Sundown, USA,* Garlic (p. 279), Ginger (p. 293), Hawthorn (p. 346)

Hebert Caramelos *Fed. Arg. de Coop. Farm., Argentina,* Senega (p. 533)

HEC *Laboratoires Chauvin Bausch & Lomb, France,* Witch Hazel (p. 601) *Bausch & Lomb Swiss AG, Switzerland,* Witch Hazel (p. 601)

Hecrosine B12 *Ortoquimica Ind. Químico Farmacêutica Ltda, Brazil,* Artichoke (p. 67)

Hederix *Laboratoires Plan SA, Switzerland,* Elecampane (p. 240), Senega (p. 533)

Heemex *G.R. Lane Health Products Ltd, UK,* Witch Hazel (p. 601)

Heilsalbe *Pharma-Natura (Pty) Ltd, South Africa,* Calendula (p. 121)

Helmontskruie *Aspen Pharmacare (Pty) Ltd, South Africa,* Aloes (p. 50), Gentian (p. 290), Ginger (p. 293), Myrrh (p. 449), Rhubarb (p. 506), Valerian (p. 580)

Hemocane *Key Pharmaceuticals P/L, Australia,* Witch Hazel (p. 601)

Hemodotti *Prodotti Laboratório Farmacêutico Ltda, Brazil,* Witch Hazel (p. 601)

Hemofissural *Farmoquimica Baldacci, SA, Portugal,* Witch Hazel (p. 601)

Hemolax *B L Hua & Co. Ltd, Thailand,* Cascara (p. 128)

Hemoral *Slovakofarma sro, Czech Republic,* Agrimony (p. 42), Yarrow (p. 604)

Hemorid For Women *Chattem Consumer Products, USA,* Aloe Vera (p. 48)

Hemorid *Pharmamagist Kft, Wagner Pharmafax Kft, Hungary,* Yarrow (p. 604)

Hemorrogel *Laboratoires Arkopharma, France,* Calendula (p. 121), Horse-chestnut (p. 363), Pilewort (p. 472)

Hemorroidex *Medic Industrial Farmacêutica Ltda, Brazil,* Horse-chestnut (p. 363), Witch Hazel (p. 601)

Hepabene *Ratiopharm Arzneimittel Vertriebs-GmbH, Austria,* Fumitory (p. 276), Milk Thistle (p. 429) *Ratiopharm CZ sro, Czech Republic,* Fumitory (p. 276), Milk Thistle (p. 429) *ratiopharm Hungária Kft, Hungary,* Fumitory (p. 276), Milk Thistle (p. 429)

Hepabene (Гепабене) *Ratiopharm Group, Russia,* Fumitory (p. 276), Milk Thistle (p. 429)

Hepabil *Instituto Sanitas SA, Chile,* Boldo (p. 91)

Hepaclem *Laboratoires Clément-Thionville, France,* Artichoke (p. 67), Boldo (p. 91)

Hepacur *Química Medical Arg. S.A.C.I., Argentina,* Artichoke (p. 67), Boldo (p. 91)

Heparfelien *G. Streuli & Co. AG, Switzerland,* Artichoke (p. 67), Boldo (p. 91), Buchu (p. 100), Dandelion (p. 204), Juniper (p. 386)

Heparin Comp *Sanidom Handels-GmbH, Austria,* Arnica (p. 64), Horse-chestnut (p. 363) *ct-Arzneimittel GmbH, Germany,* Arnica (p. 64), Horse-chestnut (p. 363)

Heparin-Gel *Pharma Funcke, Czech Republic,* Arnica (p. 64), Horse-chestnut (p. 363)

Hepatalgina *Altana Pharma SA, Argentina,* Artichoke (p. 67), Boldo (p. 91), Wild Carrot (p. 593)

Hepatodirectol *Instituto Sanitas Arg. SACIPQ y M., Argentina,* Artichoke (p. 67), Boldo (p. 91), Hawthorn (p. 346)

Hepatofalk *Jacobson Medical (Hong Kong) Ltd, Hong Kong,* Artichoke (p. 67), Dandelion (p. 204), Frangula (p. 270), Rhubarb (p. 506)

Hepatofalk Planta *JDH Pharmaceutical Division, Singapore,* Milk Thistle (p. 429)

Hepatoregius *Farmoterapica Dovalle Indústria Química Farmacêutica Ltda, Brazil,* Artichoke (p. 67), Boldo (p. 91)

Hepatos *Teofarma, Italy,* Boldo (p. 91), Cascara (p. 128)

Hepatos B12 *Teofarma, Italy,* Boldo (p. 91), Cascara (p. 128)

Hepatoum *Laboratoires Hépatoum, France,* Pulsatilla (p. 489)

Hepax *Laboratoires Tradiphar, France,* Artichoke (p. 67), Boldo (p. 91), Rosemary (p. 508)

Hepedren *Laboratorios Parggon S.A. de C.V., Mexico,* Artichoke (p. 67), Boldo (p. 91)

Herb and Honey Cough Elixir *Weleda (UK) Ltd, UK,* Aniseed (p. 57), Elder (p. 237), Marshmallow (p. 418), Thyme (p. 574)

Herbaccion Celfin *Instituto Seroterapico Argentino S.A.I.C., Argentina,* Ginkgo (p. 299), Hydrocotyle (p. 371)

Herbaccion Ginseng Y Magnesio *Instituto Seroterapico Argentino S.A.I.C., Argentina,* Ginseng, Panax (p. 325)

Herbaccion Memory *Instituto Seroterapico Argentino S.A.I.C., Argentina,* Ginkgo (p. 299)

Herbal Anxiety Formula *Mayne Pharma P/L, Australia,* Passionflower (p. 461)

Herbal Arthritis Formula *Mayne Pharma P/L, Australia,* Devil's Claw (p. 207), Ginkgo (p. 299)

Herbal Capillary Care *Mayne Pharma P/L, Australia,* Ginkgo (p. 299), Horse-chestnut (p. 363)

Herbal Cleanse *Vitaplex Products, Australia,* Aloes (p. 50), Burdock (p. 102), Clivers (p. 164), Dandelion (p. 204), Echinacea (p. 217), Ginger (p. 293), Golden Seal (p. 337), Ispaghula (p. 374), Milk Thistle (p. 429), Sarsaparilla (p. 515), Slippery Elm (p. 545), Yellow Dock (p. 608)

Herbal Cold & Flu Relief *Mayne Pharma P/L, Australia,* Echinacea (p. 217), Garlic (p. 279), Liquorice (p. 411)

Herbal Cold Relief *Jamieson Laboratories, Canada,* Ephedra (p. 243)

Herbal Digestive Formula *Mayne Pharma P/L, Australia,* Ginger (p. 293), Liquorice (p. 411)

Herbal Diuretic *Swiss Herbal Remedies Ltd, Canada,* Buchu (p. 100), Celery (p. 146), Juniper (p. 386), Parsley (p. 456), Uva-Ursi (p. 577)

Herbal Diuretic Formula *Mayne Pharma P/L, Australia,* Dandelion (p. 204), Uva-Ursi (p. 577)

Herbal Energy *Sundown, USA,* Ginger (p. 293)

Herbal Indigestion Naturtabs *The Cantassium Company, UK,* Myrrh (p. 449), Scullcap (p. 530), Valerian (p. 580)

Herbal Laxative *Swiss Herbal Remedies Ltd, Canada,* Cascara (p. 128), Gentian (p. 290), Rhubarb (p. 506), Senna (p. 537)

Herbal Laxative Tablets *Frank Roberts (Herbal Dispensaries) Ltd, UK,* Aloe Vera (p. 48), Rhubarb (p. 506)

Herbal Nerve *Swiss Herbal Remedies Ltd, Canada,* Gentian (p. 290), Liquorice (p. 411), Scullcap (p. 530), Valerian (p. 580)

Herbal Pain Relief *The Cantassium Company, UK,* Passionflower (p. 461), Valerian (p. 580), Willow (p. 598)

Herbal PMS Formula *Mayne Pharma P/L, Australia,* Bilberry (p. 79), Cohosh, Black (p. 168), Liquorice (p. 411)

Herbal Relax *Wampole Brands Inc., Canada,* Valerian (p. 580)

Herbal Sleep Aid *Wampole Brands Inc., Canada,* Hops (p. 354), Passionflower (p. 461), Valerian (p. 580)

Herbal Sleep Well *Swiss Herbal Remedies Ltd, Canada,* Hops (p. 354), Lime Flower (p. 409), Melissa (p. 425), Passionflower (p. 461), Valerian (p. 580)

Herbal Throat *Jamieson Laboratories, Canada,* Parsley (p. 456), Slippery Elm (p. 545), Thyme (p. 574)

Herbalax *Santé Naturelle (AG) Ltée, Canada,* Cascara (p. 128), Frangula (p. 270), Rhubarb (p. 506), Senna (p. 537)

Herbelix *G.R. Lane Health Products Ltd, UK,* Marshmallow (p. 418)

Herbesan *Laboratoires Pfizer, France,* Aniseed (p. 57), Couchgrass (p. 193), Senna (p. 537)

Herbheal Ointment *Potter's (Herbal Supplies) Ltd, UK,* Marshmallow (p. 418)

Herbion Drops for the Gallbladder (Гербион Капли Желчегонные) *KRKA d.d., Russia,* Agrimony (p. 42), Artichoke (p. 67)

Herbion Drops for the Heart (Гербион Сердечные Капли) *KRKA d.d., Russia,* Hawthorn (p. 346), Milk Thistle (p. 429), Valerian (p. 580)

Herbion Drops for the Stomach (Гербион Желудочные Капли) *KRKA d.d., Russia,* Centaury (p. 149), Gentian (p. 290)

Herbion Urological Drops (Гербион Урологические Капли) *KRKA d.d., Russia,* Parsley (p. 456), Uva-Ursi (p. 577)

Herbion Urtica (Гербион Уртика) *KRKA d.d., Russia,* Nettle (p. 452)

Herborex *Rolmex International Inc., Canada,* Cascara (p. 128), Yellow Dock (p. 608)

Herbulax *Chefaro UK Ltd, UK,* Dandelion (p. 204), Frangula (p. 270)

Hertz- und Kreislauftee *Abtswinder Naturheilmittel GmbH, Czech Republic,* Calendula (p. 121), Hawthorn (p. 346), Melissa (p. 425), Rosemary (p. 508), Valerian (p. 580), Yarrow (p. 604)

Heumann Beruhigungstee Tenerval *Lichtenstein Pharmazeutica GmbH & Co., Germany,* Melissa (p. 425), Valerian (p. 580)

Heumann Bronchialtee Solubifix T *Lichtenstein Pharmazeutica GmbH & Co., Germany,* Cowslip (p. 195), Liquorice (p. 411), Marshmallow (p. 418)

Heumann Magentee Solu-Vetan *Lichtenstein Pharmazeutica GmbH & Co., Germany,* Liquorice (p. 411)

Heumann Verdauungstee Solu-Lipar *Lichtenstein Pharmazeutica GmbH & Co., Germany,* Boldo (p. 91), Milk Thistle (p. 429)

Heumann's Bronchialtee *Sanova Pharma GmbH, Austria,* Cowslip (p. 195), Liquorice (p. 411), Marshmallow (p. 418)

Hevert-Blasen-Nieren-Tee N *Hevert-Arzneimittel GmbH & Co. KG, Germany,* Couchgrass (p. 193), Java Tea (p. 381)

Heweberberol-Tee *Hevert-Arzneimittel GmbH & Co. KG, Germany,* Java Tea (p. 381), Liquorice (p. 411)

Hewenephron duo *Hevert-Arzneimittel GmbH & Co. KG, Germany,* Echinacea (p. 217)

Himcolin (Химколин) *Transatlantic International, Russia,* Cinnamon (p. 162)

Himelan *Soria Natural, Spain,* Angelica (p. 53), Melissa (p. 425)

Hingfong-Essenz Hofmanns *Hofmann & Sommer GmbH & Co. KG, Germany,* Valerian (p. 580)

Hiperogyn *Madaus S.r.l., Italy,* Cohosh, Black (p. 168), St John's Wort (p. 549)

Hipoglos Cremoso *Industria Farmacéutica Andrómaco, S.A. de C.V., Mexico,* Aloe Vera (p. 48)

Histo-Fluine P *Laboratoires Richard, France,* Horse-chestnut (p. 363), Pulsatilla (p. 489), Senna (p. 537), Witch Hazel (p. 601)

Honey & Molasses *G.R. Lane Health Products Ltd, UK,* Capsicum (p. 125), Liquorice (p. 411), St John's Wort (p. 549)

Horehound and Aniseed Cough Mixture *Potter's (Herbal Supplies) Ltd, UK,* Elecampane (p. 240), Marshmallow (p. 418), Pleurisy Root (p. 477), Skunk Cabbage (p. 543)

Horseradish Plus *Swiss Bio Pharma Sdn Bhd, Malaysia,* Fenugreek (p. 260), Garlic (p. 279), Horseradish (p. 367), Liquorice (p. 411), Marshmallow (p. 418)

Hot Flashex *Natrol, USA,* Chamomile, German (p. 152), Cohosh, Black (p. 168)

Hova *Gebro Pharma GmbH, Austria,* Hops (p. 354), Valerian (p. 580) *Sager Pharma Kft, Hungary,* Hops (p. 354), Valerian (p. 580) *Gebro Pharma SA, Switzerland,* Hops (p. 354), Valerian (p. 580)

HRI Calm Life *Jessup Marketing, UK,* Hops (p. 354), Ispaghula (p. 374), Scullcap (p. 530), Valerian (p. 580)

HRI Clear Complexion *Jessup Marketing, UK,* Blue Flag (p. 87), Burdock (p. 102), Sarsaparilla (p. 515)

HRI Golden Seal Digestive *Jessup Marketing, UK,* Ginger (p. 293), Golden Seal (p. 337), Myrrh (p. 449), Rhubarb (p. 506), Valerian (p. 580)

HRI Night *Jessup Marketing, UK,* Hops (p. 354), Passionflower (p. 461), Valerian (p. 580), Vervain (p. 591), Wild Lettuce (p. 596)

HRI Water Balance *Jessup Marketing, UK,* Buchu (p. 100), Dandelion (p. 204), Parsley Piert (p. 459), Uva-Ursi (p. 577)

Huile de millepertuis A. Vogel (huile de St. Jean) *Bioforce AG, Switzerland,* St John's Wort (p. 549)

Humulus Compound *Phytomedicine P/L, Australia,* Hops (p. 354), Passionflower (p. 461), Valerian (p. 580)

Hydracur *Léro, France,* Dandelion (p. 204)

Hydrastis Complex *Blackmores Ltd, Australia,* Golden Seal (p. 337), Liquorice (p. 411), Marshmallow (p. 418)

Hyperesa *Dolorgiet GmbH & Co. KG, Germany,* St John's Wort (p. 549), Valerian (p. 580)

Hyperiforce comp *Bioforce AG, Switzerland,* Hops (p. 354), Melissa (p. 425), St John's Wort (p. 549)

Hypotonicka *Megafyt-R sro, Czech Republic,* Hawthorn (p. 346), Melissa (p. 425), Milk Thistle (p. 429)

Höfels Echinacea and Rosehip *Seven Seas Ltd, UK,* Echinacea (p. 217)

Höfels One-A-Day Cardiomax *Seven Seas Ltd, UK,* Garlic (p. 279)

Höfels One-A-Day Garlic *Seven Seas Ltd, UK,* Garlic (p. 279)

Höfels One-A-Day Garlic with Parsley *Seven Seas Ltd, UK,* Garlic (p. 279), Parsley (p. 456)

Höfels One-A-Day Ginge *Seven Seas Ltd, UK,* Ginger (p. 293)

Höfels One-A-Day Ginger, Ginkgo and Garlic *Seven Seas Ltd, UK,* Garlic (p. 279), Ginger (p. 293)

Iberogast *Steigerwald Arzneimittelwerk GmbH, Germany,* Angelica (p. 53), Liquorice (p. 411), Melissa (p. 425), Milk Thistle (p. 429) *Hänseler AG, Switzerland,* Angelica (p. 53), Liquorice (p. 411), Melissa (p. 425), Milk Thistle (p. 429)

Ideolaxyl *Laboratoires GlaxoSmithKline, France,* Aloes (p. 50), Senna (p. 537)

Ifuchol *Laboratorios Ifusa S.A., Mexico,* Artichoke (p. 67), Boldo (p. 91)

Ifupasil *Laboratorios Ifusa S.A., Mexico,* Hawthorn (p. 346), Passionflower (p. 461), Willow (p. 598)

IgeE *Les Grands Espaces Thérapeutiques, France,* Raspberry (p. 495)

Ilja Rogoff *Roche Consumer Health Deutschland GmbH, Germany,* Garlic (p. 279), Hawthorn (p. 346), Hops (p. 354), Milk Thistle (p. 429)

Imegul *Laboratoires Arkopharma, France,* Cascara (p. 128), Ispaghula (p. 374)

Immumil *Milte Italia S.p.A., Italy,* Echinacea (p. 217), Thyme (p. 574)

Immune Insurance *Healthy Direct, UK,* Echinacea (p. 217)

Immune Support *Sundown, USA,* Echinacea (p. 217), Golden Seal (p. 337)

Imugins *Schumit 1967 Co. Ltd, Thailand,* Ginseng, Panax (p. 325)

Imuvit *Boots Healthcare (Switzerland) AG, Hermal, Switzerland,* Ginseng, Panax (p. 325) *Sriprasit Dispensary R O P, Thailand,* Ginseng, Panax (p. 325)

Inconturina *OTW-Naturarzneimittel Regneri GmbH & Co KG, Germany,* Clove (p. 166)

Indian Brandee *OTC Concepts, UK,* Capsicum (p. 125) *Potter's (Herbal Supplies) Ltd, UK,* Capsicum (p. 125), Ginger (p. 293), Rhubarb (p. 506)

Indigestion and Flatulence *The Cantassium Company, UK,* Myrrh (p. 449), Valerian (p. 580)

Indigestion Mixture *Potter's (Herbal Supplies) Ltd, UK,* Gentian (p. 290), Meadowsweet (p. 423)

Indigestion Relief *Herbal Concepts Ltd, UK,* Capsicum (p. 125), Ginger (p. 293)

Infant Calm *Brauer Natural Medicine P/L, Australia,* Passionflower (p. 461)

Infant Tonic *Brauer Natural Medicine P/L, Australia,* Angelica (p. 53), Ginseng, Panax (p. 325), Nettle (p. 452), St John's Wort (p. 549)

Inflamase *Amnol Chimica Biologica S.r.l., Italy,* Horse-chestnut (p. 363)

Inflamol *Healthy Direct, UK,* Scullcap (p. 530)

Influ-Zinc *Wassen Italia S.r.l., Italy,* Echinacea (p. 217), Willow (p. 598)

Influ-Zinc Gola *Wassen Italia S.r.l., Italy,* Liquorice (p. 411)

4

Inotyol *Brady C. KG, Austria,* Witch Hazel (p. 601) *Perrigo Ltd, Israel,* Witch Hazel (p. 601)

Intim *ICIM International S.r.l., Italy,* Witch Hazel (p. 601)

Intradermi *Dr. Friedrich Eberth Arzneimittel, Germany,* Horse-chestnut (p. 363)

Intrait de Marron d'Inde P *Laboratoires Aérocid, France,* Horse-chestnut (p. 363)

Iodeto de Potassio *Sedar Indústria Farmacêutica Ltda, Brazil,* Marshmallow (p. 418)

Iodeto dePotassio *Instituto Terapeutico Delta Ltda, Brazil,* Marshmallow (p. 418)

Iol *Quimioterapica Brasileira Ltda, Brazil,* Marshmallow (p. 418)

Iolin *Quimioterapica Brasileira Ltda, Brazil,* Marshmallow (p. 418)

Ipasin *Vifor SA, Switzerland,* Hawthorn (p. 346), Horse-chestnut (p. 363)

Ipecarin *Ivax-CR as, Ivax-CR as, Czech Republic,* Liquorice (p. 411)

Iridil *Montefarmaco S.p.A., Italy,* Eyebright (p. 256), Witch Hazel (p. 601)

Irontona *Brauer Natural Medicine P/L, Australia,* Angelica (p. 53), Ginseng, Panax (p. 325), Nettle (p. 452), St John's Wort (p. 549)

Isalax Fibras *Instituto Seroterapico Argentino S.A.I.C., Argentina,* Ispaghula (p. 374)

I-Sight *Healthy Direct, UK,* Bilberry (p. 79), Ginkgo (p. 299)

Ixana *Química Medical Arg. S.A.C.I., Argentina,* Senega (p. 533)

Jacksons Herbal Laxative *Anglian Pharma Plc, UK,* Cascara (p. 128), Rhubarb (p. 506), Senna (p. 537)

Jamaican Sarsaparilla *Potter's (Herbal Supplies) Ltd, UK,* Capsicum (p. 125), Liquorice (p. 411), Sarsaparilla (p. 515)

Jaquesor *Soria Natural, Spain,* Lime Flower (p. 409), Melissa (p. 425), Willow (p. 598), Yarrow (p. 604)

Jarabe de Manzanas *Laboratorios Ifusa S.A., Mexico,* Senna (p. 537)

Jarabe Manceau *Alcor, Spain,* Senna (p. 537)

Jecopeptol *Alpharma France, France,* Boldo (p. 91)

Jengimiel *Jengimiel C.A., Venezuela,* Ginger (p. 293)

Joint & Muscle Relief Cream *Brauer Natural Medicine P/L, Australia,* Arnica (p. 64), St John's Wort (p. 549)

Jouvence de l'Abbe Soury *Laboratoires Chefaro-Ardeval, France,* Calamus (p. 118), Ispaghula (p. 374), Witch Hazel (p. 601)

Jukunda Melissen-Krautergeist N *Jukunda Naturarzneimittel Dr Ludwig Schmitt GmbH & Co. KG, Germany,* Melissa (p. 425)

Jungborn *Taro Pharmaceutical International, Israel,* Aniseed (p. 57), Lime Flower (p. 409), Senna (p. 537), Uva-Ursi (p. 577)

Jurubileno *Ibefar Inst. Brasileiro de Esp. Ftcas. Ltda, Brazil,* Artichoke (p. 67), Boldo (p. 91), Cascara (p. 128)

Kalms *G.R. Lane Health Products Ltd, UK,* Gentian (p. 290), Hops (p. 354), Valerian (p. 580)

Kalms Sleep *G.R. Lane Health Products Ltd, UK,* Hops (p. 354), Passionflower (p. 461), Valerian (p. 580), Vervain (p. 591), Wild Lettuce (p. 596)

Kamfeine *Wolfs SA, Belgium,* Marshmallow (p. 418)

Kamillan Plus *Pharma Wernigerode GmbH, Germany,* Yarrow (p. 604)

Kamilotract *Tamar Marketing, Israel,* Sage (p. 512)

Kanormal *German Remedies Ltd, India,* Frangula (p. 270)

Kas-Bah *Potter's (Herbal Supplies) Ltd, UK,* Buchu (p. 100), Clivers (p. 164), Couchgrass (p. 193), Senna (p. 537), Uva-Ursi (p. 577)

Katapekt *Vitabalans Oy, Finland,* Thyme (p. 574)

Kavatrol *Natrol, USA,* Chamomile, German (p. 152)

Keli-med *Permamed AG, Switzerland,* Garlic (p. 279)

Kelual DS *Laboratoires Pierre Fabre, France,* Saw Palmetto (p. 521)

Keppur *Drossapharm SA, Switzerland,* Comfrey (p. 188)

Keracnyl *Pierre Fabre Argentina S.A., Argentina,* Saw Palmetto (p. 521) *Laboratoires Pierre Fabre, France,* Saw Palmetto (p. 521)

Keracnyl eau nettoyante *Laboratoires Pierre Fabre, France,* Witch Hazel (p. 601)

Kernosan Elixir *E Kern AG, Pharmazeutische Krauterspezialitäten, Switzerland,* Aniseed (p. 57), Calamus (p. 118), Cowslip (p. 195), Horseradish (p. 367), Liquorice (p. 411), Plantain (p. 474)

Kernosan Heidelberger Poudre *E Kern AG, Pharmazeutische Krauterspezialitäten, Switzerland,* Aniseed (p. 57), Juniper (p. 386), Yarrow (p. 604)

Kilkof *Bell, Sons & Co. (Druggists), UK,* Capsicum (p. 125)

Kinder Em-eukal Hustensaft *Dr. C. Soldan GmbH, Germany,* Cowslip (p. 195), Thyme (p. 574)

KLB6 Fruit Diet *Natural Life S.A., Argentina,* Uva-Ursi (p. 577)

Klorane Shampooing Antipelliculaire *Laboratoires Klorane, France,* Bilberry (p. 79)

Klosterfrau Beruhigungs Forte *Maria Clementine Martin Klosterfrau Vertriebsgesellschaft mbH, Germany,* Hops (p. 354), Valerian (p. 580)

Klosterfrau Melisana *Maria Clementine Martin Klosterfrau Vertriebsgesellschaft mbH, Germany,* Angelica (p. 53), Cinnamon (p. 162), Clove (p. 166), Elecampane (p. 240), Gentian (p. 290), Ginger (p. 293), Melissa (p. 425)

Korodin *Robugen GmbH Pharmazeutische Fabrik, Germany,* Hawthorn (p. 346)

Krampdruppels *Aspen Pharmacare (Pty) Ltd, South Africa,* Valerian (p. 580)

Krauter Hustensaft *Apomedica GmbH, Austria,* Cowslip (p. 195), Elder (p. 237), Liquorice (p. 411), Thyme (p. 574)

Kronolax *Altana Pharma SA, Argentina,* Ispaghula (p. 374), Senna (p. 537)

Kruidvat Spierbalsem *Pharmethica BV, Netherlands,* Capsicum (p. 125)

KW *Lagos Laboratorios Argentina S.R.L., Argentina,* Aloe Vera (p. 48)

Kyolic 101 *Boehringer Ingelheim (Canada) Ltd, Canada,* Garlic (p. 279)

Kyolic 102 *Boehringer Ingelheim (Canada) Ltd, Canada,* Garlic (p. 279)

Kyolic 103 *Boehringer Ingelheim (Canada) Ltd, Canada,* Garlic (p. 279)

Kyolic 104 *Boehringer Ingelheim (Canada) Ltd, Canada,* Garlic (p. 279)

Kyolic 106 *Boehringer Ingelheim (Canada) Ltd, Canada,* Garlic (p. 279)

Kytta Baume *Iromedica AG, Switzerland,* Comfrey (p. 188)

Kytta-Balsam f *Merck KGaA, Germany,* Comfrey (p. 188)

Kytta-Sedativum *Merck KGaA, Germany,* Hops (p. 354), Passionflower (p. 461), Valerian (p. 580)

Laci Le Beau Super Dieter's Tea *Natrol, USA,* Marshmallow (p. 418), Senna (p. 537)

Laci Le Beau Throat Care *Natrol, USA,* Slippery Elm (p. 545)

Laci Supplement Power Time *Natrol, USA,* Echinacea (p. 217)

Laci Throat Care Soothing Citrus *Natrol, USA,* Chamomile, German (p. 152), Echinacea (p. 217)

Lacto Calamine *CSL (NZ) Ltd, New Zealand,* Witch Hazel (p. 601) *Schering-Plough Ltd, UK,* Witch Hazel (p. 601)

Lactolas *Infosint S.p.A., Italy,* Frangula (p. 270), Rhubarb (p. 506), Senna (p. 537)

Lane's Sage and Garlic Catarrh Remedy *Richard Lane's, UK,* Garlic (p. 279), Liquorice (p. 411), Sage (p. 512)

Lapidar 10 *Krauterpfarrer Kunzle AG, Switzerland,* Frangula (p. 270), Liquorice (p. 411), Senna (p. 537)

Lassatina *Kedrion S.p.A., Italy,* Aniseed (p. 57), Cascara (p. 128), Liquorice (p. 411), Rhubarb (p. 506), Senna (p. 537)

Lassativi Vetegali&xref details= *Giovanni Ogna & Figli S.p.A., Zeta Farmaceutici S.p.A., Italy,* Aloes (p. 50), Rhubarb (p. 506)

Lavandula Oligoplex *Lab. Dr. Madaus & Co. SA, Argentina,* Calendula (p. 121), Witch Hazel (p. 601)

Laxacaps *Gelcaps Exp. de Mexico SA de CV, Mexico,* Senna (p. 537)

Laxaco *Jamieson Laboratories, Canada,* Cascara (p. 128), Senna (p. 537)

Laxalpin *F. Joh. Kwizda, Austria,* Elder (p. 237), Frangula (p. 270), Liquorice (p. 411), Senna (p. 537)

Laxante Bescansa Aloico *Bescansa, Spain,* Rhubarb (p. 506)

Laxante Sanatorium *Santiveri, Spain,* Aloes (p. 50), Aniseed (p. 57), Senna (p. 537)

Laxarine *Farmion Laboratório Brasileiro de Farmacologia Ltda, Brazil,* Liquorice (p. 411), Senna (p. 537)

Laxative *Nobel Pharm Enrg, Canada,* Aloes (p. 50), Cascara (p. 128)

Laxative Comp *Teva Pharmaceuticals Ind. Ltd, Israel,* Aloes (p. 50)

Laxative Tablets *Herbal Concepts Ltd, UK,* Aloes (p. 50), Cascara (p. 128), Senna (p. 537), Valerian (p. 580)

Laxolind *Metochem-Pharma GmbH, Austria,* Frangula (p. 270), Senna (p. 537)

Laxomax *Soria Natural, Spain,* Aniseed (p. 57), Liquorice (p. 411), Senna (p. 537)

Laxtam *Merck S.A. Industrias Químicas, Brazil,* Liquorice (p. 411), Senna (p. 537)

Lefkaflam *Laboratorio Esp. Med. Knop Ltda, Chile,* Arnica (p. 64)

Lenicalm *Laboratoires Dolisos Italia S.r.l., Italy,* Hawthorn (p. 346), Lime Flower (p. 409)

Lenirose *Novogaleno S.r.l., Italy,* Calendula (p. 121)

Lepisor *Soria Natural, Spain,* Java Tea (p. 381)

Leukona-Beruhigungsbad *Dr. Atzinger Pharmazeutische Fabrik, Germany,* Hops (p. 354), Valerian (p. 580)

Leukona-Wundsalbe *Dr. Atzinger Pharmazeutische Fabrik, Germany,* Witch Hazel (p. 601)

Lewensessens *Aspen Pharmacare (Pty) Ltd, South Africa,* Aloes (p. 50), Gentian (p. 290), Ginger (p. 293), Myrrh (p. 449), Rhubarb (p. 506)

Lexat *Eagle Pharmaceuticals P/L, Australia,* Aloes (p. 50), Bloodroot (p. 84), Boldo (p. 91)

Lice Blaster *Douglas Pharmaceuticals Ltd, New Zealand,* Echinacea (p. 217)

Lidersoft *Higaté Medical Argentina, Argentina,* Hydrocotyle (p. 371)

Lido Tea *Trima, Israel,* Liquorice (p. 411), Senna (p. 537)

Life Drops *Potter's (Herbal Supplies) Ltd, UK,* Capsicum (p. 125), Elder (p. 237)

Lifechange Circulation Aid *Mayne Pharma P/L, Australia,* Ginkgo (p. 299), Hawthorn (p. 346)

Lifechange Menopause Formula *Mayne Pharma P/L, Australia,* Red Clover (p. 498)

Lifechange Mens Complex with Saw Palmetto *Mayne Pharma P/L, Australia,* Saw Palmetto (p. 521)

Lifechange Multi Plus Antioxidant *Mayne Pharma P/L, Australia,* Ginkgo (p. 299)

Lifesystem Herbal Formula 1 Arthritic Aid *Mayne Pharma P/L, Australia,* Celery (p. 146), Devil's Claw (p. 207), Juniper (p. 386), Willow (p. 598)

Lifesystem Herbal Formula 4 Women's Formula *Mayne Pharma P/L, Australia,* Agnus Castus (p. 36), Angelica (p. 53), Cohosh, Black (p. 168), Cohosh, Blue (p. 180), Pulsatilla (p. 489)

Lifesystem Herbal Formula 6 For Peripheral Circulation *Mayne Pharma P/L, Australia,* Capsicum (p. 125), Ginkgo (p. 299), Hawthorn (p. 346)

Lifesystem Herbal Formula 7 Liver Tonic *Mayne Pharma P/L, Australia,* Artichoke (p. 67), Dandelion (p. 204), Garlic (p. 279), Milk Thistle (p. 429)

Lifesystem Herbal Plus Formula 2 Valerian *Mayne Pharma P/L, Australia,* Passionflower (p. 461), Valerian (p. 580)

Lifesystem Herbal Plus Formula 5 Eye Relief *Mayne Pharma P/L, Australia,* Eyebright (p. 256), Ginkgo (p. 299)

Lifesystem Herbal Plus Formula 8 Echinacea *Mayne Pharma P/L, Australia,* Echinacea (p. 217)

Lifesystem Herbal Plus Formula 11 Ginkgo *Mayne Pharma P/L, Australia,* Ginger (p. 293), Ginkgo (p. 299)

Lightning Cough Remedy *Potter's (Herbal Supplies) Ltd, UK,* Liquorice (p. 411)

Linctus Tussi Infans *Adcock Ingram Pharmaceuticals Ltd, South Africa,* St John's Wort (p. 549)

Lindofluid N *Lindopharm GmbH, Germany,* Arnica (p. 64), Melissa (p. 425)

Linimento Naion *Puerto Galiano, Spain,* Capsicum (p. 125), Rosemary (p. 508)

Linkus (Линкас) *Herbion Pakistan PVT Ltd, Russia,* Liquorice (p. 411), Marshmallow (p. 418)

Linoforce *Bioforce AG, Switzerland,* Frangula (p. 270), Senna (p. 537)

LinoMed *Bioforce AG, Switzerland,* Frangula (p. 270), Senna (p. 537)

Lion Cleansing Herbs *Potter's (Herbal Supplies) Ltd, UK,* Elder (p. 237), Senna (p. 537)

Lipidavit *Rodisma-Med Pharma GmbH, Germany,* Garlic (p. 279)

Lipograsil *Uriach, Spain,* Artichoke (p. 67), Cascara (p. 128)

Liquid Elderberry with Ester-C *Natrol, USA,* Elder (p. 237)

Lisian *Laboratório Iodo Suma Ltda, Brazil,* Uva-Ursi (p. 577)

Lisotox *Cifarma Cientifica Farmacêutica Ltda, Brazil,* Artichoke (p. 67)

Liv 52 (Лив 52) *Transatlantic International, Russia,* Yarrow (p. 604)

Liver Formula *Natrol, USA,* Ginger (p. 293), Milk Thistle (p. 429)

Liver Formula Herbal Blend *Natrol, USA,* Burdock (p. 102), Dandelion (p. 204)

Liver Tonic Herbal Formula 6 *Mayne Pharma P/L, Australia,* Artichoke (p. 67), Dandelion (p. 204), Garlic (p. 279), Milk Thistle (p. 429)

Livstim *Mediherb P/L, Australia,* Artichoke (p. 67), Dandelion (p. 204), Milk Thistle (p. 429)

Livton Complex *Mediherb P/L, Australia,* Artichoke (p. 67), Dandelion (p. 204), Milk Thistle (p. 429)

Llantusil *Soria Natural, Spain,* Coltsfoot (p. 185), Marshmallow (p. 418)

Logicin Natural Lozenges *Sigma Pharmaceuticals P/L, Australia,* Echinacea (p. 217)

Lomal *Lomapharm, Rudolf Lohmann GmbH KG, Germany,* Drosera (p. 215), Thyme (p. 574)

Lorasil Feminine Hygeine *Medispec (M) Sdn Bhd, Malaysia,* Aloe Vera (p. 48)

Lotio Pruni Comp cum Cupro *Pharma-Natura (Pty) Ltd, South Africa,* Arnica (p. 64), Burdock (p. 102), Witch Hazel (p. 601)

Lozione Same Urto *Savoma Medicinali S.p.A., Italy,* Coltsfoot (p. 185), Yarrow (p. 604)

Lupassin *Laboratorios Elmor S.A., Venezuela,* Hops (p. 354), Passionflower (p. 461), Valerian (p. 580)

Lustys Herbalene *G.R. Lane Health Products Ltd, UK,* Elder (p. 237), Frangula (p. 270), Senna (p. 537)

Luuf-Hustentee *Apomedica GmbH, Austria,* Thyme (p. 574)

Luvased *Biocur Arzneimittel GmbH, Germany,* Hops (p. 354), Valerian (p. 580)

LX-30 *Laboratorios Sigma, Argentina,* Rhubarb (p. 506), Senna (p. 537)

Lycia Luminique *Artsana S.p.A., Italy,* Witch Hazel (p. 601)

Macro Anti-Stress *Whitehall Laboratories Australia P/L, Australia,* Valerian (p. 580)

Madecassol C *Sanofi-Synthelabo de Mexico S.A. de C.V., Mexico,* Hydrocotyle (p. 371)

Madecassol N *Sanofi-Synthelabo de Mexico S.A. de C.V., Mexico,* Hydrocotyle (p. 371)

Madecassol Neomicina *Productos Roche Ltda, Chile,* Hydrocotyle (p. 371)

Madecassol NeomycineHydrocortisone *Laboratoires Roche Nicholas, France,* Hydrocotyle (p. 371)

Mag Kottas Krauterexpress Abfuhrtee *Kottas-Heldenberg Mag. R.u. Sohn, Austria,* Frangula (p. 270), Senna (p. 537)

Mag Kottas May-Cur-Tee *Kottas-Heldenberg Mag. R.u. Sohn, Austria,* Frangula (p. 270), Senna (p. 537)

Magen- und Darmtee N *Abtswinder Naturheilmittel GmbH, Czech Republic,* Cinnamon (p. 162), Liquorice (p. 411)

Magentee St Severin *EF-EM-ES - Dr Smetana & Co., Austria,* Centaury (p. 149), Dandelion (p. 204), St John's Wort (p. 549)

Magisbile *Magis Farmaceutici S.p.A., Italy,* Boldo (p. 91), Cascara (p. 128), Rhubarb (p. 506)

Mailen *Investi Farma S.A., Argentina,* Hydrocotyle (p. 371)

Majocarmin-Tee *Hevert-Arzneimittel GmbH & Co. KG, Germany,* Aniseed (p. 57)

Makaphyt Gouttes antitussives *Gebro Pharma SA, Switzerland,* Drosera (p. 215), Liquorice (p. 411), Senega (p. 533), Thyme (p. 574)

Makaphyt Sirop *Gebro Pharma SA, Switzerland,* Drosera (p. 215), Liquorice (p. 411), Senega (p. 533), Thyme (p. 574)

Makatussin Tropfen *Altana Pharma Deutschland GmbH, Germany,* Thyme (p. 574)

Makatussin Tropfen forte *Altana Pharma Deutschland GmbH, Germany,* Drosera (p. 215)

Malvaliz *Soria Natural, Spain,* Liquorice (p. 411), Marshmallow (p. 418)

Malvatricin Natural *Laboratório Daudt Oliveira Ltda, Brazil,* Calendula (p. 121), Echinacea (p. 217)

Malvatricin Natural Organic *Laboratório Daudt Oliveira Ltda, Brazil,* Echinacea (p. 217), Witch Hazel (p. 601)

Malveol *Laboratoires Magistra SA, Switzerland,* Marshmallow (p. 418)

Manevac *Galen Ltd, UK,* Ispaghula (p. 374), Senna (p. 537)

Manolio *Brasmedica S.A. Industrias Farmacêuticas, Brazil,* Witch Hazel (p. 601)

Manzan *Lab E J Gezzi SRL, Argentina,* Witch Hazel (p. 601)

Maraslavin (Мараславин) *Sopharma AO, Russia,* Clove (p. 166), Ginger (p. 293), Thyme (p. 574)

Mariazeller *Apotheke zur Gnadenmutter, Austria,* Bogbean (p. 89), Centaury (p. 149), Cinnamon (p. 162), Clove (p. 166), Gentian (p. 290), Ginger (p. 293), Holy Thistle (p. 352), Juniper (p. 386), Melissa (p. 425), Yarrow (p. 604)

Massage Balm with Calendula *Weleda (UK) Ltd, UK,* Calendula (p. 121)

Matikomp *Laboratorio Esp. Med. Knop Ltda, Chile,* Arnica (p. 64), Calendula (p. 121)

Mavena Proctal-Gen *Psorimed AG, Switzerland,* Witch Hazel (p. 601)

Maximum Strength Flexall 454 *Chattem Consumer Products, USA,* Aloe Vera (p. 48)

Medalginan *Laboratório Medinfar, SA, Portugal,* Capsicum (p. 125)

Mediflor no 11 Draineur Renal et Digestif *Merck Lipha Santé, France,* Boldo (p. 91)

Mediflor Tisane Antirhumatismale No 2 *Merck Lipha Santé, France,* Couchgrass (p. 193), Frangula (p. 270), Juniper (p. 386), Lime Flower (p. 409), Meadowsweet (p. 423), Uva-Ursi (p. 577)

4

Mediflor Tisane Calmante Troubles du Sommeil No 14 *Merck Lipha Santé, France,* Hawthorn (p. 346), Lime Flower (p. 409), Melissa (p. 425), Passionflower (p. 461), Valerian (p. 580)

Mediflor Tisane Circulation du Sang No 12 *Merck Lipha Santé, France,* Frangula (p. 270), Hawthorn (p. 346), Horse-chestnut (p. 363), Melissa (p. 425), Milk Thistle (p. 429), Valerian (p. 580), Willow (p. 598), Witch Hazel (p. 601)

Mediflor Tisane Contre la Constipation Passagere No 7 *Merck Lipha Santé, France,* Liquorice (p. 411), Rosemary (p. 508), Senna (p. 537)

Mediflor Tisane Digestive No 3 *Merck Lipha Santé, France,* Angelica (p. 53), Aniseed (p. 57), Elecampane (p. 240), Rosemary (p. 508)

Mediflor Tisane Hepatique No 5 *Merck Lipha Santé, France,* Boldo (p. 91), Elecampane (p. 240), Liquorice (p. 411), Rosemary (p. 508), Senna (p. 537)

Mediflor Tisane No 4 Diuretique *Merck Lipha Santé, France,* Couchgrass (p. 193), Liquorice (p. 411), Marshmallow (p. 418), Meadowsweet (p. 423), Uva-Ursi (p. 577)

Medilaxan *Laboratorios Beta S.A., Argentina,* Ispaghula (p. 374)

Medinat Esten *Bioglan Ltd, Australia,* Angelica (p. 53), Cohosh, Black (p. 168), Damiana (p. 201), Ginseng, Eleutherococcus (p. 315)

Medinat PMT-Eze *Bioglan Ltd, Australia,* Buchu (p. 100), Parsley (p. 456), Uva-Ursi (p. 577)

Mefedra-N *Medipharma Ltd, Hong Kong, Hong Kong,* Euphorbia (p. 249), Senega (p. 533), St John's Wort (p. 549)

Melaton *Slovakofarma sro, Czech Republic,* Melissa (p. 425)

Melipass *Laboratorio Esp. Med. Knop Ltda, Chile,* Melissa (p. 425)

Melissa Comp. *Weleda (UK) Ltd, UK,* Angelica (p. 53), Cinnamon (p. 162), Clove (p. 166), Melissa (p. 425)

Melissengeist *Hofmann & Sommer GmbH & Co. KG, Germany,* Angelica (p. 53), Cinnamon (p. 162), Clove (p. 166), Melissa (p. 425), Rosemary (p. 508), Sage (p. 512), Thyme (p. 574) *Pharma-Natura (Pty) Ltd, South Africa,* Angelica (p. 53), Cinnamon (p. 162), Clove (p. 166), Melissa (p. 425)

Meloids *Olic (Thailand) Ltd, Thailand,* Capsicum (p. 125), Cinnamon (p. 162), Liquorice (p. 411)

Memoactive *Euroderm S.r.l., Italy,* Ginkgo (p. 299)

Memorandum *Lampugnani Farmaceutici S.p.A., Italy,* Ginkgo (p. 299)

Memovisus *Pharmacia Italia S.p.A., Italy,* Bilberry (p. 79)

Menabil Complex *Menarini, Spain,* Artichoke (p. 67), Cascara (p. 128), Rhubarb (p. 506)

Menodoron *Weleda GmbH & Co. KG, Austria,* Nettle (p. 452), Senna (p. 537), Yarrow (p. 604) *Pharma-Natura (Pty) Ltd, South Africa,* Nettle (p. 452), Senna (p. 537), Yarrow (p. 604)

Menopace Plus *Vitabiotics Ltd, UK,* Sage (p. 512)

Menopause Relief *Herbal Concepts Ltd, UK,* Lime Flower (p. 409), Motherwort (p. 447), Pulsatilla (p. 489), Valerian (p. 580) *Walgreens Finest Natural, USA,* Cohosh, Black (p. 168)

Menopause Support *Sundown, USA,* Cohosh, Black (p. 168), Ginseng, Eleutherococcus (p. 315)

Menstrunat *Soria Natural, Spain,* Calendula (p. 121), Sage (p. 512), Yarrow (p. 604)

Mental Clarity *Sundown, USA,* Bilberry (p. 79), Ginkgo (p. 299), Ginseng, Panax (p. 325)

Mentania *Laboratorios Saval SA, Chile,* Ginkgo (p. 299), Ginseng, Panax (p. 325)

Mento-O-Cap *Rekah Ltd, Israel,* Capsicum (p. 125)

Mentopin *Brady C. KG, Austria,* Capsicum (p. 125), Nettle (p. 452), Sage (p. 512)

Mepalax *Istituto Biologico Chemioterapico SpA, Italy,* Boldo (p. 91), Cascara (p. 128), Rhubarb (p. 506)

Mermelax *Lab. Argenfarma S.R.L., Argentina,* Ispaghula (p. 374)

Me-Sabona plus *Sabona GmbH, Germany,* Melissa (p. 425), St John's Wort (p. 549)

Mesatil *Soria Natural, Spain,* Lime Flower (p. 409), Melissa (p. 425), Rosemary (p. 508), Willow (p. 598)

Metiogen *Química Medical Arg. S.A.C.I., Argentina,* Artichoke (p. 67), Boldo (p. 91), Wild Carrot (p. 593)

Midalgan *Qualicare AG, Switzerland,* Capsicum (p. 125)

Midro *Laboratori Italiani Vaillant S.r.l., Italy,* Liquorice (p. 411), Senna (p. 537) *Crefar, Lda, Portugal,* Clove (p. 166), Liquorice (p. 411), Senna (p. 537)

Midro Tee *Sanova Pharma GmbH, Austria,* Liquorice (p. 411), Senna (p. 537)

Midro-Tea *ProMedico Ltd, Israel,* Liquorice (p. 411), Senna (p. 537)

Mielocol *Herbes Universelles, Canada,* Bloodroot (p. 84)

Milk Thistle *Nutravite, Canada,* Artichoke (p. 67), Milk Thistle (p. 429)

Milk Thistle Extract Formula *Boehringer Ingelheim (Canada) Ltd, Canada,* Dandelion (p. 204), Liquorice (p. 411), Milk Thistle (p. 429)

Mint-Lysoform *Lysoform Dr. Hans Rosemann GmbH, Germany,* Myrrh (p. 449)

Mirfulan *Ratiopharm Arzneimittel Vertriebs-GmbH, Austria,* Witch Hazel (p. 601) *Merckle GmbH, Germany,* Witch Hazel (p. 601)

Mirorroidin *Laboratório Sedabel Ltda, Brazil,* Horse-chestnut (p. 363), Witch Hazel (p. 601)

Miroton *Abbott GmbH & Co. KG, Germany,* St John's Wort (p. 549)

Mirtilene *Società Industria Farmaceutica Italiana S.p.A., Italy,* Bilberry (p. 79)

Mirtilus *Llorens, Spain,* Bilberry (p. 79)

Mirtilux *Mediwhite Srl, Italy,* Bilberry (p. 79)

Mist Expect Stim *Vida Laboratories Ltd, Hong Kong,* Liquorice (p. 411), Senega (p. 533), St John's Wort (p. 549)

Mithen *Fidia Farmaceutici S.p.A., Italy,* St John's Wort (p. 549)

Mixagel *Productos Naturissima de Venezuela, Venezuela,* Thyme (p. 574)

Mixed Vegetable Tablets *Dorwest Herbs Ltd, UK,* Celery (p. 146), Horseradish (p. 367), Parsley (p. 456)

MM Expectorante *Laboratório Americano de Farmacoterapia S/A, Brazil,* Marshmallow (p. 418)

Modane *Coopération Pharmaceutique Francaise, France,* Senna (p. 537)

Modern Herbals Cold & Catarrh *G.R. Lane Health Products Ltd, UK,* Echinacea (p. 217), Elder (p. 237), Marshmallow (p. 418)

Modern Herbals Cold & Congestion *G.R. Lane Health Products Ltd, UK,* Marshmallow (p. 418)

Modern Herbals Cough Mixture *G.R. Lane Health Products Ltd, UK,* St John's Wort (p. 549)

Modern Herbals Laxative *G.R. Lane Health Products Ltd, UK,* Cascara (p. 128), Senna (p. 537)

Modern Herbals Menopause *G.R. Lane Health Products Ltd, UK,* Clivers (p. 164), Parsley (p. 456), Senna (p. 537), Vervain (p. 591)

Modern Herbals Pile *G.R. Lane Health Products Ltd, UK,* Cascara (p. 128), Slippery Elm (p. 545), Witch Hazel (p. 601)

Modern Herbals Rheumatic Pain *G.R. Lane Health Products Ltd, UK,* Bogbean (p. 89), Celery (p. 146), Cohosh, Black (p. 168)

Modern Herbals Stress *G.R. Lane Health Products Ltd, UK,* Motherwort (p. 447), Passionflower (p. 461), Valerian (p. 580), Vervain (p. 591)

Modern Herbals Water Retention *G.R. Lane Health Products Ltd, UK,* Burdock (p. 102), Clivers (p. 164), Uva-Ursi (p. 577)

Montana *Pharmonta Mag. pharm. Dr Fischer, Austria,* Cinnamon (p. 162), Dandelion (p. 204), Hops (p. 354)

Montana N *Pharmonta Mag. pharm. Dr Fischer, Austria,* Centaury (p. 149), Cinnamon (p. 162), Gentian (p. 290)

Mon-tana *Pharmonta Mag. pharm. Dr Fischer, Austria,* Gentian (p. 290)

Moradorm S *Apotheker Walter Bouhon GmbH & Co. KG, Germany,* Hops (p. 354), Passionflower (p. 461), Valerian (p. 580)

Moragen *Euroderm Laboratorios S.R.L., Argentina,* Hydrocotyle (p. 371)

Moultons Herbal Extract *Pharmaceutical Enterprises (Pty) Ltd, South Africa,* Aloes (p. 50), Cascara (p. 128), Rhubarb (p. 506)

Mr Nits *Pacific Pharmaceuticals Co. Ltd, New Zealand,* Borage (p. 96), Melissa (p. 425)

MSM with Glucosamine Creme *Natrol, USA,* Aloe Vera (p. 48), Arnica (p. 64), Capsicum (p. 125), Chamomile, German (p. 152), Comfrey (p. 188)

Mucilar Avena *Spirig Pharma AG, Switzerland,* Ispaghula (p. 374)

Mucinum *Sabex Inc., Canada,* Cascara (p. 128), Senna (p. 537)

Mucinum a l'Extrait de Cascara *Laboratoires Innotech International, Sté du groupe Innothéra, France,* Aniseed (p. 57), Boldo (p. 91), Cascara (p. 128), Senna (p. 537)

Mucinum Cascara *Wing Wai Trading Co., Hong Kong,* Aniseed (p. 57), Boldo (p. 91), Cascara (p. 128), Senna (p. 537)

Muc-Sabona *Sabona GmbH, Germany,* Liquorice (p. 411), Thyme (p. 574)

Multilim RG *Atlantic Pharmaceutical Co. Ltd, Thailand,* Ginseng, Panax (p. 325)

Multi-Mam Compressas *Farmalight, Lda, Portugal,* Aloe Vera (p. 48)

Multi-Vitamin Day & Night *Mayne Pharma P/L, Australia,* Hawthorn (p. 346), Passionflower (p. 461), Valerian (p. 580)

Muscle Rub *Pharma-Natura (Pty) Ltd, South Africa,* Arnica (p. 64), Capsicum (p. 125)

Mutellon *Dr Gustav Klein, Germany,* Motherwort (p. 447), Valerian (p. 580)

My Defense *Natrol, USA,* Cranberry (p. 197)

My Favorite Multiple *Natrol, USA,* Ginger (p. 293), Hawthorn (p. 346)

My Favorite Multiple Energizer *Natrol, USA,* Alfalfa (p. 45)

My Favorite Multiple Iron-Free *Natrol, USA,* Bilberry (p. 79)

My Favorite Multiple Original *Natrol, USA,* Bilberry (p. 79)

My Favorite Multiple Prime Multi Vitamin *Natrol, USA,* Bilberry (p. 79)

My Favorite Multiple Take One *Natrol, USA,* Alfalfa (p. 45), Bilberry (p. 79)

My Favorite Multiple Take One Iron-Free *Natrol, USA,* Alfalfa (p. 45), Bilberry (p. 79)

Myrrhinil-Intest *Repha GmbH Biologische Arzneimittel, Germany,* Myrrh (p. 449)

Nadem Forte *Ivax Argentina SA, Argentina,* Horse-chestnut (p. 363)

Napiers Back Ache Tea *Culpeper and Napiers, UK,* Pulsatilla (p. 489)

Napiers Backache Tea *Culpeper and Napiers, UK,* Celery (p. 146)

Napiers Breathe Easy Tea *Culpeper and Napiers, UK,* Clivers (p. 164), Plantain (p. 474)

Napiers Cold Tablets *Culpeper and Napiers, UK,* Garlic (p. 279)

Napiers Digestion Tablets *Culpeper and Napiers, UK,* Ginger (p. 293), Myrrh (p. 449), Valerian (p. 580)

Napiers Echinacea Tea *Culpeper and Napiers, UK,* Calendula (p. 121), Echinacea (p. 217), Liquorice (p. 411), Melissa (p. 425), Nettle (p. 452), Sage (p. 512)

Napiers Monthly Calm Tea *Culpeper and Napiers, UK,* Chamomile, German (p. 152), Ginger (p. 293), Pulsatilla (p. 489)

Napiers Skin Tablets *Culpeper and Napiers, UK,* Blue Flag (p. 87), Burdock (p. 102), Sarsaparilla (p. 515)

Napiers Sleep Tablets *Culpeper and Napiers, UK,* Hops (p. 354), Valerian (p. 580), Vervain (p. 591), Wild Lettuce (p. 596)

Napiers Slimming Tablets *Culpeper and Napiers, UK,* Boldo (p. 91), Dandelion (p. 204), Fucus (p. 273)

Napiers Tension Tablets *Culpeper and Napiers, UK,* Hops (p. 354), Scullcap (p. 530), Valerian (p. 580)

Napiers Uva Ursi Tea *Natrol, UK,* Corn Silk (p. 191) *Culpeper and Napiers, UK,* Couchgrass (p. 193), Marshmallow (p. 418), Meadowsweet (p. 423), Uva-Ursi (p. 577)

Nappy Rash Relief Cream *Brauer Natural Medicine P/L, Australia,* Calendula (p. 121), St John's Wort (p. 549)

Nasal-Ease *Hi-Tech Pharmacal, USA,* Aloe Vera (p. 48), Calendula (p. 121)

Natrasleep *Chefaro UK Ltd, UK,* Hops (p. 354), Valerian (p. 580)

Natravene *Chefaro UK Ltd, UK,* Dandelion (p. 204), Frangula (p. 270)

Natrol Complete Balance for Menopause AM/PM Formula *Natrol, USA,* Cohosh, Black (p. 168)

Natudor *Dolisos SA, Belgium,* Hawthorn (p. 346), Lime Flower (p. 409), Valerian (p. 580) *Laboratoires Plantes et Médecines, France,* Hawthorn (p. 346), Passionflower (p. 461)

Natural Deep Sleep *Naturopathica, Australia,* Hops (p. 354), Melissa (p. 425), Passionflower (p. 461), Valerian (p. 580)

Natural Herb Tablets *Dorwest Herbs Ltd, UK,* Aloes (p. 50), Cascara (p. 128), Dandelion (p. 204), Senna (p. 537), Valerian (p. 580)

Natural Herbal Water Tablets *Sundown, USA,* Alfalfa (p. 45), Couchgrass (p. 193), Juniper (p. 386), Parsley (p. 456)

Natural HRT *Swiss Herbal Remedies Ltd, Canada,* Agnus Castus (p. 36), Burdock (p. 102), Cohosh, Black (p. 168), Red Clover (p. 498)

Nature Complex Reduct-Te *Laboratorio Prater SA, Chile,* Boldo (p. 91), Lime Flower (p. 409)

Nature's Garden *Worldwide Health Corp. Ltd, UK,* Bilberry (p. 79), Ginkgo (p. 299)

Naturident *Memsep sro, Czech Republic,* St John's Wort (p. 549)

Naturland Grosser Swedenbitter *Naturland Czech Republic sro, Czech Republic,* Agrimony (p. 42), Bogbean (p. 89), Centaury (p. 149), Clove (p. 166), Gentian (p. 290), Ginger (p. 293), Liquorice (p. 411), Milk Thistle (p. 429), Rosemary (p. 508)

Naturlax *Laboratorios Maver SA, Chile,* Liquorice (p. 411), Senna (p. 537)

Natursel-C *Laboratorio Ximena Polanco, Chile,* Wild Carrot (p. 593)

Natur-Zin *Laboratorio Ximena Polanco, Chile,* Wild Carrot (p. 593)

Natusor Aerofane *Soria Natural, Spain,* Melissa (p. 425)

Natusor Artilane *Soria Natural, Spain,* Nettle (p. 452)

Natusor Asmaten *Soria Natural, Spain,* Elecampane (p. 240), Thyme (p. 574)

Natusor Astringel *Soria Natural, Spain,* Agrimony (p. 42), Liquorice (p. 411)

Natusor Broncopul *Soria Natural, Spain,* Elecampane (p. 240), Marshmallow (p. 418)

Natusor Circusil *Soria Natural, Spain,* Yarrow (p. 604)

Natusor Farinol *Soria Natural, Spain,* Agrimony (p. 42), Marshmallow (p. 418), Sage (p. 512), Thyme (p. 574)

Natusor Gastrolen *Soria Natural, Spain,* Liquorice (p. 411), Marshmallow (p. 418), St John's Wort (p. 549), Yarrow (p. 604)

Natusor Gripotul *Soria Natural, Spain,* Elder (p. 237), Lime Flower (p. 409), Thyme (p. 574)

Natusor Harpagosinol *Soria Natural, Spain,* Devil's Claw (p. 207), Meadowsweet (p. 423), Willow (p. 598)

Natusor Hepavesical *Soria Natural, Spain,* Boldo (p. 91), Centaury (p. 149), Fumitory (p. 276), Rosemary (p. 508)

Natusor High Blood Pressure *Soria Natural, Spain,* Hawthorn (p. 346)

Natusor Infenol *Soria Natural, Spain,* Thyme (p. 574)

Natusor Jaquesan *Soria Natural, Spain,* Lime Flower (p. 409), Melissa (p. 425), Willow (p. 598), Yarrow (p. 604)

Natusor Low Blood Pressure *Soria Natural, Spain,* Ginseng, Eleutherococcus (p. 315), Liquorice (p. 411), Rosemary (p. 508), Sage (p. 512)

Natusor Malvasen *Soria Natural, Spain,* Marshmallow (p. 418), Senna (p. 537)

Natusor Renal *Soria Natural, Spain,* Meadowsweet (p. 423), Thyme (p. 574)

Natusor Sinulan *Soria Natural, Spain,* Elder (p. 237), Lime Flower (p. 409), Rosemary (p. 508), Thyme (p. 574)

Natusor Somnisedan *Soria Natural, Spain,* Hawthorn (p. 346), Lime Flower (p. 409), St John's Wort (p. 549), Valerian (p. 580)

Neda Fruchtewurfel *Gebro Pharma GmbH, Austria,* Senna (p. 537)

Negacne *Wierhom Pharma S.A., Argentina,* Aloe Vera (p. 48), Coltsfoot (p. 185)

Nenegloss *Laboratorios Maver SA, Chile,* Aloe Vera (p. 48)

Neo Baby Gripe Mixture *Alinter Ltd, UK,* Ginger (p. 293)

Neo Gripe Mixture *Alinter Ltd, UK,* Ginger (p. 293)

Neo Urgenin *Madaus, Spain,* Echinacea (p. 217), Saw Palmetto (p. 521)

Neo-Atropan *Laboratorios Quim-Far C.A., Venezuela,* Aniseed (p. 57)

Neo-Cleanse *GNLD International P/L, Australia,* Alfalfa (p. 45), Aniseed (p. 57), Liquorice (p. 411), Rhubarb (p. 506), Senna (p. 537)

Neo-Codion *Laboratoires Bouchara-Recordati, France,* Senega (p. 533)

Neo-Codion Babies (Нео-Кодион Для Младенцев**)** *FIC Medical, Russia,* Senega (p. 533)

Neoderma 47 *Neovita S.a.s. di G. Pirotta & C., Italy,* Vervain (p. 591)

Neoform *Pietrasanta Pharma S.r.l., Italy,* Frangula (p. 270), Rhubarb (p. 506)

Neo-Healar *Antah Pharma Sdb Bhd, Malaysia,* Aloe Vera (p. 48)

Neomyrt Plus *Baif International Products, New York S.n.c., Italy,* Bilberry (p. 79), Hydrocotyle (p. 371)

Neoplex *Austroplant-Arzneimittel GmbH, Austria,* Liquorice (p. 411)

Neoplus *Laboratorio Terapeutico M.R. S.r.l., Italy,* Ginseng, Panax (p. 325)

Neostrata *Lab Medstyle SA, Chile,* Liquorice (p. 411)

nephro-loges *Dr. Loges & Co. GmbH, Germany,* Parsley (p. 456)

Nephronorm med *Mauermann-Arzneimittel, Franz Mauermann oHG, Germany,* Calendula (p. 121), Java Tea (p. 381)

Nephrosal *Slovakofarma sro, Czech Republic,* Nettle (p. 452)

Nephroselect M *Dreluso Pharmazeutika, Dr Elten & Sohn GmbH, Germany,* Saw Palmetto (p. 521)

Nephrubin-N *Weber & Weber GmbH & Co. KG, Germany,* Java Tea (p. 381)

Nerex *Farmanova AFM S.r.l., Italy,* Bilberry (p. 79)

Nerfood Tablets *Frank Roberts (Herbal Dispensaries) Ltd, UK,* Asafoetida (p. 72), Valerian (p. 580)

Nervatona Plus *Brauer Natural Medicine P/L, Australia,* False Unicorn (p. 258), Ginseng, Panax (p. 325), Passionflower (p. 461)

Nervendragees *ratiopharm GmbH, Germany,* Hops (p. 354), Passionflower (p. 461), Valerian (p. 580)

Nerven-Dragees *ProMedico Ltd, Israel,* Hawthorn (p. 346), Hops (p. 354), Passionflower (p. 461), Valerian (p. 580)

Nervenkapseln *ratiopharm GmbH, Germany,* Hops (p. 354), Valerian (p. 580)

Nervenruh *Maria Clementine Martin Klosterfrau GmbH, Austria,* Hops (p. 354), Passionflower (p. 461), Valerian (p. 580)

Nerventee St Severin *EF-EM-ES - Dr Smetana & Co., Austria,* Hops (p. 354), St John's Wort (p. 549), Valerian (p. 580)

Nervikan *Laboratorios DHU Ibérica, S.A., Spain,* Melissa (p. 425), Valerian (p. 580)

Nervinetas *Comercial GFC SA de CV, Mexico,* Hops (p. 354), Valerian (p. 580) *Grünenthal Venezolana C.A., Venezuela,* Hops (p. 354), Valerian (p. 580)

Nervinetten *Zellaforte Vertriebsanstalt, Switzerland,* Hops (p. 354), Valerian (p. 580)

Nervinfant N *RubiePharm Vertriebs GmbH, Germany,* Hops (p. 354), Passionflower (p. 461)

Nervocalm *Lab. Garden House S.A., Argentina,* Lime Flower (p. 409), Melissa (p. 425), Passionflower (p. 461), Valerian (p. 580)

Nervoregin forte *Homöopathisches Laboratorium A. Pflüger GmbH, Germany,* Hops (p. 354), Passionflower (p. 461), Valerian (p. 580)

Nervous Dyspepsia Tablets *Frank Roberts (Herbal Dispensaries) Ltd, UK,* Dandelion (p. 204), Ginger (p. 293), Myrrh (p. 449), Rhubarb (p. 506), Valerian (p. 580)

Nervova Cajova Smes *Megafyt-R sro, Czech Republic,* Melissa (p. 425), Valerian (p. 580)

Nesfare *Madaus, Spain,* Hydrocotyle (p. 371)

Nesthakchen *Schülke & Mayr GmbH, Austria,* Aniseed (p. 57), Liquorice (p. 411)

Neurapas *Pascoe Pharmazeutische Präparate GmbH, Germany,* Passionflower (p. 461), St John's Wort (p. 549), Valerian (p. 580)

Neurocardol *Confar, Lda, Portugal,* Hawthorn (p. 346), Passionflower (p. 461), Valerian (p. 580), Willow (p. 598)

Neuroflorine *Laboratoires Fuca, France,* Hawthorn (p. 346), Passionflower (p. 461), Valerian (p. 580)

Neuropax *SERP, Monaco,* Hawthorn (p. 346), Passionflower (p. 461)

Nevaton *Mediherb P/L, Australia,* Damiana (p. 201), Scullcap (p. 530), St John's Wort (p. 549), Vervain (p. 591)

Nevril *Amnol Chimica Biologica S.r.l., Italy,* Calendula (p. 121), Devil's Claw (p. 207), Willow (p. 598), Witch Hazel (p. 601)

New Patecs A *Hong Kong Medical Supplies Ltd, Hong Kong,* Arnica (p. 64)

Newrelax *Potter's (Herbal Supplies) Ltd, UK,* Hops (p. 354), Scullcap (p. 530), Valerian (p. 580), Vervain (p. 591)

Nican *F. Uhlmann-Eyraud SA, Switzerland,* Drosera (p. 215), Thyme (p. 574)

Nico Hepatocyn *Uriach, Spain,* Aloes (p. 50), Artichoke (p. 67), Boldo (p. 91), Cascara (p. 128)

Nicoprive *Laboratoires DB Pharma, France,* Hawthorn (p. 346)

Nighttime Herb *Worldwide Health Corp. Ltd, UK,* Passionflower (p. 461), Valerian (p. 580)

Nigroids *Ernest Jackson & Co. Ltd, UK,* Liquorice (p. 411)

Ninfagin *Ricerca, Produzione e Commercializzazione di Prodotti Farmaceutici e Cosmetici Srl, Italy,* Aloe Vera (p. 48)

Nitrangin compositum *Alpharma-Isis GmbH & Co. KG, Germany,* Valerian (p. 580)

Noctis *Bouty SpA, Italy,* Hawthorn (p. 346), Passionflower (p. 461), Valerian (p. 580)

Nocvalene *Laboratoires Arkopharma, France,* Hawthorn (p. 346), Passionflower (p. 461)

Noditran *Naturland, Hungary,* Yarrow (p. 604)

Nodoff *Potter's (Herbal Supplies) Ltd, UK,* Hops (p. 354), Ispaghula (p. 374), Passionflower (p. 461), Scullcap (p. 530), Valerian (p. 580)

No-Gras *Higaté Medical Argentina, Argentina,* Hydrocotyle (p. 371)

Nontusyl *Slovakofarma sro, Czech Republic,* Agrimony (p. 42), Lime Flower (p. 409), Marshmallow (p. 418), Melissa (p. 425), Thyme (p. 574)

Nordimenty *Química Franco Mexicana Nordin S.A. de C.V., Mexico,* Melissa (p. 425), St John's Wort (p. 549)

Normacol *Schering Mexicana S.A. de C.V., Mexico,* Frangula (p. 270)

Normacol Forte *Norgine de España, Spain,* Frangula (p. 270)

Normacol Plus *Norgine P/L, Australia,* Frangula (p. 270) *Norgine SA, Belgium,* Frangula (p. 270) *Treasure Mountain Development Co. Ltd, Hong Kong,* Frangula (p. 270) *United Drug, Ireland,* Frangula (p. 270) *Angelini, Portugal,* Frangula (p. 270) *Grafton Pharmasia Pte Ltd, Singapore,* Frangula (p. 270) *Norgine (Pty) Ltd, South Africa,* Frangula (p. 270) *Norgine Pharmaceuticals Ltd, UK,* Frangula (p. 270) *CSL (NZ) Ltd, Zuellig Pharma, New Zealand,* Frangula (p. 270)

Normoprost Plus *Lab. Temis Lostaló S.A., Argentina,* Saw Palmetto (p. 521)

Nostress *Laboratoires Robert Schwartz, France,* Ginseng, Panax (p. 325), Hops (p. 354)

No-Tos Adultos *Química Medical Arg. S.A.C.I., Argentina,* Liquorice (p. 411), Senega (p. 533)

No-Tos Infantil *Química Medical Arg. S.A.C.I., Argentina,* Liquorice (p. 411), Senega (p. 533)

Notosil *Grunenthal Chilena Ltda, Chile,* Drosera (p. 215)

Novarrutina *Zurita Laboratório Farmacêutico Ltda, Brazil,* Horse-chestnut (p. 363)

Novicarbon *C.T.S. Chemical Industries Ltd, Israel,* Rhubarb (p. 506), Senna (p. 537)

Novocholin *Adler-Apotheke, Austria,* Agrimony (p. 42), Rhubarb (p. 506)

Novo-Passit *Ivax-CR as, Ivax-CR as, Czech Republic,* Elder (p. 237), Hawthorn (p. 346), Hops (p. 354), Melissa (p. 425), Passionflower (p. 461), St John's Wort (p. 549), Valerian (p. 580)

Noxivid *Biofarma Natural CMD SA de CV, Mexico,* Uva-Ursi (p. 577)

N-T-Tus *Zydus Cadila Group, India,* Liquorice (p. 411)

Nucolox *Sigma Pharmaceuticals P/L, Australia,* Ispaghula (p. 374)

Nytol Herbal *GlaxoSmithKline Consumer Healthcare, UK,* Hops (p. 354), Ispaghula (p. 374), Passionflower (p. 461), Pulsatilla (p. 489), Wild Lettuce (p. 596)

Obeflorine *Laboratoires Lehning, France,* Couchgrass (p. 193)

Oculosan *Novartis Pharma Schweiz AG, Switzerland,* Eyebright (p. 256), Witch Hazel (p. 601)

Ocusense *Natrol, USA,* Bilberry (p. 79)

Oddispasmol *Ratiopharm Arzneimittel Vertriebs-GmbH, Austria,* Fumitory (p. 276)

Odisor *Soria Natural, Spain,* Boldo (p. 91), Centaury (p. 149), Fumitory (p. 276)

Odontal *G. Streuli & Co. AG, Switzerland,* Cinnamon (p. 162), Clove (p. 166)

Odontobiotic *Higaté Medical Argentina, Argentina,* Aloe Vera (p. 48), Calendula (p. 121)

Odor Eze *Novartis New Zealand Ltd, New Zealand,* Aloe Vera (p. 48)

Odourless Garlic *Blackmores Ltd, Australia,* Garlic (p. 279), Parsley (p. 456) *Vitaplex Products, Australia,* Echinacea (p. 217), Garlic (p. 279)

Ojosbel *Dermofarm, Spain,* Witch Hazel (p. 601)

Oleum Rhinale Nasal Oil *Pharma-Natura (Pty) Ltd, South Africa,* Calendula (p. 121)

Olocynan *Makros Indústria Farmacêutica Ltda, Brazil,* Artichoke (p. 67)

Omega *Dr A & L Schmidgall, Austria,* Hawthorn (p. 346)

Omega-3 Complex *Natrol, USA,* Borage (p. 96)

Omega-3 Glucosamine *Natrol, USA,* Borage (p. 96)

One Drop Spray *Laboratorios Politecnicos Nacionales C.A., Venezuela,* Myrrh (p. 449), Sage (p. 512)

Onguent aux herbes Keller *UB Interpharm SA, Switzerland,* Arnica (p. 64), Calendula (p. 121)

Onopordon Comp B *Weleda (UK) Ltd, UK,* Cowslip (p. 195)

Onrectal *Herbes Universelles, Canada,* Witch Hazel (p. 601)

Ophtalmine *Coopération Pharmaceutique Francaise, France,* Witch Hazel (p. 601)

Opobyl *Spedrog Caillon S.A.I.y C., Argentina,* Boldo (p. 91) *Laboratoires Bailly SPEAB, France,* Aloes (p. 50), Boldo (p. 91) *Uriach, Spain,* Aloes (p. 50), Boldo (p. 91)

Opo-Veinogene *Alpharma France, France,* Horse-chestnut (p. 363)

Opplin *TNP Health Care Co. Ltd, Thailand,* Witch Hazel (p. 601)

Optimina Plus *Lab. Temis Lostaló S.A., Argentina,* Ginseng, Panax (p. 325)

Optrex *Boots Healthcare Australia P/L, Australia,* Witch Hazel (p. 601)

Optrex compresses *Boots Healthcare (Switzerland) AG, Hermal, Switzerland,* Witch Hazel (p. 601)

Optrex Red Eyes *Crookes Healthcare Ltd, UK,* Witch Hazel (p. 601)

OptrexRed-Eye Relief *Boots Healthcare New Zealand Ltd, New Zealand,* Witch Hazel (p. 601)

Orafilm *Laboratorios Rowe-Fleming C.A., Venezuela,* Rhubarb (p. 506)

Oralsone Topic *Laboratorios Gramón, Argentina,* Rhubarb (p. 506)

OraMagicRx *MPM Medical Inc., USA,* Aloe Vera (p. 48)

Original Grosser Bittner Balsam (Оригинальный Большой Бальзам Биттнера) *Herbs Trading GmbH, Russia,* Aloes (p. 50), Angelica (p. 53), Aniseed (p. 57), Bogbean (p. 89), Calamus (p. 118), Centaury (p. 149), Clove (p. 166), Elecampane (p. 240), Gentian (p. 290), Ginger (p. 293), Holy Thistle (p. 352), Liquorice (p. 411), Myrrh (p. 449), Yarrow (p. 604)

Original Herb Cough Drops *Ricola, Canada,* Cowslip (p. 195), Elder (p. 237), Marshmallow (p. 418), Sage (p. 512), Thyme (p. 574), Yarrow (p. 604)

Original Schwedenbitter *Riviera Handelsgesellschaft.m.b.h., Austria,* Angelica (p. 53), Calamus (p. 118), Dandelion (p. 204), Gentian (p. 290), Myrrh (p. 449)

Ortisan *Cabassi & Giuriati S.p.A., Italy,* Senna (p. 537)

Osmogel *Alphrema S.r.l., Italy,* Hydrocotyle (p. 371)

Ottovis *Laboratorio Fitolife S.r.l., Italy,* Ginseng, Panax (p. 325)

Out-of-Sorts *Potter's (Herbal Supplies) Ltd, UK,* Aloes (p. 50), Cascara (p. 128), Dandelion (p. 204), Senna (p. 537)

Ovumix *Laboratorio Elea S.A.C.I.F.yA., Argentina,* Hydrocotyle (p. 371)

Oxacant-sedativ *Dr Gustav Klein, Germany,* Hawthorn (p. 346), Melissa (p. 425), Motherwort (p. 447), Valerian (p. 580)

30 Plus *Ranbaxy (Malaysia) Sdn Bhd, Malaysia,* Ginseng, Panax (p. 325)

Pacifenity *Vitaplex Products, Australia,* Gentian (p. 290), Hops (p. 354), Milk Thistle (p. 429), Motherwort (p. 447), Passionflower (p. 461), Scullcap (p. 530), Valerian (p. 580)

Padma-Lax *Padma AG, Switzerland,* Aloes (p. 50), Cascara (p. 128), Frangula (p. 270), Gentian (p. 290), Ginger (p. 293), Rhubarb (p. 506)

Padmed Laxan *Padma AG, Switzerland,* Aloes (p. 50), Cascara (p. 128), Elecampane (p. 240), Frangula (p. 270), Gentian (p. 290), Ginger (p. 293), Rhubarb (p. 506)

Palatrobil *Monserrat y Eclair S.A., Argentina,* Artichoke (p. 67), Wild Carrot (p. 593)

Palmetto Plus *Usana, Singapore,* Saw Palmetto (p. 521)

Paltomiel *Laboratorio Esp. Med. Knop Ltda, Chile,* Aniseed (p. 57)

Paltomiel Plus *Laboratorio Esp. Med. Knop Ltda, Chile,* Echinacea (p. 217), Marshmallow (p. 418)

Panax Complex *Blackmores Ltd, Australia,* Alfalfa (p. 45), Fenugreek (p. 260), Ginseng, Panax (p. 325)

Pansoral Teething (Пансорал Первые Зубы) *Pierre Fabre Medicament, Russia,* Marshmallow (p. 418)

Panxeol *Laboratoires IPRAD, France,* Passionflower (p. 461)

Paracodin *Abbott GmbH, Austria,* Marshmallow (p. 418), Thyme (p. 574)

Paradenton *Austroplant-Arzneimittel GmbH, Austria,* Myrrh (p. 449), Sage (p. 512)

Parapsyllium *Laboratoires IPRAD, France,* Ispaghula (p. 374)

Paratonico *Multilab Ind. e Com. Prods. Farmacêuticos Ltda, Brazil,* Aloes (p. 50), Cinnamon (p. 162), Myrrh (p. 449)

Parche Negro Belladona *Química y Farmacia, S.A. de C.V., Mexico,* Capsicum (p. 125)

Parodium *Pierre Fabre Argentina S.A., Argentina,* Rhubarb (p. 506) *Laboratoires Pierre Fabre, France,* Rhubarb (p. 506)

Parodium (Пародиум) *Pierre Fabre Medicament, Russia,* Rhubarb (p. 506)

Parodontal *Serumwerk Bernburg AG, Germany,* Sage (p. 512)

Parodontax *GlaxoSmithKline Pharma, Austria,* Echinacea (p. 217), Myrrh (p. 449) *GlaxoSmithKline Brasil Ltda, Brazil,* Echinacea (p. 217), Myrrh (p. 449)

Parodontax Fluor *GlaxoSmithKline S.A., Argentina,* Echinacea (p. 217), Myrrh (p. 449), Sage (p. 512)

Parogencyl prevention gencives *Sanofi Synthelabo OTC, France,* Ginkgo (p. 299)

Parvisedil *Specialità Igienico Terapeutiche S.r.l., Italy,* Hawthorn (p. 346), Passionflower (p. 461), Valerian (p. 580)

Pasalix *Marjan Indústria e Comércio Ltda, Brazil,* Hawthorn (p. 346), Passionflower (p. 461), Willow (p. 598)

Pascosedon *Pascoe Pharmazeutische Präparate GmbH, Germany,* Hops (p. 354), Melissa (p. 425), Valerian (p. 580)

Pasidor *CAFAR (Compania Anonima Farmaceutica), Venezuela,* Hawthorn (p. 346), Passionflower (p. 461), Valerian (p. 580)

Pasifluidina *Productos Gache S.A., Venezuela,* Hawthorn (p. 346), Passionflower (p. 461), Valerian (p. 580)

Pasinordin *Química Franco Mexicana Nordin S.A. de C.V., Mexico,* Passionflower (p. 461)

Passacanthine *Lab. Lafage S.R.L., Argentina,* Hawthorn (p. 346), Passionflower (p. 461)

Passaneuro *Bunker Indústria Farmacêutica Ltda, Brazil,* Melissa (p. 425), Passionflower (p. 461)

Passedan *Dr Peithner KG nunmehr GmbH & Co., Austria,* Cinnamon (p. 162) *Austroplant-Arzneimittel GmbH, Austria,* Melissa (p. 425), Passionflower (p. 461)

Passelyt *Gebro Pharma GmbH, Austria,* Melissa (p. 425), Passionflower (p. 461)

Passi Catha *Laboratório Sedabel Ltda, Brazil,* Hawthorn (p. 346), Passionflower (p. 461), Willow (p. 598)

Passicalm *Laboratórios Gemballa Ltda, Brazil,* Passionflower (p. 461), Valerian (p. 580)

Passiflora *Tamar Marketing, Israel,* Hawthorn (p. 346), Passionflower (p. 461), Valerian (p. 580)

Passiflora Complex *Blackmores Ltd, Australia,* Hops (p. 354), Passionflower (p. 461), Scullcap (p. 530), Valerian (p. 580)

Passiflora Composta *Infabra Indústria Farmacêutica Brasileira Ltda, Brazil,* Hawthorn (p. 346), Passionflower (p. 461)

Passiflora Compound *Vitamed Ltd, Israel,* Passionflower (p. 461), Valerian (p. 580)

Passiflorine *Produtos Farmacêuticos Millet Roux Ltda, Brazil,* Hawthorn (p. 346), Passionflower (p. 461), Willow (p. 598) *Laboratoires Jolly-Jatel, France,* Hawthorn (p. 346) *Laboratoires Jolly-Jatel, France,* Passionflower (p. 461) *Teofarma, Italy,* Hawthorn (p. 346), Passionflower (p. 461), Willow (p. 598) *Chiesi España, Spain,* Hawthorn (p. 346), Passionflower (p. 461)

Passiflorum *Zuoz Pharma S.A., Venezuela,* Hawthorn (p. 346), Passionflower (p. 461), Willow (p. 598)

Passilex *Luper Indústria Farmacêutica Ltda, Brazil,* Melissa (p. 425), Passionflower (p. 461)

Passin *Georg Simons GmbH, Germany,* Hawthorn (p. 346), Passionflower (p. 461)

Passinevryl *Laboratoires Clément-Thionville, France,* Hawthorn (p. 346), Passionflower (p. 461), Valerian (p. 580)

4

Passionflower Plus *Eagle Pharmaceuticals P/L, Australia,* Hops (p. 354), Passionflower (p. 461), Scullcap (p. 530), Valerian (p. 580)

Pastillas Pectoral Kely *Boots Healthcare, Spain,* Liquorice (p. 411), Senega (p. 533)

Pastilles bronchiques S nouvelle formule *Hänseler AG, Switzerland,* Drosera (p. 215), Liquorice (p. 411)

Pastilles Monleon *Laboratoires Toulade, France,* Drosera (p. 215), Witch Hazel (p. 601)

Pastilles pectorales Demo N *Vifor SA, Switzerland,* Drosera (p. 215), Plantain (p. 474)

Pazbronquial *Cinfa, Spain,* Drosera (p. 215), Marshmallow (p. 418)

PC 30 V *Terra-Bio-Chemie GmbH, Germany,* Horse-chestnut (p. 363)

PC Regulax *Biovital Pty Ltd, Australia,* Ginger (p. 293), Ispaghula (p. 374), Slippery Elm (p. 545)

Pectal *Laboratório Sedabel Ltda, Brazil,* Senega (p. 533)

Pectobron *Laboratorios Sidus S.A., Argentina,* Senega (p. 533)

Pectocalmine *Vifor SA, Switzerland,* Senega (p. 533)

Pectoral N *Mepha Pharma AG, Switzerland,* Cowslip (p. 195), Plantain (p. 474), Senega (p. 533), Thyme (p. 574)

Pectoral Pasteur *Laboratorios Pasteur Ltda, Chile,* Drosera (p. 215), Liquorice (p. 411)

Pedicrem *Laboratorios Prieto S.A., Argentina,* Aloe Vera (p. 48)

Peerless Composition Essence *Potter's (Herbal Supplies) Ltd, UK,* Bayberry (p. 77)

Pegina *Potter's (Herbal Supplies) Ltd, UK,* Calamus (p. 118), Rhubarb (p. 506)

Peitoral Angico Pelotense *Companhia Industrial Farmacêutica, Brazil,* Liquorice (p. 411), Marshmallow (p. 418)

Peking Ginseng Royal Jelly N *Peking Royal Jelly Deutschland BOELL HandelsKontor, Germany,* Ginseng, Panax (p. 325)

Penaten *Johnson & Johnson/Merck Consumer Pharmaceuticals of Canada, Canada,* Witch Hazel (p. 601)

Pentol *Laboratorios Sidus S.A., Argentina,* Hydrocotyle (p. 371)

Pepsitase *B L Hua & Co. Ltd, Thailand,* Gentian (p. 290)

Peptochol *Laboratorios Grossman S.A. de C.V., Mexico,* Boldo (p. 91)

Percutane *Douglas Pharmaceuticals Australia Ltd, Australia,* Aloe Vera (p. 48), Arnica (p. 64), Burdock (p. 102)

Perdiem *Novartis Consumer Health Inc., USA,* Ispaghula (p. 374), Senna (p. 537)

Period Pain Relief *Herbal Concepts Ltd, UK,* False Unicorn (p. 258), Motherwort (p. 447), Pulsatilla (p. 489), Valerian (p. 580), Vervain (p. 591)

Peritone *Blackmores Ltd, Australia,* Aloes (p. 50), Cascara (p. 128), Ginger (p. 293), Senna (p. 537)

Perivar *Ipsen Pharma GmbH, Germany,* Ginkgo (p. 299)

Perospir *Slovakofarma sro, Czech Republic,* Coltsfoot (p. 185), Elder (p. 237), Nettle (p. 452), Thyme (p. 574), Yarrow (p. 604)

Persen *Lek Pharma sro, Czech Republic,* Melissa (p. 425), Valerian (p. 580)

Persen (Персен) *Lek, Russia,* Melissa (p. 425), Valerian (p. 580)

Perskindol Cool Arnica *Vifor SA, Switzerland,* Arnica (p. 64)

Petites Pilules Carters *Laboratoires Fumouze, France,* Aloes (p. 50)

Phlebosedol *Laboratoires Lehning, France,* Horse-chestnut (p. 363), Witch Hazel (p. 601)

Phol-Tux *Interdelta SA, Switzerland,* Senega (p. 533)

Photoderm Flush *Bioderma, France,* Ginkgo (p. 299)

Phyto Corrective Gel *Dispolab Farmaceutica SA, Chile,* Thyme (p. 574)

Phytobronchin *Steigerwald Arzneimittelwerk GmbH, Germany,* Cowslip (p. 195), Thyme (p. 574)

Phyto-Ease *Great Liaison Ltd, Hong Kong,* Saw Palmetto (p. 521)

Phytoestrin *Usana, Singapore,* Agnus Castus (p. 36), Cohosh, Black (p. 168), Liquorice (p. 411)

Phyto-Laxia *Phytopharma SA, Switzerland,* Frangula (p. 270), Senna (p. 537)

Phytolaxin *Hänseler AG, Switzerland,* Aloes (p. 50), Frangula (p. 270), Senna (p. 537)

Phytomed Cardio *Phytomed AG, Switzerland,* Hawthorn (p. 346), Passionflower (p. 461), Rosemary (p. 508)

Phytomelis *Laboratoires Lehning, France,* Horse-chestnut (p. 363), Witch Hazel (p. 601)

Phytonoctu *Steigerwald Arzneimittelwerk GmbH, Germany,* Melissa (p. 425), Passionflower (p. 461), Valerian (p. 580)

Pi-Fedrin *Laboratorios Flupal C.A., Venezuela,* Drosera (p. 215)

Pik Gel *Amnol Chimica Biologica S.r.l., Italy,* Bilberry (p. 79), Devil's Claw (p. 207), Ginger (p. 293), Ginkgo (p. 299), Horse-chestnut (p. 363), Hydrocotyle (p. 371), Meadowsweet (p. 423), Yarrow (p. 604)

Pildoras Zeninas *Puerto Galiano, Spain,* Aloes (p. 50), Cascara (p. 128)

Pileabs *G.R. Lane Health Products Ltd, UK,* Cascara (p. 128), Slippery Elm (p. 545)

Piletabs *Potter's (Herbal Supplies) Ltd, UK,* Agrimony (p. 42), Cascara (p. 128), Pilewort (p. 472), Stone Root (p. 570)

Pilka *Gebro Pharma GmbH, Austria,* Drosera (p. 215), Thyme (p. 574) *Novartis Ltd, Israel,* Drosera (p. 215), Thyme (p. 574) *Ferrer Farma, Spain,* Drosera (p. 215), Thyme (p. 574)

Pilka F *Novartis Consumer Health, Lda, Portugal,* Drosera (p. 215)

Pilka Forte *Gebro Pharma GmbH, Austria,* Drosera (p. 215), Thyme (p. 574)

Pilulas De Witt's *Companhia Industrial Farmacêutica, Brazil,* Cascara (p. 128), Juniper (p. 386), Uva-Ursi (p. 577)

Pilulas Ross *GlaxoSmithKline Brasil Ltda, Brazil,* Capsicum (p. 125)

Pinvex *Laboratorios Cofasa S.A., Venezuela,* Rhubarb (p. 506)

Piodermina *Farmachimici S.r.l., Italy,* Thyme (p. 574)

Planta Lax *Hoeveler Mag. & Co. GmbH, Austria,* Frangula (p. 270), Senna (p. 537)

Plantax *Farmion Laboratório Brasileiro de Farmacologia Ltda, Brazil,* Ispaghula (p. 374), Senna (p. 537)

Plantiodine Plus *Blackmores Ltd, Australia,* Alfalfa (p. 45)

Plantival *Laboratorios Farmasa, S.A. de C.V., Mexico,* Melissa (p. 425), Valerian (p. 580)

Plantival novo *Dr Willmar Schwabe GmbH & Co., Germany,* Melissa (p. 425), Valerian (p. 580)

Pleumolysin *Ivax-CR as, Ivax-CR as, Czech Republic,* Thyme (p. 574)

PMS Control *Natrol, USA,* Evening Primrose (p. 251), Parsley (p. 456)

PMS Support *Vitaplex Products, Australia,* Buchu (p. 100), Ginger (p. 293)

PMT Complex *Mayne Pharma P/L, Mayne Pharma P/L, Australia,* Agnus Castus (p. 36), Cohosh, Black (p. 168), Ginger (p. 293)

PMT Formula *Vitalia Health Ltd, UK,* Passionflower (p. 461), Valerian (p. 580)

Pneumopan *Gebro Pharma GmbH, Austria,* Thyme (p. 574)

Pneumopect *Gebro Pharma GmbH, Austria,* Thyme (p. 574)

Poliseng *Laboratório Teuto-Brasileiro Ltda, Brazil,* Ginseng, Panax (p. 325)

Polypirine *Laboratoires Lehning, France,* Meadowsweet (p. 423)

Pommade au Baume *Max Zeller Söhne AG, Pflanzliche Heilmittel, Switzerland,* Guaiacum (p. 344), Myrrh (p. 449), Yarrow (p. 604)

Postopyl *Laboratoires d'Evolution Dermatologique, France,* Aloe Vera (p. 48)

Potassium Iodide and Stramonium Compound *J. McGloin P/L, Australia,* Liquorice (p. 411), Marshmallow (p. 418)

Potter's Catarrh Pastilles *Ernest Jackson & Co. Ltd, UK,* Marshmallow (p. 418)

Potters Children's Cough Pastilles *Ernest Jackson & Co. Ltd, UK,* St John's Wort (p. 549)

Potters Gees Linctus *Ernest Jackson & Co. Ltd, UK,* St John's Wort (p. 549)

Potters Sugar Free Cough Pastilles *Ernest Jackson & Co. Ltd, UK,* Liquorice (p. 411)

PR21 *Laboratorios Sigma, Argentina,* Saw Palmetto (p. 521)

Prementaid *Potter's (Herbal Supplies) Ltd, UK,* Motherwort (p. 447), Pulsatilla (p. 489), Uva-Ursi (p. 577), Valerian (p. 580), Vervain (p. 591)

Preparation H Cooling Gel *Whitehall-Robins Inc., Canada,* Witch Hazel (p. 601) *Wyeth Consumer Healthcare Inc., USA,* Witch Hazel (p. 601)

Prespir *Representaciones Mex-America S.A. de C.V., Mexico,* Witch Hazel (p. 601)

Prinachol *Zurita Laboratório Farmacêutico Ltda, Brazil,* Artichoke (p. 67), Boldo (p. 91)

Pripsen *Thornton & Ross Ltd, UK,* Senna (p. 537)

Prisoventril *Laboratório Simões Ltda, Brazil,* Cascara (p. 128)

ProAktiv *Boehringer Ingelheim Austria GmbH, Austria,* Ginseng, Panax (p. 325)

Probigol *Omeofarma S.r.l., Italy,* Echinacea (p. 217)

ProBrain *Seven Seas Ltd, UK,* Ginkgo (p. 299)

Procold *Biovital Pty Ltd, Australia,* Euphorbia (p. 249), Garlic (p. 279), Horseradish (p. 367)

Proctoplex *Laboratorio Esp. Med. Knop Ltda, Chile,* Horse-chestnut (p. 363), Witch Hazel (p. 601)

Proctopure *Dermofarma Italia S.r.l., Italy,* Calendula (p. 121), Horse-chestnut (p. 363), Liquorice (p. 411), Witch Hazel (p. 601)

Proctosan *Kley Hertz SA, Brazil,* Horse-chestnut (p. 363), Witch Hazel (p. 601)

Proctosor *Soria Natural, Spain,* Golden Seal (p. 337), Senna (p. 537)

Prodiem Plus *Novartis Consumer Health Canada Inc., Canada,* Ispaghula (p. 374), Senna (p. 537)

Proesten *Biovital Pty Ltd, Australia,* Cohosh, Black (p. 168), Garlic (p. 279), Passionflower (p. 461), Sarsaparilla (p. 515)

Profelan *M & A Pharmachem Ltd, UK,* Arnica (p. 64)

Proflo *Biovital Pty Ltd, Australia,* Horse-chestnut (p. 363), Pulsatilla (p. 489), Witch Hazel (p. 601)

Profluid *Biovital Pty Ltd, Australia,* Dandelion (p. 204), Juniper (p. 386), Parsley Piert (p. 459), Uva-Ursi (p. 577)

Projimava *Megafyt-R sro, Czech Republic,* Liquorice (p. 411), Senna (p. 537), Yarrow (p. 604)

Prolax *Biovital Pty Ltd, Australia,* Senna (p. 537)

Pronervon Phyto *Dr Scheffler Nachf. GmbH & Co. KG, Germany,* Melissa (p. 425), Passionflower (p. 461), Valerian (p. 580)

Prophthal *Biovital Pty Ltd, Australia,* Bilberry (p. 79), Ginkgo (p. 299)

Prosed-X *Biovital Pty Ltd, Australia,* Hops (p. 354), Passionflower (p. 461), Valerian (p. 580)

Prosgutt *Laboratorios Farmasa, S.A. de C.V., Mexico,* Nettle (p. 452), Saw Palmetto (p. 521)

Prost-1 *Biovital Pty Ltd, Australia,* Devil's Claw (p. 207), Willow (p. 598), Yucca (p. 610)

Prosta-Caps Chassot N *Doetsch Grether AG, Switzerland,* Echinacea (p. 217), Java Tea (p. 381), Saw Palmetto (p. 521)

Prostagutt *Austroplant-Arzneimittel GmbH, Austria,* Nettle (p. 452), Saw Palmetto (p. 521)

Prostagutt forte *Dr Willmar Schwabe GmbH & Co., Germany,* Nettle (p. 452), Saw Palmetto (p. 521)

Prostagutt-F *Schwabe Pharma AG, Switzerland,* Nettle (p. 452), Saw Palmetto (p. 521)

Prostaid *Healthy Direct, UK,* Saw Palmetto (p. 521)

Prostakan Forte *Arzneimittel Schwabe International GmbH, Czech Republic,* Nettle (p. 452), Saw Palmetto (p. 521)

Prostanorm (Простанорм) *Farm Vilar ZAO, Russia,* Echinacea (p. 217), Liquorice (p. 411), St John's Wort (p. 549)

Prostaplant *Marvecs Services Srl, Italy,* Nettle (p. 452), Saw Palmetto (p. 521)

Prostate Ease *Swiss Herbal Remedies Ltd, Canada,* Saw Palmetto (p. 521)

Prostate Health *Sundown, USA,* Nettle (p. 452), Saw Palmetto (p. 521)

ProstatExcell *Natrol, USA,* Saw Palmetto (p. 521)

Prostatonin *Madaus GmbH, Austria,* Nettle (p. 452) *Boehringer Ingelheim sro, Czech Republic,* Nettle (p. 452) *Pharmaton SA, Switzerland,* Nettle (p. 452)

Prostease *Jamieson Laboratories, Canada,* Cranberry (p. 197), Saw Palmetto (p. 521) *Universal Pharmaceutical Lab Ltd, Hong Kong,* Cranberry (p. 197), Saw Palmetto (p. 521)

Prostem Plus *Laboratórios Baldacci S.A., Brazil,* Nettle (p. 452)

ProstGard *Holista Health Corp, Canada,* Saw Palmetto (p. 521)

Protecor *Duopharm GmbH, Germany,* Hawthorn (p. 346)

Protemp *Biovital Pty Ltd, Australia,* Juniper (p. 386), Parsley Piert (p. 459), Uva-Ursi (p. 577)

Protol *Biovital Pty Ltd, Australia,* Garlic (p. 279)

Proyeast *Biovital Pty Ltd, Australia,* Chaparral (p. 159), Echinacea (p. 217), Garlic (p. 279)

Pruduskova *Megafyt-R sro, Czech Republic,* Lime Flower (p. 409), Liquorice (p. 411), Marshmallow (p. 418)

Pruina *Faes Farma, Spain,* Senna (p. 537)

Prunacolon *Nycomed BV, Netherlands,* Senna (p. 537)

Prunasine *Nycomed BV, Netherlands,* Senna (p. 537)

Psor-Asist *Sunspot Products P/L, Australia,* Aloe Vera (p. 48)

Psorasolv *Potter's (Herbal Supplies) Ltd, UK,* Clivers (p. 164), Pokeroot (p. 479)

Pulmagol *Laboratorios Pasteur Ltda, Chile,* Drosera (p. 215), Marshmallow (p. 418)

Pulmofasa *Generfarma, Spain,* Senega (p. 533)

Pulmoforte *Laboratórios Osorio de Moraes Ltda, Brazil,* Marshmallow (p. 418)

Pulmoran *Leros sro, Czech Republic,* Elder (p. 237), Liquorice (p. 411), Marshmallow (p. 418), Nettle (p. 452), Sage (p. 512), Thyme (p. 574)

Pulmotin *Serumwerk Bernburg AG, Germany,* Thyme (p. 574)

Pulsalux *Novartis Farma S.p.A., Italy,* Ginkgo (p. 299)

Puma Cough Balsam *Aspen Pharmacare (Pty) Ltd, South Africa,* Liquorice (p. 411)

Puntualax *Pharbenia S.r.l., Societa del Gruppo Bayer, Italy,* Aloes (p. 50), Rhubarb (p. 506)

Puraloe *Neo Dermos S.R.L., Argentina,* Aloe Vera (p. 48)

Pykno *Biovital Pty Ltd, Australia,* Bilberry (p. 79)

Pyralvex *Laboratorio Dr. Lazar & Cia. S.A., Argentina,* Rhubarb (p. 506) *Norgine P/L, Australia,* Rhubarb (p. 506) *Norgine Pharma GmbH, Austria,* Rhubarb (p. 506) *Norgine SA, Belgium,* Rhubarb (p. 506) *Laboratoires Norgine Pharma, France,* Rhubarb (p. 506) *Faran Laboratories S.A., Greece,* Rhubarb (p. 506) *Treasure Mountain Development Co. Ltd, Hong Kong,* Rhubarb (p. 506) *United Drug, Ireland,* Rhubarb (p. 506) *Norgine Italia S.r.l., Italy,* Rhubarb (p. 506) *Norgine BV, Netherlands,* Rhubarb (p. 506) *Angelini, Portugal,* Rhubarb (p. 506) *Grafton Pharmasia Pte Ltd, Singapore,* Rhubarb (p. 506) *Norgine (Pty) Ltd, South Africa,* Rhubarb (p. 506) *Norgine AG, Switzerland,* Rhubarb (p. 506) *Zuellig Pharma Ltd, Thailand,* Rhubarb (p. 506) *Norgine Pharmaceuticals Ltd, UK,* Rhubarb (p. 506) *Grupo Farma S.A., Venezuela,* Rhubarb (p. 506) *Gervasi Farmacia, Norgine de España, Spain,* Rhubarb (p. 506)

Quelodin F *Química Ariston S.A.C.I.F., Argentina,* Dandelion (p. 204), Milk Thistle (p. 429)

Quiet Days *The Cantassium Company, UK,* Hops (p. 354), Scullcap (p. 530), Valerian (p. 580)

Quiet Life *G.R. Lane Health Products Ltd, UK,* Hops (p. 354), Motherwort (p. 447), Passionflower (p. 461), Valerian (p. 580), Wild Lettuce (p. 596)

Quiet Nite *The Cantassium Company, UK,* Hops (p. 354), Passionflower (p. 461), Valerian (p. 580), Wild Lettuce (p. 596)

Quiet Tyme *The Cantassium Company, UK,* Gentian (p. 290), Hops (p. 354), Passionflower (p. 461), Scullcap (p. 530), Valerian (p. 580)

Quinisedine *Laboratoires Sodia, France,* Hawthorn (p. 346)

Quintonine *Laboratoires GlaxoSmithKline, France,* Cinnamon (p. 162), Gentian (p. 290), Quassia (p. 491)

Rabro N *Teofarma, Italy,* Liquorice (p. 411)

Radicura *Laboratorio Walker S.R.L., Argentina,* Boldo (p. 91)

Ramend Krauter *Queisser Pharma GmbH & Co., Germany,* Aniseed (p. 57), Senna (p. 537)

Ramistos *Laboratorios Pasteur Ltda, Chile,* Drosera (p. 215), Marshmallow (p. 418)

Rapilax Fibras *Merck Química Argentina S.A.I.C., Argentina,* Ispaghula (p. 374), Senna (p. 537)

Recalm *Sanofi Aventis, Chile,* Lime Flower (p. 409), Melissa (p. 425), Passionflower (p. 461), Valerian (p. 580)

Rectovasol *Qualiphar SA, Belgium,* Horse-chestnut (p. 363), Witch Hazel (p. 601)

Red Kooga Co-Q-10 and Ginseng *Peter Black Healthcare Ltd, UK,* Ginseng, Panax (p. 325)

ReDormin *Max Zeller Söhne AG, Pflanzliche Heilmittel, Switzerland,* Hops (p. 354), Valerian (p. 580)

Redseng Polivit *Korhispana, Spain,* Ginseng, Panax (p. 325)

Reducing (Slimming) Tablets *Frank Roberts (Herbal Dispensaries) Ltd, UK,* Boldo (p. 91), Dandelion (p. 204), Fucus (p. 273)

Reduc-Te *Laboratorio Ximena Polanco, Chile,* Boldo (p. 91), Lime Flower (p. 409)

Redudiet *Laboratorio A.M. Farma Activ, Argentina,* Hydrocotyle (p. 371)

Reduktan *Leros sro, Czech Republic,* Elder (p. 237), Frangula (p. 270), Liquorice (p. 411), Senna (p. 537)

Refrane P *Neo Dermos S.R.L., Argentina,* Aloe Vera (p. 48)

Refrane Plus *Neo Dermos S.R.L., Argentina,* Aloe Vera (p. 48)

Regamint *Soria Natural, Spain,* Liquorice (p. 411)

Regina Royal Concorde *Regina Health Ltd, UK,* Damiana (p. 201), Ginseng, Panax (p. 325), Saw Palmetto (p. 521)

Regulador Xavier N-2 *Laboratório Hepacholan S.A., Brazil,* Rhubarb (p. 506)

Rekiv *Rekah Ltd, Israel,* Calamus (p. 118), Frangula (p. 270)

Relana *Cederroth, Spain,* Melissa (p. 425), Valerian (p. 580)

Relax B+ *Vitalia Health Ltd, UK,* Hops (p. 354), Passionflower (p. 461), Valerian (p. 580)

Relaxane *Max Zeller Söhne AG, Pflanzliche Heilmittel, Switzerland,* Butterbur (p. 107), Melissa (p. 425), Passionflower (p. 461), Valerian (p. 580)

Relaxaplex *Vitaplex Products, Australia,* Gentian (p. 290), Hops (p. 354), Passionflower (p. 461), Scullcap (p. 530), Valerian (p. 580)

Relaxo *UB Interpharm SA, Switzerland,* Hops (p. 354), Melissa (p. 425), Passionflower (p. 461), Valerian (p. 580)

Remifemin plus *Europharm, Austria,* Cohosh, Black (p. 168), St John's Wort (p. 549) *Schaper & Brümmer GmbH & Co. KG, Germany,* Cohosh, Black (p. 168), St John's Wort (p. 549)

4

Rendetil *Laboratorio Biotecnoquímica, Venezuela,* Valerian (p. 580)

Renob Blasen- und Nierentee *Dr R. Pfleger Chemische Fabrik GmbH, Germany,* Couchgrass (p. 193), Liquorice (p. 411)

Renusor *Soria Natural, Spain,* Corn Silk (p. 191), Couchgrass (p. 193)

Rendetil *Laboratorio Biotecnoquímica, Venezuela,* Passionflower (p. 461)

Repha-Os *Repha GmbH Biologische Arzneimittel, Germany,* Myrrh (p. 449)

Resolutivo Regium *Laboratorios Diviser-Aquilea S.L., Spain,* Boldo (p. 91), Melissa (p. 425), Rosemary (p. 508)

Resource Rhubagil *Laboratoires Novartis Nutrition, France,* Rhubarb (p. 506)

Restin *Adcock Ingram Pharmaceuticals Ltd, South Africa,* Valerian (p. 580)

Retinovit *Industria Terapeutica Splendore - Oftalmoterapica ALFA, Italy,* Bilberry (p. 79)

Retterspitz Ausserlich *Retterspitz GmbH, Germany,* Arnica (p. 64)

Retterspitz Quick *Retterspitz GmbH, Germany,* Arnica (p. 64)

Reudol *Química Franco Mexicana Nordin S.A. de C.V., Mexico,* Arnica (p. 64)

Reve *Istituto di Medicina Omeopatica S.p.A., Italy,* Passionflower (p. 461), Valerian (p. 580)

Revitan *Ranbaxy Unichem Co. Ltd, Thailand,* Ginseng, Panax (p. 325)

Revitonil *Lichtwer Pharma UK, UK,* Aniseed (p. 57), Clove (p. 166), Echinacea (p. 217), Liquorice (p. 411)

Rheuma *Weleda GmbH & Co. KG, Austria,* Arnica (p. 64)

Rheumatic Pain *The Cantassium Company, UK,* Bogbean (p. 89), Celery (p. 146), Dandelion (p. 204), Guaiacum (p. 344)

Rheumatic Pain Relief *Herbal Concepts Ltd, UK,* Bogbean (p. 89), Capsicum (p. 125), Guaiacum (p. 344)

Rheumatic Pain Remedy *Potter's (Herbal Supplies) Ltd, UK,* Bogbean (p. 89), Burdock (p. 102), Guaiacum (p. 344), Yarrow (p. 604)

Rheumatic Pain Tablets *Frank Roberts (Herbal Dispensaries) Ltd, UK,* Bogbean (p. 89), Celery (p. 146)

Rhinodoron *Laboratoires Weleda, France,* Aloe Vera (p. 48) *Weleda AG-Heilmittelbetriebe, Germany,* Aloe Vera (p. 48)

Rhuaka *OTC Concepts, UK,* Cascara (p. 128), Rhubarb (p. 506), Senna (p. 537)

Rhus Opodeldoc *Laboratorio Esp. Med. Knop Ltda, Chile,* Rosemary (p. 508), Thyme (p. 574)

Rhus-Rheuma-Gel N *Deutsche Homöopathie-Union, Germany,* Comfrey (p. 188)

Ribovir *Plants, Laboratorio della Dott.ssa Luisa Coletta, Italy,* Echinacea (p. 217)

Rilastil Dermo Solar *Dermoteca, SA, Portugal,* Uva-Ursi (p. 577)

Rob-Bron Tablets *Frank Roberts (Herbal Dispensaries) Ltd, UK,* Horehound, White (p. 361), Liquorice (p. 411)

Roberts Acidosis Tablets *Frank Roberts (Herbal Dispensaries) Ltd, UK,* Meadowsweet (p. 423)

Roberts Alchemilla Compound Tablets *Frank Roberts (Herbal Dispensaries) Ltd, UK,* Motherwort (p. 447), Pulsatilla (p. 489), Valerian (p. 580), Vervain (p. 591)

Roberts Anti-Irritant Ointment *Frank Roberts (Herbal Dispensaries) Ltd, UK,* Pilewort (p. 472)

Roberts Black Willow Compound Tablets *Frank Roberts (Herbal Dispensaries) Ltd, UK,* Buchu (p. 100), Corn Silk (p. 191), Parsley Piert (p. 459), Saw Palmetto (p. 521), Willow (p. 598)

Roidhemo *Pan Química Farmaceutica, Spain,* Horse-chestnut (p. 363), Witch Hazel (p. 601)

Romarene *Beaufour Ipsen Pharma, France,* Dandelion (p. 204), Rosemary (p. 508)

Romarinex *Laboratoires Aérocid, France,* Rosemary (p. 508)

Rooilavental *Aspen Pharmacare (Pty) Ltd, South Africa,* Cinnamon (p. 162)

Roteroblong Maagtabletten *Imgroma BV, Netherlands,* Frangula (p. 270)

Ruscimel *Soria Natural, Spain,* Horse-chestnut (p. 363), Witch Hazel (p. 601)

Rutin Compound Tablets *Frank Roberts (Herbal Dispensaries) Ltd, UK,* Ginkgo (p. 299), Yarrow (p. 604)

Rutiviscal *Sanidom Handels-GmbH, Austria,* Garlic (p. 279), Hawthorn (p. 346), Milk Thistle (p. 429)

4

S

Sabal *Pierre Fabre Argentina S.A., Argentina,* Saw Palmetto (p. 521) *Laboratoires Pierre Fabre, France,* Saw Palmetto (p. 521)

Sabatif *Apomedica GmbH, Austria,* Rhubarb (p. 506), Senna (p. 537)

Sacnel *Teofarma, Italy,* Witch Hazel (p. 601)

Sadeltan F *Hautel S.A., Argentina,* Aloe Vera (p. 48)

Sagittaproct *Sagitta Arzneimittel GmbH, Germany,* Witch Hazel (p. 601)

Salhumin *Sanova Pharma GmbH, Austria,* Capsicum (p. 125)

Salmiak *Dr. C. Soldan GmbH, Germany,* Liquorice (p. 411)

Salus Herz-Schutz-Kapseln *Salus-Haus Dr. med. Otto Greither Nachf. GmbH & Co KG, Germany,* Hawthorn (p. 346)

Salutaris *Lab. Incaico SA, Argentina,* Ispaghula (p. 374)

Salviette H *Whitehall Italia S.p.A., Italy,* Witch Hazel (p. 601)

Sambucus Complex *Blackmores Ltd, Australia,* Echinacea (p. 217), Elder (p. 237), Euphorbia (p. 249), Eyebright (p. 256), Golden Seal (p. 337)

Sanaderm *Febena Pharma GmbH, Germany,* Witch Hazel (p. 601)

Sanason *Lek Pharma sro, Czech Republic,* Hops (p. 354), Valerian (p. 580)

Sanason (Санасон) *Lek, Russia,* Hops (p. 354), Valerian (p. 580)

Sanderson's Throat Specific *Sandersons (Chemists) Ltd, UK,* Capsicum (p. 125), Quassia (p. 491), St John's Wort (p. 549)

Sanicut *Química Franco Mexicana Nordin S.A. de C.V., Mexico,* Calendula (p. 121)

Sanogencive *Laboratoires Plan SA, Switzerland,* Horseradish (p. 367), Myrrh (p. 449)

Saugella *Laboratoires Rottapharm, France,* Sage (p. 512), Thyme (p. 574)

Saugella Attiva *Rottapharm S.r.l., Italy,* Sage (p. 512), Thyme (p. 574)

Saugella Dermolatte *Rottapharm S.r.l., Italy,* Sage (p. 512)

Saugella Fitothym *Rottapharm S.r.l., Italy,* Sage (p. 512), Thyme (p. 574)

Saugella Poligyn 7 *Rottapharm S.r.l., Italy,* Thyme (p. 574)

Saugella Salviettine *Rottapharm S.r.l., Italy,* Sage (p. 512)

Saugella Solido ph 3.5 *Rottapharm S.r.l., Italy,* Sage (p. 512)

Saugella Uomo *Rottapharm S.r.l., Italy,* Clove (p. 166)

Schlaf- und Nerventee *Bad Heilbrunner Naturheilmittel GmbH & Co., Germany,* Hops (p. 354), Melissa (p. 425), Valerian (p. 580)

Schlaf-Nerventee N *Abtswinder Naturheilmittel GmbH, Czech Republic,* Hops (p. 354), Liquorice (p. 411), Melissa (p. 425), Valerian (p. 580)

Schoum *Laboratoires Pharmygiène-SCAT, France,* Fumitory (p. 276), Ispaghula (p. 374)

Schweden-Mixtur H nouvelle formulation *Hänseler AG, Switzerland,* Aloes (p. 50), Rhubarb (p. 506), Senna (p. 537)

Schwedentrunk Elixier *Pharmazeutische Fabrik Infirmarius-Rovit GmbH, Germany,* Angelica (p. 53), Cinnamon (p. 162), Gentian (p. 290), Valerian (p. 580)

Sciargo *Potter's (Herbal Supplies) Ltd, UK,* Clivers (p. 164), Senna (p. 537), Uva-Ursi (p. 577), Wild Carrot (p. 593)

Sciatica Tablets *Frank Roberts (Herbal Dispensaries) Ltd, UK,* Bogbean (p. 89), Celery (p. 146), Uva-Ursi (p. 577)

Sciroppo Berta *Berta S.r.l., Italy,* Liquorice (p. 411)

Sclerovis H *Amnol Chimica Biologica S.r.l., Italy,* Borage (p. 96), Echinacea (p. 217), Evening Primrose (p. 251)

Scottopect *Nycomed Austria GmbH, Austria,* Thyme (p. 574)

Scullcap & Gentian Tablets *Dorwest Herbs Ltd, UK,* Gentian (p. 290), Scullcap (p. 530), Valerian (p. 580), Vervain (p. 591)

SCV 300 *Laboratorios Sigma, Argentina,* Ginkgo (p. 299)

SDN 200 *Laboratorios Sigma, Argentina,* Passionflower (p. 461), Valerian (p. 580)

Sebium AKN *Dispolab Farmaceutica SA, Chile,* Ginkgo (p. 299)

Sebulex *Lab. Panalab S.A. Argentina, Argentina,* Capsicum (p. 125)

Sedacur *Schaper & Brümmer GmbH & Co. KG, Germany,* Hops (p. 354), Melissa (p. 425), Valerian (p. 580)

Sedadom *Sanidom Handels-GmbH, Austria,* Hops (p. 354), Valerian (p. 580)

Sedalin *Laboratório Dinafarma Ltda, Brazil,* Hawthorn (p. 346), Passionflower (p. 461)

Sedante Dia *La Serranita, Lab. de Esp. Medic. y Cosmet., Argentina,* Lime Flower (p. 409), Passionflower (p. 461), Valerian (p. 580)

Sedariston Konzentrat *Steiner & Co. Deutsche Arzneimittel Gesellschaft, Germany,* St John's Wort (p. 549), Valerian (p. 580)

Sedariston plus *Steiner & Co. Deutsche Arzneimittel Gesellschaft, Germany,* Melissa (p. 425), St John's Wort (p. 549), Valerian (p. 580)

Sedaselect D *Dreluso Pharmazeutika, Dr Elten & Sohn GmbH, Germany,* Hops (p. 354), Valerian (p. 580)

Sedasor *Soria Natural, Spain,* Hawthorn (p. 346), Passionflower (p. 461), Valerian (p. 580)

Sedatif Tiber *Laboratoires Phytoprevent, France,* Hawthorn (p. 346), Passionflower (p. 461)

Sedatol *EG Laboratori EuroGenerici S.p.A., Italy,* Hawthorn (p. 346), Ispaghula (p. 374), Ispaghula (p. 374), Melissa (p. 425), Passionflower (p. 461), Valerian (p. 580)

Sedinal *Melisana SA, Belgium,* Hawthorn (p. 346), Passionflower (p. 461)

Sedofit *Body Spring S.r.l., Italy,* Hawthorn (p. 346), Lime Flower (p. 409), Passionflower (p. 461)

Sedogelat *Metochem-Pharma GmbH, Austria,* Melissa (p. 425), Passionflower (p. 461), Valerian (p. 580)

Sedonat *Soria Natural, Spain,* Hawthorn (p. 346), Passionflower (p. 461), Valerian (p. 580)

Sedopal *Laboratoires Lehning, France,* Hawthorn (p. 346)

Sedopuer F *Specialità Igienico Terapeutiche S.r.l., Italy,* Hawthorn (p. 346), Passionflower (p. 461), Valerian (p. 580)

Sedotus *Laboratorios Andromaco SA, Chile,* Drosera (p. 215)

Sedovent *Pharma Schwörer GmbH, Germany,* Cinnamon (p. 162), Gentian (p. 290), Yarrow (p. 604)

Selon *Truw Arzneimittel Vertriebs GmbH, Germany,* Hops (p. 354), Valerian (p. 580)

Senagar *Sigma Pharmaceuticals P/L, Australia,* Senega (p. 533)

Senalsor *Soria Natural, Spain,* Marshmallow (p. 418), Senna (p. 537)

Sene Composta *Infabra Indústria Farmacêutica Brasileira Ltda, Brazil,* Liquorice (p. 411), Senna (p. 537)

Senega and Ammonia *J. McGloin P/L, Australia,* Liquorice (p. 411), Senega (p. 533)

Seneuval *Qualiphar SA, Belgium,* Hawthorn (p. 346), Passionflower (p. 461), Valerian (p. 580)

Senna Prompt *Konsyl Pharmaceuticals, USA,* Ispaghula (p. 374)

Senna-S *Tanta Pharmaceuticals Inc., Canada,* Senna (p. 537)

Senokot con Fibra *Grupo Farma S.A., Venezuela,* Ispaghula (p. 374)

Senokot-S *Purdue Pharma, Canada,* Senna (p. 537) *The Purdue Frederick Co., USA,* Senna (p. 537)

Sensinerv forte *Cesra Arzneimittel GmbH & Co. KG, Germany,* Hops (p. 354), Valerian (p. 580)

Se-Power *The Cantassium Company, UK,* Bilberry (p. 79), Eyebright (p. 256)

Septacord *Chemisch-Pharmazeutische Fabrik Göppingen Carl Müller, Apotheker, GmbH & Co. KG, Germany,* Hawthorn (p. 346)

Sequals G *Lagos Laboratorios Argentina S.R.L., Argentina,* Hawthorn (p. 346), Rosemary (p. 508)

Serenil *Lab. Natufarma, Argentina,* Lime Flower (p. 409), Passionflower (p. 461), Valerian (p. 580)

Serenoa Complex *Blackmores Ltd, Australia,* Buchu (p. 100), Saw Palmetto (p. 521)

Serenus *Biolab Sanus Farmacêutica Ltda, Brazil,* Hawthorn (p. 346), Passionflower (p. 461)

Seven Seas Evening Primrose Oil and Starflower Oil *Seven Seas Ltd, UK,* Evening Primrose (p. 251)

Seven Seas Ginseng *Seven Seas Ltd, UK,* Ginseng, Panax (p. 325)

Sigmafem *Laboratorios Sigma, Argentina,* Angelica (p. 53), Ginseng, Eleutherococcus (p. 315), Sage (p. 512)

Sigmafen Free *Laboratorios Sigma, Argentina,* Sage (p. 512)

Sigman-Haustropfen *Sigmapharm Arzneimittel GmbH & Co KG, Austria,* Gentian (p. 290), Liquorice (p. 411)

Sigmasedan *Laboratorios Sigma, Argentina,* Passionflower (p. 461), Valerian (p. 580)

Silberne *Brady C. KG, Austria,* Cascara (p. 128), Rhubarb (p. 506)

Silybum Complex *Blackmores Ltd, Australia,* Dandelion (p. 204), Garlic (p. 279), Milk Thistle (p. 429)

Sinotar *G.R. Lane Health Products Ltd, UK,* Echinacea (p. 217), Elder (p. 237), Marshmallow (p. 418)

Sinuforton *Lichtenstein Pharmazeutica GmbH & Co., Germany,* Cowslip (p. 195), Thyme (p. 574)

Sinupret *Austroplant-Arzneimittel GmbH, Austria,* Cowslip (p. 195), Elder (p. 237), Gentian (p. 290), Vervain (p. 591) *Arzneimittel Schwabe International GmbH, Czech Republic,* Cowslip (p. 195), Elder (p. 237), Gentian (p. 290), Vervain (p. 591) *Bionorica AG, Germany,* Cowslip (p. 195), Elder (p. 237), Gentian (p. 290), Vervain

(p. 591) *Jacobson Medical (Hong Kong) Ltd, Hong Kong,* Cowslip (p. 195), Elder (p. 237), Gentian (p. 290), Vervain (p. 591) *ASI Budapest Kft, Hungary,* Cowslip (p. 195), Elder (p. 237), Gentian (p. 290), Vervain (p. 591) *MBD Marketing (S) Pte Ltd, Singapore,* Cowslip (p. 195), Elder (p. 237), Gentian (p. 290), Vervain (p. 591) *Biomed AG, Switzerland,* Cowslip (p. 195), Elder (p. 237), Gentian (p. 290), Vervain (p. 591) *Zuellig Pharma Ltd, Thailand,* Cowslip (p. 195), Elder (p. 237), Gentian (p. 290), Vervain (p. 591)

Sinupret (Синупрет**)** *Bionorica AG, Russia,* Cowslip (p. 195), Elder (p. 237), Gentian (p. 290), Vervain (p. 591)

Sinus and Hay Fever Tablets *Frank Roberts (Herbal Dispensaries) Ltd, UK,* Echinacea (p. 217), Garlic (p. 279)

Sirop Cocillana Codeine *Laboratoire Atlas, Canada,* Euphorbia (p. 249), Senega (p. 533), St John's Wort (p. 549), Wild Lettuce (p. 596)

Sirop pectoral contre la toux S *Hänseler AG, Switzerland,* Cowslip (p. 195), Drosera (p. 215), Liquorice (p. 411)

Sirop S contre la toux et la bronchite *Hänseler AG, Switzerland,* Cowslip (p. 195), Drosera (p. 215), Liquorice (p. 411)

Skin Cleansing *The Cantassium Company, UK,* Burdock (p. 102), Clivers (p. 164), Fumitory (p. 276), Senna (p. 537)

Skin Eruptions Mixture *Potter's (Herbal Supplies) Ltd, UK,* Blue Flag (p. 87), Buchu (p. 100), Burdock (p. 102), Cascara (p. 128), Sarsaparilla (p. 515), Yellow Dock (p. 608)

Skin Hair Nails *Natrol, USA,* Burdock (p. 102)

Skin Healing Cream *Brauer Natural Medicine P/L, Australia,* Calendula (p. 121), St John's Wort (p. 549)

Sleepezy *Healthy Direct, UK,* Hops (p. 354), Passionflower (p. 461), Scullcap (p. 530)

Slippery Elm Skin Soap *Frank Roberts (Herbal Dispensaries) Ltd, UK,* Slippery Elm (p. 545)

Slippery Elm Stomach Tablets *Potter's (Herbal Supplies) Ltd, UK,* Slippery Elm (p. 545)

Slumber *Seven Seas Ltd, UK,* Hops (p. 354), Ispaghula (p. 374), Passionflower (p. 461), Wild Lettuce (p. 596)

SM-33 Adult Formula *Bayer Australia Ltd (Pharmaceutical Business Group), Australia,* Rhubarb (p. 506)

Snella Vag *Wierhom Pharma S.A., Argentina,* Aloe Vera (p. 48)

Sofderm *Cipla Ltd, India,* Aloe Vera (p. 48)

Soflax *Douglas Pharmaceuticals Australia Ltd, Australia,* Senna (p. 537)

Solarcaine Aloe Extra Burn Relief *Schering-Plough Corp., USA,* Aloe Vera (p. 48)

Solarcaine Aloe Vera Gel *Laboratorio Schering-Plough, Chile,* Aloe Vera (p. 48)

Solenil Post Solar *Lab. Fortbenton Co. S.A., Argentina,* Aloe Vera (p. 48)

Solubitrat *Sanova Pharma GmbH, Austria,* Java Tea (p. 381)

Solucion Schoum *Expanscience, Spain,* Boldo (p. 91), Fumitory (p. 276), Golden Seal (p. 337), Ispaghula (p. 374), Melissa (p. 425), Rhubarb (p. 506), Witch Hazel (p. 601)

Solution Stago Diluee *Pharma Développement, France,* Boldo (p. 91)

Soluzione Schoum *Aventis Pharma S.p.A., Italy,* Fumitory (p. 276), Ispaghula (p. 374)

Solvipect *Nycomed Pharma AS, Norway,* Liquorice (p. 411)

Solvipect comp *Nycomed Pharma AS, Norway,* Liquorice (p. 411)

Solvobil *Laboratório Americano de Farmacoterapia S/A, Brazil,* Artichoke (p. 67), Boldo (p. 91), Cascara (p. 128) *Recordati Industria Chimica e Farmaceutica S.p.a., Italy,* Boldo (p. 91), Cascara (p. 128)

Solvopret *Bionorica AG, Germany,* Cowslip (p. 195), Elder (p. 237), Gentian (p. 290) *Zuellig Pharma Ltd, Thailand,* Thyme (p. 574)

Solvopret TP *Zuellig Pharma Ltd, Thailand,* Cowslip (p. 195), Thyme (p. 574)

Sominex *EMS Ind. Farmacêutica Ltda, Brazil,* Hawthorn (p. 346), Passionflower (p. 461), Valerian (p. 580)

Sominex Herbal *Thornton & Ross Ltd, UK,* Hops (p. 354), Passionflower (p. 461), Valerian (p. 580)

Songha *F. Joh. Kwizda, Austria,* Melissa (p. 425), Valerian (p. 580) *Boehringer Ingelheim SA/NV, Belgium,* Melissa (p. 425), Valerian (p. 580) *Boehringer Ingelheim, Lda, Portugal,* Melissa (p. 425), Valerian (p. 580)

Songha Night *Boehringer Ingelheim sro, Czech Republic,* Melissa (p. 425), Valerian (p. 580) *Pharmashalom Ltd, Israel,* Melissa (p. 425), Valerian (p. 580) *Pharmaton SA, Switzerland,* Melissa (p. 425), Valerian (p. 580)

Sonhare *Boehringer Ingelheim do Brasil Quím. e Farm. Ltda, Brazil,* Melissa (p. 425), Valerian (p. 580)

Soporin *Herbamed AG, Switzerland,* Hops (p. 354), Melissa (p. 425), Passionflower (p. 461), Valerian (p. 580)

Soy Forte with Black Cohosh *Mayne Pharma P/L, Australia,* Cohosh, Black (p. 168)

Spagulax au Citrate de Potassium *Laboratoires Pharmafarm, France,* Ispaghula (p. 374)

Spagulax au Sorbitol *Laboratoires Pharmafarm, France,* Ispaghula (p. 374)

Spagymun *Spagyros AG, Switzerland,* Echinacea (p. 217)

Spagyrom *Spagyros AG, Switzerland,* Echinacea (p. 217)

Spasmine *Laboratoires Jolly-Jatel, France,* Hawthorn (p. 346), Valerian (p. 580)

Spasmo-Urgenin *Madaus GmbH, Austria,* Echinacea (p. 217), Saw Palmetto (p. 521) *Neo-Farmacéutica, Lda, Portugal,* Echinacea (p. 217), Saw Palmetto (p. 521) *Madaus, Spain,* Echinacea (p. 217), Saw Palmetto (p. 521) *Oui Heng Import Co. Ltd, Thailand,* Echinacea (p. 217), Saw Palmetto (p. 521)

Species Cholagogae Planta *Leros sro, Czech Republic,* Agrimony (p. 42), Elecampane (p. 240), Rhubarb (p. 506)

Species Diureticae Planta *Leros sro, Czech Republic,* Parsley (p. 456)

Species nervinae *F. Joh. Kwizda, Austria,* Melissa (p. 425), St John's Wort (p. 549), Valerian (p. 580)

Species Nervinae Planta *Leros sro, Czech Republic,* Hops (p. 354), Melissa (p. 425), St John's Wort (p. 549), Valerian (p. 580)

Species Pectorales Planta *Leros sro, Czech Republic,* Coltsfoot (p. 185), Liquorice (p. 411), Marshmallow (p. 418)

Species Urologicae Planta *Leros sro, Czech Republic,* Elder (p. 237), Nettle (p. 452), Parsley (p. 456), Uva-Ursi (p. 577), Yarrow (p. 604)

Speman Forte (Спеман Форте**)** *Transatlantic International, Russia,* Wild Lettuce (p. 596)

Spiritus Contra Tussim Drops *Pharma-Natura (Pty) Ltd, South Africa,* Angelica (p. 53), Cinnamon (p. 162), Clove (p. 166), Melissa (p. 425)

Sportino Akut *Harras Pharma Curarina Arzneimittel GmbH, Germany,* Arnica (p. 64)

Sportupac M *Terra-Bio-Chemie GmbH, Germany,* Horse-chestnut (p. 363)

St Bonifatius-Tee *Dr. Kolassa & Merz GmbH, Austria,* Boldo (p. 91), Juniper (p. 386), Lime Flower (p. 409)

St Johns wort Compound *Potter's (Herbal Supplies) Ltd, UK,* Scullcap (p. 530)

St Johnswort Compound *Potter's (Herbal Supplies) Ltd, UK,* Cohosh, Black (p. 168), St John's Wort (p. 549), Willow (p. 598)

St Mary's Thistle Plus *Eagle Pharmaceuticals P/L, Australia,* Bilberry (p. 79), Dandelion (p. 204), Milk Thistle (p. 429)

Steril Zeta *Zeta Farmaceutici S.p.A., Italy,* Witch Hazel (p. 601)

Stibium Comp *Pharma-Natura (Pty) Ltd, South Africa,* Horse-chestnut (p. 363), Witch Hazel (p. 601)

Stimolfit *Body Spring S.r.l., Italy,* Cascara (p. 128), Rhubarb (p. 506), Senna (p. 537)

Stodal *Boiron CZ sro, Czech Republic,* Drosera (p. 215), Senega (p. 533) *Prisfar, SA, Portugal,* Senega (p. 533)

Stoffwechseltee N *Abtswinder Naturheilmittel GmbH, Czech Republic,* Liquorice (p. 411), Nettle (p. 452)

Stomach Mixture *Potter's (Herbal Supplies) Ltd, UK,* Dandelion (p. 204), Gentian (p. 290), Rhubarb (p. 506)

Stomachysat N *Johannes Bürger Ysatfabrik GmbH, Germany,* Yarrow (p. 604)

Stomacine *Laboratoires Plan SA, Switzerland,* Quassia (p. 491)

Stomaran *Leros sro, Czech Republic,* Agrimony (p. 42), Angelica (p. 53), Calamus (p. 118), Centaury (p. 149), St John's Wort (p. 549)

Stomargil *Laboratoires Motima, France,* Bilberry (p. 79)

Stomatosan *Slovakofarma sro, Czech Republic,* Clove (p. 166), Comfrey (p. 188), Sage (p. 512), Thyme (p. 574), Vervain (p. 591), Yarrow (p. 604)

Stop-Itch Plus *Sime Darby Marketing, A Division of Sime Darby Singapore Ltd, Singapore,* Witch Hazel (p. 601)

Stoptussin-Fito (Стоптуссин-фито**)** *Ivax AC, Russia,* Thyme (p. 574)

Strath Gouttes contre la toux *Bio-Strath AG, Switzerland,* Cowslip (p. 195), Thyme (p. 574)

Strath Gouttes pour le coeur *Bio-Strath AG, Switzerland,* Hawthorn (p. 346), Passionflower (p. 461)

Strath Gouttes pour le foie et la bile *Bio-Strath AG, Switzerland,* Artichoke (p. 67)

Strath Gouttes pour le nerfs et contre l'insomnie *Bio-Strath AG, Switzerland,* Passionflower (p. 461), Valerian (p. 580)

Strath Gouttes pour les muqueuses *Bio-Strath AG, Switzerland,* Sage (p. 512)

Strath Gouttes pour les reins et la vessie *Bio-Strath AG, Switzerland,* Dandelion (p. 204), Uva-Ursi (p. 577)

Strath Gouttes pour les veines *Bio-Strath AG, Switzerland,* Cowslip (p. 195), Horse-chestnut (p. 363)

Strath Gouttes pour l'estomac *Bio-Strath AG, Switzerland,* Gentian (p. 290), Liquorice (p. 411)

Strath Gouttes Rhumatisme *Bio-Strath AG, Switzerland,* Cowslip (p. 195), Willow (p. 598)

Strength *Potter's (Herbal Supplies) Ltd, UK,* Damiana (p. 201), Saw Palmetto (p. 521)

Strength Tablets *Frank Roberts (Herbal Dispensaries) Ltd, UK,* Damiana (p. 201), Saw Palmetto (p. 521)

Strepsils Echinacea Defence *Boots Healthcare New Zealand Ltd, New Zealand,* Echinacea (p. 217)

Stress Complex *Natrol, USA,* Valerian (p. 580)

StressEez *Nature Made, USA,* Valerian (p. 580)

Stressless *DDD Ltd, UK,* Hops (p. 354), Scullcap (p. 530), Valerian (p. 580), Vervain (p. 591)

Stuidruppels *Aspen Pharmacare (Pty) Ltd, South Africa,* Asafoetida (p. 72), Valerian (p. 580)

Stullmaton *Pharma Stulln GmbH, Germany,* Arnica (p. 64), Centaury (p. 149), Melissa (p. 425)

Succus Cineraria Maritima *Walker Pharmacal, USA,* Witch Hazel (p. 601)

Sulgan 99 *Maria Clementine Martin Klosterfrau GmbH, Austria,* Witch Hazel (p. 601)

Sulgan 99 *Maria Clementine Martin Klosterfrau GmbH, Austria,* Witch Hazel (p. 601)

Summertime Tea Blend *Culpeper and Napiers, UK,* Chamomile, Roman (p. 156), Elder (p. 237), Eyebright (p. 256), Liquorice (p. 411), Nettle (p. 452)

SuNerven *G.R. Lane Health Products Ltd, UK,* Motherwort (p. 447), Passionflower (p. 461), Valerian (p. 580), Vervain (p. 591)

Supa-Tonic Tablets *Frank Roberts (Herbal Dispensaries) Ltd, UK,* Damiana (p. 201), Rosemary (p. 508), Saw Palmetto (p. 521)

Supositorio Hamamelis Composto *Laboratório Simões Ltda, Brazil,* Horse-chestnut (p. 363), Witch Hazel (p. 601)

Supradyn Vital 50+ *Bayer (Schweiz) AG, Pharma, Switzerland,* Ginseng, Panax (p. 325)

Supranettes *Alcon Pharmaceutical C.A., Venezuela,* Calendula (p. 121), Witch Hazel (p. 601)

Supranettes Naturalag *Alcon Laboratorios, S.A. de C.V., Mexico,* Calendula (p. 121), Witch Hazel (p. 601)

Supravital *Liferpal MD, S.A. de C.V., Mexico,* Garlic (p. 279)

Sure-Lax (Herbal) *Chefaro UK Ltd, UK,* Aloes (p. 50), Holy Thistle (p. 352), Valerian (p. 580)

Swarm *J. Pickles & Sons, UK,* Witch Hazel (p. 601)

Swiss Herb Cough Drops *Ricola, Canada,* Burnet (p. 105), Marshmallow (p. 418), Parsley Piert (p. 459), Thyme (p. 574)

SX-22 *Laboratorios Sigma, Argentina,* Echinacea (p. 217)

Sympaneurol *Sanofi-Aventis, France,* Hawthorn (p. 346), Passionflower (p. 461), Valerian (p. 580)

Sympathyl *Laboratoires Innotech International, Sté du groupe Innothéra, France,* Hawthorn (p. 346)

Sympavagol *Novartis Santé Familiale SA, France,* Hawthorn (p. 346), Passionflower (p. 461)

Tabritis *Potter's (Herbal Supplies) Ltd, UK,* Burdock (p. 102), Clivers (p. 164), Elder (p. 237), Senna (p. 537), Uva-Ursi (p. 577), Yarrow (p. 604)

Tabritis Tablets *Potter's Herbal Medicines, UK,* Burdock (p. 102), Clivers (p. 164), Elder (p. 237), Poplar (p. 482), Prickly Ash, Northern (p. 484), Uva-Ursi (p. 577), Yarrow (p. 604)

Talowin *Costec S.R.L. Esp. Dermatocosméticas, Argentina,* Aloe Vera (p. 48)

Tamaril *Marjan Indústria e Comércio Ltda, Brazil,* Liquorice (p. 411), Senna (p. 537)

Tamarine *Barrenne Indústria Farmacêutica Ltda, Brazil,* Liquorice (p. 411), Senna (p. 537) *Barrenne Indústria Farmacêutica Ltda, GlaxoSmithKline, Chile,* Senna (p. 537) *Laboratoires GlaxoSmithKline, France,* Senna (p. 537) *Whitehall Italia S.p. A., Italy,* Liquorice (p. 411), Senna (p. 537)

Tamarix *Hebron S.A. Indústria Química e Farmacêutica, Brazil,* Liquorice (p. 411), Senna (p. 537)

Tampositorien mit Belladonna *Provita Pharma GmbH, Austria,* Witch Hazel (p. 601)

Tandpyndruppels *Aspen Pharmacare (Pty) Ltd, South Africa,* Capsicum (p. 125)

Tea Tree & Witch Hazel Cream *G.R. Lane Health Products Ltd, UK,* Witch Hazel (p. 601)

Tealine *Laboratoires Arkopharma, France,* Java Tea (p. 381)

Tendro *Tentan AG, Switzerland,* Eyebright (p. 256), Witch Hazel (p. 601)

Tensiben *Soria Natural, Spain,* Hawthorn (p. 346)

Tereonsit *Hautel S.A., Argentina,* Sage (p. 512)

Thalgo Tonic *Lab Thalgo Nutrition, France,* Ginseng, Panax (p. 325)

The a l'avoine sauvage de Vollmer *Dr Dünner SA, Switzerland,* Nettle (p. 452), St John's Wort (p. 549)

The Chambard-Tee *Brady C. KG, Austria,* Calendula (p. 121), Marshmallow (p. 418), Melissa (p. 425), Senna (p. 537)

The Salvat *Leros sro, Czech Republic,* Agrimony (p. 42), Boldo (p. 91), Dandelion (p. 204), Frangula (p. 270)

Thermocream *Laboratoires Belges Pharmacobel SA, Belgium,* Capsicum (p. 125)

Throat Discs *GlaxoSmithKline, USA,* Capsicum (p. 125)

Thymomel *Ivax-CR as, Czech Republic,* Thyme (p. 574)

Thymoval *EF-EM-ES - Dr Smetana & Co., Austria,* Cowslip (p. 195), Thyme (p. 574), Valerian (p. 580)

Thyreogutt *Austroplant-Arzneimittel GmbH, Austria,* Motherwort (p. 447)

Tickly Cough & Sore Throat Relief *Herbal Concepts Ltd, UK,* Liquorice (p. 411), Senega (p. 533)

Tisana Kelemata *Kelemata S.p.A., Italy,* Aniseed (p. 57), Couchgrass (p. 193), Melissa (p. 425), Sarsaparilla (p. 515), Senna (p. 537)

Tisane antirhumatismale *Sidroga AG, Switzerland,* Passionflower (p. 461), Willow (p. 598)

Tisane calmante pour les enfants *Sidroga AG, Switzerland,* Hops (p. 354), Melissa (p. 425), Passionflower (p. 461), Valerian (p. 580)

Tisane contre les refroidissements *Sidroga AG, Switzerland,* Elder (p. 237), Lime Flower (p. 409)

Tisane Diuretique *Sidroga AG, Switzerland,* Nettle (p. 452)

Tisane favorisant l'allaitement *Sidroga AG, Switzerland,* Aniseed (p. 57), Melissa (p. 425)

Tisane Hepatique de Hoerdt *Laboratoires Michel Iderne, France,* Agrimony (p. 42), Bogbean (p. 89), Boldo (p. 91), Centaury (p. 149), Couchgrass (p. 193), Sage (p. 512), Yarrow (p. 604)

Tisane hepatique et biliaire *Sidroga AG, Switzerland,* Artichoke (p. 67), Boldo (p. 91), Dandelion (p. 204), Milk Thistle (p. 429), Yarrow (p. 604)

Tisane laxative *Sidroga AG, Switzerland,* Liquorice (p. 411), Senna (p. 537)

Tisane pectorale et antitussive *Sidroga AG, Switzerland,* Liquorice (p. 411), Marshmallow (p. 418), Plantain (p. 474), Sage (p. 512), Thyme (p. 574)

Tisane pectorale pour les enfants *Sidroga AG, Switzerland,* Cowslip (p. 195), Liquorice (p. 411), Marshmallow (p. 418), Plantain (p. 474), Thyme (p. 574)

Tisane pour le coeur et la circulation *Sidroga AG, Switzerland,* Hawthorn (p. 346), Melissa (p. 425), Motherwort (p. 447)

Tisane pour le sommeil et les nerfs *Sidroga AG, Switzerland,* Hops (p. 354), Melissa (p. 425), Valerian (p. 580)

Tisane pour les problemes de prostate *Sidroga AG, Switzerland,* Cinnamon (p. 162), Clove (p. 166), Ginger (p. 293), Nettle (p. 452)

Tisane pour les reins et la vessie *Sidroga AG, Switzerland,* Java Tea (p. 381), Juniper (p. 386), Uva-Ursi (p. 577)

Tisane pour l'estomac *Sidroga AG, Switzerland,* Calamus (p. 118), Centaury (p. 149), Melissa (p. 425), Yarrow (p. 604)

Tisane pour nourissons et enfants *Sidroga AG, Switzerland,* Lime Flower (p. 409), Melissa (p. 425), Vervain (p. 591)

Tisane Provencale No 1 *F. Uhlmann-Eyraud SA, Switzerland,* Marshmallow (p. 418), Senna (p. 537)

Ton Was *Chiesi España, Spain,* Ginseng, Panax (p. 325)

Tonactil *Laboratoires Arkopharma, France,* Ginseng, Panax (p. 325)

Tonimax *Soria Natural, Spain,* Ginseng, Eleutherococcus (p. 315)

Tonsilgon *Bionorica AG, Germany,* Dandelion (p. 204), Marshmallow (p. 418), Yarrow (p. 604)

Tonsilgon N (Тонзилгон Н**)** *Bionorica AG, Russia,* Dandelion (p. 204), Marshmallow (p. 418), Yarrow (p. 604)

Topaceta *G. Streuli & Co. AG, Switzerland,* Arnica (p. 64)

Tormentan *Leros sro, Czech Republic,* Bilberry (p. 79), Burnet (p. 105), Liquorice (p. 411), Sage (p. 512)

Tornix *Steierl Pharma GmbH, Germany,* Hawthorn (p. 346), Passionflower (p. 461), Valerian (p. 580)

Total Magnesiano con Ginseng *Lab. Temis Lostaló S.A., Argentina,* Ginseng, Panax (p. 325)

Total Magnesiano con Vitaminas y Minerales *Lab. Temis Lostaló S.A., Argentina,* Ginseng, Panax (p. 325)

Tranquil *Swiss Bio Pharma Sdn Bhd, Malaysia,* Capsicum (p. 125)

Total Man *Swiss Bio Pharma Sdn Bhd, Malaysia,* Damiana (p. 201), Echinacea (p. 217), Garlic (p. 279), Ginger (p. 293), Ginkgo (p. 299), Ginseng, Panax (p. 325), Hydrocotyle (p. 371), Liquorice (p. 411), Parsley (p. 456), Sarsaparilla (p. 515), Saw Palmetto (p. 521)

Tranquil *Pharmadass Ltd, UK,* Hawthorn (p. 346), Lime Flower (p. 409)

Tranquital *Novartis Santé Familiale SA, France,* Hawthorn (p. 346), Valerian (p. 580)

Trauma-cyl *Pharma Liebermann GmbH, Germany,* Arnica (p. 64), Horse-chestnut (p. 363), Witch Hazel (p. 601)

Trauma-Salbe warmend *Mayrhofer Pharmazeutika, Austria,* Capsicum (p. 125)

Traumed *Herbarium Laboratório Botanico Ltda, Brazil,* Arnica (p. 64), Ginkgo (p. 299), Horse-chestnut (p. 363)

Travelaide *Yauyip P/L, Australia,* Ginger (p. 293), Slippery Elm (p. 545)

Traveleeze *Ernest Jackson & Co. Ltd, UK,* Ginger (p. 293)

Triallin *Iromedica AG, Switzerland,* Garlic (p. 279), Ginkgo (p. 299), Ginseng, Panax (p. 325), Hawthorn (p. 346)

Trifolium Complex *Blackmores Ltd, Australia,* Burdock (p. 102), Dandelion (p. 204), Red Clover (p. 498), Yellow Dock (p. 608)

TriMune *Nature Made, USA,* Echinacea (p. 217)

Tucks *Pfizer Consumer Healthcare, Division of Pfizer Canada Inc., Canada,* Witch Hazel (p. 601) *Pfizer Inc., USA,* Witch Hazel (p. 601)

Tummy Ease *Zydus Cadila Group, India,* Asafoetida (p. 72), Ginger (p. 293)

Turulington Tincture *Aspen Pharmacare (Pty) Ltd, South Africa,* Aloes (p. 50)

Tuscalman *F. Joh. Kwizda, Austria,* Elder (p. 237), Marshmallow (p. 418) *Desma Healthcare BV, Switzerland,* Marshmallow (p. 418)

Tussamag *Montavit GmbH, Austria,* Thyme (p. 574)

Tussidoron *Laboratoires Weleda, France,* Drosera (p. 215), Thyme (p. 574)

Tussiflorin Hustensaft *Pascoe Pharmazeutische Präparate GmbH, Germany,* Cowslip (p. 195)

Tussiflorin Hustentropfen *Pascoe Pharmazeutische Präparate GmbH, Germany,* Cowslip (p. 195)

Tussilen *Ivax-CR as, Ivax-CR as, Czech Republic,* Drosera (p. 215)

Tussimont *Pharmonta Mag. pharm. Dr Fischer, Austria,* Senega (p. 533), Thyme (p. 574)

TUSSinfant N *RubiePharm Vertriebs GmbH, Germany,* Cowslip (p. 195), Thyme (p. 574)

Tussol *Amnol Chimica Biologica S.r.l., Italy,* Bilberry (p. 79), Lime Flower (p. 409), Liquorice (p. 411), Thyme (p. 574)

Tussucalman *Ibefar Inst. Brasileiro de Esp. Ftcas. Ltda, Brazil,* Liquorice (p. 411)

Tux *Pfizer SA, Belgium,* Senega (p. 533), Senna (p. 537)

Tyroseng *Eagle Pharmaceuticals P/L, Australia,* Ginseng, Eleutherococcus (p. 315)

Ulcu-Pasc *Pascoe Pharmazeutische Präparate GmbH, Germany,* Liquorice (p. 411)

Ulgastrin *Oui Heng Import Co. Ltd, Thailand,* Liquorice (p. 411)

Ultimate Antioxidant Formula *Natrol, USA,* Artichoke (p. 67), Bilberry (p. 79), Calendula (p. 121)

Ultra Quercitin *Jamieson Laboratories, Canada,* Nettle (p. 452)

Ultracal *Lab. Baliarda S.A., Argentina,* Saw Palmetto (p. 521)

Ultravisin *Farmigea Industria Chimico Farmaceutica S.p.A., Italy,* Bilberry (p. 79)

Ungolen *Slovakofarma sro, Czech Republic,* Agrimony (p. 42), Dandelion (p. 204), Holy Thistle (p. 352), Milk Thistle (p. 429), Yarrow (p. 604)

Unguentum lymphaticum *PGM Pharmazeutische Gesellschaft mbH & Co. München, Germany,* Calendula (p. 121)

Unwind Herbal Nytol *GlaxoSmithKline Consumer Healthcare, UK,* Hops (p. 354), Valerian (p. 580), Wild Lettuce (p. 596)

Urapro *Eagle Pharmaceuticals P/L, Australia,* Golden Seal (p. 337), Nettle (p. 452), Saw Palmetto (p. 521)

Urcyston Planta *Leros sro, Czech Republic,* Bilberry (p. 79), Elder (p. 237), Thyme (p. 574), Uva-Ursi (p. 577)

Urelium Neu *Europharm, Austria,* Dandelion (p. 204)

Urgenin *Thursday Plantation laboratories Ltd, Australia,* Echinacea (p. 217), Saw Palmetto (p. 521) *Madaus GmbH, Austria,* Echinacea (p. 217), Saw Palmetto (p. 521) *Madaus Pharma SA, Belgium,* Echinacea (p. 217), Saw Palmetto (p. 521) *Trinity Trading Co. Ltd, Hong Kong,* Echinacea (p. 217), Saw Palmetto (p. 521) *Salomon, Levin, & Elstein Ltd, Israel,* Echinacea (p. 217), Saw Palmetto (p. 521) *Madaus, Spain,* Echinacea (p. 217), Saw Palmetto (p. 521)

Urinase *Eagle Pharmaceuticals P/L, Australia,* Buchu (p. 100), Echinacea (p. 217), Golden Seal (p. 337), Saw Palmetto (p. 521), Uva-Ursi (p. 577)

Urinefrol *Lab. Lafage S.R.L., Argentina,* Liquorice (p. 411), Sarsaparilla (p. 515)

Urinex *E Kern AG, Pharmazeutische Krauterspezialitäten, Switzerland,* Buchu (p. 100), Calamus (p. 118), Calendula (p. 121), Meadowsweet (p. 423), Uva-Ursi (p. 577)

Urisor *Soria Natural, Spain,* Java Tea (p. 381), Uva-Ursi (p. 577)

Urologicka Cajova Smes *Megafyt-R sro, Czech Republic,* Parsley (p. 456), Uva-Ursi (p. 577)

Uromil *Laboratoires IPRAD, France,* Uva-Ursi (p. 577)

Urophytum *Laboratoires Arkopharma, France,* Buchu (p. 100), Uva-Ursi (p. 577)

Uropurat *F. Joh. Kwizda, Austria,* Uva-Ursi (p. 577)

Uvacin *Lichtwer Pharma UK, UK,* Dandelion (p. 204), Uva-Ursi (p. 577) *Medic Herb UK Ltd, UK,* Dandelion (p. 204)

Uva-Ursi Complex *Blackmores Ltd, Australia,* Buchu (p. 100), Clivers (p. 164), Dandelion (p. 204), Uva-Ursi (p. 577)

Uva-Ursi Plus *Eagle Pharmaceuticals P/L, Australia,* Dandelion (p. 204), Parsley (p. 456), Uva-Ursi (p. 577)

Uze Active *Dist. Ofar S.A., Argentina,* Quassia (p. 491)

Vagicural Plus *Lab. Raymos S.A.I.C., Argentina,* Hydrocotyle (p. 371)

Vagisil *Combe Inc., USA,* Aloes (p. 50)

Vagostabyl *Laboratoires Leurquin Mediolanum, France,* Hawthorn (p. 346), Melissa (p. 425)

Vagostesyl *Laboratório Gross S.A., Brazil,* Passionflower (p. 461)

Valdispert comp *Solvay Arzneimittel GmbH, Germany,* Hops (p. 354), Valerian (p. 580)

Valdispert Complex *Solvay Pharma, Spain,* Passionflower (p. 461), Valerian (p. 580)

Valerian *Vitaplex Products, Australia,* Capsicum (p. 125), Motherwort (p. 447), Scullcap (p. 530), Valerian (p. 580)

Valerian Plus Herbal Plus Formula 12 *Mayne Pharma P/L, Australia,* Passionflower (p. 461), Valerian (p. 580)

Valeriana comp novum *Hevert-Arzneimittel GmbH & Co. KG, Germany,* Valerian (p. 580)

Valeriana mild *Hevert-Arzneimittel GmbH & Co. KG, Germany,* Hops (p. 354), Passionflower (p. 461), Valerian (p. 580)

Valeriana Oligoplex *Lab. Dr. Madaus & Co. SA, Argentina,* Melissa (p. 425), Valerian (p. 580)

Valerina Day Time *Lichtwer Pharma UK, UK,* Melissa (p. 425), Valerian (p. 580)

Valerina Day-Time *Medic Herb UK Ltd, UK,* Melissa (p. 425), Valerian (p. 580)

Valerina Night-Time *Lichtwer Pharma UK, UK,* Hops (p. 354), Melissa (p. 425), Valerian (p. 580) *Medic Herb UK Ltd, UK,* Melissa (p. 425), Valerian (p. 580)

Valesono *Laboratório J. Neves, Lda, Portugal,* Passionflower (p. 461), Valerian (p. 580)

Valin Baldrian *Sanova Pharma GmbH, Austria,* Valerian (p. 580)

Valofyt Neo *Leros sro, Czech Republic,* Angelica (p. 53), Hawthorn (p. 346), Hops (p. 354), Melissa (p. 425), Valerian (p. 580), Willow (p. 598)

Valupass *Laboratorio Esp. Med. Knop Ltda, Chile,* Hops (p. 354), Valerian (p. 580)

Valverde Baldrian Hopfen bei Einschlafstorungen und zur Beruhigung *Novartis Consumer Health GmbH, Germany,* Hops (p. 354), Valerian (p. 580)

Valverde Coeur *Sidroga AG, Switzerland,* Hawthorn (p. 346), Hops (p. 354), Passionflower (p. 461), Valerian (p. 580)

Valverde Constipation dragees *Sidroga AG, Switzerland,* Butterbur (p. 107), Senna (p. 537)

Valverde Constipation sirop *Sidroga AG, Switzerland,* Senna (p. 537)

Valverde Detente dragees *Sidroga AG, Switzerland,* Butterbur (p. 107), Melissa (p. 425), Passionflower (p. 461), Valerian (p. 580)

Valverde Sommeil *Sidroga AG, Switzerland,* Hops (p. 354), Valerian (p. 580)

Valviska *Tentan AG, Switzerland,* Melissa (p. 425), Valerian (p. 580)

Varicell *Eversil Produtos Farmacêuticos Indústria e Comércio Ltda, Brazil,* Senna (p. 537)

Varicofit *Body Spring S.r.l., Italy,* Bilberry (p. 79), Dandelion (p. 204), Ginkgo (p. 299), Hydrocotyle (p. 371)

Varicogel *Alfa Wassermann S.p.A., Italy,* Horse-chestnut (p. 363), Witch Hazel (p. 601)

Varicose Ointment *Potter's (Herbal Supplies) Ltd, UK,* Witch Hazel (p. 601)

Varicylum-S *Pharma Liebermann GmbH, Germany,* Arnica (p. 64), Horse-chestnut (p. 363), Witch Hazel (p. 601)

Varisedan *Wierhom Pharma S.A., Argentina,* Garlic (p. 279)

Varizol *Laboratório Simões Ltda, Brazil,* Horse-chestnut (p. 363), Witch Hazel (p. 601)

Varizol *Laboratório Simões Ltda, Brazil,* Witch Hazel (p. 601)

Vasobrain *Errekappa Euroterapici S.p.A., Italy,* Ginkgo (p. 299)

Vasobrain Plus *Errekappa Euroterapici S.p.A., Italy,* Ginkgo (p. 299)

Vasopt *Bausch & Lomb Oftal SpA, Italy,* Ginkgo (p. 299)

Vegetable Cough Remover *Potter's (Herbal Supplies) Ltd, UK,* Capsicum (p. 125), Cohosh, Black (p. 168), Elecampane (p. 240), Liquorice (p. 411), Marshmallow (p. 418), Pleurisy Root (p. 477), Scullcap (p. 530), Skunk Cabbage (p. 543), Valerian (p. 580)

Vegetex *G.R. Lane Health Products Ltd, UK,* Bogbean (p. 89), Celery (p. 146), Cohosh, Black (p. 168)

Veinophytum *Laboratoires Arkopharma, France,* Horse-chestnut (p. 363)

Veinostase *Merck Lipha Santé, France,* Horse-chestnut (p. 363), Witch Hazel (p. 601)

Veinotonyl *Merck Lipha Santé, France,* Horse-chestnut (p. 363)

Venactive *Euroderm S.r.l., Italy,* Horse-chestnut (p. 363), Hydrocotyle (p. 371), Witch Hazel (p. 601)

Venen Krauter NT *Salus-Haus Dr. med. Otto Greither Nachf. GmbH & Co KG, Germany,* Horse-chestnut (p. 363)

Venengel *ratiopharm GmbH, Germany,* Arnica (p. 64), Horse-chestnut (p. 363)

Venen-Salbe N *ct-Arzneimittel GmbH, Germany,* Horse-chestnut (p. 363)

Venocur Triplex *Knoll SA Produtos Químicos e Farmacêuticos, Brazil,* Horse-chestnut (p. 363)

Venofit *Arkochim España, Spain,* Witch Hazel (p. 601)

Venoful *Lab. Garden House S.A., Argentina,* Ginkgo (p. 299), Horse-chestnut (p. 363), Hydrocotyle (p. 371), Witch Hazel (p. 601)

Venoplus *Also S.p.A., Italy,* Horse-chestnut (p. 363), Milk Thistle (p. 429), Witch Hazel (p. 601)

Ventre Livre *Companhia Industrial Farmacêutica, Brazil,* Cascara (p. 128)

ventri-loges N *Dr. Loges & Co. GmbH, Germany,* Calamus (p. 118), Gentian (p. 290)

Veracolate *Laboratorio Elea S.A.C.I.F.yA., Argentina,* Cascara (p. 128) *Pfizer (Thailand) Ltd, Thailand,* Cascara (p. 128)

Verbascum Complex *Blackmores Ltd, Australia,* Liquorice (p. 411), Pleurisy Root (p. 477)

Versterkdruppels *Aspen Pharmacare (Pty) Ltd, South Africa,* Gentian (p. 290), Quassia (p. 491)

Vertiginkgo *Midax Italia S.r.l., Italy,* Ginkgo (p. 299)

Vethoine *Wolfs SA, Belgium,* Cascara (p. 128)

Viadent *Colgate Palmolive Canada, Canada,* Bloodroot (p. 84)

Vicks Baby Balsam *Procter & Gamble Srl, Italy,* Aloe Vera (p. 48)

Vida Brown Mixture *Vida Laboratories Ltd, Hong Kong,* Liquorice (p. 411)

Vifortol *Laboratorio Elea S.A.C.I.F.yA., Argentina,* Ginseng, Panax (p. 325)

Vig *Key Pharmaceuticals P/L, Australia,* Ginkgo (p. 299), Ginseng, Panax (p. 325)

Vigilia *Les Grands Espaces Thérapeutiques, France,* Lime Flower (p. 409), Vervain (p. 591)

Vigortonic *Arkochim España, Spain,* Cinnamon (p. 162), Ginseng, Panax (p. 325)

Virgilocard *Sanova Pharma GmbH, Austria,* Hawthorn (p. 346)

Vi-Siblin S *Recip AB, Sweden,* Ispaghula (p. 374)

Visinal *Stada Pharma International os, Czech Republic,* Hops (p. 354), Passionflower (p. 461), Valerian (p. 580)

Visionom *União Química Farmacêutica Nacional S.A., Brazil,* Witch Hazel (p. 601)

Vitace *Prisfar, SA, Portugal,* Echinacea (p. 217)

Vital Eyes *Novartis Consumer Health, UK,* Eyebright (p. 256), Witch Hazel (p. 601)

VitAmour *Healthy Direct, UK,* Damiana (p. 201)

Vitanox *Mediherb P/L, Australia,* Rosemary (p. 508)

Vitatona *Brauer Natural Medicine P/L, Australia,* Angelica (p. 53), Ginseng, Panax (p. 325), Nettle (p. 452), St John's Wort (p. 549)

Vitegin Capsules *Frank Roberts (Herbal Dispensaries) Ltd, UK,* Ginseng, Panax (p. 325)

Vivinox Day *Dr Gerhard Mann, Chem.-pharm. Fabrik GmbH, Germany,* Hops (p. 354), Passionflower (p. 461), Valerian (p. 580)

VNS 45 *Laboratorios Sigma, Argentina,* Ginkgo (p. 299), Horse-chestnut (p. 363), Hydrocotyle (p. 371), Witch Hazel (p. 601)

Vocalzone *Kestrel Healthcare Ltd, UK,* Liquorice (p. 411), Myrrh (p. 449)

Vollmers praparierter gruner N *Salus-Haus Dr. med. Otto Greither Nachf. GmbH & Co KG, Germany,* Nettle (p. 452)

Vulnopur *Devergè Medicina e Medicalizzazione S.r.l., Italy,* Aloe Vera (p. 48)

Wala Echinacea *Wala Schweiz GmbH, Switzerland,* Calendula (p. 121), Echinacea (p. 217), Sage (p. 512)

Wala Pulmonium suc contre la toux *Wala Schweiz GmbH, Switzerland,* Butterbur (p. 107)

Waldheim Abfuhrdragees forte *Sanochemia Pharmazeutika AG, Austria,* Aloes (p. 50)

Waldheim Abfuhrdragees mild *Sanochemia Pharmazeutika AG, Austria,* Aloes (p. 50), Frangula (p. 270)

Wampole Bronchial Cough Syrup *Wampole Brands Inc., Canada,* Bloodroot (p. 84), Senega (p. 533)

Water Naturtabs *Larkhall Laboratories, UK,* Burdock (p. 102), Clivers (p. 164), Ground Ivy (p. 342)

Water Pill *Natrol, USA,* Buchu (p. 100), Juniper (p. 386)

Watershed *Potter's (Herbal Supplies) Ltd, UK,* Buchu (p. 100), Clivers (p. 164), Juniper (p. 386), Parsley Piert (p. 459), Uva-Ursi (p. 577), Wild Carrot (p. 593)

Wecesin *Pharma-Natura (Pty) Ltd, South Africa,* Arnica (p. 64), Calendula (p. 121), Echinacea (p. 217)

Wechseltee St Severin *EF-EM-ES - Dr Smetana & Co., Austria,* Hawthorn (p. 346), Hops (p. 354), Melissa (p. 425), Milk Thistle (p. 429), Passionflower (p. 461), St John's Wort (p. 549), Valerian (p. 580)

Weight Loss Aid *Herbal Concepts Ltd, UK,* Boldo (p. 91), Dandelion (p. 204)

Weleda Hamorrhoidalzapfchen *Weleda AG-Heilmittelbetriebe, Germany,* Horse-chestnut (p. 363), Witch Hazel (p. 601)

Well-Beeing *Panacea Biotec Ltd, India,* Ginger (p. 293), Valerian (p. 580)

Wellman *Vitabiotics Ltd, UK,* Ginseng, Panax (p. 325)

Wellwoman *Potter's (Herbal Supplies) Ltd, UK,* Lime Flower (p. 409), Motherwort (p. 447), Scullcap (p. 530), Valerian (p. 580), Yarrow (p. 604)

Winar *Apogepha Arzneimittel GmbH, Germany,* Nettle (p. 452)

Wind & Dyspepsia Relief *Herbal Concepts Ltd, UK,* Dandelion (p. 204), Ginger (p. 293), Golden Seal (p. 337), Myrrh (p. 449), Rhubarb (p. 506), Valerian (p. 580)

Wobenzimal *Vitafarma, Spain,* Thyme (p. 574)

Women's Formula Herbal Formula 3 *Mayne Pharma P/L, Australia,* Agnus Castus (p. 36), Angelica (p. 53), Cohosh, Black (p. 168), Cohosh, Blue (p. 180), Pulsatilla (p. 489)

Women's Menopause Formula *Natrol, USA,* Agnus Castus (p. 36), Cohosh, Black (p. 168), Damiana (p. 201), Raspberry (p. 495), Red Clover (p. 498)

Wonderkroonessens *Aspen Pharmacare (Pty) Ltd, South Africa,* Aloes (p. 50), Elecampane (p. 240), Gentian (p. 290), Ginger (p. 293), Rhubarb (p. 506), Valerian (p. 580)

Wood Sap Ointment *Richard Lane's, UK,* Rosemary (p. 508), Slippery Elm (p. 545)

Xarope de Macas Rainetas *Sociedade Farmacêutica Gestafarma, Lda, Portugal,* Senna (p. 537)

Xarope Iodo-Suma *Laboratório Iodo Suma Ltda, Brazil,* Gentian (p. 290)

X-Prep Bowel Evacuant Kit-1 *The Purdue Frederick Co., USA,* Senna (p. 537)

Yalu *Lab. Lacefa S.A.I.C.A., Argentina,* Quassia (p. 491)

Yerba Diet *Instituto Seroterapico Argentino S.A.I.C., Argentina,* Passionflower (p. 461)

Ymea *Chefaro UK Ltd, UK,* Hops (p. 354)

Yuyo *Lab. Incaico SA, Argentina,* Aloe Vera (p. 48), Cascara (p. 128)

Zaludecni Cajova Smes *Megafyt-R sro, Czech Republic,* Liquorice (p. 411), St John's Wort (p. 549), Yarrow (p. 604)

Zeller Sommeil *Max Zeller Söhne AG, Pflanzliche Heilmittel, Switzerland,* Hops (p. 354), Valerian (p. 580)

Zeniac *Laboratoires d'Evolution Dermatologique, France,* Burdock (p. 102)

Zeniac LP *Laboratoires d'Evolution Dermatologique, France,* Burdock (p. 102)

Zero Flush Niacin 400mg *Natrol, USA,* Alfalfa (p. 45)

Zinaxin Plus *Diethelm & Co. Ltd, Thailand,* Ginger (p. 293) *JDH Pharmaceutical Sdn Bhd, Diethelm Malaysia Sdn Bhd, Malaysia,* Ginger (p. 293)

Zinc Zenith *Eagle Pharmaceuticals P/L, Australia,* Alfalfa (p. 45)

Zinopin *Pynogin GmbH, Gee Lawson Distribution Centre, UK,* Ginger (p. 293)

Zlucnikova Cajova Smes *Megafyt-R sro, Czech Republic,* Agrimony (p. 42), Rhubarb (p. 506)

Zotrim *Sigma Chemical Co. Ltd, UK,* Damiana (p. 201)

Appendix 5
Suppliers Directory

5

A

1 A Pharma GmbH *Keltenring 1 + 3, 82041 Oberhaching, Germany.*
Tel: +49 (0) 89 61388250 Fax: +49 (0) 89 613882525
Email: medwiss@1apharma.de Web: www.1apharma.de

A. Menarini Industrie Farmaceutiche Riunite S.r.l. *Via Sette Santi 3, 50131 Florence, Italy.*
Tel: +39 055 56801 Fax: +39 055 582771
Web: www.menarini.com

A. Nikolakopoulos & Co. O.E *115 Galatsiou Ave, 111 46 Athens, Greece.*
Tel: +30 1 2918671 Fax: +30 1 2922581

aar pharma GmbH & Co. KG *Alleestr. 11, 42853 Remscheid, Germany.*
Tel: +49 (0) 2191 923013 Fax: +49 (0) 2191 923028
Email: info@aar.de Web: www.aar.de

Abbott GmbH *Perfektastrasse 86, A-1230 Vienna, Austria.*
Tel: +43 (0) 1 891220 Fax: +43 (0) 1 8912244
Web: www.abbott.com

Abbott GmbH & Co. KG *Max-Planck-Ring 2, 65205 Wiesbaden, Germany.*
Tel: +49 (0) 6122 580 Fax: +49 (0) 6122 581244
Web: www.abbott.de

Abbott Laboratories de Mexico S.A. de C.V. *Av. Coyoacan 1622, Benito Juarez del Valle, 03100 Mexico D.F., Mexico.*
Tel: +52 55 57264600 Fax: +52 55 57264601
Web: www.abbott.com

Abbott Laboratories Ltd *20/F AIA Tower, 183 Electric Rd, North Point, Hong Kong.*
Tel: +852 25668711 Fax: +852 28072917
Web: www.abbott.com

Abbott South Africa (Pty) Ltd *P.O. Box 7208, Weltevredenpark, Johannesburg 1715, South Africa.*
Tel: +27 (0) 11 8582000 Fax: +27 (0) 11 8582070
Web: www.abbott.com

Abigo Medical AB *, 436 32 Askim, Sweden.*
Tel: +46 (0) 31 7484950 Fax: +46 (0) 31 683951
Email: pharma@abigo.se Web: www.abigo.com

Abnoba Heilmittel GmbH *Hohenzollernstr. 16, 75177 Pforzheim, Germany.*
Tel: +49 (0) 7231 316478 Fax: +49 (0) 7231 358714
Email: info@abnoba.de Web: www.abnoba.de

Abtswinder Naturheilmittel GmbH *, Czech Republic.*

A.C.P. S.C *Rue Georges Moreau 174, 1070 Brussels, Belgium.*
Tel: +32 (0) 2 3848711 Fax: +32 (0) 2 3847711
Email: direx@direx.be

Adcock Ingram Pharmaceuticals Ltd *Adcock Ingram Park, 17 Harrison Ave, Bryanston 2021, South Africa.*
Tel: +27 (0) 11 7099300 Fax: +27 (0) 11 7099332
Web: www.adcock.co.za

Adler-Apotheke *Wahringer Strasse 149, A-1180 Vienna, Austria.*
Tel: +43 (0) 1 4793320 Fax: +43 (0) 1 470978430

Adroka AG *Postfach, 4123 Allschwil, Switzerland.*
Tel: +41 (0) 61 4863600 Fax: +41 (0) 61 4863636
Email: info@adroka.ch Web: www.adroka.ch

AFOM Medical S.p.A. *Via S Cristoforo 97, 20090 Trezzano S/Naviglio (MI), Italy.*
Tel: +39 02 48463151 Fax: +39 02 48401787

Alcon Cusi *Camil Fabra 58, El Masnou, 08320 El Masnou Barcelona, Spain.*
Tel: +34 93 4977000 Fax: +34 93 4977010
Web: www.alconlabs.com

Alcon Italia S.p.A. *Viale Giulio Richard 1/B, 20143 Milan, Italy.*
Tel: +39 02 818031 Fax: +39 02 8910550
Web: www.alconlabs.com

Alcon Laboratorios Argentina S.A. *Estados Unidos 5335, 1667 Tortuguitas, Buenos Aires, Argentina.*
Tel: +54 (0) 3327 443400 Fax: +54 (0) 3327 443557
Web: www.alconlabs.com

Alcon Laboratorios, S.A. de C.V. *Adolfo Prieto 1644, Benito Juarez del Valle, 03100 Mexico D.F., Mexico.*
Tel: +52 55 52001100 Fax: +52 55 55245264
Web: www.alconlabs.com

Alcon Pharmaceutical C.A. *Av. Diego Cisneros, Edificio Siemens, Torre Sur, Mezzanina, Los Ruices, Caracas 1070, Venezuela.*
Tel: +58 (0) 212 Fax: +58 (0) 212
Web: www.alconlabs.com

Alcor *P Del Prado 14 1 C, 28014 Madrid, Spain.*
Tel: +34 91 4204032 Fax: +34 91 3694788

Alfa Wassermann S.p.A. *Contrada Sant'Emidio, 65020 Alanno (PE), Italy.*
Tel: +39 085 85711 Fax: +39 085 8541625

Alinter Ltd *New Abbey Court, 51-53 Stert St, Abingdon, OX14 3HB, UK.*
Tel: +44 (0) 1235 538700 Fax: +44 (0) 1235 538800
Email: info@alinter.co.uk Web: www.alinter.co.uk

allcura Naturheilmittel GmbH *Reichendaker 7, 97877 Wertheim, Germany.*
Tel: +49 (0) 9342 96110 Fax: +49 (0) 9342 961196
Email: info@allcura.de Web: www.allcura.de

Allen Laboratorios, S.A. de C.V. *Av. Instituto Politécnico Nacional No. 4728, Gustavo A Madero, Tlacamaca, 07380 Mexico D.F, Mexico.*
Tel: +52 55 55678027 Fax: +52 55 55678027

Allens & Co. (Anglesey) Ltd *Freshwinds, Pentraeth, Isle of Anglesey, LL75 8YF, UK.*
Tel: +44 (0) 1248 450604 Fax: +44 (0) 1248 450822
Email: info@allenshealthcare.co.uk Web: www.allenshealthcare.co.uk

Allergan Produtos Farmacêuticos Ltda *Av. Cardoso de Melo 1955 13 andar, 4548005 São Paulo, Brazil.*

Alliance Boots plc *4th Floor, 361 Oxford Street, Sedley Place, London, W1C 2JL, UK.*
Web: www.allianceboots.com

Allmedica Arzneimittel GmbH *Schillerstr. 4, 37269 Eschwege, Germany.*
Tel: +49 (0) 5651 60356 Fax: +49 (0) 5651 70888

Almirall Prodesfarma S.A. *Rda Gral Mitre 151, 08022 Barcelona, Spain.*
Tel: +34 93 2913000 Fax: +34 93 2913180
Web: www.almirall.es

Alpa sro *, Velke Meziřiči, Czech Republic.*

Alpharma France *40 rue Lecuyer, 93300 Aubervilliers, France.*
Tel: +33 (0) 1 48110820 Fax: +33 (0) 1 48339662
Web: www.alpharma.fr

Alpharma-Isis GmbH & Co. KG *Elisabeth-Selbert-Str. 1, 40764 Langenfeld, Germany.*
Tel: +49 (0) 2173 16740 Fax: +49 (0) 2173 1674205
Email: info.de@alpharma.de Web: www.alpharma.de

Alphrema S.r.l. *Via 4 Novembre 92, 20021 Bollate (MI), Italy.*
Tel: +39 (0) 23506945 Fax: +39 (0) 238306418

Alsitan GmbH & Co. KG *Am Buhl 16-18, 86926 Greifenberg, Germany.*
Tel: +49 (0) 8192 93010 Fax: +49 (0) 8192 7827
Web: www.alsitan.com

Also S.p.A. *Viale Monte Rosa 96, 20149 Milan, Italy.*
Tel: +39 02 485631 Fax: +39 02 4984727

Altana Madaus Pty Ltd *1st Floor, Uplands 12, The Woodlands, ZA-2080 Woodmead, Sandton, South Africa.*
Tel: +27 (0) 11 8042914 Fax: +27 (0) 11 3152125
Web: www.altana.com

Altana Pharma Deutschland GmbH *Moltkestr. 4, 78467 Constance, Germany.*
Email: customerservice@altanapharma.de
Web: www.altanapharma.de

Altana Pharma GmbH *Ketzergasse 2000, A-1235 Vienna, Austria.*
Tel: +43 (0) 1 866530 Fax: +43 (0) 1 86653430

Altana Pharma Ltd *Bachstrasse 10, 8280 Kreuzlingen, Switzerland.*
Tel: +41 (0) 71 6771333 Fax: +41 (0) 71 6771334
Email: mail@altanapharma.ch

Altana Pharma Ltda *Rua do Estilo Barroco 721, Santo Amaro, 04709-011 São Paulo, Brazil.*
Tel: +55 (0) 11 51884400 Fax: +55 (0) 11 51834361
Web: www.altana.com

Altana Pharma SA *Tronador 4890, 1430 Buenos Aires, Argentina.*

Altana Pharma S.A. de C.V. *Av Primero de Mayo No. 130, Col. San Andres Atoto, 53519 Naucalpan de Juarez., Mexico.*
Tel: +52 55 53879330 Fax: +52 55 53590108
Web: www.altana.com

Alter *Mateo Inurria 30, 28036 Madrid, Spain.*
Tel: +34 91 3592000 Fax: +34 91 3501165
Email: informacion@alter.es Web: www.alter.es

Amerx Health Care Corp. *1150 Cleveland St, Suite 410, Clearwater, FL 33755, USA.*

Amino AG *Althofstrasse 12, 5432 Neuenhof, Switzerland.*
Tel: +41 (0) 56 4061264 Fax: +41 (0) 56 4061764
Email: info@amino.ch

Amnol Chimica Biologica S.r.l. *C.so della Vittoria 12/b, 28100 Novara (NO), Italy.*
Tel: +39 0321 499199 Fax: +39 0321 499202
Web: www.amnol.net

Amternes Laegemiddelregistreringskontor I/S *Amsträdsforeningen, Dampfaergevej 22 (postboks 2593), 2100 Copenhagen O, Denmark.*
Tel: +45 35298151 Fax: +45 35298333
Email: alis@arf.dk

Andrae GmbH *Marinonigasse 2-6, A-1210 Vienna, Austria.*
Tel: +43 (0) 1 29215590 Fax: +43 (0) 1 2921559

Aneid, Lda *Rua José Florindo, Quinta da Pedra, Bloco B, R/C A, 2750-401 Cascais, Portugal.*
Tel: +351 21 4849620 Fax: +351 21 4849629
Email: info@aneid.pt Web: www.aneid.pt

Angelini *Rua João Chagas 53, Piso 3, 1495-072 Alges, Portugal.*
Tel: +351 214 148300 Fax: +351 214 142981

Anglian Pharma Plc *P.O. Box 161, Hitchin, SG4 7WE, UK.*
Tel: +44 (0) 1438 743070 Fax: +44 (0) 1438 743080
Web: www.anglianpharma.com

Antah Pharma Sdb Bhd *3 Jln 19/1, 46300 Petaling Jaya, Malaysia.*
Tel: +60 (0) 3 79567677 Fax: +60 (0) 3 79552007

Antistress AG, Gesellschaft fur Gesundheitsschutz *Fluhstrasse 30, 8640 Rapperswil, Switzerland.*
Tel: +41 (0) 55 2201212 Fax: +41 (0) 55 2201213
Email: services@antistress.ch Web: www.antistress.ch

Apivita SA *3 Koletti St, 144 52 Metamorfosi Attikis, Greece.*
Tel: +30 210 2856350 Fax: +30 210 2843580
Web: www.apivita.com

Apogepha Arzneimittel GmbH *Kyffhauserstr. 27, 01309 Dresden, Germany.*
Tel: +49 (0) 351 33633 Fax: +49 (0) 351 3363440
Email: apo@apogepha.de Web: www.apogepha.de

Apomedica GmbH *Roseggerkai 3, A-8011 Graz, Austria.*
Tel: +43 (0) 316 823533 Fax: +43 (0) 316 82353352

Aponova Pharma Handels GmbH *Niederhart 100, A-6253 Hart, Austria.*
Tel: +43 (0) 5288 64885 Fax: +43 (0) 5288 64885-5

Apotheke zur Gnadenmutter *Hauptplatz 4, A-8630 Mariazell, Austria.*
Tel: +43 (0) 3882 2102 Fax: +43 (0) 3882 210222

Apotheker Walter Bouhon GmbH & Co. KG *Walter-Bouhan-Str 4, 90427 Nurnberg, Germany.*
Tel: +49 (0) 911 936700 Fax: +49 (0) 911 3071780
Email: info@freioel.de Web: www.freioel.de

APS Pharma GmbH *Angelsrieder Feld 22, 82234 Wessling, Germany.*
Tel: +49 (0) 8153 90810 Fax: +49 (0) 8153 908130

Ardeypharm GmbH *Loerfeldstr. 20, 58313 Herdecke, Germany.*
Tel: +49 (0) 2330 977677 Fax: +49 (0) 2330 977697
Email: office@ardeypharm.de Web: www.ardeypharm.de

Ariston Industrias Químicas e Farm. Ltda *Rua Adherbal Stresser 84, 05566-000 São Paulo, Brazil.*
Tel: +55 (0) 11 37838000

Arko Pharma GmbH *Bajurwarenring 12, 82041 Oberhaching, Germany.*
Tel: +49 (0) 89 6281710 Fax: +49 (0) 89 62817177
Email: info@arkopharma.de Web: www.arkopharma.com

Arkochim España *Meneses 2, 28045 Madrid, Spain.*
Tel: +34 91 5271512 Fax: +34 91 5279991
Email: marketing@arkochim.es Web: www.arkochim.es

Arkofarm S.r.l. *Via Limone Piemonte 13/D, 18039 Ventimiglia (IM), Italy.*
Tel: +39 0184 236611 Fax: +39 0184 230900
Web: www.arkopharma-italia.com

Arkopharma UK Ltd *6 Redlands Centre, Redlands, Coulsden, CR5 2HT, UK.*
Tel: +44 (0) 20 8763 1414 Fax: +44 (0) 20 8763 2124
Email: info@arkopharma.co.uk Web: www.arkopharma.com

Arlex de México, S.A.deC.V. *Puerto Acapulco No.35, Col. Piloto, Deleg. Alvaro Obregon, 01290 Mexico D.F., Mexico.*
Tel: +52 55 56435099 Fax: +52 55 56435099

Artesan Pharma GmbH & Co. KG *Wendlandstr. 1, 29439 Luchow, Germany.*
Tel: +49 (0) 5841 9390 Fax: +49 (0) 5841 939200
Email: artesan@t-online.de Web: www.artesan.de

Artsana S.p.A. *Via Saldarini Catelli 1, 22070 Grandate (CO), Italy.*
Tel: +39 031 382111 Fax: +39 031 382400

Arzneimittel Schwabe International GmbH Čestmirová 1, 140 00 Prague 4, Czech Republic.
Tel: +420 (0) 2 6913971 Fax: +420 (0) 2 6913541
Email: asi@login.cz

A.S.A.C. Pharma *Sagitario 14, 03006 Alicante, Spain.*
Tel: +34 96 5286700 Fax: +34 96 5286434
Email: asac@asac.net Web: www.asac.net

Ashbury Biologicals Inc. *349 Wildcat Rd, Toronto, M3J 2S3, Canada.*
Tel: +1 416 6670555 Fax: +1 416 6612108
Email: ashbury@dalton.com Web: www.ashburybio.com

ASI Budapest Kft *Üllői u 91/b I/7, 1091 Budapest, Hungary.*
Tel: +36 2150672

Aspen Pharmacare (Pty) Ltd *P. O. Box 1587, Gallo Manor 2052, South Africa.*
Tel: +27 (0) 11 2396100 Fax: +27 (0) 11 2396111
Web: www.aspenpharmacare.co.za

Asta Medica Ltda *Rua Santo Antonio 184 19 degrees andar, 01314-900 São Paulo, Brazil.*
Tel: +55 (0) 11 32436800 Fax: +55 (0) 11 31072291
Email: cac@astamedica.com.br Web: www.astamedica.com.br

AstraZeneca GmbH *, 22876 Wedel, Germany.*
Tel: +49 (0) 4103 7080 Fax: +49 (0) 4103 7083293
Email: azinfo@astrazeneca.com Web: www.astrazeneca.de

AstraZeneca Sverige AB *Storgatan 42, 151 85 Södertälje, Sweden.*
Tel: +46 (0) 8 55326000 Fax: +46 (0) 8 55328920
Web: www.astrazeneca.se

Astrid Twardy GmbH *Liebigstr. 18, 65439 Florsheim/Main, Germany.*
Tel: +49 (0) 6145 5930 Fax: +49 (0) 6145 593210
Email: info@twardy.de Web: www.twardy.de

Ativus Farmacêutica Ltda *Rua Fonte Mecia 2050, 13270000 Valinhos, Brazil.*
Tel: +55 (0) 19 38498600 Email: ativus@ativus.com.br
Web: www.ativus.com.br

Atlantic Pharmaceutical Co. Ltd *2038 Sukhumvit Rd, Bangkok 10250, Thailand.*
Tel: +66 2 311 0111 Fax: +66 2 331 5697
Email: atlantic@mozart.inet.co.th Web: www.atlanticlab.com

Atlas Farmaceutica *JV Gonzalez 2456, 1417 Buenos Aires, Argentina.*

Australian Medic-Care Co. Ltd *Suite 2810, Metroplaza Tower 2, 223 Hing Fong Rd, Kwai Fong, Kwai Chung, Hong Kong.*
Tel: +852 24804822 Fax: +852 24804866

Austroplant-Arzneimittel GmbH *Richard-Strauss-Strasse 13, A-1232 Vienna, Austria.*
Tel: +43 (0) 1 61626440 Fax: +43 (0) 1 616264418

Avanderm Mexico, S.A. de C.V. *Patricio Saenz 1582, Del Valle, 3100 Mexico D. F., Mexico.*
Tel: +52 55 55249250 Fax: +52 55 55341456

Aventis Pharma *Bijenvlucht 30, 3871 JJ Hoevelaken, Netherlands.*
Tel: +31 (0) 33 2533911 Fax: +31 (0) 33 2535017
Web: www.aventis.nl

Aventis Pharma Ltda *Avenida Marginal do Rio Pinheiros 5200, 05693-000 São Paulo, Brazil.*
Tel: +55 (0) 11 37596000 Fax: +55 (0) 11 2476640
Web: www.aventispharma.com.br

5

Aventis Pharma (Pty) Ltd *Private Bag X207, Midrand 1683, South Africa.*
Tel: +27 (0) 11 2563700 Fax: +27 (0) 11 2563722
Web: www.sanofi-aventis.com

Aventis Pharma S.A. de C.V. *Av. Universidad No. 1738, Col. Coyoacan, 04000 Mexico D.F., Mexico.*
Tel: +52 55 54844400 Fax: +52 55 54804113
Web: www.aventis.com

Aventis Pharma S.p.A. *P.le Stefano Turr 5, 20149 Milan (MI), Italy.*
Tel: +39 (0) 2937661 Fax: +39 (0) 293766046
Web: www.aventispharma.it

Aventis Pharma sro *Novodvorská 994, 142 21 Prague 4, Czech Republic.*
Tel: +420 (0) 2 44043355 Fax: +420 (0) 2 44044110
Web: www.aventis.com

Awareness Corp. *210-9087B-198th Street, Langley, V1M 3B1, Canada.*

Aziende Chimiche Riunite Angelini Francesco S.p.A. *Viale Amelia 70, 00100 Rome, Italy.*
Tel: +39 06 780531 Fax: +39 06 78053291

B

B L Hua & Co. Ltd *2 Somdej Chaopraya Rd, Klongsan, Bangkok 10600, Thailand.*
Tel: +66 2 437 0154 Fax: +66 2 437 5655

Bad Heilbrunner Naturheilmittel GmbH & Co. *Am Krebsenbach 5-7, 83670 Bad Heilbrunn, Germany.*
Tel: +49 (0) 8046 91990 Fax: +49 (0) 8046 919999
Email: info@bad-heilbrunner.de Web: www.bad-heilbrunner.de

Baif International Products, New York S.n.c. *Via XX Setembre 20/68, 16121 Genoa, Italy.*
Tel: +39 010 566251 Fax: +39 010 566252

Balmar *P.O. Box 41-014, St Lukes, Auckland, New Zealand.*
Tel: +64 (0) 9 8151020 Fax: +64 (0) 9 8151036
Web: www.balmar.co.nz

Balverda Srl *Via Robert Kock 1.2, 20152 Milan, Italy.*
Tel: +39 (0) 248381 Fax: +39 (0) 248382734

Barrenne Indústria Farmacêutica Ltda *Rua Antunes Maciel 86, São Cristovao, 20940-010 Rio de Janeiro, Brazil.*
Tel: +55 (0) 21 25898973 Fax: +55 (0) 21 25891364
Web: www.barrene.com.br

Bastian-Werk GmbH *August-Exter-Str. 4, 81245 Munich, Germany.*
Tel: +49 (0) 89 820930 Fax: +49 (0) 89 8209359
Email: bastian@bastian-werk.de Web: www.bastian-werk.de

Bausch & Lomb Oftal SpA *Corso Italia 141, 95127 Catania (CT), Italy.*
Tel: +39 (0) 957221322 Fax: +39 (0) 957223856

Bausch & Lomb Swiss AG *Sumpfstrasse 3, 6312 Steinhausen, Switzerland.*
Tel: +41 (0) 41 7471060 Fax: +41 (0) 41 7471069

Bayer Argentina S.A. *Ricardo Gutierrez 3652, 1605 Munro, Buenos Aires, Argentina.*
Tel: +54 (0) 11 47627000 Fax: +54 (0) 11 47627100
Web: www.bayer.com.ar

Bayer Australia Ltd (Pharmaceutical Business Group) *P.O. Box 903, Pymble, NSW 2073, Australia.*
Tel: +61 (0) 2 93916000 Fax: +61 (0) 2 93916061
Web: www.bayer.com

Bayer Austria GmbH *Am Heumarkt 10, Postfach 10, 1037 Vienna, Austria.*
Tel: +43 (0) 1 711460 Fax: +43 (0) 1 711462788
Web: www.bayer.at

Bayer SA *Carlos Fernandez 260, San Joaquin, Santiago, Chile.*

Bayer (Schweiz) AG, Pharma *Postfach, Grubenstrasse 6, 8045 Zurich, Switzerland.*
Tel: +41 (0) 1 4658111 Fax: +41 (0) 1 4620754
Web: www.bayer.ch

Beaufour Ipsen International *U platenice 10, 150 00 Prague 5, Czech Republic.*
Tel: +420 (0) 2 57324660 Fax: +420 (0) 2 57324660
Email: bii@tnet.cz

Beaufour Ipsen International SNC *Mosenka Park Tower, Taganskaya ul. 19, 109004 Moscow, Russia.*
Tel: +7 095 2585400 Fax: +7 095 2585401
Web: www.ipsen.com

Beaufour Ipsen Pharma *24 rue Erlanger, 75781 Paris cdx 16, France.*
Tel: +33 (0) 1 44961313 Fax: +33 (0) 1 44961199
Web: www.beaufour-ipsen.com

Beethoven-Pharma Dr Wiemann GmbH *Steinthalstr. 1, 90455 Nurnberg, Germany.*
Tel: +49 (0) 911 880044 Fax: +49 (0) 911 880255

Beiersdorf GmbH *Laxenburger Strasse 151, A-1101 Vienna, Austria.*
Tel: +43 (0) 1 614000 Fax: +43 (0) 1 61400391
Email: contact@vienna.beiersdorf.com Web: www.beiersdorf.com

Beiersdorf SA *Lo Espejo 501, Maipu, Santiago, Chile.*

Beiersdorf UK Ltd *2010 Solihull Parkway, Birmingham Business Park, Birmingham, B37 7YS, UK.*
Tel: +44 (0) 121 3298800 Fax: +44 (0) 121 329 8801
Web: www.beiersdorf.com

Bell, Sons & Co. (Druggists) *P.O. Box 62, Tanhouse Lane, Widnes, WA8 0SA, UK.*
Tel: +44 (0) 151 422 1200 Fax: +44 (0) 151 420 1211
Email: brianlunt@bells-healthcare.com Web: www.bells-healthcare.com

Benedetti S.p.A. *Vicolo de' Bacchettoni 3, 51100 Pistoia (PT), Italy.*
Tel: +39 0573 536496 Fax: +39 0573 534673
Email: ledisar@tin.it

Berlin Pharmaceutical Industry Co. Ltd *359 New Rd, Bangkok 10100, Thailand.*
Tel: +66 2 223 1011 Fax: +66 2 225 4260
Email: berlinin@lox1.loxinfo.co.th Web: www.berlinpharm.com

Berlin-Chemie Képviselet *Váci út 113, 1138 Budapest, Hungary.*
Tel: +36 3296808 Fax: +36 3409352

Berlin-Chemie Menarini Group *Komarková 27, 148 00 Prague 4, Czech Republic.*
Tel: +420 (0) 2 71913199 Fax: +420 (0) 2 7929742
Email: office@berlin-chemie.cz

Berlin-Pharma ZAO Moscow *ul. Kashirskoe 22-3, Str. 3, 115201 Moscow, Russia.*
Tel: +7 095 4928709 Fax: +7 095 7975958
Email: info@berlin-pharma.ru Web: www.berlin-chemie.ru

Berta S.r.l. *Via Andrea Doria 7, 20124 Milan, Italy.*
Tel: +39 02 6694750 Fax: +39 02 6693828

Bescansa *Pl. Inds. Tambre-via Pasteur 8, Santiago de Compostela, 15890 La Coruna, Spain.*
Tel: +34 981 958002 Fax: +34 981 552745
Email: labbescansa@telefonica.net

betapharm Arzneimittel GmbH *Kobelweg 95, 86156 Augsburg, Germany.*
Tel: +49 (0) 821 748810 Fax: +49 (0) 821 74881420
Email: info@betapharm.de Web: www.betapharm.de

Biocare Ltd *Lakeside, 180 Lifford Lane, Kings Norton, Birmingham, B30 3NU, UK.*
Tel: +44 (0) 121 433 8725 Fax: +44 (0) 121 433 8705
Email: sales@biocare.co.uk Web: www.biocare.co.uk

Biochimici PSN S.p.A. *Via Viadagola 30, 40050 Quarto Inferiore (BO), Italy.*
Tel: +39 051 767015 Fax: +39 051 767154
Email: psn@biochimici.it

Biocur Arzneimittel GmbH *Otto-von-Guericke-Allee 1, 39179 Barleben, Germany.*
Tel: +49 (0) 8024 9080 Fax: +49 (0) 8024 9081290
Email: medwiss@biocur.de Web: www.biocur.de

Bioderma *75 cours Albert-Thomas, 69447 Lyon cdx 03, France.*
Tel: +33 (0) 4 72114800 Fax: +33 (0) 4 78538254
Web: www.bioderma.com

Bio-Diät-Berlin GmbH *Selerweg 43-45, 12169 Berlin, Germany.*
Tel: +49 (0) 30 795201112 Fax: +49 (0) 30 7967233
Email: info@bio-diaet-berlin.de Web: www.bio-diaet-berlin.de

Biofarma Natural CMD SA de CV *Industria Hulera 97 Fracc. Indust., 45130 Zapopan Norte Zapopan, Mexico.*

Bioforce AG *Postfach 76, 9325 Roggwil/TG, Switzerland.*
Tel: +41 (0) 71 4546161 Fax: +41 (0) 71 4546162
Email: info@bioforce.ch Web: www.bioforce.ch

Bioforce GmbH *Bruhlstr. 15, 78465 Constance, Germany.*
Tel: +49 (0) 7533 93010 Fax: +49 (0) 7533 930130
Email: bioforce@bioforce.de Web: www.bioforce.de

Bioforce UK Ltd *2 Brewster Place, Irvine, KA11 5DD, UK.*
Tel: +44 (0) 1294 277344 Fax: +44 (0) 1294 277922
Email: enquires@bioforce.co.uk Web: www.bioforce.co.uk

Biogal-Teva Pharma Rt *Róbert Károly krt 66, 1134 Budapest, Hungary.*
Tel: +36 2886400 Fax: +36 2886410

Bio-Garten GmbH *Triesterstrasse 14/1, A-2351 Wiener Neudorf, Austria.*
Tel: +43 (0) 2236 865901 Fax: +43 (0) 2236 86590122

Bioglan Ltd *8/10 Yalgar Rd, Yalgar Business Park, Kirrawee, NSW 2232, Australia.*
Tel: +61 (0) 2 95451165 Fax: +61 (0) 2 95451067
Web: www.bioglan.com.au

Biolab Sanus Farmacêutica Ltda *Av. dos Bandeirantes 5386, Planalto Paulista, 04071-900 São Paulo, Brazil.*
Tel: +55 (0) 11 55862000 Fax: +55 (0) 11 55840376
Web: www.biolabfarma.com.br

Biomed AG *Uberlandstrasse 199, Postfach, 8600 Dubendorf 1, Switzerland.*
Tel: +41 (0) 44 8021616 Fax: +41 (0) 44 8021600
Email: biomed@biomed.ch Web: www.biomed.ch

Biomedica sro *, Prague, Czech Republic.*

biomo Pharma GmbH *Lendersbergstrasse 86, 53721 Siegburg, Germany.*
Tel: +49 (0) 2241 385081 Fax: +49 (0) 2241 387007

Bional Pharma Deutschland GmbH & Co. KG *Heidsieker Heide 144, 33739 Bielefeld, Germany.*
Tel: +49 (0) 5206 704433 Fax: +49 (0) 5206 704443
Email: info@bional.de Web: www.bional.de

Bionax Singapore Pte Ltd *99 Bukit Timah Rd, Alfa Centre 03-06, S 229835, Singapore.*
Tel: +65 6333 3432 Fax: +65 6339 7875
Email: bionax@pacific.net.sg

Bionax (Thailand) Ltd *10 Fl, Unit A, Lake Rajada Office Complex, 193/35 New Rachadapisek Rd, Kwaeng Klongtoey, Khet Klongtoey, Bangkok 10110, Thailand.*
Tel: +66 2 661 9208 Fax: +66 2 264 0316

Bionorica AG *Kerschensteinerstr. 11-15, 92318 Neumarkt/Opf, Germany.*
Tel: +49 (0) 9181 23190 Fax: +49 (0) 9181 231265
Email: info@bionorica.de Web: www.bionorica.de

Bionorica AG *Udaltsova 52, 119607 Moscow, Russia.*
Tel: +7 095 5029019 Fax: +7 095 7341200
Email: bionorica@co.ru Web: www.bionorica.de

Bio-Pharmaceuticals Sdn Bhd *C-5-8, Block C, Centre Point Business Park, 5 Jln 26/53, Seksyen 26, 400000 Shah Alam, Malaysia.*
Tel: +60 (0) 3 51011450 Fax: +60 (0) 3 51912025

Bioplanta Arzneimittel GmbH *Bahnhofstr. 5, 76275 Ettlingen, Germany.*
Tel: +49 (0) 7243 939845 Fax: +49 (0) 7243 939846

Bioprogress S.p.A. *Via Aurelia 58, 00100 Rome, Italy.*
Tel: +39 06 39383101 Fax: +39 06 39382134

Biosaúde Produtos Farmaceuticos SA *Rua Ramalho Ortigão 45A, 1070-228 Lisbon, Portugal.*
Tel: +351 21 3191280 Fax: +351 21 3191289

Bio-Strath AG *, Czech Republic.*

Bio-Strath AG *Muhlebachstrasse 25, 8032 Zurich, Switzerland.*
Tel: +41 (0) 1 258151 Fax: +41 (0) 1 2624326

biosyn Arzneimittel GmbH *Schorndorfer Str. 32, 70734 Fellbach, Germany.*
Tel: +49 (0) 711 5753200 Fax: +49 (0) 711 5753299
Email: info@biosyn.de Web: www.biosyn.de

Biovital Pty Ltd *24/10 Yalgar Road, Kirrawee, NSW 2232, Australia.*
Tel: +61 (0) 2 95451899 Fax: +61 (0) 2 95451992

Birchwood Laboratories Inc. *7900 Fuller Rd, Eden Prairie, MN 53344-2195, USA.*
Tel: +1 952 937 7943 Fax: +1 952 937 7979
Email: medical@birchlabs.com Web: www.birchlabs.com

Bittermedizin Arzneimittel Vertriebs-GmbH *Taku-Fort-Str. 20, 81827 Munich, Germany.*
Tel: +49 (0) 89 4306841 Fax: +49 (0) 89 4304043
Email: info@bittermedizin.com Web: www.bittermedizin.com

BJC Trading Co Ltd *99 Soi Rubia, Sukhumvit 42 Rd, Bangkok 10110, Thailand.*
Tel: +66 2 367 1274 Fax: +66 2 381 4551
Email: bjcpharma@berlijucker.co.th Web: www.bjc.co.th

Blackmores Ltd *P.O. Box 258, Balgowlah, NSW 2093, Australia.*
Tel: +61 (0) 2 99510111 Fax: +61 (0) 2 99491954
Web: www.blackmores.com.au

Body Spring S.r.l. *Via Parco della Rimembranza 27, 00041 Albano Laziale (RM), Italy.*
Tel: +39 (0) 718091 Fax: +39 (0) 71809440

Boehringer Ingelheim *Carlos Fernandez 260, San Joaquin, Santiago, Chile.*

Boehringer Ingelheim *Prat d ela Riba S/N, Sector Turo de Can Matas, Sant Cugat del Valles, 08190 Barcelona, Spain.*
Tel: +34 93 4045100 Fax: +34 93 4045580
Email: webmaster@boehringer-ingelheim.es
Web: www.boehringer-ingelheim.es

Boehringer Ingelheim Austria GmbH *Dr Boehringer-Gasse 5-11, A-1121 Vienna, Austria.*
Tel: +43 (0) 1 801050 Fax: +43 (0) 1 8040823
Web: www.boehringer-ingelheim.at

Boehringer Ingelheim (Canada) Ltd *5180 South Service Rd, Burlington, L7L 5H4, Canada.*
Tel: +1 905 6390333 Fax: +1 905 6393769
Web: www.boehringer-ingelheim.ca

Boehringer Ingelheim, Division Diethelm Malaysia Sdn Bhd *P.O. Box 3031, 47620 Subang Jaya, Malaysia.*
Tel: +60 (0) 3 80246088 Fax: +60 (0) 3 80249088
Web: www.boehringer-ingelheim.com

5

Boehringer Ingelheim do Brasil Quím. e Farm. Ltda *Av. Maria Coelho Aguair 215, Bl. F. 3 degrees andar, 05805-000 São Paulo, Brazil.*
Tel: +55 (0) 11 37412181 Fax: +55 (0) 11 37411678
Web: www.boehringer-ingelheim.com.br

Boehringer Ingelheim France *37-9 rue Boissière, 75116 Paris, France.*
Tel: +33 (0) 1 44346565 Web: www.boehringer-ingelheim.fr

Boehringer Ingelheim Italia S.p.A. *Via Lorenzini 8, 20139 Milan, Italy.*
Tel: +39 02 53551 Fax: +39 02 5355222
Web: www.boehringer-ingelheim.it

Boehringer Ingelheim, Lda *Av. António Augusto de Aguiar 104, 1069-029 Lisbon, Portugal.*
Tel: +351 21 3135300 Fax: +351 21 3135303
Web: www.boehringer-ingelheim.com

Boehringer Ingelheim Pharma GmbH *Moscow Office, Donskaya ul. 39/9, Str. 1, 119049 Moscow, Russia.*
Tel: +7 095 4117801 Fax: +7 095 4117802
Web: www.boehringer-ingelheim.com

Boehringer Ingelheim Pharma GmbH & Co. KG *Binger Str. 173, 55216 Ingelheim, Germany.*
Tel: +49 (0) 1805 779090 Fax: +49 (0) 6132 729999
Email: webmaster.bipd@boehringer-ingelheim.com
Web: www.boehringer-ingelheim.de

Boehringer Ingelheim Pharma Magyarországi Kereskedelmi Képviselet *Dobsinai u 19, 1124 Budapest, Hungary.*
Tel: +36 2247120 Fax: +36 2247121

Boehringer Ingelheim Promeco, S.A. de C.V. *Calle del Maiz No. 49, Col. Xaltocan, Deleg. Xochimilco, 16090 Mexico D.F., Mexico.*
Tel: +52 55 56298300 Fax: +52 55 56765866
Email: webmaster@mex.boehringer-ingelheim.com
Web: www.boehringer-ingelheim.com.mx

Boehringer Ingelheim S.A. *Av. del Libertador 7208, 1429 Buenos Aires, Argentina.*
Tel: +54 (0) 11 47048600 Fax: +54 (0) 11 47048630
Web: www.bai.boehringer-ingelheim.com

Boehringer Ingelheim SA/NV *Ave Ariane 16, 1200 Brussels, Belgium.*
Tel: +32 (0) 2 7733311 Fax: +32 (0) 2 7733300
Email: external@bru.boehringer-ingelheim.com
Web: www.boehringer-ingelheim.be

Boehringer Ingelheim sro *Lublańská 21, 120 00 Prague 2, Czech Republic.*
Tel: +420 (0) 2 21983111 Fax: +420 (0) 2 21983222
Email: info@boehringer-ingelheim.cz Web: www.boehringer-ingelheim.cz

Boehringer Ingelheim (Thai) Ltd *12 Fl, Charn Issara Tower II, 2922/207-208 New Petchburi Rd, Bangkapi, Huay Kwang, Bangkok 10310, Thailand.*
Tel: +66 2 308 8500 Fax: +66 2 308 2117
Web: www.boehringer-ingelheim.com

Boiron CZ sro *Vlková 40, 130 00 Prague 3, Czech Republic.*
Tel: +420 (0) 2 22722350 Fax: +420 (0) 2 22721139
Email: office@boiron.cz

Bolder Arzneimittel GmbH & Co. KG *Koblenzer Str. 65, 50968 Cologne, Germany.*
Tel: +49 (0) 221 376520 Fax: +49 (0) 221 3765225
Email: info@bolder.de Web: www.bolder.de

Boots Healthcare *Doctor Zamenhof 36 Dup 2, 28027 Madrid, Spain.*
Tel: +34 91 7433930 Fax: +34 91 3249527
Email: info@bhi.com Web: www.bootshealthcare.es

Boots Healthcare Australia P/L *Locked Bag 2067, North Ryde, NSW 1670, Australia.*
Tel: +61 (0) 2 98706000 Fax: +61 (0) 2 98706100
Web: www.skinexpert.net

Boots Healthcare New Zealand Ltd *P.O. Box 27-341, Wellington 1, New Zealand.*
Tel: +64 (0) 4 4733859 Fax: +64 (0) 4 4722706
Web: www.skinexpert.net

Boots Healthcare (SA) (Pty) Ltd *20 Zulberg Close, Building A, Entrance 2, Johannesburg 2198, South Africa.*
Tel: +27 (0) 11 6165544 Fax: +27 (0) 11 6160710
Web: www.skinexpert.net

Boots Healthcare S.p.A. *Via Tarantelli 13/15, 22076 Mozzate (CO), Italy.*
Tel: +39 0331 838111 Fax: +39 0331 821450
Web: www.skinexpert.net

Boots Healthcare (Switzerland) AG, Hermal *Untermuli 11, 6300 Zug, Switzerland.*
Tel: +41 (0) 41 7632575 Fax: +41 (0) 41 7632576
Web: www.skinexpert.net

Boots Trading (Malaysia) Sdn Bhd *Level 4, Wisma Samudra, 1 Jln Kontraktor U1/14, Hicom-Glenmarie Industrial Park, 40150 Shah Alam, Malaysia.*
Tel: +60 (0) 3 55695418 Fax: +60 (0) 3 55695452
Web: www.skinexpert.net

Bouty SpA *V.le Casiraghi 471, 20099 Sesto S Giovanni (MI), Italy.*
Tel: +39 02 262891 Fax: +39 02 26221305

Bouzen S.A.C,.I.F.A.F. *Calle 36 No. 165/67, 1900 La Plata, Buenos Aires, Argentina.*
Tel: +54 (0) 11 4839908 Web: www.bouzensa.com.ar

Bracco S.p.A. *Via E. Folli 50, 20134 Milan, Italy.*
Tel: +39 02 21771 Fax: +39 02 26410678
Web: www.bracco.com

Brady C. KG *Horlgasse 5, A-1092 Vienna, Austria.*
Tel: +43 (0) 1 3106960

Brasmedica S.A. Industrias Farmacêuticas *Avenida Miguel Stefano 2278, 04301-002 São Paulo, Brazil.*

Brauer Natural Medicine P/L *P.O. Box 234, Tanunda, SA 5352, Australia.*
Tel: +61 (0) 8 85632932 Fax: +61 (0) 8 85633398
Email: admin@brauer.com.au Web: www.brauer.com.au

Bristol-Myers Squibb *3 rue Joseph-Monier, 92506 Rueill-Malmaison cdx, France.*
Tel: +33 (0) 1 58836000 Fax: +33 (0) 1 58836001
Email: infomed@bms.com Web: www.bms.com

British Dispensary *272 Moo 1 Soi Pattanasuk, Teparak Rd, Samutprakarn 10270, Thailand.*
Tel: +66 (0) 2755 7300 Fax: +66 (0) 2755 7315
Email: customerservice@britishdispensary.com

British Snoring & Sleep Apnoea Association Ltd *2nd Floor Suite, 52 Albert Rd North, Reigate, RH2 9EL, UK.*
Tel: +44 (0) 1737 245638 Fax: +44 (0) 1737 248744
Email: info@britishsnoring.co.uk Web: www.britishsnoring.co.uk

Bucca *Juan Alvarez Mendizabal 43, 28008 Madrid, Spain.*
Tel: +34 91 5473463 Fax: +34 91 5473463

Bunker Indústria Farmacêutica Ltda *Rua Anibal dos Anjos Carvalho 212, 04810-050 São Paulo, Brazil.*
Tel: +55 (0) 11 56660266 Fax: +55 (0) 11 56660739

Byk Nederland BV *Weerenweg 29, 1161 AG Zwanenburg, Netherlands.*
Tel: +31 (0) 20 4079400 Fax: +31 (0) 20 4976117

C

Cabassi & Giuriati S.p.A. *Via Uruguay 20/22, Z.I. Padua, 35127 Padua, Italy.*
Tel: +39 049 8705870 Fax: +39 049 8700783
Email: giuriati@tin.it Web: www.cabassi-giuriati.it

Ca.Di.Group S.r.l. *Via Pieve Tesino 75, 00124 Rome, Italy.*
Tel: +39 06 52363403 Fax: +39 06 52363401
Email: cadigroup@cadigroup.it Web: www.cadigroup.it

Caesaro Med GmbH *Raidenstrasse 46, A-4060 Leonding, Austria.*
Tel: +43 (0) 732 677164 Fax: +43 (0) 732 6771649

CAFAR (Compania Anonima Farmaceutica) *Avenida M. Perez Pisanti, Sector Industrial Los 3 puentes, Urb. El Tambor Los Teques, Caracas, Venezuela.*
Tel: +58 (0) 212 3231811 Fax: +58 (0) 212 3231974
Email: cafar2000@cantv.net Web: www.cafar.com.ve

Capo Sole S.r.l. *Via Edison 60, 20019 Settimo Milanese (MI), Italy.*
Tel: +39 02 33512309 Fax: +39 02 33500602

Carl Hoernecke GmbH *Halberstadter Chaussee 22, 39116 Magdeburg, Germany.*
Tel: +49 (0) 391 635460 Fax: +49 (0) 391 6354627
Email: info@hoernecke.com Web: www.hoernecke.com

Carter Horner Inc. *6600 Kitimat Rd, Mississauga, L5N 1L9, Canada.*
Tel: +1 905 8266200 Fax: +1 905 8260389

Casa Granado Lab. Farmacias e Drogarias S.A. *Travessa do Comércio 17, 20010-080 Rio de Janeiro, Brazil.*
Tel: +55 (0) 21 2031212 Fax: +55 (0) 21 2215589
Web: www.granado.com.br

Cassella-med GmbH & Co. KG *Gereonsmuhlengasse 1, 50670 Cologne, Germany.*
Tel: +49 (0) 221 120157 Fax: +49 (0) 221 124495
Email: cmed@cassella-med.de

Cazi Química Farmacêutica Indústria e Comércio Ltda *Rua Antônio Lopes 17, 06600-000 Jandira, Brazil.*
Tel: +55 (0) 11 47075155 Fax: +55 (0) 11 47075144

C.B. Fleet Co. (Australia) P/L *P.O. Box 716, Braeside, VIC 3195, Australia.*
Tel: +61 (0) 3 95802755 Fax: +61 (0) 3 95802899
Email: cbfleet@hyperlink.net.au Web: www.ozpages.comcbfleet

C.B. Fleet Co. Inc. *4615 Murray Pl., P.O. Box 11349, Lynchburg, VA 24506, USA.*
Tel: +1 804 528 4000 Fax: +1 804 847 4219
Web: www.cbfleet.com

Cedar Health Ltd *Pepper Rd, Bramhall Moor Lane, Hazel Grove, Stockport, SK7 5BW, UK.*
Tel: +44 (0) 161 483 1235 Fax: +44 (0) 161 456 4321
Email: customerservices@cedarhealth.co.uk
Web: www.cedarhealth.co.uk

Cederroth *C/Jose Bardasano Baos 9, Edificio Gorbea 3, 28016 Madrid, Spain.*
Tel: +34 91 3836171 Fax: +34 91 3836197
Email: info@cederroth.es Web: www.cederroth.com

Cefak KG *Ostbahnhofstr. 15, 87437 Kempten, Germany.*
Tel: +49 (0) 831 574010 Fax: +49 (0) 831 5740148
Email: cefak@cefak.com Web: www.cefak.com

Cesam, Lda *Rua de Ceuta 4, Piso, 2795-056 Linda-a-Velha, Portugal.*
Tel: +351 21 4142880 Fax: +351 21 4199496

Cesra Arzneimittel GmbH & Co. KG *Braunmattstr. 20, 76532 Baden-Baden, Germany.*
Tel: +49 (0) 7221 95400 Fax: +49 (0) 7221 54026
Email: cesra@cesra.de Web: www.cesra.de

Ceutical Trading Co. Ltd *Rm 24, 12/F, Goldfield Industrial Ctr, 1 Sui Wo Rd, Fo Tan, Shatin, Hong Kong.*
Tel: +852 26065262 Fax: +852 26917214

Chattem Consumer Products *1715 West 38th St, Chattanooga, TN 37409, USA.*
Tel: +1 615 821 4571 Web: www.chattem.com

Chauvin ankerpharm GmbH *Brunsbutteler Damm 165-173, 13581 Berlin, Germany.*
Tel: +49 (0) 30 33093300 Fax: +49 (0) 30 33093350
Email: ankerpharm@bausch.com

Chefaro UK Ltd *1 Tower Close, St Peters Industrial Park, Huntingdon, PE29 7DH, UK.*
Tel: +44 (0) 1480 421800 Fax: +44 (0) 1480 434861
Email: enquiries@chefaro.co.uk Web: www.chefaro.com

Chemische Fabrik Dr. Hetterich GmbH & Co. KG *Gebhardtstr. 5, 90762 Furth/Bayern, Germany.*
Tel: +49 (0) 911 97706 Fax: +49 (0) 911 9770755
Web: www.hetterich.de

Chemisch-Pharmazeutische Fabrik Göppingen Carl Müller, Apotheker, GmbH & Co. KG *Bahnhofstr. 33-35 & 40, 73033 Goppingen, Germany.*
Tel: +49 (0) 7161 6760 Fax: +49 (0) 7161 676298
Email: info@mueller-goeppingen.de Web: www.mueller-goeppingen.de

Cheplapharm Arzneimittel GmbH *Bahnhofstr 1a, 17498 Mesekenhagen, Germany.*
Tel: +49 (0) 38351 53690 Fax: +49 (0) 38351536925
Web: www.cheplapharm.de

Chiesi España *Berlin 38-48, 7 planta, 08029 Barcelona, Spain.*
Tel: +34 93 4948000 Fax: +34 93 4948030
Email: chiesi@chiesi.es Web: www.chiesigroup.com

Chrisana GmbH *Ruggenstrasse 31, 8903 Birmensdorf, Switzerland.*
Tel: +41 (0) 1 7370069 Fax: +41 (0) 1 7370061
Web: www.chrisana.ch

Christo Pharmaceuticals Ltd *Blk A-D, 14/F, Stage 2, Superluck Industrial Ctr, 57 Sha Tsui Rd, Tsuen Wan, Hong Kong.*
Tel: +852 24140146 Fax: +852 24935666

Cifarma Cientifica Farmacêutica Ltda *Av. das Industrias 3651, 33040-130 Belo Horizonte, Brazil.*
Tel: +55 (0) 31 36414100 Email: cifarma@uai.com.br
Web: www.cifarma.com.br

Cimed Indústria de Medicamentos Ltda *Rua Engenheiro Prudente 119, 01550-000 São Paulo Vila Monumento, Brazil.*
Tel: +55 (0) 11 69159090 Web: www.cimed.ind.br

Cinfa *Olaz-Chipi 10, Poligono Areta, Huarte-Pamplona, 31620 Navarra, Spain.*
Tel: +34 948 335005 Fax: +34 948 330367
Email: cinfa@cinfa.com Web: www.cinfa.com

Cipan, Companhia Industrial Produtora de Antibioticos SA *Vala do Carregado, Apartado 60, 2600-733 Castanheira do Ribatejo, Portugal.*
Tel: +351 263 856800 Fax: +351 263 855020
Web: www.cipan.pt

Cipla Ltd *Mumbai Central, Mumbai 400 008, India.*
Tel: +91 (0) 22 23082891 Fax: +91 (0) 22 23070013
Web: www.cipla.com

Cipla-Medpro (Pty) Ltd *Rosen Heights, Rosen Park, Bellville 7530, South Africa.*
Tel: +27 (0) 21 9140520 Fax: +27 (0) 21 9140247
Email: medical@ciplamedpro.co.za Web: www.ciplamedpro.co.za

CNW (Hong Kong) Ltd *Rm 606, 6/F, Fo Tan Industrial Ctr, 26-28 Au Pui Wan St, Fo Tan, Shatin, Hong Kong.*
Tel: +852 23882933 Fax: +852 27712138
Email: cnw@cnw-hk.com Web: www.cnwhk.com

Colgate Palmolive Canada *99 Vanderhoof Ave, Toronto, M4G 2H6, Canada.*
Tel: +1 416 4216000 Web: www.colgate.com

Coll Farma *Napoles 166, 08013 Barcelona, Spain.*
Tel: +34 93 2314505

Combe Inc. *1101 Westchester Ave, White Plains, NY 10604, USA.*
Tel: +1 914 694 5454 Fax: +1 800 431 2610
Email: combe@combe.com Web: www.combe.com

Comercial GFC SA de CV *Blvd Juan A de Torres 220, 37360 Leon Gto Vibar, Mexico.*

Companhia Industrial Farmacêutica *Rua Figueira de Melo 301, 20941-001 Rio de Janeiro, Brazil.*
Tel: +55 (0) 21 30823535 Fax: +55 (0) 21 30823527
Web: www.cif-farmaceutica.com.br

Concept for Pharmacy Ltd *P.O. Box 2105, Kfar Sava 44643, Israel.*
Tel: +972 (0) 9 7667890 Fax: +972 (0) 9 7667899
Email: info@concept-rx.co.il Web: www.concept-rx.co.il

Concept Pharmaceuticals Ltd *167 C.S.T. Rd, Santacruz (E), Mumbai 400 098, India.*

Confar, Lda *Rua Sebastião e Silva 25, Zona Industrial de Massama, 2745-838 Queluz, Portugal.*
Tel: +351 214 371009 Fax: +351 214 387489
Email: med@confar.pt

Coopération Pharmaceutique Francaise *, 77020 Melun cdx, France.*
Tel: +33 (0) 1 64872000 Fax: +33 (0) 1 64872087

Cooperativa Farmaceutica Soc. (CoFa Farmaceutici) *Via Passione 8, 20122 Milan, Italy.*
Tel: +39 02 784141 Fax: +39 02 781308

Coradol-Pharma GmbH *Ludwig-Erhard-Str. 10, 50129 Bergheim, Germany.*
Tel: +49 (0) 2238 940251 Fax: +49 (0) 2238 940258
Email: info@coradol.de Web: www.coradol.de

Corifel SA *Via Clemente Maraini 9, 6907 Lugano 7, Switzerland.*
Tel: +41 (0) 91 9239657 Fax: +41 (0) 91 9210807

Cornelli Consulting Sas *Corso Indipendenza 1, 20129 Milan, Italy.*
Tel: +39 (0) 2714904 Fax: +39 (0) 2714904
Email: info@cornelliconsulting.it Web: www.cornelliconsulting.it

Corporacion de Salud C.A. *Av. J. M. Vargas, Edif. Artico Piso 1 Oficina 15B, Sta. Fe Norte Caracas, Caracas, Venezuela.*
Tel: +58 (0) 212 9795945 Fax: +58 (0) 212 9795945

Cosmofarma, Lda (Laboratórios Cosmos) *Rua Arco do Carvalhão 14, 1070 Lisbon, Portugal.*

Costec S.R.L. Esp. Dermatocosméticas *Av. Corrientes 1296 Piso 7 Dto.76, 1043 Buenos Aires, Argentina.*
Tel: +54 (0) 11 43818729 Fax: +54 (0) 11 43818729

Craveri S.A.I.C. *Arengreen 830, 1405 Buenos Aires, Argentina.*
Tel: +54 (0) 11 51670555 Fax: +54 (0) 11 51670505
Web: www.craveri.com.ar

Crefar, Lda *Rua da Madalena 171, 1149-032 Lisbon, Portugal.*
Tel: +351 21 8824690 Fax: +351 21 8862546
Email: mail@crefar.pt

Croma-Pharma GmbH *Industriezeile 6, A-2100 Leobendorf, Austria.*
Tel: +43 (0) 2262 684680 Fax: +43 (0) 2262 6846815

Crookes Healthcare Ltd *D6 Building, Nottingham, NG90 6BH, UK.*
Tel: +44 (0) 115 968 8922 Fax: +44 (0) 115 968 8923
Email: medicalinfo@crookes.co.uk Web: www.crookes.co.uk

CSL (NZ) Ltd *P.O. Box 62590, Central Park, Auckland 6, New Zealand.*
Tel: +64 (0) 9 5798105 Fax: +64 (0) 9 5798106
Web: www.csl.com.au

ct-Arzneimittel GmbH *Lengeder Str. 42A, 13407 Berlin, Germany.*
Tel: +49 (0) 30 4090080 Fax: +49 (0) 30 40900821
Email: office@ct-berlin.de Web: www.ct-berlin.de

C.T.S. Chemical Industries Ltd *4 Haharosh St, P.O.Box 10, Hod-Hasharon 45240, Israel.*
Tel: +972 (0) 9 7626333 Fax: +972 (0) 9 7626300
Web: www.cts.co.il

Culpeper and Napiers *Bourton Industrial Park, , Bourton-On-The-Water, GL54 2HQ, UK.*
Tel: +44 (0) 1451 812 341 Fax: +44 (0) 1451 812 349
Email: wholesale@culpeperandnapier.co.uk

CuraMED Pharma GmbH *Pforzheimer Str. 5, 76227 Karlsruhe, Germany.*
Tel: +49 (0) 721 402089 Fax: +49 (0) 721 4005530

CytoChemia AG *Im Burgerstock 7, 79241 Ihringen, Germany.*
Tel: +49 (0) 7668 99220 Fax: +49 (0) 7668 992233
Email: info@cytochemia.de Web: www.cytochemia.de

D

Darrow Laboratórios S.A. *Rua Marques de Olinda 69, 22251-040 Rio de Janeiro, Brazil.*
Tel: +55 (0) 21 25538150 Fax: +55 (0) 21 25532551

Dávi Farmacêutica, Lda *Estrada da Barrosa, Elospark, Arm. 8, Algueirão, 2725-193 Mem Martins, Portugal.*
Tel: +351 21 9229720 Fax: +351 21 9229729

DC Labs Ltd *795 Pharmacy Ave, Toronto, M1L 3K2, Canada.*

DDD Ltd *94 Rickmansworth Rd, Watford, WD1 7JJ, UK.*
Tel: +44 (0) 1923 229251 Fax: +44 (0) 1923 220728
Email: info@dddltd.co.uk Web: www.dddgroup.co.uk

De Mayo Industrias Químicas e Farmacêuticas Ltda *Rua Barão de Petrópolis 109, 20251-061 Rio de Janeiro, Brazil.*
Tel: +55 (0) 21 22931409

Defuen S.A. *Av. Dorrego 331, 1414 Buenos Aires, Argentina.*
Tel: +54 (0) 11 48551249 Fax: +54 (0) 11 48562895

Delamac Pharmaceuticals P/L *Suite 1/14 Hill Street, Spring Hill, Qld 4000, Australia.*
Tel: +61 (0) 7 38321432 Fax: +61 (0) 7 38326623
Email: delamac@healthnut.com.au

Dentinox Gesellschaft für Pharmazeutische Präparate Lenk & Schuppan *Nunsdorfer Ring 19, 12277 Berlin, Germany.*
Tel: +49 (0) 30 7200340 Fax: +49 (0) 30 7211038
Email: dentinox@dentinox.de Web: www.dentinox.de

Depofarma S.r.l. *Via Guindazzi 44/54, 80040 Pollena Trocchia (NA), Italy.*
Tel: +39 081 5305468 Fax: +39 081 5302124
Email: info@dermilia.it

Dermofarm *Can Sant Joan, Rubi, 08191 Barcelona, Spain.*
Tel: +34 93 6026026 Fax: +34 93 6026036
Email: email@dermofarm.com Web: www.dermofarm.com

Dermofarma Italia S.r.l. *Via Beata Francesca 10, 83100 Avellino, Italy.*
Tel: +39 0825 30263 Fax: +39 0825 30263

Dermoteca, SA *Estrada Nacional 117, 2720 Alfragide, Portugal.*
Tel: +351 21 4718322 Fax: +351 21 4718381

Desma Healthcare BV *Corso San Gottardo 32, 6830 Chiasso, Switzerland.*
Tel: +41 (0) 91 6831506 Fax: +41 (0) 91 6831509

Deutsche Homöopathie-Union *Ottostr. 24, 76227 Karlsruhe, Germany.*
Tel: +49 (0) 721 409301 Fax: +49 (0) 721 4093263
Web: www.dhu.de

Devergè Medicina e Medicalizzazione S.r.l. *C.so Casale 206, 10132 Turin, Italy.*
Tel: +39 011 8993844 Fax: +39 011 8995514

5

Dexxon *P.O. Box 50, Hadera 38100, Israel.*
Tel: +972 (0) 6 6364000 Fax: +972 (0) 6 6364004
Email: info@dexcel.com Web: www.dexxon.co.il

Diafarm *Avda Arraona 119-123, Barbera del Valles, 08210 Barcelona, Spain.*
Tel: +34 93 7192120 Fax: +34 93 7192104
Email: info@diafarm.es Web: www.diafarm.es

Dicofarm S.p.A. *Via Vitorchiano 151, 00100 Rome, Italy.*
Tel: +39 06 3322891 Fax: +39 06 3332172
Email: dicofarm@dicofarm.it Web: www.dicofarm.it

Diethelm & Co. Ltd *Pharmaceutical Division, 280 New Rd, Bangkok 10100, Thailand.*
Tel: +66 2 221 1121 Fax: +66 2 224 8475
Email: ditco@loxinfo.co.th Web: www.diethelmpharma-thailand.com

Diethelm Malaysia Sdn Bhd *74 Jln Universiti, 46700 Petaling Jaya, Malaysia.*
Tel: +60 (0) 3 79660288 Fax: +60 (0) 3 79576649
Web: www.diethelmkeller.com

Diethelm Singapore Pte Ltd *34 Boon Leat Terrace, S 119866, Singapore.*
Tel: +65 6471 0888 Web: www.diethelm.com.sg

Dispolab Farmaceutica SA *Santa Victoria 213, Providencia, Santiago, Chile.*

Dist. Ofar S.A. *Salom 651, 1277 Buenos Aires, Argentina.*
Tel: +54 (0) 11 43018687

DM Indústria Farmacêutica Ltda *Av. Piracema 155, 06460-030 Barueri, Brazil.*
Tel: +55 (0) 11 41952122 Fax: +55 (0) 11 41914855

DMG Italia S.r.l. *Via Campello sul Clitunno 34, 00100 Rome, Italy.*
Tel: +39 06 78359715 Fax: +39 06 78359719
Email: info@dmgit.com

Doetsch Grether AG *, 4002 Basle, Switzerland.*
Tel: +41 (0) 61 2873411 Fax: +41 (0) 61 2873413
Web: www.doetschgrether.ch

Dolisos SA *Rue Carli 5, 1140 Brussels, Belgium.*
Tel: +32 (0) 2 2406770 Fax: +32 (0) 2 2406771

Dolorgiet GmbH & Co. KG *Otto-von-Guericke-Str. 1, 53757 St. Augustin/Bonn, Germany.*
Tel: +49 (0) 2241 3170 Fax: +49 (0) 2241 317390

Donini S.r.l. *Via Ecce Homo 18, 37054 Nogara (VR), Italy.*
Tel: +39 0442 88922 Fax: +39 0442 50537

Dorwest Herbs Ltd *Shipton Gorge, Bridport, DT6 4LP, UK.*
Tel: +44 (0) 1308 987272 Fax: +44 (0) 1308 987929
Email: info@dorwest.co.uk Web: www.dorwest.co.uk

Douglas Pharmaceuticals Australia Ltd *P.O. Box 7004, Baulkham Hills Business Centre, Baulkham Hills, NSW 2153, Australia.*
Tel: +61 1800 678 302 Fax: +61 (0) 2 88182122
Web: www.douglas.com.au

Douglas Pharmaceuticals Ltd *P.O. Box 45-027, Auckland, New Zealand.*
Tel: +64 (0) 9 8350660 Fax: +64 (0) 9 8350665
Web: www.douglas.co.nz

DP-Medica SA, Pharmazeutische Produkte *Case postale 238, Fribourg, Switzerland.*
Tel: +41 (0) 26 4929370 Fax: +41 (0) 26 4929371

Dr A & L Schmidgall *Wolfganggasse 45-7, A-1121 Vienna, Austria.*
Tel: +43 (0) 1 81158 Fax: +43 (0) 1 811587

Dr A & M Kropf *Promenade, 3780 Gstaad, Switzerland.*
Tel: +41 (0) 33 7488626 Fax: +41 (0) 33 7488620
Email: apotheke.kropf@gstaad.ch

Dr. Atzinger Pharmazeutische Fabrik *Dr. Atzinger Str. 5, 94036 Passau, Germany.*
Tel: +49 (0) 851 955210 Fax: +49 (0) 851 9552155

Dr. August Wolff Arzneimittel GmbH & Co. *Sudbrackstr. 56, 33611 Bielefeld, Germany.*
Tel: +49 (0) 521 880805 Fax: +49 (0) 521 8808334
Email: info@wolff-arzneimittel.de Web: www.wolff-arzneimittel.de

Dr AW Gubler *Petersgraben 5, 4051 Basle, Switzerland.*
Tel: +41 (0) 61 2612026 Fax: +41 (0) 61 2616513

Dr. C. Soldan GmbH *Herderstr. 5-9, 90427 Nürnberg, Germany.*
Tel: +49 (0) 911 327801 Fax: +49 (0) 911 3278159
Web: www.soldan.com

Dr Dünner SA *Artherstrassec 60, 6405 Immensee, Switzerland.*
Tel: +41 (0) 41 8544600 Fax: +41 (0) 41 8544603

Dr. E. Ritsert GmbH & Co. KG *Klausenweg 12, 69412 Eberbach, Germany.*
Tel: +49 (0) 6271 92210 Fax: +49 (0) 6271 922155
Email: info@ritsert.de Web: www.ritsert.de

Dr. Falk Pharma GmbH *Leinenweberstr. 5, 79108 Freiburg, Germany.*
Tel: +49 (0) 761 15140 Fax: +49 (0) 761 1514321
Email: zentrale@drfalkpharma.de Web: www.drfalkpharma.de

Dr. Falk Pharma Portugal Lda *Av. José Gomes Ferreira 11, Edifício Atlas II - 3 Piso, Sala 33, Miraflores, 1495-139 Algés, Portugal.*
Tel: +351 21 4126170 Fax: +351 21 4126179

Dr. Friedrich Eberth Arzneimittel *Hohenburger Str. 39, 92289 Ursensollen, Germany.*
Tel: +49 (0) 9628 91368 Fax: +49 (0) 9628 91399
Email: info@eberth.de Web: www.eberth.de

Dr Gerhard Mann, Chem.-pharm. Fabrik GmbH *Brunsbutteler Damm 165-73, 13581 Berlin, Germany.*
Tel: +49 (0) 30 330930 Fax: +49 (0) 30 33093350
Email: dmp@bausch.com Web: www.mannpharma.de

Dr Grandel GmbH *Pfladergasse 7-13, 86150 Augsburg, Germany.*
Tel: +49 (0) 821 32020 Fax: +49 (0) 821 3202229
Web: www.grandel.de

Dr Grossmann AG, Pharmaca *Hardstrasse 25, Postfach 914, 4127 Birsfelden/Basle, Switzerland.*
Tel: +41 (0) 61 3775000 Fax: +41 (0) 61 3775050
Email: administration@grossmannpharma.com
Web: www.grossmannpharma.com

Dr Gustav Klein *Steinenfeld 3, 77736 Zell am Harmersbach, Germany.*
Tel: +49 (0) 7835 63550 Fax: +49 (0) 7835 634685
Email: info@klien-phytopharma.de Web: www.klein-phytopharma.de

Dr Heinz Welti AG *Althofstrasse 12, 5432 Neuenhof, Switzerland.*
Tel: +41 (0) 56 4062994 Fax: +41 (0) 56 4061764
Email: info@drwelti.ch

Dr. Hobein & Co. Nachf. GmbH Arzneimittel *Grenzstr. 2, 53340 Meckenheim, Germany.*
Tel: +49 (0) 2225 88940 Fax: +49 (0) 2225 889466
Email: info@eubos.de Web: www.eubos.de

Dr Kade Pharmazeutische Fabrik GmbH *Rigistr. 2, 12277 Berlin, Germany.*
Tel: +49 (0) 30 720820 Fax: +49 (0) 30 72082200
Email: info@kade.de Web: www.kade.de

Dr. Kolassa & Merz GmbH *Gastgebgasse 5-13, A-1230 Vienna, Austria.*
Tel: +43 (0) 1 8691604 Fax: +43 (0) 1 869160418

Dr. Loges & Co. GmbH *Schutzenstr. 5, 21423 Winsen, Germany.*
Tel: +49 (0) 4171 7070 Fax: +49 (0) 4171 707100
Email: info@loges.com Web: www.loges.com

Dr med G Knobel AG *Bahnhofstrasse 9, 8730 Uznach, Switzerland.*
Tel: +41 (0) 55 2804020

Dr Niedermaier GmbH *Taufkirchner Str. 59, 85662 Hohenbrunn bei Munich, Germany.*
Tel: +49 (0) 89 6607970 Fax: +49 (0) 89 66079750
Email: info@niedermaier-pharma.de Web: www.niedermaier-pharma.de

Dr. Ottolenghi & C. S.r.l. *Via Cuneo 5, 10028 Trofarello (TO), Italy.*
Tel: +39 011 6481028 Fax: +39 011 6497132
Email: info@ottolenghi.it Web: www.ottolenghi.it

Dr Peithner KG nunmehr GmbH & Co. *Richard-Strauss-Strasse 13, A-1232 Vienna, Austria.*
Tel: +43 (0) 1 61626440 Fax: +43 (0) 1 616264418

Dr R. Pfleger Chemische Fabrik GmbH *, 96045 Bamberg, Germany.*
Tel: +49 (0) 951 60430 Fax: +49 (0) 951 604329
Email: info@dr-pfleger.de Web: www.dr-pfleger.de

Dr Scheffler Nachf. GmbH & Co. KG *Senefelderstr. 44, 51469 Bergisch Gladbach, Germany.*
Tel: +49 (0) 2202 1050 Fax: +49 (0) 2202 105344

Dr W Schwabe *Pol Ind Francoli, Parcela 3, Nave 2, 43006 Tarragona, Spain.*
Tel: +34 977 550542 Fax: +34 977 550848
Web: www.schwabepharma.com

Dr. Werner Janssen Nachf. Chem.-pharm. Produkte GmbH *Grenzstr. 2, 53340 Meckenheim, Germany.*
Tel: +49 (0) 2225 88940 Fax: +49 (0) 2225 889466

Dr Wild & Co. AG *Lange Gasse 4, 4002 Basle, Switzerland.*
Tel: +41 (0) 61 2799000 Fax: +41 (0) 61 2799009
Email: info@wild-pharma.com Web: www.wild-pharma.com

Dr Willmar Schwabe GmbH & Co. *Willmar-Schwabe-Str. 4, 76227 Karlsruhe, Germany.*
Tel: +49 (0) 721 40050 Fax: +49 (0) 721 4005500
Web: www.schwabe.de

Dreluso Pharmazeutika, Dr Elten & Sohn GmbH *Marktplatz 5, 31840 Hessisch Oldendorf, Germany.*
Tel: +49 (0) 5152 94240 Fax: +49 (0) 5152 3408
Web: www.dreluso.de

Drossapharm SA *Postfach 2660, 4002 Basle, Switzerland.*
Tel: +41 (0) 61 7021000 Fax: +41 (0) 61 7021005
Email: info@drossapharm.ch Web: www.drossapharm.ch

Duopharm GmbH *Grassingerstr. 9, 83043 Bad Aibling, Germany.*
Tel: +49 (0) 8061 931400 Fax: +49 (0) 8061 931425
Email: info@duopharm.de Web: www.duopharm.de

Dyckerhoff Pharma GmbH & Co. *Robert-Perthel-Str. 49, 50739 Cologne, Germany.*
Tel: +49 (0) 221 9574370 Fax: +49 (0) 221 95743745
Web: www.dyckerhoff-pharma.de

Dynacren Laboratorio Farmaceutico del Dott. A. Francioni e di M. Gerosa S.r.l. *Via P Nenni 12, Loc Malpensa, 28053 Castelletto Ticino (NO), Italy.*
Tel: +39 0331 924205 Fax: +39 0331 913415
Email: dynacren@dyncren.it Web: www.dynacren.it

E

E Kern AG, Pharmazeutische Krauterspezialitäten *Hauptstrasse 23, 8867 Niederumen, Switzerland.*
Tel: +41 (0) 55 6102727 Fax: +41 (0) 55 6102508
Email: kern.pharma@bluewin.ch

Eagle Pharmaceuticals P/L *P.O. Box 927, Castle Hill, NSW 1765, Australia.*
Tel: +61 (0) 2 98999099 Fax: +61 (0) 2 98996564

Eastern Pharmaceuticals Ltd *Coomb House, St. Johns Rd, Isleworth, TW7 6NA, UK.*
Tel: +44 (0) 20 8569 8174 Fax: +44 (0) 20 8569 8175
Email: sales@eastern-pharmaceuticals.co.uk
Web: www.eastern-pharmaceuticals.co.uk

Ebewe Pharma (ASIA) Ltd *8/F Eastwood Ctr, 5 A Kung Ngam Village Rd, Shaukeiwan, Hong Kong.*
Email: asia@ebewe.com.hk

E.C. De Witt & Co. Ltd *Tudor Rd, Manor Park, Runcorn, WA7 1SZ, UK.*
Tel: +44 (0) 1928 579029 Fax: +44 (0) 1928 579712
Email: info@ecdewitt.com Web: www.ecdewitt.co.uk

EciFarma SA *Carmen Covarrubias 271, Nunoa, Santiago, Chile.*

Ecofarm Group Srl *Via F Vezzani 99/r, 16159 Genoa Rivarolo, Italy.*
Tel: +39 (0) 107261682 Fax: +39 (0) 107268296
Email: ecofarmgroup@tin.it

Ecosol AG *Hinterbergstrasse 24, 6330 Cham, Switzerland.*
Tel: +41 (0) 41 7483080 Fax: +41 (0) 41 7483081
Email: contact@ecosol.ch Web: www.ecosol.ch

Edmond Pharma S.r.l. *Via dei Giovi 131, 20037 Paderno Dugnano (MI), Italy.*
Tel: +39 02 9100111 Fax: +39 02 91001351

EF-EM-ES - Dr Smetana & Co. *Scheidlstrasse 28, A-1180 Vienna, Austria.*
Tel: +43 (0) 1 4792142 Fax: +43 (0) 1 4700746

EG Laboratori EuroGenerici S.p.A. *Via Domenico Scarlatti 31, 20124 Milan, Italy.*
Tel: +39 02 8310371 Fax: +39 02 83103776

EGIS Pharmaceuticals *Hungária krt 179-187, 1146 Budapest, Hungary.*
Tel: +36 4692222 Fax: +36 3839257

Eladon Ltd *P.O. Box 111, Bangor, LL57 1ZB, UK.*
Tel: +44 (0) 1248 370059 Fax: +44 (0) 1248 364208
Web: www.elagen.com

Elhoim S.R.L. *Independencia 2809 Piso 6 Dto. A, 1225 Buenos Aires, Argentina.*
Tel: +54 (0) 11 48151105

Ellem Läkemedel AB *Svärdvägen 13, 182 12 Danderyd, Sweden.*
Tel: +46 (0) 8 54496030 Fax: +46 (0) 8 54496049
Email: info@ellem.nu Web: www.ellem.nu

Elvetium S.A. *Catulo Castillo 2437, 1261 Buenos Aires, Argentina.*
Tel: +54 (0) 11 43081474 Fax: +54 (0) 11 49415980

Emerging Pharma Sdn Bhd *Phileo Damansara II, Lot 3A03, Block B, No 15, Jln 16/11, Off Jln Damansara, 46350 Petaling Jaya, Malaysia.*
Tel: +60 (0) 3 79560658 Fax: +60 (0) 3 79552260
Email: info@emergingp.com Web: www.emergingp.com

Emonta Pharma GmbH *Weidelstrasse 21, A-1100 Vienna, Austria.*
Tel: +43 (0) 1 6892035 Fax: +43 (0) 1 6892037

EMS Ind. Farmacêutica Ltda *Rodovia SP 101, Km 08, 13186-481 Hortolandia, Brazil.*
Tel: +55 (0) 19 38879800 Fax: +55 (0) 19 38879824
Email: departamentomedico@ems.com.br
Web: www.ems.com.br

Engelhard Arzneimittel GmbH & Co. KG *Herzbergstr. 3, 61138 Niederdorfelden, Germany.*
Tel: +49 (0) 6101 539300 Fax: +49 (0) 6101 539315
Email: info@engelhard-am.de Web: www.engelhard-am.de

ERA Medical ApS *Storeholm 25, 2670 Greve, Denmark.*
Tel: +45 46151677 Fax: +45 43600301

Ernest Jackson & Co. Ltd *29 High St, Crediton, EX17 3AP, UK.*
Tel: +44 (0) 1363 633000 Fax: +44 (0) 1363 636063
Web: www.ejackson.co.uk

Errekappa Euroterapici S.p.A. *Via C. Menotti 1/A, 20129 Milan, Italy.*
Tel: +39 02 7491345 Fax: +39 02 715734

Esp. Medicinales Northia S.A.C.I.F.I.A. *Madero 135, 1408 Buenos Aires, Argentina.*
Tel: +54 (0) 11 46440911 Fax: +54 (0) 11 46427975

esparma GmbH *Lange Gohren 3, 39171 Osterweddingen, Germany.*
Tel: +49 (0) 39205 420 Fax: +49 (0) 39205 42240
Email: info@esparma.de Web: www.esparma.de

Esplanade-Apotheke *Esplanade 18, A-4820 Bad Ischl, Austria.*
Tel: +43 (0) 6132 23427 Fax: +43 (0) 6132 2342716

Eu Rho OTC Pharma GmbH *Kamen Karree 32-34, 59174 Kamen, Germany.*
Tel: +49 (0) 2307 2020 Fax: +49 (0) 2307 202155

Euroderm Laboratorios S.R.L. *Emilio Mitre 1790/94, 1424 Buenos Aires, Argentina.*
Tel: +54 (0) 11 49213310 Fax: +54 (0) 11 49248090

Euroderm S.r.l. *V.le Italia 147, 19126 La Spezia, Italy.*
Tel: +39 0187 777276 Fax: +39 0187 778424
Web: www.euroderm.net

Euroderm-RDC S.p.A. *P.le Aquileia 8, 20144 Milan (MI), Italy.*
Tel: +39 02 335728 Fax: +39 02 33572818

Eurofarma Laboratórios Ltda *Rua Barão do Triunfo 1440, 04602-005 São Paulo, Brazil.*
Tel: +55 (0) 11 50908600 Fax: +55 (0) 11 50908742
Email: euroatende@eurofarma.com.br Web: www.eurofarmalaboratorio.com.br

Europharm *Jochen-Rindt-Strasse 23, A-1230 Vienna, Austria.*
Tel: +43 (0) 1 61684250 Fax: +43 (0) 1 616842510

Europharm Trade Kft *Kövirózsa út 5, 1163 Budapest, Hungary.*
Tel: +36 4024204 Fax: +36 4024205

Eversil Produtos Farmacêuticos Indústria e Comércio Ltda *Rua Agostinho Teixeira de Lima 344, 04826-230 São Paulo, Brazil.*
Tel: +55 (0) 11 59284199 Web: www.eversil.com.br

Expanscience *Pol. Ind. Los Olivos, Adaptación 33, Getafe, 28906 Madrid, Spain.*
Tel: +34 91 6011070 Fax: +34 91 6011076
Email: infomustela@expanscience.es Web: www.mustela.com

E-Z-EM Canada Inc. *11 065 L-H Lafontaine, Anjou, H1J 2Z4, Canada.*
Tel: +1 514 3535820 Fax: +1 514 3533450
Email: info@ezemcanada.com Web: www.ezemcanada.com

F

F. Joh. Kwizda *Effingergasse 21, A-1160 Vienna, Austria.*
Tel: +43 (0) 1 48855 Fax: +43 (0) 1 48855320

F Trenka Chemisch-Pharmazeutische Fabrik GmbH *Goldeggassee 5, A-1040 Vienna, Austria.*
Tel: +43 (0) 1 50503410 Fax: +43 (0) 1 505034131

F. Uhlmann-Eyraud SA *28 chemin du Grand-Puits, 1217 Meyrin 2/Geneva, Switzerland.*
Tel: +41 (0) 22 9893100 Fax: +41 (0) 22 9893105

Faes Farma *Alpedrete 24, 28045 Madrid, Spain.*
Tel: +34 91 4680800 Fax: +34 91 4685934
Web: www.faes.es

Falqui Prodotti Farmaceutici S.p.A. *Via Fabio Filzi 8, 20124 Milan, Italy.*
Tel: +39 02 67078288 Fax: +39 02 6694509

F.A.M.A. Istituto Chimico Biologico S.r.l. *Via A. Sauli 21, 20127 Milan, Italy.*
Tel: +39 02 2846802 Fax: +39 02 26824535

Faran Laboratories S.A. *Achaias & Troizinias, 145 64 N. Kifisia, Greece.*
Tel: +30 210 6269200 Fax: +30 210 8071688
Email: faran@faran.gr Web: www.faran.gr

5

Fardi *Grassot 16, 08025 Barcelona, Spain.*
Tel: +34 93 2073751 Fax: +34 93 4570717
Email: lab@fardi.es Web: www.fardi.es

Farm Vilar ZAO *Grina ul. 7, 117216 Moscow, Russia.*
Tel: +7 095 7121081 Fax: +7 095 7121072
Web: www.farmvilar.ru

Farma Lepori *Osi 7-9, 08034 Barcelona, Spain.*
Tel: +34 93 2534500 Fax: +34 93 3940900
Email: farmalepori@finaf92.es Web: www.farmalepori.com

Farmaceutici Ecobi s.a.s. *Via E. Bazzano 26, 16019 Ronco Scrivia (GE), Italy.*
Tel: +39 010 935280 Fax: +39 010 9350679
Email: ecobi@aleph.it

Farmaceutici G.B. Panzera S.r.l. *Via de Sanctis 71, 20141 Milan, Italy.*
Tel: +39 02 89502462 Fax: +39 02 89502459

Farmachimici S.r.l. *Via Mercanti 36, 84121 Salerno, Italy.*
Tel: +39 089 252389 Fax: +39 081 5552728
Email: info@farmachimici.it Web: www.farmachimici.it

Farmalab Industrias Químicas e Farmacêuticas Ltda *Av. BrigADEIRO Faria Lima 1811, 12 degrees andar, 01451-001 São Paulo, Brazil.*
Tel: +55 (0) 11 30970012 Fax: +55 (0) 11 30952357
Email: cientifico@farmalabchiesi.com.br Web: www.farmalabchiesi.com.br

Farmalight, Lda *Rua Padre Américo 18, Escritório 1, 1600-548 Lisbon, Portugal.*
Tel: +351 21 7122240 Fax: +351 21 7122245
Email: farmalight@farmalight.pt Web: www.farmalight.pt

Farmanova AFM S.r.l. *Via Flaminia 287 Sc. A. int.10, 00100 Rome, Italy.*
Tel: +39 06 3210307 Fax: +39 06 3212996
Email: farmanova@tiscali.it Web: www.farmanova.org

Farmasan Arzneimittel GmbH & Co. *Pforzheimer Str. 5, 76227 Karlsruhe, Germany.*
Tel: +49 (0) 721 40050 Fax: +49 (0) 721 4005500

Farmasierra S.A. *Ctra de Irun Km 26.2, San Sebastian de Los Reyes, 28100 Madrid, Spain.*
Tel: +34 91 6570659 Fax: +34 91 6539805
Email: farmasierra@farmasierra.com Web: www.farmasierra.com

Farmasur *Pol Store C/H 28-A, 41008 Seville, Spain.*

Farmigea Industria Chimico Farmaceutica S.p.A. *Via G. Oliva n. 8, 56121 Ospedaletto-Pisa, Italy.*
Tel: +39 050 31211 Fax: +39 050 3121255
Email: info@farmigea.it Web: www.farmigea.it

Farmila-Thea Farmaceutici S.p.A. *Via E. Fermi 50, 20019 Settimo Milanese (MI), Italy.*
Tel: +39 02 335501 Fax: +39 02 3285160
Web: www.farmila.it

Farmion Laboratório Brasileiro de Farmacologia Ltda *Avenida Celso dos Santos 579, 04658-240 São Paulo, Brazil.*
Tel: +55 (0) 11 55620742 Fax: +55 (0) 11 55620742

Farmo Química del Pacifico SA *Av. Grecia 2208, Nunoa, Santiago, Chile.*

Farmoquimica Baldacci, SA *Rua Duarte Galvão 44, 1549-005 Lisbon, Portugal.*
Tel: +351 21 7783031 Fax: +351 21 7785457

Farmoterapica Dovalle Indústria Química Farmacêutica Ltda *Rodovia SC 438 Km 3, 88701970 Tubarao, Brazil.*
Tel: +55 (0) 48 6280337

Febena Pharma GmbH *Oskar-Jager-Str. 115, 50825 Cologne, Germany.*
Tel: +49 (0) 221 9544770 Fax: +49 (0) 221 9544775
Email: info@febena.de Web: www.febena.de

Fed. Arg. de Coop. Farm. *Av. Pte. Peron 2742, 1754 San Justo, Buenos Aires, Argentina.*
Tel: +54 (0) 11 44825522 Fax: +54 (0) 11 44825549

Felton, Grimwade & Bickford P/L *P.O. Box 74, Oakleigh South, VIC 3167, Australia.*
Tel: +61 (0) 3 95627711 Fax: +61 (0) 3 95627291
Web: www.fgb.com.au

Ferlito Farmaceutici, Divisione Palmares S.p.A. *Via E Ramarini 31-33, 00016 Monterotondo Scalo (RM), Italy.*
Tel: +39 06 9060327 Fax: +39 06 9060932
Email: ferlitoromaced@kosmos.it Web: www.ferlitofarmaceutici.it

Ferrer Farma *Edifici L'illa, Diagonal 549. 5a planta, 08029 Barcelona, Spain.*
Tel: +34 93 6003700 Fax: +34 93 4907078
Email: ferrerfarma@ferrergrupo.com Web: www.ferrergrupo.com

Ferring Arzneimittel GmbH *Wienerbergstrasse 11, A-1100 Vienna, Austria.*
Tel: +43 (0) 1 60808 Fax: +43 (0) 1 6080880
Web: www.ferring.com

Ferring Portuguesa, Lda *Rua Professor Henrique de Barros, Edifício Sagres, 8 - Sala A, 2685-338 Prior Velho, Portugal.*
Tel: +351 21 9405190 Fax: +351 21 9405199
Web: www.ferring.com

Ferring S.A. de C.V. *Av. Nemesio Diez Riega Mza. 2 Lote 15, Col. Parque Industrial Cerrillo II, 52000 Lerma, Mexico.*
Tel: +52 728 2825636 Fax: +52 728 2825635
Web: www.ferring.com

Fher, Divisione della Boehringer Ingelheim *Casella Postale, 50100 Florence, Italy.*
Tel: +39 055 86501 Fax: +39 055 8650222

FIC Medical *Krasnopresnenskaya nab. 12, Gostinitsa International-2, Of. 742, 123610 Moscow, Russia.*
Tel: +7 095 2582006 Fax: +7 095 2582007
Email: fmv@aha.ru Web: www.aha.ru

FidesLine Biologische Heilmittel Heel GmbH *Dr.-Reckeweg-Str. 2-4, 76532 Baden-Baden, Germany.*
Tel: +49 (0) 7221 501200 Fax: +49 (0) 7221 501160
Web: www.fides.de

Fidia Farmaceutici S.p.A. *Via Ponte della Fabbrica 3/A, 35031 Abano Terme (Padua), Italy.*
Tel: +39 049 8232111 Fax: +39 049 810653

Fischer Pharmaceuticals Ltd *P.O. Box 39071, Tel Aviv 61390, Israel.*
Tel: +972 3 6772081 Fax: +972 3 6776959
Email: info@dr-fischer.com Web: www.dr-fischer.com

FIT Pharma GmbH *Humboldstr. 4, 32756 Detmold, Germany.*
Email: info@docsalbe.de Web: www.docsalbe.de

Fitobucaneve S.r.l. *Via Galvani 25/27, 20018 Sedriano (MI), Italy.*
Tel: +39 02 90111001 Fax: +39 02 90111003

Flordis Pty Ltd *Level 2, 3 Carlingford Rd, Epping, NSW 2121, Australia.*
Tel: +61 (0) 2 98694111 Fax: +61 (0) 2 98694155
Email: flordis@flordis.com.au Web: www.flordis.com.au

Floris *, Misgav 20179, Israel.*
Tel: +972 (0) 4 9991333 Fax: +972 (0) 4 9991336

Fontovit Laboratórios Ltda *Rua Antônio das Chagas 862, 04714-001 São Paulo, Brazil.*
Tel: +55 (0) 11 51829655 Fax: +55 (0) 11 51829604
Email: fontovit@fontovit.com.br Web: www.fontovit.com.br

Forder Lab. Esp. Dermatologicas *Rivadavia 5747 Piso 5 Dto.A, 1406 Cdad., Buenos Aires, Argentina.*
Tel: +54 (0) 11 44319702 Fax: +54 (0) 11 44319702

franconpharm Arzneimittel GmbH *Alexandrinenstr. 1, 96450 Coburg, Germany.*
Tel: +49 (0) 9561 20615 Fax: +49 (0) 9561 20617

Frank Roberts (Herbal Dispensaries) Ltd Frank Roberts (Herbal Dispensaries Ltd) *Dean Street, , Bristol, BS2 8FR, UK.*
Tel: +44 (0) 117 942 8704 Fax: +44 (0) 117 944 1297
Email: info@robertsherbalmedicines.co.uk
Web: www.robertsherbalmedicines.co.uk

Fritz Zilly GmbH *Eckbergstr. 18, 76534 Baden-Baden, Germany.*
Tel: +49 (0) 7221 73734 Fax: +49 (0) 7221 73733

Fujisawa Deutschland GmbH *Berg-am-Laim-Str. 129, 81673 Munich, Germany.*
Tel: +49 (0) 89 454401 Fax: +49 (0) 89 45441329
Email: info@fujisawa-deutschland.de Web: www.fujisawa-deutschland.de

Fujisawa GmbH *Linzerstrasse 221/E0.2, A-1140 Vienna, Austria.*
Tel: +43 (0) 1 87726680 Fax: +43 (0) 1 8771636
Web: www.fujisawa.at

G

G. Pohl-Boskamp GmbH & Co. *Kieler Str. 11, 25551 Hohenlockstedt, Germany.*
Tel: +49 (0) 4826 590 Fax: +49 (0) 4826 59109
Web: www.pohl-boskamp.de

G. Streuli & Co. AG *, 8730 Uznach, Switzerland.*
Tel: +41 (0) 55 2859292 Fax: +41 (0) 55 2859290

Galactopharm Hans Sanders *Sudstr. 10, 49751 Sogel, Germany.*
Tel: +49 (0) 5952 9250 Fax: +49 (0) 5952 9251
Email: infos@galactopharm.de Web: www.galactopharm.de

Galderma Mexico S.A. de C.V. *Jose Maria Ibarraran No. 20, Col. San Jose Insurgentes, 03900 Mexico D.F., Mexico.*
Tel: +52 55 55934355 Fax: +52 55 55933420
Web: www.galderma.com.mx

Galen Ltd *Seagoe Industrial Estate, Craigavon, BT63 5UA, UK.*
Tel: +44 (0) 28 3833 4974 Fax: +44 (0) 28 3835 0206
Email: galen@galen.co.uk Web: www.galenplc.com

GD Tecnologie Interdisciplinari Farmaceutiche S.r.l. *Via Augusto Gaudenzi 29, 00163 Rome, Italy.*
Tel: +39 06 66418170 Fax: +39 06 66415358
Web: www.gditalia.biz

Gebro Pharma GmbH *, A-6391 Fieberbrunn, Austria.*
Tel: +43 (0) 5354 53000 Fax: +43 (0) 5354 53500710
Email: pharma@gebro.com Web: www.gebro.com

Gebro Pharma SA *Postfach 397, 4410 Liestal, Switzerland.*
Tel: +41 (0) 61 9268833 Fax: +41 (0) 61 9268844
Email: info@gebro.ch Web: www.gebro.com

Gelcaps Exp. de Mexico SA de CV *Circuito Centro Civico 27, 53100 Naucalpan de Juarez Ciudad Satel, Mexico.*

General Nutrition Canada *6299 Airport Td, Ste 201, Mississauga, L4V 1N3, Canada.*

Generfarma *Los Centelles 7, 46006 Valencia, Spain.*
Tel: +34 96 3742212 Fax: +34 96 3951982

Georg Simons GmbH *Bunsenstr. 1, 82152 Planegg/Martinsried, Germany.*
Tel: +49 (0) 89 8991620 Fax: +49 (0) 89 8575742
Email: simons@merz.de Web: www.simons.de

Geritrex Corp. *144 Kingsbridge Rd East, Mt Vernon, NY 10550, USA.*
Tel: +1 914 668 4003 Fax: +1 914 668 4047
Email: info@geritrex.com Web: www.geritrex.com

German Remedies Ltd *Shivsagar Estate 'A', Dr Annie Besant Rd, Worli, Mumbai 400 018, India.*
Tel: +91 (0) 22 4935528 Fax: +91 (0) 22 4950327
Web: www.germanremedies.com

Germania Pharmazeutika GmbH *Schuselkagasse 8, A-1150 Vienna, Austria.*
Tel: +43 (0) 1 9823399 Fax: +43 (0) 1 982339924

Gerot-Pharmazeutika GmbH *Arnethgasse 3, A-1160 Vienna, Austria.*
Tel: +43 (0) 1 48535050 Fax: +43 (0) 1 4857773

Gervasi Farmacia *C/Juan XXIII 15-19, 08950 Brcelona, Spain.*
Tel: +34 93 4809911

Geymonat S.p.A. *Via S. Anna 2, 03012 Anagni (FR), Italy.*
Tel: +39 0775 768081 Fax: +39 0775 768082

Giovanardi Farmaceutici S.n.c. del Dr Benito Giovanardi e Figli *Via Sapeto 28, 16131 Genoa, Italy.*
Tel: +39 010 381651 Fax: +39 010 393248
Email: info@giovanardi.net Web: www.giovanardi.net

Giovanni Ogna & Figli S.p.A. *Via Figini 41, 20053 Muggio (MI), Italy.*
Tel: +39 039 2782954 Fax: +39 039 2782958
Email: ogna@ogna.it Web: www.ogna.it

Gisand AG *Schlaflistrasse 14, 3013 Berne, Switzerland.*
Tel: +41 (0) 31 3323113

Giuliani S.p.A. *Via Palagi 2, 20129 Milan, Italy.*
Tel: +39 02 20541 Fax: +39 02 2054297

GlaxoSmithKline *Av. Andres Bello 2687, Las Condes, Santiago, Chile.*

GlaxoSmithKline *Private Bag 10-6600, Downtown, Aukland, New Zealand.*
Tel: +64 (0) 9 3672900 Fax: +64 (0) 9 3672910
Web: www.gsk.co.nz

GlaxoSmithKline *Talstrasse 3-5, 3053 Münchenbuchsee, Switzerland.*
Tel: +41 (0) 31 8622111 Fax: +41 (0) 31 8622200
Web: www.glaxosmithkline.ch

GlaxoSmithKline *5 Moore Drive, P.O. Box 13398, Research Triangle Park, NC 27709, USA.*
Tel: +1 215 751 4000 Web: www.gsk.com

GlaxoSmithKline Brasil Ltda *Estrada dos Bandeirantes 8464, 22783-110 Rio de Janeiro, Brazil.*
Tel: +55 21 24446000 Fax: +55 21 24446001
Web: www.gsk.com.br

GlaxoSmithKline Consumer Healthcare *2030 Bristol Circle, Oakville, L6H 5V2, Canada.*
Tel: +1 905 8292030 Fax: +1 905 8296064
Web: www.gsk.ca

GlaxoSmithKline Consumer Healthcare *980 Great West Rd, Brentford, TW8 9BD, UK.*
Tel: +44 (0) 20 8047 5000 Fax: +44 (0) 20 8990 4328
Web: www.gsk.com

GlaxoSmithKline Consumer Healthcare GmbH & Co. KG *Bussmatten 1, 77815 Buhl, Germany.*
Tel: +49 (0) 7223 760 Fax: +49 (0) 7223 764000
Web: www.gsk-consumer.de

GlaxoSmithKline Mexico S.A. de C.V. *Calz. Mexico-Xochimilco No. 4900, Deleg. Tlalpan San Lorenzo Huipulco, 14370 Mexico D.F., Mexico.*
Tel: +52 55 54838300 Fax: +52 55 54838629
Web: www.gsk.com.mx

GlaxoSmithKline Pharma *Albert-Schweitzer-Gasse 6, A-1140 Vienna, Austria.*
Tel: +43 (0) 1 970750 Fax: +43 (0) 1 97075198
Web: www.gsk.com

GlaxoSmithKline Pharmaceuticals (India) Ltd *Dr Annie Besant Rd, Mumbai 400 025, India.*
Tel: +91 (0) 22 4933871 Fax: +91 (0) 22 4935358
Web: www.gsk.com

5

GlaxoSmithKline S.A. *Carlos Casares 3690, 1644 Victoria, Buenos Aires, Argentina.*
Tel: +54 (0) 11 47258900 Fax: +54 (0) 11 47460244
Web: www.gsk.com

Glenmark Pharmaceuticals Ltd *801-813, 8th Floor, Mahalaxmi Chambers, 22 Bhulabhai Desai Rd, Mumbai 400 026, India.*
Tel: +91 (0) 22 4964893 Fax: +91 (0) 22 4932648
Web: www.glenmarkpharma.com

GNLD International P/L *P.O. Box 419, Beenleigh, Qld 4207, Australia.*
Tel: +61 (0) 7 38053499 Fax: +61 (0) 7 38052728
Web: www.gnld.com.au

Gordon Laboratories *6801 Ludlow St, Upper Darby, PA 19082-2408, USA.*
Tel: +1 610 734 2011 Fax: +1 800 347 5678
Web: www.gordonlabs.com

Gothaplast Verbandpflasterfabrik GmbH *Postfach: 100132, 99851 Gotha/ Thuringen, Germany.*
Tel: +49 (0) 3621 30650 Fax: +49 (0) 3621 306530
Email: gothaplast@aol.com Web: www.gothaplast.de

GPL Ginsana Products Lugano SA, Tochterunternehmen der Pharmaton SA *Postfach, 6903 Lugano, Switzerland.*
Tel: +41 (0) 91 6103111 Fax: +41 (0) 91 6103211
Web: www.pharmaton-sa.ch

G.R. Lane Health Products Ltd *Sisson Rd, Gloucester, GL1 3QB, UK.*
Tel: +44 (0) 1452 524012 Fax: +44 (0) 1452 507930
Web: www.laneshealth.com

Graf Fruttasan AG *Untere Etzmatten 16, 4467 Rothenfluh/BL, Switzerland.*
Tel: +41 (0) 61 9959595 Fax: +41 (0) 61 9959590
Email: info@fruttasan.ch Web: www.fruttasan.ch

Grafton Pharmasia Pte Ltd *66 Tannery Lane, 01-05A Sindo Building, S 347805, Singapore.*
Tel: +65 6841 3606 Fax: +65 6841 7526
Web: www.grafton.com.sg

Great Eastern Healthcare Ltd *9/F, Blk A Kerry BCI Godown, 3 Kin Chuen St, Kwai Chung, Hong Kong.*
Tel: +852 24818832 Fax: +852 26101483
Email: gehl@gehl.com.hk

Great Liaison Ltd *Unit 705, Fibres & Fabrics Industrial Ctr, 7 Shing Yip St, Kwun Tong, Kowloon, Hong Kong.*
Tel: +852 28516662 Fax: +852 28505314

Greater Pharma Ltd Part *46, 46/1-2 Soi Charansanitwongs 40, Bangyikhan, Bangkok 10700, Thailand.*
Tel: +66 2 433 0256 Fax: +66 2 433 0076
Email: greater@mozart.inet.co.th

Greenpharma Química e Farmacêutica Ltda *Quadra 2-A Modulos 32/35 DAIA, 75133-600 Anapolis, Brazil.*
Tel: +55 (0) 62 3106400 Fax: +55 (0) 62 3106401
Email: greenpharma@greenpharma.com.br
Web: www.greenpharma.com.br

Group Laboratories SA (Pty) Ltd *21 Wrench Rd, Isando, South Africa.*

Grunenthal Chilena Ltda *Av. Providencia 727, Providencia, Santiago, Chile.*

Grünenthal Lda *Rua Alfredo da Silva no 16, 2610-016 Amadora, Portugal.*
Tel: +351 21 4726300 Fax: +351 21 4710910
Web: www.grunenthal.com

Grünenthal Venezolana C.A. *Av. 1, Torre Centro Profesional Los Samanes Piso 6, Urb. Los Samanes, Caracas, Venezuela.*
Tel: +58 (0) 212 9498511 Fax: +58 (0) 212 9450201
Email: info@grunenthal.com.ve Web: www.grunenthal.com.ve

Grupo Farma S.A. *Av. Principal, Los Ruices, Edif. Farma, Urb. Los Ruices, Caracas 1071, Venezuela.*
Tel: +58 (0) 212 2026200 Fax: +58 (0) 212 2377456
Web: www.grupofarma.com

Gulf Pharmaceutical Industries, Julphar *P.O. Box 997, Ras Al Khaimah, United Arab Emirates.*
Tel: +971 7 2461461 Fax: +971 7 2462462
Web: www.julphar.com

Gynea Laboratorios *Avda Cataluna 127 B, 08184 Palau-Solita i Plegamans, Barcelona, Spain.*
Tel: +34 93 8639560 Fax: +34 93 8646853
Email: gynea@gynea.com Web: www.gynea.com

5

H

Hamilton Pharmaceuticals P/L *P.O. Box 7, Adelaide, SA 5001, Australia.*
Tel: +61 (0) 8 82232957 Fax: +61 (0) 8 82321480
Email: enquire@hamiltonlabs.com.au Web: www.hamiltonlabs.com.au

Hänseler AG *Industriestrasse 35, 9100 Herisau, Switzerland.*
Tel: +41 (0) 71 3535858 Fax: +41 (0) 71 3535800
Web: www.haenseler.ch

Harras Pharma Curarina Arzneimittel GmbH *Am Harras 15, 81373 Munich, Germany.*
Tel: +49 (0) 89 7473670 Fax: +49 (0) 89 74736719
Email: mail@harraspharma.de Web: www.harraspharma.de

Hautel S.A. *Warnes 829 Dto. A, 1414 Buenos Aires, Argentina.*
Tel: +54 (0) 11 48556753

Health Imports Ltd *Binbrook Mill, Young Street, Bradford, BD8 9RE, UK.*
Tel: +44 (0) 1274 488511

Health Perception Ltd *Lakeside Business Park, Swan Lane, Sandhurst, GU47 9DN, UK.*
Tel: +44 (0) 1252 861454 Fax: +44 (0) 1252 861455
Email: queries@health-perception.co.uk Web: www.health-perception.co.uk

Healthy Direct *Unit C, Empress Park, 179 Empress Road, Southampton, SO14 0JX, UK.*
Tel: +44 (0) 800 107 5757 Fax: +44 (0) 800 011 1132
Email: customercare@healthydirect.co.uk

Hebron S.A. Indústria Química e Farmacêutica *Rua Ribeiro de Brito 573, 6 andar, 51021-310 Recife, Brazil.*
Tel: +55 (0) 81 34649294 Fax: +55 (0) 81 34649268
Email: hebron@hebron.com.br Web: www.hebron.com.br

Helago-Pharma GmbH *Rheinallee 11, 53173 Bonn, Germany.*
Tel: +49 (0) 228 956940 Fax: +49 (0) 228 956949
Email: helago@t-online.de Web: www.helago.de

Helixor Heilmittel GmbH & Co. *Fischermuhle 1, 72348 Rosenfeld, Germany.*
Tel: +49 (0) 7428 9350 Fax: +49 (0) 7428 935102
Email: mail@helixor.de Web: www.helixor.de

Hennig Arzneimittel GmbH & Co. KG *Liebigstr. 1-2, 65439 Florsheim am Main, Germany.*
Tel: +49 (0) 6145 5080 Fax: +49 (0) 6145 508140
Email: medwiss@hennig-am.de Web: www.hennig-am.de

Herbal Concepts Ltd *2 Park St., Woburn, MK17 9PG, UK.*
Tel: +44 (0) 1525 292345 Fax: +44 (0) 1525 292346
Email: contactus@herbal-concepts.co.uk Web: www.herbal-concepts.co.uk

Herbal Laboratories Ltd *Malew House, 21 Malew St., Castletown, IM9 1AD, UK.*
Tel: +44 (0) 1624 827885 Fax: +44 (0) 1624 824623
Web: www.herballaboratories.com

Herbalist & Doc Gesundheitsgesellschaft mbH *Waldseeweg 6, 13467 Berlin, Germany.*
Tel: +49 (0) 30 40008100 Fax: +49 (0) 30 40008500
Email: info@herbalist-doc.com Web: www.herbalist-doc.com

Herbamed AG *Untere Au, 9055 Buhler, Switzerland.*
Tel: +41 (0) 71 7918050 Fax: +41 (0) 71 7933720
Email: herbamed@access.ch Web: www.herbamed.ch

Herbarium Laboratório Botanico Ltda *Rua Maua 838, 80030-200 Curitiba, Brazil.*
Tel: +55 (0) 41 2545450 Fax: +55 (0) 41 2546511
Email: decex@herbarium.net Web: www.herbarium.com.br

Herbert Bregenzer *Am Damm 20, A-6820 Frastanz, Austria.*
Tel: +43 (0) 5522 51127 Fax: +43 (0) 5522 5112721

Herbes Universelles *7, 70e Ave O, Blainville, J7C 1R7, Canada.*
Tel: +1 514 4357514

Herbion Pakistan PVT Ltd *Miklukho-Maklaya ul. 8, str. 3, 117198 Moscow, Russia.*
Tel: +7 095 7812073 Fax: +7 095 7814569
Web: www.herbion.com

Herbs Trading GmbH *Novinskii boulevard, d.3, str. 1, 121099 Moscow, Russia.*
Tel: +7 095 7979660 Fax: +7 095 7979661
Web: www.bittner.ru

Hermes Arzneimittel GmbH *Georg-Kalb-Str. 5-8, 82049 Grosshesselohe/Munich, Germany.*
Tel: +49 (0) 89 791020 Fax: +49 (0) 89 79102280
Web: www.hermes-arzneimittel.de

Herron Pharmaceuticals P/L *P.O. Box 95, Brisbane Market, QLD 4106, Australia.*
Fax: +61 (0) 7 38483650 Web: www.herron.com.au

Hevert-Arzneimittel GmbH & Co. KG *In der Weiherwiese 1, 55569 Nussbaum, Germany.*
Tel: +49 (0) 6751 9100 Fax: +49 (0) 6751 910150
Email: info@hevert.de Web: www.hevert.de

Hexal AG *3, ul. Kulneva, 121170 Moscow, Russia.*
Tel: +7 095 787-85-88 Fax: +7 095 787-85-92
Email: hexal@hexal.ru Web: www.hexal.ru

Hexal Argentina S.A. *Paseo Colyn 221 Piso 7, 1063 Buenos Aires, Argentina.*
Tel: +54 (0) 11 43342080 Fax: +54 (0) 11 43342084
Web: www.hexal.com.ar

Hexal do Brasil Ltda *Av. Itaborai 1425, 04135-001 São Paulo, Brazil.*
Tel: +55 11 55917600 Fax: +55 11 55946485
Email: hexal.brasil@hexal.com.br Web: www.hexal.com.br

Hexal Hungária Kft *Tímár u 20, 1034 Budapest, Hungary.*
Tel: +36 4302890 Fax: +36 4302899

Hexal Pharma GmbH *Wilhelminenstrasse 91/II F, A-1160 Vienna, Austria.*
Tel: +43 (0) 1 4869622 Fax: +43 (0) 1 486962233
Web: www.hexal.at

Higaté Medical Argentina *Av. Eva Peron 3052, 1650 San Marten Villa Libertad, Buenos Aires, Argentina.*
Tel: +54 (0) 11 45126841

Hilary's Distribution Ltd *145 Idema Rd, Markham, L3R 1A9, Canada.*
Tel: +1 905 4755446 Fax: +1 905 4750377

Hind Wing Co. Ltd *Unit No 1103B, 11/F, Block B, Seaview Estate, 2-8 Watson Rd, North Point, Hong Kong.*
Tel: +852 25410909 Fax: +852 28540695
Email: hindwing@netvigator.com

Hi-Tech Pharmacal *369 Bayview Ave, Amityville, NY 11701, USA.*
Tel: +1 631 789 8228 Web: www.hitechpharm.com

Hoeveler Mag. & Co. GmbH *Mosham 40, A-4943 Geinberg, Austria.*
Tel: +43 (0) 7723 42305 Fax: +43 (0) 7723 4230515

Hofmann & Sommer GmbH & Co. KG *Lindenstr. 11, 07426 Konigsee, Germany.*
Tel: +49 (0) 36738 42762 Fax: +49 (0) 36738 42798
Email: hofmannundsommer@t-online.de Web: www.hofmannundsommer.de

Holista Health Corp *PO Box 57525, Coquitlam, V3K 5Y9, Canada.*
Tel: +1 604 4223500 Fax: +1 888 6684252
Web: www.holistahealth.com

Holland and Barrett *Samuel Ryder House, Townsend Drive, Attleborough Fields, Nuneaton, CV11 6XW, UK.*
Tel: +44 (0) 870 606 6606
Email: healthinformation@hollandandbarrett.com
Web: www.hollandandbarrett.com

Homöopathisches Laboratorium A. Pflüger GmbH *Bielefelder Str. 17, 33378 Rheda-Wiedenbruck, Germany.*
Tel: +49 (0) 5242 92820 Fax: +49 (0) 5242 55932
Email: info@pflueger.de Web: www.pflueger.de

Hong Kong Medical Supplies Ltd *7/F China Aerospace Centre, 143 Hoi Bun Rd, Kwun Tong, Hong Kong.*
Tel: +852 28063112 Fax: +852 28873425
Email: info@hkmedsup.com.hk

Horna Business Service *Narcisová 2/850, 106 00 Prague 10, Czech Republic.*
Tel: +420 (0) 2 72654588

Hoyer-Madaus GmbH & Co. KG *Alfred-Nobel-Str. 10, 40789 Monheim, Germany.*
Tel: +49 (0) 2173 483100 Fax: +49 (0) 2173 483198
Email: information@hoyer-madaus.de Web: www.hoyer-madaus.de

HPC Harras Pharma Curarina *Worbstrasse 221, 3073 Gumligen, Switzerland.*
Tel: +41 (0) 31 9513313 Fax: +41 (0) 31 9516465

Hubert A.C. Thomas & Co. *Burry Port, SA16 0TB, UK.*
Tel: +44 (0) 1554 835512

HWS-OTC-Service GmbH *Steindorf 65, A-5570 Mauterndorf, Austria.*
Tel: +43 (0) 6472 20076 Fax: +43 (0) 6472 2007641

Ibefar Inst. Brasileiro de Esp. Ftcas. Ltda *Rua Franca Pinto 1357, 04016-035 São Paulo, Brazil.*
Tel: +55 (0) 11 55718855 Fax: +55 (0) 11 5571 2343

ICIM International S.r.l. *Via Peloritana 28, 20024 Garbagnate Milanese (MI), Italy.*
Tel: +39 02 9947931 Fax: +39 02 99479340

ICN Czech Republic as *Truhlářská 13-15, 110 00 Prague 1, Czech Republic.*
Tel: +420 (0) 2 21434111 Fax: +420 (0) 2 21434214
Email: info@icnpharm.cz Web: www.icnpharm.cz

IDS (Hong Kong) Ltd Healthcare Division *14/F LiFung Ctr, 2 On Ping St, Siu Lek Yuen, Shatin, Hong Kong.*
Tel: +852 26355555 Fax: +852 26375818
Web: www.idsmarketing.com

Imgroma BV *Aldebert van Scharnlaan 170 A-2, 6224 JX Maastricht, Netherlands.*

Indoco Remedies Ltd *Indoco House, 166 CST Rd, Santacruz (East), Mumbai 400 098, India.*
Tel: +91 (0) 22 6541851 Fax: +91 (0) 22 6523976
Web: www.indoco.com

Industria Farmacéutica Andrómaco, S.A. de C.V. *Andrómaco No. 104, Col. Ampliación Granada, Deleg. Miguel Hidalgo, 11520 Mexico D.F., Mexico.*
Tel: +52 55 55457285 Fax: +52 55 55450727
Web: www.andromaco.com.mx

Industria Terapeutica Splendore - Oftalmoterapica ALFA *Via F.lli Bandiera 26, 80026 Casoria (NA), Italy.*
Tel: +39 081 5846060 Fax: +39 081 5842526
Email: alfaintes@alfaintes.it

Infabra Indústria Farmacêutica Brasileira Ltda *Av. das Americas 8.445 Conj.803, 22793-080 Rio de Janeiro, Brazil.*
Tel: +55 (0) 21 24876305 Fax: +55 (0) 21 24876309
Web: www.infabra.com.br

Infosint S.p.A. *C. Dir. Colleoni, Pal. Pegaso 2, 20041 Agrate Brianza (MI), Italy.*
Tel: +39 039 6892207 Fax: +39 039 6892246
Email: infosint@tiscalinet.it

Inkeysa *Juan XXIII 15, Esplugas de Llobregat, 08950 Barcelona, Spain.*
Tel: +34 93 4809911 Fax: +34 93 3726551
Email: inkeysa@inkeysa.es Web: www.inkeysa.es

Institut Biochimique SA *Via del Piano, 6915 Pambio-Noranco, Switzerland.*
Tel: +41 (0) 91 9857776 Fax: +41 (0) 91 9857686
Email: info@ibsa.ch Web: www.ibsa.ch

Instituto de Medicamentos e Alergia IMA Ltda *Rua Araujo Leitao 193, 20715-310 Rio de Janeiro, Brazil.*
Tel: +55 (0) 21 25010248 Fax: +55 (0) 21 22181651

Instituto Sanitas Arg. SACIPQ y M. *Saladillo 2452, 1440 Buenos Aires, Argentina.*
Tel: +54 (0) 11 46873663 Fax: +54 (0) 11 46874065

Instituto Sanitas SA *Avda Americo Vespucio 1260, Quilicura, Santiago, Chile.*

Instituto Seroterapico Argentino S.A.I.C. *Av. Larrazabal 1848, 1440 Buenos Aires, Argentina.*
Tel: +54 (0) 11 46838888 Fax: +54 (0) 11 46838888

Instituto Terapeutico Delta Ltda *Rua Engenheiro Guilherme Cristiano Frendez 827, 03477-000 São Paulo, Brazil.*
Tel: +55 (0) 11 67245311 Fax: +55 (0) 11 67246480

Interdelta SA *Case postale 791, 1701 Fribourg, Switzerland.*
Tel: +41 (0) 26 4665126 Fax: +41 (0) 26 4667400

Interpharm GmbH *Effingergasse 21, A-1160 Vienna, Austria.*
Tel: +43 (0) 1 48855 Fax: +43 (0) 1 48855320

Intersan GmbH *Einsteinstr. 30, 76275 Ettlingen, Germany.*
Tel: +49 (0) 7243 1840 Fax: +49 (0) 7243 18439

Investi Farma S.A. *Lisandro de la Torre 2160, 1440 Buenos Aires, Argentina.*
Tel: +54 (0) 11 43342080 Fax: +54 (0) 11 43342080

IP Farma Sas *Via Vigna 6, 80078 Pozzuoli (NA), Italy.*
Tel: +39 (0) 815269226 Fax: +39 (0) 815269899

Ipsen EpE *63 AG. Dimitriou St., 174 56 Alimos, Greece.*
Tel: +30 210 9843324 Fax: +30 210 9887911
Web: www.ipsen.com

Ipsen NV *Guldensporenpark 87, 9820 Merelbeke, Belgium.*
Tel: +32 (0) 9 2439600 Fax: +32 (0) 9 2204473
Web: www.ipsen.com

Ipsen Pharma *Ctra Laurea Miro 395, Sant Feliu de Llobregat, 08980 Barcelona, Spain.*
Tel: +34 93 6858100 Fax: +34 93 6851011
Web: www.ipsen.com

Ipsen Pharma GmbH *Einsteinstr. 30, 76275 Ettlingen, Germany.*
Tel: +49 (0) 7243 18480 Fax: +49 (0) 7243 18439
Email: info@ipsen-pharma.de Web: www.ipsen-pharma.de

5

Ipsen Portugal, SA *Rua General Ferreira Martins, Alameda Fernão Lopes 16-11, Miraflores, 1495-136 Algés, Portugal.*
Tel: +351 21 4123550 Fax: +351 21 4123551
Web: www.beaufour-ipsen.com

Iromedica AG *Haggenstrasse 45, 9014 St Gallen, Switzerland.*
Tel: +41 (0) 71 2741800 Fax: +41 (0) 71 2741801
Email: info@iromedica.ch Web: www.iromedica.ch

Isdin Chile Ltda *Carmencita 25 Of. 82, Las Condes, Santiago, Chile.*

Isdin Lda *Rua da Ilha dos Amores, Lote 4.08.01,X, Parque das Nações - Zona Norte, Santa Maria dos Olivais, 1990-118 Lisbon, Portugal.*
Tel: +351 21 8950084 Fax: +351 21 8950101

Iso-Arzneimittel GmbH & Co. KG *Bunsenstr. 6-10, 76275 Ettlingen, Germany.*
Tel: +49 (0) 7243 10603 Fax: +49 (0) 7243 106169
Email: info@iso-arznei.de Web: www.iso-arznei.de

Istituto Biologico Chemioterapico SpA *Via Crescentino 25, 10154 Turin, Italy.*
Tel: +39 (0) 112440011 Fax: +39 (0) 112485341
Email: info@abcfarmaceutici.it Web: www.abcfarmaceutici.it

Istituto di Medicina Omeopatica S.p.A. *Via Vincenzo Monti 6, 20123 Milan, Italy.*
Tel: +39 02 909313250 Fax: +39 02 909313211
Email: imo@omeoimo.it Web: www.omeoimo.it

Istituto Ganassini S.p.A. di Ricerche Biochimiche *Via Gaggia 16, 20139 Milan, Italy.*
Tel: +39 02 5357041 Fax: +39 02 534106
Email: istituto@ganassini.it Web: www.ganassini.it

Ivax AC *Dmitrovskii per. 9, Business-Centre Stoleshniki, et. 5, 103031 Moscow, Russia.*
Tel: +7 095 2349713 Fax: +7 095 2349711
Web: www.ivax.com

Ivax Argentina SA *JJ Castelli 6701, 1605 Munro, Buenos Aires, Argentina.*

Ivax Pharmaceuticals Inc. *4400 Biscayne Blvd, Miami, FL 33137, USA.*
Tel: +1 305 575 6000 Web: www.ivaxpharmaceuticals.com

Ivax Pharmaceuticals Mexico S.A. de C.V. *Calz de Hueso 859, Ex-Hacienda Coapa, 14100 Mexico D.F., Mexico.*
Tel: +52 55 5990000 Fax: +52 55 6170038
Web: www.ivax.com

Ivax-CR a s Közvetlen Kereskedelmi Képviselet *Berlini út 47-49, 1045 Budapest, Hungary.*
Tel: +36 3993343 Fax: +36 3993494

Ivax-CR as *Pod Habrovou 3, 152 00 Prague 5, Czech Republic.*
Tel: +420 (0) 2 51007111 Fax: +420 (0) 2 51007110
Web: www.ivax.cz

J. McGloin P/L *P.O. Box 294, Kings Grove, NSW 2208, Australia.*
Tel: +61 (0) 2 95023777 Fax: +61 (0) 2 95022054

J. Pickles & Sons *Beech House, 62 High St, Knaresborough, HG5 0EA, UK.*
Tel: +44 (0) 1423 867314 Fax: +44 (0) 1423 869177
Email: enquiries@jpickleshealthcare.com Web: www.jpickleshealthcare.com

Jacobson Medical (Hong Kong) Ltd *15/F China Trade Ctr, 122-124 Wai Yip St, Kwun Tong, Kowloon, Hong Kong.*
Tel: +852 28271616 Fax: +852 25072829
Email: Jacobson@jacobsonmedical.com.hk

Jamieson Laboratories *4025 Rhodes Drive, Windsor, N8W 5B5, Canada.*
Tel: +1 519 9748482 Fax: +1 519 9744742

JDH Pharmaceutical Division *279 Jalan Ahmad Ibrahim, 03-01, S 639938, Singapore.*
Tel: +65 6566 1188 Fax: +65 6861 7307
Email: jdhpharm@sg.lfdis.com

JDH Pharmaceutical Sdn Bhd *LiFung Centre, Lot 6, Persiaran Perusahaan Seksyen 23, Kawasan Perusahaan Shah Alam, 40300 Shah Alam, Malaysia.*
Tel: +60 (0) 3 55417748 Fax: +60 (0) 3 55421486

Jenapharm GmbH & Co. KG *Otto-Schott-Str. 15, 07745 Jena, Germany.*
Tel: +49 (0) 3641 645 Fax: +49 (0) 3641 646085
Email: jenapharm@jenapharm.de Web: www.jenapharm.de

Jengimiel C.A. *Calle Capitolio, Edificio Indelca, piso 3, local E, Boleita Sur, Caracas, Venezuela.*
Tel: +58 (0) 212 2354715 Fax: +58 (0) 212 2388302
Email: informacion@jengimiel.com Web: www.jengimiel.com

Jessup Marketing *27 Old Gloucester St, London, WC1N 3XX, UK.*
Tel: +44 (0) 1932 854825 Fax: +44 (0) 1923 850519
Email: mail@jessup.co.uk Web: www.jessup.co.uk

Jofadel Ind. Farmacêutica S.A. *Av. Jose da Frota Vasconcelos 100, 37062-500 Varginha, Brazil.*
Tel: +55 (0) 35 2141522 Fax: +55 (0) 35 2142380
Web: www.jofadel.com.br

Johannes Bürger Ysatfabrik GmbH *Herzog-Julius-Str. 83, 38667 Bad Harzburg, Germany.*
Tel: +49 (0) 5322 4444 Fax: +49 (0) 5322 780229
Email: info@ysat.de

Johnson & Johnson Consumer Products Co. *199 Grandview Rd, Skillman, NJ 08558-9418, USA.*
Tel: +1 732 524 0400 Web: www.jnj.com

Johnson & Johnson/Merck Consumer Pharmaceuticals of Canada *890 Woodlawn Rd W, Guelph, N1K 1A5, Canada.*
Tel: +1 519 8266300 Fax: +1 519 8266202
Web: www.jnjgateway.com

Jukunda Naturarzneimittel Dr Ludwig Schmitt GmbH & Co. KG *Hofmarkstr. 35, 82152 Planegg, Germany.*
Tel: +49 (0) 89 8993450 Fax: +49 (0) 89 89934520
Email: info@jukunda.de Web: www.jukunda.de

K

Kameliya NPP OOO *Gostinichnyi prospekt d. 6, korp. 2, 127106 Moscow, Russia.*
Tel: +7 095 2219202 Email: kamelia@astelit.ru
Web: www.kamelia.ru

Kedrion S.p.A. *Localita ai Conti Barga, 55020 Castelvecchio Pascoli (LU), Italy.*
Tel: +39 0583 19691 Fax: +39 0583 766121

Kelemata S.p.A. *Via S Quintino 28, 10121 Turin, Italy.*
Tel: +39 011 5160411 Fax: +39 011 9976512

Kemiprogress S.r.l. *Via Aurelia 58, 00100 Rome, Italy.*
Tel: +39 06 39383101 Fax: +39 06 39383131

Kestrel Healthcare Ltd *Ashfield House, Resolution Rd, Ashby de la Zouch, LE65 1HW, UK.*
Tel: +44 (0) 1530 562301 Fax: +44 (0) 1530 562430
Email: kestrel@ventiv.co.uk

Key Pharmaceuticals P/L *P.O. Box 121, Concord West, NSW 2138, Australia.*
Tel: +61 (0) 2 97363811 Fax: +61 (0) 2 97363316
Email: otc@keypharm.com.au Web: www.keypharm.com.au

Kley Hertz SA *Rua Comendador Azevedo 224, 90220-150 Porto Alegre, Brazil.*
Tel: +55 (0) 51 33468488 Fax: +55 (0) 51 33468488
Web: www.grupohertz.com

KLI Corp. *1119 Third Ave SW, Carmel, IN 46032, USA.*
Tel: +1 317 846 7452 Fax: +1 317 846 1676
Email: info@entertainers-secret.com Web: www.entertainers-secret.com

Kneipp (Schweiz) GmbH *Schwarzackerstrasse 2, 8304 Wallisellen, Switzerland.*
Tel: +41 (0) 1 8833860 Fax: +41 (0) 1 8833864
Email: info@kneipp-schweiz.ch Web: www.kneipp-schweiz.ch

Kneipp-Werke *, 97064 Wurzburg, Germany.*
Tel: +49 (0) 931 80020 Fax: +49 (0) 931 8002104
Email: info@kneipp.de Web: www.kneip.de

Knoll Australia *15 Orion Road, Lane Cove, NSW 2066, Australia.*
Tel: +61 (0) 2 94279900

Knoll Lusitana, Lda *Rua Alfredo da Silva 3 C/D, 1300-040 Lisbon, Portugal.*
Tel: +351 21 3616350 Fax: +351 21 3616378

Knoll SA Produtos Químicos e Farmacêuticos *Estrada dos Bandeirantes 2400, 27710-104 Rio de Janeiro, Brazil.*
Tel: +55 (0) 21 24442525 Fax: +55 (0) 11 24442517

Konsyl Pharmaceuticals *8050 Industrial Park Rd, Easton, MD 21601, USA.*
Tel: +1 410 822 5192 Fax: +1 410 820 7032
Email: sales@konsyl.com Web: www.konsyl.com

Korangi S.A. *Parque Empresarial Primóvel Edifício A1, r/c Albarraque, 2635-595 Rio de Mouro, Portugal.*
Tel: +351 21 9251901 Fax: +351 21 9251905

Korhispana *PSJ Can Politic 17 3, Hospitalet de Llobregat, 08907 Barcelona, Spain.*
Tel: +34 93 3358167 Fax: +34 93 3351822
Web: www.korhispana.com

Kotra Pharma (M) Sdn Bhd *No. 1 Jln TTC 12, Cheng Industrial Estate, 75250 Melaka, Malaysia.*
Tel: +60 (0) 6 3362222 Fax: +60 (0) 6 3366122
Web: www.kotrapharma.com

Kottas-Heldenberg Mag. R.u. Sohn *Bauernmarkt 24, A-1014 Vienna, Austria.*
Tel: +43 (0) 1 531210

Krauterpfarrer Kunzle AG *, 6573 Magadino, Switzerland.*
Tel: +41 (0) 91 7430340 Fax: +41 (0) 91 7434034

Krewel Meuselbach GmbH *Krewelstr. 2, 53783 Eitorf, Germany.*
Tel: +49 (0) 2243 870 Fax: +49 (0) 2243 87175
Email: medzin@krewel-meuselbach.de Web: www.krewel-meuselbach.de

Krewel Meuselbach GmbH *Nam. gen. Kutlvašra 6, 140 00 Prague 4, Czech Republic.*
Tel: +420 (0) 2 41404181 Email: krewel@vol.cz

KRKA d.d. *ul. 2-ya Zvenigorodskaya, d. 13, Str. 41, et. 5, 125009 Moscow, Russia.*
Tel: +7 095 7396600 Fax: +7 095 7396601
Email: info@krka.ru Web: www.krka.ru

Kur- und Stadtapotheke *Oberer Stadtplatz 5, A-6060 Hall in Tirol, Austria.*
Tel: +43 (0) 5223 57216 Fax: +43 (0) 5223 43316

L

La Serranita, Lab. de Esp. Medic. y Cosmet. *Calle 49 3752, 1653 Villa Ballester, Buenos Aires, Argentina.*
Tel: +54 (0) 11 47674297 Fax: +54 (0) 11 47644891

Lab. Argenfarma S.R.L. *LLavallol 2649, 1417 Buenos Aires, Argentina.*
Tel: +54 (0) 11 45029504 Fax: +54 (0) 11 45029504

Lab. Baliarda S.A. *Alberti 1283, 1247 Buenos Aires, Argentina.*
Tel: +54 (0) 11 43081450 Fax: +54 (0) 11 43080281
Web: www.baliarda.com.ar

Lab. Cevallos Salud S.R.L. *Zapiola 2836/40, 1428 Buenos Aires, Argentina.*
Tel: +54 (0) 11 45433335 Fax: +54 (0) 11 45440637

Lab. Dr. Madaus & Co. SA *Av. Luis Maria Campos 585, 1426 Buenos Aires, Argentina.*
Tel: +54 (0) 11 47711734 Fax: +54 (0) 11 47754380

Lab. Ducto Ind. Farm. Ltda *Rua VPR 3 Quadra 2-A, Modulos 20/21 DAIA, 75133-600 Anapolis, Brazil.*
Tel: +55 (0) 62 3105700 Fax: +55 (0) 62 3105757
Email: ducto@ducto.com.br Web: www.ducto.com.br

Lab E J Gezzi SRL *14 de Julio 855 OB Dto. 2, 1427 Buenos Aires, Argentina.*

Lab. Fabra S.R.L. *Carlos Villate 5271, 1605 Munro, Buenos Aires, Argentina.*
Tel: +54 (0) 11 47567293 Fax: +54 (0) 11 47564153

Lab. Ferro *Av. Mate de Luna 4333, 4000 S.M. de Tucuman, Tucuman, Argentina.*
Tel: +54 (0) 381 4350214 Fax: +54 (0) 381 4355281

Lab. Fortbenton Co. S.A. *Escalada 133, 1407 Buenos Aires, Argentina.*
Tel: +54 (0) 11 46829376 Fax: +54 (0) 11 46829314
Web: www.fortbenton.com.ar

Lab. Garden House S.A. *Estomba 1058/60, 1427 Buenos Aires, Argentina.*
Tel: +54 (0) 11 45551816 Fax: +54 (0) 11 45547749

Lab. Hexa-Medinova S.A. *Helguera 254/58, 1406 Buenos Aires, Argentina.*
Tel: +54 (0) 11 46116845 Fax: +54 (0) 11 46133013

Lab. Incaico SA *Montiel 156, 1408 Buenos Aires, Argentina.*
Tel: +54 (0) 11 46413632 Fax: +54 (0) 11 46417310

Lab. Lacefa S.A.I.C.A. *Ladines 2263/7, 1419 Buenos Aires, Argentina.*
Tel: +54 (0) 11 45740444 Fax: +54 (0) 11 45713103

Lab. Lafage S.R.L. *J. E. Uriburu 61, 1027 Buenos Aires, Argentina.*
Tel: +54 (0) 11 49539168 Fax: +54 (0) 11 49538076

Lab Medstyle SA *Monsenor Felix Cabrea 42 Of. 1, Providencia, Santiago, Chile.*

Lab. Natufarma *Av. Cordoba 1745, 3080 Esperanza, Santa Fe, Argentina.*
Tel: +54 (0) 3496 420153 Fax: +54 (0) 3496 420153
Web: www.natufarma.com.ar

Lab. Panalab S.A. Argentina *Av. Del Libertador 6250 Piso 2, 1428 Buenos Aires, Argentina.*
Tel: +54 (0) 11 47885717

Lab. Pharma del Plata S.R.L. *Valentin Torra 5450, 3100 Pque.Ind.G. Belgrano, Entre Rios, Argentina.*
Tel: +54 (0) 343 4262104

Lab. Primula S.A. *Andonaegui 1141, 1427 Buenos Aires, Argentina.*
Tel: +54 (0) 11 45230031

Lab. Raymos S.A.I.C. *Vuelta de Obligado 2775, 1428 Buenos Aires, Argentina.*
Tel: +54 (0) 11 47812552 Fax: +54 (0) 11 47882625
Web: www.raymos.com

Lab. Roux-Ocefa S.A. *Montevideo 79/81, 1019 Buenos Aires, Argentina.*
Tel: +54 (0) 11 43830067 Fax: +54 (0) 11 43814661

Lab. Serch S.R.L. *Av. Arturo Illia 668, 1706 Haedo, Buenos Aires, Argentina.*
Tel: +54 (0) 11 46588456 Fax: +54 (0) 11 46586876

Lab. Temis Lostaló S.A. *Zepita 3178, 1285 Buenos Aires, Argentina.*
Tel: +54 (0) 11 63441300 Fax: +54 (0) 11 63441390
Web: www.temislostalo.com.ar

Lab Thalgo Nutrition *Domaine des Châtaigniers, 83520 Roquebrune-sur-Argens, France.*
Tel: +33 (0) 4 94197373 Fax: +33 (0) 4 94816012
Web: www.thalgo.com

Laboratoire Atlas *900 Blvd des Sciences, Suite 200, St-Leonard, H1H 1H1, Canada.*
Tel: +1 514 2547188 Fax: +1 514 2543006

Laboratoire Golaz SA *Case postale 1067, 1701 Fribourg-Moncor, Switzerland.*
Tel: +41 (0) 26 4076111 Fax: +41 (0) 26 4011485

Laboratoire RTA SA *chemin du Signal 18, 1071 Chexbres, Switzerland.*
Tel: +41 (0) 21 9643430 Fax: +41 (0) 21 9643431
Email: rta.jlv@bluewin.ch

Laboratoires Aérocid *248 bis, rue Gabriel-Peri, 94230 Cachan, France.*
Tel: +33 (0) 1 41986700 Fax: +33 (0) 1 45479445

Laboratoires Arkopharma *B.P. 28, 06511 Carros cdx, France.*
Tel: +33 (0) 4 93291128 Fax: +33 (0) 4 93291162
Web: www.arkopharma.com

Laboratoires Asepta *17 bd Prince-Héréditaire-Albert, MC 98000, Monaco.*
Tel: +377 92057551 Fax: +377 92052484
Web: www.asepta.com

Laboratoires Bailly SPEAB *60 rue Pierre-Charron, 75008 Paris, France.*
Tel: +33 (0) 1 44951495 Fax: +33 (0) 1 44951490

Laboratoires Belges Pharmacobel SA *Ave de Scheut 46-50, 1070 Brussels, Belgium.*
Tel: +32 (0) 2 5243966 Fax: +32 (0) 2 5216071

Laboratoires Besins International *13 rue Perier, 92120 Montrouge, France.*
Tel: +33 (0) 1 47353510 Fax: +33 (0) 1 47353891

Laboratoires Bio2 *99 bvd des Belges, 69006 Lyon, France.*
Tel: +33 (0) 4 72740785 Fax: +33 (0) 4 78523890
Email: info@bio2labo.com Web: www.bio2labo.com

Laboratoires Biocom *44 bd Saint-Jacques, 75014 Paris, France.*

Laboratoires Bouchara-Recordati *68 rue Marjolin, 92302 Levallois-Perret, France.*
Tel: +33 (0) 1 45191000

Laboratoires CCD *60 rue Pierre-Charron, 75008 Paris, France.*
Tel: +33 (0) 1 44951495 Fax: +33 (0) 1 44951490
Web: www.ccd-lab.com

Laboratoires Chauvin Bausch & Lomb *416 rue Samuel-Morse, B.P. 1174, 34009 Montpellier cdx 1, France.*
Tel: +33 (0) 4 67123030 Fax: +33 (0) 4 67123031
Web: www.bausch.com

Laboratoires Chefaro-Ardeval *2-4 rue de Chaintron, 92542 Montrouge cdx, France.*

Laboratoires Clément-Thékan *2-4 rue Chaintron, B.P. 850, 92542 Montrouge cdx, France.*
Tel: +33 (0) 1 55481800 Fax: +33 (0) 1 55481801

Laboratoires Clément-Thionville *6 rue Joffre, B.P. 60028, 57101 Thionville cdx, France.*
Tel: +33 (0) 3 82827673 Fax: +33 (0) 3 82827677

Laboratoires Codifra *18 av. Dutarte, 78150 de Chesney, France.*
Tel: +33 (0) 1 39238920 Fax: +33 (0) 1 39439659

Laboratoires CS Dermatologie *35 rue d'Artois, 75008 Paris, France.*
Tel: +33 (0) 1 53761111 Fax: +33 (0) 1 53761212

Laboratoires d'Evolution Dermatologique *7 rue d'Aguesseau, 75008 Paris, France.*
Tel: +33 (0) 1 44560007 Fax: +33 (0) 1 44560008

Laboratoires DB Pharma *1 bis, rue du Cdt-Rivière, 94210 La Varenne-St-Hilaire, France.*
Tel: +33 (0) 1 48832514 Fax: +33 (0) 1 48832757

Laboratoires Dergam *6 rue Saint-Nicolas, 75012 Paris, France.*
Tel: +33 (0) 1 43437911 Fax: +33 (0) 1 43437911
Email: dergam@wnandoo.fr

Laboratoires Dermatologiques Uriage *98 av de la Republique, 92400 Courbevoie, France.*
Tel: +33 (0) 1 55701900 Web: www.labo-uriage.com

Laboratoires Dexo *179 bureaux de la Colline, 92213 Saint-Cloud cdx, France.*
Tel: +33 (0) 1 41121700 Fax: +33 (0) 1 41121701

Laboratoires Dolisos *45 place Abel Gance, 92100 Boulogne, France.*
Tel: +33 (0) 5 62477700 Web: www.dolisos.fr

Laboratoires Dolisos Italia S.r.l. *Via Pontina Vecchia km 34,200, 00040 Ardea (Rome), Italy.*
Tel: +39 06 91602810 Fax: +39 06 91821345
Email: dolisos@dolisos.it Web: www.dolisos.it

Laboratoires du Dermophil Indien *B.P. 9, 61600 La Ferte-Mace, France.*
Tel: +33 (0) 2 33306550 Fax: +33 (0) 2 33380632

Laboratoires Fournier SA *153 rue de Buzenval, 92380 Garches, France.*
Tel: +33 (0) 1 47108800 Fax: +33 (0) 1 47108801
Web: www.groupe-fournier.com

Laboratoires Fuca *1 bis, rue de Plaisance, 94732 Nogent-sur-Marne cdx, France.*
Tel: +33 (0) 1 43247070

Laboratoires Fumouze *Le Malesherbes, 110-114 rue Victor-Hugo, 92303 Levallois-Perret cdx, France.*
Tel: +33 (0) 1 49684100

Laboratoires Gabriel Lesourd *6 rue Ste-Isaure, 75018 Paris, France.*
Tel: +33 (0) 1 46064108

Laboratoires Gilbert *av. du Général-de-Gaulle, B.P.115, 14204 Hérouville-Saint-Clair cdx, France.*
Tel: +33 (0) 2 31471515 Fax: +33 (0) 2 31439500
Web: www.groupebatteur.fr

Laboratoires GlaxoSmithKline *100 rte de Versailles, 78163 Marly-le-Roi cdx, France.*
Tel: +33 (0) 1 39178000 Fax: +33 (0) 1 39171758
Web: www.gsk.fr

Laboratoires Hépatoum *B.P. 5, 03270 Saint-Yorre, France.*
Tel: +33 (0) 1 70588400

Laboratoires Holistica International *465 chemin des Jalassières, 13510 Eguilles, France.*
Tel: +33 (0) 4 42951717 Fax: +33 (0) 4 42951718
Web: www.holistica.fr

Laboratoires Innotech International, Sté du groupe Innothéra *7-9 av Francois-Vincent-Raspail, B.P. 32, 94111 Arcueil cdx, France.*
Tel: +33 (0) 1 46152920 Fax: +33 (0) 1 45464015
Email: innotech@innotechinternational.fr
Web: www.innotechinternational.fr

Laboratoires IPRAD *42-52 rue de l'Aqueduc, 75010 Paris, France.*
Tel: +33 (0) 1 40051188

Laboratoires Jaldes *10 ac de Poussan, B.P. 30, 34770 Gigean cdx, France.*
Tel: +33 (0) 4 67789898 Fax: +33 (0) 4 67781087

Laboratoires Jolly-Jatel *28 av. Carnot, 78100 Saint-Germain-en-Laye, France.*
Tel: +33 (0) 1 34510083

Laboratoires Klorane *Les Cauquillous, B.P. 100, 81506 Lavaur cdx, France.*
Tel: +33 (0) 5 63588800 Fax: +33 (0) 5 63588672

Laboratoires Legras *114 Bis, rue Michel-Ange, 75016 Paris, France.*
Tel: +33 (0) 1 47047852

Laboratoires Lehning *1-3 rue du Petit-Marais, 57640 Sainte-Barbe, France.*
Tel: +33 (0) 3 87767224 Web: www.lehning.com

Laboratoires Leurquin Mediolanum *68/88 rue Ampere, 93330 Neuilly-sur-Marne, France.*
Tel: +33 (0) 1 49442929 Fax: +33 (0) 1 49442914
Web: www.mediolanum-farma.com

5

Laboratoires Liérac *35 av Franklin-Roosevelt, 75008 Paris, France.*
Tel: +33 (0) 1 53939906 Fax: +33 (0) 1 53939901

Laboratoires Madaus *55 bis, quai de Grenelle, Immeuble Mercure III, 75015 Paris, France.*
Tel: +33 (0) 1 56771900 Fax: +33 (0) 1 56771919

Laboratoires Magistra SA *28 Chemin du Grand-Puits, Case postale 122, 1217 Meyrin 2/Geneva, Switzerland.*
Tel: +41 (0) 22 7825542 Fax: +41 (0) 22 7850443

Laboratoires Mazal Pharmaceutique *11 rue Rontgen, B.P. 1309, 29000 Quimper cdx, France.*
Tel: +33 (0) 2 98535455

Laboratoires Médix *18 rue Saint-Mathieu, 78550 Houdan, France.*
Tel: +33 (0) 1 30881600 Fax: +33 (0) 1 30881380

Laboratoires Michel Iderne *Parc d'activités Rosenmeer, 67560 Rosheim, France.*
Tel: +33 (0) 3 88480055

Laboratoires Monin-Chanteaud *Parc Euromedecine II, rue de la Valsière, 34099 Montpellier cdx 5, France.*
Tel: +33 (0) 4 67041106

Laboratoires Motima *19 rue de Passy, 75016 Paris, France.*
Tel: +33 (0) 1 42249873 Fax: +33 (0) 1 45203814
Email: motima@club-internet.fr

Laboratoires Noguès *43 rue de Neuilly, 92000 Nanterre, France.*
Tel: +33 (0) 1 47241501

Laboratoires Norgine Pharma *23 av. de Neuilly, 75116 Paris, France.*
Tel: +33 (0) 1 44174888 Fax: +33 (0) 1 44174896
Email: norgine.pharma.france@norgine.com
Web: www.norgine.com

Laboratoires Novartis Nutrition *B.P. 29, 31250 Revel, France.*
Tel: +33 (0) 5 62187283 Fax: +33 (0) 5 62187284
Web: www.novartisnutrition.com

Laboratoires Pfizer *23-25 av. du Dr-Lannelongue, 75668 Paris cdx 14, France.*
Tel: +33 (0) 1 58073000 Fax: +33 (0) 1 58073440
Web: www.pfizer.com

Laboratoires Pharmaceutiques Trenker SA *Ave Dolez 480-482, 1180 Brussels, Belgium.*
Tel: +32 (0) 2 3740253 Fax: +32 (0) 2 3746881
Email: info@trenker.be Web: www.trenker.be

Laboratoires Pharmafarm *13 av de la Porte d'Italie, 75648 Paris, France.*
Tel: +33 (0) 1 46461920 Fax: +33 (0) 1 46461922

Laboratoires Pharmygiène-SCAT *2-4 rue Chaintron, B.P. 850, 92542 Montrouge cdx, France.*
Tel: +33 (0) 1 55481800 Fax: +33 (0) 1 55481801

Laboratoires Phytomedica *ZI Les Milles, B.P. 5000, Parc d'activités de Pichaury, 13791 Aix-en-Provence cdx 3, France.*
Tel: +33 (0) 4 42245624 Fax: +33 (0) 4 42245628
Email: info@phytomedica.com Web: www.phytomedica-labo.com

Laboratoires Phytoprevent *15 av. de Segur, 75007 Paris, France.*
Tel: +33 (0) 1 53868600 Fax: +33 (0) 1 56582152

Laboratoires Pierre Fabre *45 place Abel-Gance, 92100 Boulogne, France.*
Tel: +33 (0) 5 63714500 Fax: +33 (0) 5 63725066
Web: www.pierre-fabre.com

Laboratoires Pionneau *, 33870 Vayres, France.*
Tel: +33 (0) 5 57748501

Laboratoires Plan SA *Chemin de la Verseuse 1, Case postale 208, 1219 Aire-Geneva, Switzerland.*
Tel: +41 (0) 22 7961585 Fax: +41 (0) 22 7961586
Email: pharma@plansa.com

Laboratoires Plantes et Médecines *Le Payrat, 46000 Cahors, France.*
Tel: +33 (0) 5 63516800 Fax: +33 (0) 5

Laboratoires Richard *rue du Progrès, ZI des Reys de Saulce, 26270 Saulce-sur-Rhone, France.*
Tel: +33 (0) 4 75631720 Fax: +33 (0) 4 75632007

Laboratoires Robert Schwartz *Parc d'Innovation, Illkirck, 67400 Strasbourg, France.*
Tel: +33 (0) 3 88673232 Fax: +33 (0) 3 88661129

Laboratoires Roche Nicholas *33 Rue de l'Industrie, 74240 Gaillard, France.*
Tel: +33 (0) 4 50877070 Fax: +33 (0) 4 50877077
Web: www.roche.com

Laboratoires Rosa-Phytopharma *68 rue Jean-Jaques-Rousseau, 75001 Paris, France.*
Tel: +33 (0) 1 45080242

Laboratoires Rottapharm *83-85 bd Vincent-Auriol, 75013 Paris, France.*
Tel: +33 (0) 1 56619461 Fax: +33 (0) 1 56619462
Web: www.rotta.com

Laboratoires Sodia *av. Robert Schuman, 51100 Reims, France.*
Tel: +33 (0) 3 26790000 Fax: +33 (0) 3 26790009
Email: sodia@wanadoo.fr

Laboratoires Théa *12 rue Louis-Bleriot, 63016 Clermont-Ferrand cdx 2, France.*
Tel: +33 (0) 4 73981436 Fax: +33 (0) 4 73981438
Web: www.laboratoires-thea.fr

Laboratoires Theratech *6 rue Dubais, 27000 Evreux, France.*
Tel: +33 (0) 2 32311714

Laboratoires Toulade *av. du Docteur-Aubry, 76280 Criquetot-L'Esneval, France.*
Tel: +33 (0) 2 35287874 Fax: +33 (0) 2 35287872

Laboratoires Tradiphar *176 rue de l'Arbrisseau, 59000 Lille, France.*
Tel: +33 (0) 3 20971370 Fax: +33 (0) 3 20970970
Email: contact@tradiphar.com Web: www.tradiphar.com

Laboratoires Weleda *9 rue Eugene-Jung, 68330 Huningue, France.*
Tel: +33 (0) 3 89696800 Fax: +33 (0) 3 89696899
Web: www.weleda.com

Laboratoires Zambon France *13 rue René-Jaques, 92138 Issy-les-Moulineaux, France.*
Tel: +33 (0) 1 58044141 Fax: +33 (0) 1 58044100
Web: www.zambongroup.com

Laboratori Gambar S.r.l. *Via Bolognola 45, 00138 Rome, Italy.*
Tel: +39 06 8804548 Fax: +39 06 8804537

Laboratori Guidotti S.p.A. *Via Livornese 897, 56010 Pisa La Vettola (PI), Italy.*
Tel: +39 050 971011 Fax: +39 050 9710306
Web: www.labguidotti.it

Laboratori Italiani Vaillant S.r.l. *Via Cavalieri V. Veneto 241, 21040 Cislago (VA), Italy.*
Tel: +39 02 96382620 Fax: +39 02 96380208

Laboratorio A.M. Farma Activ *Italia 743, 2000 Rosario, Argentina.*
Tel: +54 (0) 341 4255580

Laboratório Americano de Farmacoterapia S/A *Rua Nova York 245, 04560-908 São Paulo, Brazil.*
Tel: +55 (0) 11 50496200 Fax: +55 (0) 11 50496266
Web: www.farmasa.com.br

Laboratorio Biotecnoquímica *Calle 10 con 5 Edif. Walpirema, Piso 1, La Urbina, Caracas, Venezuela.*
Tel: +58 (0) 212 2410545 Fax: +58 (0) 212 2427662
Email: btq@biotecnoquimica.com Web: www.biotecnoquimica.com

Laboratório Catarinense S.A. *Rua Doutor João Colin 1053, 89204-001 Joinville, Brazil.*
Tel: +55 (0) 47 4519036 Fax: +55 (0) 47 4519090
Email: sac@labcat.com.br Web: www.labcat.com.br

Laboratório Daudt Oliveira Ltda *Rua Simões da Mota 57, 21540-100 Rio de Janeiro, Brazil.*
Tel: +55 (0) 21 24502878 Fax: +55 (0) 21 3901772
Email: odontis@odontis.com.br Web: www.odontis.com.br

Laboratorio di Chimica Medica dell' Antipiol S.n.c. *Via S. Benigno 26, 10154 Turin, Italy.*
Tel: +39 (0) 11 201141 Fax: +39 (0) 11 2428028

Laboratório Dinafarma Ltda *Avenida Major Alvim 155, 12942550 Atibaia, Brazil.*
Fax: +55 (0) 11 44131814

Laboratorio DNR Farma SRL *Hipolito Vieytes 147, 1603 Villa Martelli, Buenos Aires, Argentina.*

Laboratorio Dr. Lazar & Cia. S.A. *Av. Velez Sarsfield 5855, 1605 Carapachay, Buenos Aires, Argentina.*
Tel: +54 (0) 11 47620181 Fax: +54 (0) 11 47620181
Web: www.lazar.com.ar

Laboratorio Elea S.A.C.I.F.yA. *Sanabria 2353 Piso 1, 1417 Buenos Aires, Argentina.*
Tel: +54 (0) 11 43794300 Fax: +54 (0) 11 43794333
Web: www.laboratorioelea.com.ar

Laboratorio Esp. Med. Knop Ltda *Av. Lib. Bdo. O'higgins 1671, Santiago, Chile.*

Laboratorio Farmaceutico Master SA *Av. Irarrazaval 2821, Torre A, Of. 1001, Santiago, Chile.*

Laboratório Farmaervas Ltda *Rua Saldanha Marinho 161, 3055020 São Paulo, Brazil.*

Laboratorio Fitolife S.r.l. *Via Domiziana km 55, 80072 Arco Felice Pozzuoli (NA), Italy.*
Tel: +39 081 8042385 Fax: +39 081 8042838
Email: info@fitolife.it Web: www.fitolife.it

Laboratório Gross S.A. *Rua Padre Ildefonso Penalba 389, 20775-020 Rio de Janeiro, Brazil.*
Tel: +55 (0) 21 25973112 Fax: +55 (0) 21 25973112
Email: gross@gross.com.br Web: www.gross.com.br

Laboratório Hepacholan S.A. *Av. Manoel Monteiro de Araújo 1051, Vila Jaguara, 05113-020 São Paulo, Brazil.*
Tel: +55 (0) 11 36214122 Fax: +55 (0) 11 36219595

Laboratório Iodo Suma Ltda *Rua Maximiliano Fraga 35, 36880-000 Muriae, Brazil.*
Tel: +55 (0) 32 7223155

Laboratório J. Neves, Lda *Parque Industrial do Seixal, 2840-069 Paio Pires, Portugal.*
Tel: +351 21 2134800 Fax: +351 21 2134899
Email: evazlabjneves@mail.eunet.pt

Laboratorio Koni-Cofarm SA *Crescente Errazuriz 2077, Nunoa, Santiago, Chile.*

Laboratorio Leti S.A.V. *2a Av., Parcela 3, Manzana J Edif. Leti, Guarenas, Caracas, Venezuela.*
Tel: +58 (0) 212 3622424 Fax: +58 (0) 212 3624545
Email: myanez@leti.com.ve Web: www.leti.com.ve

Laboratório Medinfar, SA *Rua Manuel Ribeiro da Pavia 1 - 1, Venda Nova, 2700-547 Amadora, Portugal.*
Tel: +351 21 4748228 Fax: +351 21 4751736
Web: www.medinfar.pt

Laboratório Neo Química Comércio e Indústria Ltda *Rua VPR 1 Quadra 2-A, Modulo 4 DAIA, 75133-600 Anapolis, Brazil.*
Tel: +55 (0) 62 3102500 Fax: +55 (0) 62 3161022
Web: www.neoquimica.com.br

Laboratório Phos-Kola Ltda *Rua das Laranjeiras 984, 49010-000 Aracaju, Brazil.*
Tel: +55 (0) 79 2119798

Laboratorio Prater SA *Av. P Aguirre Cerda 5291, Cerrillos, Santiago, Chile.*

Laboratorio Schering-Plough *Burgos 80, Las Condes, Santiago, Chile.*

Laboratório Sedabel Ltda *Rodovia Washington Luiz 1308 Km 4.5, 25085-000 Duque de Caxias, Brazil.*
Tel: +55 (0) 21 26713636 Email: sedabel@sedabel.com.br
Web: www.sedabel.com.br

Laboratório Simões Ltda *Rua Pereira de Almeida 102, 20260-100 Rio de Janeiro, Brazil.*
Tel: +55 (0) 21 5010555 Fax: +55 (0) 21 5027000

Laboratório Sinterapico Industrial e Farmacêutico Ltda *Rua Olegario Cunha Lobo 25, 12940-000 Atibaia, Brazil.*
Tel: +55 (0) 11 44110333 Fax: +55 (0) 11 44133313

Laboratorio Terapeutico M.R. S.r.l. *Via Domenico Veneziano 13, 50143 Florence, Italy.*
Tel: +39 055 714724 Fax: +39 055 708371
Email: labtermr@tin.it Web: www.mr-online.it

Laboratório Teuto-Brasileiro Ltda *VP 7-D Modulo 11 Quadra 13, 75133-600 Anapolis, Brazil.*
Email: trade@teuto.com.br Web: www.teutointernational.com

Laboratorio Walker S.R.L. *E. Zeballos 249, 2000 Rosario, Santa Fe, Argentina.*
Tel: +54 (0) 341 4492945 Web: www.laboratoriowalker.com.ar

Laboratorio Wunderpharm S.R.L. *Remedios 5322, 1440 Buenos Aires, Argentina.*
Tel: +54 (0) 11 46356078 Fax: +54 (0) 11 46352891

Laboratorio Ximena Polanco *Dresden 4640, Santiago, Chile.*

Laboratorios Andromaco SA *Av. Quilin 5273, Penalolen, Santiago, Chile.*

Laboratorios Andrómaco S.A.I.C.I. *Ingeniero Huergo 1145, 1107 Buenos Aires, Argentina.*
Tel: +54 (0) 11 43076000 Fax: +54 (0) 11 43620725
Web: www.andromaco.com.ar

Laboratorios Bagó S.A. *Bernardo de Irigoyen 248, 1072 Buenos Aires, Argentina.*
Tel: +54 (0) 11 43442000 Fax: +54 (0) 11 43442086
Web: www.bago,com.ar

Laboratórios Baldacci S.A. *Rua Pedro de Toledo 520, 04039-001 São Paulo, Brazil.*
Tel: +55 (0) 11 50854444

Laboratorios Basi *R.do do Padrão 98, 3000-312 Coimbra, Portugal.*
Tel: +351 239 827021 Fax: +351 239 492845
Email: basi@basi.com.pt

Laboratorios Beta S.A. *Av. San Juan 2266, 1232 Buenos Aires, Argentina.*
Tel: +54 (0) 11 59216200 Fax: +54 (0) 11 59216299
Web: www.betalab.com.ar

Laboratórios Biosintetica Ltda *Av das Nações Unidas 22.428, Predio 30, 04795-916 São Paulo, Brazil.*
Tel: +55 (0) 11 55466822 Fax: +55 (0) 11 55466812
Email: biosintetica@biosintetica.com.br Web: www.biosintetica.com.br

Laboratorios Biotech C.A. *Calle del Arenal Edif. Biotech, Urb. La Trinidad, Caracas, Venezuela.*
Tel: +58 (0) 212 9035400 Fax: +58 (0) 212 9035690
Web: www.biotech.com.ve

5

Laboratorios Chile SA *Av. Marathon 1315, Nunoa, Santiago, Chile.*

Laboratorios Cofasa S.A. *Urbanización Industrial Lebrún, Edificio Cofasa, 4to. Piso, Caracas, Venezuela.*
Tel: +58 (0) 212 2566344 Fax: +58 (0) 212 2568464
Email: info@laboratoriocofasa.com Web: www.laboratoriocofasa.com

Laboratorios Columbia de Argentina SA *Cervantes 2950, Buenos Aires, Argentina.*

Laboratorios Dermatologicos Darier S.A. de C.V. *Av. Insurgentes sur 3579 Torre 3, Piso 8, M Hidalgo La Joya Olimpica, 14020 Mexico D.F., Mexico.*
Tel: +52 55 53505555 Fax: +52 55 53505538
Email: atencionaclientes@darier.com.mx Web: www.darier.com.mx

Laboratorios DHU Ibérica, S.A. *Pol Ind Francolm Parcela 3, Nave 1-2, Apartado de Correos 1082, 43006 Tarragona, Spain.*
Tel: +34 977 550542 Fax: +34 977 550848
Email: marketing@dhu.es Web: www.dhu.es

Laboratorios Diviser-Aquilea S.L. *Pont Reixat 5, Saint Just Desvern, 08960 Barcelona, Spain.*
Tel: +34 93 4733000 Fax: +34 93 4332092
Email: aquilea@aquilea.com Web: www.aquilea.com

Laboratorios Elmor S.A. *Av. Eugenio Mendoza, Centro Letonia, Piso 16, La Castellana, Apartado Postal 80444, Caracas 1062, Venezuela.*
Tel: +58 (0) 212 2638233 Fax: +58 (0) 212 2672910
Email: servicioalcliente@elmor.com.ve Web: www.laboratorioselmor.com.ve

Laboratorios Excelentia S.A. *Santo Domingo 4088, 1437 Buenos Aires, Argentina.*
Tel: +54 (0) 11 49119114 Fax: +54 (0) 11 49119114

Laboratorios Farmasa, S.A. de C.V. *Bufalo No. 27, Col. del Valle, 03100 Mexico D.F., Mexico.*
Tel: +52 55 55247451 Fax: +52 55 55246789

Laboratorios Flupal C.A. *Parcelamiento Industrial La Fe Parcel a Nro. B23, Macarao, Caracas 1000 A, Venezuela.*
Tel: +58 (0) 212 4319360 Fax: +58 (0) 212 4335482

Laboratórios Gemballa Ltda *Avenida Sete de Setembro 50, 89160-000 Rio do Sul, Brazil.*
Tel: +55 (0) 47 5318040 Fax: +55 (0) 47 5318002

Laboratórios Goulart S.A. *Rua Aguape 56, Parada de Lucas, 21010-080 Rio de Janeiro, Brazil.*
Tel: +55 (0) 21 24851960

Laboratorios Gramón *Intendente Amaro Avalos 4208, 1605 Munro, Buenos Aires, Argentina.*
Tel: +54 (0) 11 47627600 Fax: +54 (0) 11 47627605
Web: www.gramon.com.ar

Laboratorios Grisi Hermanos, S.A. de C.V. *Calle Amores No. 1746, Col. del Valle, Deleg. Benito Juarez, 03100 Mexico D.F., Mexico.*
Tel: +52 55 56299902 Fax: +52 55 55341003
Web: www.grisi.com.mx

Laboratorios Grossman S.A. de C.V. *Blvd Manuel Avila Camacho 40, P.20 T.Es, Miguel Hidalgo Lomas de Chapulte, 11000 Mexico D.F., Mexico.*

Laboratorios Hochstetter SA *Dardignac 6, Santiago, Chile.*

Laboratorios Hormona S.A. de C.V. *Blvd. M. Avila Camacho No.470, Col. San Andres Atoto, 53500 Naucalpan de Juarez, Mexico.*
Tel: +52 55 55762511 Fax: +52 55 55765467

Laboratorios Ifusa S.A. *Francisco Lorenzana 20, Col. San Rafael, Deleg. Cuauhtemoc, 06470 Mexico D.F., Mexico.*
Tel: +52 55 57051410 Fax: +52 55 55353961

5

Laboratórios Inibsa, SA *Sintra Business Park, Zona Industrial da Abrunheira, Edifício 1 - 2, 2710-089 Sintra, Portugal.*
Tel: +351 219 112730 Fax: +351 219 112023
Email: inibsa@inibsa.pt Web: www.inibsa.com

Laboratorios Intra S.A. *Av. Principal 50-75, Barrio Los Estanques Maracaibo, Zulia, Venezuela.*
Tel: +58 (0) 61 348826 Fax: +58 (0) 61 343357

Laboratórios Klinger do Brasil Ltda *Rua Assahy 45, Rudge Ramos, 09633-010 São Bernardo do Campo, Brazil.*
Tel: +55 (0) 11 43624660 Email: marketing@labklinger.com.br
Web: www.labklinger.com.br

Laboratorios L.O. Oftalmi C.A. *Edificio Santo Domingo, Calle 6, Zona Industrial La Urbina, Apto 66285, Caracas 1061-A, Venezuela.*
Tel: +58 (0) 212 2424747 Fax: +58 (0) 212 2427446
Web: www.oftalmi.com

Laboratorios Maver SA *Emilio Vaisse 574, Providencia, Santiago, Chile.*

Laboratorios Millet-Franklin S.A. *Thames 121 Piso 1 of. 2, 1609 Boulogne, Buenos Aires, Argentina.*
Tel: +54 (0) 11 47665848 Fax: +54 (0) 11 47664774
Web: www.milletfranklin.com

Laboratórios Osorio de Moraes Ltda *Avenida Cardeal Eugenio Pacelli 2281, 32210-001 Contagem, Brazil.*
Tel: +55 (0) 31 33610844 Fax: +55 (0) 31 33618045

Laboratorios Parggon S.A. de C.V. *Av. Vallarta 7000, Zapopan San Juan de Ocotan, 45019 Jalisco, Mexico.*
Tel: +52 33 36820388

Laboratorios Pasteur Ltda *Ignacio Serrano 568, Concepción, Santiago, Chile.*

Laboratorios Phoenix S.A.I.C.F. *Humahuaca 4065, 1192 Buenos Aires, Argentina.*
Tel: +54 (0) 11 43794200 Fax: +54 (0) 11 43794244
Web: www.phoenix.com.ar

Laboratorios Politecnicos Nacionales C.A. *Cipreses a Hoyo 109-11, Pso.1 Edif. El Viejo, Urb. Sta. Rosalía Caracas, Caracas, Venezuela.*
Tel: +58 (0) 212 5423384 Fax: +58 (0) 212 5423548

Laboratorios Prieto S.A. *Maza 1869/73, 1240 Buenos Aires, Argentina.*
Tel: +54 (0) 11 49210365 Fax: +54 (0) 11 49210419

Laboratórios Prima Ltda *Rua Juparana 62, 20510-040 Rio de Janeiro, Brazil.*
Tel: +55 (0) 21 25723855 Fax: +55 (0) 21 25713198
Email: sac@primalab.com.br Web: www.laboratoriosprima.com.br

Laboratorios Quim-Far C.A. *Chacaíto-Quinta Nueva Segovia, Urb. Bello Monte Caracas, Caracas, Venezuela.*
Tel: +58 (0) 212 9512679 Fax: +58 (0) 212 9513246

Laboratorios Recalcine SA *San Eugenio 567, Santiago, Chile.*

Laboratorios Rider SA *Placer 1348, Santiago, Chile.*

Laboratorios Rowe-Fleming C.A. *Av.La Habana con calle Quito Edif. Vizcaya, Los Caobos Entrada B Pent House, Caracas, Venezuela.*
Tel: +58 (0) 212 7932080 Fax: +58 (0) 212 7933404

Laboratorios Saval SA *Avenida Presidente Eduardo Frei Montalva 4600, Santiago, Chile.*
Email: lab@saval.cl Web: www.saval.cl

Laboratorios Sidus S.A. *Av. del Libertador 742, 1638 Vicente Lopez, Buenos Aires, Argentina.*
Tel: +54 (0) 11 47966800 Fax: +54 (0) 11 47966860
Web: www.sidus.com.ar

Laboratorios Sigma *Chaco 667, 5000 Cordoba Capital, Argentina.*
Tel: +54 (0) 351 4224716

Laboratorios Silesia SA *Av. Chile Espana 325, Santiago, Chile.*

Laboratorios SMB Farma SA *Av. Bulnes 377, Dpto 305, Santiago, Chile.*

Laboratorios Vincenti C.A. *Urb. Industrial Santa Cruz, Calle Roma, Edif., Centro Proa, Piso 2 Guarenas, Caracas, Venezuela.*
Tel: +58 (0) 212 3632455 Fax: +58 (0) 212
Email: info@vincentilab.com Web: vincentilab.com

Laboritorios Felipe Bajer S.A.I.C. *Alfredo R. Bufano 1265, 1416 Buenos Aires, Argentina.*
Tel: +54 (0) 11 45827920 Web: www.bajer.com.ar

Lacer *Sardenya 350, 08025 Barcelona, Spain.*
Tel: +34 93 4465300 Fax: +34 93 3479009
Web: www.lacer.es

Laclede Inc. *2030 East University Drive, Rancho Dominguez, CA 90220, USA.*
Web: www.laclede.com

Lagos Laboratorios Argentina S.R.L. *Jorge Newbery 1829, 1426 Buenos Aires, Argentina.*
Tel: +54 (0) 11 47727599 Fax: +54 (0) 11 47747587
Web: www.lagoslab.com.ar

Lampugnani Farmaceutici S.p.A. *Via Gramsci 4, 20014 Nerviano (Milan), Italy.*
Tel: +39 0331 587354 Fax: +39 0331 585588
Email: info@lampugnanifarmaceutici.it

Larkhall Laboratories *Forest Road, Charlbury, Chipping Norton, OX7 3HH, UK.*
Tel: +44 (0) 1608 811539 Fax: +44 (0) 1608 811834

Lavipharm Group *Agias Marinas St, 190 02 Peania Attica, Greece.*
Tel: +30 210 6691106 Fax: +30 210 6691208
Email: comm@lavipharm.gr Web: www.lavipharm.gr

Leciva as *U Kabelorny 130, 10237 Prague 10, Czech Republic.*
Tel: +420 (0) 2 67241111 Fax: +420 (0) 2 72702402
Email: leciva@leciva.cz Web: www.leciva.cz

Lek *Starokonyushennyi per. 10/10 str. 1, 119002 Moscow, Russia.*
Tel: +7 095 2588484 Fax: +7 095 2588485

Lek Pharma sro *Jeseniová 30, 130 00 Prague 3, Czech Republic.*
Tel: +420 (0) 2 21421611 Fax: +420 (0) 2 21421629
Email: lekpharma@lek-cz.cz

Leo Pharma A/S *Industriparken 55, 2750 Ballerup, Denmark.*
Tel: +45 44923800 Fax: +45 44943040
Web: www.leo-pharma.com

Léro *65 bd du Mal-de-Lattre-de-Tassigny, 92150 Suresnes, France.*
Tel: +33 (0) 1 40991433 Fax: +33 (0) 1 45062764

Leros sro *U Narodni galerie 460, 156 15 Prague 5, Czech Republic.*
Tel: +420 (0) 2 57898111 Fax: +420 (0) 2 57922200
Email: leros@leros.cz Web: www.leros.cz

Les Grands Espaces Thérapeutiques *B.P. 6054, 34030 Montpellier cdx 01, France.*
Tel: +33 (0) 4 67070071

Les Laboratoires Bio-Santé *3564 Griffith St, St-Laurent, H4C 1A7, Canada.*
Tel: +1 514 7377343 Fax: +1 514 7376878

Lichtenstein Pharmazeutica GmbH & Co. *Industriestrasse 26, 56218 Mulheim-Karlich, Germany.*
Tel: +49 (0) 261 809030 Fax: +49 (0) 261 8090321
Web: www.lichtenstein-pharma.de

Lichtwer Pharma *145 Idema Road, Markham, Ontario, L3R 1A9, Canada.*
Tel: +1 905 475 5446 Fax: +1 905 475 0377
Web: www.lichtwer.de

Lichtwer Pharma AG *Wallenroder Str. 8-10, 13435 Berlin, Germany.*
Tel: +49 (0) 30 403700 Fax: +49 (0) 30 40370103
Email: info@lichtwer.de Web: www.lichtwer.de

Lichtwer Pharma UK *Regency House, Mere Park, Dedmere Rd, Marlow, SL7 1FJ, UK.*
Tel: +44 (0) 1628 487780 Fax: +44 (0) 1628 487781
Web: www.lichtwer.co.uk

Liferpal MD, S.A. de C.V. *Refineria No. 1266, Col. Alamo Industrial, 44490 Guadalajara, Jalisco, Mexico.*
Tel: +52 33 36661228 Fax: +52 33 36661073

Lindopharm GmbH *Neustr. 82, 40721 Hilden, Germany.*
Tel: +49 (0) 2103 2065 Fax: +49 (0) 2103 206600
Web: www.lindopharm.de

Liptis Pharmaceuticals Inc. *8941 Atlanta Ave., Huntington Beach, CA 92648, USA.*
Email: mail@liptis.com Web: www.liptis.com

Lisapharma S.p.A. *Via Licinio 11, 22036 Erba (Como), Italy.*
Tel: +39 031 641257 Fax: +39 031 644182
Email: lisapharma@lisapharma.it

Lizofarm S.r.l. *Via S. Gottardo 37, 20052 Monza (MI), Italy.*
Tel: +39 039 3900277 Fax: +39 039 389671

Llorens *Ciudad de Balaguer 7-11, 08022 Barcelona, Spain.*
Tel: +34 93 2125312 Fax: +34 93 4174741

Lomapharm, Rudolf Lohmann GmbH KG *Langes Feld 5, 31860 Emmerthal, Germany.*
Tel: +49 (0) 5155 63200 Fax: +49 (0) 5155 63210
Email: service@lomapharm.de Web: www.lomapharm.de

Lopes Produtos Farmaceuticos S.A. *Rodovia BR 491, Km 5, Caixa Postal:62, 37002-970 Varginha, Brazil.*
Tel: +55 (0) 35 32221233 Fax: +55 (0) 35 32221429

LPC Medical (UK) Ltd *30 Chaul End Lane, Luton, LU4 8EZ, UK.*
Tel: +44 (0) 1582 560393 Fax: +44 (0) 1582 560395
Email: info@lpcpharma.com Web: www.lpcpharma.com

Luper Indústria Farmacêutica Ltda *Rua Doutor Clementino 608, 03059-030 São Paulo, Brazil.*
Tel: +55 (0) 11 2917344 Fax: +55 (0) 11 66930498
Email: luper@luper.com.br Web: www.luper.com.br

Lysoform Dr. Hans Rosemann GmbH *Kaiser-Wilhelm-Str. 133, 12247 Berlin, Germany.*
Tel: +49 (0) 30 779920 Fax: +49 (0) 30 77992219
Email: kontakt@lysoform.de Web: www.lysoform.de

M

M & A Pharmachem Ltd *Allenby Laboratories, Wigan Rd, Westhoughton, Bolton, BL6 2LA, UK.*
Tel: +44 (0) 1942 816184 Fax: +44 (0) 1924 813937
Email: buy@mapharmachem.co.uk Web: www.mapharmachem.co.uk

Madariaga *Electronica, 7, Poligono Urtinsa II, Alcorcon, 28923 Madrid, Spain.*
Tel: +34 91 6437500 Fax: +34 91 6433990

Madaus *FOC 68-82, 08038 Barcelona, Spain.*
Tel: +34 93 2988200 Fax: +34 93 2231652
Email: info@madaus.es Web: www.madaus.es

Madaus AG *Colonia-Allee 15, 51067 Cologne, Germany.*
Tel: +49 (0) 221 89980 Fax: +49 (0) 221 8998701
Email: info@madaus.de Web: www.madaus.de

Madaus GmbH *Lienfeldergasse 91-93, A-1171 Vienna, Austria.*
Tel: +43 (0) 1 48016000 Fax: +43 (0) 1 480160025

Madaus Pharma SA *Rue des Trois Arbres 16, 1180 Brussels, Belgium.*
Tel: +32 (0) 2 3704777 Fax: +32 (0) 2 3704774
Email: madaus.pharma@skynet.be Web: www.masaus.com

Madaus S.r.l. *Rivera Francia 3/A, 35127 Padua, Italy.*
Tel: +39 0496989211 Fax: +39 0496989204
Email: info@madaus.it

Mag. Dr. Till Strallhofer *St-Veit-Gasse 56, A-1130 Vienna, Austria.*
Tel: +43 (0) 1 8770699 Fax: +43 (0) 1 877069916

Magis Farmaceutici S.p.A. *Via Cacciamali 34-36-38, Zona Ind. (Loc. Noce), 25125 Brescia, Italy.*
Tel: +39 030 349761 Fax: +39 030 349352

Makros Indústria Farmacêutica Ltda *Rua Riachuelo 410, 20230-013 Rio de Janeiro, Brazil.*
Tel: +55 (0) 21 22325851

Manx Pharma Ltd *Manx House, Spectrum Business Estate, Bircholt Rd, Maidstone, ME15 9YP, UK.*
Tel: +44 (0) 1622 766389 Fax: +44 (0) 1622 761435
Web: www.manxhealthcare.com

Marco Antonetto S.p.A. *Via Arsenale 29, 10121 Turin, Italy.*
Tel: +39 011 5613031 Fax: +39 011 5628190

Maria Clementine Martin Klosterfrau GmbH *Doerenkampgasse 11, A-1105 Vienna, Austria.*
Tel: +43 (0) 1 6882161 Fax: +43 (0) 1 688216127

Maria Clementine Martin Klosterfrau Vertriebsgesellschaft mbH *, 50606 Cologne, Germany.*
Tel: +49 (0) 221 16520 Fax: +49 (0) 221 1652430
Web: www.klosterfrau.de

Marjan Indústria e Comércio Ltda *Rua Gibraltar 165, 04755-070 São Paulo, Brazil.*
Tel: +55 (0) 11 56429888 Fax: +55 (0) 11 56416009
Email: sac@marjan.com.br Web: www.marjan.com.br

Marvecs Services Srl *Via Paracelso 26, 20041 Agrate Brianza, Italy.*
Tel: +39 039684641 Fax: +39 039664300

Mauermann-Arzneimittel, Franz Mauermann oHG *Heinrich-Knote-Str. 2, 82343 Pocking, Germany.*
Tel: +49 (0) 8157 1002 Fax: +49 (0) 8157 4208
Email: info@mauermann-arznei.de

Mavena AG *Birkenweg 1-8, 3123 Belp, Switzerland.*
Tel: +41 (0) 31 8185588 Fax: +41 (0) 31 8185590

Mavena GmbH *Haubachstrasse 33, 10585 Berlin, Germany.*
Tel: +49 (0) 30 3450693 Fax: +49 (0) 30 34506950
Web: www.mavena.com

Max Zeller Söhne AG, Pflanzliche Heilmittel *Seeblickstrasse 4, Postfach 29, 8590 Romanshorn, Switzerland.*
Tel: +41 (0) 71 4660500 Fax: +41 (0) 71 4635007
Email: zeller@zellerag.ch Web: www.zellerag.ch

MaxMedic Pharma GmbH & Co. KG *Amalienstr. 71, 80799 Munich, Germany.*
Tel: +49 (0) 89 2889060 Fax: +49 (0) 89 28890620
Email: info@maxmedic.de Web: www.maxmedic.de

Mayne Pharma P/L *Level 6, 390 St Kilda Road, Melbourne, VIC 3004, Australia.*
Tel: +61 (0) 3 98680700 Web: www.maynegroup.com

Mayrhofer Pharmazeutika *Melissenweg 15, A-4021 Linz, Austria.*
Tel: +43 (0) 732 76590 Fax: +43 (0) 732 7659100

MBD Marketing (S) Pte Ltd *371 Beach Rd, 03-30 KeyPoint, S 199597, Singapore.*
Tel: +65 6391 5915 Fax: +65 6392 3929
Email: mbdmktg@singnet.com.sg

MD Pharmaceuticals Pte Ltd *896 Dunearn Rd, 04-03 Sime Darby Centre, S 589472, Singapore.*
Tel: +65 6460 2753 Fax: +65 6469 8979
Email: md777@singnet.com.sg

Meda AB *Box 906, 170 09 Solna, Sweden.*
Tel: +46 (0) 8 6301900 Fax: +46 (0) 8 6301950
Email: info@meda.se Web: www.meda.se

Meda A/S *Bjerkas Industriomrade, 3470 Slemmestad, Norway.*
Tel: +47 31294500 Fax: +47 31294545
Web: www.meda.se

Meda Oy *Lemminkäisenkatu 32, 20520 Turku, Finland.*
Tel: +358 (0) 2 2849900 Fax: +358 (0) 2 2849929
Web: www.meda.fi

Medibrands *P.O. Box 531, Yokneam 20692, Israel.*
Tel: +972 (0) 4 9590131 Fax: +972 (0) 4 9590028

Medic Herb UK Ltd *PO Box 2835, Brewery Courtyard, Draymans Lane, Marlow, SL7 2XG, UK.*
Tel: +44 (0) 1628 400 608 Fax: +44 (0) 1628 891 701
Email: customercare@medicherb.co.uk Web: www.medicherb.co.uk

Medic Industrial Farmacêutica Ltda *Rua Conselheiro Mayrink 362, 20960-140 Rio de Janeiro, Brazil.*
Tel: +55 (0) 21 22414436

Medice, Arzneimittel Pütter GmbH & Co. KG *Kuhloweg 37, 58638 Iserlohn, Germany.*
Tel: +49 (0) 2371 9370 Fax: +49 (0) 2371 937329
Email: info@medice.de Web: www.medice.de

Medichemie AG *Bruhlstrasse 50, 4107 Ettingen, Switzerland.*
Tel: +41 (0) 61 7262200 Fax: +41 (0) 61 7262205

Mediherb P/L *P.O. Box 713, Warwick, QLD 4370, Australia.*
Tel: +61 (0) 7 46610700 Fax: +61 (0) 7 46610788
Web: www.mediherb.com.au

Medika Lizenz Pharmaz. Präparate *Am Alten Weg 20, 82041 Oberhaching, Germany.*
Tel: +49 (0) 89 6131786 Fax: +49 (0) 89 2606384

Medipharma Homburg GmbH *Michelinstr. 10, 66424 Homburg, Germany.*
Tel: +49 (0) 6841 709246 Fax: +49 (0) 6841 709265

Medipharma Ltd, Hong Kong *Unit 2409, Tsuen Wan Industrial Ctr, 220-248 Texaco Rd, Tsuen Wan, Hong Kong.*
Tel: +852 24089171 Fax: +852 24076092

Medispec (M) Sdn Bhd *No 55 & 57 Lorong Sempadan 2, Off Boundary Rd, 11400 Ayer Itam, Malaysia.*
Tel: +60 (0) 4 827 3450 Fax: +60 (0) 4 827 3453
Web: www.medispec.com.my

Meditec/Sam-On Ltd *P.O. Box 1224, Bat-Yam 59602, Israel.*
Tel: +972 (0) 3 5511925 Fax: +972 (0) 3 5526453
Web: www.meditec.co.il

Medi-Test *Imm Azur, 4 rue Rene-Razel, 91400 Saclay, France.*
Tel: +33 (0) 1 69411000 Fax: +33 (0) 1 69412241
Web: www.medi-test.fr

Mediwhite Srl *Via del Forte Bravetta 98, 00100 Rome, Italy.*

Medopharm Arzneimittel GmbH & Co. KG *Grunwalderstr. 22, 79098 Freiburg, Germany.*
Tel: +49 (0) 7633 909500 Fax: +49 (0) 7633 909505
Email: info@medopharm.de Web: www.medopharm.de

5

medphano Arzneimittel GmbH *Maienbergstr. 10, 15562 Rudersdorf, Germany.*
Tel: +49 (0) 33638 7490 Fax: +49 (0) 33638 74977
Email: info@medphano.de Web: www.medphano.de

MedPointe Healthcare Inc *265 Davidson Ave , Suite 300 , Somerset , NJ 08873-4120 , USA.*
Tel: +1 732 564 2200 Web: www.medpointeinc.com

Medtech Lab *120 Harry Walker Parkway N, New Market, L3Y 7B2, Canada.*

Megafyt-R sro *, Vrané nad Vltavou, Czech Republic.*

Melisana AG *Ankerstrasse 53, Postfach, 8026 Zurich, Switzerland.*
Tel: +41 (0) 44 2454350 Fax: +41 (0) 44 2454355

Melisana SA *Ave du Four à Briques 1, 1140 Brussels, Belgium.*
Tel: +32 (0) 2 7261565 Fax: +32 (0) 2 7262970
Email: webmaster@melisana.be Web: www.melisana.be

Memsep sro *Strakonická 1134/13, 150 00 Prague 5, Czech Republic.*
Tel: +420 (0) 2 57321621

Menarini *Alfonso XII 587, Badalona, 08918 Barcelona, Spain.*
Tel: +34 93 4628800 Fax: +34 93 4628820
Email: info@menarini.es Web: www.menarini.es

Mentholatum Inc. *707 Sterling Dr., Orchard Park, NY 14127, USA.*
Tel: +1 716 677 2500 Web: www.mentholatum.com

Mentholatum South Africa (Pty) Ltd *80 Bonza Bay Rd, Beacon Bay 5241, South Africa.*
Web: www.mentholatum.com

Mepha Pharma AG *Postfach 445, 4147 Aesch/BL, Switzerland.*
Tel: +41 (0) 61 7054343 Fax: +41 (0) 61 7054385
Email: contact@mepha.ch Web: www.mepha.ch

Merck & Co. *1 Merck Dr, White House Station, NJ 08889-1000, USA.*
Tel: +1 908 423 1000 Web: www.merck.com

Merck dura GmbH *Postfach: 100635, 64206 Darmstadt, Germany.*
Tel: +49 (0) 6151 723400 Fax: +49 (0) 6151 723409
Email: merck-dura@merck.de Web: www.merck-dura.de

Merck GmbH *Zimbagasse 5, A-1147 Vienna, Austria.*
Tel: +43 (0) 1 57600 Fax: +43 (0) 1 5773370
Email: merck-wien@merck.at Web: www.merck.at

Merck KGaA *Frankfurter Str. 250, 64271 Darmstadt, Germany.*
Tel: +49 (0) 6151 720 Fax: +49 (0) 6151 723250
Email: medizinpartner@merck.de Web: www.medizinpartner.de

Merck Lipha Santé *37 rue St-Romain, 69008 Lyon, France.*
Tel: +33 (0) 4 72782525 Fax: +33 (0) 4 78753905
Web: www.mercksante.fr

Merck Química Argentina S.A.I.C. *Panamericana Plaza Tronador 4890 Piso 5, 1430 Buenos Aires, Argentina.*
Tel: +54 (0) 11 45468100 Fax: +54 (0) 11 45468199
Web: www.merck.com.ar

Merck Química Chilena Ltda *Francisco de Paula Taforo 1981, Nunoa, Santiago, Chile.*

Merck S.A. *Hans Neumann Ed.Corimon p3, Los Cortijos de Lou., Caracas, Venezuela.*
Tel: +58 (0) 212 2351379 Fax: +58 (0) 212 2377632
Web: www.merck.com

Merck S.A. Industrias Químicas *Estrada dos Bandeirantes 1099, 22710-571 Rio de Janeiro, Brazil.*
Tel: +55 (0) 21 24442000 Fax: +55 (0) 21 24452263
Email: farma@merck.com.br Web: www.merck.com.br

Merckle GmbH *Graf-Arco-Str. 3, 89079 Ulm, Germany.*
Tel: +49 (0) 731 4027426 Fax: +49 (0) 731 4024141
Email: service@merckle.de Web: www.merckle.de

Merz Pharma (Schweiz) AG *Postfach, 4123 Allschwil, Switzerland.*
Tel: +41 (0) 61 4863600 Fax: +41 (0) 61 4863636
Email: info@merz.ch Web: www.merz.ch

Merz Pharmaceuticals GmbH *Eckenheimer Landstr. 100, 60318 Frankfurt (Main), Germany.*
Tel: +49 (0) 69 15031 Fax: +49 (0) 69 5962150
Email: arzneimittelservice@merz.de Web: www.merz.de

Metochem-Pharma GmbH *Jochen-Rindt-Strasse 23, A-1230 Vienna, Austria.*
Tel: +43 (0) 1 61684250 Fax: +43 (0) 1 616842510

Meyer Productos Terapéuticos S.A. *Urb. Ind. Boleíta Norte Calle E, Edif. Meyer, Aptdo. 70008, Caracas 1071-A, Venezuela.*
Tel: +58 (0) 212 2382633 Fax: +58 (0) 212 2341918
Email: general@meyer.com.ve Web: www.meyer.com.ve

Microsules y Bernabo S.A. *Terrada 2346, 1416 Buenos Aires, Argentina.*
Tel: +54 (0) 11 45013278 Fax: +54 (0) 11 45016426
Web: www.microsulesybernabo.com.ar

Midax Italia S.r.l. *Via Piave 5, 35010 San Pietro in Gu (PD), Italy.*
Tel: +39 049 9455636 Fax: +39 049 9459434

Midro Lörrach GmbH *Barenfelser Str. 7, 79539 Lörrach, Germany.*
Tel: +49 (0) 7621 46415 Fax: +49 (0) 7621 87664
Email: mail@midro.de Web: www.midro.de

Midro Vertrieb AG *Uferstrasse 90, 4019 Basle, Switzerland.*
Tel: +41 (0) 61 3027036 Fax: +41 (0) 61 3020750
Web: www.midro.com

Milte Italia S.p.A. *Via Tadino 29/A, 20124 Milan, Italy.*
Tel: +39 02 29517803 Fax: +39 02 29517938
Web: www.milte.it

Monserrat y Eclair S.A. *Virrey Cevallos 1625/7, 1135 Buenos Aires, Argentina.*
Tel: +54 (0) 11 43044524

Montavit GmbH *Salzbergstrasse 96, A-6060 Absam, Austria.*
Tel: +43 (0) 5223 57926 Fax: +43 (0) 5223 5792611
Web: www.montavit.com

Montefarmaco S.p.A. *Via G. Galilei 7, 20016 Pero (MI), Italy.*
Tel: +39 02 39171 Fax: +39 02 33911205
Email: info@montefarmaco.com Web: www.montefarmaco.com

MPL, Marching Pharmaceutical Ltd *Units 2,4,8-12, 9/F Block B Vigor Ind Bldg, 14-20 Cheung Tat Rd, Tsing Yi, Hong Kong.*
Tel: +852 24326993 Fax: +852 24323522
Email: info@marching.com.hk Web: www.marching.com.hk

MPM Medical Inc. *2301 Crown Ct, Irving, TX 75038, USA.*
Web: www.mommedicalinc.com

Mr J W Wenig GmbH *Van der Nullgasse 22, A-1100 Vienna, Austria.*
Tel: +43 (0) 1 604149018

Multilab Ind. e Com. Prods. Farmacêuticos Ltda *RS 401 Km 30 No. 1009, 96700-000 São Jeronimo, Brazil.*
Tel: +55 (0) 51 32304006 Fax: +55 (0) 51 32304007
Web: www.multilab.com.br

mundipharma AS *Postboks 218, 1326 Lysaker, Norway.*
Tel: +47 67518900 Fax: +47 67518901
Web: www.mundipharma.com

Mundipharma GmbH *Apollogasse 16-18, A-1072 Vienna, Austria.*
Tel: +43 (0) 1 52325050 Fax: +43 (0) 1 523250544
Web: www.mundipharma.co.uk

Mundipharma GmbH *Turisticka 36, 621 00 Brno, Czech Republic.*
Tel: +420 (0) 5 775062 Email: mundipharma@iol.cz

Mundipharma GmbH *Mundipharma Str. 2, 65549 Limburg (Lahn), Germany.*
Tel: +49 (0) 6431 7010 Fax: +49 (0) 6431 74272
Email: mundipharma@mundipharma.de Web: www.mundipharma.de

Mundipharma Medical Co *St Alban-Rheinweg 74, 4020 Basle, Switzerland.*
Tel: +41 (0) 61 2051111 Fax: +41 (0) 61 2051187
Email: info@mundipharma.ch Web: www.mundipharma.ch

Mundipharma Oy *Rajatorpantie 41 B, 01640 Vantaa, Finland.*
Tel: +358 (0) 9 85202065 Fax: +358 (0) 9 85202062
Web: www.mundipharma.com

N

NAM Neukönigsförder Arzneimittel GmbH *Moorbeker Strasse 35, 26197 Grossenkneten, Germany.*
Tel: +49 (0) 4435 5067 Fax: +49 (0) 4435 6166
Email: info@nam.de Web: www.nam.de

Natrol *21411 Prairie Street, , Chatsworth, CA 91311, USA.*
Tel: +1 818 739 6000 Email: customer-service@natrol.com
Web: www.natrol.com

Natural Life S.A. *Tucuman 3516, 1189 Buenos Aires, Argentina.*
Tel: +54 (0) 11 41279300 Fax: +54 (0) 11 41279317

Nature Made *PO Box 9606, , Mission Hills, CA 91346-9606, USA.*
Tel: +1 800 276 2878 Web: www.naturemade.com

Nature's Bounty *90 Orville Drive, , Bohemia, NY 11716, USA.*
Tel: +1 800 433 2990 Email: info@naturesbounty.com
Web: www.naturesbounty.com

Nature's Resources *, , USA.*
Nature Made

Naturland *Csillagvirág u 8, 1106 Budapest, Hungary.*
Tel: +36 4312040

Naturland Czech Republic sro *Kartouzská 4/200, 15 000 Prague 5, Czech Republic.*

Naturopathica *P.O. Box 7096, Sydney, NSW 2001, Australia.*
Fax: +61 (0) 2 92790464 Web: www.naturopathica.com.au

Naturpharma SA *5d route des Jeunes, Case postale 8, 1211 Geneva 26, Switzerland.*
Tel: +41 (0) 22 3004740 Fax: +41 (0) 22 3001396

Naturprodukt Kft *DEPO Pf: 8, 2046 Törökbálint, Hungary.*
Tel: +36 23 336331 Fax: +36 23 336333

Naturwaren OHG *, Czech Republic.*

Naytsal *C/ Molino 2, Meco, 28880 Madrid, Spain.*
Tel: +34 91 8876055 Fax: +34 91 8876054
Email: natysal@pasanet.es Web: www.natysal.com

Neckerman Indústria Farmacêutica Ltda *Rua das Perobeiras 157, 05879-470 São Paulo, Brazil.*
Tel: +55 (0) 11 58732890 Fax: +55 (0) 11 58734788

Neo Dermos S.R.L. *Francisco Bilbao 1927, 1406 Buenos Aires, Argentina.*
Tel: +54 (0) 11 46320717 Fax: +54 (0) 11 46335670

Neo-Farmacêutica, Lda *Avenida D João II, 1990-090 Lisbon, Portugal.*
Tel: +351 21 7812300 Fax: +351 21 7812390
Email: neofarmaceutica@mail.telepac.pt Web: www.neo-farmaceutica.pt

Neopharm Ltd *8 Hashiloach St, P.O. Box 7063, Petach Tikva 49170, Israel.*
Tel: +972 (0) 3 9373737 Fax: +972 (0) 3 9373770
Email: hana.c@neopharmisrael.com Web: www.neopharmisrael.com

Neopharma GmbH & Co. KG *Kirchstr. 10, 83229 Aschau i. Chiemgau, Germany.*
Tel: +49 (0) 8052 306 Fax: +49 (0) 8052 5429
Email: neopharma@t-online.de

Neovita S.a.s. di G. Pirotta & C. *Via Solferino 4, 21040 Uboldo (VA), Italy.*
Tel: +39 02 96780394 Fax: +39 02 96780394
Email: neogiul@tin.it

Neutrogena Corp. *5760 W 96th St, Los Angeles, CA 90045-5595, USA.*
Tel: +1 310 647 1150 Web: www.neutrogena.com

Nippon Shinyaku Co. Ltd *14 Nishinosho-Monguchi-cho, Kisshoin, Minami-ku, Kyoto 601-8550, Japan.*
Tel: +81 (0) 75 3211111 Fax: +81 (0) 75 3210678

Nizhpharm OAO *7 Salganskaya ul., GSP-459, 603950 Nizhny Novgorod, Russia.*
Tel: +7 8312 788000 Fax: +7 8312 307213
Email: med@nizhpharm.ru Web: www.nizhpharm.com

Nobel Pharm Enrg *2615 pl. Chasse, Montreal, H1Y 2C3, Canada.*
Tel: +1 514 5223187

Norgine AG *Neue Bahnhofstrasse 160, 4132 Muttenz, Switzerland.*
Tel: +41 (0) 61 4610868 Fax: +41 (0) 61 4610875
Email: norgine.switzerland@norgine.com Web: www.norgine.com

Norgine BV *Hogehilweg 7, 1101 CA Amsterdam Zuid-Oost, Netherlands.*
Tel: +31 (0) 20 5670900 Fax: +31 (0) 20 5670999
Email: norgine.netherlands@norgine.com Web: www.norgine.com

Norgine de España *Maudes, 51 8 Pl., 28003 Madrid, Spain.*
Tel: +34 91 3956350 Fax: +34 91 3956396
Email: norgine.spain@norgine.com Web: www.norgine.com

Norgine GmbH *Im Schwarzenborn 4, 35041 Marburg, Germany.*
Tel: +49 (0) 6421 98520 Fax: +49 (0) 6421 985230
Email: info@norgine.de Web: www.norgine.de

Norgine Italia S.r.l. *Via Prina 15, 20154 Milan (MI), Italy.*
Tel: +39 02 33614476 Fax: +39 02 315625
Email: norgine.italy@norgine.com Web: www.norgine.com

Norgine Pharma GmbH *Haidestrasse 4, A-1110 Vienna, Austria.*
Tel: +43 (0) 1 8178120 Fax: +43 (0) 1 7436370
Email: norgine.pharma.austria@norgine.com
Web: www.norgine.com

Norgine Pharmaceuticals Ltd *Chaplin House, Moorhall Rd, Harefield, Uxbridge, UB9 6NS, UK.*
Tel: +44 (0) 1895 826600 Fax: +44 (0) 1895 825865
Email: norgine.uk@norgine.com Web: www.norgine.com

Norgine P/L *3/14 Rodborough Road, Frenchs Forest, NSW 2086, Australia.*
Tel: +61 (0) 2 99727500 Web: www.norgine.com

Norgine (Pty) Ltd *P.O. Box 781247, Gauteng, Sandton 2146, South Africa.*
Tel: +27 (0) 11 8835630 Fax: +27 (0) 11 7831712
Email: norgine.south.africa@norgine.com
Web: www.norgine.com

Norgine SA *Haasrode Research Park, Romeinsestraat 10, 3001 Heverlee, Belgium.*
Tel: +32 (0) 16 392710 Fax: +32 (0) 16 392720
Email: norgine_info@norgine.com Web: www.norgine.com

Normon S.A. *Ronda de Valdecarrizo 6, Tres Cantos, 28760 Madrid, Spain.*
Tel: +34 91 8065240 Fax: +34 91 8065256
Web: www.normon.com

Novag Infancia S.A. de C.V. *Claz. de Tlalpan No. 3417, Col. Sta. Ursula Coapa-Coyoacan, 04650 Mexico D.F., Mexico.*
Tel: +52 55 56664120 Fax: +52 55 56067076

Novaquimica Sigma Pharma-Nature's Plus Ltda *Rodovia SP101 (Campinas a Monte Mor) Km 08, 13186-481 Hortolandia, Brazil.*
Tel: +55 (0) 19 8871209 Fax: +55 (0) 19 8872242

Novartis Argentina S.A. *Ramallo 1851, 1429 Buenos Aires, Argentina.*
Tel: +54 (0) 11 47037000 Fax: +54 (0) 11 47037251
Web: www.ar.novartis.com

Novartis Consumer Health *Wimblehurst Rd, Horsham, RH12 4AB, UK.*
Tel: +44 (0) 1403 210211 Fax: +44 (0) 1403 323939
Web: www.novartis.co.uk

Novartis Consumer Health Canada Inc. *2233 Argentia Rd, Suite 205, Mississauga, L5N 2X7, Canada.*
Tel: +1 905 8124100 Fax: +1 905 8214058
Web: www.ca.novartis.com

Novartis Consumer Health GmbH *Zielstattstr. 40, 81379 Munich, Germany.*
Tel: +49 (0) 89 78770 Fax: +49 (0) 89 7877444
Email: munich_de@ch.novartis.com Web: www.novartis-consumerhealth.de

Novartis Consumer Health Inc. *200 Kimball Drive, Parsippany, NJ 07054-0622, USA.*
Tel: +1 973 503 8000 Fax: +1 973 503 8400
Web: www.novartis.com

Novartis Consumer Health, Lda *Av Poeta Mistral 2-2, 1069-172 Lisbon, Portugal.*
Tel: +351 21 7811010 Fax: +351 21 7811011
Web: www.consumer-health.novartis.com

Novartis Consumer Health Schweiz AG *Monbijoustrasse 118, 3001 Berne, Switzerland.*
Tel: +41 (0) 31 3776111 Fax: +41 (0) 31 3776100
Web: www.novartis-consumer-health.ch

Novartis Farma S.p.A. *Largo Umberto Boccioni 1, 21040 Origgio (VA), Italy.*
Tel: +39 02 96541 Fax: +39 02 96542910
Web: www.novartis.it

Novartis Farmaceutica *Gran Via Corts Catalanes 764, 08013 Barcelona, Spain.*
Tel: +34 93 3064200 Fax: +34 93 3064290
Web: www.es.novartis.com

Novartis Finland Oy *Metsänneidonkuja 10, 02130 Espoo, Finland.*
Tel: +358 (0) 9 61332211 Fax: +358 (0) 9 61332200
Web: www.novartis.fi

Novartis (Hellas) A.E.B.E. *12o chlm. Ethnikis Odou Athinon-Lamias, 144 51 Metamorfosi, Greece.*
Tel: +30 210 2811712 Fax: +30 210 2812014
Web: www.novartis.gr

Novartis Ltd *Hasivim 23, Petach Tikva, Israel.*
Tel: +972 (0) 3 9201111 Fax: +972 (0) 3 9229230
Web: www.novartis.com

Novartis New Zealand Ltd *Private Bag 19-999, Avondale, Auckland, New Zealand.*
Tel: +64 (0) 9 8283149 Fax: +64 (0) 9 8286565
Web: www.novartis.com

Novartis Pharma Schweiz AG *Monbijoustrasse 118, Postfach, 3001 Berne, Switzerland.*
Tel: +41 (0) 31 3775111 Fax: +41 (0) 31 3775211
Web: www.novartis.ch

Novartis Pharmaceuticals Corp. *One Health Plaza, East Hanover, NJ 07936-1080, USA.*
Tel: +1 862 778 8300 Fax: +1 973 781 8265
Web: www.pharma.us.novartis.com

Novartis Santé Familiale SA *14 bd Richelieu, B.P. 440, 92845 Rueil-Malmaison cdx, France.*
Tel: +33 (0) 1 55478000

Novartis South Africa (Pty) Ltd *P.O. Box 92, ZA-Kempton Park, Isando 1600, South Africa.*
Tel: +27 (0) 11 9299111 Fax: +27 (0) 11 9292544
Web: www.novartis.com

5

Novartis Sverige AB *Box 1150, 183 11 Täby, Sweden.*
Tel: +46 (0) 8 7323200 Fax: +46 (0) 8 7323201
Email: info.se@pharma.novartis.com Web: www.novartis.se

Novipharm GmbH *Klagenfurter Strasse 164, A-9210 Portschach, Austria.*
Tel: +43 (0) 4272 2751 Fax: +43 (0) 4272 3119

Novogaleno S.r.l. *Largo Sermoneta 24, 80123 Naples, Italy.*
Tel: +39 081 7613117 Fax: +39 081 7613117
Email: novogaleno@hotmail.com

Novogen Laboratories P/L *140 Wicks Rd, North Ryde, NSW 2113, Australia.*
Tel: +61 (0) 2 98780088 Fax: +61 (0) 2 98780055
Web: www.novogen.com

Novopharm Ltd *30 Novopharm Court, Toronto, M1B 2K9, Canada.*
Tel: +1 416 2918888 Fax: +1 416 2911874
Web: www.novopharm.com

Nucleopharm SRL *Av. Remedios 5341/49, 1440 Buenos Aires, Argentina.*

Numark Laboratories Inc. *164 North Field Ave, Edison, NJ 08818, USA.*
Tel: +1 732 417 1870 Web: www.numarklabs.com

Nutravite *1470 Leathead Rd, Unit 2, Kelowna, V1X 7J6, Canada.*
Tel: +1 250 7120600 Fax: +1 250 7120617
Web: www.nutravite.com

Nutridiver SL *C/del Pont Reixat 5, 08960 Sant Just Desvern, Barcelona, Spain.*

Nycomed Austria GmbH *St Peter-Strasse 25, A-4020 Linz, Austria.*
Tel: +43 (0) 732 69190 Fax: +43 (0) 732 655568

Nycomed BV *Nikkelstraat 5, 4823 AE Breda, Netherlands.*
Tel: +31 (0) 76 5481600 Fax: +31 (0) 76 5412197
Web: www.nycomed.nl

Nycomed Christiaens *Chris Juliam, Gentsesteenweg 615, 1080 Brussels, Belgium.*
Tel: +32 (0) 2 4640611 Fax: +32 (0) 2 4640699
Web: www.nycomed.be

Nycomed Pharma AS *Hagalokkv. 13, Postboks 205, 1372 Asker, Norway.*
Tel: +47 67763030 Fax: +47 67763040
Web: www.nycomed.no

OBA Pharma ApS *Kronprinsessegade 26 A (postboks 117), 1004 Copenhagen K, Denmark.*
Tel: +45 33326647 Fax: +45 33126647

Officina Farmaceutica Fiorentina S.r.l. Istituto Biochimico *Quart. Varignano 12-14, 55049 Viareggio (Lucca), Italy.*
Tel: +39 0584 392353 Fax: +39 0584 388374
Email: info@off-biolabs.it

Olic (Thailand) Ltd *280 New Rd, Bangkok 10100, Thailand.*
Tel: +66 (0) 2220 9000 Fax: +66 (0) 2220 9009
Email: info@olic-thailand.com Web: www.olic-thailand.com

Omegin Dr Schmidgall GmbH & Co. KG *Industriepark 210, 78244 Gottmadingen, Germany.*
Tel: +49 (0) 7731 98250 Web: www.omegin.de

Omeofarma S.r.l. *Via di Morena 12/a, 00043 Ciampino (Rome), Italy.*
Tel: +39 06 7903101 Fax: +39 06 79031208
Email: omeofarmaciampino@tiscalinet.it

Orient Europharm Pte Ltd *1 Sophia Rd, 04-12 Peace Centre, S 228149, Singapore.*
Tel: +65 6339 8820 Fax: +65 6339 5272
Email: orienteuro@pacific.net.sg

Orion-yhtymä Oyj *Kalkkipellontie 2, 02601 Espoo, Finland.*
Tel: +358 (0) 10 4291 Fax: +358 (0) 10 4293939
Email: etunimi.sukunimi@orionpharma.com
Web: www.orionpharma.com

Ortoquimica Ind. Químico Farmacêutica Ltda *Av. Magalhães de Castro 800, 05502-001 São Paulo, Brazil.*
Tel: +55 (0) 11 38135052

OTC Concepts *, UK.*

OTW-Naturarzneimittel Regneri GmbH & Co KG *Carl-Zeiss-Str. 4, 76275 Ettlingen, Germany.*
Tel: +49 (0) 7243 5100 Fax: +49 (0) 7243 510100

Oui Heng Import Co. Ltd *46, 46/2 Soi Charansanitwongs 40, Charansanwitwongs Rd, Bangkok 10700, Thailand.*
Tel: +66 2 433 0061 Fax: +66 2 883 1842

Oy Leiras Finland AB *PL 1406, 00101 Helsinki, Finland.*
Tel: +358 (0) 20 7465000 Fax: +358 (0) 20 7465090
Email: etunimi.sukunimi@leirasfinland.fi Web: www.leiras.fi

Pacific Healthcare (Thailand) Co. Ltd *229/1 South Sathorn Rd, Bangkok 10120, Thailand.*
Tel: +66 2 211 5142 Fax: +66 2 212 5323
Email: phc@phc.co.th Web: www.phc.co.th

Pacific Pharmaceuticals Co. Ltd *P.O. Box 11-183, Ellerslie, Auckland, New Zealand.*
Tel: +64 (0) 9 5792792 Fax: +64 (0) 9 5797072

Padma AG *Wiesenstrasse 5, 8603 Schwerzenbach, Switzerland.*
Tel: +41 (0) 43 3434444 Fax: +41 (0) 43 3434443
Email: mail@padma.ch Web: www.padma.com

Pan Química Farmaceutica *Rufino Gonzalez 50, 28037 Madrid, Spain.*
Tel: +34 91 3756230 Fax: +34 91 3047881

Panacea Biotec Ltd *B-1 Extn. A-27,, Mohan Co-op. Industrial Estate, Mathura Rd, New Delhi 110 044, India.*
Tel: +91 (0) 11 26945270 Fax: +91 (0) 11 26974600
Web: www.panacea-biotec.com

Paradise Promotions Ltd *13 George St, Novar, P0A 1R0, Canada.*

Parsenn-Produkte AG, Abt. Pharmazeutik *Klus, 7240 Kublis, Switzerland.*
Tel: +41 (0) 81 3003333 Fax: +41 (0) 81 3003339

Pascoe Pharmazeutische Präparate GmbH *Schiffenberger Weg 55, 35394 Giessen, Germany.*
Tel: +49 (0) 641 79600 Fax: +49 (0) 641 7960119
Email: webmaster@pascoe.de Web: www.pascoe.de

Peking Royal Jelly Deutschland BOELL HandelsKontor *Am Kirchberg 3, 86666 Burgheim, Germany.*
Tel: +49 (0) 8432 94010 Fax: +49 (0) 8432 940126
Email: info@boell-peking.de Web: www.boell-peking.de

Pentamedical S.r.l. *Via G. Mazzini 1, 20021 Bollate (MI), Italy.*
Tel: +39 02 38302445 Fax: +39 02 38302790

Permamed AG *Ringstrasse 29, Postfach 360, 4106 Therwil, Switzerland.*
Tel: +41 (0) 61 7252020 Fax: +41 (0) 61 7252040
Email: permamed@permamed.ch Web: www.permamed.ch

Perrigo *Wrafton Laboratories Ltd., Wrafton, Braunton, EX33 2DL, UK.*
Tel: +44 (0) 1271 815815 Fax: +44 (0) 1271 818997
Web: www.wrafton.com

Perrigo Ltd *29 Lehi Street, Bnei Brak 51200, Israel.*
Tel: +972 (0) 3 5773700 Fax: +972 (0) 3 5773500
Web: www.perrigo.com

Personal Care Group Inc. *225 Summit Ave, Montvale, NJ 07645-1574, USA.*
Tel: +1 201 573 5633

Peter Black Healthcare Ltd *William Nadin Way, Swadlincote, DE11 0BB, UK.*
Tel: +44 (0) 1283 228300 Fax: +44 (0) 1283 228328
Email: info.pbh@peterblack.co.uk Web: www.peterblack.co.uk

Peter Italia sas *Via Tommaso Silvestri 22, 00135 Rome, Italy.*
Tel: +39 06 3380459 Fax: +39 06 30601489
Email: peteritalia@linet.it Web: www.medicinaestetica.it

Pfeiffer Company *65-71 University Ave, P.O. Box 4447, Atlanta, GA 30302, USA.*
Tel: +1 404 614 0255 Web: www.pfeifferpharmaceuticals.com

Pfizer ApS Danmark *Lautrupvang 8, 2750 Ballerup, Denmark.*
Tel: +45 44201100 Fax: +45 44201101
Web: www.pfizer.dk

Pfizer AS *Postboks 3, 1324 Lysaker, Norway.*
Tel: +47 67526100 Fax: +47 67526196
Web: www.pfizer.no

Pfizer BV *Roer 266, 2908 AA Capelle a/d Ijssel, Netherlands.*
Tel: +31 (0) 10 4064200 Fax: +31 (0) 10 4064299
Web: www.pfizer.com

Pfizer Consumer Healthcare, Division of Pfizer Canada Inc. *2200 Eglinton Ave E, Toronto, M1L 2N3, Canada.*
Tel: +1 416 2882200 Fax: +1 416 2882588
Web: www.pfizer.ca

Pfizer GmbH *Pfizerstr. 1, 76139 Karlsruhe, Germany.*
Tel: +49 (0) 721 61019000 Fax: +49 (0) 721 62039000
Email: info@pfizer.de Web: www.pfizer.de

Pfizer Inc. *235 East 42nd St, New York, NY 10017-5755, USA.*
Tel: +1 212 733 2323 Web: www.pfizer.com

Pfizer Italiana S.r.l. *Via Valbondione 113, 00188 Rome, Italy.*
Tel: +39 06 331821 Fax: +39 06 33626019
Web: www.pfizer.it

Pfizer Laboratories (Pty) Ltd *P.O. Box 2271, Cape Town 8000, South Africa.*
Tel: +27 (0) 21 4063224 Fax: +27 (0) 21 4063459
Web: www.pfizer.co.za

Pfizer Ltd *Walton Oaks, Dorking Rd, Tadworth, KT20 7NS, UK.*
Tel: +44 (0) 1304 616161 Fax: +44 (0) 1304 656221
Web: www.pfizer.co.uk

Pfizer Oy *PL 36, 00331 Helsinki, Finland.*
Tel: +358 (0) 9 430040 Fax: +358 (0) 9 43004400
Web: www.pfizer.fi

Pfizer P/L *P.O. Box 57, West Ryde, NSW 2114, Australia.*
Tel: +61 (0) 2 98503333 Fax: +61 (0) 2 98581347
Web: www.pfizer.com.au

Pfizer Pte Ltd *152 Beach Rd, 29-00 Gateway East, S 189721, Singapore.*
Tel: +65 6311 3688 Fax: +65 6311 3698
Web: www.pfizer-singapore.com

Pfizer SA *Boulevard de la Plaine 17, 1050 Brussels, Belgium.*
Tel: +32 (0) 2 5546211 Fax: +32 (0) 2 5546660
Web: www.pfizer.com

Pfizer SA *Scharenmoosstrasse 99, 8052 Zurich, Switzerland.*
Tel: +41 (0) 43 4957111 Fax: +41 (0) 43 4957280
Web: www.pfizer.ch

Pfizer (Thailand) Ltd *36-38 Fl, 42 Fl, United Center Building, 323 Silom Rd, Kwang Silom, Khet Bangrak, Bangkok 10500, Thailand.*
Tel: +66 (0) 2665 4666 Fax: +66 (0) 2635 5471
Web: www.pfizer.co.th

PGM Pharmazeutische Gesellschaft mbH & Co. München *Fürstenstr 6, 80333 Munich, Germany.*
Tel: +49 (0) 89 284633 Fax: +49 (0) 89 2809703
Email: info@pgm-muenchen.de Web: www.pgm-muenchen.de

Pharbenia S.r.l., Societa del Gruppo Bayer *V'le Certosa 130, 20156 Milan, Italy.*
Tel: +39 02 39781 Fax: +39 02 39782109

Pharma Développement *40 rue des Bergers, 75015 Paris, France.*
Tel: +33 (0) 1 45752200

Pharma Fabre Hellas S.A. *85 Lavriou Ave , , 190 02 Paiania , Greenland.*
Tel: +30 210 6683000 Fax: +30 210 6683250

Pharma Funcke *, Czech Republic.*

Pharma Guri *P.O. Box 15164, Rishon Le Zion 75105, Israel.*
Tel: +972 (0) 8 9205888 Fax: +972 (0) 8 9205999
Email: pharma_g@inter.net.il Web: www.pharmaguri.co.il

Pharma Italia Laboratori Farmaceutici S.r.l. *Via Vittor Pisani 93, 70033 Corato (BA), Italy.*
Tel: +39 080 3593060 Fax: +39 080 3580238
Email: info@pharmaitalia.com Web: www.pharmaitalia.com

Pharma Liebermann GmbH *Hauptstr. 27, 89423 Gundelfingen/Do., Germany.*
Tel: +49 (0) 9073 958930 Fax: +49 (0) 9073 9589355
Email: info@pharma-liebermann.de Web: www.pharma-liebermann.de

Pharma Schwörer GmbH *Goethestr. 29, 69257 Wiesenbach, Germany.*
Tel: +49 (0) 6223 4347 Fax: +49 (0) 6223 47438
Email: info@pharma-schwoerer.de Web: www.pharma-schwoerer.de

Pharma Selz GmbH *Leininger Ring 65a, 67278 Bockenheim, Germany.*
Tel: +49 (0) 6359 943610 Fax: +49 (0) 6359 943636
Web: www.pharmaselz.de

Pharma Stulln GmbH *Werksstr. 3, 92551 Stulln, Germany.*
Tel: +49 (0) 9435 30080 Fax: +49 (0) 9435 300899
Email: info@pharmastulln.de Web: www.pharmastulln.de

Pharma Wernigerode GmbH *Dornbergsweg 35, 38855 Wernigerode/Harz, Germany.*
Tel: +49 (0) 3943 5540 Fax: +49 (0) 3943 554183
Email: info@pharmawernigerode.de Web: www.pharmawernigerode.de

Pharmaceutical Enterprises (Pty) Ltd *Howards Drive, Pinelands, Howard Place 7405, South Africa.*
Tel: +27 (0) 21 5311341 Fax: +27 (0) 21 5312692

Pharmachemie BV *Swensweg 5, 2031 GA Haarlem, Netherlands.*
Tel: +31 (0) 23 5147147 Fax: +31 (0) 23 5312879
Web: www.pharmachemie.com

Pharmachoice (Pty) Ltd *P.O. Box 291, Fourways 2055, South Africa.*
Tel: +27 (0) 11 4653647 Fax: +27 (0) 11 4653696
Email: info@pharmachoice.co.za Web: www.pharmachoice.co.za

Pharmacia Asia Ltd *16/F Stanhope House, 738 Kings Rd, North Point, Hong Kong.*
Tel: +852 28119711 Fax: +852 25790599
Web: www.pharmacia.com

Pharmacia GmbH *Am Wolfsmantel 46, 91058 Erlangen, Germany.*
Tel: +49 (0) 9131 620 Fax: +49 (0) 9131 621202
Web: www.pharmacia.de

Pharmacia Italia S.p.A. *Via Robert Koch 1.2, 20152 Milan, Italy.*
Tel: +39 02 48381 Fax: +39 02 48382734
Web: www.pharmaciaitalia.it

Pharmacia Singapore Pte Ltd *101 Thomson Rd, 31-04/05 United Square, S 307591, Singapore.*
Tel: +65 6354 9828 Fax: +65 6354 9501
Web: www.pharmacia.com

Pharmacie du Collège, Dr Cl & A Behringer *rue du Lac 42, 1400 Yverdons-les-Bains, Switzerland.*
Tel: +41 (0) 24 4252107 Fax: +41 (0) 24 4258910

Pharmadass Ltd *HealthAid House, Marlborough Hill, Harrow, HA1 1UD, UK.*
Tel: +44 (0) 20 8426 3400 Fax: +44 (0) 20 8426 3434
Email: sales@pharmadass.com Web: www.pharmadass.com

Pharmalab, Division de Stonglass SA *Av. Santa Fe 3312, Piso 7 C, 1425 Buenos Aires, Argentina.*

Pharmamagist Kft *Patakhegyi út 83-85, 1028 Budapest, Hungary.*
Tel: +36 3975174 Fax: +36 3975175

Pharma-Natura (Pty) Ltd *P.O. Box 494, Bergvlei 2012, South Africa.*
Tel: +27 (0) 11 4456000 Fax: +27 (0) 11 4456089
Email: healthcare@pharma.co.za Web: www.pharma.co.za

Pharmanex Inc. *74 West Center, Provo, UT 84601, USA.*
Tel: +1 801 345 9800 Fax: +1 801 345 2850
Email: productsupport@pharmanex.com Web: www.pharmanex.com

Pharmaniaga Marketing Sdn Bhd *P.O. Box 2030, Pusat Business Bukit Raja, 40800 Shah Alam, Malaysia.*
Tel: +60 (0) 3 33429999 Fax: +60 (0) 3 33417777
Web: www.pharmaniaga.com.my

Pharmascience Inc. *6111 Royalmount Ave, Suite 100, Montreal, H4T 2T4, Canada.*
Tel: +1 514 3401114 Fax: +1 514 3427764
Web: www.pharmascience.com

Pharmasette di Paolo Donati e C. S.a.s. *Via Lusitania 15/A, 00183 Rome, Italy.*
Tel: +39 06 58232820 Fax: +39 06 58232820

Pharmashalom Ltd *21 Hamelaha St, Park Afek, Rosh Ha'ayin, Israel.*
Tel: +972 (0) 3 9031424 Fax: +972 (0) 3 9031358

Pharmastra, Usines Chimiques et Pharmaceutiques de Strasbourg *40 rue du Canal, 67460 Souffelweyersheim, France.*
Tel: +33 (0) 3 88200212 Fax: +33 (0) 3 88339347
Email: info@pharmastra.com Web: www.pharmastra.com

Pharmateam Marketing *P.O. Box 405, Jerusalem, Israel.*
Tel: +972 (0) 2 5712140 Fax: +972 (0) 2 5712235
Email: ptm@pharmateam-mktg.co.il Web: www.pharmateam.co.il

Pharmaton SA *, 6934 Bioggio, Switzerland.*
Tel: +41 (0) 91 6103111 Fax: +41 (0) 91 6103211

Pharmatrix, Div. de Therabel Pharma S.A. *Arenales 259, 1704 Ramos Mejia, Buenos Aires, Argentina.*
Tel: +54 (0) 11 46561816 Fax: +54 (0) 11 46583557
Web: www.pharmatrix.com.ar

Pharmazeutische Fabrik Evers & Co. GmbH *Siemensstr. 4, 25421 Pinneberg, Germany.*
Tel: +49 (0) 4101 73800 Fax: +49 (0) 4101 73889
Email: evco@pharmaevers.de Web: www.pharmaevers.de

Pharmazeutische Fabrik Infirmarius-Rovit GmbH *Eislinger Str. 66, 73084 Salach, Germany.*
Tel: +49 (0) 7162 930800 Fax: +49 (0) 7162 9308091
Email: info@infirmarius-rovit.de Web: www.infirmarius-rovit.de

Pharmethica BV *Ronde Tocht 11, 1507 CC Zaandam, Netherlands.*

Pharmia Oy *Kalliotie 2, 04360 Tuusula, Finland.*
Tel: +358 (0) 9 8254030 Fax: +358 (0) 9 8709715
Email: info@pharmia.fi Web: www.pharmia.fi

Pharmonta Mag. pharm. Dr Fischer *Montanastrasse 7, A-8112 Gratwein, Austria.*
Tel: +43 (0) 3124 51368 Fax: +43 (0) 3124 5136821
Email: pharmonta@sime.at Web: www.pharmonta.com

5

Phytomed AG *Tschamerie 25, 3415 Hasle/Burgdorf, Switzerland.*
Tel: +41 (0) 34 4602211 Fax: +41 (0) 34 4614163
Email: info@phytomed.ch

Phytomedicine P/L *P.O. Box 1995, Dee Why, NSW 2099, Australia.*
Tel: +61 (0) 2 99391380 Fax: +61 (0) 2 99391333
Email: cust.serv@phytomedicine.com.au Web: www.phytomedicine.com.au

Phytopharma SA *Chemin des Golettes 4a, 1666 Grandvillard, Switzerland.*
Tel: +41 (0) 26 9281549 Fax: +41 (0) 26 9282149
Email: phytopharma@bluewin.ch Web: www.phytopharma.ch

Phytotec Hungária Kft *Lotz Károly u 3, 1026 Budapest, Hungary.*
Tel: +36 3920385 Fax: +36 3980192

Pierre Fabre Argentina S.A. *Marcelo T de Alvear 684, piso 7, 1058 Buenos Aires, Argentina.*
Tel: +54 (0) 11 43189600 Fax: +54 (0) 11 43189626
Web: www.pierre-fabre.com.ar

Pierre Fabre Farma de Mexico S.A. de C.V. *Blvd Manuel Avila Camacho 191, Piso 4 In, Polanco Los Morales, 11510 Mexico D.F., Mexico.*
Tel: +52 55 21223700 Web: www.pierre-fabre.com

Pierre Fabre Iberica *Ramon Trias Fargas 7-11, Edifico Marina Village, 08005 Barcelona, Spain.*
Tel: +34 93 4833000 Fax: +34 93 4833059
Email: info@pierre-fabre.es Web: www.pierre-fabre.es

Pierre Fabre Italia S.p.A. *Via G.G. Winckelmann 1, 20146 Milan, Italy.*
Tel: +39 02 477941 Fax: +39 02 425589
Web: www.pierre-fabre.com

Pierre Fabre Medicament *Usacheva ul. 33, 119048 Moscow, Russia.*
Tel: +7 095 7452650 Fax: +7 095 7452654
Web: www.pierre-fabre.com

Pierre Fabre Médicament Portugal, Lda *Rua Rodrigo da Fonseca 178 - 2 Esq, 1099-067 Lisbon, Portugal.*
Tel: +351 21 3815320 Fax: +351 21 3860370
Web: www.pierre-fabre.com

Pierre Fabre Medicament sro *Radimová 36, 160 00 Prague 6, Czech Republic.*
Tel: +420 (0) 2 20516778 Fax: +420 (0) 2 20517415
Email: all@pfm.cz

Pietrasanta Pharma S.r.l. *Loc. S. Rocchino, 55054 Massarosa (LU), Italy.*
Tel: +39 0584 49855 Fax: +39 0584 45190
Email: pietrasantapharma@interbusiness.it
Web: www.pietrasantapharma.it

Plantina Biologische Arzneimittel AG *Jochbergweg 1, 82418 Murnau, Germany.*
Tel: +49 (0) 8841 48880 Fax: +49 (0) 8841 488820
Email: info@plantina.de Web: www.plantina.de

Plants, Laboratorio della Dott.ssa Luisa Coletta *Viaria C, Zona Industriale, 98040 Giammoro (ME), Italy.*
Tel: +39 090 9387033 Fax: +39 090 9387237

Polymedic Trading Enterprise Pte Ltd *150 Kampong Ampat, 06-07 KA Centre, S 368324, Singapore.*
Tel: +65 6283 6826 Fax: +65 6382 4948
Email: polymed@starhub.net.sg

Polypharm GmbH *Bad Nauheimer Str. 4, 64289 Darmstadt, Germany.*
Tel: +49 (0) 6151 601980 Fax: +49 (0) 6151 6019820
Email: email@polypharm.de

Ponce & Benzo Sucesores C.A. *Edificio Ponce & Benzo, 2da. Avenida, Urb. Santa Eduvigis, Caracas, Venezuela.*
Tel: +58 (0) 212 2863822 Fax: +58 (0) 212 2833389
Email: info@ponce-benzo.com Web: www.ponce-benzo.com

Potter's Herbal Medicines *1 Botanic Court, Martland Park, Wigan, WN5 0JZ, UK.*
Tel: +44 (0) 1942 219 960 Fax: +44 (0) 1942 219 966
Email: info@pottersherbals.co.uk Web: www.pottersherbals.co.uk

Potter's (Herbal Supplies) Ltd *Unit 5b, Chipchase Court, Seaham Grange Industrial Estate, Seaham, SR7 0PP, UK.*
Tel: +44 (0) 191 5236578 Fax: +44 (0) 191 5236059
Email: info@herbal-direct.com Web: www.herbal-direct.com

Presselin-Arzneimittel GmbH & Co. KG *Heinkelstr. 8a, 76461 Muggensturm, Germany.*
Tel: +49 (0) 7222 96930 Fax: +49 (0) 7222 969325
Email: webmaster@presselin.de Web: www.presselin.de

Primal Chemical Co. Ltd *Flat A, 7/F, Hoi Bun Industrial Bldg, 6 Wing Yip St, Kwun Tong, Kowloon, Hong Kong.*
Tel: +852 23433212 Fax: +852 27978595

Prisfar, SA *Rua Antero de Quentel 629, 4200-068 Porto, Portugal.*
Tel: +351 22 5573600 Fax: +351 22 5504207
Web: www.prisfar.pt

Procter & Gamble *1 or 2, Procter & Gamble Plaza, Cincinnati, OH 45201, USA.*
Tel: +1 513 983 1100 Web: www.pg.com

Procter & Gamble AG *47 rue de Saint-Georges, 1213 Petit-Lancy 1, Switzerland.*
Tel: +41 (0) 22 7096111 Fax: +41 (0) 22 7096855
Web: www.pg.com

Procter & Gamble Australia P/L *Locked Bag 75, Parramatta, NSW 2124, Australia.*
Tel: +61 (0) 2 96854400 Fax: +61 (0) 2 96854777
Web: www.pg.com

Procter & Gamble Austria GmbH *Guglgasse 7-9, A-1030 Vienna, Austria.*
Tel: +43 (0) 1 58857400 Fax: +43 (0) 1 588575400
Web: www.pg.com

Procter & Gamble de Mexico S.A. de C.V. *Loma Florida 32, Lomas de Vistahermosa, Del. Cuajimalpa, 05100 Mexico D.F., Mexico.*
Tel: +52 55 57242000 Fax: +52 55 57242331
Web: www.pg.com.mx

Procter & Gamble do Brasil S.A. *Av. Maria Coelho Aguiar 251, Bloco E- Andares 4./5, Jd São Luiz, 05805-000 Paulo, Brazil.*
Tel: +55 (0) 11 37480264 Fax: +55 (0) 11 37480244
Web: www.procter.com.br

Procter & Gamble (Health & Beauty Care) Ltd *The Heights, Brooklands, Weybridge, KT13 0XP, UK.*
Tel: +44 (0) 1923 896000 Fax: +44 (0) 1923 896200
Email: ukmisc.im@pg.com Web: www.uk.pg.com

Procter & Gamble Inc. *P.O. Box 355, Station A, Toronto, M5W 1C5, Canada.*
Tel: +1 416 7304711 Fax: +1 416 7306049
Web: www.pg.com

Procter & Gamble Interamericanos Inc. *Suipacha 664 Piso 2, 1008 Buenos Aires, Argentina.*
Tel: +54 (0) 11 43230600 Fax: +54 (0) 11 43230781
Web: www.pg.com

Procter & Gamble NPD, Inc. *7th Floor, Acer Building, 10-12 Scotia Place, Auckland, New Zealand.*
Tel: +64 (0) 9 3561800 Fax: +64 (0) 9 3561818
Web: www.pg.com

Procter & Gamble Pharmaceuticals *Watermanweg 100, 3067 GG Rotterdam, Netherlands.*
Tel: +31 (0) 10 2863100 Fax: +31 (0) 10 2863131
Web: www.pg.com

Procter & Gamble Pharmaceuticals UK Ltd *Rusham Park Technical Centre, Whitehall Lane, Egham, TW20 9NW, UK.*
Tel: +44 (0) 1784 474900 Fax: +44 (0) 1784 495253
Email: ukmisc.im@pg.com Web: www.uk.pg.com

Procter & Gamble Srl *Viale C Pavese 385, 00100 Rome, Italy.*
Tel: +39 06 50971 Fax: +39 06 5011881
Web: www.pg.com

Procter Gamble *Av. del Partenon 16-18, Campo de las Naciones, 28042 Madrid, Spain.*
Tel: +34 91 7222100 Fax: +34 91 7222411
Web: www.pg.com

Prodotti Laboratório Farmacêutico Ltda *Avenida João Dias 1084, Santo Amaro, 04724-001 São Paulo, Brazil.*
Tel: +55 (0) 11 55419344 Fax: +55 (0) 11 55228718

Productos Farmaceuticos Collins S.A. de C.V. *Cipres No. 1677, Col. del Fresno, 44900 Guadalajara, Jalisco, Mexico.*
Tel: +52 33 38115171 Fax: +52 33 38115i71
Web: www.collins.com.mx

Productos Gache S.A. *Calle La Industria, Ed. Lemar P.B., Urb. Palo Verde, Caracas, Venezuela.*
Tel: +58 (0) 212 2510964 Fax: +58 (0) 212 2512662

Productos Maver S.A. de C.V. *Av. Oleoducto No. 2804, Fracc. Industrial El Alamo, 44490 Tlaquepaque, Jalisco, Mexico.*
Tel: +52 33 36661873 Fax: +52 33 36662773

Productos Medix S.A. de C.V. *Calz. del Hueso No. 39, Col. Ejido Santa Ursula Coapa, Deleg. Coyoacan, 04910 Mexico D.F., Mexico.*
Tel: +52 55 55992800 Fax: +52 55 56795652

Productos Naturissima de Venezuela *Calle del Arenal Edif. Biotech, Urb. La Trinidad, Caracas, Venezuela.*
Tel: +58 (0) 212 9035400 Fax: +58 (0) 212 9035690

Productos Roche Ltda *Av. Quilin 3750, Macul, Santiago, Chile.*

Productos Roche S.A. *Edificio Roche, Av. Diego Cisneros/Los Ruices, Caracas 1062, Venezuela.*
Tel: +58 (0) 212 2734611 Fax: +58 (0) 212 2398191
Web: www.roche.com.ve

Productos Ronava C.A. *Final calle Mara, Edif.Ronava Zona Ind. El Marqué, Caracas, Venezuela.*
Tel: +58 (0) 212 2396413 Fax: +58 (0) 212 2397186
Email: ventas@ronava.com.ve Web: www.ronava.com.ve

Produtos Farmacêuticos Millet Roux Ltda *Praia de Botafogo 440, 25 andar, 22250-040 Rio de Janeiro, Brazil.*
Tel: +55 (0) 21 25390608 Fax: +55 (0) 21 22861076
Email: milletroux@milletroux.com.br Web: www.milletroux.com.br

ProMedico Ltd *4 Baltimor St, Petach Tikva 49510, Israel.*
Tel: +972 (0) 3 9265965 Fax: +972 (0) 3 9248548
Web: www.promedico.co.il

Protina Pharmazeutische Gesellschaft mbH *Adalperostr. 90, 85737 Ismaning, Germany.*
Tel: +49 (0) 89 9965530 Fax: +49 (0) 89 963446
Email: info@protina.de Web: www.protina.de

Provita Pharma GmbH *Seidengasse 33-35, A-1070 Vienna, Austria.*
Tel: +43 (0) 1 4709631 Fax: +43 (0) 1 4796463

Psorimed AG *Postfach, 5401 Baden, Switzerland.*

Puerto Galiano *Calle 'S', 4, Parque Europolis, Las Rozas, 28230 Madrid, Spain.*
Tel: +34 91 7105047 Fax: +34 91 6371989
Email: okal@puertogaliano.com Web: www.puertogaliano.com

Purdue Pharma *575 Granite Court, Pickering, L1W 3W8, Canada.*
Tel: +1 905 4206400 Fax: +1 905 4200385

Pynogin GmbH, Gee Lawson Distribution Centre *Unit 15 South Nottingham & Wilford Industrial Estate, Wilford, Nottingham, NG11 7EP, UK.*

Qualicare AG *Florenz-Strasse 7, 4142 Münchenstein, Switzerland.*
Tel: +41 (0) 61 3330085 Fax: +41 (0) 61 3330086
Email: mail@qualicare.ch Web: www.qualicare.ch

Qualiphar SA *Rijksweg 9, 2880 Bornem, Belgium.*
Tel: +32 (0) 3 8891721 Fax: +32 (0) 3 8896913
Web: www.qualiphar.be

Queisser Pharma GmbH.& Co. *Lyusinovskaya ul. 36, Of. 73, 113093 Moscow, Russia.*
Tel: +7 095 3635051 Fax: +7 095 3635057
Email: office@queisser.ru Web: www.queisser.ru

Queisser Pharma GmbH & Co. *Schleswiger Str. 74, 24941 Flensburg, Germany.*
Tel: +49 (0) 461 99960 Fax: +49 (0) 461 9996110
Email: lorenzen@queisser.de Web: www.queisser.de

Quest Vitamins Ltd *8 Venture Way, Aston Science Park, Birmingham, B7 4AP, UK.*
Tel: +44 (0) 121 359 0056 Fax: +44 (0) 121 359 0313
Email: info@questvitamins.co.uk Web: www.questvitamins.co.uk

Química Ariston S.A.C.I.F. *O'Connor 550/5, 1707 V. Sarmiento, Buenos Aires, Argentina.*
Tel: +54 (0) 11 46583051 Fax: +54 (0) 11 46587290

Química E Farmacêutica Nikkho do Brasil Ltda *Rua Jaime Perdigao 431-435, 21920-240 Ilha do Governador, Brazil.*
Tel: +55 (0) 21 3934266 Fax: +55 (0) 21 3931343

Química Franco Mexicana Nordin S.A. de C.V. *Paseo Lomas Atlas No. 292, Col. Lomas del Valle, 45120 Zapopan, Jal., Mexico.*
Tel: +52 33 36423030 Fax: +52 33 36428833
Web: www.nordin.com.mx

Química Knoll de Mexico S.A. de C.V. *La Candelaria No.186, Col. Atlantida, Deleg. Coyoacan, 04370 Mexico D.F., Mexico.*
Tel: +52 55 55493740 Fax: +52 55 56898256

Química Medical Arg. S.A.C.I. *Int. Amaro Avalos 4208, 1605 Munro, Buenos Aires, Argentina.*
Tel: +54 (0) 11 47627600 Fax: +54 (0) 11 47627664

Química y Farmacia, S.A. de C.V. *Av. Insurgentes sur 619 Desp 602, Benito Juarez Napoles, 3810 Mexico D.F., Mexico.*
Tel: +52 55 53402230

Quimifar *Comadran 37, Pol Ind Can Salvatella, Barbera del Valles, 08210 Barcelona, Spain.*
Tel: +34 93 7297900 Fax: +34 93 7297901
Email: info@quimifar.es Web: www.quimifar.es

Quimioterapica Brasileira Ltda *Rua São Januario 712, Tubalina, 38400-410 Uberlandia, Brazil.*
Tel: +55 (0) 34 32383111

Ranbaxy (Malaysia) Sdn Bhd *Box #8, Wisma Selangor Dredging, 5th Floor, South Block, 142-A Jalan Ampang, 50450 Kuala Lumpur, Malaysia.*
Tel: +60 (0) 3 21614181 Fax: +60 (0) 3 21627589
Web: www.ranbaxy.com

Ranbaxy Unichem Co. Ltd *3 Fl, Rm 314-8, Phayathai Building, 31 Phayathai Rd, Rajathevi, Bangkok 10400, Thailand.*
Tel: +66 2 246 3300 Fax: +66 2 246 4727
Email: saleserv@ranbaxy.co.th Web: www.ranbaxy.com

5

Ratiopharm Arzneimittel Vertriebs-GmbH *Albert-Schweitzer-Gasse 3, A-1140 Vienna, Austria.*
Tel: +43 (0) 1 97007 Fax: +43 (0) 1 9700766
Web: www.ratiopharm.at

Ratiopharm CZ sro *Bělehradská 54, 120 00 Prague 2, Czech Republic.*
Tel: +420 (0) 2 51021122 Fax: +420 (0) 2 51021123
Email: ratiopharm@ratiopharm.cz

ratiopharm GmbH *Graf-Arco-Str. 3, 89079 Ulm/Donautal, Germany.*
Tel: +49 (0) 731 40202 Fax: +49 (0) 731 4027329
Email: info@ratiopharm.de Web: www.ratiopharm.de

Ratiopharm Group *Vspolny per. 19/20, str. 2, 123001 Moscow, Russia.*
Tel: +7 095 2321247 Fax: +7 095 2321369
Email: moscow@ranbaxy.ru Web: www.ranbaxy.com

ratiopharm Hungária Kft *Uzsoki u 36/a, 1145 Budapest, Hungary.*
Tel: +36 2732730 Fax: +36 2732731

Recip AB *Bränningevägen 12, 120 54 Årsta, Sweden.*
Tel: +46 (0) 8 6025200 Fax: +46 (0) 8 818703
Email: info@recip.se Web: www.recip.se

Reckitt Benckiser *Pharmapark, Chapelizod, Dublin 20, Ireland.*
Tel: +353 (0) 1 630 5420 Fax: +353 (0) 1 630 5430
Web: www.reckittbenckiser.com

Reckitt Benckiser Hong Kong Ltd *1203-5 Allied Kajima Bldg, 138 Gloucester Rd, Hong Kong.*
Tel: +852 25980328 Fax: +852 25980808
Web: www.reckitt.com

Reckitt Benckiser (Overseas) Ltd *Unit No 1101, Level 11, Uptown 2, 2 Jln SS 21-37, Damansara Uptown, 47400 Petaling Jaya, Malaysia.*
Tel: +60 (0) 3 77253042 Fax: +60 (0) 3 77253008
Web: www.reckittbenckiser.com

Reckitt Benckiser Pharmaceuticals *P.O. Box 138, West Ryde, NSW 2114, Australia.*
Tel: +61 (0) 2 93254000 Fax: +61 (0) 2 93254018
Web: www.reckittbenckiser.com

Reckitt Benckiser Pharmaceuticals (Pty) Ltd *P.O. Box 164, Isando 1600, South Africa.*
Tel: +27 (0) 11 8711611 Fax: +27 (0) 11 8711831
Web: www.reckittbenckiser.com

Reckitt Benckiser plc *Dansom House, Hull, HU8 7DS, UK.*
Tel: +44 (0) 1482 326151 Fax: +44 (0) 1482 582526
Email: miu@reckittbenckiser.com Web: www.reckittbenckiser.com

Reckitt Benckiser SA/NV *Allée de la Recherche 20, 1070 Brussels, Belgium.*
Tel: +32 (0) 2 5261811 Fax: +32 (0) 2 5200230
Email: reckitt@skynet.be Web: www.reckittbenckiser.com

Reckitt Benckiser (Thailand) Ltd *9 Fl, Vanissa Building, 29 Soi Chidlom, Ploenchit Rd, Patumwan, Bangkok 10330, Thailand.*
Tel: +66 2 252 3149 Fax: +66 2 252 3195
Web: www.reckittbenckiser.com

Recordati Industria Chimica e Farmaceutica S.p.a. *Via Civitali 1, 20148 Milan, Italy.*
Tel: +39 02 487871 Fax: +39 02 40073747

Regina Health Ltd *NLA Tower, 12-16 Addiscombe Rd, Croydon, CR0 0XT, UK.*
Tel: +44 (0) 20 8410 2550 Fax: +44 (0) 20 8686 0807
Email: regina@netcom.uk.co.uk Web: www.reginahealthcare.com

Regional Health Ltd *P.O. Box 101-104, North Shore Mail Centre, Auckland, New Zealand.*
Tel: +64 (0) 9 9686688 Fax: +64 (0) 9 9686689
Email: info@regional.co.nz Web: www.regional.co.nz

Reig Jofre *Gran Capitan 10, Sant Joan Despi, 08970 Barcelona, Spain.*
Tel: +34 93 4806715 Fax: +34 93 4806721
Web: www.reigjofre.com

5

Rekah Ltd *P.O. Bos 25, Azor 58190, Israel.*
Tel: +972 (0) 3 5581233 Fax: +972 (0) 3 5565919
Email: info@rekah.co.il Web: www.rekah.co.il

Repha GmbH Biologische Arzneimittel *Alt-Godshorn 87, 30855 Langenhagen, Germany.*
Tel: +49 (0) 511 786100 Fax: +49 (0) 511 7861099
Email: info@repha.de Web: www.repha.de

Representaciones Mex-America S.A. de C.V., *Diagonal 20 de Noviembre No. 264, Col. Obrera, Deleg. Cuauhtemoc, 06800 Mexico D.F., Mexico.*
Tel: +52 55 55783570 Fax: +52 55 55783090
Web: www.remexa.com

Retterspitz GmbH *Laufer Str. 17-19, 90571 Schwaig, Germany.*
Tel: +49 (0) 911 507000 Fax: +49 (0) 911 5070045
Web: www.retterspitz.de

Ricerca, Produzione e Commercializzazione di Prodotti Farmaceutici e Cosmetici Srl *Via Grottole 80/B, 81020 Castel Morrone (CE), Italy.*
Tel: +39 (0) 823399187 Fax: +39 (0) 823399870

Richard Lane's *47 Mayflower Street, , Plymouth, PL1 1QL, UK.*
Tel: +44 (0) 1752 665 175 Fax: +44 (0) 1752 255 212
Email: herbals@richardlanes.co.uk Web: www.richardlanes.co.uk

Richter Pharma *Feldgasse 19, A-4600 Wels, Austria.*
Tel: +43 (0) 7242 4900 Fax: +43 (0) 7242 49015

Ricola *, Canada.*

Ridupharm *Emil Frey-Strasse 99, 4142 Münchenstein, Switzerland.*
Tel: +41 (0) 61 4114385 Fax: +41 (0) 61 4139757

Riemser Arzneimittel AG *An der Wiek 7, 17493 Greifswald/Insel Riems, Germany.*
Tel: +49 (0) 38351 760 Fax: +49 (0) 38351 308
Email: info@riemser.de Web: www.riemser.de

Riviera Handelsgesellschaft.m.b.h. *Penzingerstrasse 54, A-1140 Vienna, Austria.*
Tel: +43 (0) 1 8943366 Fax: +43 (0) 1 894336622

Robapharm España *Ramon Trias Fargas 7-11, Edificio Marina Village, 08005 Barcelona, Spain.*
Tel: +34 93 4833000 Fax: +34 93 4833059

Robapharm SA *Gewerbestrasse 18, 4123 Allschwil, Switzerland.*
Tel: +41 (0) 61 4878888 Fax: +41 (0) 61 4878899
Email: info@robapharm.ch Web: www.robapharm.ch

Robugen GmbH Pharmazeutische Fabrik *Alleenstr. 22-6, 73730 Esslingen, Germany.*
Tel: +49 (0) 711 366016 Fax: +49 (0) 711 367450
Email: robugen@robugen.de Web: www.robugen.de

Roche Consumer Health Deutschland GmbH *Valterweg 24-5, 65817 Eppstein-Bremthal, Germany.*
Tel: +49 (0) 6198 3000 Fax: +49 (0) 6198 30035
Email: rch.deutschland-gmbh@roche.com
Web: www.roche.de

Roche (Magyarország) Kft *Edison u 1, 2040 Budaörs, Hungary.*
Tel: +36 23 446800 Fax: +36 23 446860

Roche SA/NV *Rue Dante 75, 1070 Brussels, Belgium.*
Tel: +32 (0) 2 5258211 Fax: +32 (0) 2 5258201
Email: brussels.internet@roche.com Web: www.roche.be

Roche S.p.A. *Viale G.B. Stucchi 10, 20052 Monza (MI), Italy.*
Tel: +39 039 2471 Fax: +39 039 2474328
Web: www.roche.com

Rodisma-Med Pharma GmbH *Kölner Str. 48, 51149 Cologne, Germany.*
Tel: +49 (0) 2203 91200 Fax: +49 (0) 2203 9120300
Web: www.rodisma.de

roha Arzneimittel GmbH *Rockwinkeler Heerstr. 100, 28355 Bremen, Germany.*
Tel: +49 (0) 421 25790 Fax: +49 (0) 421 2579280
Web: www.roha-bremen.de

Rolmex International Inc. *1351 rue Gay-Lussac, Boucherville, J4B7K1, Canada.*

Rottapharm S.r.l. *Via Valosa di Sopra 9, 20052 Monza (MI), Italy.*
Tel: +39 039 73901 Fax: +39 039 7390446
Web: www.rotta.com

Rovi *Julian Camarillo 35, 28037 Madrid, Spain.*
Tel: +34 91 3756230 Fax: +34 91 3047881
Email: rovi@rovi.es Web: www.rovi.es

Roxane Laboratories Inc., a Subsidiary of Boehringer Ingelheim *P.O. Box 16532, Columbus, OH 43216, USA.*
Tel: +1 614 276 4000 Fax: +1 614 279 5517
Web: www.roxane.com

RubiePharm Vertriebs GmbH *Brüder-Grimm-Str. 121, 36396 Steinau an der Strasse, Germany.*
Tel: +49 (0) 6663 96040 Fax: +49 (0) 6663 960432
Email: hallo@rubiepharm.de Web: www.rubiepharm.de

Rye Pharmaceuticals *Unit 1, Block F, 25-7 Paul St North, North Ryde, NSW 2113, Australia.*
Tel: +61 (0) 2 98573830 Fax: +61 (0) 2 98573831
Email: rye@ryepharmaceuticals.com Web: www.ryepharmaceuticals.com

S

Sabex Inc. *145 Jules-Leger St, Boucherville, J4B 7K8, Canada.*
Tel: +1 514 5960000 Fax: +1 514 5960003

Sabona GmbH *Gutenbergstr. 1, 83052 Bruckmühl, Germany.*
Tel: +49 (0) 8062 904837 Fax: +49 (0) 8062 904827
Email: sabona@t-online.de Web: www.sabona.de

Sager Pharma Kft *Pálya u 9, 1012 Budapest, Hungary.*
Tel: +36 2146559 Fax: +36 2146561

Sagitta Arzneimittel GmbH *Frühlingstr. 7, Postfach: 1262, 83618 Feldkirchen-Westerham, Germany.*
Tel: +49 (0) 8063 97010 Fax: +49 (0) 8063 970111

Salomon, Levin, & Elstein Ltd *P.O. Box 8077, Kiryat Nordau, Netanya, Israel.*
Tel: +972 (0) 9 8927878 Fax: +972 (0) 9 8854766

Salus France *B.P. 104 Principal, 83403 Hyères cdx, France.*
Tel: +33 (0) 4 94126060 Fax: +33 (0) 4 94574724
Email: salus.france@wanadoo.fr

Salus-Haus Dr. med. Otto Greither Nachf. GmbH & Co KG *Bahnhofstr. 24, 83052 Bruckmühl/Mangfall (Obb.), Germany.*
Tel: +49 (0) 8062 9010 Fax: +49 (0) 8062 901352
Email: info@salus.de Web: www.salus.de

Salutas Pharma GmbH *Otto-von-Guericke-Allee 1, 39179 Barleben, Germany.*
Tel: +49 (0) 39203 710 Fax: +49 (0) 39203 71777

Sanamed GmbH *Rudolf Waisenhorngasse 32, A-1230 Vienna, Austria.*
Tel: +43 (0) 1 8886338 Fax: +43 (0) 1 8898395

Sandersons (Chemists) Ltd *37 Oakwood Rise, Heaton, Bolton, BL1 5EE, UK.*
Tel: +44 (0) 1204 841285

Sandoz Pharmaceuticals GmbH *Carl-Zeiss-Ring 3, 85737 Ismaning, Germany.*
Tel: +49 (0) 89 244040 Fax: +49 (0) 89 24404100
Email: info@sandoz.de Web: www.sandoz.de

Sanidom Handels-GmbH *Sundlweg 2, A-8045 Graz, Austria.*
Tel: +43 (0) 316 694944 Fax: +43 (0) 316 6949444

Sanitalia S.n.c. di Battaglia & C. *Strada dei Tadini 5, 10131 Turin, Italy.*
Tel: +39 011 6603246

Sankyo Pharma Italia S.p.A. *Via Reno 5, 00100 Rome, Italy.*
Tel: +39 06 852551 Fax: +39 06 85255235
Email: sankyo@sankyo-pharma.it Web: www.sankyo-pharma.com

Sanochemia Pharmazeutika AG *Boltzmanngasse 9a-11, A-1091 Vienna, Austria.*
Tel: +43 (0) 1 31914560 Fax: +43 (0) 1 319145644
Email: office@sanochemia.at Web: www.sanochemia.at

Sanofi Aventis *Coyancura 2283 Piso 13, Providencia, Santiago, Chile.*

Sanofi Synthelabo OTC *9 rue du President-Allende, 94258 Gentilly cdx, France.*
Tel: +33 (0) 8 25088352 Web: www.sanofi-synthelabo.com

Sanofi-Aventis *174 av de France, 75013 Paris, France.*
Tel: +33 1 53774000 Fax: +33 1 53779157
Web: www.sanofi-aventis.fr

Sanofi-Aventis *Ulansky Pereulok 4, 101000 Moscow, Russia.*
Tel: +7 095 9265703 Fax: +7 095 9265710
Web: www.sanofi-aventis.com

Sanofi-Aventis (Schweiz) AG *11 rue de Veyrot, 1217 Meyrin 1/GE, Switzerland.*
Tel: +41 (0) 22 9890147 Fax: +41 (0) 22 7839255
Web: www.sanofi-aventis.ch

Sanofi-Synthelabo de Mexico S.A. de C.V. *Km 37.5 Autopista Mexico-Qro, 54730 Cuautitlan Izcali, Mexico.*
Tel: +52 55 50623300 Fax: +52 55 50627514
Email: contacto@sanofi-synthelabo.com.mx
Web: www.sanofi-synthelabo.com.mx

Sanofi-Synthelabo GmbH *Potsdamer Str. 8, 10785 Berlin, Germany.*
Tel: +49 (0) 30 25752000 Fax: +49 (0) 30 25752001
Email: info.deutschland@de.sanofi-synthelabo.com
Web: www.sanofi-synthelabo.de

Sanofi-Synthelabo S.p.A. *Via GB Piranesi 38, 20137 Milan, Italy.*
Tel: +39 02 73941 Fax: +39 02 76110389
Web: www.sanofi-synthelabo.com

Sanol GmbH *Alfred-Nobel-Str. 10, 40789 Monheim, Germany.*
Tel: +49 (0) 2173 485857 Fax: +49 (0) 2173 485851
Web: www.sanol.de

Sanopharm AG *Via dei Ciossi 8, 6648 Minusio, Switzerland.*
Tel: +41 (0) 91 7446862 Fax: +41 (0) 91 7446863
Email: sanopharm@econophone.ch

Sanova Pharma GmbH *Postfach 3, A-1110 Vienna, Austria.*
Tel: +43 (0) 1 801040 Fax: +43 (0) 1 8042904

Santé Naturelle (AG) Ltée *369 Charles Péguy, La Prairie, J5R 3E8, Canada.*
Tel: +1 450 6597723 Fax: +1 450 6599791
Web: www.santenaturelle.ca

Santiveri *Encuny 8, 08038 Barcelona, Spain.*
Tel: +34 93 2986800 Fax: +34 93 2986819
Email: informacion@santiveri.es Web: www.santiveri.es

Sanum-Kehlbeck GmbH & Co. KG *Hasseler Steinweg 9-12, 27318 Hoya, Germany.*
Tel: +49 (0) 4251 93520 Fax: +49 (0) 4251 935290
Email: sanum-kehlbeck@t-online.de Web: www.sanum.com

Saros Laboratorios *FOC 68, 08038 Barcelona, Spain.*
Tel: +34 93 2988200 Fax: +34 93 2231652

Savoma Medicinali S.p.A. *Via Baganza 2/A, 43100 Parma, Italy.*
Tel: +39 0521 963890 Fax: +39 0521 968408
Email: savoma@tin.it

Schaper & Brümmer GmbH & Co. KG *Bahnhofstr. 35, 38259 Salzgitter (Ringelheim), Germany.*
Tel: +49 (0) 5341 3070 Fax: +49 (0) 5341 307124
Email: info@schaper-bruemmer.de Web: www.schaper-bruemmer.de

Schering Mexicana S.A. de C.V. *Calz. Mexico Xochimilco No. 5019, Tlalpan San Lorenzo Huipulco, 14370 Mexico D.F., Mexico.*
Tel: +52 55 56277000 Fax: +52 55 56717053
Email: info@scheringmexicana.com Web: www.schering.com.mx

Schering (NZ) Ltd *P.O. Box 101-691, North Shore Mail Centre, Auckland 10, New Zealand.*
Tel: +64 (0) 9 4152850 Fax: +64 (0) 9 4156497
Web: www.schering.com

Schering P/L *27-31 Doody Street, Alexandria, NSW 2015, Australia.*
Tel: +61 (0) 2 93178666 Fax: +61 (0) 2 93172138
Web: www.schering.com

Schering sro *Šafaříková 17, 120 00 Prague 2, Czech Republic.*
Tel: +420 (0) 2 71730661 Fax: +420 (0) 2 71730657
Email: schering@mbox.vol.cz

Schering-Plough Central East AG *Usacheva ul. 33, str.1, 119048 Moscow, Russia.*
Tel: +7 095 9167100 Fax: +7 095 9167094
Web: www.schering-plough.ru

Schering-Plough Corp. *Galloping Hill Rd, Kenilworth, NJ 07033-0530, USA.*
Tel: +1 908 298 4000 Web: www.schering-plough.com

Schering-Plough Healthcare Products Canada Inc. *6400 Northam Drive, Mississauga, L4V 1J1, Canada.*
Tel: +1 905 6736242 Fax: +1 905 6710686
Web: www.schering-plough.com

Schering-Plough Ltd *Schering-Plough House, Shire Park, Welwyn Garden City, AL7 1TW, UK.*
Tel: +44 (0) 1707 363636 Fax: +44 (0) 1707 363763
Email: medinfo@spcorp.com Web: www.schering-plough.com

Schering-Plough S.A. de C.V. *Av. 16 de Septiembre No. 301, Col. Xaltocan, Deleg. Xochimilco, 16090 Mexico D.F., Mexico.*
Tel: +52 55 57284444 Fax: +52 55 56530926
Web: www.schering-plough.com

Schöning Pharmazeutische Präparate GmbH & Co. KG *Porschestr. 22-24, 12107 Berlin, Germany.*
Tel: +49 (0) 30 7007760 Fax: +49 (0) 30 7417003
Email: schoeningberlin@aol.com Web: www.schoeningberlin.de

Schuck GmbH *Industriestr. 11, 90571 Schwaig b. Nürnberg, Germany.*
Tel: +49 (0) 911 500185 Fax: +49 (0) 911 508802
Email: info@schuck-arzneimittel.de Web: www.schuck-arzneimittel.de

Schülke & Mayr GmbH *Zieglergasse 8/3, A-1070 Vienna, Austria.*
Tel: +43 (0) 1 5232501 Fax: +43 (0) 1 523903579
Web: www.schuelke-mayr.com

Schumit 1967 Co. Ltd *13 Soi Latphrao 91, Latphrao Rd, Wangthonglaeng, Bangkok 10310, Thailand.*
Tel: +66 2 542 1791 Fax: +66 2 542 0325
Email: schumit@ksc.th.com

Schwabe Pharma AG *Erlistrasse 2, Postfach, 6403 Kussnacht a.R., Switzerland.*
Tel: +41 (0) 41 8541860 Fax: +41 (0) 41 8541861
Email: info@schwabepharma.ch Web: www.schwabepharma.com

Schwabe S.A.C.I. *Tte. Gral. Peron 1666, 1037 Buenos Aires, Argentina.*
Tel: +54 (0) 11 43727772 Fax: +54 (0) 11 43826267

Schwarzwälder Natur-Heilmittel *Marktplatz 4, 93183 Kallmunz, Germany.*
Tel: +49 (0) 9473 457 Fax: +49 (0) 9473 8769

Seber Portuguesa Farmacêutica, SA *Rua Norberto de Oliveira 1-5, 2620-111 Póvoa de St Adrião, Portugal.*
Tel: +351 21 9381500 Fax: +351 21 9374237
Email: medicamentos@seber-farmaceutica.pt

5

Sedar Indústria Farmacêutica Ltda *Rodovia BR 101 Sul Km 18, Distr. Ind. dos Prazeres, 50950-000 Recife, Brazil.*

Self-Care Products Ltd *30 Sycamore Rd, Amersham, HP6 5DR, UK.*
Tel: +44 (0) 1494 722741

Sella A. Lab. Chim. Farm. S.r.l. *Via Vicenza 67, 36015 Schio (Vicenza), Italy.*
Tel: +39 0445 670088 Fax: +39 0445 673537
Email: info@sellafarmaceutici.it Web: www.sellafarmaceutici.it

SERP *le Triton, 5 rue du Gabian, MC 98000, Monaco.*
Tel: +377 97778705 Fax: +377 92167827
Email: serp@monaco377.com

Sertürner Arzneimittel GmbH *Wallenroder Str. 8-10, 13435 Berlin, Germany.*
Tel: +49 (0) 30 4037070 Fax: +49 (0) 30 40370103
Email: info@sertuerner.de Web: www.sertuerner.de

Serumwerk Bernburg AG *Hallesche Landstr. 105 b, 06406 Bernburg, Germany.*
Tel: +49 (0) 3471 8600 Fax: +49 (0) 3471 860130
Email: swb-ag@t-online.de Web: www.serum-werk.de

Seven Seas Ltd *Hedon Rd, Marfleet, Hull, HU9 5NJ, UK.*
Tel: +44 (0) 1482 375234 Fax: +44 (0) 1482 374345
Email: info@seven-seas.ltd.uk Web: www.seven-seas.ltd.uk

Shaklee Canada Inc. *952 Century Dr, Burlington, L7L 5P2, Canada.*
Tel: +1 905 681 1422 Web: www.shaklee.ca

Shire Pharmaceuticals *725 Chesterbrook Blvd, Wayne, PA 19087-5637, USA.*
Tel: +1 484 595 8800 Fax: +1 484 595 8900
Email: medinfo@us.shire.com Web: www.shire.com

Sidefarma SA *Rua da Guine 26, 2689-514 Prior Velho, Portugal.*
Tel: +351 21 9426100 Fax: +351 21 9416205

Sidone Indústria e Comércio Ltda. *Rua São Francisco Xavier 930, 38412-080 Uberlandia, Brazil.*
Tel: +55 (0) 34 32175352

Sidroga AG *Postfach, 4800 Zofingen, Switzerland.*
Tel: +41 (0) 62 7461777 Fax: +41 (0) 62 7461707
Email: administration@sidroga.com Web: www.sidroga.com

Sigma Chemical Co. Ltd *1 Colonial Way, North Watford Industrial Estate, North Watford, WD2 4PJ, UK.*
Tel: +44 (0) 1923 444999 Fax: +44 (0) 1923 444998
Email: info@sigpharm.co.uk Web: www.sigpharm.co.uk

Sigma Pharmaceuticals P/L *96 Merrindale Drive, Croydon, VIC 3136, Australia.*
Tel: +61 (0) 3 98392800 Fax: +61 (0) 3 98392801
Web: www.sigmaco.com.au

Sigma Tau Espana *Poligono Azque, Apt. do 1144, Alcalá de Henares, 28815 Madrid, Spain.*
Tel: +34 91 8883600 Fax: +34 91 8883616
Email: sigmatau@nauta.es Web: www.sigma-tau.com

Sigma Tau S.p.A. *Via Pontina Km. 30,400, 00040 Pomezia (Rome), Italy.*
Tel: +39 06 91391 Fax: +39 06 91393980
Web: www.sigma-tau.it

Sigmapharm Arzneimittel GmbH & Co KG *Leystrasse 129, A-1204 Vienna, Austria.*
Tel: +43 (0) 1 3300671 Fax: +43 (0) 1 330067138
Email: sigmapharm@sigmapharm.at Web: www.sigmapharm.at

Sigma-Tau Arzneimittel GmbH *Shadowstr. 44, 40212 Dusseldorf, Germany.*
Tel: +49 (0) 211 3694993 Fax: +49 (0) 211 161527
Email: sigmatau@cww.de Web: www.sigma-tau.it

Sigma-Tau Ethifarma B.V. *Postbus 10072, 9400 CB Assen, Netherlands.*
Tel: +31 (0) 592 333000 Fax: +31 (0) 592 333009
Web: www.sigma-tau.it

5

Sime Darby Marketing, A Division of Sime Darby Singapore Ltd *896 Dunearn Rd, 04-03 Sime Darby Centre, S 589472, Singapore.*
Tel: +65 6469 8877 Fax: +65 6468 4928
Email: simemktg@singnet.com.sg

Skills in Farmacia S.r.l. *Piazza Buonarroti 32, 20145 Milan, Italy.*
Tel: +39 02 4675111 Fax: +39 02 46751160
Email: info@skillsfarmacia.it Web: www.skillsfarmacia.it

Slovakofarma sro *Machová 18, 120 00 Prague 2, Czech Republic.*
Tel: +420 (0) 2 96530102 Fax: +420 (0) 2 96530112
Email: info@slofa.sk

Sociedade Farmacêutica Gestafarma, Lda *Rua Dr. Álvaro de Castro 65-7, 1600-058 Lisbon, Portugal.*
Tel: +351 21 7961158

Società Industria Farmaceutica Italiana S.p.A. *Via Ercole Patti 36, 95025 Lavinao-Aci S. Antonio (CY), Italy.*
Tel: +39 095 7922111 Fax: +39 095 7893435

Solara Farmaceutica SA de CV *Av Paseo de las Palmas 330 PB, 11000 Lomas de Chapultepec, Mexico.*

Solvay Arzneimittel GmbH *Hans-Bockler-Allee 20, 30173 Hannover, Germany.*
Tel: +49 (0) 511 8572400 Fax: +49 (0) 511 8573120
Email: solvay.arzneimittel@solvay.com Web: www.solvay-arzneimittel.de

Solvay Farma Ltda *Rua Sergipe 120, 1243000 São Paulo, Brazil.*

Solvay Pharma *Avda Diagonal 507-509, 08029 Barcelona, Spain.*
Tel: +34 93 4954500 Fax: +34 93 4052492
Email: atencli.pharma@solvay.com Web: www.solvaypharma.es

Solvay Pharma & Cie S.N.C. *Blue Planet Building, Ave Bourgemestre E. Demunter 3, 1090 Brussels, Belgium.*
Tel: +32 (0) 2 4222711 Fax: +32 (0) 2 4222799
Email: pharma.be@solvay.com Web: www.solvaypharmaceuticals.com

Solvay Pharma AB *Sisjö Kullegata 8, 421 32 Västra Frölunda, Sweden.*
Tel: +46 (0) 31 689030 Fax: +46 (0) 31 689040
Email: info@solvay-pharma.se Web: www.solvaypharmaceuticals.com

Solvay Pharma AG *Untermattweg 8, 3027 Bern, Switzerland.*
Tel: +41 (0) 31 9969600 Fax: +41 (0) 31 9969699
Email: solvay-bern@solvay.com Web: www.solvaypharmaceuticals.com

Solvay Pharma BV *C J Van Houtenlaan 36, 1381 CP Weesp, Netherlands.*
Tel: +31 (0) 294 479000 Fax: +31 (0) 294 432189
Web: www.solvaypharmaceuticals.com

Solvay Pharma GmbH *Donaustrasse 106, A-3400 Klosterneuburg, Austria.*
Tel: +43 (0) 2243 25620 Fax: +43 (0) 2243 2562040
Web: www.solvaypharma.at

Solvay Pharma (Pty) Ltd *P.O. Box 5278, halfway House 1685, South Africa.*
Tel: +27 (0) 11 3139803 Fax: +27 (0) 11 3139804
Web: www.solvaypharmaceuticals.com

Solvay Pharma S.p.A. *Via della Liberta 30, 10095 Grugliasco (TO), Italy.*
Tel: +39 011 4027911 Fax: +39 011 783955
Web: www.solvaypharmaceuticals.com

Solvay Pharma sro *Bieblová 19, 150 00 Prague 5, Czech Republic.*
Tel: +420 (0) 2 51562156 Fax: +420 (0) 2 51561588
Email: solvay@solvay-pharma.cz

Solvayfarma, Lda *Av. Marechal Gomes da Costa 33, 1800-255 Lisbon, Portugal.*
Tel: +351 21 8315800 Fax: +351 21 8315860
Web: www.solvaypharmaceuticals.com

Sopharma AO *Taganskaya ul. 19, et. 10, 109147 Moscow, Russia.*
Tel: +7 095 7995511

Soria Natural *Pol Ind La Sacea 1, Garray, 42162 Soria, Spain.*
Tel: +34 975 252046 Fax: +34 975 252267
Email: soria@sorianatural.es Web: www.sorianatural.es

Spagyros AG *Tannackerstrasse 7, 3073 Gumlingen, Switzerland.*
Tel: +41 (0) 31 9595580 Fax: +41 (0) 31 9595581

Specialità Igienico Terapeutiche S.r.l. *C.so Cavour 70, 27035 Mede (Pavia), Italy.*
Tel: +39 0384 820416 Fax: +39 0384 822133
Email: sit@sit-farmaceutici.com

Spedrog Caillon S.A.I.y C. *Alte. Fco. J. Segui 2106, 1416 Buenos Aires, Argentina.*
Tel: +54 (0) 11 45820411 Fax: +54 (0) 11 45852929

Spineda, Pérez y Hnos. Y Cia SRL *Zado 3735, 1431 Villa Urquiza, Buenos Aires, Argentina.*
Tel: +54 (0) 11 45722902 Fax: +54 (0) 11 45730529

Spirig Pharma AG *Postfach 111, 4622 Egerkingen, Switzerland.*
Tel: +41 (0) 62 3878787 Fax: +41 (0) 62 3878799

Sriprasit Dispensary R O P *617 Charoen Rath Rd, Klongsarn, Bangkok 10600, Thailand.*
Tel: +66 2 437 0343 Fax: +66 2 438 8060
Email: sipasit@tcc.or.th

Stada GmbH *Stadastr. 2-18, 61118 Bad Vilbel, Germany.*
Tel: +49 (0) 6101 6030 Fax: +49 (0) 6101 603259
Email: info@stada.de Web: www.stada.de

Stada Pharma International os *Hnevkovská 58, 148 00 Prague 4, Czech Republic.*

Stanley Pharmaceuticals Ltd, Division of Vita Health Products Ltd *150 Beghin Ave, Winnipeg, R2J 3W2, Canada.*
Tel: +1 204 6618386 Fax: +1 204 6638386

Steierl Pharma GmbH *Muhlfelder Str. 48, 82211 Herrsching, Germany.*
Tel: +49 (0) 8152 93220 Fax: +49 (0) 8152 932244
Email: info@steierl.de Web: www.steierl.de

Steigerwald Arzneimittelwerk GmbH *Havelstr. 5, 64295 Darmstadt, Germany.*
Tel: +49 (0) 6151 33050 Fax: +49 (0) 6151 3305410
Web: www.steigerwald.de

Steiner & Co. Deutsche Arzneimittel Gesellschaft *Ostpreussendamm 72/74, 12207 Berlin, Germany.*
Tel: +49 (0) 30 710940 Fax: +49 (0) 30 7125012
Email: info@steinerarznei-berlin.de Web: www.steinerarznei-berlin.de

Stella Pharmaceutical Canada Inc. *407-220 Duncan Mill Rd, Don Mills, M3B 3J5, Canada.*
Tel: +1 416 4430636 Fax: +1 416 4438504
Web: www.nutribar.com

Strathmann AG & Co. *Sellhopsweg 1, 22459 Hamburg, Germany.*
Tel: +49 (0) 40 559050 Fax: +49 (0) 40 5509253
Email: info@strathmann.de Web: www.strathmann.de

Strathmann Ag & Co Képviselete *Ipoly u 5/f, 1133 Budapest, Hungary.*
Tel: +36 3202865 Fax: +36 3202867

Sundown *6111 Broken Sound Parkway NW, , Boca Raton, FL 33487, USA.*
Tel: +1 561 241 9400 Email: info@sundownnutrition.com
Web: www.sundownnutrition.com

Sunspot Products P/L *Level 3, Suite 303, 20 Bungan St, Mona Vale, NSW 2103, Australia.*
Tel: +61 (0) 2 99797333 Fax: +61 (0) 2 99978647
Email: enquires@sunspot.com.au Web: www.sunspot.com.au

Super Mayoreo Naturista S.A. de C.V. *Calle 3 No. 13 Local 4, Fracc. Industrial Alce Blanco, Naucalpan de Juarez, 53370 Mexico D.F., Mexico.*
Tel: +52 55 53594180 Fax: +52 55 53594181
Web: www.smn.com.mx

Swiss Bio Pharma Sdn Bhd *2nd Fl, Blk E, No 10, Jln Bersatu 13/4, 46200 Petaling Jaya, Malaysia.*
Tel: +60 (0) 3 79573873 Email: enquiries@vitahealth.com.my

Swiss Herbal Remedies Ltd *35 Leek Cres, Richmond Hill, L4B 4C2, Canada.*
Tel: +1 905 8869500 Fax: +1 905 8865434
Web: www.swissherbal.com

SwissHealth *, UK.*

Synco (HK) Ltd *Blk D, 3/F, Sun View Industrial Bldg, 3 On Yip St, Chaiwan, Hong Kong.*
Tel: +852 25560157 Fax: +852 28972582
Email: info@synco.com.hk Web: www.synco-pharma.com

Syxyl GmbH & Co. KG *Gereonsmühlengasse 5, 50670 Cologne, Germany.*
Tel: +49 (0) 221 1652630 Fax: +49 (0) 221 1652631

T

TAD Pharma GmbH *Heinz-Lohmann-Str. 5, 27472 Cuxhaven, Germany.*
Tel: +49 (0) 4721 6060 Fax: +49 (0) 4721 606333
Email: info@tad.de Web: www.tad.de

Tamar Marketing *, Rishon-Lezion 75652, Israel.*

Tanning Research Labs Inc. *P.O. Box 265111, Daytone Beach, FL 32126-5111, USA.*
Tel: +1 386 677 9559 Fax: +1 386 677 9595
Web: www.htropic.com

Tanta Pharmaceuticals Inc. *1009 Burns St East, Whitby, L1N 6A6, Canada.*
Tel: +1 905 4308440 Fax: +1 905 4308449

Taro Pharmaceutical International *14 Hakitor St, P.O. Box 10347, Haifa Bay 26110, Israel.*
Tel: +972 (0) 4 8475700 Web: www.taro.co.il

Techni-Pharma *7 rue de l'Industrie, B.P. 717, MC 98014, Monaco.*
Tel: +377 92057510 Fax: +377 92057710

Teclapharm GmbH *Heilgenthalar Str. 4, 21335 Luneburg, Germany.*
Tel: +49 (0) 4131 404100 Fax: +49 (0) 4131 43380
Web: www.teclapharm.de

Tecnifar, SA *Rua Tierno Galvan, Torre 3, 12 Piso, 1099-036 Lisbon, Portugal.*
Tel: +351 21 0330700 Fax: +351 21 0330709

Tecnonat S.A. *24 de Noviembre 368, 1170 Buenos Aires, Argentina.*
Tel: +54 (0) 11 49322600 Web: www.tecnonat.com

Tender Corporation *, Czech Republic.*

Tentan AG *Brunnliweg 16, 4433 Ramlinsburg, Switzerland.*
Tel: +41 (0) 61 9313874 Fax: +41 (0) 61 9313876
Email: info@tentan.ch Web: www.tentan.ch

Teofarma *Via F.lli Cervi 5, 27100 Valle Salimbene (PV), Italy.*
Tel: +39 0382 422008 Fax: +39 0382 525845
Web: www.teofarma.it

Terra-Bio-Chemie GmbH *Lindenbergstr. 5, 79199 Kirchzarten, Germany.*
Tel: +49 (0) 7661 90320 Fax: +49 (0) 7661 903279
Email: info@terra-bio.de Web: www.terra-bio.de

tetesept Pharma GmbH *Marschnerstr. 10, 60318 Frankfurt, Germany.*
Tel: +49 (0) 69 15031 Fax: +49 (0) 69 5962150
Email: merzpr@merz.de Web: www.merz.de

Tetra Pharm *1 Azrieli Center, Round Bldg, 24 floor, Tel Aviv 67021, Israel.*
Tel: +972 (0) 3 6911688 Fax: +972 (0) 3 6911686
Email: info@sebocalm.co.il Web: www.sebocalm.co.il

Teva Pharmaceuticals Ind. Ltd *P.O. Box 8077, Kiryat Nordau, Netanya, Israel.*
Tel: +972 (0) 9 8639777 Fax: +972 (0) 9 8653764
Web: www.tevapharm.com

The Boots Company (Far East) Pte Ltd *180-B Bencoolen St, 09-03 The Bencoolen, S 189648, Singapore.*
Tel: +65 6332 9230 Fax: +65 6837 0285

The Cantassium Company *Larkhill Farm, Putney, UK.*

The Purdue Frederick Co. *One Stamford Forum, 201 Tresser Blvd, Stamford, CT 06901-3431, USA.*
Tel: +1 203 588 8000 Fax: +1 203 588 8850
Web: www.pharma.com

Therabel Pharma SA *Rue Egide Van Ophem 108, 1180 Brussels, Belgium.*
Tel: +32 (0) 2 3704611 Fax: +32 (0) 2 3704690
Web: www.therabel.com

Therasophia *630 route des Dolines, 06560 Valbonne, France.*
Tel: +33 (0) 4 93755955 Fax: +33 (0) 4 93755716
Email: infos@therasophia.com Web: www.therasophia.com

Thornton & Ross Ltd *Linthwaite Laboratories, Huddersfield, HD7 5QH, UK.*
Tel: +44 (0) 1484 842217 Fax: +44 (0) 1484 847301
Email: mail@thorntonross.com Web: www.thorntonross.com

Thuna Herbal Remedies Ltd *298 Danforth Ave, Toronto, M4K 1N6, Canada.*
Tel: +1 416 4653511

Thursday Plantation laboratories Ltd *Pacific Highway, Gallen's Road, Ballina, NSW 2478, Australia.*
Tel: +61 (0) 2 66867273 Fax: +61 (0) 2 66867458
Web: www.thursdayplantation.com.au

Tilman SA/NV *Zoning Industriel 15, 5377 Baillonville, Belgium.*
Tel: +32 (0) 84 320360 Fax: +32 (0) 84 320375
Email: export@tilman.be Web: www.tilman.be

TNP Health Care Co. Ltd *94/7 Soi Yimprakrob, Ngamwongwan Rd, Nonthaburi 11000, Thailand.*
Tel: +66 (0) 2951 8008 Fax: +66 (0) 2589 2729
Email: thainakorn@thainakorn.com Web: www.thainakorn.com

Torrex Pharma GmbH *Lange Gasse 76/12, A-1080 Vienna, Austria.*
Tel: +43 (0) 1 4073919 Fax: +43 (0) 1 40739194

Tramedico BV *Postbus 192, 1380 AD Weesp, Netherlands.*
Tel: +31 (0) 294 461122 Fax: +31 (0) 294 461170
Web: www.tramedico.nl

Transatlantic International *Ulof Palme ul. 1, Section 5, 119590 Moscow, Russia.*
Tel: +7 095 7753938 Fax: +7 095 5141054
Email: office@transatlantic.ru Web: www.transatlantic.ru

Treasure Mountain Development Co. Ltd *19/F Chit Lee Commercial Bldg, 30-36 Shaukeiwan Rd, Hong Kong.*
Tel: +852 25677983 Fax: +852 25672600
Email: tmdcl@netvigator.com Web: www.tmdcl.com.hk

Trima *, Kibbutz Ma'abarot 40230, Israel.*
Tel: +972 (0) 9 8982862 Fax: +972 (0) 9 8982879
Email: info@trima.co.il Web: www.trima.co.il

Trinity Trading Co. Ltd *Unit 7A-B, 39/F Cable TV Tower, 9 Hoi Shing Rd, Tsuen Wan, Hong Kong.*
Tel: +852 23856044 Fax: +852 27701508

Truw Arzneimittel Vertriebs GmbH *Ziethenstr. 8, 33330 Gutersloh, Germany.*
Tel: +49 (0) 5241 300740 Fax: +49 (0) 5241 3007415
Email: info@truw.de Web: www.truw.de

Tubilux Pharma S.p.A. *Via Costarica 20/22, 00040 Pomezia (RM), Italy.*
Tel: +39 06 911831 Fax: +39 06 91183410
Email: tubilux@tubilux.it

Typharm Ltd *14D Wendover Rd, Rackheath Industrial Estate, Norwich, NR13 6LH, UK.*
Tel: +44 (0) 1603 735200 Fax: +44 (0) 1603 735217
Email: customerservices@typharm.com Web: www.typharm.com

U

UB Interpharm SA *36 av Cardinal-Mermillod, 1227 Carouge/GE, Switzerland.*
Tel: +41 (0) 22 3001734 Fax: +41 (0) 22 3003679

Ubepharm *Bodor u 8 I/6, 1138 Budapest, Hungary.*
Tel: +36 3597113

UCB Pharma BV *Druivenstraat 5, 4816 KB Breda, Netherlands.*
Tel: +31 (0) 76 5879222 Fax: +31 (0) 76 5875264
Web: www.ucbpharma.com

União Química Farmacêutica Nacional S.A. *Avenida dos Bandeirantes 5386, 04071-900 São Paulo, Brazil.*
Tel: +55 (0) 11 55862000 Fax: +55 (0) 11 55859755
Email: faleconosco@uniaoquimica.com.br
Web: www.uniaoquimica.com.br

Uniderm Farmaceutici S.r.l. *P.le F. il Macedone 140, 00124 Casalpalocco (RM), Italy.*
Tel: +39 06 50930618 Fax: +39 06 50930587
Email: uniderm@uniderm.it Web: www.uniderm.it

Union Medical (Thailand) Co. Ltd *513/199-200 Jaransanitwong Rd, Soi 37 Bangkoknoi, Bangkok 10700, Thailand.*
Tel: +66 2 412 1915 Fax: +66 2 412 5927
Email: umc@unionmedical.co.th Web: www.unionmedical.co.th

Unipharm de Mexico SA de CV *Tamarindos XV-A Lote 10 y 11, 91697 Veracruz C Ind. Bruno Pagliai, Mexico.*

Uni-Pharma Kleon Tsetis, Pharmaceutical Laboratories S.A. *14th km National Rd 1, 145 64 Kifissia, Greece.*
Tel: +30 210 8072512 Fax: +30 210 8078907
Email: unipharma@uni-pharma.gr Web: www.uni-pharma.gr

Unique Pharmaceutical Laboratories *Sadovaya-Kudrinskaya ul. 3, 123242 Moscow, Russia.*
Tel: +7 095 2547579 Fax: +7 095 2548382
Email: unique@relline.ru

United Drug *United Drug House, Belgard Rd, Tallaght, Dublin 24, Ireland.*
Tel: +353 (0) 1 459 8877 Fax: +353 (0) 1 459 6893
Email: info@united-drug.ie Web: www.united-drug.ie

Universal Pharmaceutical Lab Ltd *Eastern Ctr, G/F & 1/F, Unit 1-5, 1065 King's Rd, Quarry Bay, Hong Kong.*
Tel: +852 25628131 Fax: +852 25657913

Universal Pharmaceuticals (Pty) Ltd *7 Browning St, Jeppe, Johannesburg, South Africa.*

Upsifarma, Lda *S. Domingos à Lapa 8, Letra H, 1200-835 Lisbon, Portugal.*
Tel: +351 21 3953644 Fax: +351 21 3954765

Uriach *Avdaa. Cami Real 51-57, Pol. Industrial Riera de Caldes, Palau-Solita i Plegamans, 08184 Barcelona, Spain.*
Tel: +34 93 3471511 Fax: +34 93 8646606
Email: corp@uriach.com Web: www.uriach.com

Ursapharm Arzneimittel GmbH & Co. KG *Industriestr., 66129 Saarbrucken, Germany.*
Tel: +49 (0) 6805 92920 Fax: +49 (0) 6805 929288
Email: info@ursapharm.de Web: www.ursapharm.de

Usana *, Singapore.*

Usana Hong Kong Ltd *Unit 2504-06, 25/F, World Trade Centre, 280 Gloucester Rd, Causeway Bay, Hong Kong.*
Tel: +852 21621818 Fax: +852 21621228

5

V

Valuge S.A. *Cuyo 2870, 1640 Martinez, Buenos Aires, Argentina.*
Tel: +54 (0) 48363636

Verla-Pharm, Arzneimittelfabrik, Apotheker H.J.v. Ehrlich GmbH & Co. KG *Hauptstr. 98, 82327 Tutzing, Germany.*
Tel: +49 (0) 8158 2570 Fax: +49 (0) 8158 257250
Email: info@verla.de Web: www.verla.de

Vianex S.A. *Tatoiou Str., 18th Km Lamia National Rd, 146 10 Nea Erythrea, Greece.*
Tel: +30 210 8009111 Fax: +30 210 8071573
Email: mailbox@vianex.gr Web: www.vianex.gr

Viatris *Av J.F. Kennedy, 33701 Mérignac cdx, France.*
Tel: +33 (0) 5 56553535 Fax: +33 (0) 5 56341328
Email: info@viatris.fr Web: www.viatris.fr

Viatris BV *Verrijn Stuartweg 60, 1112 AX Diemen, Netherlands.*
Tel: +31 (0) 20 5198300 Fax: +31 (0) 20 6906435
Email: info@viatris.nl Web: www.viatris.nl

Viatris Farmacêutica SA *Rua do Centro Cultural 13, 1749-066 Lisbon, Portugal.*
Tel: +351 21 8420300 Fax: +351 21 8492042
Email: info@viatris.pt Web: www.viatris.pt

Viatris Pharma GmbH *Liesinger Flur-Gasse 2C, A-1230 Vienna, Austria.*
Tel: +43 (0) 1 863900 Fax: +43 (0) 1 863903161
Email: info@viatris.at Web: www.viatris.at

Viatris S.p.A. *Viale Brenta 18, 20139 Milan, Italy.*
Tel: +39 02 700671 Fax: +39 02 716574
Email: info@viatris.it Web: www.viatris.com

Vicis Pharma Kft *Kapás u 11-15, Buda Business Center, 1027 Budapest, Hungary.*
Tel: +36 4579921

Vida Laboratories Ltd *Unit 919 Vanta Industrial Ctr, 21 Tai Lin Pai Rd, Kwai Chung, Hong Kong.*
Tel: +852 24236333 Fax: +852 24236232
Email: mail-box@vidalab.com Web: www.vidalab.com

Vifor SA *Route de Moncor 10, 1752 Villars-sur-Glâne, Switzerland.*
Tel: +41 (0) 26 4076111 Fax: +41 (0) 26 4011485
Email: info@vifor.ch Web: www.vifor.ch

Viñas *Provenza 386, 08025 Barcelona, Spain.*
Tel: +34 93 2070512 Fax: +34 93 2071932

Vita Health Care AG *, 3177 Laupen, Switzerland.*

Vita Healthcare Ltd *Palladium House, 1-4 Argyll St, London, W1V 2LD, UK.*
Tel: +44 (0) 20 73289797 Fax: +44 (0) 20 73288555
Email: addresse@vitahealthcare.com

Vitabalans Oy *Varastokatu 8, 13500 Hämeenlinna, Finland.*
Tel: +358 (0) 3 615600 Fax: +358 (0) 3 6183902
Email: etunimi.sukunimi@vitabalans.fi Web: www.vitabalans.fi

Vitabiotics Ltd *1 Apsley Way, , London, NW2 7HF, UK.*
Tel: +44 (0) 20 8955 2600 Fax: +44 (0) 20 8955 2601
Web: www.vitabiotics.com

Vitafarma *C/Florida 29, Hernani, 20120 Guipuzcoa, Spain.*
Tel: +34 943 335273 Fax: +34 943 335269
Email: d.comercial@vitafarma.es Web: www.vitafarma.es

Vitalia Health Ltd *P.O. Box 2492, Marlow, SL7 2WW, UK.*
Tel: +44 (0) 1628 898366 Fax: +44 (0) 1628 898367
Email: information@vitalia-health.co.uk Web: www.vitalia-health.co.uk

Vitamed Ltd *P.O. Box 114, Binyamina 30550, Israel.*
Tel: +972 (0) 4 6189000 Fax: +972 (0) 4 6189029
Email: ricki@vitamed.co.il

Vitaplex Products *P.O. Box 270, Gymea, NSW 2227, Australia.*
Tel: +61 (0) 2 95452633 Fax: +61 (0) 2 95452642

Viternat Laboratórios Ltda *Av Dr Luis Arrobas Martins 759, 04781-001 São Paulo, Brazil.*
Tel: +55 (0) 11 56862661

VSM Belgium *Prins Boudewijnlaan 17 unit 7, 2550 Kontich, Belgium.*
Tel: +32 (0) 3 4508166 Fax: +32 (0) 3 4583624
Email: info@vsm.be Web: www.vsm.nl

VSM Geneesmiddelen BV *Postbus 9321, 1800 GH Alkmaar, Netherlands.*
Tel: +31 (0) 72 5661122 Fax: +31 (0) 72 5623883
Web: www.vsm.nl

W. Spitzner, Arzneimittelfabrik GmbH *Bunsenstr. 6-10, 76275 Ettlingen, Germany.*
Tel: +49 (0) 7243 10601 Fax: +49 (0) 7243 106333
Web: www.spitzner.de

Wagner Pharmafax Kft *Gyógyszer Business Center, Kassai u 56-58/b, 1041 Budapest, Hungary.*
Tel: +36 3804596 Fax: +36 3708633

Wala Schweiz GmbH *Waaghausgasse 3, 3011 Berne, Switzerland.*
Tel: +41 (0) 31 8493901 Fax: +41 (0) 31 8493902

Walgreens Finest Natural *200 Wilmot Road, , Deerfield, IL 60015, USA.*
Tel: +1 847 914 2500 Web: www.walgreens.com

Walker Pharmacal *4200 Laclede Ave, St Louis, MO 63108, USA.*
Tel: +1 314 533 9600

Wallace Pharmaceuticals Ltd *101/2 Floral Deck Plaza, Off Central MIDC Rd, Andheri (East), Mumbai 400 093, India.*
Tel: +91 (0) 22 8390681 Fax: +91 (0) 22 8390733
Web: www.wallacepharma.net

Wampole Brands Inc. *5950 Cote-de-Liesse, Montreal, H4T 1E2, Canada.*
Tel: +1 866 2219267

Wassen Italia S.r.l. *Via Canova 25, 20145 Milan, Italy.*
Tel: +39 02 3191061 Fax: +39 02 33100935
Email: wassen@wassen.it Web: www.wassen.it

Watson Pharmaceuticals Inc. *311 Bonnie Circle, Corona, CA 91720, USA.*
Tel: +1 951 493 5300 Fax: +1 951 493 5842
Web: www.watsonpharm.com

Weber & Weber GmbH & Co. KG *Herrschinger Str. 33, 82266 Inning/Ammersee, Germany.*
Tel: +49 (0) 8143 9270 Fax: +49 (0) 8143 7084
Email: service@weber-weber.de Web: www.weber-weber.de

Weleda AG *Stollenrain 11, 4144 Arlesheim, Switzerland.*
Tel: +41 (0) 61 7052121 Fax: +41 (0) 61 7052310
Email: info@weleda.ch Web: www.weleda.ch

Weleda AG-Heilmittelbetriebe *Mohlerstr. 3-5, 73525 Schwabisch Gmund, Germany.*
Tel: +49 (0) 7171 9190 Fax: +49 (0) 7171 919362
Email: med-wiss@weleda.de Web: www.weleda.de

Weleda GmbH & Co. KG *Hosenedelgasse 27, A-1220 Vienna, Austria.*
Tel: +43 (0) 1 2566060 Fax: +43 (0) 1 2594204
Web: www.weleda.at

Weleda (UK) Ltd *Heanor Rd, Ilkeston, DE7 8DR, UK.*
Tel: +44 (0) 115 944 8200 Fax: +44 (0) 115 944 8210
Email: info@weleda.co.uk Web: www.weleda.co.uk

Wellchem Pharmaceuticals Pte Ltd *221 Henderson Rd, 04-15 Henderson Building, S 159557, Singapore.*
Tel: +65 6276 6533 Fax: +65 6276 5672
Email: wellchem@singnet.com.sg Web: www.wellchem.com

Weston Pharmaceutical Ltd *Unit 26, 8/F Tower A, Southmark, 11 Yip Hing St, Wong Chuk Hang, Hong Kong.*
Tel: +852 25528122 Fax: +852 25526799
Email: westonph@netvigator.com

WF Young Inc. *1225 rue Volta, Boucherville, J4B 7M7, Canada.*
Tel: +1 450 6416496 Fax: +1 450 6419347

Whitehall *P.O. Box 12736, Penrose, Auckland, New Zealand.*
Tel: +64 (0) 9 5253807 Fax: +64 (0) 9 5257971

Whitehall Italia S.p.A. *Via Puccini 3, 20121 Milan, Italy.*
Tel: +39 02 8069181 Fax: +39 02 80691871

Whitehall Laboratories Australia P/L *Private Mailbag 1, Punchbowl, NSW 2196, Australia.*
Tel: +61 (0) 2 95341000 Fax: +61 (0) 2 95333980

Whitehall-Much GmbH *Regina-Protmann-Str. 16, 48159 Münster, Germany.*
Tel: +49 (0) 251 92718 Fax: +49 (0) 251 92713099
Email: wh-medwiss@wyeth.com Web: www.whitehall-much.de

Whitehall-Robins AG *Grafenauweg 10, 6301 Zug 7, Switzerland.*
Tel: +41 (0) 41 7290250 Fax: +41 (0) 41 7290255

Whitehall-Robins Inc. *5975 Whittle Rd, Mississauga, L4Z 3M6, Canada.*
Tel: +1 905 5077000 Fax: +1 905 5077111

Wick Pharma Zweigniederlassung der Procter & Gamble GmbH *Sulzbacher Str. 40, 65824 Schwalbach, Germany.*
Tel: +49 (0) 6196 8901 Fax: +49 (0) 6196 894929
Web: www.wickpharma.de

Wiedemann Pharma GmbH *Pilotyweg 14, 82541 Munsing, Germany.*
Tel: +49 (0) 8177 93140 Fax: +49 (0) 8177 931414
Email: mail@wiedemann-pharma.de Web: www.wiedemann-pharma.de

Wierhom Pharma S.A. *Arismendi 2441, 1427 Buenos Aires, Argentina.*
Tel: +54 (0) 11 45234815

Will-Pharma SA *Rue du Manil 80, 1301 Wavre, Belgium.*
Tel: +32 (0) 10 243838 Fax: +32 (0) 10 243377
Email: willpharma@willpharma.com Web: www.willpharma.com

Wing Wai Trading Co. *Unit E, 2/F Freder Ctr, 3 Mok Cheong St, Kowloon, Hong Kong.*
Tel: +852 23346228 Fax: +852 23344665

Woelm Pharma GmbH & Co. *Rhondorfer Str. 80, 53604 Bad Honnef, Germany.*
Tel: +49 (0) 2224 7740 Fax: +49 (0) 2224 774170
Email: kontakt@woelm.com Web: www.woelm.com

Wolfs SA *Industriepark West 68, 9100 Sint-Niklaas, Belgium.*
Tel: +32 (0) 3 7806390 Fax: +32 (0) 3 7806391
Email: info@wolfsnv.be

Worldwide Health Corp. Ltd *Freepost, Alderney, Guernsey, Channel Islands, GY1 555, UK.*
Tel: +44 (0) 800 952 9952 Fax: +44 (0) 1481 824 878
Email: info@wwhonline.com Web: www.wwhonline.com

Wörwag Pharma GmbH & Co *Pod Zameckem 1372, 500 12 Hradec Králové, Czech Republic.*
Tel: +420 (0) 49 5267157 Fax: +420 (0)
Email: woerwag@traveller.cz

Wörwag Pharma GmbH & Co. KG *Calwer Str. 7, 71034 Böblingen, Germany.*
Tel: +49 (0) 7031 62040 Fax: +49 (0) 7031 620431
Email: info@woerwagpharma.de Web: www.woerwagpharma.de

Wyeth Consumer Healthcare *Del Inca 4446, Of. 201, Las Condes, Santiago, Chile.*

Wyeth Consumer Healthcare Inc. *5 Giralda Farms, Madison, NJ 07940, USA.*
Tel: +1 973 660 5500 Fax: +1 973 660 7111
Web: www.wyeth.com

Wyeth Laboratories *Huntercombe Lane South, Taplow, Maidenhead, SL6 0PH, UK.*
Tel: +44 (0) 1628 604377 Fax: +44 (0) 1628 666368
Web: www.wyeth.co.uk

Wyeth Pharmaceuticals, Division of Wyeth Australia P/L *Locked Bag 5002, Baulkham Hills BC, NSW 2153, Australia.*
Tel: +61 (0) 2 88508200 Fax: +61 (0) 2 90230000
Web: www.wyeth.com.au

Wyeth-Lederle Pharma GmbH *Storchengasse 1, A-1150 Vienna, Austria.*
Tel: +43 (0) 1 891140 Fax: +43 (0) 1 89114399
Web: www.wyeth.at

Yauyip P/L *Suite 503 Cliveden, 4 Bridge Street, NSW 2000, Australia.*
Tel: +61 (0) 2 92474160

Y.S.P. Industries (M) Sdn Bhd *18 Jln Wan Kadir, Taman Tun Dr Ismail, 60000 Kuala Lumpur, Malaysia.*
Tel: +60 (0) 3 77276390 Fax: +60 (0) 3 77276701
Web: www.ysp.com.my

Yung Shin Pharmaceutical (S) Pte Ltd *8 Kaki Bukit Rd 2, 02-26 Ruby Warehouse Complex, S 417841, Singapore.*
Tel: +65 6741 2466 Fax: +65 6747 6009
Email: yspsin@singnet.com.sg Web: www.ysp.com.tw

Z

Zambon Group SpA *Glazovskii per. 7, of. 17, 119002 Moscow, Russia.*
Tel: +7 095 9333830 Fax: +7 095 9333831
Email: zambin@zambon.ru Web: www.zambon.ru

Zambon SA *Ave Bourgemestre E. Demunter 1 boite 9, 1090 Brussels, Belgium.*
Tel: +32 (0) 2 7719936 Fax: +32 (0) 2 7718570
Web: www.zambongroup.com

Zellaforte Vertriebsanstalt *Austrasse 52, FL-9490 Vaduz, Switzerland.*
Tel: +41 (0) 75 2322617

Zeppenfeldt Pharma GmbH *Weiler Str. 19-21, 79540 Lorrach, Germany.*
Tel: +49 (0) 7621 919290 Fax: +49 (0) 7621 9192930
Email: mail@zeppenfeldt.de Web: www.zeppenfeldt.de

Zeta Farmaceutici S.p.A. *Via Galvani 10, 36066 Sandrigo (VI), Italy.*
Tel: +39 0444 461911 Fax: +39 0444 658351
Email: info@zetafarm.it

Ziethen *Tengstr. 26, 80798 Munich, Germany.*
Tel: +49 (0) 89 2714759 Fax: +49 (0) 89 339558

Zuellig Pharma *316-318 Richmond Road, Grey Lynn, Auckland, New Zealand.*
Tel: +64 (0) 9 3610403 Fax: +64 (0) 9 3610445
Web: www.zuelligpharma.com

Zuellig Pharma Ltd *8-9 Ploenchit Center, 2 Sukhumvit Rd, Kwang Klongtoey, Khet Klongtoey, Bangkok 10110, Thailand.*
Tel: +66 2 656 9800 Fax: +66 2 656 9801
Email: info@zuelligpharma.co.th Web: www.zuelligpharma.com

Zuellig Pharma Pte Ltd *19 Loyang Way, 08-20, S 508724, Singapore.*
Tel: +65 6546 8188 Fax: +65 6546 8288
Email: enquiry@zuelligpharma.com Web: www.zuelligpharma.com

Zuellig Pharma Sdn Bhd *Level 3A, No 10, Jln Bersatu 13/4, 46200 Petaling Jaya, Malaysia.*
Tel: +60 (0) 3 79856688 Fax: +60 (0) 3 79551388
Web: www.zuelligpharma.com

Zuoz Pharma S.A. *Esquina Puente Restaurador a Río, Av. Oeste 20, Santa Teresa, Caracas, Venezuela.*
Tel: +58 (0) 212 4818833 Fax: +58 (0) 212 4846401
Email: clientes@zuoz.com Web: www.zuozpharma.com.ve

Zurita Laboratório Farmacêutico Ltda *Rua Domingos Graziano 104, 13600-000 Araras, Brazil.*
Tel: +55 (0) 19 5411611 Fax: +55 (0) 19 5412052
Email: zurita@zurita.com.br Web: www.zurita.com.br

Zydus Cadila Group *Zydus Tower, Satellite Cross Roads, Ahmedabad 380 015, India.*
Tel: +91 (0) 79 6868100 Fax: +91 (0) 79 6862366
Web: www.cadila-zydus.com

Zyfas Medical Co *102E Pasir Panjang Rd, 02-10/11 Citilink Warehouse Complex, S 118529, Singapore.*
Tel: +65 6275 7757 Fax: +65 6275 2287
Email: zyfas@singnet.com.sg

Index

Page numbers in **bold** refer to monographs.

I

C

D

E

F

G

H

I

J

Q

R

S

I

U

V

W

Yellowcard

COMMISSION ON HUMAN MEDICINES

In Confidence

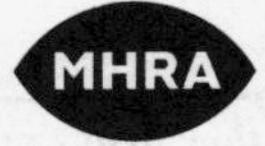

SUSPECTED ADVERSE DRUG REACTIONS

If you suspect that an adverse reaction may be related to a drug, or a combination of drugs, you should complete this Yellow Card or complete a report on the website at www.yellowcard.gov.uk. For *intensively monitored medicines* (identified by ▼) report **all** suspected reactions (including any considered not to be serious). For *established drugs* and *herbal remedies* report **all serious** adverse reactions in adults; report **all serious and minor** adverse reactions in **children** (under 18 years). You do not have to be certain about causality: if in doubt, please report. Do not be put off reporting just because some details are not known. See BNF (page 10) or the MHRA website (www.yellowcard.gov.uk) for additional advice.

PATIENT DETAILS Patient Initials: ________ Sex: M / F Weight if known (kg): ________

Age (at time of reaction): ________ Identification (Your Practice / Hospital Ref.)*: ________

SUSPECTED DRUG(S)

Give brand name of drug and batch number if known	Route	Dosage	Date started	Date stopped	Prescribed for

SUSPECTED REACTION(S)

Please describe the reaction(s) and any treatment given:

Outcome
- Recovered ☐
- Recovering ☐
- Continuing ☐
- Other ☐

Date reaction(s) started: ________ Date reaction(s) stopped: ________

Do you consider the reaction to be serious? Yes / No

If *yes*, please indicate why the reaction is considered to be serious (please tick all that apply):

- Patient died due to reaction ☐
- Life threatening ☐
- Congenital abnormality ☐
- Involved or prolonged inpatient hospitalisation ☐
- Involved persistent or significant disability or incapacity ☐
- Medically significant; please give details:

* This is to enable you to identify the patient in any future correspondence concerning this report

Yellowcard

COMMISSION ON HUMAN MEDICINES

In Confidence

MHRA

SUSPECTED ADVERSE DRUG REACTIONS

If you suspect that an adverse reaction may be related to a drug, or a combination of drugs, you should complete this Yellow Card or complete a report on the website at www.yellowcard.gov.uk. For *intensively monitored medicines* (identified by ▼) report **all** suspected reactions (including any considered not to be serious). For *established drugs* and *herbal remedies* report **all serious** adverse reactions in adults; report **all serious and minor** adverse reactions in **children** (under 18 years). You do not have to be certain about causality: if in doubt, please report. Do not be put off reporting just because some details are not known. See BNF (page 10) or the MHRA website (www.yellowcard.gov.uk) for additional advice.

PATIENT DETAILS Patient Initials: ________ Sex: M / F Weight if known (kg): ________

Age (at time of reaction): ________ Identification (Your Practice / Hospital Ref.)*: ________

SUSPECTED DRUG(S)

Give brand name of drug and batch number if known	Route	Dosage	Date started	Date stopped	Prescribed for

SUSPECTED REACTION(S)

Please describe the reaction(s) and any treatment given:

Outcome
- Recovered ☐
- Recovering ☐
- Continuing ☐
- Other ☐

Date reaction(s) started: ________ Date reaction(s) stopped: ________

Do you consider the reaction to be serious? Yes / No

If *yes*, please indicate why the reaction is considered to be serious (please tick all that apply):

- Patient died due to reaction ☐
- Life threatening ☐
- Congenital abnormality ☐
- Involved or prolonged inpatient hospitalisation ☐
- Involved persistent or significant disability or incapacity ☐
- Medically significant; please give details:

* This is to enable you to identify the patient in any future correspondence concerning this report

Please attach additional pages if necessary

Please list other drugs taken in the last 3 months prior to the reaction (including self-medication & herbal remedies)

Was the patient on any other medication? Yes / No If *yes*, please give the following information if known:

Drug (Brand, if known)	Route	Dosage	Date started	Date stopped	Prescribed for

Additional relevant information e.g. medical history, test results, known allergies, rechallenge (if performed), suspected drug interactions. For congenital abnormalities please state all other drugs taken during pregnancy and the date of the last menstrual period.

REPORTER DETAILS

Name and Professional Address: ________

Post code: ________ Tel No: ________

Speciality: ________

Signature: Date:

CLINICIAN (if not the reporter)

Name and Professional Address: ________

Post code: ________

Tel No: ________ Speciality: ________

If you would like information about other adverse reactions associated with the suspected drug, please tick this box ☐

If you report from an area served by a Yellow Card Centre (YCC), MHRA may ask the Centre to communicate with you, on its behalf, about your report. See BNF (page 10) for further details on YCCs. If you want only MHRA to contact you, please tick this box. ☐

Send to **Medicines and Healthcare products Regulatory Agency, CHM FREEPOST, LONDON SW8 5BR**

Please attach additional pages if necessary

Please list other drugs taken in the last 3 months prior to the reaction (including self-medication & herbal remedies)

Was the patient on any other medication? Yes / No If *yes*, please give the following information if known:

Drug (Brand, if known)	Route	Dosage	Date started	Date stopped	Prescribed for

Additional relevant information e.g. medical history, test results, known allergies, rechallenge (if performed), suspected drug interactions. For congenital abnormalities please state all other drugs taken during pregnancy and the date of the last menstrual period.

REPORTER DETAILS

Name and Professional Address: ________

Post code: ________ Tel No: ________

Speciality: ________

Signature: Date:

CLINICIAN (if not the reporter)

Name and Professional Address: ________

Post code: ________

Tel No: ________ Speciality: ________

If you would like information about other adverse reactions associated with the suspected drug, please tick this box ☐

If you report from an area served by a Yellow Card Centre (YCC), MHRA may ask the Centre to communicate with you, on its behalf, about your report. See BNF (page 10) for further details on YCCs. If you want only MHRA to contact you, please tick this box. ☐

Send to **Medicines and Healthcare products Regulatory Agency, CHM FREEPOST, LONDON SW8 5BR**

Yellowcard

COMMISSION ON HUMAN MEDICINES

In Confidence

MHRA

SUSPECTED ADVERSE DRUG REACTIONS

If you suspect that an adverse reaction may be related to a drug, or a combination of drugs, you should complete this Yellow Card or complete a report on the website at www.yellowcard.gov.uk. For *intensively monitored medicines* (identified by ▼) report **all** suspected reactions (including any considered not to be serious). For *established drugs* and *herbal remedies* report **all serious** adverse reactions in adults; report **all serious and minor** adverse reactions in **children** (under 18 years). You do not have to be certain about causality: if in doubt, please report. Do not be put off reporting just because some details are not known. See BNF (page 10) or the MHRA website (www.yellowcard.gov.uk) for additional advice.

PATIENT DETAILS Patient Initials: ______ Sex: M / F Weight if known (kg): ______

Age (at time of reaction): ______ Identification (Your Practice / Hospital Ref.)*: ______

SUSPECTED DRUG(S)

Give brand name of drug and batch number if known	Route	Dosage	Date started	Date stopped	Prescribed for

SUSPECTED REACTION(S)

Please describe the reaction(s) and any treatment given:

Outcome

Recovered ☐
Recovering ☐
Continuing ☐
Other ☐

Date reaction(s) started: ______ Date reaction(s) stopped: ______

Do you consider the reaction to be serious? Yes / No

If *yes*, please indicate why the reaction is considered to be serious (please tick all that apply):

Patient died due to reaction ☐ Involved or prolonged inpatient hospitalisation ☐

Life threatening ☐ Involved persistent or significant disability or incapacity ☐

Congenital abnormality ☐ Medically significant; please give details:

* This is to enable you to identify the patient in any future correspondence concerning this report

Yellowcard

COMMISSION ON HUMAN MEDICINES

In Confidence

MHRA

SUSPECTED ADVERSE DRUG REACTIONS

If you suspect that an adverse reaction may be related to a drug, or a combination of drugs, you should complete this Yellow Card or complete a report on the website at www.yellowcard.gov.uk. For *intensively monitored medicines* (identified by ▼) report **all** suspected reactions (including any considered not to be serious). For *established drugs* and *herbal remedies* report **all serious** adverse reactions in adults; report **all serious and minor** adverse reactions in **children** (under 18 years). You do not have to be certain about causality: if in doubt, please report. Do not be put off reporting just because some details are not known. See BNF (page 10) or the MHRA website (www.yellowcard.gov.uk) for additional advice.

PATIENT DETAILS Patient Initials: ______ Sex: M / F Weight if known (kg): ______

Age (at time of reaction): ______ Identification (Your Practice / Hospital Ref.)*: ______

SUSPECTED DRUG(S)

Give brand name of drug and batch number if known	Route	Dosage	Date started	Date stopped	Prescribed for

SUSPECTED REACTION(S)

Please describe the reaction(s) and any treatment given:

Outcome

Recovered ☐
Recovering ☐
Continuing ☐
Other ☐

Date reaction(s) started: ______ Date reaction(s) stopped: ______

Do you consider the reaction to be serious? Yes / No

If *yes*, please indicate why the reaction is considered to be serious (please tick all that apply):

Patient died due to reaction ☐ Involved or prolonged inpatient hospitalisation ☐

Life threatening ☐ Involved persistent or significant disability or incapacity ☐

Congenital abnormality ☐ Medically significant; please give details:

* This is to enable you to identify the patient in any future correspondence concerning this report

Please attach additional pages if necessary

Please list other drugs taken in the last 3 months prior to the reaction (including self-medication & herbal remedies)

Was the patient on any other medication? Yes / No If *yes*, please give the following information if known:

Drug (Brand, if known)	Route	Dosage	Date started	Date stopped	Prescribed for

Additional relevant information e.g. medical history, test results, known allergies, rechallenge (if performed), suspected drug interactions. For congenital abnormalities please state all other drugs taken during pregnancy and the date of the last menstrual period.

REPORTER DETAILS

Name and Professional Address: __________

Post code: __________ Tel No: __________

Speciality: __________

Signature: Date:

CLINICIAN (if not the reporter)

Name and Professional Address: __________

Post code: __________

Tel No: __________ Speciality: __________

If you would like information about other adverse reactions associated with the suspected drug, please tick this box ☐

If you report from an area served by a Yellow Card Centre (YCC), MHRA may ask the Centre to communicate with you, on its behalf, about your report. See BNF (page 10) for further details on YCCs. If you want only MHRA to contact you, please tick this box. ☐

Send to **Medicines and Healthcare products Regulatory Agency, CHM FREEPOST, LONDON SW8 5BR**

Please attach additional pages if necessary

Please list other drugs taken in the last 3 months prior to the reaction (including self-medication & herbal remedies)

Was the patient on any other medication? Yes / No If *yes*, please give the following information if known:

Drug (Brand, if known)	Route	Dosage	Date started	Date stopped	Prescribed for

Additional relevant information e.g. medical history, test results, known allergies, rechallenge (if performed), suspected drug interactions. For congenital abnormalities please state all other drugs taken during pregnancy and the date of the last menstrual period.

REPORTER DETAILS

Name and Professional Address: __________

Post code: __________ Tel No: __________

Speciality: __________

Signature: Date:

CLINICIAN (if not the reporter)

Name and Professional Address: __________

Post code: __________

Tel No: __________ Speciality: __________

If you would like information about other adverse reactions associated with the suspected drug, please tick this box ☐

If you report from an area served by a Yellow Card Centre (YCC), MHRA may ask the Centre to communicate with you, on its behalf, about your report. See BNF (page 10) for further details on YCCs. If you want only MHRA to contact you, please tick this box. ☐

Send to **Medicines and Healthcare products Regulatory Agency, CHM FREEPOST, LONDON SW8 5BR**